In Silico Approaches in Drug Design

In Silico Approaches in Drug Design

Editor

Osvaldo Santos-Filho

MDPI • Basel • Beijing • Wuhan • Barcelona • Belgrade • Manchester • Tokyo • Cluj • Tianjin

Editor
Osvaldo Santos-Filho
Instituto de Pesquisas de
Produtos Naturais Walter
Mors
Universidade Federal do Rio
de Janeiro
Rio de Janeiro
Brazil

Editorial Office
MDPI
St. Alban-Anlage 66
4052 Basel, Switzerland

This is a reprint of articles from the Special Issue published online in the open access journal *Pharmaceuticals* (ISSN 1424-8247) (available at: www.mdpi.com/journal/pharmaceuticals/special_issues/Silico_Approaches_Drug).

For citation purposes, cite each article independently as indicated on the article page online and as indicated below:

LastName, A.A.; LastName, B.B.; LastName, C.C. Article Title. *Journal Name* **Year**, *Volume Number*, Page Range.

ISBN 978-3-0365-5384-9 (Hbk)
ISBN 978-3-0365-5383-2 (PDF)

Contents

About the Editor

Osvaldo Santos-Filho

Osvaldo Andrade Santos-Filho is a computational physical chemist and professor at the Federal University of Rio de Janeiro, Brazil, where he is the director the Laboratory of Molecular Modeling and Computational Structural Biology. Before assuming his position as a university professor, he worked as an analytical chemist in aeronautical and chemical companies (1988-1993); postdoctoral researcher at the Institute of Chemistry of the Federal University of Rio de Janeiro (2000-2002); postdoctoral researcher at the College of Pharmacy of the University of Illinois at Chicago, USA (2002-2006); research associate at the Faculty of Medicine of the University of British Columbia, Vancouver, Canada (2006-2008); senior scientist at the Department of Drug Synthesis of Farmanguinhos/Fiocruz (2009-2013), Brazil; and visiting scientist at the Inflammation Laboratory of IOC/Fiocruz (2014-2015), Brazil. His research is mainly focused on the application of Molecular Modeling and Computational Chemistry in Medicinal Chemistry, Structural Biology, Protein Engineering, and Enzymatic Catalysis.

Preface to "In Silico Approaches in Drug Design"

Mainly due to the development of new hardware architectures and software technologies, Computational Chemistry has achieved maturity and, nowadays is one of the central scientific fields in the pharmaceutical industry. In particular, in silico approaches have been shown to be fundamental for the development of drugs and the study of biological systems, not only at the molecular level, but also at the cellular level.

Applications of in silico tools are crucial in the early stages of drug design, such as planning more efficient and economic synthetic routes for chemical administration, screening of huge databases, as well as proposing hypotheses for probable mechanisms of action of drugs in macromolecular targets. Such endeavors are extremely complex and require the usage of modern and sophisticated approaches, such as artificial intelligence, data mining, computational molecular simulations through classical mechanics and quantum mechanics, molecular docking, chemoinformatics, applied mathematics, and biostatistics.

To celebrate the success story and advances in the important synergistic combination of drug design and in silico investigation, I accepted the challenge of editing a Special Issue for the prestigious journal *Pharmaceuticals*, which is now assembled into a reprint. The text is a collection of 31 original articles and four reviews, published from 2021 to 2022, focused on the application of a wide range of computational tools in medicinal chemistry projects: from molecular docking to artificial intelligence approaches.

I am grateful to Mr. Owen Shu from MDPI for his dedication and wonderful professional support for organizing this work, and, of course, I cannot forget to thank my lovely wife, Claudia Valeria, for encouraging me all the time.

I hope that this reprint makes for interesting reading and will be useful to fellow scientists and graduate students interested in Computational Medicinal Chemistry.

This book is dedicated to:
Prof. Dr. J. Daniel Figueroa-Villar
Prof. Dr. Anton J. Hopfinger, *in memoriam*
Prof. Dr. Ricardo Bicca de Alencastro, *in memoriam*

Osvaldo Santos-Filho
Editor

pharmaceuticals

MDPI

Article

Identification of Potential Allosteric Site Binders of Indoleamine 2,3-Dioxygenase 1 from Plants: A Virtual and Molecular Dynamics Investigation

Vitor Martins de Almeida and Osvaldo Andrade Santos-Filho *

Laboratório de Modelagem Molecular e Biologia Estrutural Computacional, Instituto de Pesquisas de Produtos Naturais Walter Mors, Centro de Ciências da Saúde, Universidade Federal do Rio de Janeiro, Av. Carlos Chagas Filho, 373, Bloco H, Cidade Universitária, Rio de Janeiro 21941-599, RJ, Brazil

* Correspondence: osvaldo@ippn.ufrj.br

Abstract: Ligand and structure-based computational screenings were carried out to identify flavonoids with potential anticancer activity. Kushenol E, a flavonoid with proven anticancer activity and, at the same time, an allosteric site binder of the enzyme indoleamine 2,3-dioxygenase-1 (IDO1), was used as the reference compound. Molecular docking and molecular dynamics simulations were performed for the screened flavonoids with known anticancer activity. The following two of these flavonoids were identified as potential inhibitors of IDO1: dichamanetin and isochamanetin. Molecular dynamics simulations were used to assess the conformational profile of IDO1-flavonoids complexes, as well as for calculating the bind-free energies.

Keywords: cancer; immunology; flavonoids; IDO1; virtual screening; molecular docking; molecular dynamics; free energy

Citation: de Almeida, V.M.; Santos-Filho, O.A. Identification of Potential Allosteric Site Binders of Indoleamine 2,3-Dioxygenase 1 from Plants: A Virtual and Molecular Dynamics Investigation. *Pharmaceuticals* **2022**, *15*, 1099. https://doi.org/10.3390/ph15091099

Academic Editor: Mary J. Meegan

Received: 13 July 2022
Accepted: 31 August 2022
Published: 2 September 2022

1. Introduction

1.1. Tryptophan Metabolism and the Kynurenine Pathway

Studies show that tumor tissues within a chronic inflammatory context (presence of pro-inflammatory cytokines for a long time) catabolize in large proportions the amino acid L-tryptophan in the cell matrix and synthesize metabolites from one of the main degradation pathways of tryptophan, the pathway of kynurenine [1,2].

Almost all metabolites of the kynurenine pathway affect immune activity through various mechanisms. Figure 1 illustrates the effects of kynurenine pathway metabolites on the immune system. The determining step of the kynurenine pathway is the formation of N-formylkynurenine, regulated by the family of dioxygenase enzymes known as tryptophan 2,3-dioxygenase (TDO) and indolamine 2,3-dioxygenase (IDO), which may exist in the following two isoforms: IDO1 and IDO2 [3].

TDO, IDO1, and IDO2 are heme-bearing enzymes and catalyze the rate-limiting step of tryptophan catabolization. TDO is mainly expressed in the liver and oxidizes excess tryptophan in the body, generating ATP and especially NAD+. The expression of TDO is stimulated by the concentration of blood tryptophan as well as by the synthesis of the heme cofactor [4].

IDO1 can be expressed by many different cells, including antigen-presenting cells (APCs), such as monocyte-derived macrophages, dendritic cells (DCs), and fibroblasts. Its expression is mainly induced by inflammatory cytokines, such as IFN-γ, TNF-α, IL-1, and IL-2, secreted by Th1-type lymphocytes, as well as TGF-β, IL-10, and adenosine secreted by regulatory T lymphocytes [5]. IDO1 expression is further stimulated by its own product, kynurenine, via the aryl hydrocarbon receptor (AhR) [6,7].

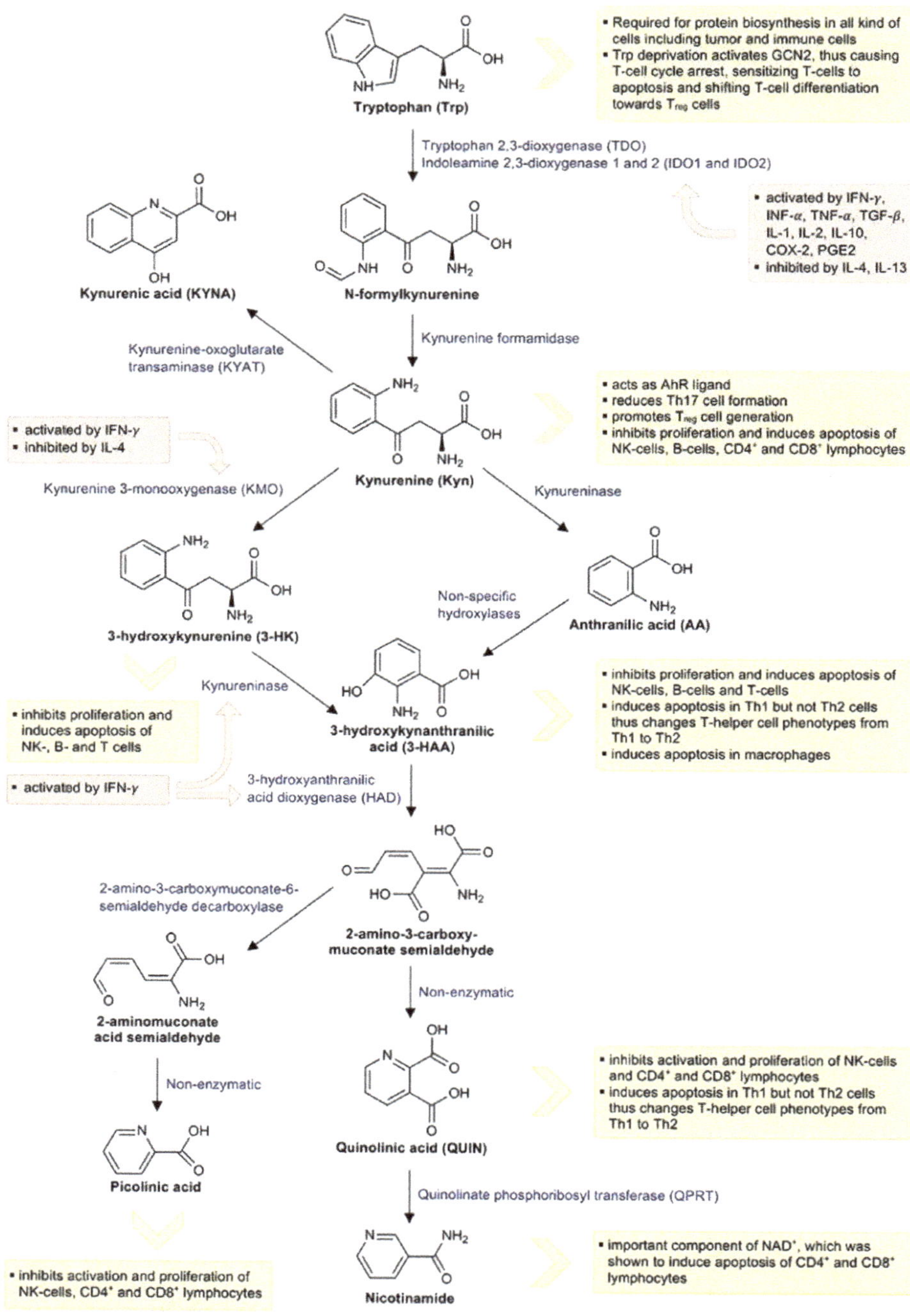

Figure 1. Catabolization of tryptophan via the kynurenine pathway and its interactions with the immune system. Orange boxes indicate the effects of immune mediators on the kynurenine pathway and yellow boxes indicate the effects of tryptophan metabolites on the immune system. Adapted from Lanser et al. [4].

IDO2 is significantly less active than IDO1 [8]. Similar to IDO1, its expression is stimulated by the activation of AhR [9]. Although IDO2 is expressed by cancer cells, when compared to IDO1, it contributes little to the accumulation of kynurenine pathway metabolites [10,11].

In healthy patients, IDO1 expression is restricted to endothelial cells in the placenta, lung, mature dendritic cells in secondary lymphoid organs, and in epithelial cells scattered in the female genital tract [12]. Whereas, under inflammatory conditions, IDO1 expression is strongly induced by INF-γ [13]. Furthermore, it is highly expressed at inflammatory sites, where it may contribute to negative feedback against local immune response activity [12]. Inflamed tumors may also express IDO1 as an adaptive resistance mechanism, in which it is induced by IFN-γ produced by dendritic cells and tumor-infiltrated macrophages [14].

Given the physiological importance of the IDO1 enzyme within the tumor microenvironment, the need for structural studies and the development of increasingly efficient inhibitors has become an attractive approach to treating cancer patients.

1.2. IDO1: Structure

The human IDO1 is a monomeric α-helical dioxygenase enzyme containing an N-terminal minor domain (residues 1–154) and a C-terminal major domain (residues 155–403), where the catalytic site and a cofactor heme are located (Figure 2).

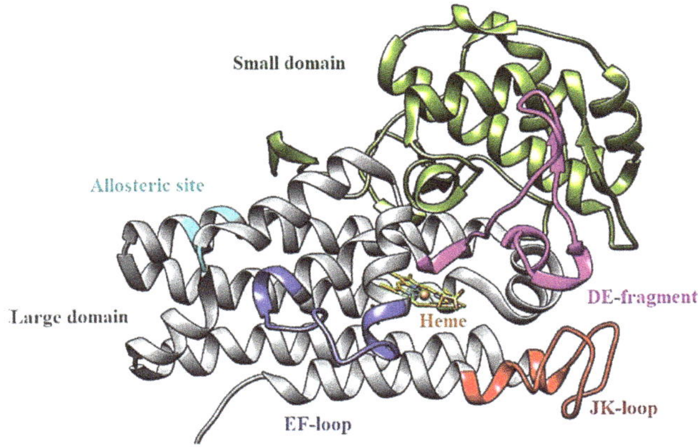

Figure 2. Structure of indoleamine deoxygenase 1 (IDO1) with highlighted regions: minor domain (green) and major domain (grey, magenta, red, blue, and cyan). Contained in the larger domain are: the DE fragment, composed of the DE hairpin and the DE loop; JK loop; EF loop; the heme cofactor (orange); the allosteric site.

The minor domain or N-terminal domain, shown in green in Figure 2, contains residues Gly11 to Asp158, consisting of six α-helices (involving amino acids Tyr36 to His45, His45 to Ser52, Gln54 to Lys61, Asp72 to Gly93, Pro104 to Glu119 and Val125 to Val130 or helix A, contributing to the active site), four 3_{10}-helices (Ser12 to His16, Pro33 to Phe35, Ser66 to Leu70 and Thr144 to Glu146) and a small antiparallel β-sheet formed by residues Lys135 to Lys136 and Met148 to Asp149. Such a domain makes up part of the upper region of the catalytic site and acts as structural support for the enzyme [15].

The major domain or C-terminal domain, shown in grey in Figure 2, contains residues Cys159 to Gly403, being constituted by 9 α-helices [15]. This domain performs functions related to conversion, positioning, and displacement of substrates/products in the enzyme and is where the catalytic site is located. There are also regions with specific functionalities that are important for the enzymatic reaction to occur. Among them, there is the "access" tunnel for the entrance of small molecules from the external environment (ligand delivery tunnel) and the JK loop (red), with the function of conducting and maintaining the substrate (tryptophan) inside the catalytic site [16].

Finally, there is the DE fragment, consisting of the DE-hairpin (Ser235 to Tyr249) and the DE loop (Glu250 to Gly262) (magenta), the EF loop (Gly278 to His287) (blue), and the JK loop (Gln360 to Gly380) [17].

IDO1 has the following two non-competitive natural substrates: tryptophan and molecular oxygen (O_2). Moreover, the enzyme has the following four states:

- apo-IDO1: without the heme cofactor;
- holo-IDO1: containing the iron atom of the heme group in the ferric state (Fe^{3+});
- holo-IDO1 with the iron atom of the heme group in the ferrous state (Fe^{2+});
- O_2-linked holo-IDO1 complex.

Despite not being the active form of the enzyme, apo-IDO1 is a promising macromolecular target since cellular studies have shown that this form is the most abundant in the cell medium, about 85% [18]. Therefore, it is likely that there is a binding site where potential inhibitors of the apo form can interact with this form of the enzyme. The main objective of this project was to apply molecular modeling methods in order to investigate this possibility.

1.3. IDO1: Inhibitors

Over the past decade, the scientific academy has been making efforts for the development of IDO1 inhibitors [2]. Röhrig and collaborators classified existing test-phase inhibitors into the following four categories: type I, II, III, and IV inhibitors [19].

Type I inhibitors are classified as competitive inhibitors of tryptophan. In general, type I inhibitors target the molecular oxygen-bound holo-IDO1 form and do not form a direct bond with heme iron [17]. The 1-LMT and 1-DMT are classified within this category of inhibitors [20].

Type II inhibitors are classified as competitive inhibitors of molecular oxygen by binding to the iron atom in its ferrous state of the heme group, acting in the ferrous holo-IDO1 form. Inhibitors such as β-carboline [21], and Epacadostat [22] fall into this category.

Type III inhibitors are noncompetitive inhibitors of tryptophan. New inhibitors in this class are being studied, such as 4PI, Navoximod, and MMG-0358 [19].

Type IV inhibitors are the most recently described class of inhibitors in the literature, including inhibitors such as the clinical compound BMS-986205, which targets the apo-IDO1 form [23].

The structures of the mentioned inhibitors are shown in Figure 3.

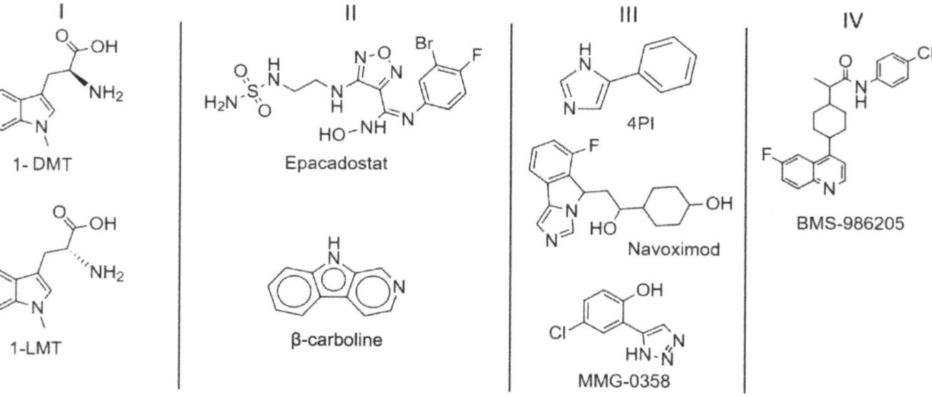

Figure 3. IDO1 inhibitors.

Kwon and collaborators [24] determined the amino acid residues that define an allosteric site for the action of apo-IDO1 inhibitors (Ser12, Tyr15, Ile17, Ile178, Lys179, Ile181, Pro182, Phe185, Lys186, Phe306, Ser309, Leu310, Ser312, Asn313, and Pro314), and found that the flavonoid obtained from plants of the species *Sophora flavescens*, known as Kushenol E, acts as an inhibitor of this site (Figure 4). The authors described the amino acids Pro182 and Phe185, located in the larger domain of the enzyme, as the main components of the allosteric site for inhibitory activity. Site-directed mutagenesis experiments were performed on these residues, and in vitro enzyme inhibition assays were performed. The results proved the contribution of these amino acids to enzymatic function and indicate this allosteric site as a target for new inhibitors [24].

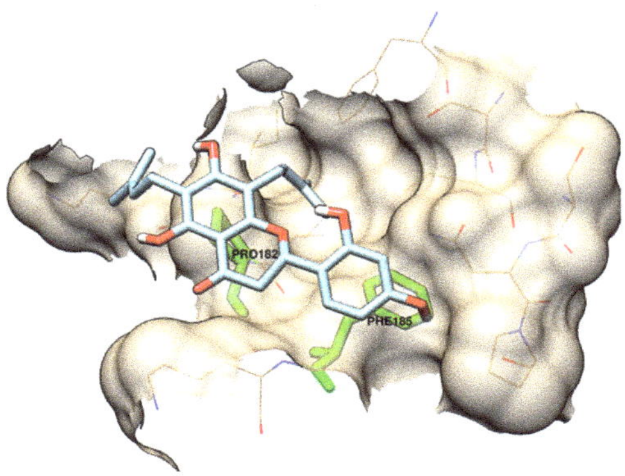

Figure 4. Allosteric site described by Kwon and colleagues [24]. The docked flavonoid Kushenol E, as well as Pro182, and Phe185 are shown in detail.

Most IDO1 inhibitors are obtained from a natural source; however, as shown by Kwon, flavonoids may inhibit IDO1 [24]. The diverse variety of natural products can make the screening of these compounds a time-consuming and expensive task. Due to the development of more powerful computers, virtual screening of chemical compounds and pharmacodynamic validation of ligand-receptor interactions can accelerate the process of discovering potential new drugs. In this context, we focused our work on the identification of potential inhibitors of the naturally occurring apo-IDO1 allosteric site.

2. Results and Discussion

2.1. Ligand-Based Virtual Screening

In order to identify potential IDO1 inhibitors capable of interacting with its allosteric site, the following two virtual screening tools were used: the Mcule platform [25] and the ZINC 15 database [26]. At this stage of the work, the flavonoid Kushenol E (Figure 5) was used as the reference compound, due to its proven effectiveness as a non-competitive inhibitor that binds to the allosteric site of the enzyme [24]. Tanimoto's coefficient was used as the sampling criterium [27], and 172 compounds were sampled.

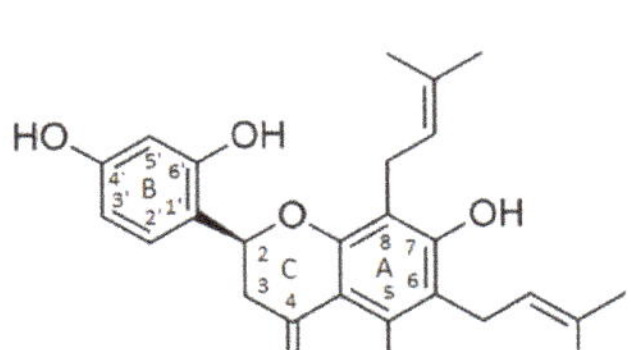

Figure 5. Kushenol E.

2.2. Structure-Based Virtual Screening and Molecular Docking

Besides the ligand-based virtual screening mentioned above, a structure-based virtual screening was also carried out (Figure 6). In this approach, the previously sampled compounds, including Kushenol E, were docked into the allosteric site of the IDO1.

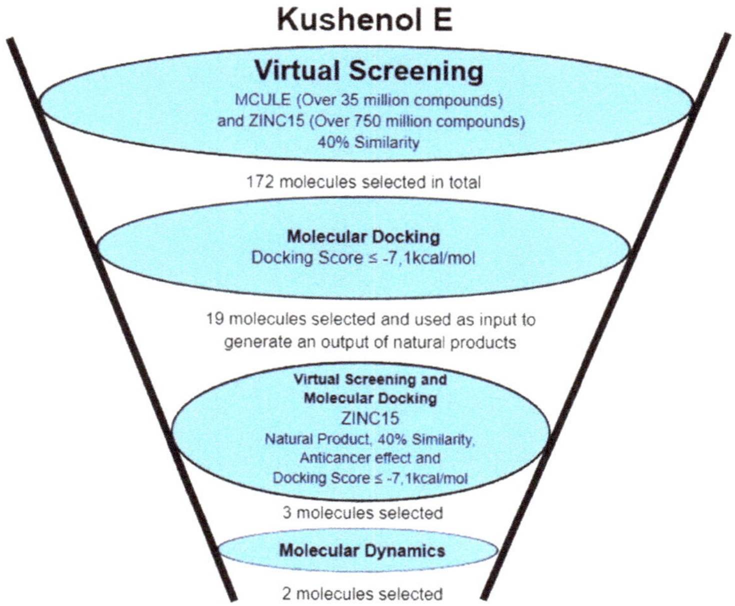

Figure 6. Workflow of ligand-based and structure-based virtual approaches.

The calculated docking energies of each compound are shown in Supplementary Material (Table S1). The range of calculated energies varied from −8.1 kcal/mol to −5.3 kcal/mol. The docking energy for Kushenol E is equal to −6.6 kcal/mol. We realized that most of the sampled compounds were not from natural sources. Since the focus of this research was the identification of substances obtained from natural products with the potential ability to inhibit the biological response of the enzyme IDO1 through interaction at the allosteric site, a new virtual screening was carried out. The strategy was to use each compound that presented interaction energies equal to or lower than −7.1 kcal/mol (19 compounds; represented in red in Supplementary Materials, Table S1) as reference compounds in new ligand-based virtual screenings. The ZINC 15 database was the chosen tool. In this context, 28 natural products were selected, which were later docked to the allosteric site of the IDO1 enzyme. The result of this second-round structure-based virtual screening is shown in Table 1. While, in this investigation, Kushenol E (shown in bold red) works as the positive control, it is also important to consider a compound that would work as a negative control. In this context, as in the paper by Kwon [24], steppogenin was chosen as such a compound. As shown in the table, among all compounds, steppogenin shows the least favorable docking energy (shown in light red).

In this second molecular docking calculation, two additional criteria were used for the final screening as follows: (a) compounds that presented docking energies equal to or lower than −7.1 kcal/mol; (b) compounds that showed some anticancer activity (as described in the literature). Consequently, the following three flavonoids were selected: dichamanetin, isochamanetin, and chamaejasmin B, shown in bold black.

Table 1. Structure-based (second) virtual screening.

Compound	Docking (kcal/mol)	Compound	Docking (kcal/mol)
chamuvaritin	−7.9	Kushenol C	−6.5
chamaejasmin B	**−7.9**	butin	−6.5
dichamanetin	**−7.8**	estrobopinin	−6.4
chamaejasmin	−7.7	rhamnocitrin	−6.4
neochamaejasmin A	−7.6	7-benziloxicumarin	−6.3
obovatine	−7.5	naringenin	−6.3
isochamanetin	**−7.5**	uvaretin	−6.2
β-naftoflavone	−6.9	pinocembrin	−6.1
pinobanksine	−6.9	genkwanin	−6.1
tectocrisina	−6.8	glabranin	−6.0
soforaflavanone B	−6.7	7-hidroxiflavanone	−6.0
strobopinin-7-methyl-ether	−6.7	apigenin-4′,7-dimethyl-ether	−6.0
diuvaretin	−6.6	2-hidroxiflavanone	−6.0
izalpinin	−6.6	asebogenine	−5.9
Kushenol E	**−6.6**	steppogenin	−5.8

Dichamanetin is a C-benzylated flavanone that can be obtained from several Southeast Asian plant species, such as the following: *Uvaria alba*, *Uvaria chamae*, *Piper sarmentosum*, and *Xylopia pierrei* [28–30]. Isochamanetin, another C-benzylated flavanone, was obtained from several plant species such as *Sphaeranthus amaranthoides*, *Xylopia pierrei*, and *Ulvaria chamae* [28,31,32]. Chamaejasmin B is a dimeric biflavonoid formed by two isosacuranetin subunits linked by C3-C3 carbons, and obtained from Southwest Asian plant species, such as *Stellera chamaejasme L.* [33].

Table 2 and Figure 7 show the intermolecular interactions formed with specific residues of the allosteric site of IDO1.

As shown in Table 2 and Figure 7, the flavonoids interact with amino acid residues from the allosteric site, as defined by Kwon [24] (Ser12, Tyr15, Ile17, Ile178, Lys179, Ile181, Pro182, Phe185, Lys186, Phe306, Ser309, Leu310, Ser312, Asn313, Pro314). Since flavonoids are compounds that have several aromatic rings, the main interactions formed with the enzyme are of the pi and van der Waals types. The screened flavonoids (Table 2) have a significant number of oxygens; consequently, they can work as hydrogen bond donors and acceptors. Furthermore, according to Kwon [24], residues Pro182 and Phe185 are essential for the structural and functional integrity of the IDO1 enzyme system.

Dichamanetin and isochamanetin A rings interact via pi-sigma interaction with Pro182. According to Kwon [24], this residue would be important for the structural and functional integrity of the IDO1 system. In chamaejasmin B, which is a biflavonoid, one of the A rings interacts with Pro182 (pi-alkyl) and Phe185 (pi-pi) with the assistance of van der Waals interactions with neighboring residues; the second ring A interacts with Phe185 (hydrogen bond) and with Pro314 (pi-alkyl), in addition to van der Waals interactions.

Focusing on substituents attached to the A ring of flavonoids, some structural features must be considered. The hydroxyl group attached to carbon 7 of the A rings of isochamanetin, dichamanetin, and Kushenol E forms strong hydrogen bond interactions with Ser12. Phenyl groups linked to the A ring of dichamanetin and isochamanetin probably help in the stability of the interaction of these compounds with the allosteric site. As shown in Table 2, dichamanetin interacts more strongly with IDO1 than with isochamanetin (−7.8 kcal/mol and −7.5 kcal/mol, respectively), with the first compound forming two pi-alkyl interactions with Pro182. It is also noted that the participation of a weak hydrogen bond interaction with Gly11. Isochamanetin, on the other hand, forms only one interaction. As will be shown in the next section, referring to molecular dynamics simulations, both Ser12 and Pro182 residues contribute significantly to the energetic stabilization of the formed complex.

Table 2. The interacting amino acid residues of IDO1 with chamaejasmin B, dichamanetin, isochamanetin, Kushenol E, and steppogenin.

Compound	Molecular Structure	H Bond	van der Waals	Pi-Alkyl	Pi-Sigma	Pi-Pi	Alkyl	Unfavorable
chamaejasmin B	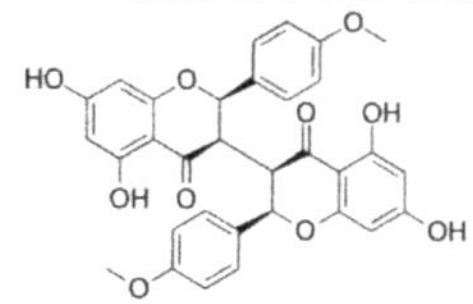	Phe185, Asn313	Tyr15, Ile181, Gln189, Met188, Phe306, Ser309, Leu310	Pro182, Pro314	-	Phe185	Lys186, Pro182	-
dichamanetin	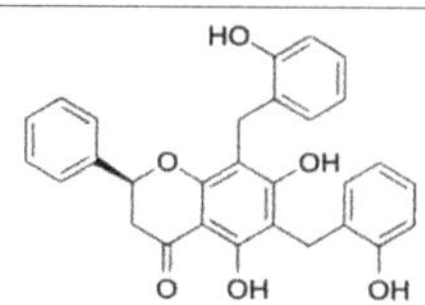	Ser12, Gly11	Ala13, Tyr15, Lys179, Ile181, Lys186, Gln189, Phe306, Ser309, Leu310, Asn313, Pro314	Pro182	Pro182	Phe185	-	-
isochamanetin	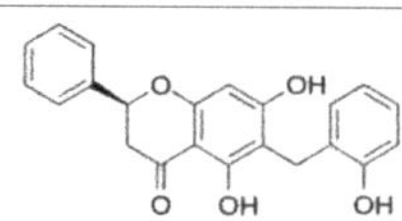	Ser12,	Gly11, Ala13, Lys179, Lys186, Gln189, Asn313, Pro314	Pro182	Pro182	Phe185	-	-
Kushenol E	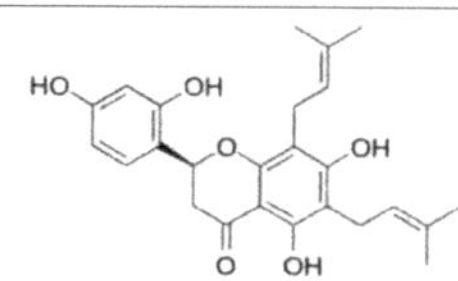	Ser12	Gly11, Lys179, Phe185, Lys186, Gln189, Asn313, Pro314	Pro182	Pro182	-	Ile181, Pro182, Phe306, Leu310	-
steppogenin	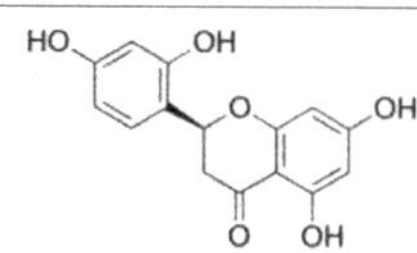	Asn313	Ser12, Tyr15, Phe185, Lys186, Phe306, Ser309, Leu310, Pro314	Pro182	-	-	-	Gln189

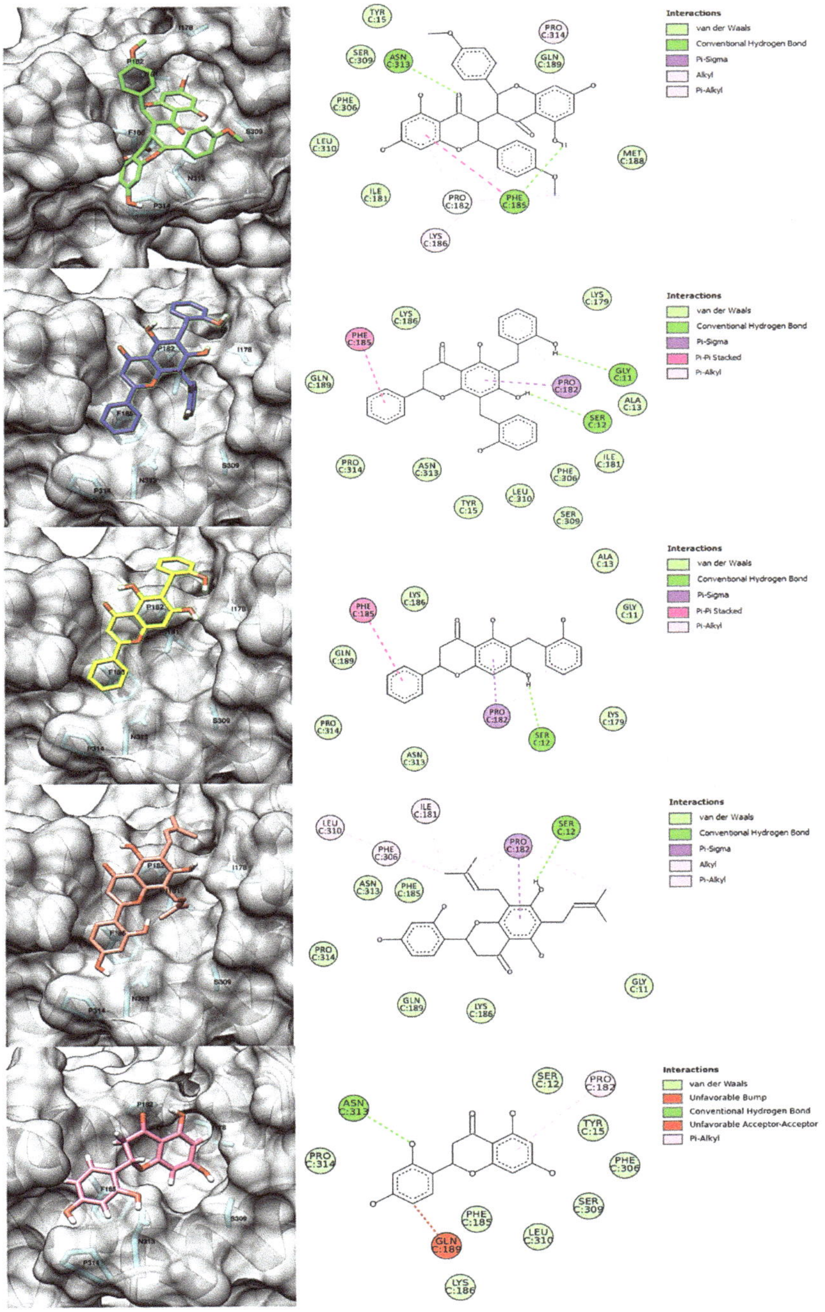

Figure 7. Intermolecular interactions formed with specific residues from the allosteric site of IDO1: chamaejasmin B, dichamanetin, isochamanetin, Kushenol E, and steppogenin, respectively.

Rings B of both dichamanetin and isochamanetin interact via pi-pi stacking with Phe185. Ring B of chamaejasmin B interacts with Pro182 and Lys186 (pi-alkyl interaction). The methoxyl group attached to the C4′ carbon of the ring B of chamaejasmin B forms an alkyl interaction with Pro182. Of all the flavonoids, the only one that interacts with IDO1 from the C ring is chamaejasmin B. This occurs through a hydrogen bond with a carbonyl group on carbon 4 of the C ring. It is worthy of note the fact that steppogenin is the only compound that shows unfavorable bump and acceptor-acceptor interactions.

Pro182 interacts through pi interactions or with the A ring of flavanones or with phenolic groups attached to the same ring. It is known that the proline ring faces are partially positively charged [34]. As shown in Figure 8, hydrogens adjacent to the carbonyl and nitrogen of the amide (Hα and Hδ, respectively) are the most partially positive. The proline side chain is also conformationally restricted, allowing interaction with aromatic residues with minimal entropic or steric penalty [34].

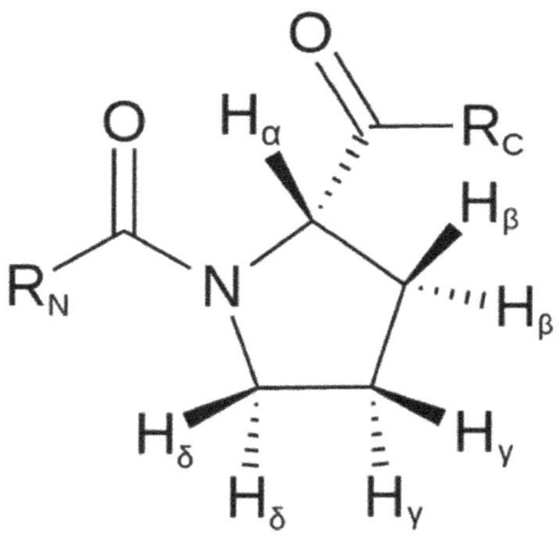

Figure 8. Hydrogens in proline.

Phe185, an aromatic residue (Figure 9), interacts with flavonoids through pi-pi and pi-pi/T stacking, and van der Waals interactions [35], which are very important for the stabilization of the structural energy of protein complexes with flavonoids.

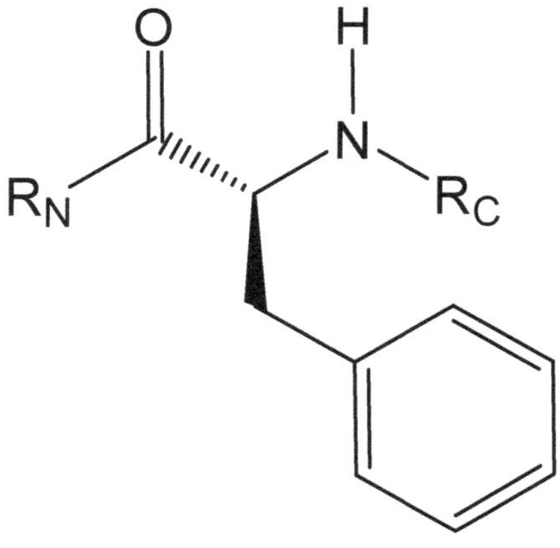

Figure 9. Hydrogens in phenilalanine.

Comparing our docking modeling of Kushenol E (Figure 7) with the docking modeling proposed by Kwon [24] (Figure 10), we can see that our simulation shows this compound in a different orientation in the cavity of the allosteric site, with a deviation of the longitudinal axis towards the B direction for the prenyl group attached to the C6 carbon of the A ring. According to Kwon, the B ring of the flavonoid is positioned inside the cavity formed by the amino acids Leu178, Ile181, and Phe306 (Figure 10). Differently, we found the same ring located next to residues Leu178, Ile181, and Phe306. Furthermore, according to Kwon, A and C rings interact with Ser309 and Asn313. Instead, in our model, this interaction takes place with the Pro182, and there is assistance from a few van der Waals interactions. The Kwon model shows the prenyl group attached to carbon 6 of the ring interacting with Pro314, whereas our model shows interaction with Pro182. Since the structure of the IDO1-Kushenol E complex has not been experimentally determined to date, a definitive answer about the correct orientation of Kushenol E will only be inferred after the structural elucidation study by X-ray crystallography, nuclear magnetic resonance, or cryo-electron microscopy.

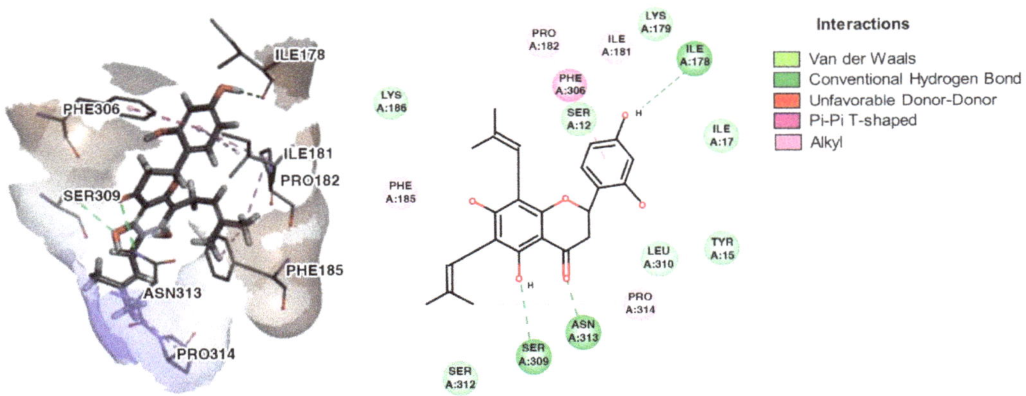

Figure 10. Kwon's docking model of Kushenol E—IDO1 complex [24].

2.3. Molecular Dynamics Simulations and Free Energy Calculation

To further refine and investigate the ability of molecular docking simulation to predict the conformational profile of the IDO1-flavonoid complexes, and to calculate the respective binding free energies, molecular dynamics simulations were carried out.

Three-dimensional structures of the IDO1-flavonoid complexes at 20 ns, 40 ns, 60 ns, 80 ns, and 100 ns are shown in Figure 11. With the exception of chamaejasmin B, which detaches from the allosteric site cavity after 40 ns, all other flavonoids remained docked. Interestingly, after detaching from the allosteric site, chamaejasmin B stabilizes next to the JK loop. Furthermore, only one of the isosacuranetin subunits interacts with the allosteric site, while the other subunit is exposed to the solvent. Moreover, Figure 11 also shows that after 80 ns, steppogenin is almost completely detached from the allosteric site.

It is worthy of note that although the interactions of chamaejasmin B were not strong enough to keep it docked in place during 100 ns, this flavonoid showed the "best" docking energy. It is possible that its isosacuranetin subunit (Figure 12) be a good candidate for future studies of docking and molecular dynamics.

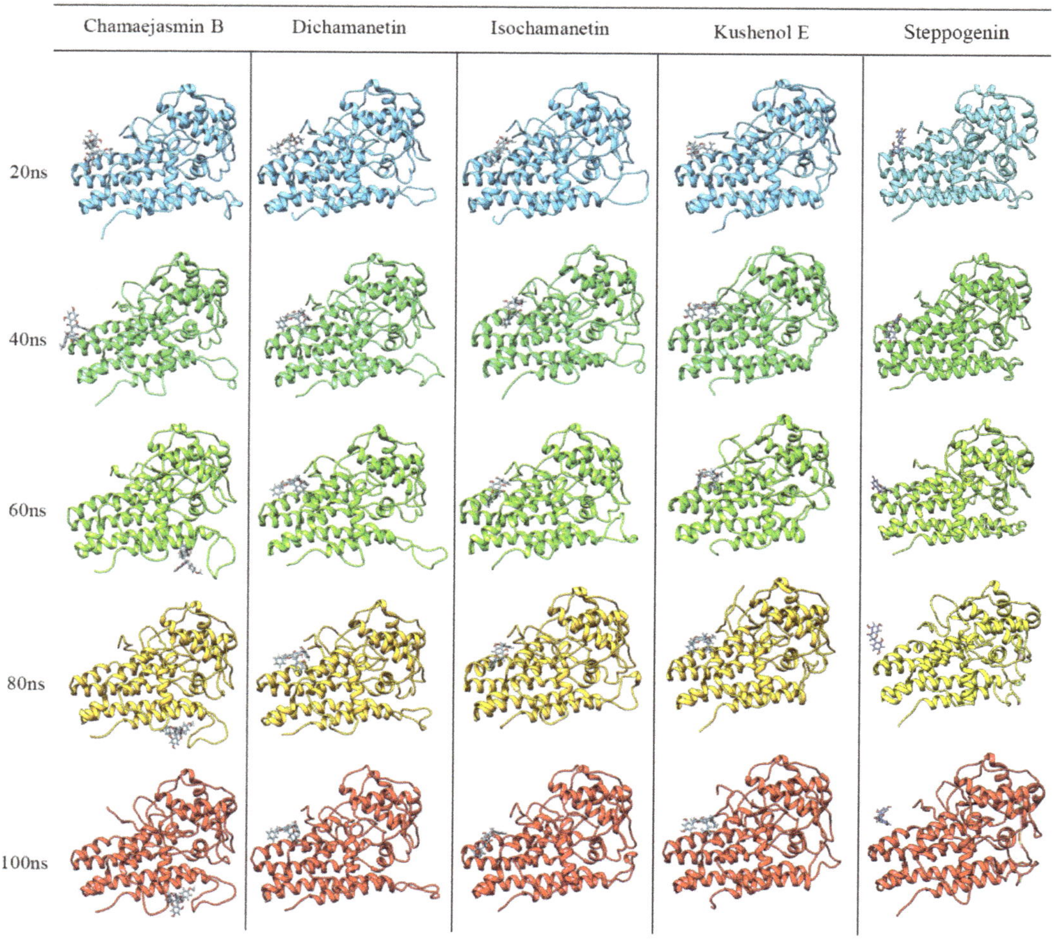

Figure 11. Conformational profile of the complexes formed by the interaction of IDO1 with chamaejasmin B, dichamanetin, isochamanetin, Kushenol E, and steppogenin, respectively, up to 100 ns molecular dynamic simulations.

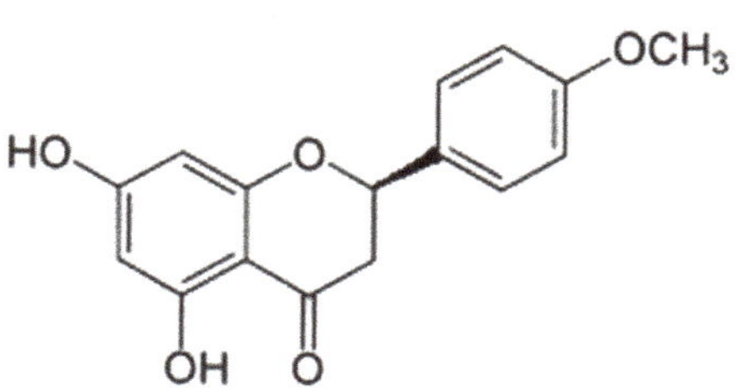

Figure 12. Isosacuranetin.

In order to verify how flavonoids could alter the conformational profile (packing/folding) of IDO1, radii of gyration (Rg) plots were calculated not only for IDO1 in its apo form but also for each IDO1-flavonoid complex. The corresponding plots are shown in Supplementary Material (Figure S1). In molecular dynamics, the radius of gyration is a measure of the stability of a system consisting of several particles and describes the variation in density as a function of the center of mass over time. According to Figure S1, the IDO1-steppogenin complex is the one with the highest degree of energetic-structural destabilization when compared to the other complexes. The IDO1-dichamanetin complex was the most stable. These stability data are supported by the values of relative molecular docking energies, shown in Table 1, and by the values of free energy of interaction between the flavonoids and IDO1, shown in Table 3.

Table 3. Free energy of interaction of each flavonoid with IDO1.

Energy Component	Kushenol E ΔG (kcal/mol)	Steppogenin ΔG (kcal/mol)	Dichamanetin ΔG (kcal/mol)	Isochamanetin ΔG (kcal/mol)
van der Waals	−33.4464 +/− 2.7222	−12.6589 +/− 5.4591	−38.7571 +/− 2.8011	−33.1692 +/− 2.6773
Electrostatic	−0.4995 +/− 2.3494	−9.5176 +/− 5.6553	−8.1238 +/− 3.5253	−2.7772 +/− 2.1816
Polar Solvation	16.2786 +/− 3.5898	18.1821 +/− 8.5497	25.4326 +/− 4.2624	17.7325 +/− 2.3312
SASA	−3.9866 +/− 0.2390	−1.7428 +/− 0.7148	−4.4861 +/− 0.2483	−3.8790 +/− 0.3585
Free energy of interaction	−21.6563 +/− 3.1142	−5.7373 +/− 5.2005	−25.9345 +/− 3.1214	−22.0960 +/− 3.1859

Based on Figure S2, one can assess how each flavonoid changes the conformation of IDO1 (its apo conformation). In this context, Kushenol E and isochamanetin distort the IDO1 structure more significantly. Whereas dichamanetin is the flavonoid that less intensely distorts IDO1.

In addition to the radius of gyration and RMSD plots, root means square fluctuation (RMSF) for Cα of each enzyme residue was calculated (Figure S3). This measure is described by means of a two-dimensional graph where the abscissa shows each Cα associated with a given residue and the ordinate shows the average value of the fluctuations. It is verified that helices B (residues Cys159 to Met190) and G (residues Pro300 to Asn313), important for the formation of the allosteric site, do not undergo significant fluctuations due to the interaction of flavonoids. The EF loop (residues Gly278 to His287), significatively fluctuates due to the interaction of Kushenol E, steppogenin, and isochamanetin. Such an effect is less significant when dichamanetin is the interacting flavonoid. As mentioned before, residues between 251 and 300 and the EF loop are part of the molecular oxygen access tunnel structure. Figure S3 indicates that, of the three flavonoids, only dichamanetin does not "stiffen" the tunnel. The JK loop did not fluctuate significantly under the action of flavonoids.

RMSF plots were also constructed for each docked flavonoid into the allosteric site of IDO1 along with the molecular dynamic simulations (Figure S4). As can be seen, dichamanetin and isochamanetin showed lower atomic fluctuations than Kushenol E and steppogenin do. These results reinforce, once again, the relative stability of the interactions of each flavonoid with the allosteric site.

The complexes were also analyzed for the frequency of hydrogen bonds formed during the molecular dynamics simulation (Figure S5). Dichamanetin has a higher frequency of hydrogen bonds than isochamanetin and Kushenol E. These data demonstrate that hydrogen bonds are important for the stabilization of the IDO1-flavonoid complexes, mainly for dichamanetin and isochamanetin. However, steppogenin shows an "anomalous" hydrogen bond frequency. Perhaps that should be due to the highest degree of freedom ("pose fluctuations"), since, as shown in Figure 11, that compound seems to be slightly bound to the allosteric site.

The MM-PBSA method evaluates conformational fluctuations as a function of the simulation trajectory and, consequently, it is a useful approach for inferring the entropic profile of the formed complexes, as well as for calculating the free energy of binding of each flavonoid with the IDO1. The results are shown, respectively, in Tables 3 and 4. According to Table 3, the affinity of each flavonoid with IDO1 increases in the following order: steppogenin (−5.73 kcal/mol); Kushenol E (−21.65 kcal/mol); isochamanetin (−22.09 kcal/mol); dichamanetin (−25.93 kcal/mol). It is worth noting the calculated affinity value for steppogenin (the negative control), testifying once again, and in accordance with the experimental data [24], that steppogenin forms the least stable complex with IDO1. The free energy contributions of each constituent residue of the allosteric site are shown in Table 4.

Table 4. Distributed binding energies per amino acid for each modeled IDO1-flavonoid complex.

Alloesteric Site	Kushenol E ΔG (kcal/mol)	Steppogenin ΔG (kcal/mol)	Dichamanetin ΔG (kcal/mol)	Isochamanetin ΔG (kcal/mol)
Lys179	−5.6572 +/− 0.009	0.0522 +/− 0.0146	−10.2480 +/− 0.0138	−0.1242 +/− 0.0023
Ile181	−5.5043 +/− 0.003	−0.0478 +/− 0.0006	−7.1328 +/− 0.0045	−5.9646 +/− 0.0042
Pro182	−2.7174 +/− 0.009	−0.6856 +/− 0.0075	−2.9304 +/− 0.0094	−0.9383 +/− 0.0058
Phe185	−9.7036 +/− 0.0064	−0.1037 +/− 0.0017	−10.9729 +/− 0.0063	−2.6943 +/− 0.0152
Lys186	−0.0069 +/− 0.0271	−0.6023 +/− 0.0201	−12.8116 +/− 0.0194	−3.0506 +/− 0.0093
Met188	−0.1075 +/− 0.0007	−0.0451 +/− 0.0006	−0.1199 +/− 0.0006	−6.0922 +/− 0.0049
Gln189	−4.2292 +/− 0.0045	−0.0770 +/− 0.0020	−4.7260 +/− 0.0061	−7.7712 +/− 0.0108
Phe306	−13.3145 +/− 0.0084	−0.0055 +/− 0.0003	−14.2844 +/− 0.0076	−7.4103 +/− 0.0070
Ser309	0.0639 +/− 0.0090	0.0004 +/− 0.0012	0.1190 +/− 0.0077	2.6300 +/− 0.0092
Leu310	−6.0265 +/− 0.0047	−0.0027 +/− 0.0004	−6.1063 +/− 0.0043	−6.0442 +/− 0.0048
Asn313	3.2576 +/− 0.0086	−0.0099 +/− 0.0015	−0.0466 +/− 0.0065	−0.0041 +/− 0.0150
Pro314	−0.0440 +/− 0.0013	−0.0007 +/− 0.0007	−0.0231 +/− 0.0009	−5.5250 +/− 0.0143

3. Materials and Methods

3.1. IDO1

The crystallographic structure of IDO1 in its holo form, with a resolution of 2.44 Å (PDB ID: 7A62) [15], was obtained from the Protein Data Bank [36]. The enzyme preparation steps were carried out as follows: (1) non-essential water molecules were removed; (2) polar hydrogens were added to the enzyme; (3) partial charges were calculated using both Kollman and Gasteiger's approaches [37,38].

3.2. Virtual Screening

For the virtual screening of compounds, Mcule platform [25], ZINC 15 database [26], and AutoDock Vina 1.1.2 program [39] were used.

3.3. Molecular Docking

Molecular docking simulations were performed with the AutoDock Vina 1.1.2 program [39]. This tool uses a hybrid scoring function, i.e., it is a combination of empirical and knowledge-based functions [39]. The binding energy is predicted as the sum of distance-dependent atom pair interactions as follows:

$$E = \sum e_{pair}\,(d)$$

Here d is the surface distance calculated as follows, where r is the interatomic distance and R_i and R_j are the radii of the atoms in the pairs:

$$d = r - R_i - R_j$$

Every atom pair interacts through a steric interaction given by the first three terms of the equation shown below. Moreover, depending on the atom type, there could be hydrophobic and non-directional H-bonding interactions, given by the last two terms.

$$e_{pair}(d) = \begin{cases} + w_1 * Gauss_1(d) \\ + w_2 * Gauss_2(d) \\ + w_3 * Repulsion(d) \\ + w_4 * Hydrophobic(d) \\ + w_5 * HBond(d) \end{cases}$$

The combination of an attractive Gaussian function with a repulsive parabolic function reproduces the general shape of a typical Lennard-Jones interaction, provided the Gaussian term is negative and the parabolic positive.

3.4. Molecular Dynamics Simulations and Free Energy Calculation

All molecular dynamics simulations were performed with the CHARMM36 force field [40] implemented in the GROMACS 2018.1 program [41]. The parameterization of flavonoids was performed using the CHARMM General Force Field (CGenFF) program [42]. Subsequently, a dodecahedral simulation box, including solvent inside (TIP3P water model) was created. Sodium and chlorine ions were added to the system, aiming to electronically neutralize it. Periodic boundary conditions were used.

Each complex was submitted to energy minimization using the steepest descent algorithm, involving 50,000 steps and the convergence criterion of less than 2.39 kcal/mol. Subsequently, two 100 ps molecular dynamics simulations were performed, aiming to balance the IDO1-flavonoid complexes. In the first simulation, the NVT ensemble was used, and in the second one, the NPT ensemble was used. In both cases, the simulation temperature was kept constant at 300 K and, when performing the NPT ensemble, the pressure was kept constant at 1 bar.

After the equilibration of the complexes, 100 ns molecular dynamics simulations were performed, aiming to calculate the free energies of interaction of each flavonoid with IDO1 (production stage). The running conditions were the following: ensemble NPT, where temperature was maintained, using the V-rescale implementation of Berendsen's thermostat [43]. A molecular frame was sampled every 10 ps. To keep the pressure constant, the Parrinello-Rahman pressure coupling method was used [44]; for the long-range treatment, the PME method was used [45].

Free energy calculations were calculated with the g_mmpbsa tool [46]. The binding energy can be individually decomposed as a function of the constituent residues of the macromolecular target. Initially, the E_{MM}, $G_{polar,}$ and $G_{nonpolar}$ energy components of the individual atoms of each residue are calculated in the bound, as well as the unbound form. Subsequently, the contribution to the interaction energy ΔR_x^{BE} of the residue x is calculated as follows:

$$\Delta R_x^{BE} = \sum_{i=0}^{n} \left(A_i^{bound} - A_i^{free} \right)$$

where, A_i^{bound} and A_i^{free} are the energy of atom i of residue x in bonded and unbonded states, respectively, and n is the total number of atoms in the residue. The energy contribution added to all residues is equal to the interaction energy, that is, $\Delta G_{binding} = \sum_{x=0}^{m} \Delta R_x^{BE}$, where m is the total number of residues that make up the ligand-protein complex [46].

3.5. Visualization Tools and Plots

Molecular Visualization Programs BIOVIA Discovery Studio 2021 [47], UCSF Chimera [48], and AutoDock Tools [49] were used. Grace plotting tool was used for graphical analysis [50].

4. Conclusions

IDO1, one of the enzymes that participate in the immune modulation process, is an interesting macromolecular target for anticancer action. From a known drug (Kushenol E), with proven anticancer activity, extensive virtual screening studies were carried out in digital databases. Both ligand- and structure-based approaches were performed. In this context, three natural products, isolated from plants, were identified as potential allosteric site binders of IDO1. Two of which, dichamanetin and isochamanetin, were shown to be promising IDO1 inhibitors and, in our opinion, should be considered in future studies of biological activity, molecular optimization, organic synthesis, and enzymatic assays. From the point of view of structural biology (conformational characteristics of IDO1), it was found that helices constituting the allosteric site did not undergo significant modifications; the same happened for the JK loop (located at the entrance of the catalytic site). In order to investigate, if the presence of the identified allosteric binders could weaken the binding of orthosteric binders (O_2, tryptophan), as well as weaken the binding of the heme cofactor, further simulations, involving multiscale quantum mechanics/molecular mechanics (QM/MM) are being performed in the laboratory.

Supplementary Materials: The following supporting information can be downloaded at: https://www.mdpi.com/article/10.3390/ph15091099/s1, Figure S1: Radius of gyration plots of apo IDO1 (black), IDO1-Kushenol E (red), IDO1-steppogenin (magenta), IDO1-dichamanetin (blue), and IDO1-isochamanetin (yellow) systems.; Figure S2: RMSD plots. Apo IDO1 (black), IDO1-Kushenol E (red), IDO1-steppogenin (magenta), IDO1-dichamanetin (blue), and IDO1-isochamanetin (yellow); Figure S3: RMSF plots. Apo IDO1 (black), IDO1- Kushenol E (red), IDO1-steppogenin (magenta), IDO1-dichamanetin (blue), and IDO1-isochamanetin (yellow); Figure S4: RMSF plots for the flavonoids: Kushenol E (red), steppogenin (magenta), dichamanetin (blue), and isochamanetin (yellow); Figure S5: Hydrogen bond frequency. IDO1 Kushenol E (red), IDO1-steppogenin (magenta), IDO1-dichamanetin (blue) and IDO1-isochamanetin (yellow); Table S1: Screened compounds using Mcule and ZINC 15 databases.

Author Contributions: Conceptualization, O.A.S.-F.; methodology, O.A.S.-F. and V.M.d.A.; software, O.A.S.-F.; validation, O.A.S.-F. and V.M.d.A.; formal analysis, O.A.S.-F. and V.M.d.A.; investigation, V.M.d.A.; resources, O.A.S.-F.; data curation, V.M.d.A.; writing—original draft preparation, O.A.S.-F.; writing—review and editing, O.A.S.-F.; visualization, V.M.d.A.; supervision, O.A.S.-F.; project administration, O.A.S.-F.; funding acquisition, O.A.S.-F. All authors have read and agreed to the published version of the manuscript.

Funding: This study was financed in part by the Coordenação de Aperfeiçoamento de Pessoal de Nível superior—Brasil (CAPES)—Finance Code 001. Resources of the Laboratório de Modelagem Molecular e Biologia Estrutural Computacional (LMMBEC) were used in this research.

Institutional Review Board Statement: Not applicable.

Informed Consent Statement: Not applicable.

Data Availability Statement: Data is contained within the article and supplementary material.

Conflicts of Interest: The authors declare no conflict of interest.

References

1. Esfahani, K.; Roudaia, L.; Buhlaiga, N.; Del Rincon, S.V.; Papneja, N.; Miller, W.H. A review of cancer immunotherapy: From the past, to the present, to the future. *Curr. Oncol.* **2020**, *27*, 87–97. [CrossRef]
2. Platten, M.; Nollen, E.A.A.; Röhrig, U.F.; Fallarino, F.; Opitz, C.A. Tryptophan metabolism as a common therapeutic target in cancer, neurodegeneration and beyond. *Nat. Rev. Drug Discov.* **2019**, *18*, 379–401. [CrossRef] [PubMed]
3. Le Floc'h, N.; Otten, W.; Merlot, E. Tryptophan metabolism, from nutrition to potential therapeutic applications. *Amino Acids* **2011**, *41*, 1195–1205. [CrossRef] [PubMed]
4. Lanser, L.; Kink, P.; Egger, E.M.; Willenbacher, W.; Fuchs, D.; Weiss, G.; Kurz, K. Inflammation-Induced Tryptophan Breakdown is Related with Anemia, Fatigue, and Depression in Cancer. *Front. Immunol.* **2020**, *11*, 249. [CrossRef]
5. Hornyák, L.; Dobos, N.; Koncz, G.; Karányi, Z.; Páll, D.; Szabó, Z.; Halmos, G.; Székvölgyi, L. The role of indoleamine-2,3-dioxygenase in cancer development, diagnostics, and therapy. *Front. Immunol.* **2018**, *9*, 151. [CrossRef] [PubMed]
6. Nguyen, N.T.; Kimura, A.; Nakahama, T.; Chinen, I.; Masuda, K.; Nohara, K.; Fujii-Kuriyama, Y.; Kishimoto, T. Aryl hydrocarbon receptor negatively regulates dendritic cell immunogenicity via a kynurenine-dependent mechanism. *Proc. Natl. Acad. Sci. USA* **2010**, *107*, 19961–19966. [CrossRef]
7. Pallotta, M.T.; Fallarino, F.; Matino, D.; Macchiarulo, A.; Orabona, C. AhR-mediated, non-genomic modulation of IDO1 function. *Front. Immunol.* **2014**, *5*, 497. [CrossRef]
8. Prendergast, G.C.; Malachowski, W.J.; Mondal, A.; Scherle, P.; Muller, A.J. Indoleamine 2,3-Dioxygenase and Its Therapeutic Inhibition in Cancer. *Int. Rev. Cell Mol. Biol.* **2018**, *336*, 175–203. [CrossRef]
9. Vogel, C.F.A.; Goth, S.R.; Dong, B.; Pessah, I.N.; Matsumura, F. Aryl hydrocarbon receptor signaling mediates expression of indoleamine 2,3-dioxygenase. *Biochem. Biophys. Res. Commun.* **2008**, *375*, 331–335. [CrossRef]
10. Hascitha, J.; Priya, R.; Jayavelu, S.; Dhandapani, H.; Selvaluxmy, G.; Sunder Singh, S.; Rajkumar, T. Analysis of Kynurenine/Tryptophan ratio and expression of IDO1 and 2 mRNA in tumour tissue of cervical cancer patients. *Clin. Biochem.* **2016**, *49*, 919–924. [CrossRef]

11. Löb, S.; Königsrainer, A.; Zieker, D.; Brücher, B.L.D.M.; Rammensee, H.G.; Opelz, G.; Terness, P. IDO1 and IDO2 are expressed in human tumors: Levo-but not dextro-$_1$-methyl tryptophan inhibits tryptophan catabolism. *Cancer Immunol. Immunother.* **2009**, *58*, 153–157. [CrossRef] [PubMed]
12. Theate, I.; Van Baren, N.; Pilotte, L.; Moulin, P.; Larrieu, P.; Renauld, J.C.; Herve, C.; Gutierrez-Roelens, I.; Marbaix, E.; Sempoux, C.; et al. Extensive profiling of the expression of the indoleamine 2,3-dioxygenase 1 protein in normal and tumoral human tissues. *Cancer Immunol. Res.* **2015**, *3*, 161–172. [CrossRef] [PubMed]
13. Sook, Y.; Hamdy, H. Involvement of Two Regulatory Elements in Interferon-7-Regulated Expression of Human Indoleamine 2,3-Dioxygenase Gene. *J. Interferon Cytokine Res.* **1995**, *15*, 517–526.
14. Prendergast, G.C.; Jaffee, E.M. *Cancer Immunotherapy: Immune Suppression and Tumor Growth*, 2nd ed.; Academic Press: Cambridge, MA, USA, 2013.
15. Mirgaux, M.; Leherte, L.; Wouters, J. Influence of the presence of the heme cofactor on the JK-loop structure in indoleamine 2,3-dioxygenase 1. *Acta Crystallogr. Sect. D: Struct. Biol.* **2020**, *76*, 1211–1221. [CrossRef]
16. Liu, X.; Zhang, Y.; Duan, H.; Luo, Q.; Liu, W.; Liang, L.; Wan, H.; Chang, S.; Hu, J.; Shi, H. Inhibition Mechanism of Indoleamine 2, 3-Dioxygenase 1 (IDO1) by Amidoxime Derivatives and Its Revelation in Drug Design: Comparative Molecular Dynamics Simulations. *Front. Mol. Biosci.* **2020**, *6*, 164. [CrossRef]
17. Lewis-Ballester, A.; Pham, K.N.; Batabyal, D.; Karkashon, S.; Bonanno, J.B.; Poulos, T.L.; Yeh, S.R. Structural insights into substrate and inhibitor binding sites in human indoleamine 2,3-dioxygenase 1. *Nat. Commun.* **2017**, *8*, 1–8. [CrossRef]
18. Nelp, M.T.; Kates, P.A.; Hunt, J.T.; Newitt, J.A.; Balog, A.; Maley, D.; Zhu, X.; Abell, L.; Allentoff, A.; Borzilleri, R.; et al. Immune-modulating enzyme indoleamine 2,3-dioxygenase is effectively inhibited by targeting its apo-form. *Proc. Natl. Acad. Sci. USA* **2018**, *115*, 3249–3254. [CrossRef]
19. Röhrig, U.F.; Reynaud, A.; Majjigapu, S.R.; Vogel, P.; Pojer, F.; Zoete, V. Inhibition Mechanisms of Indoleamine 2,3-Dioxygenase 1 (IDO1). *J. Med. Chem.* **2019**, *62*, 8784–8795. [CrossRef]
20. Opitz, C.A.; Litzenburger, U.M.; Opitz, U.; Sahm, F.; Ochs, K.; Lutz, C.; Wick, W.; Platten, M. The indoleamine-2,3-dioxygenase (IDO) inhibitor 1-methyl-d-tryptophan upregulates IDO1 in human cancer cells. *PLoS ONE* **2011**, *6*, e19823. [CrossRef]
21. Wang, N.; Zhang, J.; Li, Q.; Xu, H.; Chen, G.; Li, Z.; Liu, D.; Yang, X. Discovery of potent indoleamine 2,3-dioxygenase (IDO) inhibitor from alkaloids in *Picrasma quassioides* by virtual screening and in vitro evaluation. *Fitoterapia* **2019**, *133*, 137–145. [CrossRef] [PubMed]
22. Yue, E.W.; Sparks, R.; Polam, P.; Modi, D.; Douty, B.; Wayland, B.; Glass, B.; Takvorian, A.; Glenn, J.; Zhu, W.; et al. INCB24360 (Epacadostat), a Highly Potent and Selective Indoleamine-2,3-dioxygenase 1 (IDO1) Inhibitor for Immuno-oncology. *ACS Med. Chem. Lett.* **2017**, *8*, 486–491. [CrossRef] [PubMed]
23. Ortiz-Meoz, R.F.; Wang, L.; Matico, R.; Rutkowska-Klute, A.; De la Rosa, M.; Bedard, S.; Midgett, R.; Strohmer, K.; Thomson, D.; Zhang, C.; et al. Characterization of Apo-Form Selective Inhibition of Indoleamine 2,3-Dioxygenase. *ChemBioChem* **2021**, *22*, 516–522. [CrossRef] [PubMed]
24. Kwon, M.; Ko, S.K.; Jang, M.; Kim, G.H.; Ryoo, I.J.; Son, S.; Ryu, H.W.; Oh, S.R.; Lee, W.K.; Kim, B.Y.; et al. Inhibitory effects of flavonoids isolated from Sophora flavescens on indoleamine 2,3-dioxygenase 1 activity. *J. Enzym. Inhib. Med. Chem.* **2019**, *34*, 1481–1488. [CrossRef]
25. Kiss, R.; Sandor, M.; Szalai, F.A. http://Mcule.com: A public web service for drug discovery. *J. Cheminformatics* **2012**, *4*, 17. [CrossRef]
26. Sterling, T.; Irwin, J.J. ZINC 15-Ligand Discovery for Everyone. *J. Chem. Inf. Modeling* **2015**, *55*, 2324–2337. [CrossRef]
27. Tanimoto, T.T. *Elementary Mathematical Theory of Classification and Prediction*, 1st ed.; International Business Machines Corporation: New York, NY, USA, 1958.
28. Chokchaisiri, R.; Kunkaewom, S.; Chokchaisiri, S.; Ganranoo, L.; Chalermglin, R.; Suksamrarn, A. Potent cytotoxicity against human small cell lung cancer cells of the heptenes from the stem bark of Xylopia pierrei Hance. *Med. Chem. Res.* **2017**, *26*, 1291–1296. [CrossRef]
29. Quimque, M.T.; Notarte, K.I.; Letada, A.; Fernandez, R.A.; Pilapil, D.Y.; Pueblos, K.R.; Agbay, J.C.; Dahse, H.M.; Wenzel-Storjohann, A.; Tasdemir, D.; et al. Potential Cancer- And Alzheimer's Disease-Targeting Phosphodiesterase Inhibitors from Uvaria alba: Insights from in Vitro and Consensus Virtual Screening. *ACS Omega* **2021**, *6*, 8403–8417. [CrossRef]
30. Yong, Y.; Matthew, S.; Wittwer, J.; Pan, L.; Shen, Q.; Kinghorn, A.D.; Swanson, S.M.; Blanco, E.J.C.D. Dichamanetin Inhibits Cancer Cell Growth by Affecting ROS-related Signaling Components through Mitochondrial-mediated Apoptosis. *Anticancer. Res.* **2013**, *33*, 5349–5355.
31. Swarnalatha, Y.; Vidhya, V.G.; Murugan, A. Isochamanetin is a Selective Inhibitor for CyclinD1 in SKOV3 Cell Lines. *Nutr. Cancer* **2019**, *71*, 657–667. [CrossRef] [PubMed]
32. Lasswell, W.L., Jr.; Hufford, C.D. Cytotoxic C-Benzylated Flavonoids from Uvaria chamae. *J. Org. Chem.* **1976**, *42*, 4–11.
33. Zhang, C.; Zhou, S.S.; Feng, L.Y.; Zhang, D.Y.; Lin, N.M.; Zhang, L.H.; Pan, J.P.; Wang, J.B.; Li, J. In vitro anti-cancer activity of chamaejasmenin B and neochamaejasmin C isolated from the root of *Stellera chamaejasme* L. *Acta Pharmacol. Sin.* **2013**, *34*, 262–270. [CrossRef]
34. Zondlo, N.J. Aromatic-Proline Interactions: Electronically Tunable CH/π Interactions. *Acc. Chem. Res.* **2012**, *46*, 1039–1049. [CrossRef] [PubMed]
35. Martinez, C.R.; Iverson, B.L. Rethinking the term "pi-stacking". *Chem. Sci.* **2012**, *3*, 2191–2201. [CrossRef]

36. Berman, H.M.; Westbrook, J.; Feng, Z.; Gilliland, G.; Bhat, T.N.; Weissig, H.; Shindyalov, I.N.; Bourne, P.E. The Protein Data Bank. *Nucleic Acids Res.* **2000**, *28*, 235–242. [CrossRef] [PubMed]
37. Bayly, C.I.; Cieplak, P.; Cornell, W.D.; Kollman, P.A. A well-behaved electrostatic potential based method using charge restraints for deriving atomic charges: The RESP model. *J. Phys. Chem.* **1993**, *97*, 10269–10280. [CrossRef]
38. Gasteiger, J.; Marsili, M. Iterative partial equalization of orbital electronegativity-a rapid access to atomic charges. *Tetrahedron* **1980**, *36*, 3219–3228. [CrossRef]
39. Trott, O.; Olson, A.J. AutoDock Vina: Improving the speed and accuracy of docking with a new scoring function, efficient optimization, and multithreading. *J. Comput. Chem.* **2009**, *31*, 455–461. [CrossRef]
40. Huang, J.; Rauscher, S.; Nawrocki, G.; Ran, T.; Feig, M.; De Groot, B.L.; Grubmüller, H.; MacKerell, A.D. CHARMM36m: An improved force field for folded and intrinsically disordered proteins. *Nat. Methods* **2016**, *14*, 71–73. [CrossRef]
41. Abraham, M.J.; Murtola, T.; Schulz, R.; Páll, S.; Smith, J.C.; Hess, B.; Lindah, E. Gromacs: High performance molecular simulations through multi-level parallelism from laptops to supercomputers. *SoftwareX* **2015**, *1–2*, 19–25. [CrossRef]
42. Vanommeslaeghe, K.; Hatcher, E.; Acharya, C.; Kundu, S.; Zhong, S.; Shim, J.; Darian, E.; Guvench, O.; Lopes, P.; Vorobyov, I.; et al. CHARMM General Force Field (CGenFF): A force field for drug-like molecules compatible with the CHARMM all-atom additive biological force fields. *J. Comput. Chem.* **2010**, *31*, 671–690. [CrossRef]
43. Berendsen, H.J.C.; Postma, J.P.M.; Van Gunsteren, W.F.; Dinola, A.; Haak, J.R. Molecular dynamics with coupling to an external bath. *J. Chem. Phys.* **1984**, *81*, 3684–3690. [CrossRef]
44. Parrinello, M.; Rahman, A. Polymorphic transitions in single crystals: A new molecular dynamics method. *J. Appl. Phys.* **1981**, *52*, 7182–7190. [CrossRef]
45. Essmann, U.; Perera, L.; Berkowitz, M.L.; Darden, T.; Lee, H.; Pedersen, L.G. A smooth particle mesh Ewald method. *J. Chem. Phys.* **1995**, *103*, 8577–8593. [CrossRef]
46. Kumari, R.; Kumar, R.; Lynn, A. G-mmpbsa-A GROMACS tool for high-throughput MM-PBSA calculations. *J. Chem. Inf. Modeling* **2014**, *54*, 1951–1962. [CrossRef] [PubMed]
47. *BIOVIA, Dassault Systèmes*; 21.1.0; Discovery Studio Visualizer; Dassault Systèmes: San Diego, CA, USA, 2021.
48. Pettersen, E.F.; Goddard, T.D.; Huang, C.C.; Couch, G.S.; Greenblatt, D.M.; Meng, E.C.; Ferrin, T.E. UCSF Chimera—a visualization system for exploratory research and analysis. *J. Comput. Chem.* **2004**, *13*, 1605–1612. [CrossRef]
49. Morris, G.M.; Ruth, H.; Lindstrom, W.; Sanner, M.F.; Belew, R.K.; Goodsell, D.S.; Olson, A.J. Software news and updates AutoDock4 and AutoDockTools4: Automated docking with selective receptor flexibility. *J. Comput. Chem.* **2009**, *30*, 2785–2791. [CrossRef]
50. Grace. Available online: https://plasma-gate.weizmann.ac.il/Grace/ (accessed on 12 July 2022).

pharmaceuticals

Review

In Silico Approaches: A Way to Unveil Novel Therapeutic Drugs for Cervical Cancer Management

Diana Gomes [1,2,3], Samuel Silvestre [1,4,5,6], Ana Paula Duarte [1,4,6], Aldo Venuti [7], Christiane P. Soares [8], Luís Passarinha [1,2,3,4,*] and Ângela Sousa [1,*]

1 CICS-UBI—Health Sciences Research Centre, Universidade da Beira Interior, 6201-506 Covilhã, Portugal; dianarouca@gmail.com (D.G.); sms@ubi.pt (S.S.); apcd@ubi.pt (A.P.D.)
2 Associate Laboratory i4HB—Institute for Health and Bioeconomy, Faculdade de Ciências e Tecnologia, Universidade NOVA, 2819-516 Caparica, Portugal
3 UCIBIO—Applied Molecular Biosciences Unit, Departamento de Química/Departamento Ciências da Vida, Faculdade de Ciências e Tecnologia, Universidade NOVA de Lisboa, 2829-516 Caparica, Portugal
4 Laboratório de Fármaco-Toxicologia-UBIMedical, Universidade da Beira Interior, 6200-284 Covilhã, Portugal
5 CNC—Center for Neuroscience and Cell Biology, University of Coimbra, 3004-504 Coimbra, Portugal
6 C4—Cloud Computing Competence Centre, UBIMedical, Universidade da Beira Interior, Estrada Municipal 506, 6200-284 Covilhã, Portugal
7 HPV-UNIT-UOSD Tumor Immunology and Immunotherapy, IRCCS Regina Elena National Cancer Institute, 00144 Rome, Italy; aldo.venuti@ifo.gov.it
8 Department of Clinical Analysis, School of Pharmaceutical Sciences, São Paulo State University (UNESP), Campus Ville, Araraquara 14800-903, São Paulo, Brazil; soarescp@fcfar.unesp.br
* Correspondence: lpassarinha@fcsaude.ubi.pt (L.P.); angela@fcsaude.ubi.pt (Â.S.); Tel.: +35-12-7532-9069 (L.P.); +35-12-7532-9052 (Â.S.)

Citation: Gomes, D.; Silvestre, S.; Duarte, A.P.; Venuti, A.; Soares, C.P.; Passarinha, L.; Sousa, Â. In Silico Approaches: A Way to Unveil Novel Therapeutic Drugs for Cervical Cancer Management. *Pharmaceuticals* **2021**, *14*, 741. https://doi.org/10.3390/ph14080741

Academic Editor: Osvaldo Andrade Santos-Filho

Received: 1 July 2021
Accepted: 27 July 2021
Published: 29 July 2021

Abstract: Cervical cancer (CC) is the fourth most common pathology in women worldwide and presents a high impact in developing countries due to limited financial resources as well as difficulties in monitoring and access to health services. Human papillomavirus (HPV) is the leading cause of CC, and despite the approval of prophylactic vaccines, there is no effective treatment for patients with pre-existing infections or HPV-induced carcinomas. High-risk (HR) HPV E6 and E7 oncoproteins are considered biomarkers in CC progression. Since the E6 structure was resolved, it has been one of the most studied targets to develop novel and specific therapeutics to treat/manage CC. Therefore, several small molecules (plant-derived or synthetic compounds) have been reported as blockers/inhibitors of E6 oncoprotein action, and computational-aided methods have been of high relevance in their discovery and development. In silico approaches have become a powerful tool for reducing the time and cost of the drug development process. Thus, this review will depict small molecules that are already being explored as HR HPV E6 protein blockers and in silico approaches to the design of novel therapeutics for managing CC. Besides, future perspectives in CC therapy will be briefly discussed.

Keywords: cervical cancer management; computer-aided drug design; E6 inhibitors; in silico studies; human papillomavirus

1. Introduction

Cancers are some of the deadliest pathologies, and according to Globocan, the global cancer burden in 2020 increased to 19.3 million cases and 10 million cancer deaths. With these new data, it is estimated that 1 in 5 people will develop cancer during their lifetime, and 1 in 8 men and 1 in 11 women will die from the disease [1]. Thereby, as logical consequence, novel pharmacotherapy approaches have increased in the recent years [2]. In particular, cervical cancer (CC) is considered the fourth cause of death among women worldwide with its establishment being associated with human papillomavirus (HPV) infection [3]. Considering the data available by Globocan regarding this pathology, there were 341,831 deaths in 2020 with a higher incidence in low-income countries (LIC). In fact, in less developed regions such as Africa, Asia, and South America, CC is the primary cancer found in women, which can be due to the lack of screening programs, limited resources and access to health care, or even anti-vaccination movements [4,5]. In developed countries, the incidence of CC cases is lower due to better health services and the high availability of HPV prophylactic vaccines, which constitutes a great step in the prevention of HPV-associated cancers. However, the prophylactic vaccines have only been effective when administered in healthy patients, and they are not able to exert a therapeutic effect or treat an established infection [6].

The current treatments for CC are based on excisional or ablative procedures, surgical resection, radiotherapy, or chemotherapy, which do not specifically target the oncogenic properties of HPV, and therefore lesion recurrence can occur [7]. In addition, most of these procedures can affect normal tissues and can have potential side effects, including bleeding, which cause patient discomfort and can reduce life quality [5]. These constraints highlight the need to improve the current therapeutic approaches by combining strategies or proposing new compounds to offer more specific and less invasive treatments, without affecting healthy tissues. Hence, the scientific community has been focused on different ways to combat CC. A strategy with great potential consists of finding new anticancer agents by targeting the major oncoproteins responsible for HPV-driven carcinogenesis, E6 and E7. In fact, the discovery of the E6 protein X-ray crystal structure, available in protein data bank (PDB ID: 4GIZ and 4XR8, accessed on 20th May 2021), led to an increase in the use of in silico approaches to uncover potential E6 inhibitors [8].

Drug discovery and development is a very expensive and time-consuming process, which can take 10 to 15 years until a drug reaches the market. In the last decades, the pharmaceutical industry has been employing computer-aided drug design (CADD) techniques to accelerate drug development, intending to reduce time, costs, and failures, namely in the final stage [9,10]. This analysis is based on calculated properties and prediction models for drug therapeutic targets and identification of safety liabilities. Typically, CADD can be divided into three categories: structure-based, ligand-based, and hybrid methods [11,12]. The structure-based approaches, including docking and the application of molecular dynamics simulations, use the 3D structure of the target molecule to screen potential ligands. These methods evaluate ligand recognition by the target molecule and the prediction and characterization of binding sites as well as binding affinity [9,12]. For instance, molecular docking is one of the most applied techniques to select promising molecules from large libraries by predicting the orientation of a compound towards the target and characterizing ligand–target interactions. Molecular dynamics techniques entail the motion principles to molecules and are frequently used to perform binding mode studies and to predict the stability of a ligand–target complex, giving a deeper understanding to the researchers on the interaction of a ligand to a biomolecular target [9,11–13]. On the other hand, ligand-based methods, including similarity searching, pharmacophore modeling, and quantitative structure–activity relationship (QSAR) studies, use the information of groups of small molecules with different structures capable of interacting with the target to identify new and powerful compounds [12,14]. These methods are usually applied when the 3D structure of the target is not available and assume that analogous compounds show similar biological activity and interaction with the target. QSAR modeling allows understanding the effects of structural variables on biological activity to develop compounds with enhanced and optimal pharmacological profiles. Another ligand-based method is similarity searching, which is mostly applied in filtering compounds from big libraries based on the assumption that compounds with structural similarity can have similar bioactivity [9]. When the 3D structure of the target is available, as well as the ligands' structure, it is possible to use hybrid methods. This means combining structure-based and ligand-based methods to perform some types of pharmacophore modeling or to predict the activity considering the biological profile of tested compounds against several targets [12]. In fact, combining CADD methods can be more effective once their advantages complement one another [11,12]. Given the importance of pharmacokinetics and toxicity properties of selected compounds, in silico ADMET (Absorption, Distribution, Metabolism, Excretion, and Toxicity) filters can also be applied to eliminate compounds with potential undesirable physiological qualities [9]. With the improvement of technology and bioinformatic tools, the use of in silico approaches for drug development, mainly in preliminary studies, has increased over the years.

Hence, in this review, we intend to summarize the current treatment used for CC stages induced by HPV persistent infection, present the small molecules that are already being explored as inhibitors/blockers for E6 protein, and retrospectively analyze the studies published in the last years that applied in silico approaches to the design of novel therapeutics for CC treatment. In addition, we will concisely discuss the future perspectives for CC management.

2. HPV, CC Development, and Clinical Treatment

HPV is the etiological agent associated with CC. There are about 200 HPV genotypes of high-risk (HR HPV) and low-risk (LR HPV) identified. HPV16 and 18 are responsible for more than 70% of invasive CC. The HPV genome presents tropism for epithelial cells, and the infections appear mainly in the anogenital tract [3,5,15] and head and neck anatomic sites. While HPV is the hallmark of CC development [15], the classic major risk factors to head and neck cancer are tobacco and alcohol, but in the past few decades, human papillomavirus (HPV) has emerged as a novel risk factor [16,17]. The biology and life cycle of human papillomavirus have been reviewed elsewhere [18]. However, we considered it helpful to readers to give a brief insight into the HPV life cycle that may lead to carcinogenesis.

The HPV genome encodes eight genes; the L1 and L2 structural proteins constitute the capsid that protects the viral genome, and the E1, E2, E4, E5, E6, and E7 proteins are involved in replication, transcription regulation, and oncogenesis. E6 and E7 oncoprotein expression disrupt the cell repair mechanisms by degradation or inhibition of the tumor suppressor proteins p53 and retinoblastoma protein (pRB), respectively, resulting in the immortalization and cellular transformation of infected cells [19–21]. The viral life cycle begins with viral particles arriving in the basal layer of the squamous epithelia via micro-abrasions. After reaching the nucleus the viral DNA is replicated, and low quantities of E1, E2, E6, and E7 proteins are produced early in the infection, halting normal keratinocyte development. Then, E2 recruits E1 to increase the number of viral episome copies, which continue to rise as the epithelium differentiates. E6 and E7 proteins are abundantly expressed in the top differentiating epithelial layers, resulting in uncontrolled cell proliferation, and the viral life cycle is completed when L1 and L2 proteins are expressed in the epithelium's highest layer. As a result, the viral genome is encapsulated, and mature virions are released [22,23]. Although many women contract HPV, most infections are eliminated or controlled by the immune system after 1–2 years [24]. The establishment of persistent infection is associated with the appearance of cervical lesions, since the accumulation of DNA damage caused by HR HPV E6 and E7 interactions with tumor suppressors, p53 and pRb, causes apoptosis suppression and uncontrolled proliferation. The chronically infected cells lead to the establishment of cervical intraepithelial neoplasia (CIN), as CIN grade I, which over time can evolve to CIN grade II, III, or invasive carcinoma [23,24].

CC is staged according to different systems. The most widely used is the FIGO system proposed by the International Federation of Gynecology and Obstetrics in collaboration with the International Union Against Cancer (IUCC) [7]. Table 1 summarizes the different stages of FIGO's system with the current treatment for managing CC.

Table 1. CC stages according to the FIGO system and the recommended treatment.

Stage	Substage	Description	Recommended Treatment
I	IA1	The disease is only found in the cervix	Conization or cone biopsy; simple hysterectomy
	IA2		Conization; simple hysterectomy with pelvic lymphadenectomy; radical hysterectomy
	IB1		Radical hysterectomy or radical trachelectomy with lymphadenectomy
	IB2		
II	IIA1	Outside the cervix, cancer has progressed to the upper vaginal wall or tissue next to the cervix (parametrium), but not to the pelvic sidewall(s)	Radical hysterectomy or radical trachelectomy with lymphadenectomy
	IIA2		Radiotherapy (RT) with or without chemotherapy
	IIB		Cisplatin-based chemotherapy and concurrent radiation (CRT)
III	IIIA	Cancer has advanced to the lower region of the vagina and through the parametrium until the pelvic sidewall(s)	Cisplatin-based chemotherapy and concurrent radiation
	IIIB		
IV	IVA	Cancer has advanced to adjacent organs or distant tissue, such as lungs and distant lymph nodes	Palliative radiotherapy or palliative systemic cytotoxic chemotherapy
	IVB		

All surgical interventions can cause side effects or complications, including bleeding and damage in the tissue nearby, and simple or radical hysterectomy results in infertility or bladder/bowel dysfunction [25]. With the spread of cancer to other tissues (metastasis), surgery is no longer a viable possibility. Radiation therapy (RT) uses radiation to destroy cancer cells, and it is possible to affect mainly the zones with the tumor in the lower abdomen in CC cases. Some side effects can be infertility, discomfort, and menopause. Chemotherapy involves the administration of cytotoxic drugs to interfere with cell proliferation, killing rapidly dividing cells. The currently approved drugs by the FDA for CC treatment include, among others, bleomycin sulfate, topotecan, pembrolizumab, bevacizumab, cisplatin, paclitaxel, vinorelbine, ifosfamide, fluorouracil, and gemcitabine [26]. Nevertheless, these treatments are unable to effectively distinguish healthy from cancer cells, affecting several types of dividing cells throughout the entire body. This effect can result, namely, in a higher risk of anemia, bleeding, and infections [3,25]. Hence, the design and development of therapeutic agents that are efficient, non-toxic, and capable of distinguishing cancerous from healthy tissue are essential. In addition, for managing early-stage CC, the employment of less invasive methods to improve quality of life and decrease treatment-related sexual dysfunction is a necessity.

3. E6 Protein

As mentioned before, E6 and E7 proteins of HR HPV play a major role in CC development once its growth is dependent on sustained E6/E7 expression. The interest in HR HPV E6 protein as a potential therapeutic target has arisen in the past years. This protein is essentially found in the cell nucleus and is constituted by 150–160 amino acids and two zinc-binding motifs. In 2013, Zanier and co-workers published in PDB the 3D structure of HPV16 E6 protein bound to the E6AP interaction domain (ID: 4GIZ) [27]. More recently, the same research group also published the 3D structure of the E6-E6AP-p53 trimeric complex (ID: 4XR8) [28]. The wild-type (wt) HPV16 E6 protein forms intermolecular disulphide bonds, which makes it very difficult, if not impossible, to purify [29]. Thus, Zanier and colleagues used an E6 nonfull-sequence structure (4C/4S mutant) to achieve its crystallization, where four cysteines were replaced with four serine residues. The E6 4C/4S mutant maintains the ability to degrade p53 in a very similar way to that of HPV16 wt E6 [30]. These crystallographic findings determine the identification and design of novel compounds to block the HR HPV E6 oncoprotein action with higher efficiency. As the E7 protein 3D structure is still unknown/resolved, this explains why researchers are mainly directing their efforts in developing strategies to block E6 to the detriment of E7.

The E6 protein binds to E6AP (E6-associated protein), a ubiquitin ligase required for the interaction with p53 protein. The formation of the trimeric E6-E6AP-p53 complex is responsible for the ubiquitination and degradation of p53, resulting in p53-dependent apoptosis blockage. The crystallization data revealed that HPV16 E6 is composed of an N-terminal and a C-terminal connected by an alpha helix, forming the hydrophobic binding pocket for E6AP [27]. E6 targets other structures that are involved in several molecular pathways, bringing down some cancer hallmarks. For example, HR HPV E6 protein is able to activate telomerase by transcriptional up-regulation of TERT (reverse transcriptase component of telomerase). There are two mechanisms proposed for this phenomenon, and both require the E6-E6AP complex formation. Briefly, one of the models proposes that the E6-E6AP complex can bind to NFX1-91 (repressor of TERT transcription) causing its degradation and releasing the transcriptional repression at the TERT promoter. On the other model, the E6-E6AP complex binds to c-myc, which may displace the inhibitory USF transcriptional repressor from the E box in the TERT promoter. Other mechanisms are possible once the telomerase activation is not well understood. Besides telomere elongation, TERT can participate in apoptosis inhibition and allow cell proliferation, which increases the probability of malignant conversion [31]. Besides E6AP binding, E6 only from high-risk HPV can bind to the PDZ-domain family of proteins through its C-terminal, although this region is not necessary for p53 interaction [28,32,33]. Thus, HR HPV E6 protein complexes, along with the different proteins that bind to E6, affect several biological functions such as cell survival, DNA damage, and cell cycle progression. Considering the problems associated with current treatments for CC and the important role of E6 oncoprotein in the progression of HR HPV infection towards cervical lesions, the inhibition/blockage of its function could be a promising and specific therapeutic strategy. Indeed, several authors have shown that decreased HR HPV E6 expression by RNA interference, flavonoids, and intracellular antibodies could restore p53 levels and induce apoptosis in HPV-positive cell lines [34,35]. Hence, a presentation of the advances made in anticancer drug design and development for the HR HPV E6 protein using computational methods will be performed. For that, three databases (PubMed, Web of Science, and ScienceDirect) were used to search articles published after 2015 with the following keywords: E6 inhibitors AND in silico; E6 inhibitors AND molecular docking; E6 protein AND in silico; E6 protein AND molecular docking.

3.1. E6-E6AP Complex Inhibitors

The HR HPV E6 protein has different binding pockets, including the hydrophobic pocket where the LxxLL motif of E6AP binds, the PDZ-binding domain, and the p53 binding site, Figure 1 [27,28]. Until recently, the most explored area to achieve inhibition has been the hydrophobic pocket, to the detriment of the HR HPV E6PDZ domain.

Researchers have been taking advantage of the E6/E6AP complex 3D structure available on PDB (ID: 4GIZ) to understand the interactions involved between both proteins and to apply in silico methods to design potential inhibitors. E6AP is required to induce E6-mediated p53 degradation by inducing structural changes in the E6 protein, which allow the formation of the trimeric complex E6/E6AP/p53 [28]. The hydrophobic pocket able to recognize the LxxLL motif is mainly constituted by the following amino acid residues: Leu100, Leu50, Cys51, Val53, Val62, Leu67, Tyr32, Tyr70, and Ile73 [27].

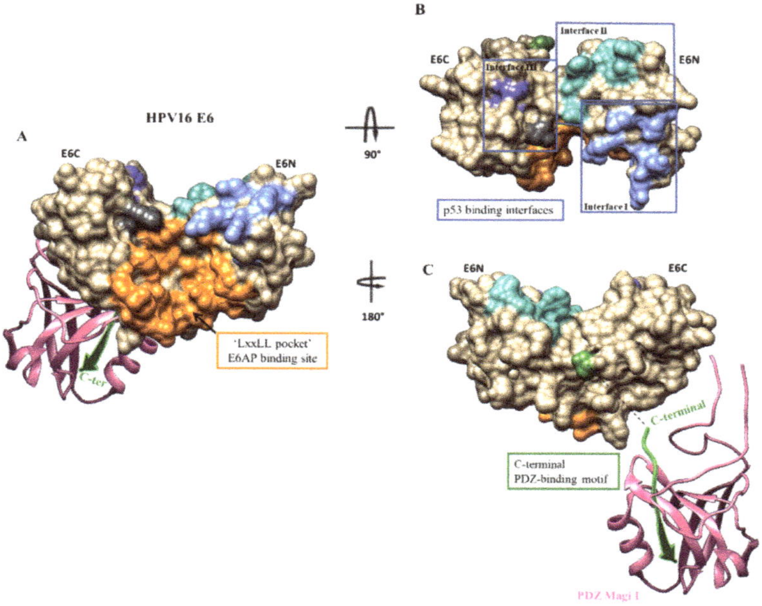

Figure 1. A map of different binding sites of the HPV16 E6 protein using PDB ID 4XR8 and 2KPL on Chimera software. Surface representation of E6 residues that participate in the binding with E6AP (**A**), p53 (**B**), and the PDZ domain (**C**). **A**—Orange residues participate in E6AP binding; **B**—The three interfaces of contact between E6 and p53 are colored in light, medium, and dark blue. **C**—The C-terminal PDZ binding motif is represented in green. E6N: N-terminal; E6C: C-terminal.

3.1.1. Synthetic Compounds

Ricci-López and co-workers developed an in silico pipeline to propose potential inhibitors of E6/E6AP interaction [36]. For this, the HPV16 E6 sequence (UniProt ID: P03126) and the template retrieved from the ternary complex E6/E6AP/p53 (PDB ID: 4XR8) were used to obtain the full-length structure of the HPV-16 E6 protein by homology modeling once the E6 protein was crystallized by using a 4C/4S mutant, as mentioned earlier. Twenty-six compounds described in the literature as capable of binding to E6 were used as reference molecules and queries in the Zinc15 database to build a compound library with almost 35,000 molecules using a structural similarity approach. ZINC15 is a public access database provided by the Irwin and Schoichet Laboratories in the Department of Pharmaceutical Chemistry at the University of California, San Francisco (UCSF). It contains over 230 million purchasable compounds in ready-to-dock, 3D formats and over 750 million purchasable compounds, and it is possible to search for analogues. It is widely used for virtual screening, ligand discovery, and pharmacophore screens, among others. Compounds were then filtered considering ADME properties, and those with the highest potential were submitted to molecular docking studies considering the hydrophobic pocket as the binding site. After the binding free energy calculations of the best-docked complexes, compound **1** (ZINC111606147), compound **2** (ZINC362643639), and compound **3** (ZINC96096545) (Figure 2) were selected for further evaluation through molecular dynamics simulations. When compared to luteolin (reference ligand), these three compounds had higher affinity to the E6 protein, and all docked complexes were stable and capable of inhibiting E6/E6AP interaction [36].

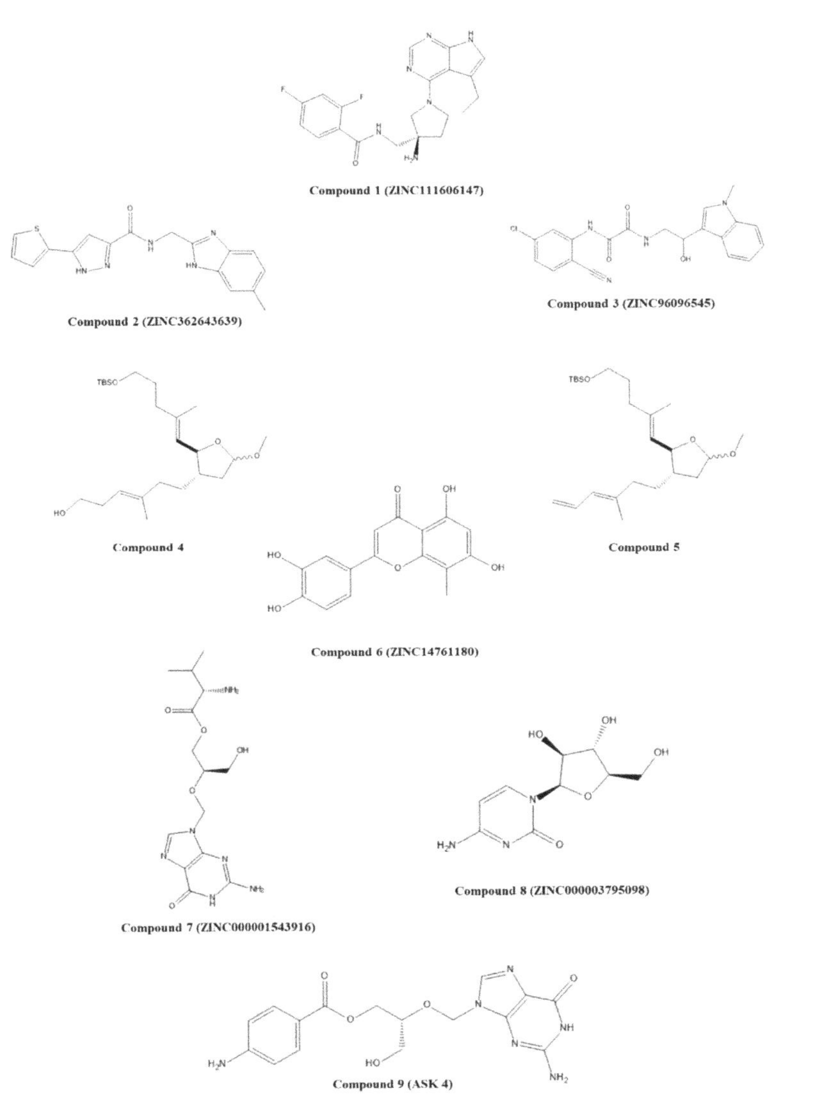

Figure 2. Structures of studied synthetic compounds as E6/E6AP inhibitors. IUPAC name of compounds—compound **1**: (*S*)-*N*-((3-amino-1-(5-ethyl-7*H*-pyrrolo [2,3-*d*]pyrimidin-4-yl)pyrrolidin-3-yl)methyl)-2,4-difluorobenzamide; compound **2**: *N*-((6-methyl-1*H*-benzo[*d*]imidazol-2-yl)methyl)-5-(thiophen-2-yl)-1*H*-pyrazole-3-carboxamide; compound **3**: N^1-(5-chloro-2-cyanophenyl)-N^2-(2-hydroxy-2-(1-methyl-1*H*-indol-3-yl)ethyl)oxalamide; compound **4**: (*E*)-6-((2*S*,3*S*)-2-((*E*)-5-((*tert*-butyldimethylsilyl)oxy)-2-methylpent-1-en-1-yl)-5-methoxytetrahydrofuran-3-yl)-4-methylhex-3-en-1-ol; compound **5**: *tert*-butyl(((*E*)-5-((2*S*,3*S*)-5-methoxy-3-((*E*)-3-methylhexa-3,5-dien-1-yl)tetrahydrofuran-2-yl)-4-methylpent-4-en-1-yl)oxy)dimethylsilane; compound **6**: 2-(3,4-dihydroxyphenyl)-5,7-dihydroxy-8-methyl-4*H*-chromen-4-one; compound **7**: (*S*)-(*R*)-2-((2-amino-6-oxo-1*H*-purin-9(6*H*)-yl)methoxy)-3-hydroxypropyl 2-amino-3-methylbutanoate; compound **8**: 4-amino-1-((2*R*,3*S*,4*S*,5*R*)-3,4-dihydroxy-5-(hydroxymethyl)tetrahydrofuran-2-yl)pyrimidin-2(1*H*)-one; compound **9**: (*R*)-2-((2-amino-6-oxo-1*H*-purin-9(6*H*)-yl)methoxy)-3-hydroxypropyl 4-aminobenzoate.

Senthilkumar and colleagues described ansiomelic acid (AA), a compound isolated from the plant *Anisomeles malabarica*, as being able to inhibit E6 and E7 protein expression and induce apoptosis in HPV-positive cancer cells. Then, they decided to perform a structure–activity relationship study with several AA analogues to identify potent inhibitors of HPV E6 and E7 oncoproteins [37]. Molecular docking was used to predict the affinity of 26 AA-derived compounds towards the hydrophobic pocket of the E6 protein (PDB ID: 4GIZ) using AA as control. Of these, compounds **4** and **5** (Figure 2) showed the highest docking scores −65.74 Kcal/mol and −63.66 Kcal/mol, respectively, and lower IC_{50} values (HPV-positive cell lines, SiHa and HeLa) were observed when compared to AA and other compounds. In addition, they displayed less toxicity towards fibroblasts than commercial drugs and were able to inhibit p53 degradation mediated by the E6 protein, according to the in vitro studies performed [37].

Rietz and his team followed a different approach. For this, small-molecule probes, which can modulate protein interactions, were used to evaluate the recognition features of the E6 protein by means of binding and functional assays [38]. In this context, authors intended to understand the contribution of the substituents in positions 2 and 6 on the benzopyranone scaffold explored and to determine which E6 features are involved in binding. Interestingly, it was observed that charged groups in position 6 and non-polar substituents in position 2 displayed higher activity. Molecular dynamics simulations with analogs of these small molecules and exploring a set of mutations in different amino acid residues allowed the authors to conclude that a group of arginines (Arg10, Arg55, Arg102, Arg129, and Arg131) play a major role in the shape of the E6 helical binding groove, as well as in molecular recognition of the binding partners. Therefore, these last results can be of relevance for structure-based targeting of HPV E6 [38].

Another strategy was developed by Kumar and colleagues using ligand-based and structure-based methods [39]. They built an e-pharmacophore model for virtual screening based on the amino acid residues involved in the interaction of E6 (ID: 4GIZ) and a peptide reported by Zanier and co-workers [35]. The ligands were selected based on literature information, and 2-aminobenzothiazole and the luteolin chromone moiety were used as query molecules to found potential compounds on the ZINC 15 database. Then, 6000 compounds were screened using the pharmacophore model developed, and molecular docking studies predicted the best compounds based on dock scores and interactions with amino acid residues of the binding site. In addition, ADME analysis and molecular dynamics simulations were performed to find the best hit. The chromone derivative, compound **6**, ZINC14761180 (Figure 2) showed the most relevant interactions, and molecular dynamics of the complex ZINC14761180-E6 protein evidenced good stability in the binding pocket [39]. These findings can be a starting point for further design and synthesis of new E6 inhibitors. Following this work, the authors decided to explore a different approach but with the same objective [40]. For this, a drug repurposing approach based on the FDA-approved drugs library was applied. This methodology consists of identifying a different therapeutic use for an available or approved drug. Approved drugs have acceptable ADMET properties; therefore, this is an effective method as it involves less time, lower costs, and reduces the probability of an undesirable ADMET profile in clinical trials [10]. After the compounds' screening through a pharmacophore model, docking, molecular dynamics simulations, and ADME analysis, the selected hits with the highest potential were compound **7** (ZINC000001543916—valganciclovir; anti-viral drug) and compound **8** (ZINC000003795098—cytarabine; anticancer drug) (Figure 2). Both drugs are purine or pyrimidine nucleoside analogues, which showed that these scaffolds can be applied to design novel E6 inhibitors. Interestingly, compound **9**, ASK4 (Figure 2), which is a valganciclovir derivative, also showed promising results. Molecular dynamics simulations indicated that these ligands could form a stable complex with E6 protein, and it was also evidenced that they have an acceptable ADME profile [40].

The zinc-finger motif was proposed as strictly necessary for E6 protein function. Therefore, mutations in zinc-fingers interfere with E6/E6AP complex formation and cellular transformation. Concerning these data, Choudhury and co-workers selected specific disulfide (C13, C14, C16, R2, R15, R19) and azoic (C4) compounds, as controls based on their ability to eject zinc from the zinc finger motif of E6 protein and inhibit E6/E6AP interaction, proved by in vitro studies. Then, derivatives of these compounds were generated, and their ADME properties were predicted to exclude undesired compounds. Molecular docking, using the 3D structure of the C-terminal zinc-binding domain of the E6 protein (PDB ID: 2FK4), was performed for the selected ligands. Afterward, ligands with the highest binding score, such as compound **10**, *(E)-N*-(2-amino-2-methylpropyl)-*N*-(thiophen-2-yl)diazene-1,2-dicarboxamide, and compound **11**, (*E*)-*N*-(2-amino-2-oxoethyl)-*N*-(4-chlorophenyl)diazene-1,2-dicarboxamide, both azoic derivatives (Figure 3), were used for pharmacophore modeling (ligand-based method). The predicted amino acid residues involved in the interaction with the ligands are Tyr15, Trp55, Asn50, Leu23, Leu33, Ser5, Ile24, Ile51, Arg47, Arg54, Arg25, Lys45, Lys38, Phe48, Cys26, and Ala1. Some of these residues are found to be conserved among HPV6, HPV11, HPV16, and HPV18 zinc fingers. This demonstrates the possibility of the zinc finger domain to be a drug target [41].

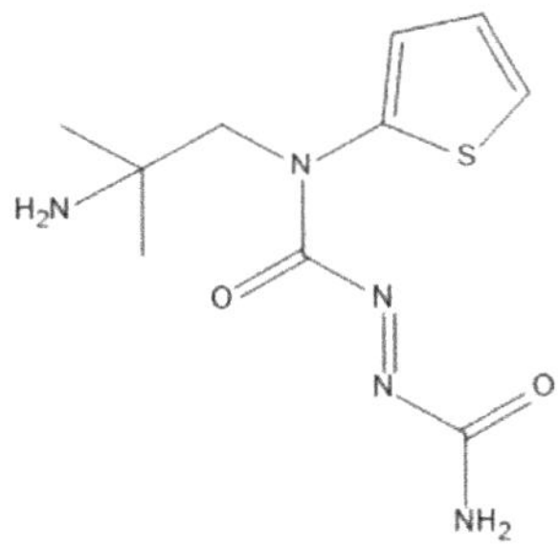

Compound 10

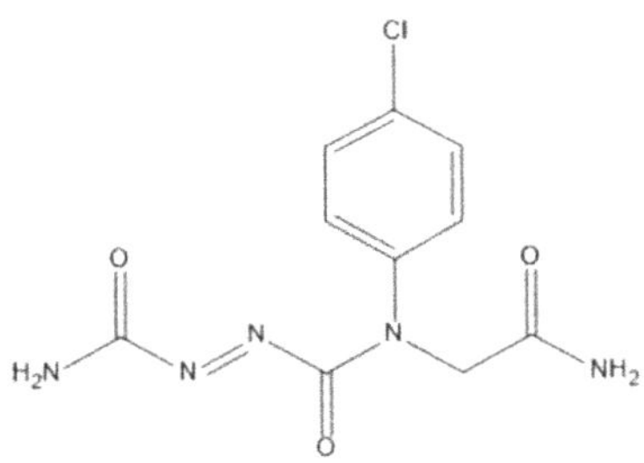

Compound 11

Figure 3. Structures of studied synthetic compounds as E6/E6AP inhibitors acting by ejecting zinc ions. IUPAC name of compounds—compound **10**: (*E*)-N^1-(2-amino-2-methylpropyl)-N^1-(thiophen-2-yl)diazene-1,2-dicarboxamide; compound **11**: (E)-N^1-(2-amino-2-oxoethyl)-N^1-(4-chlorophenyl)diazene-1,2-dicarboxamide.

3.1.2. Natural Compounds

Plant-derived compounds have been used in the prevention and treatment of different clinical conditions, and several of these natural products possess beneficial effects against several types of cancers, including cervical, colon, skin, breast, and prostate cancers [42]. In addition, many natural products are abundantly available and therefore can constitute a cost-effective way to obtain active pharmaceutical ingredients, including for cancer treatment [43]. Therefore, some researchers have focused on investigating the potential of natural compounds as E6 inhibitors. Clemente-Soto and his research team studied the ability of quercetin, compound **12** (Figure 4), a flavonol belonging to the flavonoid group, to inhibit p53 degradation mediated by E6 through in silico and in vitro studies [44]. According to molecular docking results, quercetin was able to bind in three different sites of E6 (ID: 4GIZ). Interestingly, it was predicted that the lowest energy (−7.08 Kcal/mol) and interactions with crucial amino acids for E6-E6AP formation (such as L50, L100, R102, R131) occurred in site II (corresponds to the hydrophobic pocket). As reference ligands, CAF24, C170, and luteolin were used because it was previously demonstrated that they were able to bind the E6 protein and disrupt the E6AP association [34]. Additionally, in vitro studies demonstrated that quercetin was capable to reactivate p53 and induce G2 phase cell cycle arrest and apoptosis in HPV-positive cancer cell lines [44].

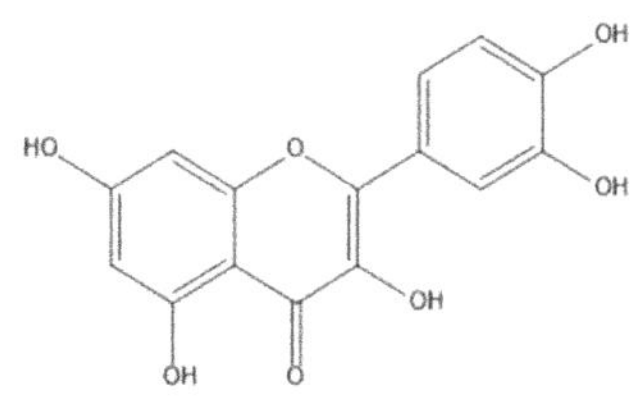

Compound 12 (Quercetin)

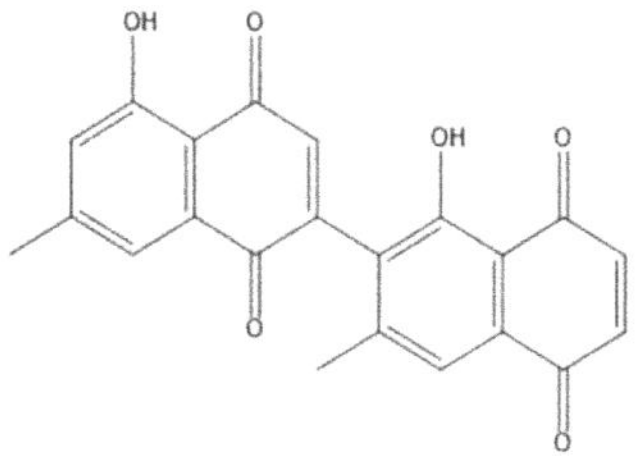

Compound 13 (Diospyrin)

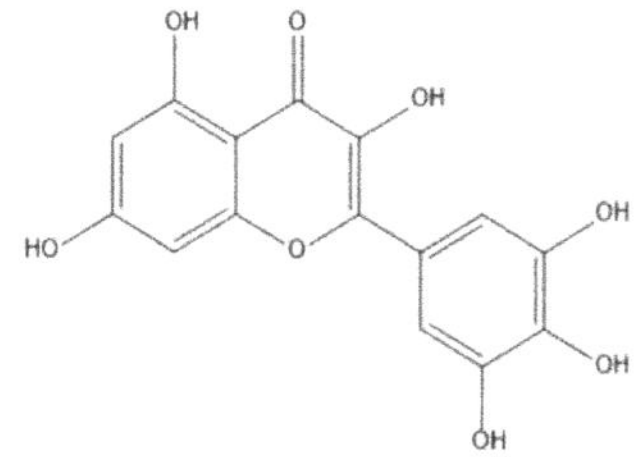

Compound 14 (Myricetrin)

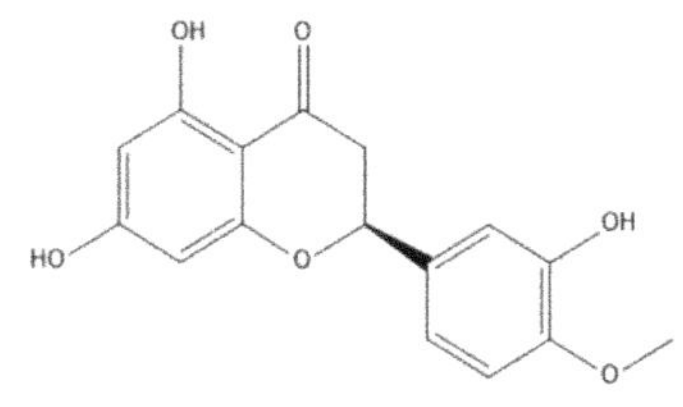

Compound 15 (Hesperetin)

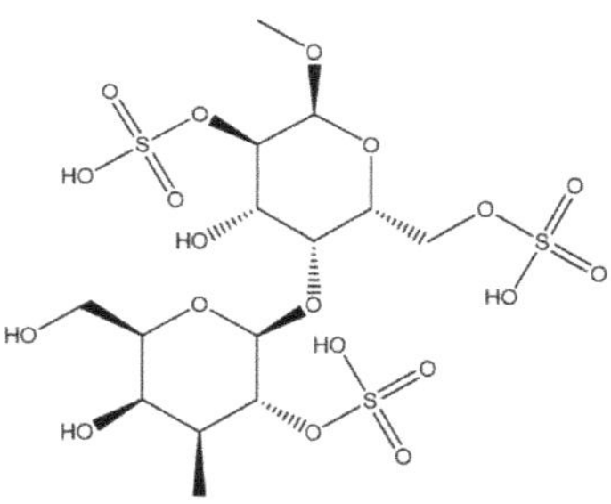

Compound 16 (Carrageenan)

Figure 4. Structures of the studied natural compounds as E6/E6AP inhibitors. IUPAC name of compounds—compound **12**: 2-(3,4-dihydroxyphenyl)-3,5,7-trihydroxy-4*H*-chromen-4-one; compound **13**: 1′,5-dihydroxy-3′,7-dimethyl-[2,2′-binaphthalene]-1,4,5′,8′-tetraone; compound **14**: (*S*)-5,7-dihydroxy-2-(3-hydroxy-4-methoxyphenyl)chroman-4-one; compound **15**: (*S*)-5,7-dihydroxy-2-(3-hydroxy-4-methoxyphenyl)chroman-4-one; compound **16**: ((2*R*,3*R*,4*S*,5*R*,6*S*)-4-hydroxy-3-(((2*S*,3*R*,4*S*,5*R*,6*R*)-5-hydroxy-6-(hydroxymethyl)-4-methyl-3-(sulfooxy)tetrahydro-2*H*-pyran-2-yl)oxy)-6-methoxy-5-(sulfooxy)tetrahydro-2*H*-pyran-2-yl)methyl hydrogen sulfate.

Kumar's research group took advantage of both 3D structures of the E6 protein available on PDB (ID: 4GIZ and 4XR8) to perform a protein–protein alignment and identify the amino acid residues that suffer conformational changes when the E6/E6AP complex recruits p53 [45]. The residues Arg8, Tyr32, Cys51, Tyr70, Ser74, and Arg131 demonstrated conformational changes when the E6/E6AP complex bound to the p53 protein. Then, an e-pharmacophore model was built based on the amino acid residues present in the predicted cavity and screened against 27,354 compounds. Molecular docking and molecular dynamics approaches were used to study the hits previously selected, where compound **13**, diospyrin (Figure 4), was identified as the best hit. H-bond interactions with Tyr32, Cys51, Ser74, and Arg131 amino acid residues were predicted, which might be important for an inhibitor to interact with the E6 protein [45].

Kolluru and his research team stated that E6 can inhibit the apoptotic pathway by binding to adaptor molecule FADD (Fas-associated death domain); therefore, the inhibition of this interaction could be a promising strategy for CC treatment [46]. As there is no information about the FADD binding site on the E6 protein, the authors decided to identify the flavonol binding pocket on HPV 16 E6 (ID: 4GIZ) protein by studying six flavonols reported in the literature as E6 inhibitors. First, a blind docking was performed to identify different pockets, followed by the determination of amino acid residues involved in interactions with ligands. Amino acids Cys51, Leu50, Arg102, Arg131, Leu67, Val62, and Gln107 were the most common among binding pockets that have scores correlated with the previously described IC_{50} (determined by the interaction of GST-E6 and His-caspase 8), indicating their importance in E6 inhibition. Compound **14**, myricetin (Figure 4), demonstrated the highest docking score in most of the binding pockets, which agrees with the IC_{50} reported in the literature. The efficacy of these ligands may be increased by conjugation with multivalent glycocalixarenes, which are known to interact with biological macromolecules [46].

Other researchers, such as Prakash and his team, studied the anticancer effect of compound **15**, hesperetin (Figure 4), a plant-isolated flavonoid, on CC via in vitro and molecular docking studies [47]. First, a preliminary study of hesperetin's effective cytotoxicity towards HeLa cells was performed. Then, molecular docking with crystal structure PDB ID: 4XR8 was applied to understand the binding mode and interaction of the hesperetin–E6 protein complex. The binding energy score was −5.58 Kcal/mol, and different bonds were established with the active site of the E6 protein, specifically H-bonds with Trp132 and Asp98, carbon–hydrogen bond with Arg102 and Leu100, and hydrophobic pi-alkyl interaction with Arg102, Arg131, and Leu100. These results demonstrated that hesperetin can bind in the hydrophobic pocket of E6 and hinder the interaction of E6 with p53 [47].

Kamma and co-workers focused on ligands available on natural sources, including carrageenan, curcumin, and papain, to target the E6 protein (PDB ID: 6SIV) [48]. Molecular docking revealed minimal binding energy (−10.7 Kcal/mol) for compound **16**, carrageenan, being considered the best ligand of this group. However, this is a preliminary study, and it is fundamental to perform in vitro studies to confirm the carrageenan behavior towards CC and non-cancer cells.

Although plant-derived compounds present many advantages as anticancer agents, their usual low availability on tumor sites could represent a drawback. Thus, their administration using adequate drug delivery systems or combination with approved drugs could be a promising way to improve their bioavailability and allow their delivery to target cells, including for CC management [43,49].

The activation of interferon regulatory factor 3 (IRF3) is dependent on the kinase binding site within the autoinhibitory domain (AD), which is blocked by E6 protein [50]. The interaction of E6 with E6AP prevents apoptosis after p53 degradation causing cell cycle disruption. Both IRF3 and E6AP E6 have specific leucine-rich motifs. In the IRF3 case, it is the N-terminal that participates in E6 binding, where for the E6AP it is the C-terminal. Therefore, HPV escape from the antiviral response is suggested to be possible through the interaction of E6 protein with IRF3 [50]. However, the mechanism of IRF3 inactivation by E6 is not completely understood. Thus, Shah and colleagues used in silico approaches to explore this mechanism [51]. The N-terminal of IRF3 comprises two leucine-rich clusters that are assumed as E6-specific binding motifs. The binding affinity of these motifs towards the E6 protein was evaluated through protein–protein docking and molecular dynamics simulations using the E6/E6AP complex structure (PDB ID:4GIZ), as a control to corroborate the protocol described by the authors. After investigation of IRF3 stable residues and identification of E6 residues with high binding energy, the binding mode of E6 inhibitors reported in the literature was explored. Molecular docking with 20 ligands (natural and synthetic compounds) into the hydrophobic pocket of E6 was performed, and their binding affinities and behaviors were evaluated through computational mutagenesis and drug resistance scanning. Computational mutagenesis was applied to study the stability of each ligand-bound E6 complex, where the polar arginine residues of the E6 pocket were mutated into alanine residues. Then, the drug resistance of E6 was determined considering the difference of binding affinities of using wild-type or mutant residues. It was noticed that the stability was compromised when Arg131 was mutated into alanine, whereas Arg102 Ala mutation reduced the ligand-binding affinities. The change in the binding affinities suggests that E6 might become more resistant to drugs when Arg131 and Arg102 are mutated into neutral amino acid residues. The data obtained indicated that the LxxLL motifs of IRF3 bind within the hydrophobic pocket of E6 and the polar areas (Arg55, Arg102, and Arg131), significantly affecting the stability of the LxxLL-E6 complex. Despite the new findings where the E6 binding to IRF3 might inhibit the kinase-mediated protein activation, the fact that the polar patches are inconsistent among HR HPV species may compromise an unsuccessful treatment due to point mutation that could make drugs ineffective [51].

3.2. *E6-p53 Complex Inhibitors*

CC satisfies the criteria of "oncogene addiction", which means that tumor cell development occurs due to the activity of one or some genes [52]. As E6 is the main protein responsible for p53 degradation, several researchers recently focused their attention on designing and developing potential inhibitors of E6/p53 binding by employing in silico methods. In fact, the direct disruption of the p53 binding site to E6 can be useful in the development and optimization of specific inhibitors, improving the likelihood of preventing off-target effects.

3.2.1. Natural Compounds

Kumar and co-workers explored natural compounds described in the literature as able to block HPV infection towards the E6 protein of HPV18 [53]. The 3D structure of E6 HPV18 was obtained by homology modeling using the amino acid sequence available in NCBI (GenBank ID: NP_040310.1), and the E6 HPV16 protein (PDB ID: 4GIZ) was employed as a structure template. After structure validation, molecular docking with 12 ligands was performed to elucidate the interactions with E6 HPV18. The binding site of p53 to E6 HPV18 was revealed by sequence comparison with E6 HPV16 and set on the residues 108–117 (CQKPLNPAEK). All studied compounds interacted with the p53 binding site on the E6 protein. However, the lowest binding energy (−5.85 Kcal/mol) was predicted for compound **17**, withaferin A (Figure 5) interacting through H-bonds with four amino acid residues of E6 (Glu116, Asn113, Asn122, and Ser140) [53]. Following this work, Atabaki and colleagues performed in silico and in vitro studies to evaluate the behavior of phytochemicals of *Jurinea macrocephala* subsp. *Elbursensis* in CC cell lines and their interaction with E6 HPV18 [54]. From this plant, three compounds were isolated, namely, 4-hydroxypectorolide-14-*O*-acetate, 4-hydroxy pectorolide, and pinoresinol monomethyl ether-β-D-glucoside (PMG), and their toxicity toward cancer cells was investigated. Of these, compound **18**, PMG (Figure 5), displayed significant toxicity on HeLa cells; therefore, molecular docking was performed to understand if it could be a potential E6 inhibitor. Using doxorubicin as control, the PMG showed higher binding energy (−4.75 Kcal/mol) and interacted through H-bonds with three amino acid residues (Arg119, Leu112, and Tyr99) [54].

Mamgmain and co-workers explored five natural compounds—colchicine, curcumin, daphnoretin, ellipticine, and epigallocatechin-3-gallate—as potential E6 inhibitors [55]. The 3D structure of the E6 protein was built through homology modeling and the crystal structure PDB ID: 4GIZ as a template. The binding sites predicted were chosen for molecular docking studies. The highest binding affinity, −8.3 Kcal/mol, was attributed to compound **19**, daphnoretin (Figure 5), which interacts through H-bonds with E6 amino acid residues Tyr39, Cys58, Ser78, Gln114, and Arg138 [55].

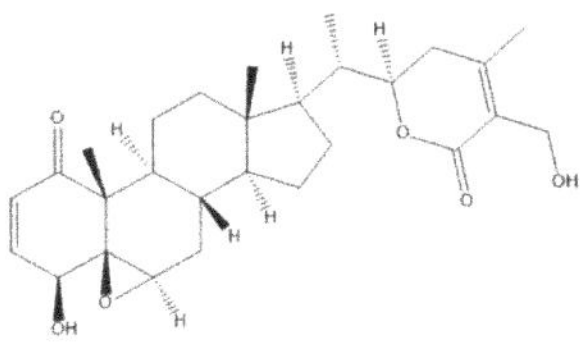

Compound 17 (Withaferin A)

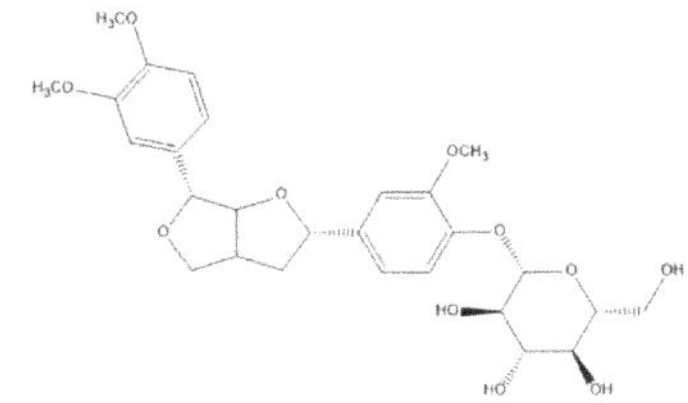

Compound 18 (PMG)

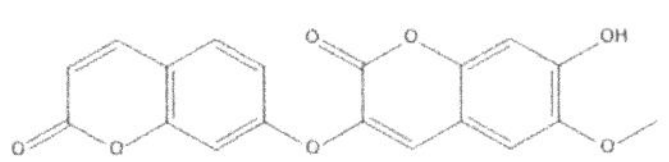

Compound 19 (Daphnoretin)

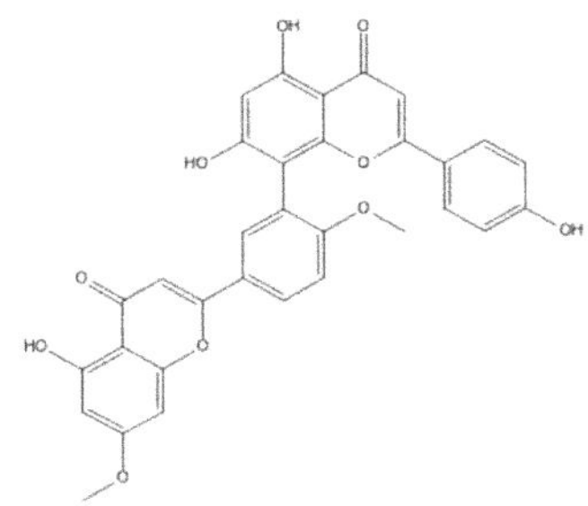

Compound 20 (Ginkgetin)

Figure 5. Structures of the studied natural compounds as E6/p53 inhibitors. IUPAC name of compounds—compound **17**: (4*S*,4a*R*,5a*R*,6a*S*,6b*S*,9*R*,9a*S*,11a*S*,11b*R*)-4-hydroxy-9-((*S*)-1-((*R*)-5-(hydroxymethyl)-4-methyl-6-oxo-3,6-dihydro-2*H*-pyran-2-yl)ethyl)-9a,11b-dimethyl-5a,6,6a,6b,7,8,9,9a,10,11,11a,11b-dodecahydrocyclopenta[1,2]phenanthro[8a,9-b]oxiren-1(4*H*)-one; compound **18**: (2*S*,3*R*,4*S*,5*S*,6*R*)-2-(4-((2*S*,6*R*)-6-(3,4-dimethoxyphenyl)hexahydrofuro[3,4-*b*]furan-2-yl)-2-methoxyphenoxy)-6-(hydroxymethyl)tetrahydro-2*H*-pyran-3,4,5-triol; compound **19**: 7-hydroxy-6-methoxy-3-((2-oxo-2*H*-chromen-7-yl)oxy)-2*H*-chromen-2-one; compound **20**: 5,7-dihydroxy-8-(5-(5-hydroxy-7-methoxy-4-oxo-4*H*-chromen-2-yl)-2-methoxyphenyl)-2-(4-hydroxyphenyl)-4*H*-chromen-4-one.

Considering the different molecules/proteins (E6AP, p53, and c-Myc) that bind to E6 protein and can interfere with normal cell function, Nabati and co-workers investigated more than 100 already described plant-derived compounds with anticancer and antiviral properties for the different protein binding sites [56]. These compounds were filtered based on their ADMET properties, and twenty compounds were selected for molecular docking studies. The crystal structure of the E6 protein PDB ID: 4GIZ was used. Compound **20**, ginkgetin (GK, Figure 5), extracted from *Gingko biloba* leaves, was the most effective in binding to all sites (E6AP, p53, and Myc) on the E6 protein, and the lowest binding energy was determined. In particular, it was predicted that GK forms five H-bonds with Arg55, Cys51, Val53, and Tyr60 on the E6AP binding site; on the p53 binding site it should form H-bonds with the same amino acid residues of the E6AP binding site; on Myc binding site, it can interact with Pro5 and Arg8 by forming four H-bonds. Considering the GK bioactivities described in the literature, including antitumor and antiviral properties, and ability to induce apoptosis in cancer cells, this study could be a starting point for the development of potential E6 inhibitor in vitro studies [56].

With the crystallization of the ternary complex E6/E6AP/p53 by Zanier and co-workers in 2016, it was possible to achieve a better structural understanding of the amino acid (aa) residues that participate in the binding interface of E6-p53. Actually, the aa residues described in the literature before 2016, or used as the binding site of p53 to E6 in some of the studies mentioned above, were predicted by computational methods since there was no information about the real binding site [28,57,58]. Even now, some authors chose to use computational methods for this purpose, while other authors used the information of the p53 binding site discovered in 2016. According to this study, the E6AP C-terminal does not substantially contribute to contacts with p53, and the E6/p53 interface can be divided into three sub-interfaces. In sub-interface I the E6 residues Glu7 and Glu18 establish interaction with p53 residues, where mutations in Glu18 impair the ternary complex formation and p53 degradation. Likewise, the hydrogen bond formed through Gln104 and Gly105 of p53 to Arg8 and Gln6 of E6 alters the conformation of the E6 N-terminal. Mutagenesis in the amino acid residues Phe2, Pro5, Arg8, or Pro9 prevented the ternary complex formation and p53 degradation. Sub-interface II has the aa residues that mediate vital contacts to p53 and are important for p53 degradation. The residues consist of Phe47, Asp44, and Asp49, which correspond to the most conserved positions in HR HPV. In addition, Ile23, His24, and Tyr43 provide hydrophobic contacts with p53. Finally, sub-interface III involves hydrophobic interactions between Leu114 and Trp146 of p53 and Leu100 and Pro112 of the E6 C-terminal [28].

3.2.2. Synthetic Compounds

Celegato and colleagues used the crystal structure of the E6/E6AP/p53 complex (PDB ID: 4XR8) to perform an in silico screening of small-molecule libraries against the central region of the p53-binding cleft of E6 [58]. This region was chosen due to its significant role in p53 binding and degradation as well as the high conservation among HR HPVs. A structure-based screening of three databases of commercially compounds was performed using chain F of the complex, and a filter step was applied considering the interactions with the residues Asp49 and Phe47 of E6. Twenty-nine compounds were selected and tested through their ability to rescue p53 by in vitro studies. This strategy allowed the selection of three compounds, but only pyrimidinone 21 (Figure 6) affected the viability of CC cells without affecting healthy cells. It was also found that this compound could re-establish p53 intracellular levels and transcriptional activity, reduce the viability and proliferation of HPV-positive cancer cells, and block 3D cervospheres formation [58]. Molecular dynamics simulations with E6-compound 20 complex were performed to gain further insight into the binding mode of compound **20**. The complex showed stability by the formation of a double H-bond with Asp49 and by hydrophobic interactions with Phe47 and established other interactions with Leu12, Cys16, and Ile23. This study suggested that compound **21** can be a starting point for the development of specific anti-HPV drugs.

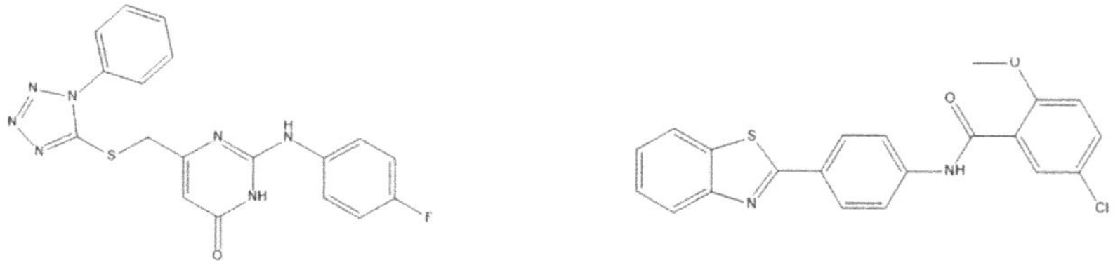

Compound 21 **Compound 22 (A-07)**

Figure 6. Structures of the studied synthetic compounds as E6/p53 inhibitors. IUPAC name of compounds—compound **21**: 2-((4-fluorophenyl)amino)-6-(((1-phenyl-1*H*-tetrazol-5-yl)thio)methyl)pyrimidin-4(3*H*)-one; compound **22**: *N*-(4-(benzo[*d*]thiazol-2-yl)phenyl)-5-chloro-2-methoxybenzamide.

Modi and co-workers explored the anticancer properties of 10 benzothiazole derivatives in CC cell lines. Later, by in silico and in vitro studies, they aimed to identify the molecular pathways involved in the apoptosis induced by *N*-(4-(benzo[d]thiazol-2-yl)phenyl)-5-chloro-2-methoxybenzamide (compound **22** or A-07, Figure 6) [59]. To perform in silico analysis in this context, the E6 and p53 crystal structures were obtained from PDB (ID: 4GIZ and 4XR8, respectively). Then, A-07 was evaluated by molecular docking against each protein where the active site was identified by the metaPocket server. It was predicted that this benzothiazolyl derivative was able to interact with both proteins, specifically with 10 amino acids of E6 and 14 amino acids of p53. These results suggest that A-07 (Figure 6) can hinder ternary complex formation and prevent p53-mediated intrinsic apoptosis in SiHa cells, as demonstrated by in vitro studies [59].

The natural and synthetic compounds presented here as HR HPV E6 protein inhibitors by either target E6/E6AP complex or the E6/E6AP/p53 complex formation are a valid starting point for drug design and development in cervical cancer management. However, strategies that combine both targets, the hydrophobic pocket and the p53-binding cleft of E6 protein, could result in an effective way to disrupt the E6/E6AP/p53 complex to specifically affect the viability of HPV-positive cancer cell lines and proposing specific anti-HPV therapies.

4. Future Perspectives

CC management still needs improvements, as current therapies are mainly surgery, chemotherapy, or radiotherapy. Several drugs have been proposed for treating patients with CC, but most do not overcome clinical trials due to low efficacy [36]. Bearing in mind the role of HR HPV E6 protein in the development and progression of HPV infection to cervical lesion or even invasive carcinoma, the inhibition of E6 function could be useful for treating CC. Results reported in this review support the idea that combining in silico approaches and in vitro studies could lead to a rise in the number of molecules understudy to block/inhibit E6 protein. According to Franconi and co-workers and Duenas-Gonzalez and co-workers, there are no clinical studies using natural or synthetic compounds as E6 or E7 inhibitors yet [43,60], due to low affinity and/or potency on in vitro and in vivo studies. Thus, the employment of in silico methodologies in the drug development process can be a great help to quickly find potential inhibitors and circumvent possible undesirable properties of compounds. Therefore, identification and functional evaluation of proteins associated with E6 could provide an insight into CC carcinogenesis and thus allow the design of specific strategies towards tumor cells. Moreover, it is essential to search and find cost-effective treatment options that could bring better outcomes for the patients. A strategy in this context could explore the potential use of plant-derived compounds, usually associated with lower toxicity and side effects when compared with classic anticancer agents. In addition, considering that drug distribution to the tumor site is low, the use of suitable drug delivery systems (DDS) compatible with the anticancer agents could be explored to achieve better clinical response with lower toxicity, as DDS could be functionalized with ligands that are specifically recognized by cancer cells [49]. Thinking about the fact that HPV infection is localized in the anatomical regions that can be easily reached for topical treatment, the possibility of locally delivering small molecules or natural compounds could be a valid option. Indeed, in low-income countries where women only can reach health facilities a few times in a lifetime, the combination of HR HPV test positivity and treatment in a single visit could be fundamental. A "screen-and-treat" approach allows reducing travel time, minimizing the number of visits, transport, childcare needs, and reducing the cost [61]. In places where is difficult to reach people and a return visit is not an option, self-sampling for HPV screening and mobile treatment for precancer could be applied [62]. Moreover, visual inspection with acetic acid (VIA) can be applied as a triage method for LIC, once it is low-cost and offers the option of treatment immediately or shortly after diagnostic testing. One of the biggest problems of cervical neoplasia is the resistance of tumor cells to chemotherapy and radiotherapy. Thus, the combination of anticancer agents in DDS with conventional chemotherapy or radiotherapy could also be a solution. This represents another line of investigation that needs to be explored in the near future. In terms of CC management, it would be interesting to explore a combinatory approach targeting E6 and E7 oncoproteins. In this case, the aim consists of exploiting molecules able to interact with E6 and E7 proteins, once both have a relevant role on CC progression. From this point forward, the use of in silico methods would be the key to pursue this approach.

Overall, our research group aims to propose a more specific, efficient, and non-toxic/invasive therapeutic approach for cervical cancer management. Thus, in silico approaches, such as those described in the present manuscript, will be used to select promising compounds as E6 potential inhibitors. Additional studies will be conducted with HPV E6 recombinant proteins and the selected compounds to characterize the kinetic magnitude and affinity constants of the compound–protein interaction. Then, the most promising compounds will be applied in in vitro studies with HPV-positive and HPV-negative cell lines to confirm the inhibitor/blocker effects of the E6 oncoprotein. In addition, drug delivery systems can be developed to circumvent a possible high toxicity and low availability of the compounds and, for instance, to combine this approach of E6 inhibitors with gene therapy to supplement p53 content and induce the cancer cell apoptosis.

5. Conclusions

The high impact that CC has in developing countries is undeniable. This review has briefly discussed the role of HPV in CC carcinogenesis as well as its different stages and current treatments. Subsequently, the potential of natural and synthetic small molecules in HR HPV E6 protein inhibition, mainly by targeting the E6/E6AP complex or the E6/E6AP/p53 complex, was discussed. The drug development process is a very expensive and time-consuming process until achieving regulatory agency approval. In silico methods represent a viable solution to these current problems by allowing a fast screening and identification of potential drugs and effective predictions. In terms of impact, in silico methodologies can help to increase the speed of acceptance of potential antiviral drugs with ADMET acceptable profiles for CC management. Moreover, in silico methods have been applied in the medical field, representing the therapeutic response of drugs on virtual organs and body systems and predicting patients' biological responses to the treatment, and this significantly improves outcomes. Computational-based approaches hold a great promise for improving drug development and revolutionizing clinical research by providing a specific treatment for women diagnosed with cervical cancer. Considering the costs of screening and treatment of CC, and knowing that the highest incidence occurs in developing countries, a more cost-effective treatment is needed. Thus, exploring natural compounds with the ability to impair E6-p53 interaction could be a specific and promising strategy for CC management in a more economical way.

Author Contributions: Conceptualization, D.G.; software, D.G.; validation, S.S., A.P.D., A.V., C.P.S., L.P. and Â.S.; writing—original draft preparation, D.G.; writing—review and editing, S.S., A.P.D., A.V., C.P.S., L.P. and Â.S.; supervision, C.P.S., L.P. and Â.S.; funding acquisition, A.P.D., L.P., Â.S. All authors have read and agreed to the published version of the manuscript.

Funding: This work was supported by the Foundation for Science and Technology (FCT), through funds from the State Budget and by the European Regional Development Fund through the "Programa Operacional Regional do Centro (Centro 2020)—Sistema de Apoio à Investigação Científica e Tecnológica—Programas Integrados de IC&DT" (Project Centro-01-0145-FEDER-000019—C4—Centro de Competências em Cloud Computing) and the project ref: UIDB/00709/2020. This work was also supported by national funds from FCT—Fundação para a Ciência e a Tecnologia, I.P., in the scope of the project UIDP/04378/2020 and UIDB/04378/2020 of the Research Unit on Applied Molecular Biosciences—UCIBIO and the project LA/P/0140/2020 of the Associate Laboratory Institute for Health and Bioeconomy—i4HB. D. Gomes also acknowledges the doctoral fellowship from FCT ref: 2020.06792.BD.

Institutional Review Board Statement: Not applicable.

Informed Consent Statement: Not applicable.

Data Availability Statement: Data sharing not applicable.

Conflicts of Interest: The authors declare no conflict of interest.

References

1. GLOBOCAN 2020: New Global Cancer Data. Available online: https://www.uicc.org/news/globocan-2020-new-global-cancer-data (accessed on 25 May 2021).
2. Bober, P.; Alexovič, M.; Tomková, Z.; Kilík, R.; Sabo, J. RHOA and mDia1 promotes apoptosis of breast cancer cells via a high dose of doxorubicin treatment. *Open Life Sci.* **2019**, *14*, 619–627. [CrossRef] [PubMed]
3. Almeida, A.M.; Queiroz, J.A.; Sousa, F.; Sousa, A. Cervical cancer and HPV infection: Ongoing therapeutic research to counteract the action of E6 and E7 oncoproteins. *Drug Discov. Today* **2019**, *24*, 2044–2057. [CrossRef] [PubMed]
4. Pal, A.; Kundu, R. Human Papillomavirus E6 and E7: The Cervical Cancer Hallmarks and Targets for Therapy. *Front. Microbiol.* **2019**, *10*, 3116. [CrossRef] [PubMed]
5. Prigge, E.S.; von Knebel Doeberitz, M.; Reuschenbach, M. Clinical relevance and implications of HPV-induced neoplasia in different anatomical locations. *Mutat. Res. Rev. Mutat. Res.* **2017**, *772*, 51–66. [CrossRef]
6. Cordeiro, M.N.; Lima, R.D.C.P.D.; Paolini, F.; Melo, A.R.S.; Campos, A.P.F.; Venuti, A.; De Freitas, A.C. Current research into novel therapeutic vaccines against cervical cancer. *Expert Rev. Anticancer Ther.* **2018**, *18*, 365–376. [CrossRef]
7. Barra, F.; Lorusso, D.; Leone Roberti Maggiore, U.; Ditto, A.; Bogani, G.; Raspagliesi, F.; Ferrero, S. Investigational drugs for the treatment of cervical cancer. *Expert Opin. Investig. Drugs* **2017**, *26*, 389–402. [CrossRef]
8. Kumar, A.; Rathi, E.; Hariharapura, R.C.; Kini, S.G. Is viral E6 oncoprotein a viable target? A critical analysis in the context of cervical cancer. *Med. Res. Rev.* **2020**, *40*, 2019–2048. [CrossRef]
9. Macalino, S.J.; Gosu, V.; Hong, S.; Choi, S. Role of computer-aided drug design in modern drug discovery. *Arch. Pharm Res.* **2015**, *38*, 1686–1701. [CrossRef]
10. Yella, J.K.; Yaddanapudi, S.; Wang, Y.; Jegga, A.G. Changing Trends in Computational Drug Repositioning. *Pharmaceuticals* **2018**, *11*, 57. [CrossRef]
11. Katsila, T.; Spyroulias, G.A.; Patrinos, G.P.; Matsoukas, M.T. Computational approaches in target identification and drug discovery. *Comput. Struct Biotechnol. J.* **2016**, *14*, 177–184. [CrossRef]
12. Prieto-Martínez, F.D.; López-López, E.; Eurídice Juárez-Mercado, K.; Medina-Franco, J.L. Computational Drug Design Methods—Current and Future Perspectives. In *In Silico Drug Design*; Elsevier: Amsterdam, The Netherlands, 2019; pp. 19–44. [CrossRef]
13. Bernetti, M.; Bertazzo, M.; Masetti, M. Data-Driven Molecular Dynamics: A Multifaceted Challenge. *Pharmaceuticals* **2020**, *13*, 253. [CrossRef]
14. Cruz-Vicente, P.; Passarinha, L.A.; Silvestre, S.; Gallardo, E. Recent Developments in New Therapeutic Agents against Alzheimer and Parkinson Diseases: In-Silico Approaches. *Molecules* **2021**, *26*, 2193. [CrossRef]
15. McBride, A.A. Oncogenic human papillomaviruses. *Phil. Trans. R. Soc. B* **2017**, *372*, 20160273. [CrossRef]
16. Sabatini, M.E.; Chiocca, S. Human papillomavirus as a driver of head and neck cancers. *Br. J. Cancer* **2020**, *122*, 306–314. [CrossRef]
17. Leemans, C.R.; Snijders, P.J.F.; Brakenhoff, R.H. The molecular landscape of head and neck cancer. *Nat. Rev. Cancer* **2018**, *18*, 269–282. [CrossRef]
18. Doorbar, J.; Quint, W.; Banks, L.; Bravo, I.G.; Stoler, M.; Broker, T.R.; Stanley, M.A. The biology and life-cycle of human papillomaviruses. *Vaccine* **2012**, *30* (Suppl. 5), F55–F70. [CrossRef]
19. Doorbar, J.; Egawa, N.; Griffin, H.; Kranjec, C.; Murakami, I. Human papillomavirus molecular biology and disease association. *Rev. Med. Virol.* **2016**, *25*, 2–23. [CrossRef]
20. De Freitas, N.L.; Deberaldini, M.G.; Gomes, D.; Pavan, A.R.; Sousa, Â.; Dos Santos, J.L.; Soares, C.P. Histone Deacetylase Inhibitors as Therapeutic Interventions on Cervical Cancer Induced by Human Papillomavirus. *Front. Cell Dev. Biol.* **2021**, *8*, 1–22. [CrossRef]
21. Farthing, A.J.; Vousden, K.H. Functions of human papillomavirus E6 and E7 oncoproteins. *Trends Microbiol.* **1994**, *2*, 170–173. [CrossRef]
22. Mittal, S.; Banks, L. Molecular mechanisms underlying human papillomavirus E6 and E7 oncoprotein-induced cell transformation. *Mutat. Res. Rev. Mutat. Res.* **2017**, *772*, 23–35. [CrossRef]
23. Martinez-Ramirez, I.; Carrillo-Garcia, A.; Contreras-Paredes, A.; Ortiz-Sanchez, E.; Cruz-Gregorio, A.; Lizano, M. Regulation of Cellular Metabolism by High-Risk Human Papillomaviruses. *Int. J. Mol. Sci.* **2018**, *19*, 1839. [CrossRef]
24. Viarisio, D.; Gissmann, L.; Tommasino, M. Human papillomaviruses and carcinogenesis: Well-established and novel models. *Curr. Opin. Virol.* **2017**, *26*, 56–62. [CrossRef] [PubMed]
25. World Health Organization. Diagnosis and treatment of invasive cervical cancer. In *Comprehensive Cervical Cancer Control: A Guide to Essential Practice*, 2nd ed.; World Health Organization: Geneva, Switzerland, 2014.
26. Liontos, M.; Kyriazoglou, A.; Dimitriadis, I.; Dimopoulos M-Athanasios, A.B. Systemic therapy in cervical cancer: 30 years in review. *Crit. Rev. Oncol. Hematol.* **2019**, *137*, 9–17. [CrossRef]
27. Zanier, K.; Charbonnier, S.; Sidi, A.O.; McEwen, A.G.; Ferrario, M.G.; Poussin-Courmontagne, P.; Cura, V.; Brimer, N.; Babah, K.O.; Ansari, T.; et al. Structural basis for hijacking of cellular LxxLL motifs by papillomavirus E6 oncoproteins. *Science* **2013**, *339*, 694–698. [CrossRef]
28. Martinez-Zapien, D.; Ruiz, F.X.; Poirson, J.; Mitschler, A.; Ramirez, J.; Forster, A.; Cousido-Siah, A.; Masson, M.; Vande Pol, S.; Podjarny, A.; et al. Structure of the E6/E6AP/p53 complex required for HPV-mediated degradation of p53. *Nature* **2016**, *529*, 541–545. [CrossRef]

29. Nomine, Y.; Ristriani, T.; Laurent, C.; Lefèvre, J.O.; Weiss, É.; Travé, G. A strategy for optimizing the monodispersity of fusion proteins: Application to purification of recombinant HPV E6 oncoprotein. *Protein Eng.* **2001**, *14*, 297–305. [CrossRef]
30. Zanier, K.; Sidi, A.o.M.h.o.; Boulade-Ladame, C.; Rybin, V.; Chappelle, A.; Atkinson, A.; Kieffer, B.; Travé, G. Solution structure analysis of the HPV16 E6 oncoprotein reveals a self-association mechanism required for E6-mediated degradation of p53. *Structure* **2012**, *20*, 604–617. [CrossRef]
31. Pol, S.B.V.; Klingelhutz, A.J. Papillomavirus E6 oncoproteins. *Virology* **2013**, *445*, 115–137. [CrossRef]
32. Grm, H.S.; Banks, L. Degradation of hDlg and MAGIs by human papillomavirus E6 is E6-AP-independent. *J. Gen. Virol.* **2004**, *85*, 2815–2819. [CrossRef]
33. Charbonnier, S.; Nominé, Y.; Ramírez, J.; Luck, K.; Chapelle, A.; Stote, R.H.; Travé, G.; Kieffer, B.; Atkinson, R.A. The Structural and Dynamic Response of MAGI-1 PDZ1 with Noncanonical Domain Boundaries to the Binding of Human Papillomavirus E6. *J. Mol. Biol.* **2011**, *406*, 745–763. [CrossRef] [PubMed]
34. Cherry, J.J.; Rietz, A.; Malinkevich, A.; Liu, Y.; Xie, M.; Bartolowits, M.; Davisson, V.J.; Baleja, J.D.; Androphy, E.J. Structure based identification and characterization of flavonoids that disrupt human papillomavirus-16 E6 function. *PLoS ONE* **2013**, *8*, e84506. [CrossRef] [PubMed]
35. Zanier, K.; Stutz, C.; Kintscher, S.; Reinz, E.; Sehr, P.; Bulkescher, J.; Hoppe-Seyler, K.; Trave, G.; Hoppe-Seyler, F. The E6AP binding pocket of the HPV16 E6 oncoprotein provides a docking site for a small inhibitory peptide unrelated to E6AP, indicating druggability of E6. *PLoS ONE* **2014**, *9*, e112514. [CrossRef] [PubMed]
36. Ricci-Lopez, J.; Vidal-Limon, A.; Zunniga, M.; Jimenez, V.A.; Alderete, J.B.; Brizuela, C.A.; Aguila, S. Molecular modeling simulation studies reveal new potential inhibitors against HPV E6 protein. *PLoS ONE* **2019**, *14*, e0213028. [CrossRef]
37. Senthilkumar, R.; Brusentsev, Y.; Paul, P.; Marimuthu, P.; Cheng, F.; Eklund, P.C.; Eriksson, J.E. Synthesis and Evaluation of Anisomelic acid-like Compounds for the Treatment of HPV-Mediated Carcinomas. *Sci. Rep.* **2019**, *9*, 20295. [CrossRef]
38. Rietz, A.; Petrov, D.P.; Bartolowits, M.; DeSmet, M.; Davisson, V.J.; Androphy, E.J. Molecular Probing of the HPV-16 E6 Protein Alpha Helix Binding Groove with Small Molecule Inhibitors. *PLoS ONE* **2016**, *11*, e0149845. [CrossRef]
39. Kumar, A.; Rathi, E.; Kini, S.G. E-pharmacophore modelling, virtual screening, molecular dynamics simulations and in-silico ADME analysis for identification of potential E6 inhibitors against cervical cancer. *J. Mol. Struct.* **2019**, *1189*, 299–306. [CrossRef]
40. Kumar, A.; Rathi, E.; Kini, S.G. Drug repurposing approach for the identification and designing of potential E6 inhibitors against cervical cancer: An in silico investigation. *Struct. Chem.* **2019**, *31*, 141–153. [CrossRef]
41. Choudhury, A.D.; Choudhury, M.D.; Chetia, P.; Chowdhury, A.; Talukdar, A.D. An In Silico Appraisal of Azoic and Disulphide Derivatives for Anticancer Activity Against HPV E6 Oncoprotein to Medicate Cervical Cancer. *Comb. Chem. High. Throughput Screen.* **2014**, *17*, 38–46. [CrossRef]
42. Tan, B.L.; Norhaizan, M.E. Plant-Derived Compounds in Cancer Therapy: Traditions of Past and Drugs of Future. In *Anticancer Plants: Properties and Application*; Akhtar, M., Swamy, M., Eds.; Springer: Singapore, 2018. [CrossRef]
43. Franconi, R.; Massa, S.; Paolini, F.; Vici, P.; Venuti, A. Plant-Derived Natural Compounds in Genetic Vaccination and Therapy for HPV-Associated Cancers. *Cancers* **2020**, *12*, 3101. [CrossRef]
44. Clemente-Soto, A.F.; Salas-Vidal, E.; Milan-Pacheco, C.; Sanchez-Carranza, J.N.; Peralta-Zaragoza, O.; Gonzalez-Maya, L. Quercetin induces G2 phase arrest and apoptosis with the activation of p53 in an E6 expressionindependent manner in HPVpositive human cervical cancerderived cells. *Mol. Med. Rep.* **2019**, *19*, 2097–2106. [CrossRef]
45. Kumar, A.; Rathi, E.; Kini, S.G. Identification of E6 Inhibitors Employing Energetically Optimized Structure-Based Pharmacophore Modelling, Ligand Docking and Molecular Dynamics Simulations Studies. *ChemistrySelect* **2019**, *4*, 10701–10708. [CrossRef]
46. Kolluru, S.; Momoh, R.; Lin, L.; Mallareddy, J.R.; Krstenansky, J.L. Identification of potential binding pocket on viral oncoprotein HPV16 E6: A promising anti-cancer target for small molecule drug discovery. *BMC Mol. Cell Biol.* **2019**, *20*, 30. [CrossRef]
47. Prakash, S.; Elavarasan, N.; Subashini, K.; Kanaga, S.; Dhandapani, R.; Sivanandam, M.; Kumaradhas, P.; Thirunavukkarasu, C.; Sujatha, V. Isolation of hesperetin—A flavonoid from Cordia sebestena flower extract through antioxidant assay guided method and its antibacterial, anticancer effect on cervical cancer via in vitro and in silico molecular docking studies. *J. Mol. Struct.* **2020**, *1207*. [CrossRef]
48. Rajasekhar, P.; Dhrub Kumar, Y.; Prasad, G.; Srinivasulu, K. In Silico Analysis of HPV E6 as Drug Target with Natural Antioxidants. *Int. J. Pharma Bio Sci.* **2020**, *10*. [CrossRef]
49. Medina-Alarcón, K.P.; Voltan, A.R.; Fonseca-Santos, B.; Moro, I.J.; Souza, F.D.O.; Chorilli, M.; Soares, C.P.; dos Santos, A.G.; Giannini, M.J.M.; Fusco-Almeida, A.M. Highlights in nanocarriers for the treatment against cervical cancer. *Mater. Sci. Eng. C* **2017**, *80*, 748–759. [CrossRef]
50. Ronco, L.V.; Karpova, A.Y.; Vidal, M.; Howley, P.M. Human papillomavirus 16 E6 oncoprotein binds to interferon regulatory factor-3 and inhibits its transcriptional activity. *Genes Dev.* **1998**, *12*, 2061–2072. [CrossRef]
51. Shah, M.; Anwar, M.A.; Park, S.; Jafri, S.S.; Choi, S. In silico mechanistic analysis of IRF3 inactivation and high-risk HPV E6 species-dependent drug response. *Sci. Rep.* **2015**, *5*, 13446. [CrossRef]
52. Weinstein, B.; Joe, A. Oncogene Addiction. *Cancer Res.* **2008**, *68*. [CrossRef]
53. Kumar, S.; Jena, L.; Mohod, K.; Daf, S.; Varma, A.K. Virtual Screening for Potential Inhibitors of High-Risk Human Papillomavirus 16 E6 Protein. *Interdiscip. Sci.* **2015**, *7*, 136–142. [CrossRef]
54. Atabaki, V.; Pourahmad, J.; Hosseinabadi, T. Phytochemical compounds from Jurinea macrocephala subsp.elbursensis and their cytotoxicity evaluation. *S. Afr. J. Bot.* **2021**, *137*, 399–405. [CrossRef]

55. Mamgain, S.; Sharma, P.; Pathak, R.K.; Baunthiyal, M. Computer aided screening of natural compounds targeting the E6 protein of HPV using molecular docking. *Bioinformation* **2015**, *11*, 236–242. [CrossRef]
56. Nabati, F.; Moradi, M.; Mohabatkar, H. In silico analyzing the molecular interactions of plant-derived inhibitors against E6AP, p53, and c-Myc binding sites of HPV type 16 E6 oncoprotein. *Mol. Biol. Res. Commun.* **2020**, *9*, 71–82. [CrossRef]
57. Kumar, S.; Jena, L.; Sahoo, M.; Kakde, M.; Daf, S.; Varma, A.K. In Silico Docking to Explicate Interface between Plant-Originated Inhibitors and E6 Oncogenic Protein of Highly Threatening Human Papillomavirus 18. *Genom. Inf.* **2015**, *13*, 60–67. [CrossRef]
58. Celegato, M.; Messa, L.; Goracci, L.; Mercorelli, B.; Bertagnin, C.; Spyrakis, F.; Suarez, I.; Cousido-Siah, A.; Trave, G.; Banks, L.; et al. A novel small-molecule inhibitor of the human papillomavirus E6-p53 interaction that reactivates p53 function and blocks cancer cells growth. *Cancer Lett.* **2020**, *470*, 115–125. [CrossRef]
59. Modi, A.; Singh, M.; Gutti, G.; Shanker, O.R.; Singh, V.K.; Singh, S.; Singh, S.K.; Pradhan, S.; Narayan, G. Benzothiazole derivative bearing amide moiety induces p53-mediated apoptosis in HPV16 positive cervical cancer cells. *Investig. New Drugs* **2020**, *38*, 934–945. [CrossRef]
60. Duenas-Gonzalez, A.; Gonzalez-Fierro, A. Pharmacodynamics of current and emerging treatments for cervical cancer. *Expert Opin. Drug Metab. Toxicol.* **2019**, *15*, 671–682. [CrossRef]
61. Kunckler, M.; Schumacher, F.; Kenfack, B.; Catarino, R.; Viviano, M.; Tincho, E.; Tebeu, P.M.; Temogne, L.; Vassilakos, P.; Petignat, P. Cervical cancer screening in a low-resource setting: A pilot study on an HPV-based screen-and-treat approach. *Cancer Med.* **2017**, *6*, 1752–1761. [CrossRef]
62. Kamath Mulki, A.; Withers, M. Human Papilloma Virus self-sampling performance in low- and middle-income countries. *BMC Women's Health* **2021**, *21*, 12. [CrossRef]

pharmaceuticals

MDPI

Review

Opportunities and Challenges for In Silico Drug Discovery at Delta Opioid Receptors

Yazan J. Meqbil [1] and Richard M. van Rijn [2,3,*]

[1] Department of Medicinal Chemistry and Molecular Pharmacology, Computational Interdisciplinary Graduate Program, Purdue University, West Lafayette, IN 47907, USA; ymeqbil@purdue.edu

[2] Department of Medicinal Chemistry and Molecular Pharmacology, Purdue Institute for Drug Discovery, Purdue Institute for Neuroscience, Purdue University, West Lafayette, IN 47907, USA

[3] Septerna Inc., South San Francisco, CA 94080, USA

* Correspondence: rvanrijn@purdue.edu; Tel.: +1-765-494-6461

Abstract: The delta opioid receptor is a Gi-protein-coupled receptor (GPCR) with a broad expression pattern both in the central nervous system and the body. The receptor has been investigated as a potential target for a multitude of significant diseases including migraine, alcohol use disorder, ischemia, and neurodegenerative diseases. Despite multiple attempts, delta opioid receptor-selective molecules have not been translated into the clinic. Yet, the therapeutic promise of the delta opioid receptor remains and thus there is a need to identify novel delta opioid receptor ligands to be optimized and selected for clinical trials. Here, we highlight recent developments involving the delta opioid receptor, the closely related mu and kappa opioid receptors, and in the broader area of the GPCR drug discovery research. We focus on the validity and utility of the available delta opioid receptor structures. We also discuss the increased ability to perform ultra-large-scale docking studies on GPCRs, the rise in high-resolution cryo-EM structures, and the increased prevalence of machine learning and artificial intelligence in drug discovery. Overall, we pose that there are multiple opportunities to enable in silico drug discovery at the delta opioid receptor to identify novel delta opioid modulators potentially with unique pharmacological properties, such as biased signaling.

Keywords: mutagenesis; artificial intelligence; computer-aided drug design; molecular dynamic simulation; biased signaling; G protein-coupled receptor

Citation: Meqbil, Y.J.; van Rijn, R.M. Opportunities and Challenges for In Silico Drug Discovery at Delta Opioid Receptors. *Pharmaceuticals* **2022**, *15*, 873. https://doi.org/10.3390/ph15070873

Academic Editor: Osvaldo Andrade Santos-Filho

Received: 23 June 2022
Accepted: 13 July 2022
Published: 15 July 2022

1. Introduction

The δ opioid receptor (δOR) is a Gi-protein-coupled receptor with a broad expression pattern both in the central nervous system and the periphery. The endogenous agonists for the δOR are pentapeptide enkephalins, particularly Leu^5-enkephalin, but other peptides that originate from plants and other species, like frogs can also bind and activate the δOR [1,2]. Similar to the μ opioid receptor (μOR), which is activated by small molecules from natural products like opium and kratom and fully synthetic small molecules like fentanyl, the δOR can be activated by a variety of naturally occurring and (semi-) synthetic small molecules [3–6].

The δOR has been a potential candidate to treat a variety of diseases and disorders. Front and center have been the ability of δOR selective agonists to reduce chronic pain, be it inflammatory, neuropathic, or migraine [7]. δOR agonists have shown promise in preventing cardiac and cerebral ischemia [8], as a potential treatment for neurodegenerative diseases [9–13], and both δOR agonists and antagonists have been proposed as mechanisms for the treatment of alcohol use disorder [5,14–16]. Outside the central nervous system, δOR antagonism and positive allosteric modulation of δOR has been proposed as a treatment for gastrointestinal motility disorders, such as irritable bowel syndrome [17,18].

Early attempts by SmithKline Beecham to synthesize δOR agonists to suppress cough (SB 227122), or to treat inflammatory pain without causing seizure activity (SB 235863) [19–21]

did not progress to clinical trials. While δOR-selective agonists, including ADL5859 and AZD2327, have previously entered clinical trials for the treatment of pain and depression, no δOR selective drugs have ultimately been approved for human use. [22–24] Both ADL5859 and AZD2327 failed to advance beyond phase II clinical trials, which are designed to establish efficacy in patients within the therapeutic indication space. ADL5859 and AZD2327 are part of a class of diethylbenzamides that include the prototypical δOR-selective agonist SNC80. However, SNC80 and multiple other δOR agonists have been reported to reduce seizure threshold and induce convulsions [25–27], and this has reduced enthusiasm for δOR agonists as a therapeutic area of research.

Around the same time that ADL5859 and AZD2327 were in clinical trials, Johnson and Johnson developed the anti-hyperalgesic δOR agonists, JNJ-20788560 and RWJ-394674 [28,29], but they did not take these into clinical trials, potentially due to the failure of the aforementioned clinical trial compounds. Prior to becoming insolvent, Ardent Pharmaceuticals, also produced multiple δOR agonists, with mixed μOR activity in their DPI series (DPI-221, DPI-125, DPI-289) in hopes of producing an analgesic drug with fewer adverse effect liabilities relative to the clinically used μOR agonists [12,30,31].

Recent studies suggest that β-arrestins, multifunctional proteins that can promote receptor desensitization and intracellular signaling, are involved in the mechanism of seizure activity of SNC80 [26]. This insight has spurt efforts to develop G-protein-biased δOR agonists to reduce adverse effects including seizures, paralleling similar efforts for increasing the therapeutic window through G-protein-biased agonism at other GPCRs, including the μOR. These endeavors have generated a multitude of peptides with reduced β-arrestin recruitment potency/efficacy [3,32–35]. Similarly, small molecule biased agonists have also been developed including TAN-67, KNT-127, TRV250, and most recently PN6047. Indeed, these G-protein-biased δOR agonists appear to suffer less from detrimental side effects including no seizure activity, no hyperlocomotion, and no rewarding effect [36–39]. Positive and negative allosteric modulators (PAM, NAM) and bitopic opioids that act as 'Ago-PAM' or 'Ago-NAM' have been identified and modeled in the δOR binding pocket. The benefit of pure allosteric modulators is that they are inert in the absence of enkephalin and only amplify (PAM) or inhibit (NAM) δOR signaling and/or binding when, for example, enkephalins are synaptically released. Allosteric modulators may promote a particular signaling conformation and bias the endogenous peptide; such a strategy could reduce the risk of tachyphylaxis, off-target effects, and even on-target side effects. Less than ten years ago now, Bristol Meyers Squibb identified a number of μOR and δOR Ago-PAMs [40–42] and more recently, novel δOR agonists lacking a basic nitrogen, including a novel chemotype and bitopic ligand, were also identified [43,44]. As these molecules are very recent their clinical utility has not been explored in much depth, but δOR PAM activity may, for example, aid the treatment of irritable bowel syndrome [18].

Still, except for TRV250, which has undergone phase I clinical trials for migraine, no real progress has occurred towards the production of δOR-based clinical candidates. Thus, there both remains a need and a large opportunity for discovering and developing novel δOR agonists as potential therapeutic agents. Here, we present a summary of current structural data that has been generated for the δOR; we first will provide an overview of available resolved structures and insights gained from mutagenesis studies and MD simulations. We will then discuss the limitations of the current structural knowledge. We conclude this review by presenting exciting opportunities for computer-aided drug design at the δOR.

2. Current Structural Insight in δOR Binding Pocket and Activation Mechanism

Early mutagenesis studies following the cloning of the δOR [45,46] hypothesized the involvement of certain amino acids in ligand recognition, selectivity, and overall receptor activation. One of the earliest mutagenesis studies investigated the role of Asp2.50 (Ballesteros-Weinstein numbering, [47]) in regulating ligand binding at the δOR where they demonstrated that Asp2.50Asn diminishes binding of peptide agonists with minimal effects on alkaloid agonists and antagonist [48]. Additionally, the authors hypothesized that Asp2.50 is in close proximity to the Na^+ binding site [48]. This was followed by another study, where Asp3.32 was investigated due to its conservation across many GPCRs that are activated via cationic neurotransmitters (protonated amines) [49]. The removal or replacement of that residue affects the binding of several δOR modulators. Unlike the alanine scanning mutations, the replacement of Asp3.32 with Asn3.32 resulted in modifications to the receptor's pharmacology and affected the binding potency of alkaloid and peptide-agonists. The authors hypothesized that the main reason for such dramatic change may be attributed to the increase in the size of the Asn3.32 side chain compared to the WT residue. Asp3.32 acts as a proton donor only whereas Asn3.32 can act as a hydrogen donor or acceptor. Additionally, the authors noted that the "Na^+ -induced low-affinity state" lowered the affinity of δOR peptide agonists such as DTLET and DADLE but did not affect the binding affinity of SNC-80 or BW373U86 (SNC-86) in agreement with the work by Kong et al. [48]. Interestingly, when the authors tested the δOR agonists DTLET, DADLE, and SNC-86 in the presence of sodium chloride, the binding affinity was reduced dramatically indicating a role for Asp2.50 in receptor activation to counteract the negative allosteric effects of the Na^+.

The same group later used single-point mutagenesis to investigate the involvement of aromatic amino acid residues (Tyr, Trp, and Phe) in transmembrane helices III–VI in ligand recognition [50]. To identify which aromatic residues to target, they used computational modeling to construct a 3D homology model for the δOR based on the human rhodopsin and hamster β2-adrenergic receptors. They showed that mutations Tyr mutations (Tyr3.33, Tyr7.42) had the most impact on the binding of deltorphin II [50]. They concluded that each ligand-receptor complex has unique binding and conformation where mutations do not have the same effect equally across various δOR ligands [50].

Another research team created a chimeric protein, DMDD, by replacing the area around the 1st extra-cellular loop 1 (ECL1) with the corresponding residues of μOR which significantly enhanced DAMGO binding to δOR [51]. A subsequent study replaced seven non-conserved residues in transmembrane domain (TM2) and TM3 with the corresponding residues in μOR and found that one residue only, Lys2.63 (replaced by Asn2.63) showed a high affinity for DAMGO. Replacement of Lys2.63 with nineteen different amino acid residues resulted in fourteen mutant receptors that could bind to DAMGO with comparable affinity to the DMDD chimera indicating a role for Lys2.63 to act as a recognition switch for δOR agonists [52]. A similar approach of using chimeric constructs for δOR in a different study demonstrated the importance of the ECL3 in the binding of selective peptide and small molecule agonists to the δOR. In the same study, the authors showed that three residues, Trp6.58, Val7.30, and Val7.31 are necessary for the binding of δOR agonists [53].

These mutagenesis studies have provided valuable insight into ligand recognition and receptor selectivity of the δOR some of which have been verified in recent structural studies (discussed below). However, these studies did not provide insight into the effect that the investigated mutations have on downstream signaling cascades at δOR. More importantly, there is a gap in knowledge with respect to the impact of most of these mutations on biased agonism.

Over the past decade, several moderate to high-resolution structures of the δOR have been produced and have confirmed older evaluations of the δOR binding pocket performed by mutagenesis and computational modeling (Figure 1, Table 1) [49,54,55]. In the first such structure (3.4Å, PDB:4EJ4), δOR was bound to the antagonist naltrindole [56]. The structure confirmed the important interaction between Asp3.32 with the protonated amine of naltrindole, which mimics the amine of Tyr[1] in endogenous OR peptides. As mentioned, this Asp3.32 was already known to be crucial for opioid affinity from mutagenesis studies [49]. In this structure, anchors are provided by hydrogen bonds (potentially including water molecules) with His6.52 and Tyr3.33 [56]. Additional amino acids surrounding the binding pocket were Met3.36, Trp6.48, Ile6.51, Val6.55, Trp6.58, Leu7.35, and Tyr7.43 [56]. A higher resolution structure (1.8Å, PDB:4N6H) of naltrindole-bound δOR was able to resolve an allosteric binding site for a sodium ion (Figure 2B) [57]. The sodium site consists of Asp2.50, Asn3.35, Asn7.45, and Asn7.49 and sits below the conserved 'message' site ['message' = part of the molecule that recognizes ORs, 'address' = part that renders the drug subtype selective] of the opioid receptor binding pocket [58]. In 2015, a third δOR structure (2.7Å, PDB:4RWD) was resolved, but this time bound to the δOR peptide antagonist Dmt[1]-Tic[2]-Phe[3]-Phe[4] (DIPP-NH2, Dmt = 2,6,-dimethyl-l-tyrosine) (Figure 2D) [59].

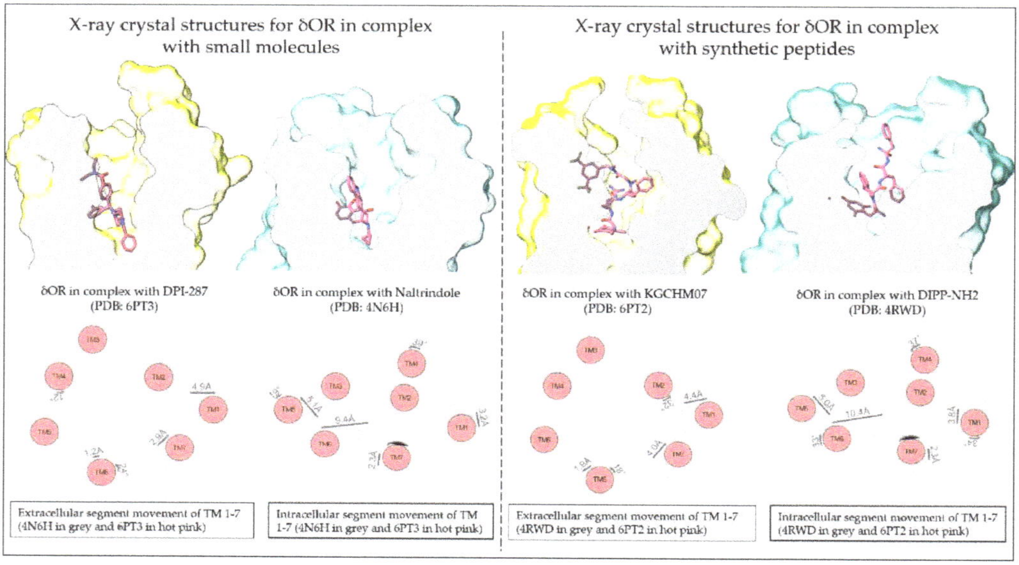

Figure 1. Resolved structures of the δOR in complex with small molecules and peptides. Schematic depiction of the small molecule agonist DPI-287 and antagonist naltrindole and the peptide agonist KGCHM07 and antagonist DIPP-NH2 bound to the δOR (Top panels; active-like structures in yellow and inactive structures in sea green). The difference in TM domain positions between the antagonist- and agonist-bound structures (Lower panels; antagonist-bound in grey and agonist bound in hot pink). TM domain positions produced using the structure comparison tool from GPCRdb.

Table 1. Overview of resolved x-ray crystal structures of the δOR. Table produced using the GPCRdb.

Structure						**Auxiliary Protein**	**Structure Ligand**		
Method	**PDB**	**Resolution**	**State**	**Degree Active (%)**	**% of Seq**	**Fusion**	**Name**	**Type**	**Function**
X-ray	6PT2	2.8	Active	76	78	BRIL	KGCHM07	peptide	Agonist
X-ray	6PT3	3.3	Active	76	78	BRIL	DPI-287	small-molecule	Agonist
X-ray *	4RWD	2.7	Inactive	7	79	BRIL	DIPP-NH2	peptide	Antagonist
X-ray	4RWA	3.3	Inactive	7	77	BRIL	DIPP-NH2	peptide	Antagonist
X-ray	4N6H	1.8	Inactive	7	81	BRIL	Naltrindole	small-molecule	Antagonist
X-ray	4EJ4	3.4	Inactive	7	76	T4-Lysozyme	Naltrindole	small-molecule	Antagonist

* 4RWD structure was obtained using the XFEL method.

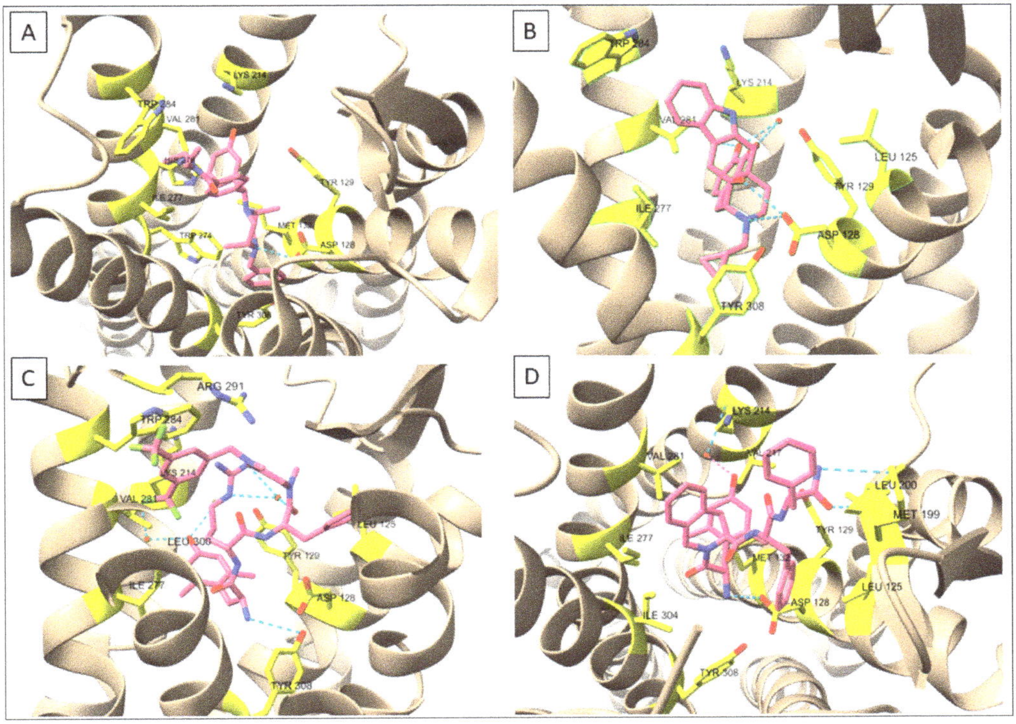

Figure 2. Receptor-ligand interactions at δOR deduced by X-ray crystallography. (**A**) δOR-DPI287 (PDB: 6PT3) (**B**) δOR-NTI (PDB: 4N6H (**C**) δOR-KGCHM07 (PDB: 6PT2) (**D**) δOR-DIPP-NH2 (PDB: 4RWD). Figures made in ChimeraX 1.1.

The DIPP-NH2 binding pocket utilized the same 'message' binding pocket residues as naltrindole with slight movements of Val6.55 and Trp6.58. As expected, the Dmt[1] residue interacted with Tyr3.33, Ile6.51, and Val6.55 with the N-terminal amine forming a salt bridge with Asp3.32 [57]. The Tic[2] side group resided in a hydrophobic pocket made up of Ile6.51, Val6.55, Trp6.58, Leu7.35, and Ile7.39. Importantly, the larger surface of DIPP-NH2 extended further into the 'address' portion of the δOR binding pocket, with Phe[3] interacting with Leu3.29, Asp3.32, and Tyr3.33. Phe[4] interacted with a Met and Leu in ECL2. In the μOR, the corresponding amino acids are charged/polar, making this a possible region important for selectivity [59,60] (Table 2).

In 2019, two agonist-bound X-ray crystal structures produced novel insight into δOR in the active-like state: the δOR bound to the peptide KGCHM07 (PDB:6PT2) and bound to the SNC80-like small molecule DPI-287 (PDB:6PT3) [61] (Figure 2A,C). Relative to the naltrindole-bound structure, the agonist structure shows the movement of TM6 (Figures 1 and 2), particularly, Phe6.44, Cys6.47, and Trp6.58, all of which had been previously linked to δOR activation [55,61]. Arg291 in ECL3 changes location in the KGCHM07 structure and forms a lid on the binding pocket and is part of a hydrophobic pocket that also includes, Ile6.51, Phe6.54, Val6.55, Trp6.58, and Leu7.35, which fits the benzyl moiety of KGCHM07 (Figure 2). Three water molecules interacted with Dmt[1] of KGCHM07 through Tyr3.33, Lys5.39 and His6.52. Water molecules also aid in forming a water-mediated salt-bridge between D-Arg[2] and Asp5.35. Slight differences were observed between the peptide and small molecule structures particularly in relation to the polar network, involving Thr2.56, Glu2.60, and Tyr7.43 the latter being part of a hydrophobic pocket that fits Phe[3] in the peptide-bound structure. Tyr7.43 stabilizes the primary amine of KGCHM07 but does not interact with DPI-287. On the other hand, Thr2.56 stabilizes the polar network for DPI-287 but not KGCHM07 [61]. Overall, the antagonist structures confirmed many predicted and experimentally established key amino acids within the δOR binding pocket. Paired with the addition of the agonist-bound structures this provides new avenues and opportunities for in silico drug discovery at the δOR.

Table 2. Receptor-ligand interactions of the δOR in complex with peptide and small-molecule agonists and antagonists. Table produced in part using the GPCRdb. [62,63]. This table does not reflect the full extent of receptor-ligand interactions, especially with regards to the involvement of the amino acid residues forming hydrophobic sub-pockets of the orthosteric site that are necessary for ligand binding. Additional amino acid residues such as Asp2.50, Asn3.35, and Ser3.39 which form the sodium binding site are also not included in this table.

				Agonist		Antagonist			
				6PT2	6PT3	4RWD	4RWA	4N6H	4EJ4
Amino Acid	**Sequence Number**	**Generic Number**	**Segment**	**KGCHM07**	**DPI-287**	**DIPP-NH2**		**Naltrindole**	
A	98	2.53	TM2						
1-10 L	125	3.29	TM3						
1-10 D	128	3.32	TM3						
1-10 Y	129	3.33	TM3						
1-10 M	132	3.36	TM3						
1-10 M	199	ECL2	ECL2						
1-10 L	200	ECL2	ECL2						
D	210	5.35	TM5						
1-10 K	214	5.39	TM5						
1-10 V	217	5.42	TM5						
1-10 W	274	6.48	TM6						
1-10 I	277	6.51	TM6						
1-10 H	278	6.52	TM6						
1-10 V	281	6.55	TM6						
1-10 W	284	6.58	TM6						
1-10 R	291	ECL3	ECL3						
1-10 L	300	7.35	TM7						
1-10 I	304	7.39	TM7						
1-10 Y	308	7.43	TM7						
Color legend:		Hydrophobic		Aromatic (face to edge)		Aromatic (face to face)		Accessible	
polar (charge-assisted hydrogen bond)			polar (charge-charge)		polar (hydrogen bond)		polar (hydrogen bond with backbone)		

3. Limitations of Current δOR Structures

All the current δOR structures have been resolved using X-ray crystallography (Table 1). The nature of X-ray crystallography relies heavily on producing a receptor that is stable and does not show a lot of movement. On the other hand, cryo-electron microscopy (cryo-EM) is more forgiving in this regard, and thereby provides more opportunities to generate a structure of a wild-type/non-thermostabilized receptor to overcome the current hurdle that the available δOR agonist structures are mutated. Importantly, the Sexton group at Monash University has made significant improvements in the workflow for generating cryo-EM structures, such that structures with resolutions below 3Å can now be routinely resolved [64].

Another limitation for in silico drug discovery at the δOR is that none of the δOR structures were co-crystallized with an effector protein. The ability of cryo-EM to determine the structures of large complexes of macromolecules gained attraction over the past decade following advancements in electron detectors and data software used to reconstruct the 3D structures from the 2D images [64]. For GPCRs in complex with downstream effector proteins, such as G-protein, β-arrestin, or GRKs, cryo-EM is increasingly becoming the method of choice for structure determination. This is in part because protein structures obtained using cryo-EM overcome some of the limitations such as thermostabilizing mutations and fusion proteins which are commonly introduced in X-ray crystallography structures [65]. The increasing number of cryo-EM structures that are being obtained in complex with downstream effector proteins can provide valuable insight into the molecular basis of GPCR signaling, potentially biased signaling, which then informs the structure-based drug discovery process.

Thus far, three cryo-EM structures of the μOR and one structure for the κ-opioid receptor (κOR) have been resolved [66–68]. Nonetheless, with respect to the δOR, the absence of X-ray crystal structures or cryo-EM structure of the δOR in complex with downstream effector proteins represents a challenge for structure-based drug discovery. Overcoming this hurdle requires careful and extensive molecular modeling that integrates the available crystal structures of the δOR in their inactive- and active-like states (Table 1) with the structures of other opioid receptors that are in complex with Gi-proteins, β-arrestins, nanobodies. This is especially crucial when using the active-like crystal structures of δOR due to the presence of thermostabilizing mutations. This method of computational structure determination was applied at the κOR where molecular dynamics (MD) simulations and an enhanced sampling method called meta-dynamics simulations were used to determine the structure of the κOR in complex with the Gi-protein. To obtain the optimized active structure, the authors started with optimizing the nb39 stabilized crystal structure of the κOR in complex with the agonist MP1104 (PDB: 6B73) then used the μOR-DAMGO-nucleotide free Gi-protein cryo-EM structure to couple the Gi-protein to the κOR [66,67,69]. Then, they used meta-dynamics simulations to optimize the κOR-Gi complex interactions before examining its stability using MD simulations. Their approach was applicable to the crystal structure of the μOR (5C1M) which they used to construct μOR-BU72-Gi and confirm the structural determinants of G-protein coupling.

To obtain the active-like δOR x-ray crystal structures bound to a peptide agonist and to a small molecule agonist, the δOR was thermostabilized by nine point mutations that negatively impacted the native pharmacology [61]. This was unsurprising, as the impact of mutations on receptor function can compound with increasing numbers [55]. Particularly, the mutations impacted the allosteric sodium binding pocket that has been implicated in β-arrestin signaling [57,61]. Thus, the crystallized conformation may not be optimal to identify signal-biased agonists reducing the utility of the current agonist-bound δOR structures.

4. Opportunities for Computer-Aided Drug Discovery at the δOR

Over the last ten years, an increasing number of opioid receptors structures have been elucidated in unbound (apo-state), antagonist bound, or agonist bound states, either stabilized with thermostabilizing mutations, G_i-protein, or nanobodies. These structures, even the antagonist-bound ones, have proven useful for performing docking studies on large virtual libraries. For example, a screen of 3M molecules on the inactive μOR (4DKL) led to the identification of a hit that was optimized in three steps to the novel G-biased agonist PZM21 [70]. Recent advances in docking have enabled the screening of libraries of nearly two magnitudes larger in size; thus far, this approach has been successfully employed to screen 138 million compounds using an antagonist-bound dopamine D_4 receptor [71], and 150 million compounds at a thermostabilized agonist-bound melatonin MT1 receptor [72]. These screens relied on the ZINC database [73] to provide decoys and screening molecules. The ZINC database is an ever-increasing repository for accessible molecules, currently holding about one billion compounds [74,75]. The increase in the size of the ZINC database is largely supported by the increase in catalog size of commercially available compounds from Enamine (https://enamine.net/news-events/press-releases/807-enamine-expands-collaboration-with-ucsf, accessed on 12 July 2022). Indeed, commercially available make-on demand chemical libraries such as Enamine's REAL Space collection which comprises 22.7 billion compounds as of the time of writing this review, make it feasible to identify novel chemotypes that could induce novel pharmacology. It comes as no surprise that high throughput virtual screening campaigns are expected to further expand the utilized ligand chemical space which will result in the identification of an increasing number of novel hit compounds. This expansion in the utilized chemical space can be effectively leveraged for structure-based drug discovery using currently available, and future, structures of δOR to virtually dock and screen more compounds than ever before.

Efforts in virtual screening of chemical libraries have used structure-based drug discovery to expand the available chemical space for various GPCR targets [72,76]. This approach has yielded many novel chemotypes across several targets that could provide useful starting points for medicinal chemists to modify and improve selectivity among other properties. However, in screening campaigns that aim to identify biased agonists in-silico, this approach represents a potential bottleneck to the discovery process and might not be sufficient to identify functionally selective ligands. Thus far, the method of choice in identifying biased agonists at the δOR and other GPCRs has relied on the functional characterization of known and novel binders using cell-based assays to establish pharmacological and SAR profiles for future hit identification and lead optimization campaigns. However, the recent advances in computational tools and enhanced sampling methods such as molecular dynamics simulations which enable the dynamic modeling of the δOR and other GPCRs should be leveraged to unravel the structural determinants of biased signaling. In other words, the structural and conformational changes induced by agonist binding at δOR that appear in an MD simulation could be correlated with pharmacological data and mutagenesis analyses. Such an approach could be used to generate structural models or snapshots of the δOR in different conformational states which would increase the ability of docking campaigns to identify novel and biased agonists (Figure 3).

Until recently, GPCRs' structures in general, including those of the opioid receptors, still do not appear to provide a clear picture of the underlying signaling mechanisms given the complexity of the involved signaling network, the limited number of available structures bound to G-proteins, β-arrestins, or GRKs, and the diversity of the chemical space interacting with these receptors [77]. The tremendous success of cryo-EM structure determination and the increasing number of high-resolution structures when coupled with MD simulations could provide insights into GPCRs in action. Hence, developing and utilizing computational methods and workflows to model ensembles of structural conformations and then combining such methods with resolving GPCR structures in complex with G-proteins, β-arrestins, and GRKs should provide a strong approach to alleviate current limitations. This could also minimize the misinterpretations that stem from comparisons and analyses that are based on static GPCR structures that suffer from the limitations mentioned above.

A similar approach was applied recently at the μOR, where Wang et al. highlighted how the implementation of molecular dynamics could be helpful in lead optimization campaigns [68]. The authors implemented a structure-based lead optimization approach to generate PZM21 analogs with improved CNS penetration and higher G-protein bias with lower β-arrestin recruitment compared to fentanyl. In the study, the authors resolved a high-resolution cryo-EM structure of PZM21 bound to the μOR in a complex with the trimeric Gi-protein (PDB: 7SBF). The resolved cryo-EM structure showed that PZM21 forms a salt bridge between its basic amine and Asp3.32 of μOR which confirmed previous findings [67,78]. To confirm the stability of the PZM21's binding pose, and characterize the water-mediated interactions with μOR, the authors performed all-atom MD simulations which showed that PZM21 formed water-mediated interactions with His6.52 and Lys5.39. Intriguingly, the authors used insights from structural and dynamic analyses for lead optimization, guided by MD simulations and the cryo-EM structure of μOR in complex with Gi-protein. The resulting PZM21 analogs were μOR-selective with improved functional selectivity. Translating such an approach at the δOR will allow for more successful hit-to-lead and lead-optimization campaigns. Recently resolved cryo-EM structures of mitragynine pseudoindoxyl, which has very low arrestin recruitment, and lofentanil, a potent arrestin recruiter demonstrate the involvement of distinct orthosteric sub-pockets in determining arrestin recruitment at the μOR. The authors demonstrated that each agonist has distinct moieties that bind in two distinct sub-pockets while sharing a central binding pocket with DAMGO [79]. Such findings support previous predictions and lead optimization strategies that have been applied to modulate biased agonism at the μOR and κOR [80,81].

Another promising area that has been on the rise recently is using machine learning and artificial intelligence in protein structure prediction and drug discovery. These advances present an exciting avenue for the discovery of novel and potential therapeutic agents at the δOR. Undeniably, the integration of machine learning and deep learning with current computational and pharmacological approaches presents a valuable opportunity to accelerate drug discovery campaigns at δOR. Machine learning models could be trained using high-quality datasets to predict drug properties, toxicity, target selectivity, and potentially ligand-receptor interactions. This has been made possible in part due to the GPCR community's efforts to provide access to curated datasets such as GPCRdb.org [62,82] and open-source machine learning packages such as DeepChem and AMPL, which allows researchers to build, train and deploy machine learning models for drug discovery [83]. Additionally, the rapid increase in high-performance cloud computing, improved Graphics Processing Units (i.e., GPUs), and increasingly efficient machine learning algorithms provide an opportunity to expand the screening of ultra-large chemical libraries or the de-novo drug design in a more efficient manner.

The significant improvement in structure prediction provided by AlphaFold 2 [84], may provide avenues for obtaining a wild-type thermostable δOR structure, that could be used for docking studies. There are significant limitations, in particular the current lack of Alphafold to predict how a protein will change conformation upon binding of a specific ligand [85]. Future machine learning algorithms may learn how to do this and further reduce the initial requirement of wet-lab science to obtain potent and selective novel molecules for a receptor target including the δOR.

MD simulations are another area that is expected to benefit from recent advances in machine learning and artificial intelligence. In fact, work is already underway to develop machine learning force fields that could increase the accuracy of MD simulations while reducing the computational cost [86]. Deep learning frameworks such as TorchMD [87] and neural networks such as graph convolutional neural networks (GCNNs) have been used for geometry optimization [88], acceleration of MD simulations, or even in improving force fields [89]. Such advances should be carefully utilized and expanded to complement the available structural and experimental data and accelerate the identification of therapeutic agents at the δOR.

To accelerate future large-scale drug discovery efforts at the δOR, well-trained and validated machine learning models should be combined with physics-based scoring functions to reduce the computational cost of docking and screening ultra-large chemical libraries. In this instance, a machine learning model could serve as a filter that could be incorporated into a docking workflow to prioritize which molecules move on to the next phase and ultimately which molecules are to be tested pharmacologically. Moreover, this approach allows the incorporation of structural and pharmacological parameters to build, train, and deploy multi-task learning models that could increase the selectivity and novelty of the identified compounds.

Despite the optimistic outlook and promising advances in computer-aided drug design, it is important to know the limits of the utilized tools. Furthermore, it is worth noting that there are numerous challenges and potential pitfalls associated with the incorporation of machine learning or deep learning models, especially with respect to the availability of large and high-quality datasets for the drug target [90,91]. For the δOR and other GPCRs, the diversity of cell-based assays that are used to characterize their pharmacology and the inconsistent practices between different research labs, or in some instances within the same lab, are two major limitations that need to be addressed before we can reliably use machine learning in GPCR drug discovery. Hence, future efforts should also focus on the standardization of experimental data collection and computational data curation and modeling.

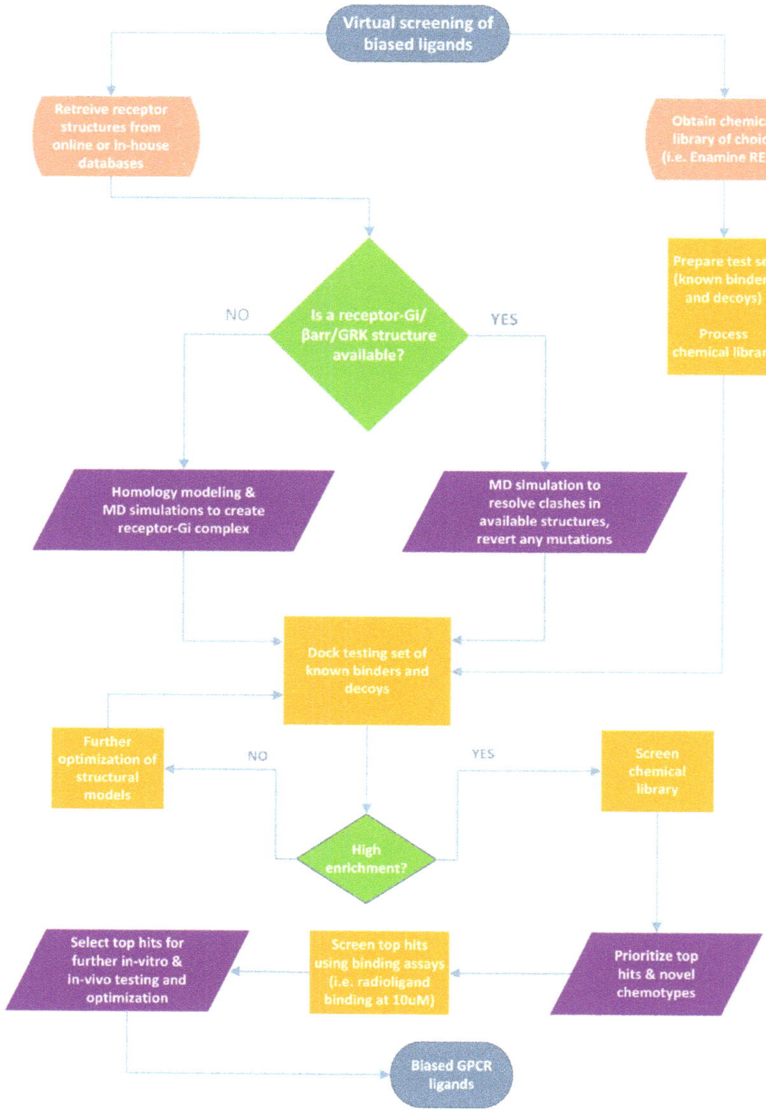

Figure 3. Proposed workflow for screening large chemical libraries to identify G-protein biased agonists at the δOR and other GPCRs. A similar workflow could be applied to identify GRK- or β-arrestin-biased small molecules given that high-quality crystal or cryo-EM structures are available. In cases where distinct interactions or sub-pockets specific to biased agonists or in cases where we know that an allosteric site/pocket could lead to biased effects, we could restrict ligand docking to that specific site to screen a given chemical library. The most accurate way to confirm such interactions would be to resolve high-quality structures and/or perform mutagenesis studies. Alternatively, enhanced sampling computational modeling to model receptor-effector complexes could be useful if computational cost is not a limiting factor.

5. Conclusions

For the identification of novel, functionally selective, and potentially therapeutic agonists at δOR, future efforts should aim to expand our understanding of the effect of various mutations on the structure and function of δOR utilizing the constantly improving *in-vitro* and *in-silico* approach. Additionally, producing multiple wild-type agonist-bound high-resolution structures of δOR will allow for a more efficient expansion of its chemical space in virtual screening campaigns or in computer-aided lead optimization. Consequently, these efforts will provide high-quality datasets that could allow for the incorporation of ML and DL tools in opioid drug discovery. Overall, we think there are more opportunities than that there are challenges to carry out a high yield in silico screen at the δOR to generate novel chemical matter that hopefully can be translated into meaningful therapeutics.

Author Contributions: Conceptualization, Y.J.M. and R.M.v.R.; writing—original draft preparation, Y.J.M. and R.M.v.R.; writing—review and editing, Y.J.M. and R.M.v.R.; visualization, Y.J.M.; funding acquisition, R.M.v.R. All authors have read and agreed to the published version of the manuscript.

Funding: This research was funded by the National Institute on Alcohol Abuse and Alcoholism, grant number R01AA025368 (R.M.v.R.).

Institutional Review Board Statement: Not applicable.

Informed Consent Statement: Not applicable.

Data Availability Statement: Not applicable.

Conflicts of Interest: van Rijn is currently employed as a Principal Scientist at Septerna Inc. and holds stock options in the company. van Rijn holds a US patent (10,954,224) describing novel delta opioid receptor agonists. YM has no conflict of interest to declare. The funders had no role in the design of the study; in the collection, analyses, or interpretation of data; in the writing of the manuscript, or in the decision to publish the results.

References

1. Erspamer, V.; Melchiorri, P.; Falconieri-Erspamer, G.; Negri, L.; Corsi, R.; Severini, C.; Barra, D.; Simmaco, M.; Kreil, G. Deltorphins: A family of naturally occurring peptides with high affinity and selectivity for delta opioid binding sites. *Proc. Natl. Acad. Sci. USA* **1989**, *86*, 5188–5192. [CrossRef] [PubMed]
2. Fricker, L.D.; Margolis, E.B.; Gomes, I.; Devi, L.A. Five Decades of Research on Opioid Peptides: Current Knowledge and Unanswered Questions. *Mol. Pharmacol.* **2020**, *98*, 96–108. [CrossRef] [PubMed]
3. Cassell, R.J.; Mores, K.L.; Zerfas, B.L.; Mahmoud, A.H.; Lill, M.A.; Trader, D.J.; van Rijn, R.M. Rubiscolins are naturally occurring G protein-biased delta opioid receptor peptides. *Eur. Neuropsychopharmacol.* **2019**, *29*, 450–456. [CrossRef] [PubMed]
4. Gutridge, A.M.; Robins, M.T.; Cassell, R.J.; Uprety, R.; Mores, K.L.; Ko, M.J.; Pasternak, G.W.; Majumdar, S.; van Rijn, R.M. G protein-biased kratom-alkaloids and synthetic carfentanil-amide opioids as potential treatments for alcohol use disorder. *Br. J. Pharmacol.* **2019**, *177*, 1497–1513. [CrossRef] [PubMed]
5. Gutridge, A.M.; Chakraborty, S.; Varga, B.R.; Rhoda, E.S.; French, A.R.; Blaine, A.T.; Royer, Q.H.; Cui, H.; Yuan, J.; Cassell, R.J.; et al. Evaluation of Kratom Opioid Derivatives as Potential Treatment Option for Alcohol Use Disorder. *Front. Pharmacol.* **2021**, *12*, 764885. [CrossRef] [PubMed]
6. Gendron, L.; Cahill, C.M.; von Zastrow, M.; Schiller, P.W.; Pineyro, G. Molecular Pharmacology of delta-Opioid Receptors. *Pharmacol. Rev.* **2016**, *68*, 631–700. [CrossRef]
7. Pradhan, A.A.; Befort, K.; Nozaki, C.; Gaveriaux-Ruff, C.; Kieffer, B.L. The delta opioid receptor: An evolving target for the treatment of brain disorders. *Trends Pharmacol. Sci.* **2011**, *32*, 581–590. [CrossRef]
8. Grant Liska, M.; Crowley, M.G.; Lippert, T.; Corey, S.; Borlongan, C.V. Delta Opioid Receptor and Peptide: A Dynamic Therapy for Stroke and Other Neurological Disorders. *Handb. Exp. Pharmacol.* **2017**, *247*, 277–299.
9. Mabrouk, O.S.; Marti, M.; Salvadori, S.; Morari, M. The novel delta opioid receptor agonist UFP-512 dually modulates motor activity in hemiparkinsonian rats via control of the nigro-thalamic pathway. *Neuroscience* **2009**, *164*, 360–369. [CrossRef]
10. Sarajarvi, T.; Marttinen, M.; Natunen, T.; Kauppinen, T.; Makinen, P.; Helisalmi, S.; Laitinen, M.; Rauramaa, T.; Leinonen, V.; Petaja-Repo, U.; et al. Genetic Variation in delta-Opioid Receptor Associates with Increased beta- and gamma-Secretase Activity in the Late Stages of Alzheimer's Disease. *J. Alzheimers Dis.* **2015**, *48*, 507–516. [CrossRef]
11. Crist, R.C.; Clarke, T.K. OPRD1 Genetic Variation and Human Disease. *Handb. Exp. Pharmacol.* **2018**, *247*, 131–145. [PubMed]
12. Johnston, T.H.; Versi, E.; Howson, P.A.; Ravenscroft, P.; Fox, S.H.; Hill, M.P.; Reidenberg, B.E.; Corey, R.; Brotchie, J.M. DPI-289, a novel mixed delta opioid agonist/mu opioid antagonist (DAMA), has L-DOPA-sparing potential in Parkinson's disease. *Neuropharmacology* **2018**, *131*, 116–127. [CrossRef] [PubMed]

13. Xu, Y.; Zhi, F.; Mao, J.; Peng, Y.; Shao, N.; Balboni, G.; Yang, Y.; Xia, Y. delta-opioid receptor activation protects against Parkinson's disease-related mitochondrial dysfunction by enhancing PINK1/Parkin-dependent mitophagy. *Aging* **2020**, *12*, 25035–25059. [CrossRef] [PubMed]
14. Alongkronrusmee, D.; Chiang, T.; van Rijn, R.M. Delta Opioid Pharmacology in Relation to Alcohol Behaviors. *Handb. Exp. Pharmacol.* **2016**, *247*, 199–225.
15. Chiang, T.; Sansuk, K.; van Rijn, R.M. beta-Arrestin 2 dependence of delta opioid receptor agonists is correlated with alcohol intake. *Br. J. Pharmacol.* **2016**, *173*, 332–343. [CrossRef]
16. Robins, M.T.; Chiang, T.; Mores, K.L.; Alongkronrusmee, D.; van Rijn, R.M. Critical Role for Gi/o-Protein Activity in the Dorsal Striatum in the Reduction of Voluntary Alcohol Intake in C57Bl/6 Mice. *Front. Psychiatry* **2018**, *9*, 112. [CrossRef]
17. Corsetti, M.; Whorwell, P. New therapeutic options for IBS: The role of the first in class mixed micro- opioid receptor agonist and delta-opioid receptor antagonist (mudelta) eluxadoline. *Expert Rev. Gastroenterol. Hepatol.* **2017**, *11*, 285–292. [CrossRef]
18. DiCello, J.J.; Carbone, S.E.; Saito, A.; Pham, V.; Szymaszkiewicz, A.; Gondin, A.B.; Alvi, S.; Marique, K.; Shenoy, P.; Veldhuis, N.A.; et al. Positive allosteric modulation of endogenous delta opioid receptor signaling in the enteric nervous system is a potential treatment for gastrointestinal motility disorders. *Am. J. Physiol. Gastrointest. Liver Physiol.* **2022**, *322*, G66–G78. [CrossRef]
19. Dondio, G. Development of novel pain relief agents acting through the selective activation of the delta-opioid receptor. *Farmaco* **2000**, *55*, 178–180. [CrossRef]
20. Kotzer, C.J.; Hay, D.W.; Dondio, G.; Giardina, G.; Petrillo, P.; Underwood, D.C. The antitussive activity of delta-opioid receptor stimulation in guinea pigs. *J. Pharmacol. Exp. Ther.* **2000**, *292*, 803–809.
21. Petrillo, P.; Angelici, O.; Bingham, S.; Ficalora, G.; Garnier, M.; Zaratin, P.F.; Petrone, G.; Pozzi, O.; Sbacchi, M.; Stean, T.O.; et al. Evidence for a selective role of the delta-opioid agonist [8R-(4bS*,8aalpha,8abeta, 12bbeta)]7,10-Dimethyl-1-methoxy-11-(2-methylpropyl)oxycarbonyl 5,6,7,8,12,12b-hexahydro-(9H)-4,8-methanobenzofuro[3,2-e]pyrrolo[2,3-g]isoquinoli ne hydrochloride (SB-235863) in blocking hyperalgesia associated with inflammatory and neuropathic pain responses. *J. Pharmacol. Exp. Ther.* **2003**, *307*, 1079–1089. [PubMed]
22. Richards, E.M.; Mathews, D.C.; Luckenbaugh, D.A.; Ionescu, D.F.; Machado-Vieira, R.; Niciu, M.J.; Duncan, W.C.; Nolan, N.M.; Franco-Chaves, J.A.; Hudzik, T.; et al. A randomized, placebo-controlled pilot trial of the delta opioid receptor agonist AZD2327 in anxious depression. *Psychopharmacology* **2016**, *233*, 1119–1130. [CrossRef] [PubMed]
23. Cubist Pharmaceuticals LLC. Analgesic Efficacy and Safety of ADL5859 in Subjects With Acute Dental Pain After Third Molar Extraction. Available online: https://clinicaltrials.gov/ct2/show/NCT00993863 (accessed on 12 July 2022).
24. Cubist Pharmaceuticals LLC. Study to Assess the Efficacy, Safety, and Tolerability of ADL5747 in Participants With Postherpetic Neuralgia. Available online: https://clinicaltrials.gov/ct2/show/NCT01058642 (accessed on 12 July 2022).
25. Broom, D.C.; Jutkiewicz, E.M.; Folk, J.E.; Traynor, J.R.; Rice, K.C.; Woods, J.H. Convulsant activity of a non-peptidic delta-opioid receptor agonist is not required for its antidepressant-like effects in Sprague-Dawley rats. *Psychopharmacology* **2002**, *164*, 42–48. [CrossRef] [PubMed]
26. Vicente-Sanchez, A.; Dripps, I.J.; Tipton, A.F.; Akbari, H.; Akbari, A.; Jutkiewicz, E.M.; Pradhan, A.A. Tolerance to high-internalizing delta opioid receptor agonist is critically mediated by arrestin 2. *Br. J. Pharmacol.* **2018**, *175*, 3050–3059. [CrossRef]
27. Jutkiewicz, E.M.; Rice, K.C.; Traynor, J.R.; Woods, J.H. Separation of the convulsions and antidepressant-like effects produced by the delta-opioid agonist SNC80 in rats. *Psychopharmacology* **2005**, *182*, 588–596. [CrossRef] [PubMed]
28. Codd, E.E.; Carson, J.R.; Colburn, R.W.; Stone, D.J.; Van Besien, C.R.; Zhang, S.P.; Wade, P.R.; Gallantine, E.L.; Meert, T.F.; Molino, L.; et al. JNJ-20788560 [9-(8-azabicyclo[3.2.1]oct-3-ylidene)-9H-xanthene-3-carboxylic acid diethylamide], a selective delta opioid receptor agonist, is a potent and efficacious antihyperalgesic agent that does not produce respiratory depression, pharmacologic tolerance, or physical dependence. *J. Pharmacol. Exp. Ther.* **2009**, *329*, 241–251.
29. Codd, E.E.; Carson, J.R.; Colburn, R.W.; Dax, S.L.; Desai-Krieger, D.; Martinez, R.P.; McKown, L.A.; Neilson, L.A.; Pitis, P.M.; Stahle, P.L.; et al. The novel, orally active, delta opioid RWJ-394674 is biotransformed to the potent mu opioid RWJ-413216. *J. Pharmacol. Exp. Ther.* **2006**, *318*, 1273–1279. [CrossRef]
30. Holt, J.D.; Watson, M.J.; Chang, J.P.; O'Neill, S.J.; Wei, K.; Pendergast, W.; Gengo, P.J.; Chang, K.J. DPI-221 [4-((alpha-s)-alpha-((2s,5r)-2,5-dimethyl-4-(3-fluorobenzyl)-1-piperazinyl)benzyl)-N,N-diethylbenzamide]: A novel nonpeptide delta receptor agonist producing increased micturition interval in normal rats. *J. Pharmacol. Exp. Ther.* **2005**, *315*, 601–608. [CrossRef]
31. Yi, S.P.; Kong, Q.H.; Li, Y.L.; Pan, C.L.; Yu, J.; Cui, B.Q.; Wang, Y.F.; Wang, G.L.; Zhou, P.L.; Wang, L.L.; et al. The opioid receptor triple agonist DPI-125 produces analgesia with less respiratory depression and reduced abuse liability. *Acta Pharmacol. Sin.* **2017**, *38*, 977–989. [CrossRef]
32. Cassell, R.J.; Sharma, K.K.; Su, H.; Cummins, B.R.; Cui, H.; Mores, K.L.; Blaine, A.T.; Altman, R.A.; van Rijn, R.M. The Meta-Position of Phe(4) in Leu-Enkephalin Regulates Potency, Selectivity, Functional Activity, and Signaling Bias at the Delta and Mu Opioid Receptors. *Molecules* **2019**, *24*, 4542. [CrossRef]
33. Vezzi, V.; Onaran, H.O.; Molinari, P.; Guerrini, R.; Balboni, G.; Calo, G.; Costa, T. Ligands raise the constraint that limits constitutive activation in G protein-coupled opioid receptors. *J. Biol. Chem.* **2013**, *288*, 23964–23978. [CrossRef] [PubMed]
34. Bella Ndong, D.; Blais, V.; Holleran, B.J.; Proteau-Gagné, A.; Cantin-Savoie, I.; Robert, W.; Nadon, J.-F.; Beauchemin, S.; Leduc, R.; Piñeyro, G.; et al. Exploration of the fifth position of leu-enkephalin and its role in binding and activating delta (DOP) and mu (MOP) opioid receptors. *Pept. Sci.* **2019**, *111*, e24070. [CrossRef]

35. Sharma, K.K.; Cassell, R.J.; Meqbil, Y.J.; Su, H.; Blaine, A.T.; Cummins, B.R.; Mores, K.L.; Johnson, D.K.; van Rijn, R.M.; Altman, R.A. Modulating beta-arrestin 2 recruitment at the delta- and mu-opioid receptors using peptidomimetic ligands. *RSC Med. Chem.* **2021**, *12*, 1958–1967. [CrossRef] [PubMed]
36. Conibear, A.E.; Asghar, J.; Hill, R.; Henderson, G.; Borbely, E.; Tekus, V.; Helyes, Z.; Palandri, J.; Bailey, C.; Starke, I.; et al. A Novel G Protein-Biased Agonist at the delta Opioid Receptor with Analgesic Efficacy in Models of Chronic Pain. *J. Pharmacol. Exp. Ther.* **2020**, *372*, 224–236. [CrossRef]
37. Crombie, A.; Arezzo, J.; Cowan, C.; DeWire, S.; Gowen-McDonald, W.; Hawkins, M.; Jutkiewicz, E.; Kramer, M.; Koblish, M.; Lark, M.; et al. TRV250: A novel G protein-biased ligand at the delta receptor for the potential treatment of migraine. *Postgrad. Med.* **2015**, *127* (Suppl. 1), S61.
38. Nagase, H.; Nemoto, T.; Matsubara, A.; Saito, M.; Yamamoto, N.; Osa, Y.; Hirayama, S.; Nakajima, M.; Nakao, K.; Mochizuki, H.; et al. Design and synthesis of KNT-127, a delta-opioid receptor agonist effective by systemic administration. *Bioorg. Med. Chem. Lett.* **2010**, *20*, 6302–6305. [CrossRef]
39. Knapp, R.J.; Landsman, R.; Waite, S.; Malatynska, E.; Varga, E.; Haq, W.; Hruby, V.J.; Roeske, W.R.; Nagase, H.; Yamamura, H.I. Properties of TAN-67, a nonpeptidic delta-opioid receptor agonist, at cloned human delta- and mu-opioid receptors. *Eur. J. Pharmacol.* **1995**, *291*, 129–134. [CrossRef]
40. Burford, N.T.; Clark, M.J.; Wehrman, T.S.; Gerritz, S.W.; Banks, M.; O'Connell, J.; Traynor, J.R.; Alt, A. Discovery of positive allosteric modulators and silent allosteric modulators of the mu-opioid receptor. *Proc. Natl. Acad. Sci. USA* **2013**, *110*, 10830–10835. [CrossRef]
41. Burford, N.T.; Livingston, K.; Canals, M.; Ryan, M.; Budenholzer, L.; Han, Y.; Shang, Y.; Herbst, J.J.; O'Connell, J.; Banks, M.; et al. Discovery, Synthesis and Molecular Pharmacology of Selective Positive Allosteric Modulators of the delta-Opioid Receptor. *J. Med. Chem.* **2015**, *58*, 4220–4229. [CrossRef]
42. Stanczyk, M.A.; Livingston, K.E.; Chang, L.; Weinberg, Z.Y.; Puthenveedu, M.A.; Traynor, J.R. The delta-opioid receptor positive allosteric modulator BMS 986187 is a G-protein-biased allosteric agonist. *Br. J. Pharmacol.* **2019**, *176*, 1649–1663. [CrossRef]
43. Fujii, H.; Uchida, Y.; Shibasaki, M.; Nishida, M.; Yoshioka, T.; Kobayashi, R.; Honjo, A.; Itoh, K.; Yamada, D.; Hirayama, S.; et al. Discovery of delta opioid receptor full agonists lacking a basic nitrogen atom and their antidepressant-like effects. *Bioorg. Med. Chem. Lett.* **2020**, *30*, 127176. [CrossRef] [PubMed]
44. Meqbil, Y.J.; Su, H.; Cassell, R.J.; Mores, K.L.; Gutridge, A.M.; Cummins, B.R.; Chen, L.; van Rijn, R.M. Identification of a Novel Delta Opioid Receptor Agonist Chemotype with Potential Negative Allosteric Modulator Capabilities. *Molecules* **2021**, *26*, 7236. [CrossRef] [PubMed]
45. Evans, C.J.; Keith, D.E., Jr.; Morrison, H.; Magendzo, K.; Edwards, R.H. Cloning of a delta opioid receptor by functional expression. *Science* **1992**, *258*, 1952–1955. [CrossRef] [PubMed]
46. Kieffer, B.L.; Befort, K.; Gaveriaux-Ruff, C.; Hirth, C.G. The delta-opioid receptor: Isolation of a cDNA by expression cloning and pharmacological characterization. *Proc. Natl. Acad. Sci. USA* **1992**, *89*, 12048–12052. [CrossRef]
47. Ballesteros, J.A.; Weinstein, H. Integrated methods for the construction of three-dimensional models and computational probing of structure-function relations in G protein-coupled receptors. *Methods Neurosci.* **1995**, *25*, 366–428.
48. Kong, H.; Raynor, K.; Yasuda, K.; Moe, S.T.; Portoghese, P.S.; Bell, G.I.; Reisine, T. A single residue, aspartic acid 95, in the delta opioid receptor specifies selective high affinity agonist binding. *J. Biol. Chem.* **1993**, *268*, 23055–23058. [CrossRef]
49. Befort, K.; Tabbara, L.; Bausch, S.; Chavkin, C.; Evans, C.; Kieffer, B. The conserved aspartate residue in the third putative transmembrane domain of the delta-opioid receptor is not the anionic counterpart for cationic opiate binding but is a constituent of the receptor binding site. *Mol. Pharmacol.* **1996**, *49*, 216–223.
50. Befort, K.; Tabbara, L.; Kling, D.; Maigret, B.; Kieffer, B.L. Role of aromatic transmembrane residues of the delta-opioid receptor in ligand recognition. *J. Biol. Chem.* **1996**, *271*, 10161–10168. [CrossRef]
51. Onogi, T.; Minami, M.; Katao, Y.; Nakagawa, T.; Aoki, Y.; Toya, T.; Katsumata, S.; Satoh, M. DAMGO, a mu-opioid receptor selective agonist, distinguishes between mu- and delta-opioid receptors around their first extracellular loops. *FEBS Lett.* **1995**, *357*, 93–97. [CrossRef]
52. Minami, M.; Nakagawa, T.; Seki, T.; Onogi, T.; Aoki, Y.; Katao, Y.; Katsumata, S.; Satoh, M. A single residue, Lys108, of the delta-opioid receptor prevents the mu-opioid-selective ligand [D-Ala2,N-MePhe4,Gly-ol5]enkephalin from binding to the delta-opioid receptor. *Mol. Pharmacol.* **1996**, *50*, 1413–1422.
53. Valiquette, M.; Vu, H.K.; Yue, S.Y.; Wahlestedt, C.; Walker, P. Involvement of Trp-284, Val-296, and Val-297 of the human delta-opioid receptor in binding of delta-selective ligands. *J. Biol. Chem.* **1996**, *271*, 18789–18796. [CrossRef] [PubMed]
54. Strahs, D.; Weinstein, H. Comparative modeling and molecular dynamics studies of the delta, kappa and mu opioid receptors. *Protein Eng.* **1997**, *10*, 1019–1038. [CrossRef] [PubMed]
55. Decaillot, F.M.; Befort, K.; Filliol, D.; Yue, S.; Walker, P.; Kieffer, B.L. Opioid receptor random mutagenesis reveals a mechanism for G protein-coupled receptor activation. *Nat. Struct. Biol.* **2003**, *10*, 629–636. [CrossRef] [PubMed]
56. Granier, S.; Manglik, A.; Kruse, A.C.; Kobilka, T.S.; Thian, F.S.; Weis, W.I.; Kobilka, B.K. Structure of the delta-opioid receptor bound to naltrindole. *Nature* **2012**, *485*, 400–404. [CrossRef] [PubMed]
57. Fenalti, G.; Giguere, P.M.; Katritch, V.; Huang, X.P.; Thompson, A.A.; Cherezov, V.; Roth, B.L.; Stevens, R.C. Molecular control of delta-opioid receptor signalling. *Nature* **2014**, *506*, 191–196. [CrossRef]

58. Chavkin, C.; Goldstein, A. Specific receptor for the opioid peptide dynorphin: Structure—Activity relationships. *Proc. Natl. Acad. Sci. USA* **1981**, *78*, 6543–6547. [CrossRef]
59. Fenalti, G.; Zatsepin, N.A.; Betti, C.; Giguere, P.; Han, G.W.; Ishchenko, A.; Liu, W.; Guillemyn, K.; Zhang, H.; James, D.; et al. Structural basis for bifunctional peptide recognition at human delta-opioid receptor. *Nat. Struct. Mol. Biol.* **2015**, *22*, 265–268. [CrossRef]
60. Varga, E.V.; Li, X.; Stropova, D.; Zalewska, T.; Landsman, R.S.; Knapp, R.J.; Malatynska, E.; Kawai, K.; Mizusura, A.; Nagase, H.; et al. The third extracellular loop of the human delta-opioid receptor determines the selectivity of delta-opioid agonists. *Mol. Pharmacol.* **1996**, *50*, 1619–1624.
61. Claff, T.; Yu, J.; Blais, V.; Patel, N.; Martin, C.; Wu, L.; Han, G.W.; Holleran, B.J.; Van der Poorten, O.; White, K.L.; et al. Elucidating the active delta-opioid receptor crystal structure with peptide and small-molecule agonists. *Sci. Adv.* **2019**, *5*, eaax9115. [CrossRef]
62. Kooistra, A.J.; Mordalski, S.; Pandy-Szekeres, G.; Esguerra, M.; Mamyrbekov, A.; Munk, C.; Keseru, G.M.; Gloriam, D.E. GPCRdb in 2021: Integrating GPCR sequence, structure and function. *Nucleic Acids Res.* **2021**, *49*, D335–D343. [CrossRef]
63. Munk, C.; Harpsoe, K.; Hauser, A.S.; Isberg, V.; Gloriam, D.E. Integrating structural and mutagenesis data to elucidate GPCR ligand binding. *Curr. Opin. Pharmacol.* **2016**, *30*, 51–58. [CrossRef] [PubMed]
64. Danev, R.; Belousoff, M.; Liang, Y.L.; Zhang, X.; Eisenstein, F.; Wootten, D.; Sexton, P.M. Routine sub-2.5 A cryo-EM structure determination of GPCRs. *Nat. Commun.* **2021**, *12*, 4333. [CrossRef] [PubMed]
65. Draper-Joyce, C.J.; Khoshouei, M.; Thal, D.M.; Liang, Y.L.; Nguyen, A.T.N.; Furness, S.G.B.; Venugopal, H.; Baltos, J.A.; Plitzko, J.M.; Danev, R.; et al. Structure of the adenosine-bound human adenosine A1 receptor-Gi complex. *Nature* **2018**, *558*, 559–563. [CrossRef] [PubMed]
66. Che, T.; Majumdar, S.; Zaidi, S.A.; Ondachi, P.; McCorvy, J.D.; Wang, S.; Mosier, P.D.; Uprety, R.; Vardy, E.; Krumm, B.E.; et al. Structure of the Nanobody-Stabilized Active State of the Kappa Opioid Receptor. *Cell* **2018**, *172*, 55–67.e15. [CrossRef]
67. Koehl, A.; Hu, H.; Maeda, S.; Zhang, Y.; Qu, Q.; Paggi, J.M.; Latorraca, N.R.; Hilger, D.; Dawson, R.; Matile, H.; et al. Structure of the micro-opioid receptor-Gi protein complex. *Nature* **2018**, *558*, 547–552. [CrossRef]
68. Gmeiner, P.; Wang, H.; Hetzer, F.; Huang, W.; Qu, Q.; Meyerowitz, J.; Kaindl, J.; Hubner, H.; Skiniotis, G.; Kobilka, B.K. Structure-based Evolution of G protein-biased mu-opioid Receptor Agonists. *Angew. Chem. Int. Ed. Engl.* **2022**, *61*, e202200269.
69. Mafi, A.; Kim, S.K.; Goddard, W.A., 3rd. The atomistic level structure for the activated human kappa-opioid receptor bound to the full Gi protein and the MP1104 agonist. *Proc. Natl. Acad. Sci. USA* **2020**, *117*, 5836–5843. [CrossRef]
70. Manglik, A.; Lin, H.; Aryal, D.K.; McCorvy, J.D.; Dengler, D.; Corder, G.; Levit, A.; Kling, R.C.; Bernat, V.; Hubner, H.; et al. Structure-based discovery of opioid analgesics with reduced side effects. *Nature* **2016**, *537*, 185–190. [CrossRef]
71. Lyu, J.; Wang, S.; Balius, T.E.; Singh, I.; Levit, A.; Moroz, Y.S.; O'Meara, M.J.; Che, T.; Algaa, E.; Tolmachova, K.; et al. Ultra-large library docking for discovering new chemotypes. *Nature* **2019**, *566*, 224–229. [CrossRef]
72. Stein, R.M.; Kang, H.J.; McCorvy, J.D.; Glatfelter, G.C.; Jones, A.J.; Che, T.; Slocum, S.; Huang, X.P.; Savych, O.; Moroz, Y.S.; et al. Virtual discovery of melatonin receptor ligands to modulate circadian rhythms. *Nature* **2020**, *579*, 609–614. [CrossRef]
73. Irwin, J.J.; Shoichet, B.K. ZINC–a free database of commercially available compounds for virtual screening. *J. Chem Inf Model.* **2005**, *45*, 177–182. [CrossRef] [PubMed]
74. Sterling, T.; Irwin, J.J. ZINC 15–Ligand Discovery for Everyone. *J. Chem. Inf. Model.* **2015**, *55*, 2324–2337. [CrossRef] [PubMed]
75. Irwin, J.J.; Tang, K.G.; Young, J.; Dandarchuluun, C.; Wong, B.R.; Khurelbaatar, M.; Moroz, Y.S.; Mayfield, J.; Sayle, R.A. ZINC20-A Free Ultralarge-Scale Chemical Database for Ligand Discovery. *J. Chem. Inf. Model.* **2020**, *60*, 6065–6073. [CrossRef]
76. Sadybekov, A.A.; Sadybekov, A.V.; Liu, Y.; Iliopoulos-Tsoutsouvas, C.; Huang, X.P.; Pickett, J.; Houser, B.; Patel, N.; Tran, N.K.; Tong, F.; et al. Synthon-based ligand discovery in virtual libraries of over 11 billion compounds. *Nature* **2022**, *601*, 452–459. [CrossRef] [PubMed]
77. Seyedabadi, M.; Gharghabi, M.; Gurevich, E.V.; Gurevich, V.V. Structural basis of GPCR coupling to distinct signal transducers: Implications for biased signaling. *Trends Biochem. Sci.* **2022**, *47*, 570–581. [CrossRef] [PubMed]
78. Huang, W.; Manglik, A.; Venkatakrishnan, A.J.; Laeremans, T.; Feinberg, E.N.; Sanborn, A.L.; Kato, H.E.; Livingston, K.E.; Thorsen, T.S.; Kling, R.C.; et al. Structural insights into micro-opioid receptor activation. *Nature* **2015**, *524*, 315–321. [CrossRef]
79. Qu, Q.; Huang, W.; Aydin, D.; Paggi, J.M.; Seven, A.B.; Wang, H.; Chakraborty, S.; Che, T.; DiBerto, J.F.; Robertson, M.J.; et al. Structural insights into distinct signaling profiles of the μOR activated by diverse agonists. *bioRxiv* **2021**. [CrossRef]
80. Uprety, R.; Che, T.; Zaidi, S.A.; Grinnell, S.G.; Varga, B.R.; Faouzi, A.; Slocum, S.T.; Allaoa, A.; Varadi, A.; Nelson, M.; et al. Controlling opioid receptor functional selectivity by targeting distinct subpockets of the orthosteric site. *Elife* **2021**, *10*, e56519. [CrossRef]
81. de Waal, P.W.; Shi, J.; You, E.; Wang, X.; Melcher, K.; Jiang, Y.; Xu, H.E.; Dickson, B.M. Molecular mechanisms of fentanyl mediated beta-arrestin biased signaling. *PLoS Comput. Biol.* **2020**, *16*, e1007394. [CrossRef]
82. Pandy-Szekeres, G.; Esguerra, M.; Hauser, A.S.; Caroli, J.; Munk, C.; Pilger, S.; Keseru, G.M.; Kooistra, A.J.; Gloriam, D.E. The G protein database, GproteinDb. *Nucleic Acids Res.* **2022**, *50*, D518–D525. [CrossRef]
83. Minnich, A.J.; McLoughlin, K.; Tse, M.; Deng, J.; Weber, A.; Murad, N.; Madej, B.D.; Ramsundar, B.; Rush, T.; Calad-Thomson, S.; et al. AMPL: A Data-Driven Modeling Pipeline for Drug Discovery. *J. Chem. Inf. Model.* **2020**, *60*, 1955–1968. [CrossRef] [PubMed]

84. Jumper, J.; Evans, R.; Pritzel, A.; Green, T.; Figurnov, M.; Ronneberger, O.; Tunyasuvunakool, K.; Bates, R.; Zidek, A.; Potapenko, A.; et al. Highly accurate protein structure prediction with AlphaFold. *Nature* **2021**, *596*, 583–589. [CrossRef] [PubMed]
85. Callaway, E. What's next for AlphaFold and the AI protein-folding revolution. *Nature* **2022**, *604*, 234–238. [CrossRef] [PubMed]
86. Unke, O.T.; Chmiela, S.; Sauceda, H.E.; Gastegger, M.; Poltavsky, I.; Schutt, K.T.; Tkatchenko, A.; Muller, K.R. Machine Learning Force Fields. *Chem Rev.* **2021**, *121*, 10142–10186. [CrossRef]
87. Doerr, S.; Majewski, M.; Perez, A.; Kramer, A.; Clementi, C.; Noe, F.; Giorgino, T.; De Fabritiis, G. TorchMD: A Deep Learning Framework for Molecular Simulations. *J. Chem. Theory Comput.* **2021**, *17*, 2355–2363. [CrossRef]
88. Yang, Y.; Jimenez-Negron, O.A.; Kitchin, J.R. Machine-learning accelerated geometry optimization in molecular simulation. *J. Chem. Phys.* **2021**, *154*, 234704. [CrossRef]
89. Fonseca, G.; Poltavsky, I.; Vassilev-Galindo, V.; Tkatchenko, A. Improving molecular force fields across configurational space by combining supervised and unsupervised machine learning. *J. Chem. Phys.* **2021**, *154*, 124102. [CrossRef]
90. Guedes, I.A.; Pereira, F.S.S.; Dardenne, L.E. Empirical Scoring Functions for Structure-Based Virtual Screening: Applications, Critical Aspects, and Challenges. *Front. Pharmacol.* **2018**, *9*, 1089. [CrossRef]
91. Jiménez-Luna, J.; Grisoni, F.; Schneider, G. Drug discovery with explainable artificial intelligence. *Nat. Mach. Intell.* **2020**, *2*, 573–584. [CrossRef]

pharmaceuticals

MDPI

Article

Computational Investigations of Traditional Chinese Medicinal Compounds against the Omicron Variant of SARS-CoV-2 to Rescue the Host Immune System

Ziad Tareq Naman [1], Salim Kadhim [2], Zahraa J. K. Al-Isawi [3], Christopher J. Butch [4,5,*] and Ziyad Tariq Muhseen [4,6,*]

1 Department of Medical Laboratory Techniques, Al-Ma'Moon University College, Aladhamia, Baghdad 72029, Iraq; msczaid86@gmail.com
2 College of Pharmacy, University of Alkafeel, Najaf 61001, Iraq; sfk8@leicester.ac.uk
3 Department of Pharmacology and Toxicology, College of Pharmacy, University of Kufa, Najaf 61001, Iraq; zahraaj.kadhim@uokufa.edu.iq
4 Department of Biomedical Engineering, College of Engineering and Applied Sciences, Nanjing University, Nanjing 210093, China
5 State Key Laboratory of Analytical Chemistry for Life Science, Jiangsu Key Laboratory of Artificial Functional Materials, Nanjing University, Nanjing 210093, China
6 Department of Pharmacy, Al-Mustaqbal University College, Hillah, Babylon 51001, Iraq
* Correspondence: chrisbutch@gmail.com (C.J.B.); ziyad.tariq82@gmail.com (Z.T.M.)

Citation: Naman, Z.T.; Kadhim, S.; Al-Isawi, Z.J.K.; Butch, C.J.; Muhseen, Z.T. Computational Investigations of Traditional Chinese Medicinal Compounds against the Omicron Variant of SARS-CoV-2 to Rescue the Host Immune System. *Pharmaceuticals* **2022**, *15*, 741. https://doi.org/10.3390/ph15060741

Academic Editor: Osvaldo Andrade Santos-Filho

Received: 4 May 2022
Accepted: 31 May 2022
Published: 13 June 2022

Abstract: Macrodomain-I of the NSP3 (non-structural protein 3) is responsible for immune response hijacking in the SARS-CoV-2 infection known as COVID-19. In the omicron variant (B.1.1.529), this domain harbors a new mutation, V1069I, which may increase the binding of ADPr and consequently the infection severity. This macrodomain-I, due to its significant role in infection, is deemed to be an important drug target. Hence, using structural bioinformatics and molecular simulation approaches, we performed a virtual screening of the traditional Chinese medicines (TCM) database for potential antiviral drugs. The screening of 57,000 compounds yielded the 10 best compounds with docking scores better than the control ADPr. Among the top ten, the best three hits—TCM42798, with a docking score of −13.70 kcal/mol, TCM47007 of −13.25 kcal/mol, and TCM30675 of −12.49 kcal/mol—were chosen as the best hits. Structural dynamic features were explored including stability, compactness, flexibility, and hydrogen bonding, further demonstrating the anti-viral potential of these hits. Using the MM/GBSA approach, the total binding free energy for each complex was reported to be −69.78 kcal/mol, −50.11 kcal/mol, and −47.64 kcal/mol, respectively, which consequently reflect the stronger binding and inhibitory potential of these compounds. These agents might suppress NSP3 directly, allowing the host immune system to recuperate. The current study lays the groundwork for the development of new drugs to combat SARS-CoV-2 and its variants.

Keywords: SARS-CoV-2; COVID-19; NSP3; TCM; MD simulations

1. Introduction

Coronavirus disease-2019 (COVID-19) is defined as a disease caused by a novel coronavirus called severe acute respiratory syndrome coronavirus 2 (SARS-CoV-2) [1]. SARS CoV-2 rapidly spread from person to person, and serious human disease was in recent times described in the city of Wuhan, Hubei Province, China. Coronavirus causes headache, fever, and respiratory disease, e.g., cough and shortness of breathing. SARS-CoV-2 infects humans through direct binding to host cell entry proteins (spike). The six functional open reading frames (ORFs) are well-arranged in order from 5′ to 3′ replicas (ORF1a/ORF1b), membrane (M), envelope (E), spike (S), and nucleocapsid (N), whereas nonstructural protein include3-chymotrypsin-like protease, papain-like protease, and RNA-dependent RNA polymerase, is encoded by the ORF region [2,3].

A SARS-CoV-2-associated global pandemic, with unceasing chaos, has now reported many variants of the virus [4]. Among the reported variants, many are particularly associated with immune response evasion, higher transmissibility, increased morbidity, and re-infection. Until now, these variants have been deemed either as variants of interest (VOIs) or variants of concern (VOCs) based on the threat they pose to public health. For instance, the alpha variant, also known as B.1.1.7, with 40–80% increased transmission, includes 69–70 del, N501Y, and P681H mutations, while beta, also called B.1.1.351, gamma, delta, and B.1.1.529 variants are classified as VOCs [5,6]. Moreover, a new version of B.1.1.7 supplemented with the E484K mutation was reported to be associated with 39 confirmed patients [7]. Moreover, B.1.351, which was reported in South Africa and harbors K417N, E484K, and N501Y variations, which were reported to increase the transmission and decrease the T cell-triggered immune response against COVID-19 infection, was recorded. In early 2021, P.1 variant was discovered in Brazil with K417T, E484K, and N501Y mutations in the RBD with transmission increased by 38% and mortality by 50% [8]. A molecular modelling study based on protein coupling deciphered the mechanism of higher infection associated with these variants of SARS-CoV-2 [9]. The binding variations were deeply discovered by demonstrating the interaction pattern and dynamic features of the complexes. In October 2020, India detected a more lethal strain of SARS-CoV-2, officially known as B.1.617.2. This variation has L452R, T478K, and P681R in the RBD, resulting in an 87 percent increase in transmissibility, an 85 percent increase in hospitalizations, and a 137 percent rise in death. Later, in India and the United Kingdom, a novel variant known as "Delta plus" was discovered with an additional mutation, K417N [10]. Similarly, a novel variant termed as Mu or B.1.621 was discovered to have spike protein alterations, some of which are shared with other VOCs. R346K, Y144T, Y145S, and insertion at position 146N are among the new mutations in this variant [11]. L452Q and F490S mutations in RBD are found in a unique VOI known as C.37 or its variant, which lowers antibody-mediated neutralization [12]. The B.1.617.1 strain with the L452R mutation in the (RBD) receptor-binding domain, on the other hand, has been attributed to decreased antibody neutralization by altering the corresponding conformational epitopes. Furthermore, the VOI Iota (lineage B.1.526) carries the mutation E484K, which confers resistance to therapeutic monoclonal antibodies and makes it more resistant to neutralization [13].

The most recent omicron strain, formally known as B.1.1.529, was discovered in November 2019 in South Africa and has 30 mutations in the spike protein including A^{67V}, Δ69–70, T^{95I}, G^{142D}, Δ143–145, Δ211, L^{212I}, ins214EPE, G^{339D}, S^{371L}, S^{373P}, S^{375F}, K^{417N}, N^{440K}, G^{446S}, S^{477N}, T^{478K}, E^{484A}, Q^{493R}, G^{496S}, Q^{498R}, N^{501Y}, Y^{505H}, T^{547K}, D^{614G}, H^{655Y}, N^{679K}, P^{681H}, N^{764K}, D^{796Y}, N^{856K}, Q^{954H}, N^{969K}, and L^{981F}, among which 15 mutations lie in the RBD [14]. Other proteins also reported mutations, such as NSP3 (K^{38R}, V^{1069I}, Δ1265, L^{1266I}, A^{1892T}), NSP4 (T^{492I}), NSP5 (P^{132H}), NSP6 (Δ105–107, A^{189V}), and NSP12 (P^{323L}), while I^{42V} was reported in NSP14. Furthermore, sub-lineages, i.e., BA.1/B.1.1.529.1, BA.2/B.1.1.529.2, and BA.3/B.1.1.529.3, were reported by WHO (World Health Organization) as a threat to public health [15]. The variant is a major health concern all around the globe, and the therapeutic effectiveness of existing vaccines against it is yet unknown [16,17]. More research is needed to determine the molecular basis of pathogenicity in the omicron variant. Furthermore, new therapies against the recently emerging SARS-CoV-2 strains would require the use of advanced techniques.

The novel coronavirus-2019 genome encodes four structural proteins (S, M, E, and N), in which the S-protein gives the virus its corona-like shape, which is mainly responsible for the attachment to host cell receptors (ACE2s) or surface proteins, and 16 non-structural proteins (NSP1 to NSP16). The binding of spike protein to ACE2 (Angiotensin-Converting Enzyme 2) of the host initiates the infection in cells. The ACE2 is mainly expressed in the lungs, kidney, and small intestine, leading to serious illness [18]. During infection, the host cell protease cleaves the S-protein at the S1/S2 cleavage site. This priming (cleavage of S-protein) results in the division of protein into the S1 ectodomain at the N-terminal and the S2 membrane-anchored domain at the C-terminal. The S1 subunit recognizes the associated cell surface receptor, while the latter assists viral entry [19]. The SARS-CoV S1 subunit of the spike protein has conserved 14 aa in the RBD, which functions to recognize ACE2 and can infect both humans and bats. Among this conserved 14 aa in SARS-CoV, eight residues are highly conserved in 2019-nCoV, supporting the assumption that ACE2 is also the receptor of this new virus [20]. Among these proteins, the main proteins, PLpro, spike, and RdRp, are deemed to be direct drug and vaccine targets, but other proteins are also essential for drug design [21]. For instance, the Mac-I of the largest protein, NSP3, has also been deemed as an attractive drug target because of its role in disrupting the innate immune reaction and increasing of virulent properties of the virus [22]. NSP3 is comprised of three macrodomains and two adjacent SUD-M-like domains that have been reported to be associated with NSP3 functional modulation. Mac-I has a significant role in viral pathogenesis and increases interferons' responses for viral neutralization [23]. Further reports have also disclosed the hijacking of the host immune response by Mac, which is carried out through interference with the IFN (Interferons) pathway and malfunctioning of STAT1 (signal transducer and activator of transcription 1) [24,25]. This hijacking of the IFN and STAT1 pathways has been reported to be possibly linked with the cytokines storm phenomena [26,27].

More research is needed to cope with this alarming pandemic situation in order to create safe and effective treatments swiftly. In this context, the macrodomain is thought to be the most druggable target for the development of COVID-19 therapy [28,29]. As a result, we used computational molecular screening to investigate the binding affinity of drugs against the macrodomain-I of the omicron (B.1.1.529) variant. The current study employs molecular docking and simulation-based methods [30–32] to identify potential anti-viral compounds from the TCM database against SARS-CoV-2. The findings provide crucial information on the antiviral effectiveness of the evaluated drugs against SARS-CoV-2. The findings will aid in the development and identification of potential medicinal solutions for the treatment of COVID-19.

2. Results and Discussion

2.1. Macrodomain of Omicron (B.1.1.529) and Structural Modelling

The continuously emerging variants of SARS-CoV-2 are a greater threat to public health [33]. These variants are associated with high infection, transmission, and re-infection. Moreover, some of the previous variants such as B.1.1.7, B.1.617, P.1, and A.30 have also been reported to escape the immune response. Recently, B.1.1.529, or the omicron variant, first identified in South Africa with the highest number of mutations ever, has been reported to be associated with higher transmissibility than other variants. All the proteins encoded by the genome of SARS-CoV-2 are responsible for essential roles in virulence and replication in different stages of infection [34–36]. Among these proteins, the largest and multi-domain protein called non-structural protein 3 or NSP3 is an essential factor for efficient translational and replication processes. NSP3 has eight functional domains that also include macrodomains, which play significant roles in viral escaping when attacked by the innate immune response. Among the macrodomains, macrodomain-I (X-domain) in particular also shares high sequence and structural conservation. Mac-I binds ADPr, and the strength of binding is directly associated with the pathogenicity level [37]. For instance, binding strength reduction or the complete loss of ADPr binding has been reported to be related to less or no infection in the IBV model [38]. Any mutation in the structure is associated with functional variations induced by conformation changes in the protein structures. For instance, K38R, V1069I, L1266I, and A1892T, as well as a deletion (Δ1266I) have recently been reported in the NSP3 protein of the omicron variant, as shown in Figure 1A. The Mac-I in the NSP3 starts from 1025–1194, and a single V1096I has been reported in this region, which may increase the binding of ADPr and consequently increase the pathogenesis by hijacking the innate immune response given in Figure 1A. Mac-I is also a potential therapeutic target; therefore, finding small molecule inhibitors for this domain might aid in the restoration of the host immunological innate response. For instance, a carbazole-based drug known as GeA-69 has been previously tested to target the human macrodomain to treat various types of cancers [39]. Similarly, structure-based approaches are being used to find drugs that target viral macrodomains [40]. New powerful therapies are needed to block Mac-I involvement in SARS-CoV-2 pathogenesis. Hence, our research combines structure-based drug discovery with molecular modelling to find new compounds that effectively target the Mac-I and salvage the innate response. The wild-type structure was used to construct a V1069I mutant of the Mac-I from the omicron variant (Figure 1B). The modelled V1069I-Mac-I, as shown in Figure 1C, demonstrated an RMSD (root mean square deviation) difference of 0.132 Å. The minimal RMSD difference demonstrated the accurate folding and distribution of secondary structural elements.

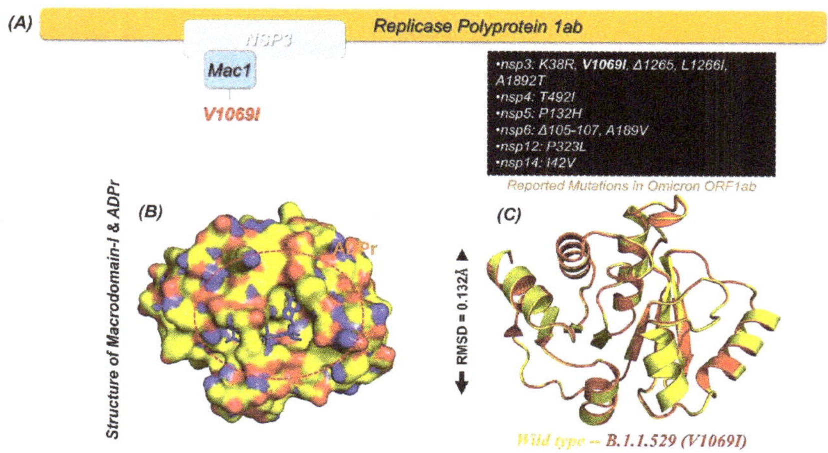

Figure 1. (**A**) NSP3 and reported mutations in the omicron variant. (**B**) Surface representation of Mac-I in complex with ADPr. (**C**) Superimposed wild type a V1069I mutation in Mac-I.

2.2. *Virtual Screening and Re-Docking of TCM*

Using EasyVS, an online web tool, the entire TCM database was screened against the Mac-I of the omicron variant. Prior to screening, the RO5 filter was applied, which reported 20,124 drugs that violated Lipinski's rule of five. Among the total of 57,000 compounds, 36,876 compounds were screened against the binding site of ADPr. Among these, 14,255 compounds reported a docking score less than −4.0 kcal/mol, and 16,453 compounds reported a docking score less than −8.0 kcal/mol. Among the remaining compounds, 5221 compounds reported a docking score of less than −9.0 kcal/mol. Among the remaining 947 compounds, only 356 were reported to have docking scores greater than −9.5 kcal/mol. Compounds with docking scores greater than −9.50 kcal/mol were considered as the threshold, because for ADPr the docking score was previously reported to be −9.46 kcal/mol. The top scoring 50 compounds were selected for re-docking using AutoDock Vina. Among these 50 compounds, 10 compounds reported the best docking score and are given in Table 1. Among the top 10 compounds, TCM42798 had a docking score of −13.70 kcal/mol, TCM47007 of −13.25 kcal/mol, TCM30675 of −12.49 kcal/mol, TCM27763 of −11.93 kcal/mol, TCM33425 of −11.72 kcal/mol, TCM28788 of −11.46 kcal/mol, TCM42159 of −11.45 kcal/mol, TCM47184 of −11.36 kcal/mol, TCM31603 of −11.04 kcal/mol, and TCM31784 of −11.02 kcal/mol. Among the top 10 compounds reported to have higher docking scores than ADPr, only the top three were selected for further analysis, such as interactions, simulation, and post-simulation analysis. In addition to the top three compounds, TCM27763 and apigenin-bioside have been previously reported to have anti-adenovirus activity, which confirms the anti-viral activity of these compounds [41]. It was reported that apigenin reduces adenovirus replication and associated cellular toxicity. For instance, TCM28788 and TCM42159 have been reported to have anti-dengue viral properties, which demonstrate the anti-viral potential of these molecules [42]. The anti-herpes simplex virus type 2 infection activity of tibeticanol and the other compounds are well documented, and it has been reported that these compounds halt viral replication [43].

Table 1. List of top 11 scoring compounds with their TCM IDs, compounds names, 3D structures, and docking scores.

TCM Database ID	Compound Names	2D Structures	Docking Scores
TCM42798	Mucic_acid_1-methyl_ester_2-O-gallate	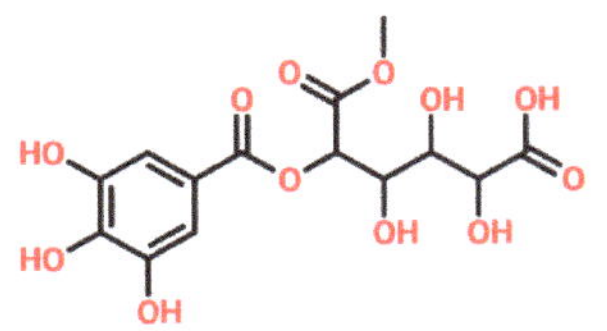	−13.70
TCM47007	(2S)-5,7,2′,5′-Tetrahydroxyflavanone_7-O--D-glucuronopyranoside	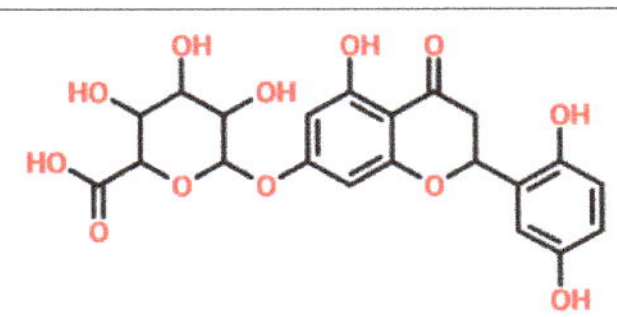	−13.25
TCM30675	(5S,6S,7S,8R)-5,6,7,8-Tetrahydroxy-2-[2-(3-hydroxy-4-methoxyphenyl)ethyl]-5,6,7,8-tetrahydro-4H-chromen-4-one	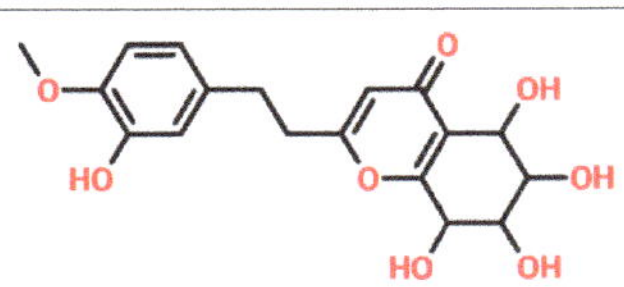	−12.49
TCM27763	30389	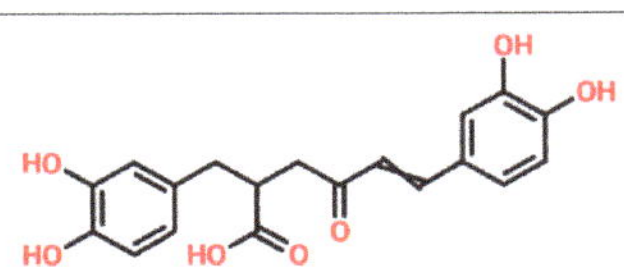	−11.93
TCM33425	Apigenin-bioside	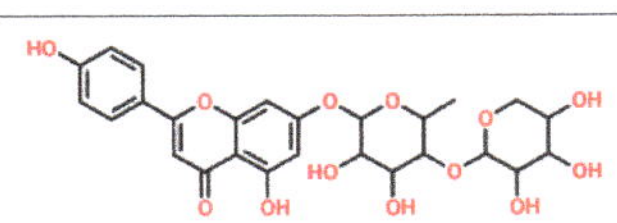	−11.72
TCM28788	31943	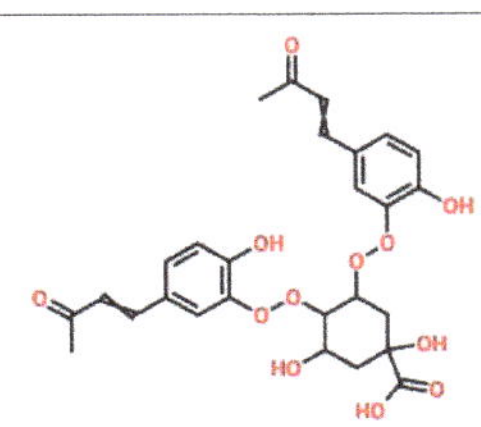	−11.46
TCM42159	(-)-5′-Methoxyisolariciresinol-2-O-D-xylopyranoside_(D2)	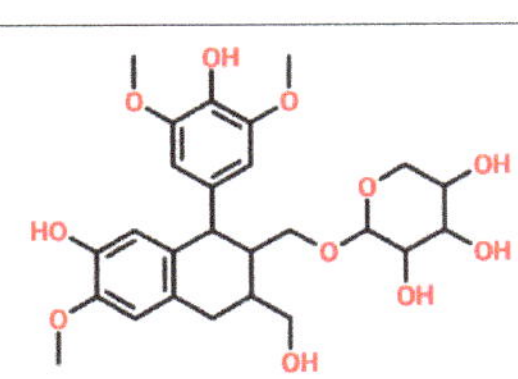	−11.45

Table 1. *Cont.*

TCM Database ID	Compound Names	2D Structures	Docking Scores
TCM47184	Tibeticanol	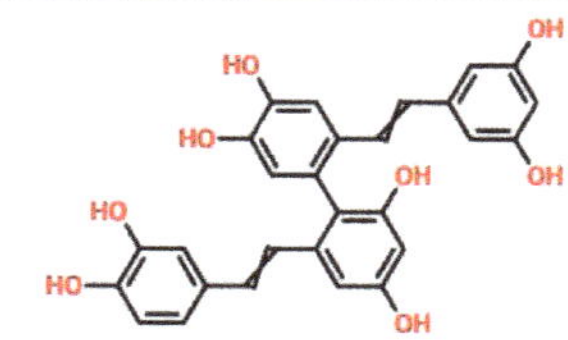	−11.36
TCM31603	36132	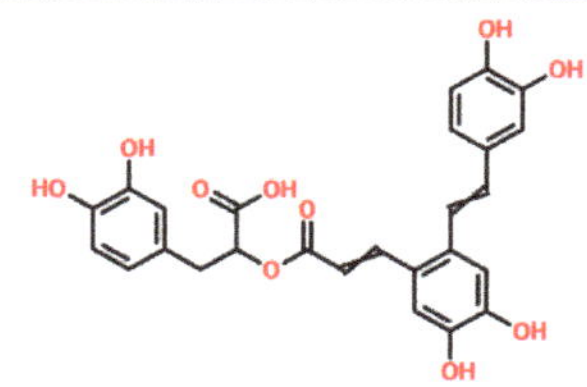	−11.04
TCM31784	36381	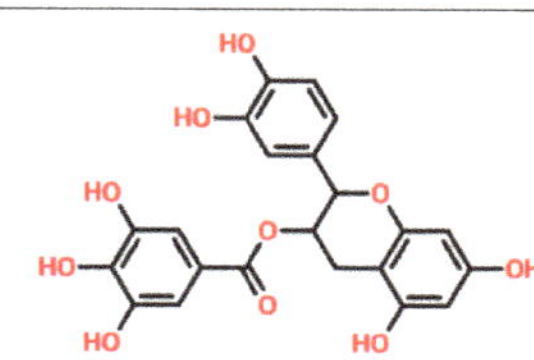	−11.02

TCM42798, or *mucic acid 1-methyl ester 2-O-gallate*, was reported to have the best docking score of −13.70 kcal/mol. Mucic acid 1-methyl ester 2-O-gallate established a total of nine hydrogen bonds with Ala1060, Asn1062, Gly1068, Val1071, Ala1072, Leu1148, Ala1176, and Phe1178. For instance, these residues were previously reported to have an important role in the binding of ADPr. Comparatively, the docking score for ADPr has been reported to be −9.46 kcal/mol [22]. This shows the strongest binding of TCM42798 and consequently produces an inhibitory effect on Mac-I. The binding pattern of TCM42798 is given in Figure 2.

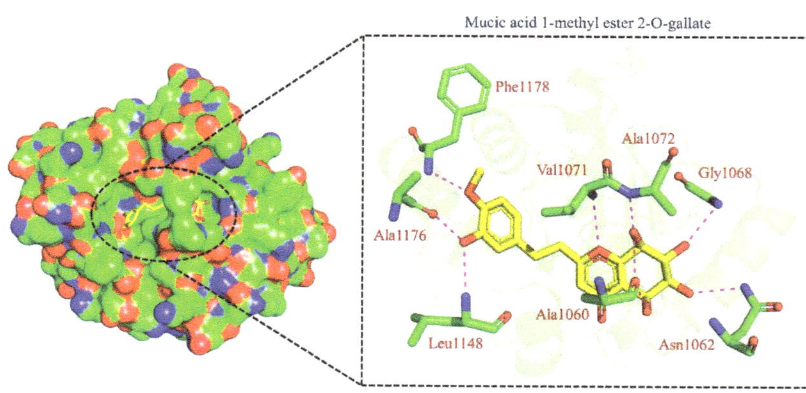

Figure 2. Binding of TCM42798 in the cavity of Mac-I. The right surface representation shows the binding mode of *mucic acid 1-methyl ester 2-O-gallate* (yellow sticks) inside the binding cavity. The right panel represent the 3D interaction pattern, where the TCM42798 is shown as yellow sticks, while the interacting residues are given in green sticks. The interactions (hydrogen bonds) are shown in pink color.

On the other hand, TCM47007, or *(2S)-5,7,2′,5′-Tetrahydroxyflavanone 7-O–D-glucuronopyranoside*, also demonstrated a good interaction profile by predicting the docking score of −13.25 kcal/mol. Unlike TCM42798, this complex reported only seven hydrogen bonds with the key residues required for interaction with ADPr. As shown in Figure 3, Ala1043, Ala1060, Gly1068, Val1071, Ala1072, and Ala1176 are involved in hydrogen bonding interactions. This shows the strongest binding of TCM47007 and consequently produces an inhibitory effect on Mac-I. Moreover, the interaction pattern for TCM30675, or *(5S,6S,7S,8R)-5,6,7,8-Tetrahydroxy-2-[2-(3-hydroxy-4-methoxyphenyl)ethyl]-5,6,7,8-tetrahydro-4H-chromen-4-1*, was also analyzed to demonstrate the binding mode of TCM30675. Residues such as Ala1060, Val1176, Phe1178, and Asp1179 are involved in direct interactions with the Mac-I. This shows the strongest binding of TCM30675 and consequently produces an inhibitory effect on Mac-I. The binding pattern of TCM42798 is given in Figure 4.

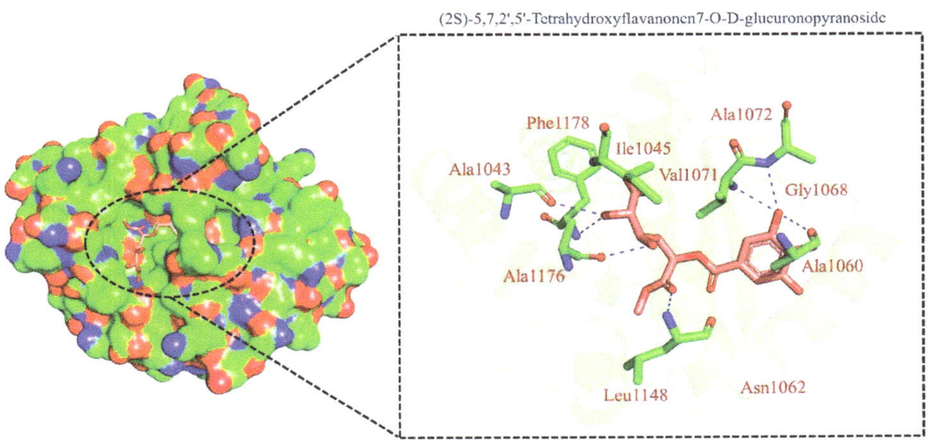

Figure 3. Binding of TCM47007 in the cavity of Mac-I. The right surface representation shows the binding mode of TCM47007 or *(2S)-5,7,2′,5′-Tetrahydroxyflavanone 7-O–D-glucuronopyranoside* (orange sticks) inside the binding cavity. The right panel represents the 3D interaction pattern, where the TCM47007 or *(2S)-5,7,2′,5′-Tetrahydroxyflavanone 7-O–D-glucuronopyranoside* is shown as orange sticks, while the interacting residues are given in green sticks. The interactions (hydrogen bonds) are shown in blue color.

2.3. Dynamic Stability Analysis of the Top Compounds

Analysis of the drug-bound protein complexes to decipher the structural stability is a key process in determining the inhibitory potential of the interacting compound. To foresee the dynamic stability of each top-scoring compound, we calculated the root mean square deviation (RMSD) for all of the simulation trajectories. As given in Figure 5A–C, all the complexes attained equilibrium at the earlier simulation and reached stability at 1.0 Å. In the case of *mucic acid 1-methyl ester 2-O-gallate*, the complex demonstrated overall stable dynamics with no significant deviation, except at the start of the simulation (1–10 ns) when the structure reported minor acceptable deviation and then reached the equilibrium point with a uniform RMSD graph. The average RMSD reported for the *mucic acid 1-methyl ester 2-O-gallate* complex was reported to be 1.0 Å. The RMSD for *mucic acid 1-methyl ester 2-O-gallate* is given in Figure 5A. The RMSD for TCM47007 or *(2S)-5,7,2′,5′-Tetrahydroxyflavanone 7-O–D-glucuronopyranoside* reported comparatively small unstable dynamics until 15 ns, but then RMSD stabilized and attained equilibrium. As given in Figure 5B, after 15 ns the structure attained stability and demonstrated an average RMSD of 1.1 Å. Furthermore, the RMSD of TCM30675 or *(5S,6S,7S,8R)-5,6,7,8-Tetrahydroxy-2-[2-(3-hydroxy-4-methoxyphenyl)ethyl]-5,6,7,8-tetrahydro-4H-chromen-4-1* demonstrated more similar behavior to the *mucic acid 1-methyl ester 2-O-gallate* complex. The RMSD initially increased until 10 ns and then attained equilibrium. The complex reported no significant deviation except a small deviation between 10 and 20 ns, and then it stabilized again. An average RMSD of 1.2 Å was reported for TCM30675 or *(5S,6S,7S,8R)-5,6,7,8-Tetrahydroxy-2-[2-(3-hydroxy-4-methoxyphenyl)ethyl]-5,6,7,8-tetrahydro-4H-chromen-4-1*, as given in Figure 5C. Consequently, this shows the stronger binding and inhibitory potential of these compounds to rescue the host immune response against the COVID-19 infection.

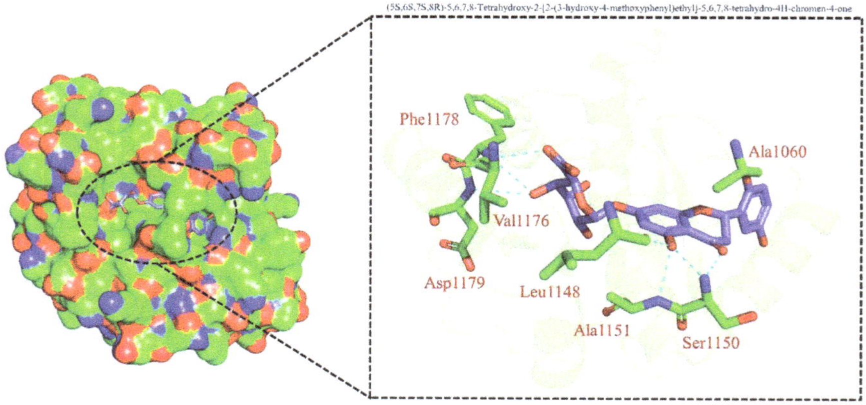

Figure 4. Binding of TCM30675 or *(5S,6S,7S,8R)-5,6,7,8-Tetrahydroxy-2-[2-(3-hydroxy-4-methoxyphenyl)ethyl]-5,6,7,8-tetrahydro-4H-chromen-4-1* in the cavity of Mac-I. The right surface representation shows the binding mode of TCM30675 or *(5S,6S,7S,8R)-5,6,7,8-Tetrahydroxy-2-[2-(3-hydroxy-4-methoxyphenyl)ethyl]-5,6,7,8-tetrahydro-4H-chromen-4-1* (blue sticks) inside the binding cavity. The right panel represent the 3D interaction pattern, where the TCM30675 or *(5S,6S,7S,8R)-5,6,7,8-Tetrahydroxy-2-[2-(3-hydroxy-4-methoxyphenyl)ethyl]-5,6,7,8-tetrahydro-4H-chromen-4-1* is shown as orange sticks, while the interacting residues are given in green sticks. The interactions (hydrogen bonds) are shown in blue color.

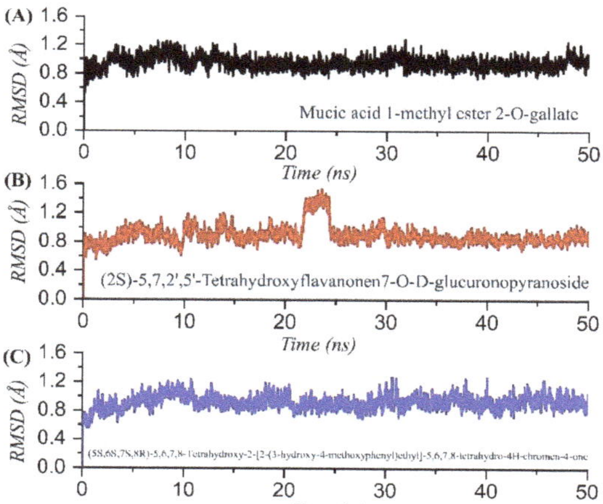

Figure 5. Dynamic stability analysis of the TCM42798, TCM47007, and TCM30675 complexes. (**A**) The RMSD graph for mucic acid 1-methyl ester 2-O-gallate. (**B**) The RMSD graph for TCM47007 or (2S)-5,7,2′,5′-Tetrahydroxyflavanone 7-O–D-glucuronopyranoside. (**C**) The RMSD graph for TCM30675 or (5S,6S,7S,8R)-5,6,7,8-Tetrahydroxy-2-[2-(3-hydroxy-4-methoxyphenyl)ethyl]-5,6,7,8-tetrahydro-4H-chromen-4-1 complex.

2.4. Structural Compactness Analysis

Analysis of structural compactness in a dynamic environment is essential to understand the binding and unbinding events that happened during the simulation. These events demonstrated significant information regarding the binding stability and could be used to select the best compounds for the inhibition potential determination in the experimental setup. Thus, to determine the structural compactness, we calculated radius of gyration (Rg) over the simulation time as a function of time for each complex. As given in Figure 6A–C, all the complexes followed a similar pattern as RMSD. The TCM42798 complex demonstrated a uniform pattern of Rg with no increase or decrease over the simulation time. The structure reported no significant deviation, and the average Rg was reported to be 14.90 Å. The Rg for TCM42798 is shown in Figure 6A. On the other hand, TCM47007 demonstrated a small deviation between 23 and 28 ns and then reported a stable straight graph, which showed the stable binding steered by different kinds of bonds between TCM47007 and Mac-I. The TCM47007-Mac-I complex reported an average Rg of 14.96 Å. The Rg for TCM47007 is shown in Figure 6B. Furthermore, TCM30675 also reported a similar pattern of Rg as RMSD with no major significant deviation. A straight uniform Rg graph can be seen in Figure 6C, where a small fluctuation between 20 and 22 ns can be observed, while the Rg then stabilized and no significant deviation was reported. An average Rg of 15.90 Å was also reported for TCM30675. The Rg for TCM30675 is shown in Figure 6C.

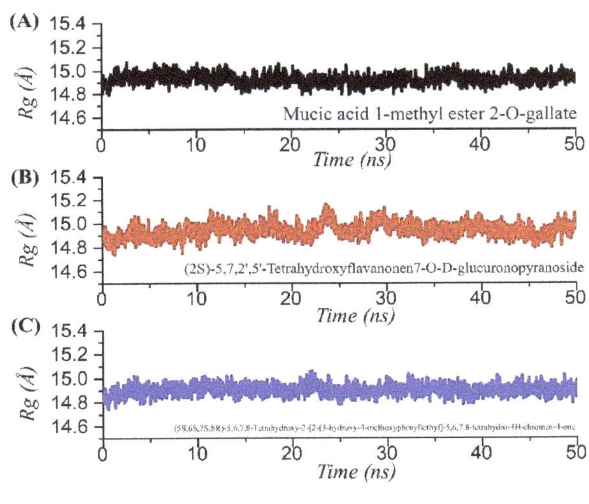

Figure 6. Structural compactness analysis in a dynamic environment of the TCM42798, TCM47007, and TCM30675 complexes calculated as Rg. (**A**) The Rg graph for mucic acid 1-methyl ester 2-O-gallate. (**B**) The Rg graph for TCM47007 or (2S)-5,7,2′,5′-Tetrahydroxyflavanone 7-O–D-glucuronopyranoside. (**C**) The Rg graph for TCM30675 or (5S,6S,7S,8R)-5,6,7,8-Tetrahydroxy-2-[2-(3-hydroxy-4-methoxyphenyl)ethyl]-5,6,7,8-tetrahydro-4H-chromen-4-1 complex.

2.5. Residues Flexibility Profiling

Residue flexibility is strongly correlated with the functional relevance of a protein, as it confers strength to the binding between the interacting molecules. Assessment of residue flexibility for the key residues demonstrates the impact of the small molecule binding. Thus, to determine how the residue flexibility is affected by the binding of these drugs, we calculated the root mean square fluctuation (RMSF) for each complex. As given in Figure 7, all the complexes demonstrated a similar pattern of residue flexibility. All the residues in each complex displayed minimal fluctuation, which showed the stronger binding of these compounds. The regions between 40 and 50, 90 and 100, and 120 and 140 demonstrated comparatively higher fluctuations due to the loop distribution.

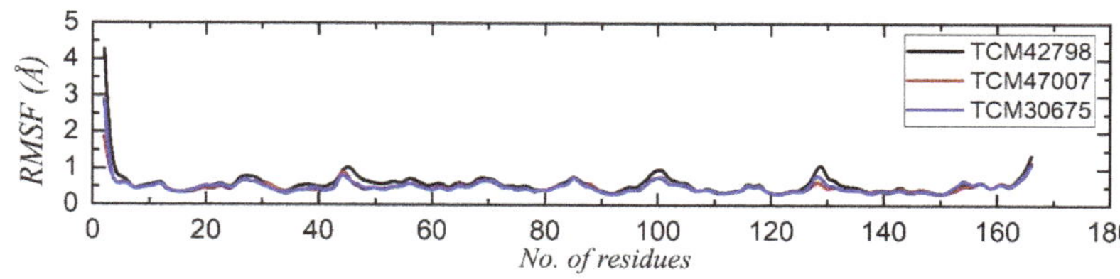

Figure 7. Residual flexibility analysis of the TCM42798, TCM47007, and TCM30675 complexes.

2.6. Hydrogen Bonding Analysis

Hydrogen bonds confer strength to the binding of small molecules. The binding of small molecules is steered by hydrogen and many other bonds, which consequently show the inhibitory features. To determine the binding strength, we calculated the total number of hydrogen bonds and the population, and the simulation trajectories were analyzed. In TCM42798 or mucic acid 1-methyl ester 2-O-gallate, the average number of hydrogen bonds was reported to be 82, while in the case of TCM47007 or (2S)-5,7,2′,5′-Tetrahydroxyflavanone 7-O–D-glucuronopyranoside, the average number of hydrogen bonds was also reported to be 79, while TCM30675 or the (5S,6S,7S,8R)-5,6,7,8-Tetrahydroxy-2-[2-(3-hydroxy-4-methoxyphenyl)ethyl]-5,6,7,8-tetrahydro-4H-chromen-4-1 complex reported 78 average hydrogen bonds. The total number of hydrogen bonds in each complex is shown in Figure 8A–C. Moreover, the hydrogen bonding population for the key interacting residues was estimated and revealed in each complex, namely Ala1060 (63%, 74%, 58%), Asn1062 (66%, 53%, 61%), Gly1068 (51%, 43%, 34%) Val1071 (32%, 24%, 23%), Ala1072 (4%, 17%, 13%), Leu1148 (1%, 6%, 12%), Ala1176 (0%, 0%, 7%), and Phe1178 (0.36%, 2%, 11%) in TCM42798, TCM47007, and TCM30675 complexes, respectively. Together these results show that these compounds bind more strongly to the Mac-I and thus produce inhibitory properties that could help to rescue the host immune response against COVID-19 infection.

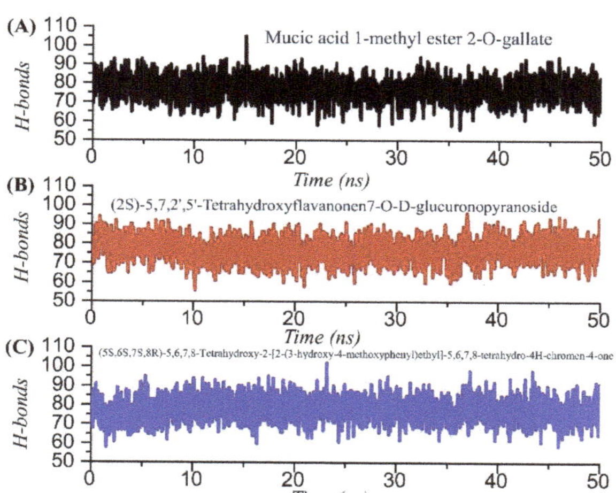

Figure 8. Hydrogen bonding analysis of the TCM42798, TCM47007, and TCM30675 complexes. (**A**) The H-bonds graph for mucic acid 1-methyl ester 2-O-gallate. (**B**) The H-bonds graph for TCM47007 or (2S)-5,7,2′,5′-Tetrahydroxyflavanone 7-O–D-glucuronopyranoside. (**C**) The H-bonds graph for TCM30675 or (5S,6S,7S,8R)-5,6,7,8-Tetrahydroxy-2-[2-(3-hydroxy-4-methoxyphenyl)ethyl]-5,6,7,8-tetrahydro-4H-chromen-4-1 complex.

2.7. Binding Free Energy Estimation

The binding strength of small molecules using the binding free energy method, MM-GBSA, is a widely used method for re-demonstrating docking stability and correct binding. The above-mentioned MM-GBSA technique is more computationally economical than the more expensive alchemical free energy method. When compared to rational scoring functions, it is one of the most accurate techniques. Keeping in mind the implementation of this approach, we also employed the same method to compute the binding free energy for TCM42798, TCM47007, and TCM30675 complexes. The vdWs for these complexes were reported to be −84.26 kcal/mol, −59.79 kcal/mol, and −53.24 kcal/mol, respectively, while the electrostatic energies were reported to be −12.22 kcal/mol, −13.22 kcal/mol, and −15.66 kcal/mol, respectively. Moreover, the ESURF values were reported to be 17.45 kcal/mol, 14.68 kcal/mol, and 12.25 kcal/mol, respectively. The total binding free energy for these complexes was reported to be −69.78 kcal/mol, −50.11 kcal/mol, and −47.64 kcal/mol, respectively, which consequently reflected the stronger binding and inhibitory potential of these compounds. The MM/GBSA results are given in Table 2.

Table 2. Binding free energy calculated as MM/GBSA. All the values are given in kcal/mol.

MM/GBSA	TCM42798	TCM47007	TCM30675
vdW	−84.26	−59.79	−53.24
electrostatic	−12.22	−13.22	−15.66
ESURF	17.45	14.68	12.25
EGB	9.25	8.22	9.01
ΔG Bind	−69.78	−50.11	−47.64

3. Material and Methods

3.1. Modelling of the Macrodomain-I (Mac-I) of B.1.1.529 Variant

The experimentally reported structure in the protein database was collected through accession number 6W02 to model the V1069I mutations reported in the Mac-I of NSP3 of the omicron variant [44]. For this purpose, the amino acid sequence using P0DTD1 accession number was obtained from UniProt, European union [45]. For modelling of the variant structure, AlphaFold 2.0 Seoul National University, Seoul, South Korea, was used, which is currently the best and most accurate approach for 3D structural modelling [46].

3.2. Virtual Screening of Traditional Chinese Medicine Database

The Traditional Chinese Medicine Database (TCM) currently holds 57,000 entries of different medicinal compounds isolated from Chinese herbs. It is considered as an important medicinal repository for discovering novel treatments that are safe and effective. Thus, we screened the complete TCM database against Mac-I of the B.1.1.529 variant. For screening, we used the EasyVS (http://biosig.unimelb.edu.au/easyvs, accessed on 10 April 2022) webserver [47]. Custom parameters were used and defined, such as the active site, and the RO5 filter was enabled for the filtration and removal of molecules that violated Lipinski's rules. Furthermore, for the top 100 hits, a second round of screening was performed using the Auto Dock Vina algorithm [48]. Finally, the top-selected compounds were used for the Induced-Fit docking (IFD) approach to remove the false-positive results. The top hits were identified based on the docking score for ADPr, taken as a control, as previously reported [22].

3.3. Molecular Dynamics Simulation (MDS)

Characterization of dynamic features to accurately portray the inhibitory potential of the top hits was studied by performing molecular dynamics simulation [49]. The top three hits were investigated by using AMBER20 simulation software by adding an optimal point charge water model and sodium ions for neutralizing the effect of any charge. Protein and drug parameterization was achieved by recruiting FF19SB and GAFF forcefields. Each system after gentle minimization was subjected to heating followed by equilibration. The production runs for 50 ns each were completed. For any long-range electrostatic interactions (10.0 Å cutoff), the PME (particle mesh Ewald algorithm) was used, while covalent bonds were treated with the SHAKE algorithm.

3.4. Trajectories Analysis Using CPPTRAJ and PTRAJ

Evaluation of the simulation trajectories to forecast the dynamic stability, flexibility index, hydrogen bonding, structural compactness, and other parameters was completed by using CPPTRAJ and PTRAJ modules [50]. Root mean square deviation (RMSD) was estimated for stability, root mean square fluctuation (RMSF) to index the flexibility of each residue, radius of gyration (Rg) to foresee the compactness, and hydrogen bonding analysis to estimate the bonding population.

3.5. Estimation of Post-Simulation Binding Energy

The most generally utilized strategy in many related studies is to evaluate the strength of small molecule binding by employing the binding free energy (BFE) approach [51–54]. We also adopted the MMPBSA.py script to compute the binding free energy of the protein–ligand complexes by evaluating 2500 snapshots, keeping in mind the relevance of this strategy in re-ranking the binding conformations. For this purpose, the following equation was used to estimate the BFE:

$$``\Delta Gbind = \Delta Gcomplex - [\Delta Greceptor + \Delta Gligand]"$$

The ΔG_{bind} represents the total binding energy, while $\Delta G_{receptor}$, ΔG_{ligand}, and $\Delta G_{complex}$ represent the binding energy of protein, drug, and complex, respectively. The following equation was used to estimate individual binding energies such as bonded (G_{bond}), electrostatic (G_{ele}), polar (G_{pol}), and non-polar (G_{npol}), which contribute to the total binding free energy.

$$``G = GbondGelectrostatic - Gvan\ der\ Waal - GpolarGnon - polar"$$

4. Conclusions

The present study employs molecular modelling and MD simulation approaches to target the macrodomain-I of the B.1.1.529 variant of SARS-CoV-2. Three novel compounds, namely TCM42798, TCM47007, and TCM30675, were identified as potential inhibitors of Mac-I. These agents may suppress NSP3 directly, allowing the host immune system to recuperate. The current study lays the groundwork for the development of new drugs to combat SARS-CoV-2 and its variants.

Author Contributions: Conceptualization, C.J.B. and Z.T.M.; Data curation, Z.T.N.; S.K. and Z.J.K.A.-I.; Formal analysis, Z.T.N. and Z.T.M.; Funding acquisition, C.J.B.; Investigation, Z.T.N.; Methodology, S.K. and Z.J.K.A.-I.; Project administration, C.J.B. and Z.T.M.; Resources, C.J.B. and Z.T.M.; Software, Z.T.M.; Supervision, C.J.B.; Validation, S.K.; Z.J.K.A.-I. and C.J.B.; Visualization, Z.T.N. and Z.T.M.; Writing—original draft, Z.T.N. and Z.T.M.; Writing—review and editing, S.K.; Z.J.K.A.-I. and C.J.B. All authors have read and agreed to the published version of the manuscript.

Funding: This research work was supported by the Nanjing University startup research funds.

Institutional Review Board Statement: Not applicable.

Informed Consent Statement: Not applicable.

Data Availability Statement: The data presented in this study are available within the article.

Acknowledgments: The authors would like to acknowledge Nanjing University, China, for providing facilities for this research.

Conflicts of Interest: The authors declare no conflict of interest.

References

1. ul Qamar, M.T.; Alqahtani, S.M.; Alamri, M.A.; Chen, L.-L. Structural basis of SARS-CoV-2 3CLpro and anti-COVID-19 drug discovery from medicinal plants. *J. Pharm. Anal.* **2020**, *10*, 313–319. [CrossRef] [PubMed]
2. V'kovski, P.; Kratzel, A.; Steiner, S.; Stalder, H.; Thiel, V.J.N.R.M. Coronavirus biology and replication: Implications for SARS-CoV-2. *Nat. Rev. Microbiol.* **2021**, *19*, 155–170. [CrossRef]
3. Fontanet, A.; Autran, B.; Lina, B.; Kieny, M.P.; Karim, S.S.A.; Sridhar, D.J.T.L. SARS-CoV-2 variants and ending the COVID-19 pandemic. *Lancet* **2021**, *397*, 952–954. [CrossRef]
4. Tao, K.; Tzou, P.L.; Nouhin, J.; Gupta, R.K.; de Oliveira, T.; Kosakovsky Pond, S.L.; Fera, D.; Shafer, R.W. The biological and clinical significance of emerging SARS-CoV-2 variants. *Nat. Rev. Genet.* **2021**, *22*, 757–773. [CrossRef] [PubMed]
5. Duong, D. Alpha, Beta, Delta, Gamma: What's important to know about SARS-CoV-2 variants of concern? *Can. Med. Assoc.* **2021**, *193*, E1059–E1060. [CrossRef]
6. Meng, B.; Kemp, S.A.; Papa, G.; Datir, R.; Ferreira, I.A.; Marelli, S.; Harvey, W.T.; Lytras, S.; Mohamed, A.; Gallo, G. Recurrent emergence of SARS-CoV-2 spike deletion H69/V70 and its role in the Alpha variant B. 1.1. 7. *Cell Rep.* **2021**, *35*, 109292. [CrossRef]
7. Han, P.; Su, C.; Zhang, Y.; Bai, C.; Zheng, A.; Qiao, C.; Wang, Q.; Niu, S.; Chen, Q.; Zhang, Y. Molecular insights into receptor binding of recent emerging SARS-CoV-2 variants. *Nat. Commun.* **2021**, *12*, 6103. [CrossRef]
8. Lauring, A.S.; Malani, P.N. Variants of SARS-CoV-2. *JAMA* **2021**, *326*, 880. [CrossRef]
9. Khan, A.; Waris, H.; Rafique, M.; Suleman, M.; Mohammad, A.; Ali, S.S.; Khan, T.; Waheed, Y.; Liao, C.; Wei, D.Q. The Omicron (B.1.1.529) variant of SARS-CoV-2 binds to the hACE2 receptor more strongly and escapes the antibody response: Insights from structural and simulation data. *Int. J. Biol. Macromol.* **2022**, *200*, 438–448. [CrossRef]
10. Mlcochova, P.; Kemp, S.A.; Dhar, M.S.; Papa, G.; Meng, B.; Ferreira, I.A.; Datir, R.; Collier, D.A.; Albecka, A.; Singh, S. SARS-CoV-2 B. 1.617. 2 Delta variant replication and immune evasion. *Nature* **2021**, *599*, 114–119. [CrossRef]
11. Messali, S.; Bertelli, A.; Campisi, G.; Zani, A.; Ciccozzi, M.; Caruso, A.; Caccuri, F. A cluster of the new SARS-CoV-2 B. 1.621 lineage in Italy and sensitivity of the viral isolate to the BNT162b2 vaccine. *J. Med. Virol.* **2021**, *93*, 6468–6470. [CrossRef]
12. Romero, P.E.; Dávila-Barclay, A.; Salvatierra, G.; González, L.; Cuicapuza, D.; Solís, L.; Marcos-Carbajal, P.; Huancachoque, J.; Maturrano, L.; Tsukayama, P. The emergence of SARS-CoV-2 variant lambda (C. 37) in South America. *Microbiol. Spectr.* **2021**, *9*, e00789-21. [CrossRef] [PubMed]
13. Khan, A.; Khan, M.T.; Saleem, S.; Junaid, M.; Ali, A.; Ali, S.S.; Khan, M.; Wei, D.-Q. Structural Insights into the mechanism of RNA recognition by the N-terminal RNA-binding domain of the SARS-CoV-2 nucleocapsid phosphoprotein. *Comput. Struct. Biotechnol. J.* **2020**, *18*, 2174–2184. [CrossRef]
14. He, X.; Hong, W.; Pan, X.; Lu, G.; Wei, X. SARS-CoV-2 Omicron variant: Characteristics and prevention. *MedComm* **2021**, *2*, 838–845. [CrossRef]
15. Karim, S.S.A.; Karim, Q.A. Omicron SARS-CoV-2 variant: A new chapter in the COVID-19 pandemic. *Lancet* **2021**, *398*, 2126–2128. [CrossRef]
16. Wilhelm, A.; Widera, M.; Grikscheit, K.; Toptan, T.; Schenk, B.; Pallas, C.; Metzler, M.; Kohmer, N.; Hoehl, S.; Helfritz, F.A. Reduced neutralization of SARS-CoV-2 Omicron variant by vaccine sera and monoclonal antibodies. *MedRxiv* **2021**. [CrossRef]
17. Roessler, A.; Riepler, L.; Bante, D.; von Laer, D.; Kimpel, J. SARS-CoV-2 B. 1.1. 529 variant (Omicron) evades neutralization by sera from vaccinated and convalescent individuals. *MedRxiv* **2021**. [CrossRef]
18. Duchene, S.; Featherstone, L.; Haritopoulou-Sinanidou, M.; Rambaut, A.; Lemey, P.; Baele, G. Temporal signal and the phylodynamic threshold of SARS-CoV-2. *Virus Evol.* **2020**, *6*, veaa061. [CrossRef] [PubMed]
19. Wrapp, D.; Wang, N.; Corbett, K.S.; Goldsmith, J.A.; Hsieh, C.L.; Abiona, O.; Graham, B.S.; McLellan, J.S. Cryo-EM structure of the 2019-nCoV spike in the prefusion conformation. *Science* **2020**, *367*, 1260–1263. [CrossRef]
20. Li, W.; Moore, M.J.; Vasilieva, N.; Sui, J.; Wong, S.K.; Berne, M.A.; Somasundaran, M.; Sullivan, J.L.; Luzuriaga, K.; Greenough, T.C. Angiotensin-converting enzyme 2 is a functional receptor for the SARS coronavirus. *Nature* **2003**, *426*, 450–454. [CrossRef]
21. Khan, A.; Ali, S.S.; Khan, M.T.; Saleem, S.; Ali, A.; Suleman, M.; Babar, Z.; Shafiq, A.; Khan, M.; Wei, D.-Q. Combined drug repurposing and virtual screening strategies with molecular dynamics simulation identified potent inhibitors for SARS-CoV-2 main protease (3CLpro). *J. Biomol. Struct. Dyn.* **2020**, *39*, 4659–4670. [CrossRef] [PubMed]
22. Hussain, I.; Pervaiz, N.; Khan, A.; Saleem, S.; Shireen, H.; Wei, D.-Q.; Labrie, V.; Bao, Y.; Abbasi, A.A. Evolutionary and structural analysis of SARS-CoV-2 specific evasion of host immunity. *Genes Immun.* **2020**, *21*, 409–419. [CrossRef] [PubMed]
23. Brosey, C.A.; Houl, J.H.; Katsonis, P.; Balapiti-Modarage, L.P.F.; Bommagani, S.; Arvai, A.; Moiani, D.; Bacolla, A.; Link, T.; Warden, L.S.; et al. Targeting SARS-CoV-2 Nsp3 macrodomain structure with insights from human poly(ADP-ribose) glycohydrolase (PARG) structures with inhibitors. *Prog. Biophys. Mol. Biol.* **2021**, *163*, 171–186. [CrossRef] [PubMed]
24. Lin, M.-H.; Chang, S.-C.; Chiu, Y.-C.; Jiang, B.-C.; Wu, T.-H.; Hsu, C.-H. Structural, biophysical, and biochemical elucidation of the SARS-CoV-2 nonstructural protein 3 macro domain. *ACS Infect. Dis.* **2020**, *6*, 2970–2978. [CrossRef]
25. Srinivasan, S.; Cui, H.; Gao, Z.; Liu, M.; Lu, S.; Mkandawire, W.; Narykov, O.; Sun, M.; Korkin, D. Structural genomics of SARS-CoV-2 indicates evolutionary conserved functional regions of viral proteins. *Viruses* **2020**, *12*, 360. [CrossRef]
26. Hoch, N.C. Host ADP-ribosylation and the SARS-CoV-2 macrodomain. *Biochem. Soc. Trans.* **2021**, *49*, 1711–1721. [CrossRef]
27. Molaei, S.; Dadkhah, M.; Asghariazar, V.; Karami, C.; Safarzadeh, E. The immune response and immune evasion characteristics in SARS-CoV, MERS-CoV, and SARS-CoV-2: Vaccine design strategies. *Int. Immunopharmacol.* **2021**, *92*, 107051. [CrossRef] [PubMed]
28. Li, F. Structure, function, and evolution of coronavirus spike proteins. *Annu. Rev. Virol.* **2016**, *3*, 237–261. [CrossRef]

29. Li, F.; Li, W.; Farzan, M.; Harrison, S.C. Structure of SARS coronavirus spike receptor-binding domain complexed with receptor. *Science* **2005**, *309*, 1864–1868. [CrossRef] [PubMed]
30. Islam, S.; Hosen, M.A.; Ahmad, S.; ul Qamar, M.T.; Dey, S.; Hasan, I.; Fujii, Y.; Ozeki, Y.; Kawsar, S.M. Synthesis, antimicrobial, anticancer activities, PASS prediction, molecular docking, molecular dynamics and pharmacokinetic studies of designed methyl α-D-glucopyranoside esters. *J. Mol. Struct.* **2022**, *1260*, 132761. [CrossRef]
31. Tahir ul Qamar, M.; Mirza, M.U.; Song, J.-M.; Rao, M.J.; Zhu, X.; Chen, L.-L. Probing the structural basis of Citrus phytochrome B using computational modelling and molecular dynamics simulation approaches. *J. Mol. Liq.* **2021**, *340*, 116895. [CrossRef]
32. Ahmad, F.; Albutti, A.; Tariq, M.H.; Din, G.; Tahir ul Qamar, M.; Ahmad, S. Discovery of Potential Antiviral Compounds against Hendra Virus by Targeting Its Receptor-Binding Protein (G) Using Computational Approaches. *Molecules* **2022**, *27*, 554. [CrossRef]
33. Abbas, K.; Khan, T.; Ali, S.; Aftab, S.; Wang, Y.; Qiankun, W.; Khan, M. SARS-CoV-2 new variants: Characteristic features and impact on the efficacy of different vaccines. *Biomed. Pharmacother.* **2021**, *143*, 112176.
34. Magrane, M. UniProt Knowledgebase: A hub of integrated protein data. *Database* **2011**, *2011*, bar009. [CrossRef] [PubMed]
35. Jumper, J.; Evans, R.; Pritzel, A.; Green, T.; Figurnov, M.; Ronneberger, O.; Tunyasuvunakool, K.; Bates, R.; Žídek, A.; Potapenko, A. Highly accurate protein structure prediction with AlphaFold. *Nature* **2021**, *596*, 583–589. [CrossRef]
36. Pires, D.E.V.; Veloso, W.N.P.; Myung, Y.; Rodrigues, C.H.M.; Silk, M.; Rezende, P.M.; Silva, F.; Xavier, J.S.; Velloso, J.P.L.; da Silveira, C.H.; et al. EasyVS: A user-friendly web-based tool for molecule library selection and structure-based virtual screening. *Bioinformatics* **2020**, *36*, 4200–4202. [CrossRef]
37. Trott, O.; Olson, A.J. AutoDock Vina: Improving the speed and accuracy of docking with a new scoring function, efficient optimization, and multithreading. *J. Comput. Chem.* **2010**, *31*, 455–461. [CrossRef]
38. Muneer, I.; Ahmad, S.; Naz, A.; Abbasi, S.W.; Alblihy, A.; Aloliqi, A.A.; Alkhayl, F.F.; Alrumaihi, F.; Ahmad, S.; El Bakri, Y. Discovery of Novel Inhibitors from Medicinal Plants for V-Domain Ig Suppressor of T-Cell Activation (VISTA). *Front. Mol. Biosci.* **2021**, *8*, 716735. [CrossRef]
39. Roe, D.R.; Cheatham, T.E., III. PTRAJ and CPPTRAJ: Software for processing and analysis of molecular dynamics trajectory data. *J. Chem. Theory Comput.* **2013**, *9*, 3084–3095. [CrossRef]
40. ul Qamar, M.T.; Ahmad, S.; Khan, A.; Mirza, M.U.; Ahmad, S.; Abro, A.; Chen, L.-L.; Almatroudi, A.; Wei, D.-Q. Structural probing of HapR to identify potent phytochemicals to control Vibrio cholera through integrated computational approaches. *Comput. Biol. Med.* **2021**, *138*, 104929. [CrossRef]
41. Altharawi, A.; Ahmad, S.; Alamri, M.A.; ul Qamar, M.T. Structural insight into the binding pattern and interaction mechanism of chemotherapeutic agents with Sorcin by docking and molecular dynamic simulation. *Colloids Surf. B Biointerfaces* **2021**, *208*, 112098. [CrossRef] [PubMed]
42. Suleman, M.; ul Qamar, M.T.; Shoaib Saleem, S.A.; Ali, S.S.; Khan, H.; Akbar, F.; Khan, W.; Alblihy, A.; Alrumaihi, F.; Waseem, M. Mutational landscape of Pirin and elucidation of the impact of most detrimental missense variants that accelerate the breast cancer pathways: A computational modelling study. *Front. Mol. Biosci.* **2021**, *8*, 692835. [CrossRef] [PubMed]
43. Arif, R.; Ahmad, S.; Mustafa, G.; Mahrosh, H.S.; Ali, M.; Tahir ul Qamar, M.; Dar, H.R. Molecular Docking and Simulation Studies of Antidiabetic Agents Devised from Hypoglycemic Polypeptide-P of Momordica charantia. *BioMed Res. Int.* **2021**, *2021*, 5561129. [CrossRef]
44. Mehmood, I.; Ijaz, M.; Ahmad, S.; Ahmed, T.; Bari, A.; Abro, A.; Allemailem, K.S.; Almatroudi, A.; Tahir ul Qamar, M. SARS-CoV-2: An update on genomics, risk assessment, potential therapeutics and vaccine development. *Int. J. Environ. Res. Public Health* **2021**, *18*, 1626. [CrossRef] [PubMed]
45. Alamri, M.A.; ul Qamar, M.T.; Mirza, M.U.; Alqahtani, S.M.; Froeyen, M.; Chen, L.-L. Discovery of human coronaviruses pan-papain-like protease inhibitors using computational approaches. *J. Pharm. Anal.* **2020**, *10*, 546–559. [CrossRef]
46. Muhseen, Z.T.; Hameed, A.R.; Al-Hasani, H.M.; ul Qamar, M.T.; Li, G. Promising terpenes as SARS-CoV-2 spike receptor-binding domain (RBD) attachment inhibitors to the human ACE2 receptor: Integrated computational approach. *J. Mol. Liq.* **2020**, *320*, 114493. [CrossRef] [PubMed]
47. Alamri, M.A.; Tahir Ul Qamar, M.; Mirza, M.U.; Bhadane, R.; Alqahtani, S.M.; Muneer, I.; Froeyen, M.; Salo-Ahen, O.M. Pharmacoinformatics and molecular dynamics simulation studies reveal potential covalent and FDA-approved inhibitors of SARS-CoV-2 main protease 3CLpro. *J. Biomol. Struct. Dyn.* **2021**, *39*, 4936–4948. [CrossRef] [PubMed]
48. Han, W.; Li, X.; Fu, X. The macro domain protein family: Structure, functions, and their potential therapeutic implications. *Mutat. Res./Rev. Mutat. Res.* **2011**, *727*, 86–103. [CrossRef] [PubMed]
49. Leung, A.K.; McPherson, R.L.; Griffin, D.E. Macrodomain ADP-ribosylhydrolase and the pathogenesis of infectious diseases. *PLoS Pathog.* **2018**, *14*, e1006864. [CrossRef]
50. Schuller, A.P.; Wu, C.C.-C.; Dever, T.E.; Buskirk, A.R.; Green, R. eIF5A functions globally in translation elongation and termination. *Mol. Cell* **2017**, *66*, 194–205.e5. [CrossRef]
51. Babar, Z.; Khan, M.; Zahra, M.; Anwar, M.; Noor, K.; Hashmi, H.F.; Suleman, M.; Waseem, M.; Shah, A.; Ali, S. Drug similarity and structure-based screening of medicinal compounds to target macrodomain-I from SARS-CoV-2 to rescue the host immune system: A molecular dynamics study. *J. Biomol. Struct. Dyn.* **2020**, *40*, 523–537. [CrossRef] [PubMed]
52. Kanerva, A.; Raki, M.; Ranki, T.; Särkioja, M.; Koponen, J.; Desmond, R.A.; Helin, A.; Stenman, U.H.; Isoniemi, H.; Höckerstedt, K.; et al. Chlorpromazine and apigenin reduce adenovirus replication and decrease replication associated toxicity. *J. Gene Med.* **2007**, *9*, 3–9. [CrossRef] [PubMed]

53. Shimu, M.S.S.; Mahmud, S.; Tallei, T.E.; Sami, S.A.; Adam, A.A.; Acharjee, U.K.; Paul, G.K.; Emran, T.B.; Zaman, S.; Uddin, M.S.; et al. Phytochemical Compound Screening to Identify Novel Small Molecules against Dengue Virus: A Docking and Dynamics Study. *Molecules* **2022**, *27*, 653. [CrossRef] [PubMed]
54. Zhang, C.-J.; Li, W.; Li, H.-Y.; Wang, Y.-L.; Yun, T.; Song, Z.-P.; Song, Y.; Zhao, X.-W. In vivo and in vitro antiviral activity of five Tibetan medicinal plant extracts against herpes simplex virus type 2 infection. *Pharm. Biol.* **2009**, *47*, 598–607. [CrossRef]

pharmaceuticals

Article

In Silico Antiprotozoal Evaluation of 1,4-Naphthoquinone Derivatives against Chagas and Leishmaniasis Diseases Using QSAR, Molecular Docking, and ADME Approaches

Lina S. Prieto Cárdenas [1], Karen A. Arias Soler [1], Diana L. Nossa González [1], Wilson E. Rozo Núñez [1], Agobardo Cárdenas-Chaparro [1], Pablo R. Duchowicz [2] and Jovanny A. Gómez Castaño [1,*]

[1] Grupo Química-Física Molecular y Modelamiento Computacional (QUIMOL), Facultad de Ciencias, Universidad Pedagógica y Tecnológica de Colombia (UPTC), Avenida Central del Norte, Tunja 050030, Colombia; lina.prieto02@uptc.edu.co (L.S.P.C.); karen.arias02@uptc.edu.co (K.A.A.S.); dlissethn@gmail.com (D.L.N.G.); wilson.rozo@uptc.edu.co (W.E.R.N.); agobardo.cardenas01@uptc.edu.co (A.C.-C.)

[2] Instituto de Investigaciones Fisicoquímicas Teóricas y Aplicadas, (CONICET—Universidad Nacional de La Plata), Diagonal 113 y Calle 64, C.C. 16, Sucursal 4, La Plata 1900, Argentina; pabloducho@gmail.com

* Correspondence: jovanny.gomez@uptc.edu.co

Citation: Prieto Cárdenas, L.S.; Arias Soler, K.A.; Nossa González, D.L.; Rozo Núñez, W.E.; Cárdenas-Chaparro, A.; Duchowicz, P.R.; Gómez Castaño, J.A. In Silico Antiprotozoal Evaluation of 1,4-Naphthoquinone Derivatives against Chagas and Leishmaniasis Diseases Using QSAR, Molecular Docking, and ADME Approaches. *Pharmaceuticals* **2022**, *15*, 687. https://doi.org/10.3390/ph15060687

Academic Editor: Osvaldo Andrade Santos-Filho

Received: 30 April 2022
Accepted: 27 May 2022
Published: 31 May 2022

Publisher's Note: MDPI stays neutral with regard to jurisdictional claims in published maps and institutional affiliations.

Abstract: Chagas and leishmaniasis are two neglected diseases considered as public health problems worldwide, for which there is no effective, low-cost, and low-toxicity treatment for the host. Naphthoquinones are ligands with redox properties involved in oxidative biological processes with a wide variety of activities, including antiparasitic. In this work, in silico methods of quantitative structure–activity relationship (QSAR), molecular docking, and calculation of ADME (absorption, distribution, metabolism, and excretion) properties were used to evaluate naphthoquinone derivatives with unknown antiprotozoal activity. QSAR models were developed for predicting antiparasitic activity against *Trypanosoma cruzi*, *Leishmania amazonensis*, and *Leishmania infatum*, as well as the QSAR model for toxicity activity. Most of the evaluated ligands presented high antiparasitic activity. According to the docking results, the family of triazole derivatives presented the best affinity with the different macromolecular targets. The ADME results showed that most of the evaluated compounds present adequate conditions to be administered orally. Naphthoquinone derivatives show good biological activity results, depending on the substituents attached to the quinone ring, and perhaps the potential to be converted into drugs or starting molecules.

Keywords: chagas; leishmaniasis; naphthoquinones; antiprotozoal evaluation; QSAR; molecular docking; ADME

1. Introduction

Chagas and leishmaniasis are two parasitic infectious diseases endemic to Latin America, considered by the World Health Organization (WHO) as neglected tropical diseases, for which there is currently no effective, safe, and economical chemotherapy treatment. For chagas, the WHO estimates that between 7 and 8 million people are infected, with 12,000 deaths and 70 million people at risk of contracting it per year [1,2], while for leishmaniasis, there is an estimated figure of 12 million infected people, 1.6 million new cases each year, and 350 million people at risk of acquiring it [3–5]. In response to this problem, a growing number of investigations, mainly in Latin America, are being carried out to find new powerful anti-chagas and anti-leishmaniasis agents with low toxicity.

Chagas disease is a zoonosis caused by the protozoan *Trypanosoma cruzi*, which affects around 150 species of mammals, including humans, and is mainly vector-borne by hematophagous insects of the *Tritominidae* subfamily (popularly known as kissing bugs, bed bugs, and whistles, among other names). Since 1970, the treatment against this pathology has been based mainly on the antiparasitic drugs Nifurtimox (NFX) and Benznidazole (BNZ). These medicines have an effectiveness of 70% during the acute phase, where the prevailing parasitic form is blood trypomastigotes, and decreases to 20% in the chronic phase, where the predominant form corresponds to the intracellular phase of amastigotes [6,7]. It has been proven that NFX and BNZ have a high toxicity for mammalian cells, with serious side effects, such as peripheral neuropathies, anorexia, nausea, and vomiting, as well as neurological reactions such as anxiety and disorientation, among others [8]. On the other hand, leishmaniasis encompasses a group of infectious diseases caused by at least 20 species of the *Leishmania* genus, including *L. braziliensis*, *L. amazonensis*, *L. infantum*, *L. guyanensis*, *L. panamensis*, and *L. mexicana*, which are the species that affect humans. Its transmission is mainly through vectors via insect bites of the *Psychodidae* family. This disease presents three different clinical forms in humans, canines, and several wild vertebrates: cutaneous, mucocutaneous, and visceral [3]. Current treatment against leishmaniasis is based on the use of pentavalent antimonials, such as Miltefosine, Amphotericin B (AmB), Paromomycin, and Pentamidine; however, there are restrictions on the use of these drugs due to their side effects, which include hepatic, cardiac, and renal toxicity [5]. Additionally, they present limitations, such as high production cost and increased resistance by the parasite [9].

Naphthoquinones stand out among the most studied natural compounds and synthetic derivatives for their anti-chagas and anti-leishmaniasis (mainly against *L. infantum* and *L. amazonensis*) activity. β-lapachone derivatives have exhibited potential anticancer, antiviral, antiparasitic (including anti-chagas and anti-leishmanial activity), antimicrobial, anti-inflammatory, anti-obesity, antioxidant, and neuroprotective activity, while showing low levels of toxicity to normal cells [10]. Naphthoimidazoles derived from β-lapachone have been prepared, and their trypanocidal activity has been evaluated using electron microscopy, flow cytometry, and biochemical techniques, indicating that some compounds lead to an oxidative imbalance, which generates the production of ROS and the death of the parasite [10–13]. De Silva et al. carried out molecular docking studies on two cysteine proteases: cruzin and rhodesain, which are fundamental in the metabolism of the *T. cruzi* parasite [14]. This allowed for the identification of 14 naphthoquinone derivatives with potential antiprotozoal activity, which were synthesized and tested in vitro. On the other hand, 2,3-diphenyl-1,4-naphthoquinone (DPNQ) is considered a potential chemotherapeutic agent against *T. cruzi* due to its high trypanocidal activity in phenotypic screening and experimental murine infection by *T. cruzi*. Treatment with DPNQ in infected female mice promoted a halving of the parasite load, and ensured a 60% survival rate of the animal [15]. In 2021, Becerra et al. used pharmacophoric models based on different studies to design and subsequently synthesize nine phenolic derivatives, which were tested against *T. cruzi* strains, most of which showed good activity compared to BNZ, and the best prospects showed low toxicity [16]. Plumbagin is a plant-derived naphthoquinone metabolite (5-hydroxy-2-methyl-1,4-naphthaquinone) that inhibits trypanothione reductase, and has been validated as a drug which is responsible for promoting oxidative stress in *Leishmania* [9]. Similarly, naphtherocarpanquinone (LQB-118), which has been evaluated against cutaneous leishmaniasis, showed activity against intracellular amastigotes of *L. amazonensis*. It is proposed, through an anti-leishmanial model, that a good level of administration could counteract this clinical form of leishmaniasis [17]. The leishmanicidal activity of a series of substituted bis-2-hydroxy-1,4-naphthoquinones prepared from lawsone with aliphatic and aromatic aldehydes has also been evaluated [18]. Overall, four of the bis-lawsone analogs showed results similar to Pentamidine, but without cytotoxicity to host cells. Other studies demonstrated the high activity and low toxicity for host cells of derivatives of nor-α-lapachone and α-lapachone fused with triazole; despite them, however, resistance similar to that presented by the reference drug (Pentamidine) was observed [19]. Likewise, α-lapachone has shown a similar inhibition to sodium stibogluconate (Pentostam) [20]. Acetylisolapachol showed greater activity against *L. amazonensis* and does not exhibit a risk to the host [21].

Continuing with our search for novel structures with high antiparasitic activity and low toxicity [22], in this work, we have carried out an extensive in silico study of substituted derivatives of 1,4-naphthoquinone as potential anti-chagas and anti-leishmanial candidates. QSAR modeling of anti-*T. cruzi* in trypomastigotes, anti-*L. amazonensis*, *anti-L. infantum*, and toxicity has been carried out, based on the antiparasitic derivatives of naphthoquinone and other related structures reported in the literature. The best QSAR models were used to evaluate the predictive antiparasitic and toxicity activity of 68 1,4-naphthoquinone derivatives with hitherto unknown biological activity. This study was complemented by the evaluation of the 68 candidates against 5 macromolecular targets related to vital processes for the survival of these protozoa. In the case of *T. cruzi*, trypanothione reductase (*Tc*TR) and lanosterol α-demethylase (*Tc*LαD) proteins were selected. For the *Leishmania* genus in general, trypanothione reductase (*L*TR) protein was selected, while for the *L. amazonensis* and *L. infantum* strains, arginase (*La*A) and tyrosine aminotransferase (*Li*TA) were selected, respectively. Additionally, the ADME (absorption, distribution, metabolism, and excretion) properties of the 68 naphthoquinone derivatives were evaluated. The best anti-chagas and anti-leishmanial candidates derived from this in silico study are currently in the organic synthesis stage at our lab for their subsequent in vitro evaluation.

2. Results and Discussion

2.1. QSAR Modeling

In total, four QSAR models were performed based on in vitro reports of naphthoquinone derivatives and related structures with anti-*T. cruzi* (in trypomastigotes) [23–31], anti-*L. amazonensis* [18,32–39], and anti-*L. infantum* [40–45] activities, as well as toxicity [30,46–51] evaluation. For each QSAR study, the top seven models were generated, which are shown in Tables S1 and S2 in the Supplementary Materials. In turn, the best model (in bold) among the seven was selected, which was performed considering high homogeneity (fitting, R^2) between the calibration and validation groups with the lowest root mean square error (RMSE), thereby avoiding over-adjusted models. For selecting the best model, the Ockham's principle of parsimony was also considered, which states that if there are models with statistical parameters of equal quality, the simplest one should be selected [52].

2.1.1. QSAR Model for Anti-chagas Activity

Equation (1) shows the best QSAR model for the anti-chagas activity predicted as $LogIC_{50}$, which was developed based on 153 derivatives of 1,2-naphthoquinone and 1,4-naphthoquinone (Figure A1) evaluating in vitro blood trypomastigotes of strain Y of *T. cruzi*. A description of the molecular descriptors that define this model is listed in Table 1.

$$\mathrm{LogIC}_{50} = 4.5112 + 0.3637a_1 + 1.1416a_2 - 0.1003a_3 + 0.9440a_4 + 0.1929a_5 - 1.8425 \times 10^{-4}a_6 \quad (1)$$

Table 1. Molecular descriptors of the best anti-chagas QSAR model as defined by Equation (1).

Descriptor	Name	Short Description	Type
a_1	frag16	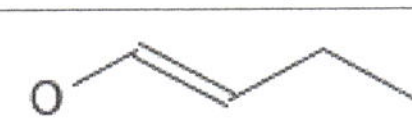	Fingerprint
a_2	MACCSFP72	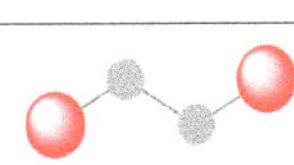 (Any bond; Red: Oxygen; Gray:Any atom)	Fingerprint
a_3	K_Q_AB_nCi_2_SS10_T_KA_r_MAS	Refractivity	2D
a_4	K_B_AB_nCi_2_DS7_C_KA_e-p_MAS	Electronegativity/Polarizability	2D
a_5	K_B_AB_nCi_2_DS2_X_KA_r-c_MAS	Refractivity/Charge	2D
a_6	N2_F_AB_nCi_2_NS7_P_KA_m_MAS	Mass	2D

The descriptors a_1 and a_2 are fingerprints calculated in Fragmentor [53], and refer to the presence of oxygen followed by an unsaturation; while the second was calculated in PaDeL [54], and belongs to the MACCS keys, a group of 166 free access fragments [55], which involves an oxygen–oxygen arrangement at a distance equal to three bonds and two intermediate atoms of any type. According to this QSAR model (Equation (1)), these molecular descriptors contribute negatively to the evaluated activity (i.e., they decrease the activity). The other descriptors of the model were calculated in the program QUBILS-MAS [56]. The descriptors a_3, a_4, and a_5 are calculated from the Kurtosis, which is a statistical invariant, while a_6 belongs to the Minkowski indicators. a_3 is a quadratic index, a_4 and a_5 are bilinear, and a_6 is linear. The descriptor a_3 is a global index that contributes to the biological activity. This is related to molar refractivity, which can sometimes be used to model London dispersion forces or attractive van der Waals interactions; these are factors related to the presence of strong interactions between a ligand and the active sites of a given macromolecular receptor. However, refractivity is the consequence of repulsive nonbonding interactions, and is highly dependent on the flexibility of the ligand [57]. The descriptor a_4 describes the electronegativity and polarizability of the fragment of carbon atoms in aliphatic chains, while a_5 is associated with the refractivity and charge of the subset of heteroatoms in the molecule [4]. Both descriptors contribute negatively to the anti-chagas activity. Considering the nature of descriptors a_4 and a_5, it is hypothesized that the anti-chagas activity could be related to the ability of the ligands to dock and inhibit essential macromolecules in the metabolism of *T. cruzi*. For its part, the descriptor a_6 provides a positive contribution to the biological activity, and is a function of the mass of aromatic carbon atoms, which suggests that the presence of aromatic systems improves activity.

Table S3 in the Supplementary Materials shows the intercorrelation relationship between each pair of descriptors included in the anti-chagas QSAR model, while Table S4 lists the values of each descriptor for each molecule. Table S5 shows the experimental values together with those predicted by the anti-chagas activity model as log IC_{50}.

2.1.2. QSAR Model for Anti-*L. amazonensis* Activity

For the anti-*L. amazonensis* (cutaneous and mucocutaneous leishmaniasis) activity (expressed as LogIC_{50}), the QSAR model with four descriptors was selected (Table S1), which is described according to Equation (2). This model was developed based on 60 ligands (Figure A2), with in vitro anti-leishmanial activity reported as IC_{50}:

$$\mathrm{LogIC}_{50} = 0.26 - 1.00b_1 + 0.24b_2 + 0.42b_3 - 0.05b_4, \quad (2)$$

where b_1, b_2, b_3, and b_4 are described as shown in Table 2.

Table 2. Molecular descriptors in the anti-*L. amazonensis* QSAR model, as described by Equation (2).

Descriptor	Name	Short Description	Type
b_1	KRFP2	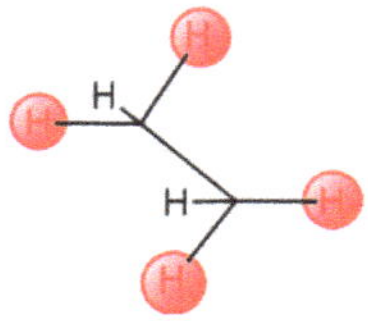 (Klekota–Roth fingerprint, presence of chemical substructures)	Fingerprint
b_2	minHBint9	Electro-topological state atom type descriptor (minimal strength E-state type descriptor for potential hydrogen bonds of path length 9)	2D
b_3	IC3	Information content index (3-order neighborhood symmetry)	2D
b_4	MDEC-23	Molecular edge distance	2D

The b_1 descriptor refers to the Klekota–Roth fingerprint KRFP2, and it comprises part of six of the seven anti-*L. amazonensis* QSAR models considered (Table S1). This descriptor provides a measure of chemical similarity related to a bond between two carbon atoms, where each carbon atom has, as its substituents, a hydrogen atom and two nonhydrogen atoms [54,58]. On the other hand, b_2, b_3, and b_4 refer to 2D type descriptors. The minHBint9 (b_2) descriptor describes the topological state of the atom's environment, such as the electronic interactions present in the atoms of the molecule at a topological distance of nine with each atom. According to Equation (2), this characteristic decreases the IC_{50}, that is, the less topological distance there is between the atoms that make up the structure, the better its antiprotozoal activity [59]. The IC3 descriptor (b_3) is based on the three-order neighborhood symmetry. This means that molecules with lower symmetry will have a better predictive activity [60]. Finally, the descriptor MDEC-23 (b_4) refers to the information regarding the edge of the molecular distance among all secondary and tertiary carbons. The presence and value of b_4 enhance the anti-leishmaniasis activity predicted by the model, indicating that the presence of secondary and tertiary carbon atoms in these molecules is related to their biological activity [61–63].

2.1.3. QSAR Model for anti-*L. infantum* Activity

For predicting anti-*L. infantum* (visceral leishmaniasis) activity such as $LogIC_{50}$, the model with six descriptors was selected (Table S1), which is represented according to Equation (3). The molecules used for constructing this QSAR model are shown in Figure A3:

$$\text{LogIC}_{50} = -1.51 + 6.83c_1 + 0.29c_2 - 3.88 \times 10^{-6}c_3 + 0.04c_4 - 3.72c_5 - 3.68 \times 10^{-6}c_6 \quad (3)$$

where $c_n (n = 1 \text{ to } 6)$ are 2D descriptors described as shown in Table 3.

Table 3. Molecular descriptors in the anti-*L. infantum* QSAR model, as described by Equation (3).

Descriptor	Name	Short Description	Type
c_1	MATS3c	Moran Correlation—lag 3/load-weighted	2D
c_2	nHBint7	Atom-like electro-topological state	2D
c_3	AM_F_AB_nCi_2_NS12_T_KA_a_MAS	Alog P (partition)	2D
c_4	AM_B_AB_nCi_2_NS2_C_KA_psa-v_MAS	C atoms in aliphatic chain Topological area of the polar surface/Vdw volume	2D
c_5	AM_B_AB_nCi_2_SS1_C_KA_v-c_MAS	Volume of Vdw/Charge	2D
c_6	AM_Q_AB_nCi_2_NS15_X_KA_a_MAS	Heteroatom–Partitioning Algorithm (Alog P)	2D

The MATS3c (c_1) descriptor refers to Moran's autocorrelation, which expresses the partial charge values of atoms separated by three distances, that is, it estimates the correlation of charges divided into three bonds [64,65]. The descriptor nHBint7 (c_2) counts resistance E-state descriptors for hydrogen bonds with a path length of seven. The c_3–c_6 descriptors are part of the QuBiLS-MAS program [66]. The c_3 descriptor refers to the partition algorithm, which is used to calculate estimates of most neutral organic compounds that have C, H, O, N, S, Se, P, B, Si, and halogen atoms. This descriptor is based on AlogP, which can also estimate local hydrophobicity, visualize molecular hydrophobicity maps, and evaluate hydrophobic interactions when protein–ligand complexes are formed [67,68]. The c_4 descriptor considers bilinear indices and aliphatic chain carbon atoms, and correlates the topological area of the polar surface and the van der Waals volume. The polar surface area (PSA) is a molecular descriptor widely used in the study of drug transport properties, related to the penetration of the blood–brain barrier and its intestinal absorption. Additionally, the descriptor c_4 alludes to the sum of the contributions of polar atoms such as oxygen, nitrogen, and hydrogen to the molecular surface area [69,70]. The descriptor c_5 correlates the carbon atoms of aliphatic chains with the van der Waals volume and charge. Molecular volume is defined as a measure of the space around electron-filled atomic nuclei, and is geometrically interpreted as the combined volume of the superimposed spheres centered on the nuclei, similar to a space-filling molecular model [71,72]. Finally, the descriptor c_6 presents a nonstochastic matrix of order 15; in this case, the descriptor considers the heteroatoms different from C and H, correlating them with the partition algorithm and estimating the different atoms. This descriptor includes most of the zwitterionic compounds that have amine, carboxylic acids, and ammonium halide salts. The c_6 descriptor is also based on an intrinsically atomistic model, which is useful for drug design, since it makes estimates of the local or general hydrophobicity of a molecule [66,68].

Table S7 in the Supporting Materials shows the intercorrelation relationship between each pair of descriptors included in the anti-leishmanial QSAR models (Equations (2) and (3)), while Table S8 (*L. amazonensis*) and Table S7 (*L. infantum*) show the values of each descriptor calculated for each molecule used in the development of these QSAR models. Tables S10 and S11 list the experimental and model-predicted values of anti-leishmanial activity as log IC_{50}.

2.1.4. QSAR Model for Toxicity

From the QSAR study for toxicity (expressed as $LogIC_{50}$), a model with five descriptors was selected (Table S2), which is represented in Equation (4). This model was developed based on 76 naphthoquinone derivatives, as shown in Figure A4.

$$\mathrm{LogIC}_{50} = 0.37 + 0.11d_1 - 0.21d_2 + 0.36d_3 - 0.05d_4 - 0.17d_5, \tag{4}$$

where $d_n (n = 1 \text{ to } 5)$ are 2D descriptors described as shown in Table 4.

Table 4. Molecular descriptors in the QSAR model of toxicity as described by Equation (4).

Descriptor	Name	Short Description	Type
d_1	K_B_AB_nCi_2_NS3_T_KA_psa-r_MAS	Topological polar surface area; refractivity	2D
d_2	K_B_AB_nCi_2_DS7_P_KA_c-p_MAS	Aromatic C atoms. Charge; polarization	2D
d_3	N2_B_AB_nCi_2_MP4_P_KA_psa-p_MAS	Aromatic C atoms. Topological polar surface area; polarization	2D
d_4	K_B_AB_nCi_2_DS3_X_KA_a-e_MAS	Heteroatoms. Partition algorithm (Log P); electronegativity	2D
d_5	K_Q_AB_nCi_2_SS14_C_KA_c_MAS	C atoms in aliphatic chain. Charge.	2D

The toxicity model descriptors were calculated using the QUBILS-MAS program [66]. The descriptors d_1, d_2, d_4, and d_5 are calculated from the Kurtosis, which is a statistical invariant of distribution. The d_1 descriptor correlates with physicochemical properties, polarized topological surface area, and refractivity. As indicated above, the topological polar surface area of a molecule depends on the sum of the surface area of polar atoms, such as oxygen, nitrogen, and hydrogen, and facilitates the ability of a molecule to penetrate cells. According to this, the greater the value of the polar topological surface in a molecule, the greater its probability of being transported [73]. Meanwhile, refractivity is a measure of the volume occupied by an atom or a group of atoms [69]. These last two properties allow for a theoretical prediction of the pharmacological potential of a molecule in a biological environment [74]. The descriptor d_2 correlates the polarization with the charge of aromatic carbon atoms because it facilitates the distortion of the atomic or molecular charge in electromagnetic fields. This descriptor refers to an electronic parameter, which impacts chemical–biological interactions [75]. The descriptor d_3 correlates the polar surface area with the polarization of the carbon atoms of the aromatic moiety and the heteroatoms attached to this moiety. The d_4 descriptor is associated with the partition algorithm, heteroatoms, and electronegativity. This descriptor is based on the tendency of a heteroatom or functional group to attract electrons and estimate the local or general hydrophobicity of a molecule [67–74,76,77]. Finally, the descriptor d_5 refers to the charge and the carbon atoms in the aliphatic chains.

Table S13 in Supporting Materials shows the intercorrelation relationship between each pair of descriptors included in the QSAR model of toxicity, while Table S15 shows the experimental and predicted values in log IC_{50} used for constructing of the QSAR model of toxicity.

2.1.5. Validation of QSAR Models

Table 5 contains a compilation of the statistical parameters used for the internal and external validation of the four QSAR models developed. From Y-randomization, it was found that $RMSE_{cal} < RMSE_{rand}$, thus indicating that all QSAR models are robust due to the absence of random correlation [78] Internal validation by the Leave-One-Out (LOO) method yielded a value of the squared correlation coefficient (R^2_{loo}) ≥ 0.5 [78,79], which ensures the statistical stability of each model. In addition to presenting good internal validation parameters, all of the QSAR models are predictive, since they meet the following requirements: the slopes k and k' of the plots of observed and predicted values are in the range 0.85–1.15 (with k corresponding to the case when the predicted values are plotted on the x-axis and the experimental values on the y-axis, while k' is the inverse graph). The CCC statistically evaluates the models, this parameter verifies the difference between the experimental and predicted values. The squared correlation coefficients have values greater than 0.5, which validate the models [80].

Table 5. Internal and external validation parameters for each best QSAR model.

Parameter	QSAR Models				
	Anti-Chagas (Ec. 1)	anti-*L. amazonensis* (Ec. 2)	Anti-*L. infantum* (Ec. 3)	Toxicity (Ec. 4)	
				98%	100%
N_{train}	107	48	72	60	60
N_{val}	23	6	9	8	8
N_{test}	23	6	9	7	8
R^2_{test}	0.83	0.78	0.66	0.91	0.70
RMS_{test}	0.48	0.38	0.35	0.22	0.32
R^2_{ijmax}	0.40	0.19	0.79	0.44	0.44
R^2_{loo}	0.71	0.70	0.66	0.92	0.92
RMS_{loo}	0.54	0.35	0.46	0.18	0.18
R^2_{Rand}	0.06	0.09	0.08	0.08	0.09
RMS_{Rand}	0.10	0.59	0.74	0.74	0.95
k	1.12	1.03	1.03	0.96	0,97
k'	0.86	0.88	0.92	1.03	1.00
Q^2_{F1}	0.80	0.80	0.71	0.89	0.75
Q^2_{F2}	0.76	0.77	0.65	0.82	0.63
Q^2_{F3}	0.77	0.65	0.80	0.88	0.75
CCC	0.86	0.86	0.79	0.89	0.83
O_3	0	0	0	0	1

Figure 1 shows the dispersion diagram of the experimental values of anti-chagas and anti-*Leishmania* (*L. amazonensis* and *L. infantum*) activity and toxicity expressed as $Log(IC_{50})$ as a function of the values predicted by each model. In all cases, it is observed how points adopt a linear trend around the line of perfect fit (in green), which confirms a multivariate linear relationship.

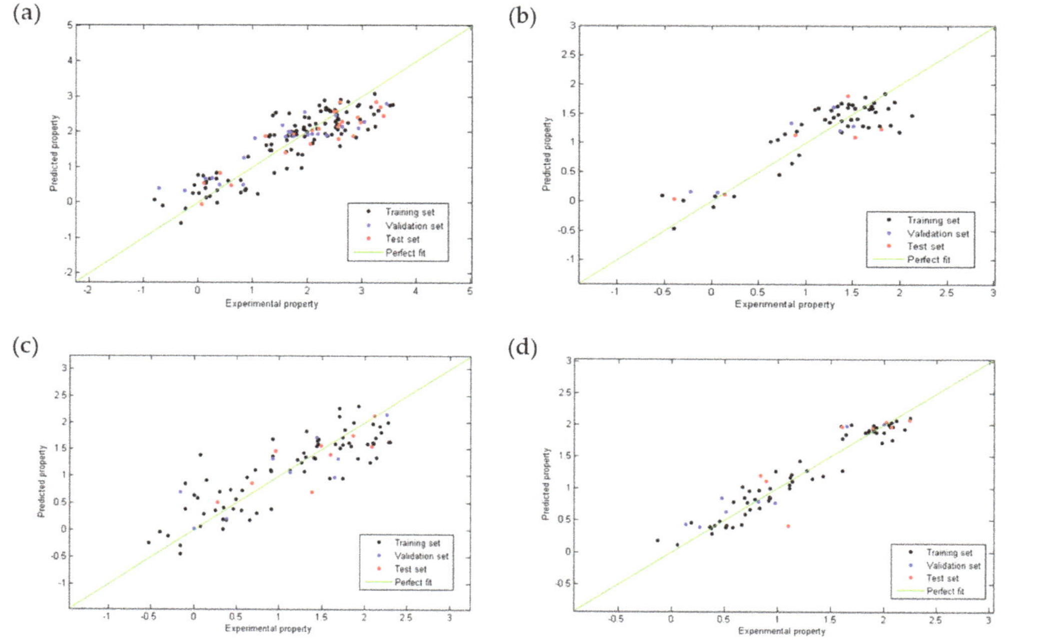

Figure 1. Linear correlation plots between the experimental and the predicted values obtained using the QSAR Equations (1) (**a**), (2) (**b**), (3) (**c**) and (4) (**d**).

Figure 2 shows the plots of the residuals for the four QSAR models developed. It was observed that for anti-chagas (Figure 2a) and anti-leishmaniasis (Figure 2b,c) activity, no residual is greater than three times the standard deviation (3S) of the model (outliers), while the toxicity model (Figure 2d) presented one outlier of the test group. In all QSAR models, the points follow a random distribution around the line at $y = 0$, which suggests that these properties are modeled using of multiple linear regression.

Due to the low diversity of molecules considered in the development of the QSAR models, the acceptable predictions are restricted to structural analogs derived from naphthoquinone, whose influence value is less than the critical influence value (h^*) in each model (Figure 3). As shown in Figure 3a,c, for anti-chagas and anti-*L. infantum* activity, all molecules of the validation group and of the test group are within the domain of applicability, and molecules of the calibration group are considered outside the value of h^*, a fact that reinforces the predictive capacity of these models. For the anti-*L. amazonensis* activity model, Figure 3b shows how a molecule of the test group is rejected, thus demonstrating its ability to reject molecules with large differences. For its part, the toxicity model shows that all molecules considered for its development and validation are within the domain of applicability.

2.1.6. Molecular Design and Applicability of QSAR Models

Both *ortho*-naphthoquinone (1,2-substituted) and *para*-naphthoquinone (1,4-substituted) are recognized as highly active cores due to the synergy between its acid base and oxidation reduction properties [81], whose derivatives have exhibited several tunable antiparasitic effects according to the substitutions made in their fused rings [82]. As can be verified from the structural compilation used for constructing our QSAR antiprotozoal models (Figures A1–A3 in Appendix A), a high in vitro anti-chagas or anti-leishmanial effect is achieved when substitutions with heterocyclic, aromatic, or aliphatic groups are made at the 2 and 3 positions, for the case of the *para*-naphthoquinone, or at the 3 and 4 positions, for the case of the *ortho*-naphthoquinone nucleus.

The molecular design of our selection group was based on the following principles: (i) restriction to only derivatives of the 1,4-naphthoquinone nucleus at positions 2 and 3; (ii) use of open-chain and heterocyclic substituents at these positions; (iii) use of nitrogenous derivatives in position 2; (iv) variation in position 3 with electro-withdrawing and electro-donor groups; and (v) substitution in the amino nitrogen, located in position 2, with both highly functionalized aromatic and heterocycle rings. Due to this strategy, four families of 1,4-naphthoquinone derivatives (Figure 4) were selected for in silico evaluation: (a) 2-chloro-3-arylamino family (NQ–Chlorine); (b) 2-amino-3-arylamino family (NQ–Amine); (c) 2-amino-3-triazolamino family (NQ–Triazole); and (d) phenazine family (NQ–Phenazine). In particular, the use of triazoles and phenazines as substituents was established based on the high intrinsic activity of these groups, as well as their enhancing effect when incorporated into other active nucleus [23,82–84].

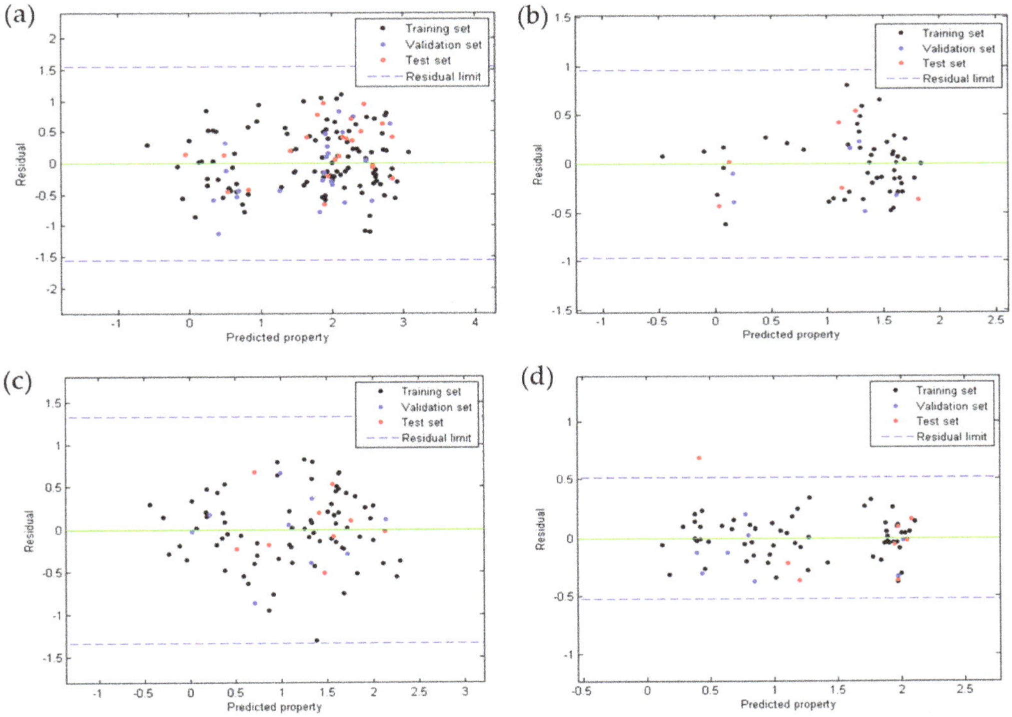

Figure 2. Dispersion of residues according to QSAR Equations (1) (**a**), (2) (**b**), (3) (**c**), and (4) (**d**).

QSAR models established according to Equations (1)–(4) were used to predict anti-chagas (IC_{50} in trypomastigotes), anti-*L. amazonensis* (cutaneous and mucocutaneous leishmaniasis), and anti-*L. infantum* (visceral leishmaniasis) activity, as well as toxicity, of the 68 derivatives of 1,4-naphthoquinone shown in Figure 4, which are structures that do not present experimental anti-chagas or anti-leishmanial activity (in vitro or in vivo) reported so far.

Figure 5a shows the prediction values of anti-chagas activity (IC_{50}) for the 68 1,4-naphthoquinone derivatives evaluated using QSAR Equation (1). As a result, 47 (69%) of the 68 evaluated molecules had a better predicted IC_{50} than the experimental value of the reference drug BNZ. Overall, 10 of these derivatives (structures 17, 43, 53–60) were not within the applicability domain of the model, so their predicted activity should be considered unreliable. High anti-chagasic activity was found for the NQ–Phenazine derivatives substituted with the isopropyl group (structures 61 and 62), as well as for the NQ–Chlorine and NQ–Amine derivatives containing the same substituent (structures 24–26 and 51–52, respectively). Additionally, the derivatives coupled to the triazole ring (NQ–Triazole family) show a slightly better predicted activity than BNZ. According to this QSAR model, those amino derivatives with electron-withdrawing substituents (nitro and fluorine, structures 34–36 and 40–42, respectively) present the less parasitic activity toward *T. cruzi* trypomastigotes.

The predicted IC_{50} values of anti-*Leishmania* activity (*L. amazonensis* and *L. infantum*) for the 68 naphthoquinone derivatives evaluated with QSAR Equations (2) and (3) are presented in Figure 5b,c respectively. According to the influence value (h^*), 63 (93%) of the 68 naphthoquinone derivatives showed reliable anti-*Leishmania* activity, and five molecules (42, 43, 64, 67 and 68) did not show reliable activity. It was found that all molecules belonging to NQ–Phenazine family, as well as some derivatives of the NQ–Chloro (structures 1, 20, 24, and 26), and NQ–Amine families (structures 27, 36, 39, 44–47, 50–51), presented a better anti-*L. amazonensis* effect than the reference drugs Miltefosine and Glucantime (see Figure 5b), unlike the all of NQ–Triazole derivatives that had lower results than the reference drugs. According to Equation (3), 51 derivatives presented a reliable predictive anti-*L. infantum* activity, while the other 17 molecules were not found within the influence parameter (0.24). Among the molecules that presented a reliable activity, the best activity was that of molecule 6 together with several other NQ–Chloro derivatives (structures 1, 3, 6–7, 9–10, 12, 14–17, and 19–26), one NQ–Phenazine derivative (structure 56), and four of the NQ–Triazole derivatives (structures 63–65 and 67), all of which presented better activity than the reference drug. All of the NQ–Amine derivatives presented lower anti-*L. infantum* activity than the two reference drugs.

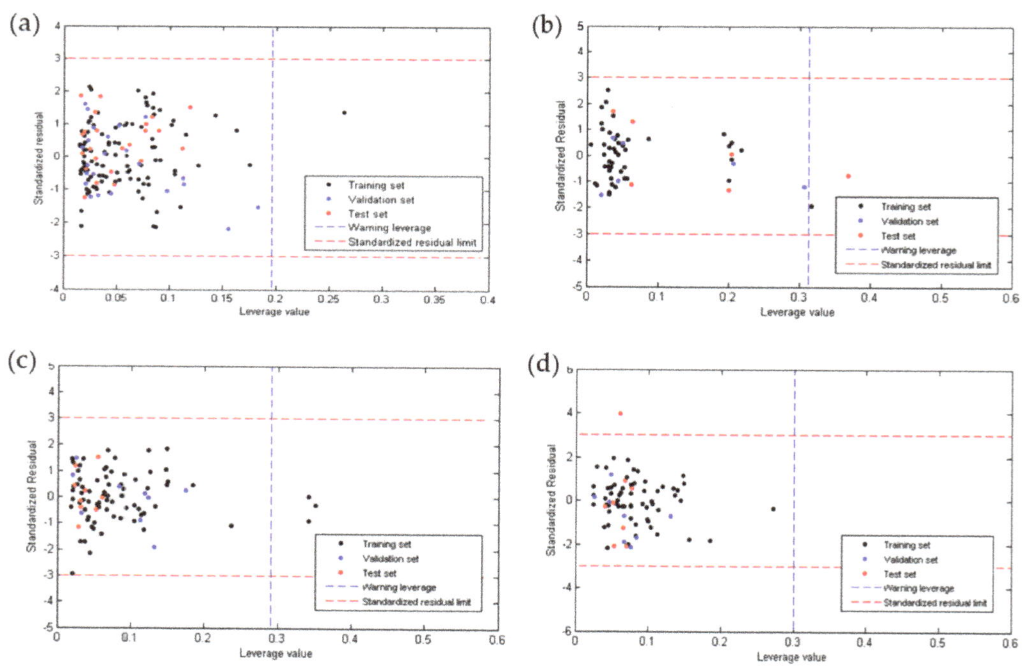

Figure 3. h^{lim} values for (**a**) anti-chagas (Table S5); (**b**) anti-*L. amazonensis* (Table S10); (**c**) anti-*L. infantum* (Table S11) activity, and (**d**) toxicity (Table S15).

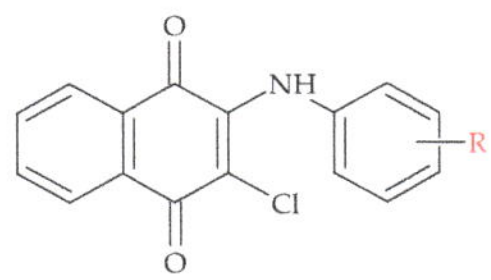

R= (1) H, (2) 2-OCH$_3$, (3) 3-OCH$_3$, (4) 4-OCH$_3$, (5) 2-OCH$_2$CH$_3$, (6) 3-OCH$_2$CH$_3$, (7) 4-OCH$_2$CH$_3$, (8) 2-F, (9) 3-F, (10) 4-F, (11) 2-Cl, (12) 3-Cl, (13) 4-Cl, (14) 2-NO$_2$, (15) 3-NO$_2$, (16) 4-NO$_2$, (17) 2,4-NO$_2$,NO$_2$ (18) 2-CH$_3$, (19) 3-CH$_3$, (20) 4-CH$_3$, (21) 2-CH$_2$CH$_3$, (22) 3-CH$_2$CH$_3$, (23) 2-CH$_2$CH$_3$, (24) 2-CH(CH$_3$)$_2$, (25) 3-CH(CH$_3$)$_2$, (26) 4-CH(CH$_3$)$_2$.

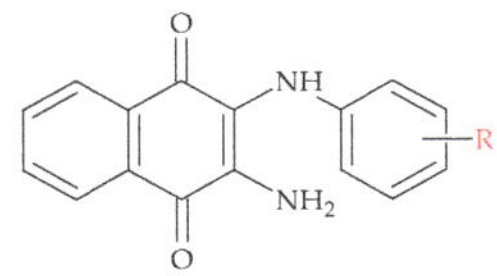

R= (27) H, (28) 2-OCH$_3$, (29) $_3$-OCH$_3$, (30) 4-OCH$_3$, (31) 2-OCH$_2$CH$_3$, (32) 3-OCH$_2$CH$_3$, (33) 4-OCH$_2$CH$_3$, (34) 2-F, (35) 3-F, (36) 4-F, (37) 2-Cl, (38) 3-Cl, (39) 4-Cl, (40) 2-NO$_2$, (41) 3-NO$_2$, (42) 4-NO$_2$, (43) 2,4-di-NO$_2$ (44) 2-CH$_3$, (45) 3-CH$_3$, (46) 4-CH$_3$, (47) 2-CH$_2$CH$_3$, (48) 3-CH$_2$CH$_3$, (49) 2-CH$_2$CH$_3$, (50) 2-CH(CH$_3$)$_2$, (51) 3-CH(CH$_3$)$_2$, (52) 4-CH(CH$_3$)$_2$.

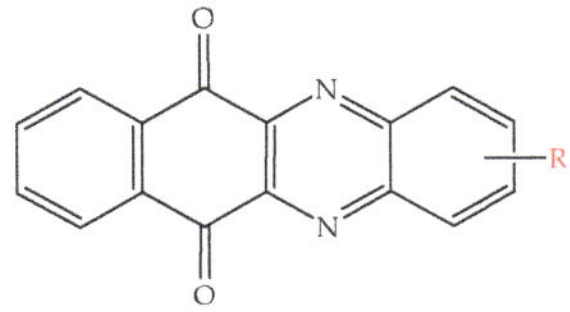

R= (53) 2-OCH$_3$, (54) 3-OCH$_3$, (55) 2-OCH$_2$CH$_3$, (56) 3-OCH$_2$CH$_3$, (57) 2-CH$_3$, (58) 3-CH$_3$, (59) 2-CH$_2$CH$_3$, (60) 3-CH$_2$CH$_3$, (61) 2-CH(CH$_3$)$_2$, (62) 3-CH(CH$_3$)$_2$

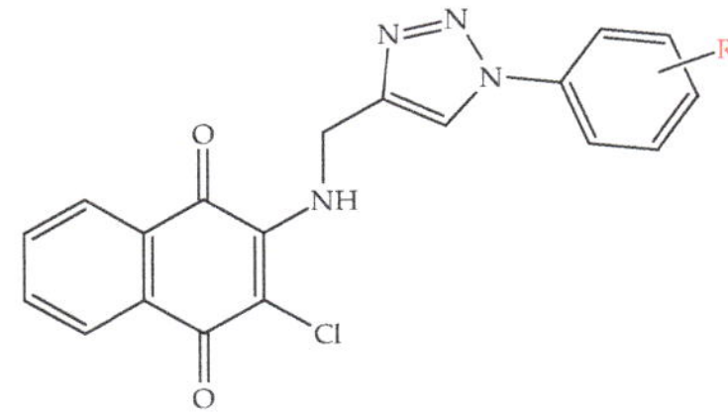

R= (63) H, (64) 4-F, (65) 3-F, (66) 2-F, (67) 3,4-di-F; (68) 2,4-di-F

Figure 4. Molecular design of 1,4-naphthoquinone derivatives with potential antiparasitic activity (chagas and leishmaniasis). (**top-left**) (NQ–Chlorine family), (**top-right**) (NQ–Amine family), (**bottom-left**) (NQ–Phenazine), and (**bottom-right**) (NQ–Triazole family).

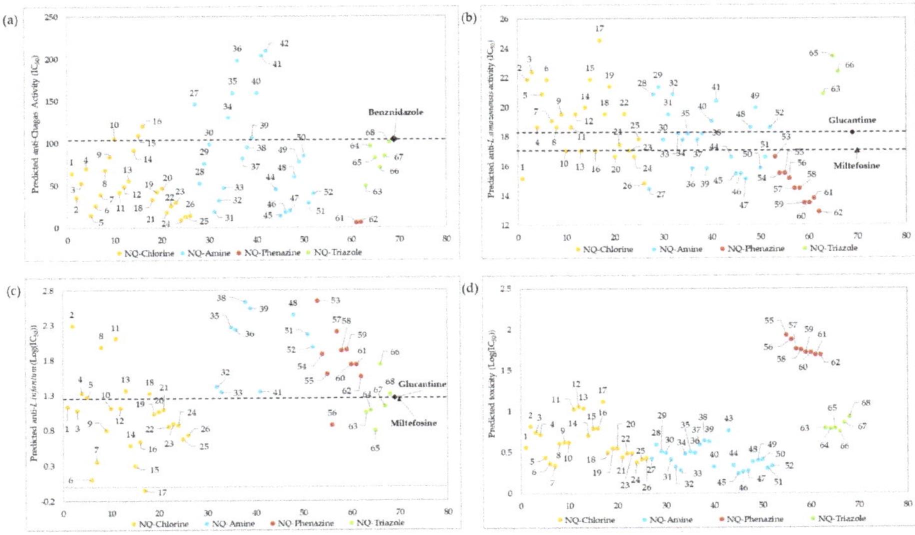

Figure 5. Prediction of anti-chagas (IC$_{50}$) (Table S6) (**a**), anti-*L. amazonensis* (IC$_{50}$) (**b**), and anti-*L. infantum* (LogIC$_{50}$) (Table S12) (**c**) activity, as well as toxicity (LogIC$_{50}$) (Table S16) (**d**), for the 68 1,4-naphthoquinone derivatives (*x*-axis) evaluated using QSAR Equations (1)–(4), respectively. Only structures with reliable activity, as determined by the influence value (*h**), are presented. The predicted values for anti-*L. infantum* and toxicity are presented in LogIC$_{50}$ because of the wide dispersion of the data.

The toxicity values (LogIC_{50}) predicted by QSAR Equation (4) for the 68 naphthoquinone derivatives are shown in Figure 5d. A total of 64 molecules presented a reliable predicted activity, while 4 of them (structures 41–42, 53 and 54) were outside of the influence parameter (h^*). Among the 68 molecules evaluated, all of the structures belonging to the NQ–Phenazine family presented the lowest toxicity values.

2.2. Molecular Docking

Ligand–protein docking simulations were carried out to determine the most effective binding mode of each of the 68 1,4-naphthoquinone derivatives within the catalytic sites of the 5 chosen molecular targets (*Tc*TR, *Tc*LαD, *L*TR, *La*R, and *Li*TA). These macromolecular receptors were selected due to their relevance in the processes of survival, metabolism, reproduction, and proliferation of the parasites *T. cruzi*, *L. amazonensis*, and *L. infantum*. Conformational flexibility was allowed in all rotational bonds of the ligand, while the protein was used as a rigid structure. The best poses were selected according to the MVD scoring function, which helped to elucidate the electronic and structural aspects of the binding mode of the ligands in the active site of each protein.

2.2.1. Docking in Trypanothione Reductase and Lanosterol α-Demethylase Proteins of *T. Cruzi*

For the *Tc*TR protein a 496 Å^3 cavity was used, while for the *Tc*LαD protein, a 481 Å^3 cavity was used (Figure S1). The results of the ligand–protein coupling are shown in Figure 6a,b, where the 68 1,4-naphthoquinone derivatives show a good interaction (from −128.75 to −79.68 kcal/mol) with the two selected molecular targets. In this study, as the interaction energy decreases, the affinity of the compounds with the enzyme improves.

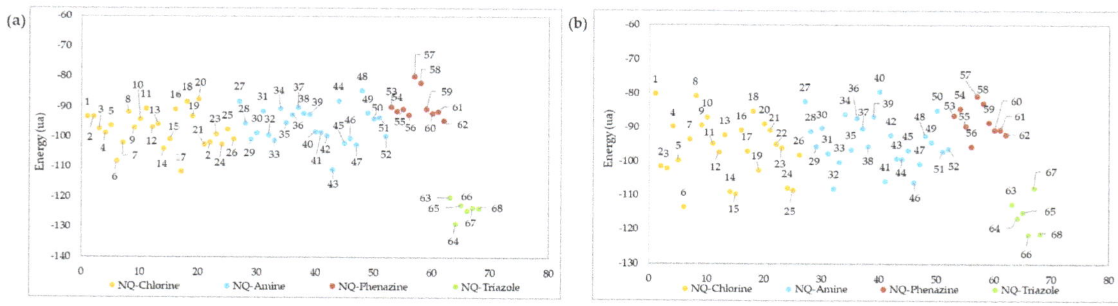

Figure 6. Ligand–protein docking energies of 1,4-naphthoquinone derivatives against (**a**) *Tc*TR and (**b**) *Tc*LαD receptors.

As shown in Figure 6a, the triazole-fused naphthoquinone derivatives had better interaction energy (from −128.75 to −120.03 kcal/mol) with the active site of the *Tc*TR. Among these, NQ–Triazole structure 64 had the best affinity, presenting 4 hydrogen bonds: 1 with the Asn 340 A residue, another with the Arg 355 A residue, and 1 with the Gly 459 B residue (Figure 7a), with the latter 2 not present in its triazole analogs; as well as steric interactions with the amino acids His 461, Thr 335, Ile 339, Glu 466, Glu 19, Pro 336, and Ser 470. Chacón et al. [85] also reported that the hydrogen bond interaction with the Gly 459 residue provided the best affinity energy to the quinoxaline derivative of the group they evaluated; and reported for this compound the same hydrophobic interactions. Similarly, the natural substrate co-crystallized in the active site of the *Tc*TR protein presented interactions with residues Glu 19 A, Gly 459 B, Pro 336 A, Ile 339 A, and His 461 B [86]. NQ–Triazole 66 presented an energy close to that of molecule 64, and in addition to the same hydrophobic interactions, it presented unions with the amino acids Leu 18 A, Tyr 111 A, and Val 54, which are also part of the *Tc*TR-trypanothione union (Figure 7b). The only hydrogen bond that this derivative presents together with the other NQ–triazole molecules is with the Ser 15 A residue, which is a solvent-mediated hydrogen bond interaction [86]. Note that this interaction occurs only in this series of compounds. Table S17 in the Supporting Materials shows the interaction energy of each ligand, as well as the hydrogen bonds with the different amino acid residues of the active site of the *Tc*TR and *Tc*LαD proteins.

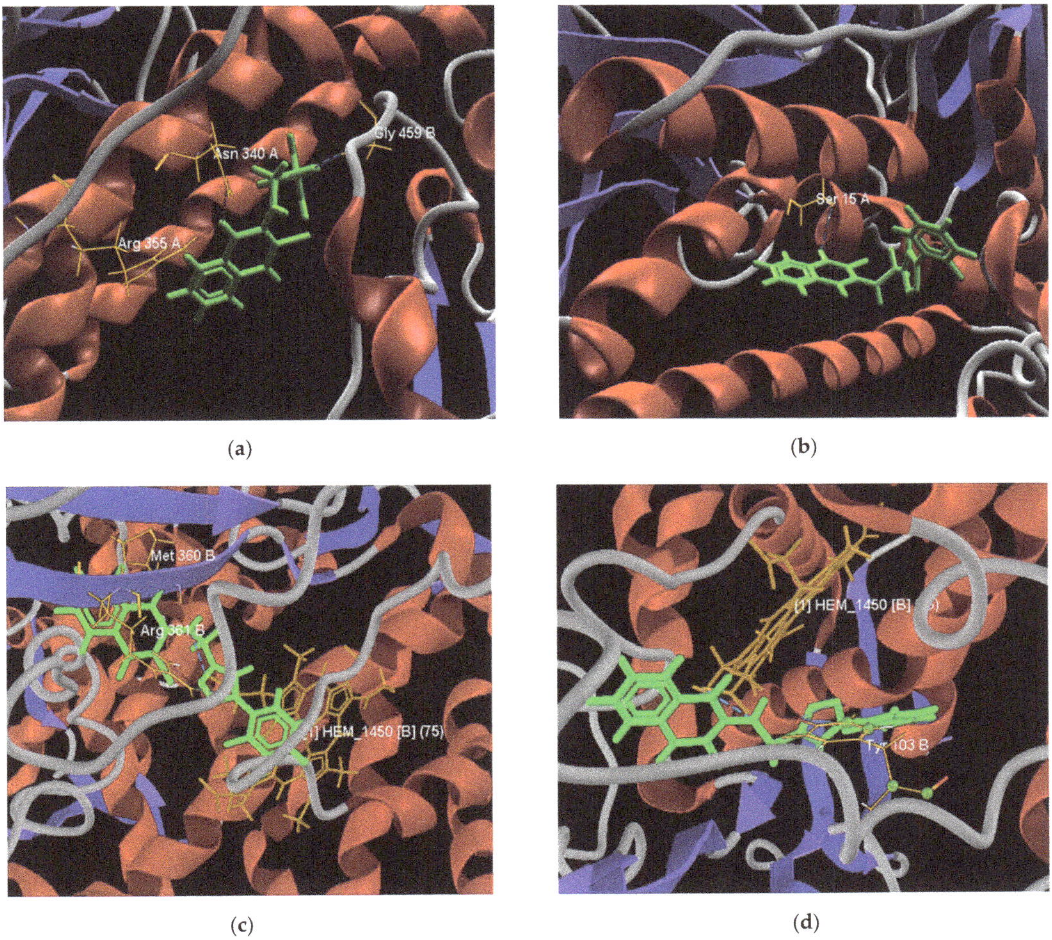

Figure 7. Best poses of derivatives 64 (**a**) and 66 (**b**) in the active site of the *Tc*TR protein. Best poses of derivatives 66 (**c**) and 68 (**d**) in the active site of the *Tc*LαD protein.

NQ–Chlorine derivatives 6 (−108.09 kcal/mol), and 17 (−111.59 kcal/mol), as well as NQ–Amine derivative 43 (−110.87 kcal/mol), also presented high ligand–protein interaction energies. Although these compounds have hydrogen bonds in the *Tc*TR active site (Figure 7c), the strength of these hydrogen bonds is comparable to those in compounds that have the least favored interaction energies, i.e., NQ–Phenazine structures 57 (−79.68 kcal/mol) and 58 (−81.93 kcal/mol). From the above, it follows that the compounds 6, 17, and 43 achieve their highest affinity and stability through other types of interactions.

The molecular docking evaluation against the *Tc*LαD protein showed that molecule 66 was again the ligand with the best affinity (−121.60 kcal/mol), followed by molecule

68 (−121.18 kcal/mol). Both structures belong to the family of triazoles substituted with fluorine atoms in the terminal aromatic ring, in this case, in the *meta* and *ortho-para* positions, respectively. Derivative 66 presents three hydrogen bonds between the three nitrogen atoms of the triazole ring with the donor oxygen atom of the Tyr 103 (B) residue; this type of interaction was also found in the binding site of Fluconazole and Posaconazole with a single hydrogen bond [87]. Ligand 66 also exhibits hydrophobic interactions with residues Tyr 116 (B), Ala 291 (B), Ala 287 (B), Met 460 (B), Phe 290 (B), Met 106 (B), and Met 40 (B). A capture the pose of compound 66 at the active site of the *Tc*LαD target is presented in Figure 7c. Structure 68 presents two hydrogen bonds, the strongest with the iron protoporphyrin IX enzymatic cofactor (HEM_1450 or Heme) co-crystallized in the amino acid chain B, and the other with the Tyr 103 residue (B) (Figure 7d), which is consistent with the interactions reported for this receptor with Fluconazole and Posaconazole [87]. The steric interactions that stabilize ligand 68, also present in the two azoles mentioned [87], occur with residues Ala 291 (B), Ala 287 (B), Tyr 116 (B), and Phe 110 (B). Cardoso et al. reported a hydrogen bond between their furan–naphthoquinones with the Tyr 116 residue in the binding site of this protein [88]; however, for molecules 66 and 68, the interactions with this residue are of the steric type. These same authors report cation-π interactions with the Fe of the Heme group, which were not observed in any 1,4-naphthoquinone derivative tested here.

Other structures that presented favorable interaction energies with the active site of the *Tc*LαD protein were the NQ–Amine derivatives 32 (−107.97 kcal/mol), 41 (−105.71 kcal/mol), and 46 (−106.12 kcal/mol), and the NQ–Chlorine derivatives 6 (−113.43 kcal/mol), 14 (−108.92 kcal/mol), 15 (−109.63 kcal/mol), 24 (−107.88 kcal/mol), and 25 (−108.50 kcal/mol). Among these, the lowest energy was found for the derivative substituted with an ethoxide group in the *meta* position of the phenylamino aromatic ring (structure 6), which did not present hydrogen bond interactions. The other 30 molecules did not present formation of hydrogen bonds with any amino acid residue of the active site.

2.2.2. Docking in Trypanothione Reductase, Arginase, and Aminotransferase Proteins of *Leismania* Genus

The docking evaluation of the 68 1,4-naphptoquinone derivatives in the catalytic sites of the proteins trypanothione reductase (*L*Tr), arginase (*La*A), and aminotransfera (*Li*AT) was carried out using cavities of 705, 305, and 1171 Å^3, respectively (Figure S2).

The ligand–protein interaction energies for the best pose of each of the 68 derivatives evaluated are shown in Figure 8. In all cases, the most effective interactions against the three macromolecular receptors of the *Leishmania* genus were obtained for derivatives belonging to the NQ–triazoles. Molecules 65, 66, and 67 showed the best interaction energies (−158,024, −121,516, and −121,426 kcal/mol) against *L*Tr, *La*A, and *Li*At active sites, respectively, while derivative 64 showed the second-best interaction energy (−155,221, −116,708, and −119,504 kcal/mol) in all three docking studies. Only in the case of the docking evaluation against the *La*A site (Figure 8b) did derivative 17, belonging to the NQ–Chlorine family, and derivatives 32, 33, 40, 41, and 43 of the NQ–amino family, show a better affinity interaction than member 63 of the NQ–triazole family.

These results conform with some studies of drugs used to combat parasitic diseases based on triazoles or azoles. These compounds lead to alterations in the mitochondria and accumulation of lipid bodies, thus interfering with the biosynthesis of the cell membrane [89], and leading to cell death of the parasite [90,91]. Thus, triazole-substituted naphthoquinone derivatives have potential antiparasitic activity against *Leishmania*, since they have also been shown to be a type of compound tolerable by patients [89].

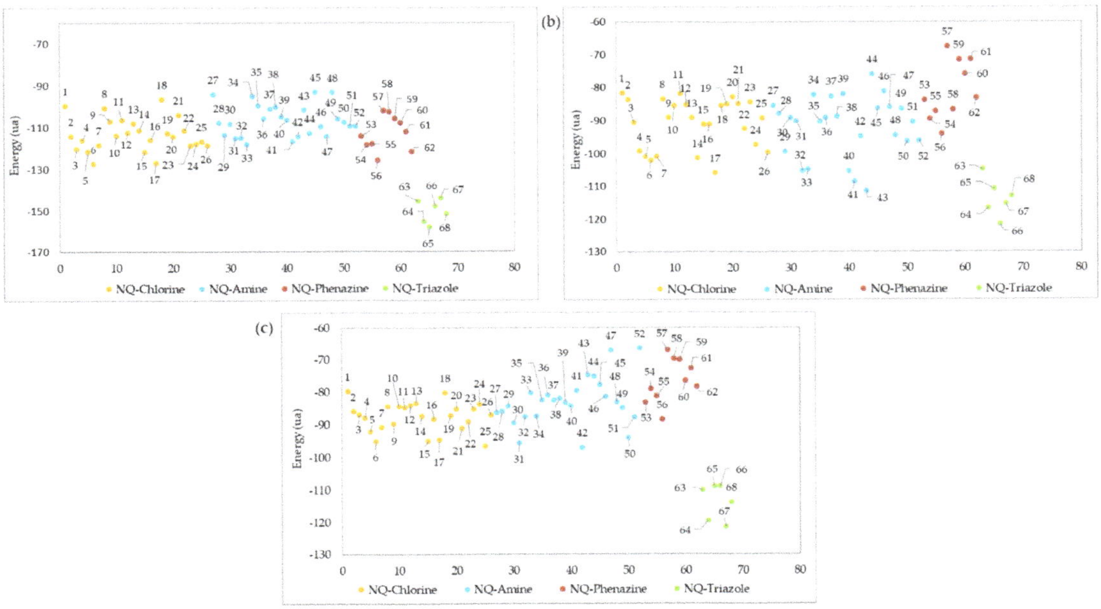

Figure 8. Ligand–protein docking energies of 1,4-naphthoquinone derivatives against (**a**) *L*Tr (Table S18), (**b**) *La*A (Table S19), and (**c**) *Li*AT (Table S20) receptors.

The two best poses adopted within the active site for each docking evaluation are presented in Figure 9. In the case of the poses of derivatives 64 and 65 against the *L*Tr protein (Figure 9a,b), both present interactions by hydrogen bonds with the amino acid residues Ser 14, Thr 335, Cys 52, and Lys 60 of *L*Tr. The two cysteine residues (Cys52 and Cys57) present in the active site form the disulfide bond in the oxidized form of the protein [92], which is a bond critical in the parasite's defense mechanism, while the interactions with the residues Thr 335 and Lys 60 are destined exclusively to the binding domain of FAD [93]. In this way, the binding of the ligands to these last residues prevents the binding of FAD and its orientation toward the active site during the reduction, which inhibits the *L*Tr enzyme [93].

The best positions of structures 64 and 66 in the active site of the *La*A protein (Figure 9c,d) presented both interactions by hydrogen bonds with residues Ser 150, Thr 148, and Val 149. Structure 64 presented hydrogen bonds with residues Gly151 and Asn 152, while structure 66 formed an interaction with residue Asn 143. In similar studies [94,95], some flavonoid ligands showed interactions with amino acid residues Ser150, Asn 152, and Asn153 within the active site, exhibited high in vitro activity against L. *amazonensis* cultures, and low toxicity in mammalian cells. Residues Ser150 and Asn143 are involved in the Mn(II) metal bridge in coordination with the active site of arginase, which is required to conduct its catalytic activity [95,96]. According to this, molecules 64 and 66 inhibit the coupling of the metallic bridge, and would be good inhibitors of the arginase protein.

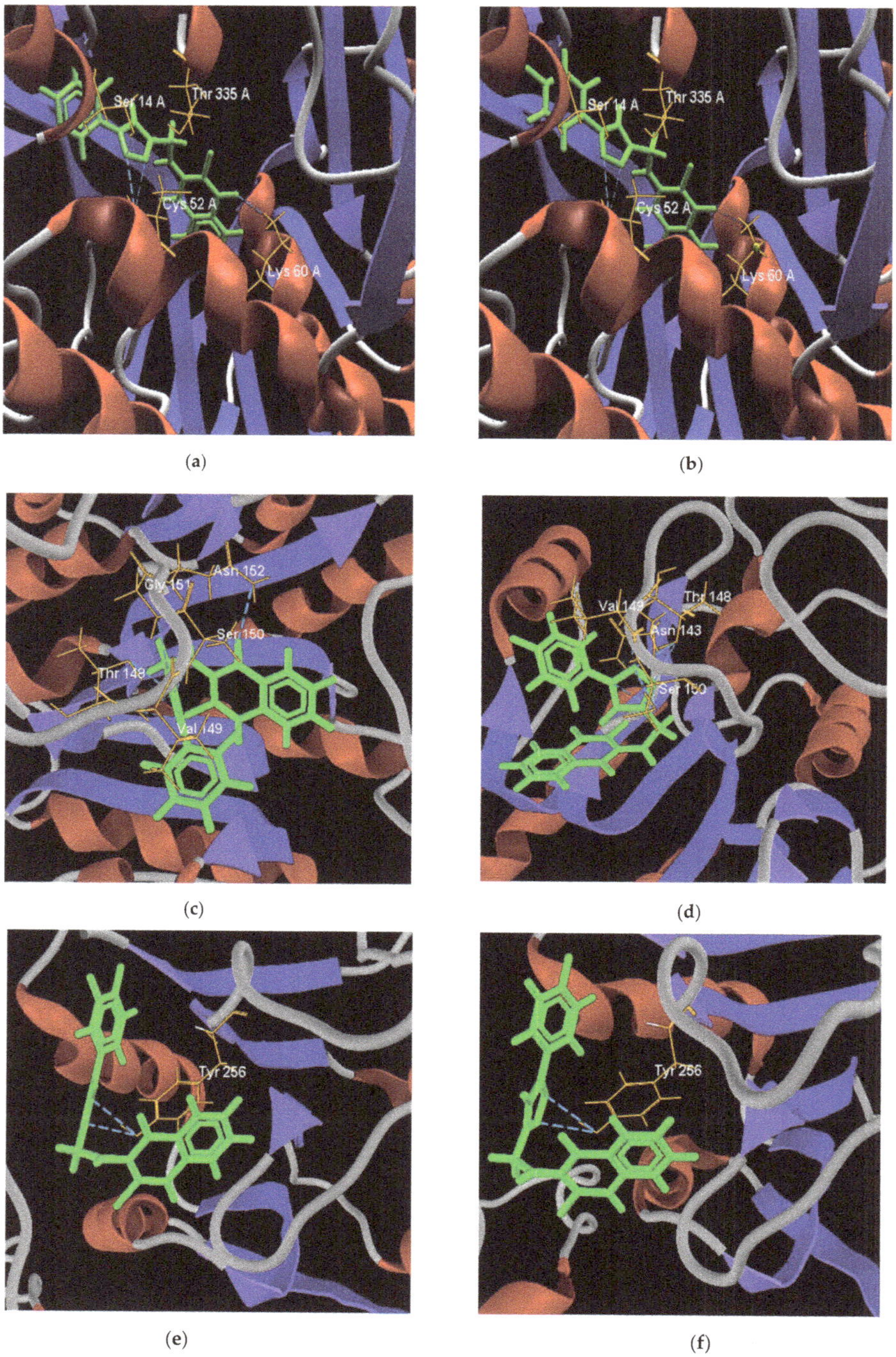

Figure 9. Best poses of derivatives: 64 (**a**) and 65 (**b**) in the active site of the *L*Tr protein; 64 (**c**) and 66 (**d**) in the active site of the *La*A protein; and 64 (**e**) and 67 (**f**) in the active site of the *Li*At protein.

The poses of structures 64 and 67 facing the *Li*At receptor are presented in Figure 9e,f. Both structures present interaction by hydrogen bonds with the residue Tyr 256. It has been shown that this residue prevents the rotation of the pyridine ring of the pyridoxal phosphate cofactor until the entrance of the amino acid, avoiding its stability [97].

2.3. ADME Analysis

Theoretical early estimation of ADME properties for the series of 68 1,4-naphthoquinone derivatives was performed in the free SwissADME web tool [98]. The data of lipophilicity, solubility, pharmacokinetic properties, and skin permeability parameters are collected in Table S21.

Figure 10 shows the estimated lipophilicity values of the 68 ligands, expressed as the logarithm of the octanol–water partition coefficient (Log $P_{o/w}$). This parameter makes it possible to determine hydrophobicity, which is a parameter considered in the initial phases of drug development, and which allows inferring how the compound will behave in biological fluids and its possible diffusion through biological membranes [77,99]. The lipophilic results show that the 68 derivatives have a Log $p < 5$ [100], so according to the Lipinski Rules, they can be administered orally [101]. NQ–Amine derivative 43 presented the lowest value (log $P_{o/w}$ = 0.49), that is, it is more hydrophilic than the rest.

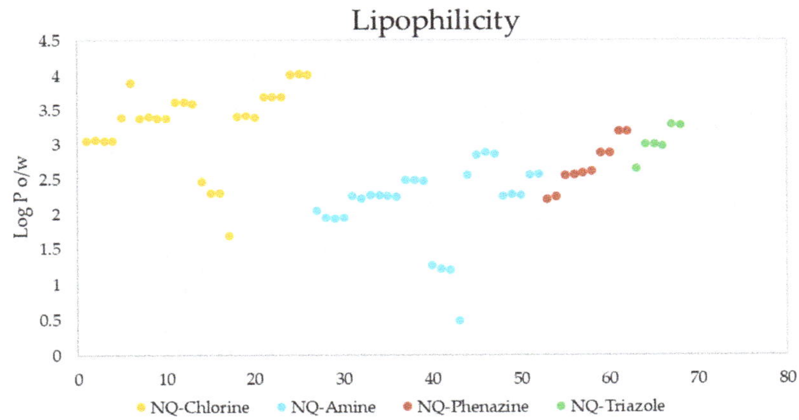

Figure 10. Lipophilicity values of the 68 naphthoquinone derivatives.

Figure 11 shows the SWISSADME solubility values (expressed as log S) of the 68 derivatives according to the ESOL (Estimated SOLubility), solubility adapted by Ali et.al., and SILICO-IT [102] methods. The ESOL method estimates the solubility in water directly from the molecular structure, followed by its weight [103]; the Ali method incorporates the effect of the topological polar surface area [104]; and the SILICO-IT method is calculated using a fragmented procedure [102]. The solubility (Log S) scales used are insoluble < -10, poor < -6, moderate < -4, soluble < -2, and high < 0. The calculated solubility data presented ESOL values of $-5.42 < \text{Log S} < -3.57$, Ali values of $-7.04 < \text{Log S} < -3.9$ and SILICO-IT values of $-8.33 < \text{Log S} < -4.28$, indicating that all 68 compounds have moderate to poor water solubility.

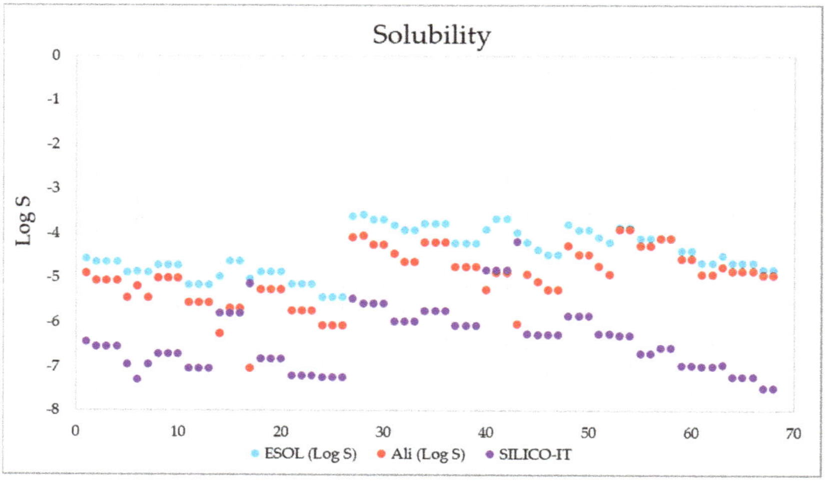

Figure 11. Solubility data (in Log S) calculated for the 68 1,4-naphthoquinone derivatives using the ESOL (blue), Ali-adapted (orange), and SILICO-IT (magenta) methods.

The evaluation of pharmacokinetic parameters of gastrointestinal (GI) absorption, P-gp substrate, and cytochrome P450 (CYP) inhibition or interaction for all 68 derivatives is presented in Figure 12.

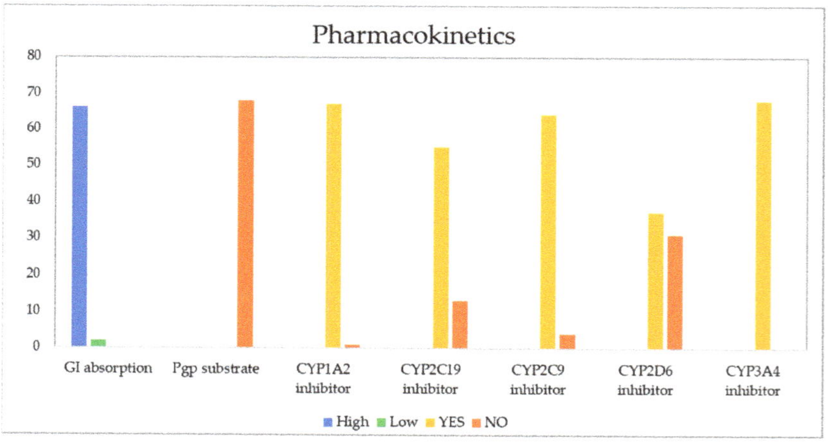

Figure 12. Pharmacokinetic properties calculated for the 68 naphthoquinone derivatives.

The GI barrier has a complex structure given the characteristics of a semi-permeable membrane, which allows fat-soluble molecules to penetrate it through a diffusion process, as is the case with most drugs [105]. As Figure 13 shows, passive human gastrointestinal (GI) absorption data estimate that 97% of the 68 compounds present high absorption in the digestive tract, while the remaining 3%, corresponding to structures 17 and 43, would present low intestinal absorption. For its part, P-glycoprotein (PGP) is a permeability protein that pumps substances out of the body and prevents their absorption, which causes drug resistance to form [105,106]. It was found that none of the compounds behaved as a substrate for P-gp; therefore, they could conduct the function without any resistance [107].

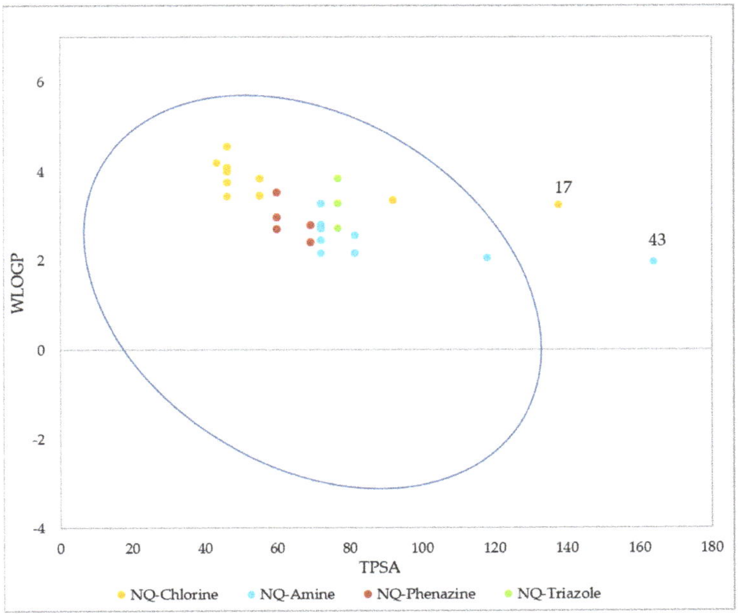

Figure 13. BOILED-Egg (adapted with permission from Ref. [108]) evaluation of gastrointestinal absorption for the 68 1,4-naphthoquinone derivatives. Molecules inside the oval indicate that they have GI permeability.

Another form of drug administration is through the skin (transdermal distribution), which allows the transport of substances through the epidermis. This parameter is related to the skin permeability coefficient (Kp), whose values indicate that the more negative the log Kp (with Kp in cm/s), the less permeant the molecule is [109,110]. Figure 14 shows the skin permeability of the 68 evaluated compounds, where it is evident that the best candidates to be administered transdermally are NQ–Chloro derivatives; among them, the best are 25, 26, and 27, while the ligand with the lowest permeability is 43.

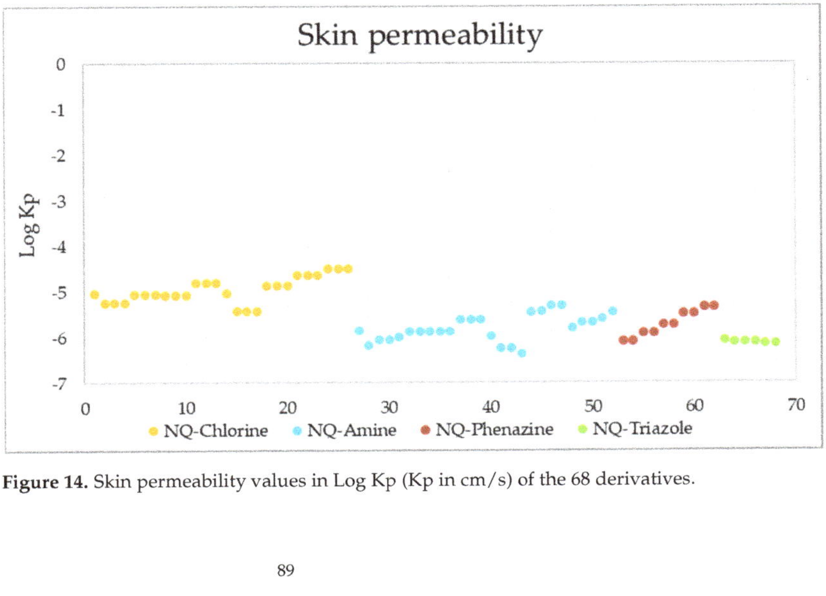

Figure 14. Skin permeability values in Log Kp (Kp in cm/s) of the 68 derivatives.

The main enzyme isoforms CYP1A2, CYP2C19, CYP2C9, CYP2D6, and CYP3A4 [98] are involved in drug metabolism, and inhibitors block their metabolic activity in a dose-dependent manner. Structure 43 was found to be the only derivative unable to inhibit CYP1A2, while 13 derivatives (36–38, 40–43, and 54–58), 4 derivatives (35–37, and 57), and 31 derivatives (11–16, 24–30, 40–43, 55–68) projected a negative inhibitory response of CYP2C19, CYP2C9, and CYP2D6, respectively. In each of these cases, the activity of the remaining molecules would be affected by their metabolism, due to their ability to bind to these enzymes, which may generate adverse effects such as high toxicity [111–113]. None of the 68 molecules reported the inhibition of CYP3A4.

Based on a similarity to drugs, filters based on Lipinski (Pfizer) [101], Ghose (Amgen) [114], Veber (GSK) [115], Egan (Pharmacia) [116], and Muegge (Bayer) [117] rules were also evaluated, as well as the bioavailability score. These filters qualitatively define the feasibility of a compound to become an oral drug candidate. The results show that 100% of the 1,4-naphthoquinone derivatives comply with the Lipinski and Ghose rules, and 98.5% comply with the Veber and Egan rules. For these last two cases, molecule 43 presented a violation, caused by a value of TPSA = 163.83 Å^2 that is above the established ranges (TPSA $\leq$ 140 and TPSA $\leq$ 131.6, respectively). Finally, the Muegge filter indicated that 90% of the derivatives present valid conditions to become oral drugs. The remaining 10% presented a violation since their XLOGP value is outside of the allowed range ($-2 \leq$ XLOGP ≤ 5) (structures 21–26), while the TPSA value of structure 43 is again above the range settled down. All compounds had a bioavailability value of 0.55, indicating oral bioavailability based on Lipinski's rules. Additionally, it was established that an AB score of 0.55 is required to be considered a sufficiently absorbable molecule orally [118].

3. Materials and Methods

3.1. QSAR Modelling

3.1.1. In Vitro Anti-Chagas and Anti-Leishmaniasis Data

All of the in vitro data used for constructing of the antiparasitic and toxicity QSAR models were taken from the literature. For constructing the anti-chagasic activity model, 153 structures derived from naphthoquinone were used, some of which were fused with triazoles and oxanes, among other heterocycles (Figure A1). All of these derivatives showed anti-*T. cruzi* activity, evaluated in vitro under the following experimental conditions. The stock solutions of the compounds were prepared in DMSO. Strain Y trypomastigotes were obtained at the peak of parasitemia from albino mice, then isolated through differential centrifugation, and resuspended in Dulbecco's Modified Eagle Medium (DME), with a concentration of 107 parasite cells/mL in the presence of 10% mouse blood. A total of 100 µL of this solution was added to 100 µL of the compound solutions. The cell count was determined in a Neubauer chamber, and the trypanocidal activity was expressed as IC_{50}, which corresponds to a concentration that allows the lysis of 50% of the parasites [23–31].

For the QSAR modeling of cutaneous anti-leishmaniasis (*L. amazonensis*) activity, 60 molecules (Figure A2) containing functional groups such as quinone, triazole, indole, and amine with high trypanocidal activity reported as IC_{50} were used. The anti-leishmanial activity of these structures was evaluated by tests with 3-(4,5-dimethylthiazol-2-yl)-2,5-diphenyltetrazolium (MTT) bromide. In these bioassays, promastigotes were seeded in RPMI medium supplemented with 10% FBS, and cultured in a 96-well plate with a concentration of 10 5 cells/plate at 37 °C. After the seeding period, the MTT solution was added, the formed complex was dissolved in DMSO, the supernatant was removed, and the cells were incubated under the same seeding conditions in the presence of various concentrations of the compounds. The concentration that inhibited 50% of parasite growth was determined as IC_{50} by linear regression [18,32–39].

For constructing the QSAR model of anti-visceral leishmaniasis (*L. infantum*) activity, 90 molecules (Figure A3) derived from quinone, triazole, and indole with activity reported as IC_{50} were used. The anti-leishmanial activity evaluation for these molecules was conducted using incubation in RPMI medium with 12% fetal calf serum (FBS), at a concentration of 105 cells/mL, for 48 h at 25 °C. After the incubation process, promastigote growth was estimated by counting the parasites with a Neubauer hemocytometer. The 50% inhibitory concentration (IC_{50}) was defined as the drug concentration required to inhibit 50% of the parasite growth [40–45].

The QSAR model of toxicity was built from 76 structures (Figure A4) derived from naphthoquinone, some fused with triazoles, pyrazoles, imidazoles, and aromatic rings, with experimental data measured according to the following parameters. Mouse fibroblasts (L929) were used and determined by the reduction of 3-(4,5-dimethyl-2-thiazol)-2,5-diphenyl-2H-tetrazolium bromide (MTT), expressed as IC_{50} [30,46–51].

3.1.2. Development of Antiprotozoal QSAR Models

All molecules were processed in MDL mol (V2000) format using the ACD/I-Lab software version 11.0 13 [119]. The calculation of 83,180 fingerprint-type, one-dimensional, and two-dimensional molecular descriptors was performed in the programs PaDEL-Descriptor [54], Mold2 [120], QuBiLS-MAS [56], and Fragmentor [121] (all free access). By using the balanced subsets method, the data sets were divided into calibration, validation, and test groups, using 70, 15, and 15%, for the anti-chagas activity model, 80%, 10%, and 10% for the anti-leishmanial activity models, and 70, 15, and 15% for toxicity, respectively. Subsequently, the Replacement Method (RM) [122], which is available in the MatLab programming language, was applied to explore the set of descriptors. RM is an unequivocal algorithm based on multivariable linear regression (MLR), which searches for the best subsets of descriptors in large databases. By using the RM algorithm, multivariable regression models of up to seven descriptors were generated for each model, which was carried out in the MATLAB software version 7.12.0 [123].

3.1.3. Validation of the QSAR Models

Validation of all QSAR models was performed through both internal and external validation processes. Internal validation was performed using the LOO (Leave-One-Out) validation method. For the internal validation of each QSAR model, the statistical parameters R2 LOO (square correlation coefficient of LOO) and SLOO (standard deviation of LOO) were determined. Additionally, the statistical robustness of the models was determined using randomization Y [124,125]. For its part, the external validation verified the predictive capacity, applying the methodology proposed by Golbraikh and Tropsha [78], where the correlation coefficients between the predicted and experimental properties of the compounds in the test set are estimated.

3.2. *Molecular Docking*

The structures of the macromolecular targets used for molecular docking were extracted from the Protein Data Bank (PDB). In the case of *T. cruzi*, trypanothione reductase (*Tc*TR) [86] and lanosterol α-demethylase (*Tc*LαD) [87] proteins were selected, with 1BZL and 2WUZ coding and a resolution of 2.40 Å and 2.45 Å, respectively. For the *Leishmania* genus in general, the protein trypanothione reductase (*L*TR) [126,127] with code 2JK6 and a resolution of 2.95 Å was selected, while for the strains *L. amazonensis* and *L. infantum* arginase (*La*A) [128] and tyrosine aminotransferase (*Li*TA) [129] were selected, with codes 4IU0 and 4IX8 and resolutions of 1.77 Å and 2.35 Å, respectively.

Before the molecular docking simulations, the proteins were prepared in the Molegro Virtual Docker (MVD) program [130], where bond assignment, bond order, hybridization, missing hydrogens, charge assignment, and atom tripos were performed. To validate the software and optimize the molecular docking parameters, a re-docking procedure of the co-crystallized ligands was carried out. For each protein, a cavity was created by delimiting the coupling space of the co-crystallized ligand, and the best pose (Figure 15) was selected based on the lowest RMSD value (<2) [131].

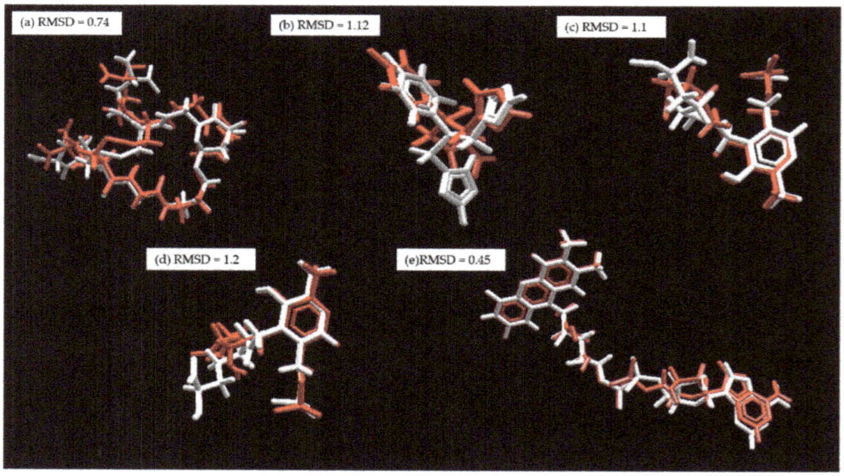

Figure 15. Re-coupling, white: co-crystallized substrate. Red: Substrate coupled using MVD. (**a**) *Tc*TR; (**b**) *Tc*LαD, (**c**) *Li*TA, (**d**) *La*A, and (**e**) *L*TR.

For the preparation of the ligands, the structures of the naphthoquinone derivatives (68) were built in the ACD-Labs program, and saved as .mol files. These structures were then optimized in the Gaussian 09W program [132] by simultaneously relaxing all geometric parameters to the theoretical level B3LYP/6–31 + G(d).

For the molecular docking simulations, 5 poses (conformation and orientation) were generated for each of the 68 ligands evaluated, using the search algorithm MolDock Optimizer, which was executed with 10 repetitions. The data analysis was performed in the Molegro Virtual Modeller (MVM) program, where the best pose in each case was selected, and the data were plotted based on the energy calculated using the scoring function (Equation (5)).

$$E_{score} = E_{inter} + E_{intra} \tag{5}$$

where E_{inter} is the intermolecular interaction energy of the ligand–protein, and the E_{intra} is the internal energy of the ligand. The E_{inter} is shown in Equation (6):

$$E_{inter} = \sum_{i \in ligand} \sum_{i \in ligand} \left[E_{PLP}(r_{ij})\right] + 332.0 \frac{q_i q_j}{4r_{ij}^2} \tag{6}$$

where the EPLP term represents the PLP (piecewise linear potential) energy, which consists of the use of two different parameter sets, described as follows: one for approximation of the steric term (van der Waals) among atoms, and the other potential for the hydrogen binding. The second term ($332.0\ \frac{q_i q_j}{4r_{ij}^2}$) is related to the electrostatic interactions among overloaded atoms. It is a Coulomb potential with a dielectric constant dependent on the distance (D(r) = 4r). The numerical value of 332.0 is responsible for the electrostatic energy unit to be given in kilocalories per mol. The q_i and q_j terms represent the charges of the atoms i and j, respectively. The r_{ij} term indicates the interatomic distance between the atoms i and j [133].

The E_{intra} is shown in Equation (7).

$$E_{inter} = \sum_{i \in ligand} \sum_{i \in ligand} \left[E_{PLP}(r_{ij})\right] + \sum_{flexible\ bonds} A[1 - cos(m.\theta - \theta_0)] + E_{Clash} \tag{7}$$

The first part of the equation (double summation) is among all pairs of atoms in the ligand, taking off those which are connected by two bonds. The second term characterizes the torsional energy, where θ is the torsional angle of the bond and θ_0 is its corresponding value in the equilibrium. The average of the torsional energy bond contribution is used if several torsions could be determined. The last term, E_{clash}, assigns a penalty of 1.000 if the distance between two heavy atoms (more than two bonds apart) is shorter than 2.0 Å, not considering infeasible ligand conformations [134]. The docking search algorithm that is applied in the MVD program considers an evolutionary algorithm, the interactive optimization techniques which are inspired by Darwinian evolution theory, and a new hybrid search algorithm called guided differential evolution. This hybrid combines the differential evolution optimization technique with a cavity prediction algorithm during the search process, thereby allowing for fast and accurate identification of potential binding modes (poses) [133–135].

3.3. ADME Analysis

The ADME study was conducted using the SWISSADME web tool of the Swiss Institute of Bioinformatics [98]. This free web tool allows you to calculate properties, such as lipophilicity, water solubility, pharmacokinetics, and drug similarity, based on the structure or SMILE of the molecule.

4. Conclusions

A total of four QSAR models based on naphthoquinone derivative structures were developed and validated, three of them for antiprotozoal activity against *T. cruzi, L. amazonensis*, and *L. infantum*, and one for toxicity prediction. All QSAR models were built using in vitro inhibitory concentrations (IC_{50}) which were previously reported. The anti-*T. cruzi* model was developed based on 153 molecules, the anti-*L. amazonensis* used 60 molecules, the anti-*L. infantum* model used 90 structures, and the toxicity model was built with 76. According to the anti-*T. cruzi* QSAR model, the anti-chagasic activity is favored by the refractivity, electronegativity, and polarizability of the molecules. These characteristics possibly give them a better binding capacity and inhibition of essential macromolecules in the metabolism of the parasite. Additionally, it was found that the presence of aromatic fragments in these structures increases their antiparasitic activity. Of the proposed molecules, structures 61 and 62, belonging to the derivatives fused with phenazine, and 24, 25, and 54, which are phenylamino derivatives, presented a better activity against *T. cruzi* predicted by the QSAR model compared to that of the reference drug. The QSAR anti-*L. amazonensis* predicts that molecules with less symmetry and with the presence of secondary and tertiary carbons will be more active. Thus, phenazines 62, 60, 59, 61, 58, and 57 showed a predicted potential activity against *L. amazonensis*, as well as derivatives 56, 27, and 26 of the phenylamine family. A total of 22 structures showed better predicted activity than Miltefosine, and 37 demonstrated better results than Glucantime. According to the anti-*L. infantum* QSAR model, the activity is a function of LogP, which is an essential characteristic for ligands to be considered drugs, since it gives them the ability to permeate biological membranes. Similarly, the activity increases with PSA, which is related to the penetration of the blood–brain barrier and its intestinal absorption. The derivatives with the best predicted anti-*L. infantum* activity were 6, 15, 7, 14, and 16, which belong to the phenylamino family. Additionally, it is highlighted that 23 molecules were more active than the reference drugs (Miltefosine and Glucantime).

According to the results of molecular docking, all the evaluated compounds present very favorable interaction energies with the selected receptors, which are essential in the metabolism of both *T. cruzi* and *Leishmania*. In the *Tc*TR protein, the derivatives fused with triazole stand out. The best of these was structure 64, which, unlike its analogs, features two hydrogen bonds between the triazole ring and the Gly 459 residue. Similarly, the triazole derivatives presented the best interaction energies for the *Tc*LαD protein. The best of them was structure 66. This derivative presents three interactions of hydrogen bonds between the triazole ring and the Tyr 103 residue, which is a fundamental residue in the active site of said receptor. The triazole derivatives 65, 66, and 67 presented the best interaction affinities against the catalytic sites of all leishmania proteins evaluated (Trypanothione reductase, Arginase, and Tyrosine Aminotransferase). These types of derivatives have a wide variety of biological activities, and according to our results, they are considered potent inhibitors of macromolecular targets. Ligands belonging to this type of molecules are currently used as active principles of antiparasitic drugs because they generate cell deformation and alterations in the mitochondria, thus interfering with the biosynthesis of the parasite's cell membrane, causing cell death.

The results of ADME showed that the 68 evaluated compounds met the requirements to be administered orally. ADME calculations included lipophilicity, solubility, pharmacokinetics, and drug-likeness.

Supplementary Materials: The following supporting information can be downloaded at: https://www.mdpi.com/article/10.3390/ph15060687/s1, Figure S1: Cavities in the active site of TcTR (a) and TcLαD (b) proteins; Figure S2: Cavities in the active site of LTR (a). LaA (b). and LiTA (c) proteins; Table S1: Antiparasitic QSAR models for chagas and leishmaniasis protozoa based on naphthoquinone derivatives obtained by the replacement method; Table S2: Toxicity QSAR models based on naphthoquinone derivatives obtained by the replacement method; Table S3: Intercorrelation matrix of the QSAR model descriptors for anti-chagas activity; Table S4: Numerical values of the QSAR anti-chagas model descriptors; Table S5: Experimental and predicted values of anti-chagas activity. Residuals and influence values h (h^lim = 0.196) are reported. ^ validation group and * test group; Table S6: Values predicted by the QSAR model of anti-chagas activity of the 68 naphthoquinone derivatives (prediction group); Table S7: Intercorrelation matrix of the QSAR model descriptors for anti-leishmanial activity; Table S8: Numerical values of the QSAR anti-L. amazonensis model descriptors; Table S9: Numerical values of the QSAR anti-L. infantum model descriptors; Table S10: Experimental and predicted values of anti-L. amazonensis activity. Residuals and influence values h (h^lim = 0.3125) are reported. ^ validation group and * test group; Table S11: Experimental and predicted values of anti-L. infantum activity. Residuals and influence values h (h^lim = 0.24) are reported. ^ validation group and * test group; Table S12: Values predicted by the QSAR models of anti-leishmanial activity of the 68 naphthoquinone derivatives (prediction group); Table S13: Intercorrelation matrix of the QSAR model descriptors for toxicity; Table S12: Numerical values of the QSAR toxicity model descriptors Table S14. Numerical values of the QSAR toxicity model descriptors; Table S15: Experimental and predicted values of toxicity. Residuals and influence values h (h^lim = 0.3125) are reported. ^ validation group and * test group; Table S16: Values predicted by the QSAR model of toxicity of the 68 naphthoquinone derivatives (prediction group); Table S17: Results of the coupling of naphthoquinone derivatives in the active site of the TcTR and TcLαD proteins. Table S18: Results of the docking of naphthoquinone derivatives in the active site of the LTR protein; Table S19: Results of the docking of naphthoquinone derivatives in the active site of the LaA protein; Table S20: Results of the docking of naphthoquinone derivatives in the active site of the LiTA protein; Table S21: ADME parameters.

Author Contributions: Conceptualization, J.A.G.C., D.L.N.G. and A.C.-C.; methodology, L.S.P.C., K.A.A.S., J.A.G.C. and D.L.N.G.; software, L.S.P.C., K.A.A.S., J.A.G.C., D.L.N.G. and P.R.D.; validation, L.S.P.C., K.A.A.S., D.L.N.G. and P.R.D.; formal analysis, L.S.P.C., K.A.A.S., J.A.G.C., D.L.N.G. and P.R.D.; investigation, L.S.P.C., K.A.A.S. and D.L.N.G.; resources, J.A.G.C.; data curation, L.S.P.C., K.A.A.S. and D.L.N.G.; writing—original draft preparation, L.S.P.C., K.A.A.S. and J.A.G.C.; writing—review and editing, L.S.P.C., K.A.A.S., J.A.G.C., D.L.N.G., P.R.D., A.C.-C. and W.E.R.N.; visualization, L.S.P.C., K.A.A.S. and J.A.G.C.; supervision, J.A.G.C.; project administration, J.A.G.C.; funding acquisition, J.A.G.C. All authors have read and agreed to the published version of the manuscript.

Funding: This research was funded by the Universidad Pedagógica y Tecnológica de Colombia (UPTC) through projects SGI2033, SGI2949, SGI3038, and SGI3188 of the Dirección de Investigaciones (DIN).

Institutional Review Board Statement: Not applicable.

Informed Consent Statement: Not applicable.

Data Availability Statement: Data is contained within the article and Supplementary Material.

Acknowledgments: The authors greatly acknowledge the financial support provided by the Universidad Pedagógica y Tecnológica de Colombia (UPTC) and Ministerio de Ciencia, Tecnología e Innovación de Colombia (Minciencias). K.A.A.S. especially thanks the Ministerio de Ciencia, Tecnología e Innovación de Colombia (Minciencias) for awarding a Young Researcher Scholarship through call 891 of 2020. P.R.D. gives thanks to Ministerio de Ciencia, Tecnología e Innovacion Productiva de Argentina for the electronic library facilities. P.R.D. is a member of the scientific researcher career of CONICET.

Conflicts of Interest: The authors declare no conflict of interest. The funders had no role in the design of the study; in the collection, analyses, or interpretation of data; in the writing of the manuscript, or in the decision to publish the results.

Appendix A

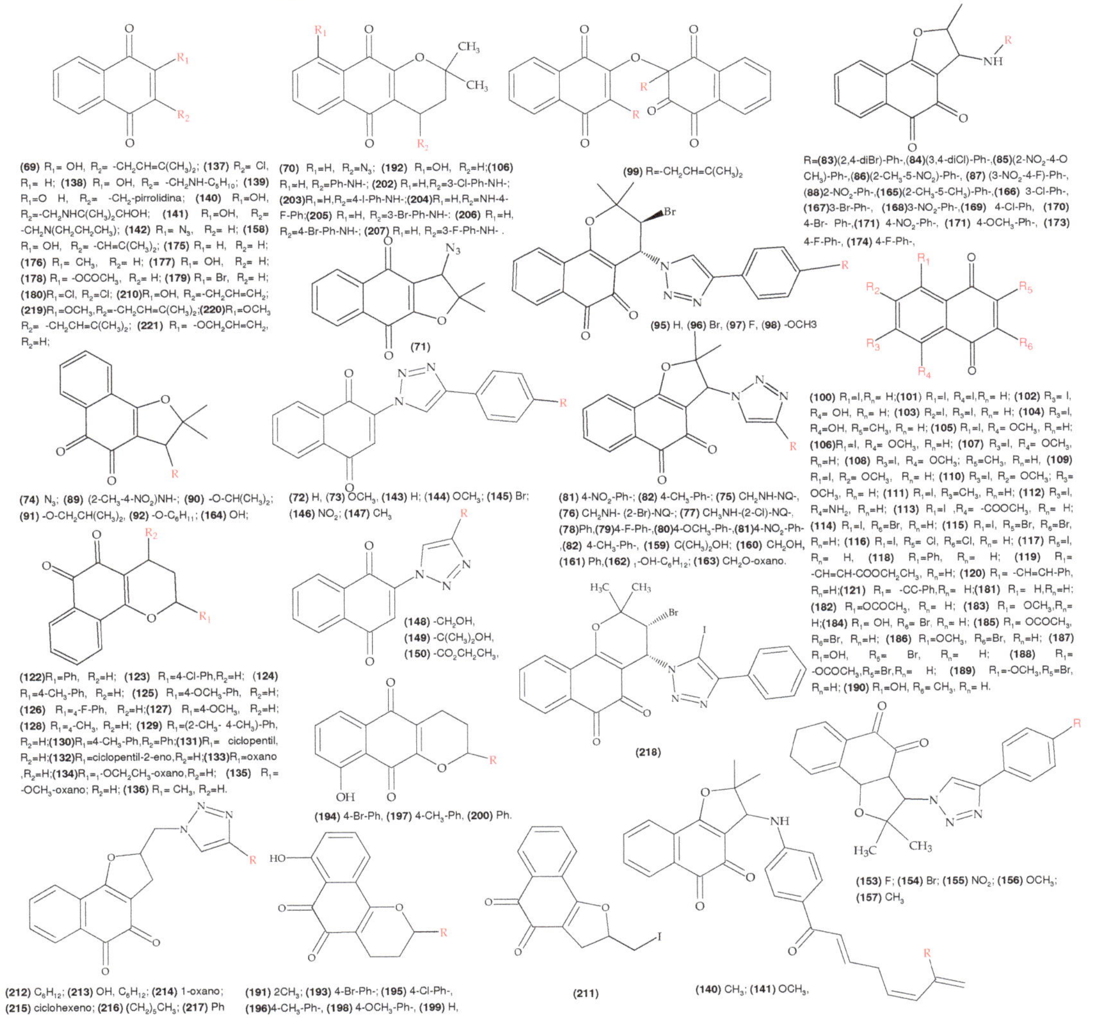

Figure A1. Molecules with reported biological activity (IC_{50}) used for the development of the QSAR anti-*T. cruzi*.

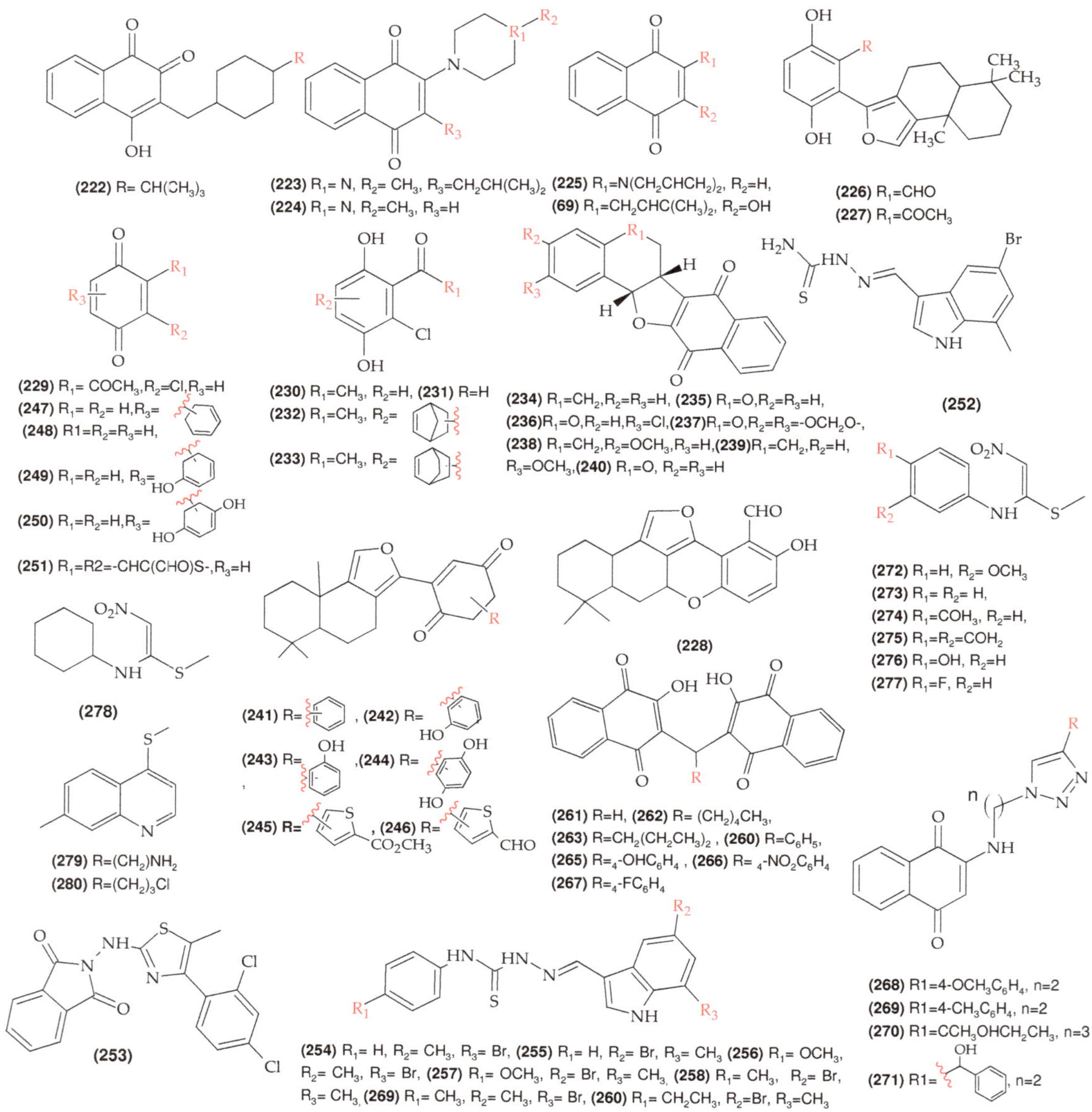

Figure A2. Molecules with reported biological activity used for the development of the anti-L. amazonensis QSAR model.

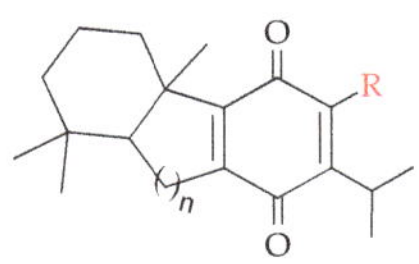

(281) R= Br, **(282)** R=-OCH_3
(286) R= H, n=2.

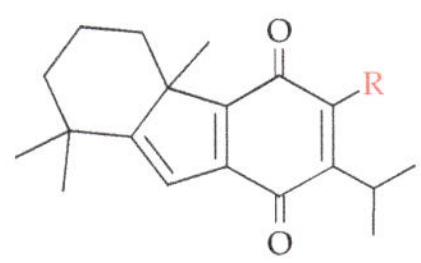

(283) R=H, **(284)** R=Br,
(285) OH

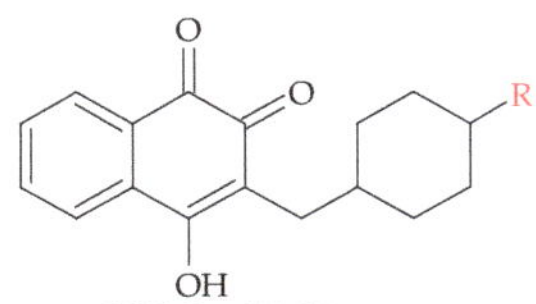

(222) R= -$CH(CH_3)_3$

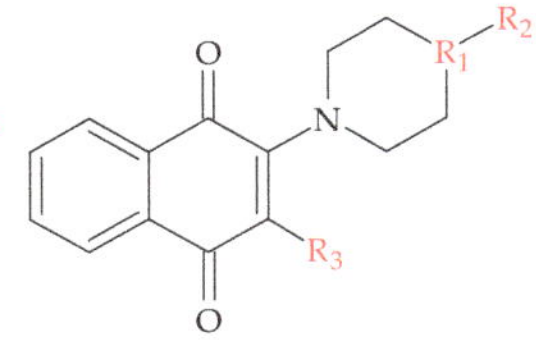

(223)R_1=N,R_2=CH_3, R_3=-$CH_2CH(CH_3)_2$,**(287)** R_1=O, R_3=H,**(288)** R_1= S,R_3=H,**(224)**R_1=N, R_2=CH_3, R_3=H

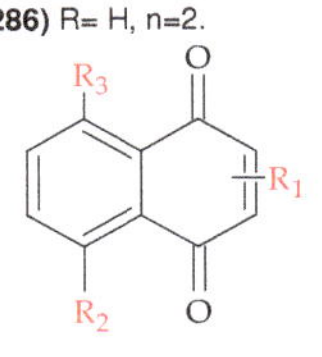

(225) R_1=3-H,2-N(CH_2CHCH_2)$_2$, R_2=R_3=H,
(289) R_1=3-H,2-$NHCH_3$,R_2=R_3=H,
(69) R_1=3-OH,2-$CH_2CHC(CH_3)_2$,R_2=R_3=H,
(290) R_1= 3-H,2-CH_3, R_2= OH, R_3= H,
(291) R_1=2-CH(Ph)$_2$,3-H, R_2,R_3=H,
(292) R_1= 2,3-diCH_3, R_2=R_3= OH,
(293) R_1= -$CH_2(CH_2)_2CH_2$-, R_2=R_3=OH,

(294) R_2=R_3=H, R_1= 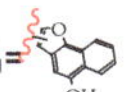

(295) R_2=R_3=H, R_1= 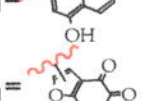

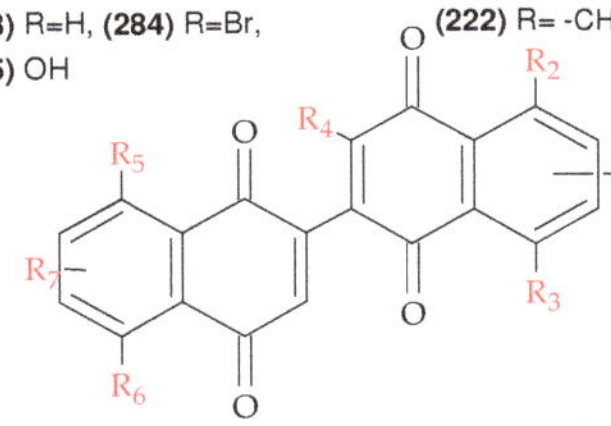

(296)R_1=-Ph-,$R_{2,3}$=$R_{5,6}$=OCH_3,R_4=H,R_7=-C_6H_4-
(298)R_1=R_3=R_4=R_5=R_7=H,R_2=R_6=CH_3,
(299)R_1=2-OCH_2CH_3, R_2,R_6=H, R_7=2OCH2CH,
(300) R1=R_2=R_4=R_6=R_7=H, R_3=R_5=OH
(297)R_2=R_6=H,R_3=R_5=OH,R_4=OCH_3,
R_1= 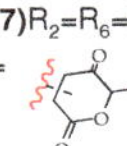 , R_7= 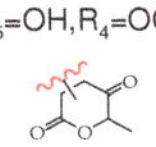

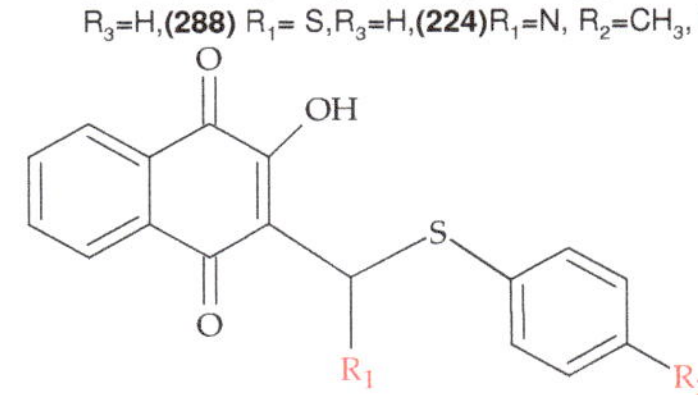

(301) R_1= R_2 =H, **(302)** R_1=H, R_2 =-OCH_3,**(303)** R_1=H, R_2=Cl, **(304)** R_1=H, R_2=F, **(305)** R_1=H, R_2=CH_3 **(306)** R_1=H, R_2=NO_2, **(307)** R_1=H,R_2 =OH

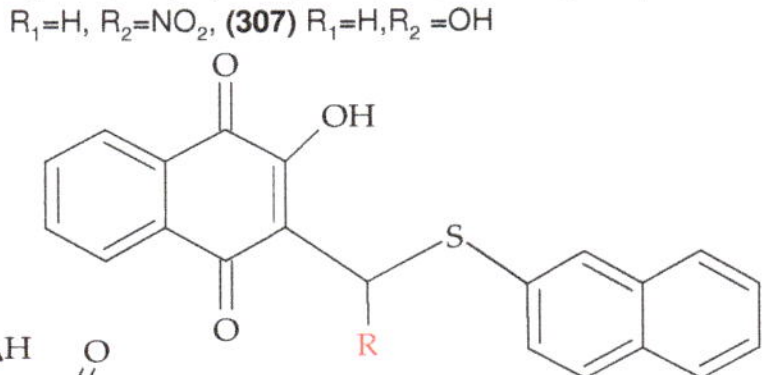

(318) R= C_6H_5

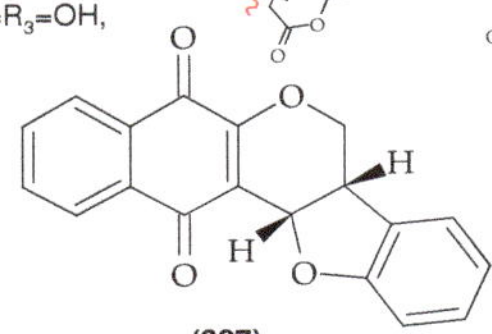

(327)

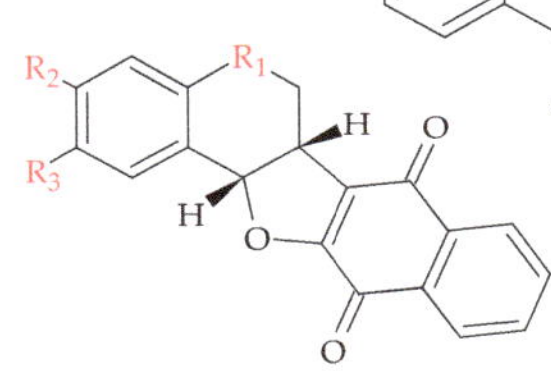

(234) R_1= CH_2, R_2= R_3 = H, **(235)** R_1= O, R_2 = R_3 = H, **(236)** R_1= O, R_2 = H, R_3 = Cl, **(237)** R_1=O, R_2= R_3= -OCH_2O-, **(238)** R_1=CH_2, R_2= OCH_3, R_3= H,
(239) R_1=CH_2, R_2= H, R_3= OCH_3

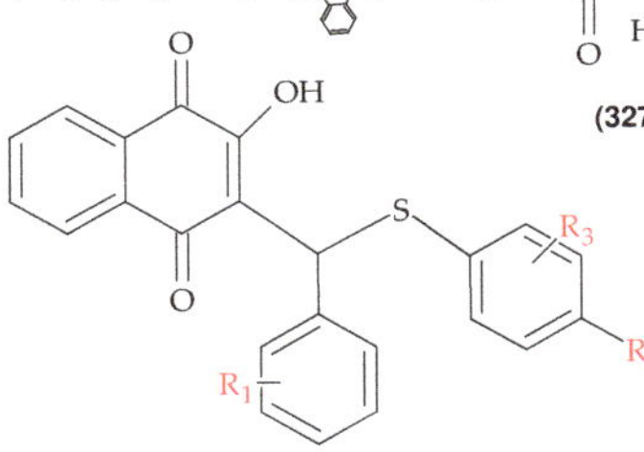

(308) R_1=R_3=H, R_2=Cl, **(309)** R_1=R_3=H,R_2=F,**(310)** R_1=R_3=H, R_2=SCH_3, **(311)** R_1=R_3=H, R_2=CH_3, **(312)** R_1=R_3=H, R_2=CH_3 **(313)** R_1=R_3=H, R_2=4-OHC_6H_4, **(314)** R_1=R_3=H, R_2=4-$NO_2C_6H_4$, **(315)** R_1=R_3=H, R_2=3-$CH_3C_6H_5$, **(316)** R_1=R_3=H, R_2=C_6H_5, **(317)** R_1=R_3=H, R_2=2-$CH_3C_6H_5$, **(319)** R_1=4-NO_2,R_2=CH_3, R_3=H, **(320)** R_1=4-NO_2, R_2=Cl,R_3=H **(321)** R_1=4-NO_2, R_2=F, R_3=H, **(322)** R_1=4-NO_2, R_2=R_3=H, **(323)** R_1=4-NO_2, R_2=SCH_3,R_3=H, **(324)** R_1=R_2=NO_2,R_3=H **(325)** R_1=4-NO_2, R_2=OCH_3 , R_3=H,**(326)** R_1=4-NO_2, R_2=H, R_3=3-CH_3, **(327)** R_1=4-NO_2, R_2=2-CH_3

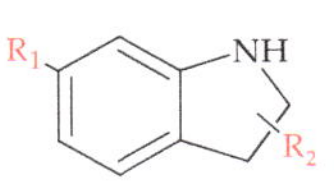

(348) R_1=H, R_2= 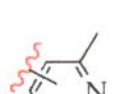

(349) R_1=OCH_3, R_2= 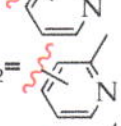

(350) R_1=OCH_3, R_2= 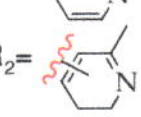

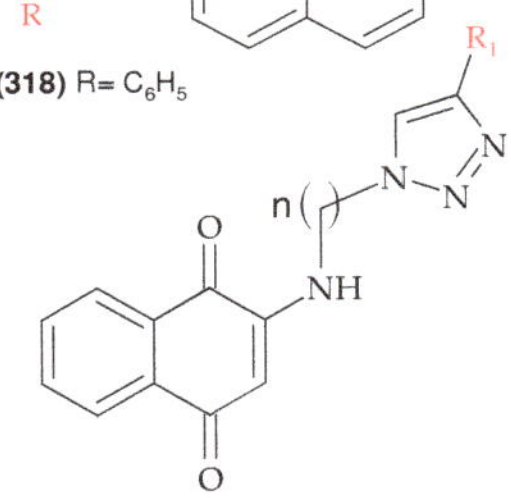

(269) R_1=4-$OCH_3C_6H_4$, n=2
(352) R_1=C$(CH_3)_2$OH, n=2
(353) R_1=C$(CH_3)_2$OH, n=3
(355) R_1=$CCH_3OHCH_2CH_3$, n= 2
(356) R_1=$(CH_2)_3CH_3$, n= 2

(354) R_1= 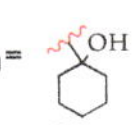 n= 2

(357) R_1= 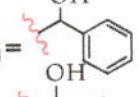 , n= 2

(358) R_1= 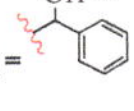 , n= 3

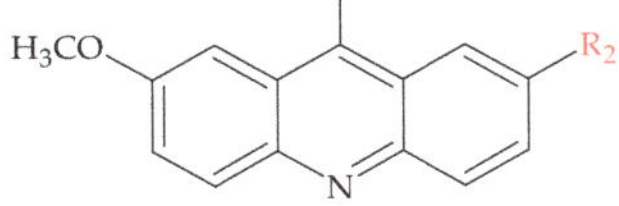

(329) R_1=NH_2, R_2=CH_3, **(330)** R_1=NH_2, R_2=-CH_2OH, **(331)** R_1=NH_2, R_2=-CH_2Br, **(332)** R_1=NH_2, R_2=-$C_4H_8O_3$, **(333)** R_1=NH_2, R_2=-$C_6H_{12}O_2$, **(334)** R_1=NH_2,R_2=-$C_7H_{14}O_2$, **(335)** R_1=NH_2, R_2=-$C_9H_{10}O_2$, **(336)** R_1=NH_2, R_2=-$C_9H_9FO_2$, **(337)** R_1=NH_2, R_2=$C_{10}H_{12}O_3$, **(338)** R_1=Cl, R_2=CH_3, **(339)**R_1=Cl, R_2=CH_3OH, **(340)** R_1=Cl, R_2= CH_3Br, **(341)**R_1=Cl, R_2=$C_4H_8O_3$, **(342)**R_1=Cl, R_2= $C_6H_{12}O_2$, **(343)**R_1=Cl, R_2=$C_7H_{14}O_2$, **(344)**R_1=Cl, R_2=-$C_9H_{10}O_2$, **(345)**R_1=Cl, R_2=-$C_9H_9FO_2$, **(346)**R_1=Cl, R_2=-$C_9H_9ClO_2$, **(347)** R_1=Cl, R_2=-$C_{10}H_{12}O_3$

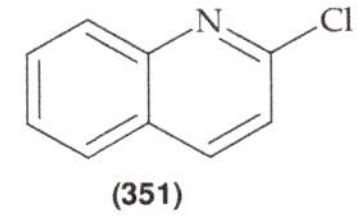

(351)

Figure A3. Molecules with reported biological activity used for the development of the anti-L. infantum QSAR model.

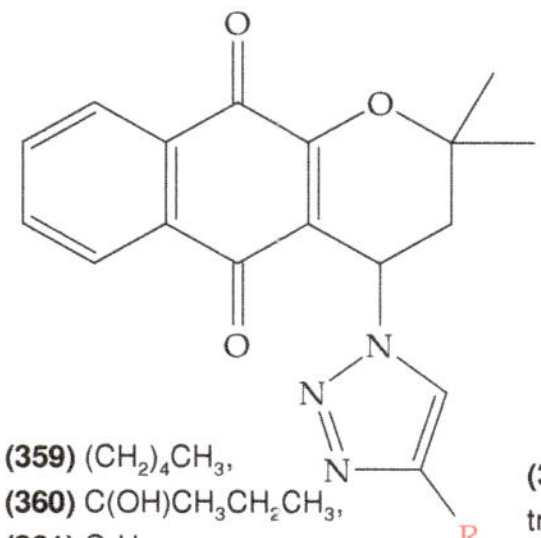

(359) $(CH_2)_4CH_3$, **(360)** $C(OH)CH_3CH_2CH_3$, **(361)** C_6H_{12}.

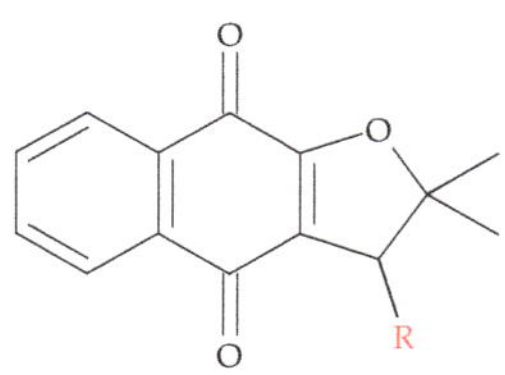

(362) triazol-$(CH_2)_5CH_3$, **(363)** triazol-Ph, **(364)** triazol-C_6H_{12}, **(375)** S-Ph.

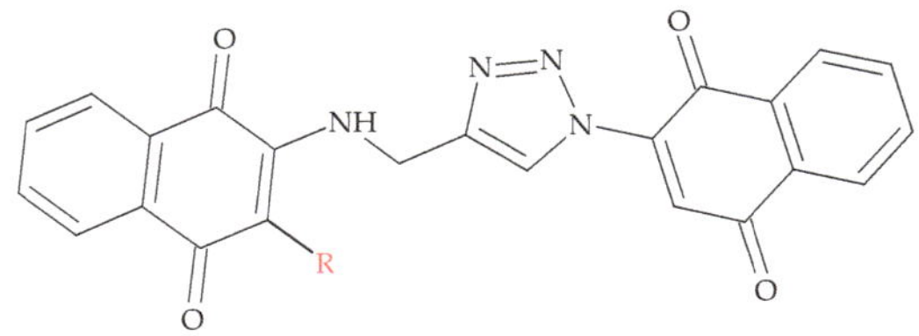

(365) H, **(366)** Cl

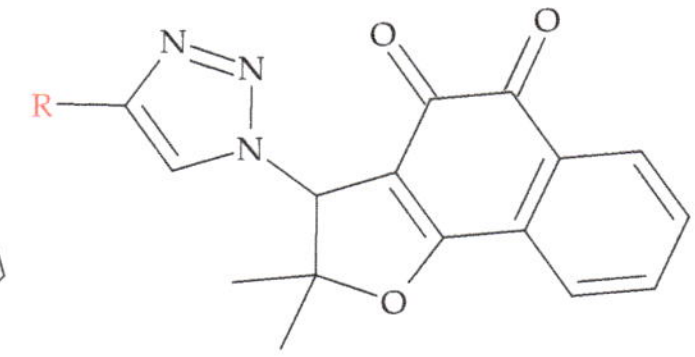

(160) CH_2OH, **(78)** Ph, **(162)** OH and C_6H_{12}

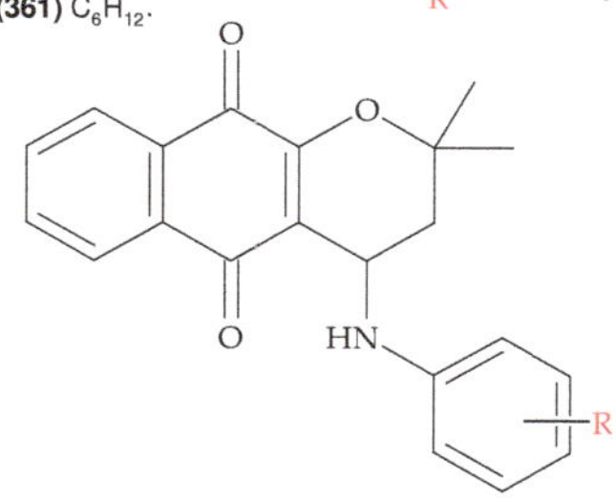

(367) 4-NO_2, **(368)** 4-Br, **(369)** 4-I, **(370)**4-Cl, **(371)** 4-OCH_3, **(372)** 3-F, **(373)** 3-NO_2, **(374)** 3-Br.

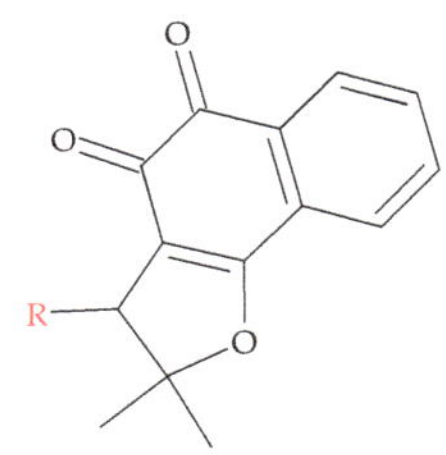

(376) N_3, **(377)** triazol-$C(OH)(CH_3)_2$,**(425)**NH-(4-F)-Ph, **(426)** NH-(4-Cl)-Ph, **(427)** NH-(4-Br)-Ph, **(428)** NH-(4-NO_2)- Ph, **(429)** NH-Ph.

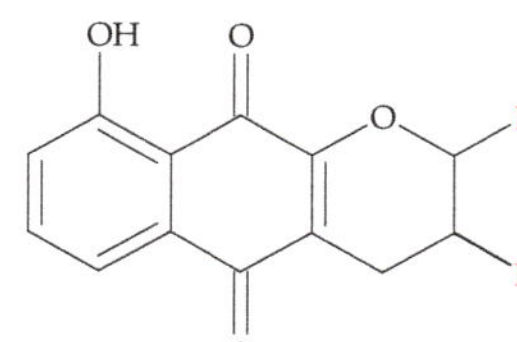

(413) R_1= 2-CH_3, R_2=H, **(414)** R_1= H, R_2=CH_3, **(415)** R_1= CH_3, R_2=H, **(416)** R_1= $(CH_2)_2CH_3$, R_2=H,

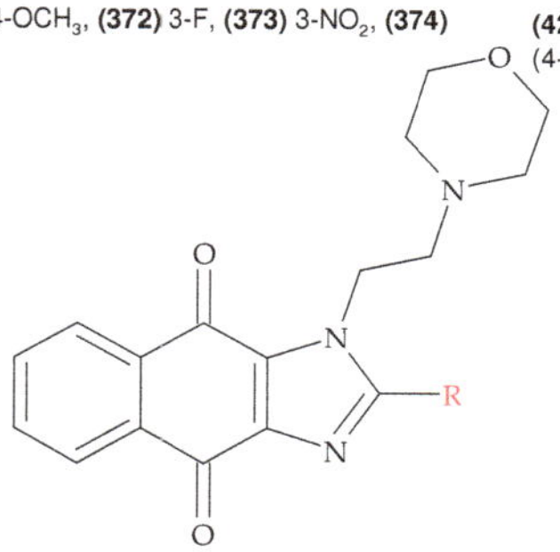

(378) CH_3,**(379)** CH_2CH_3, **(380)** $(CH_2)_2CH_3$, **(381)** $CH(CH_3)_2$, **(382)**$C(CH_3)_3$,**(383)**$C(F)_3$,**(384)**$H(CH_3)CH_2CH_3$,**(385)**$CH_2CHCH_3)_2$, **(386)**$CH(CH_2CH_3)_2$,**(387)**$(CH_2)_2$-furan-CH_3,CH_3,**(388)** C_3H_5 **(389)** C_4H_7**(390)**CH_2-C_6H_{10},**(391)**CH=CH-Ph,**(392)**Ph**(393)** naphtalene, **(394)** 2-CH_3-Ph, **(395)** 4-$(CH(CH_3)_2)$-Ph, **(396)** 4-OCH_3-Ph, **(397)** 3-Cl-4-OCH_3-Ph, **(398)** 3-F-Ph, **(399)** 3-Cl-4-F-Ph, **(400)** 3-$C(F)_3$-Ph, **(401)** (4-Cl-$_3$-$C(F)_3$)-Ph, **(402)** 1-thiophene. **(403)** furan, **(404)** 2-thiophene, **(405)**pyridin, **(406)** 2-pyridin, **(407)** 3-pyridin, **(408)** pyrazine.

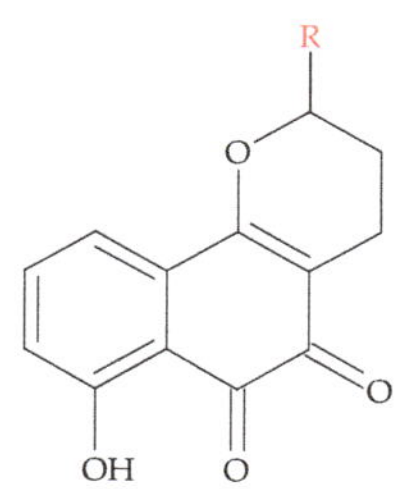

(191) $2CH_3$; **(417)** CH_3; **(418)** $(CH_2)_2CH_3$; **(193)** 4-Br-Ph;**(195)** 4-Cl-Ph, **(196)** 4-CH_3-Ph, **(198)** 4-OCH_3-Ph,**199)** H, **(201)** CH_3, Ph

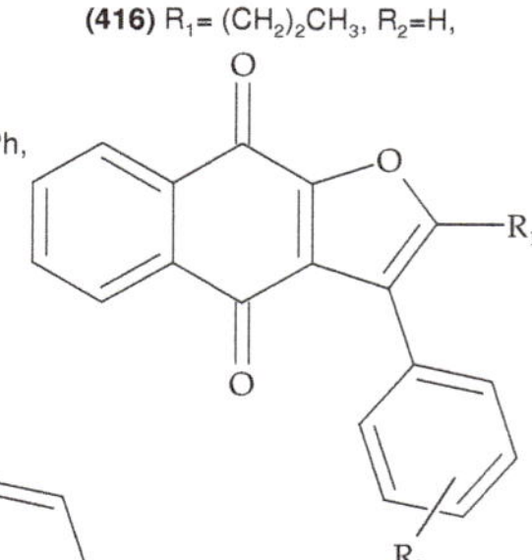

(422) R_1=H, R_2= 4-F, **(423)** R_1=H, R_2= Ph, **(424)** R_1=$CH_2COOCH_2CH_3$, R_2= 3,4-OCH_3,

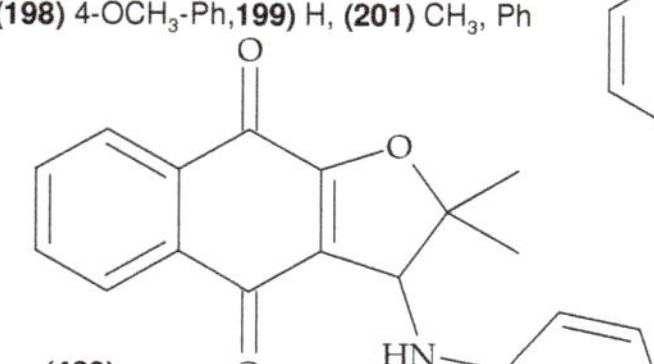

(430)

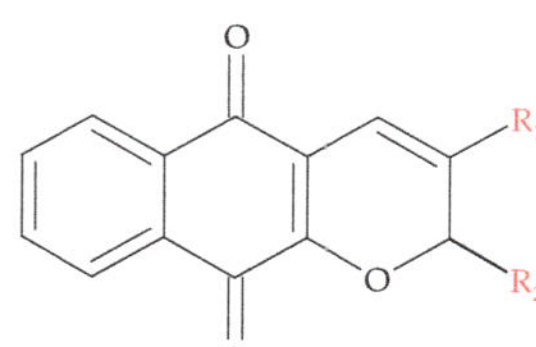

(419) R_1=CH_3, R_2=H, **(420)** R_1=CH_3, R_2= $_2CH_3$, **(421)** R_1=Br, R_2= $_2CH_3$,

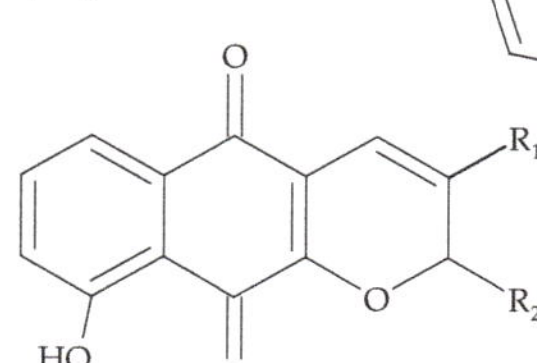

(409) R_1=H, R_2= 2-CH_3, **(410)**R_1=CH_3, R_2=H, **(411)** R_1=H, R_2=CH_3, **(412)** R_1=H, R_2=$(CH_2)_2CH_3$.

Figure A4. Molecules with reported toxicity in mouse fibroblasts (L929) used for the development of the QSAR model of toxicity.

References

1. Enfermedad de Chagas—OPS/OMS. Available online: https://www.paho.org/es/temas/enfermedad-chagas (accessed on 5 April 2022).
2. Dos Santos Naujorks, A.A.; Da Silva, A.O.; Da Silva Lopez, R.; De Albuquerque, S.; Beatriz, A.; Marquez, M.R.; Pires De Lima, D. Novel naphthoquinone derivatives and evaluation of trypanocidal and leishmanicidal activities. *J. Mater. Chem. B* **2018**, *6*, 1–3. [CrossRef]
3. Alonso-Padilla, J.; Rodríguez, A. High Throughput Screening for Anti–Trypanosoma cruzi Drug Discovery. *PLoS Negl. Trop. Dis.* **2014**, *8*, e3259. [CrossRef] [PubMed]
4. Coura, J.R. Present situation and new strategies for Chagas disease chemotherapy: A proposal. *Mem. Inst. Oswaldo Cruz* **2009**, *104*, 549–554. [CrossRef]
5. Schmunis, G.A.; Yadon, Z.E. Chagas disease: A new worldwide challenge. *Acta Trop.* **2010**, *115*, 14–21. [CrossRef] [PubMed]
6. Arias, D.G.; Garay, A.S.; Rodrigues, D.; Forastieri, P.S.; Luna, L.E.; Bürgui, M.D.L.M.; Prieta, C.; Iglesia, A.A.; Cravero, R.M.; Guerrero, S.A. Rational design of nitrofuran derivatives: Synthesis and valuation as inhibitors of Trypanosoma cruzi trypanothione reductase. *Eur. J. Med. Chem.* **2017**, *125*, 1088–1097. [CrossRef] [PubMed]
7. Urbina, J.A. Ergosterol biosynthesis and drug development for Chagas disease. *Mem. Inst. Oswaldo Cruz* **2009**, *104*, 311–318. [CrossRef]
8. Valdez, R.H.; Düsman Tonin, L.T.; Ueda-Nakamura, T.; Dias Filho, B.P.; Monrgado-Diaz, J.A.; Sarragitto, M.H.; Vataru Nakamura, C. Biological activity of 1,2,3,4-tetrahydro-β-carboline-3-carboxamides against Trypanosoma cruzi. *Acta Trop.* **2009**, *110*, 7–14. [CrossRef]
9. De Souza, E.M.; Lansiaux, A.; Bailly, C.; Wilson, W.D.; Hu, Q.; Boykin, D.W.; Batista, M.M.; Araújo-Jorge, T.C.; Soerio, M.N.C. Phenyl substitution of furamidine markedly potentiates its anti-parasitic activity against Trypanosoma cruzi and Leishmania amazonensis. *Biochem. Pharmacol.* **2004**, *68*, 593–600. [CrossRef]
10. Rolim Neto, P.J.; Luiz Gomes, C.; Wanderley Sales, V.D.A.; de Melo, C.G.; Ferreira da Silva, R.M.; Vicente Nishimura, R.H.; Araújo, R. Beta-lapachone: Natural occurrence, physicochemical properties, biological activities, toxicity and synthesis. *Phytochemistry* **2021**, *186*, 112713. [CrossRef]
11. Menna-Barreto, R.F.S.; Henriques-Pons, A.; Pinto, A.V.; Morgado-Diaz, J.A.; Soares, M.J.; De Castro, S.L. Effect of a β-lapachone-derived naphthoimidazole on Trypanosoma cruzi: Identification of target organelles. *J. Antimicrob. Chemother.* **2005**, *56*, 1034–1041. [CrossRef]
12. Menna-Barreto, R.F.S.; Corrêa, J.R.; Pinto, A.V.; Soares, M.J.; De Castro, S.L. Mitochondrial disruption and DNA fragmentation in Trypanosoma cruzi induced by naphthoimidazoles synthesized from β-lapachone. *Parasitol. Res.* **2007**, *101*, 895–905. [CrossRef] [PubMed]
13. Menna-Barreto, R.F.S.; Correa, J.R.; Cascabulho, C.M.; Fernandes, M.C.; Pinto, A.V.; Soares, M.J.; De Castro, S.L. Naphthoimidazoles promote different death phenotypes in Trypanosoma cruzi. *Parasitology* **2009**, *136*, 499–510. [CrossRef] [PubMed]
14. Silva, L.R.; Souza Guimaraes, A.; Do Nascimento, J.; Do Santo Nascimento, I.J.; Barbosa da Silva, E.; McKerrow, J.H.; Cardoso, S.H.; da Silva-Júnior, E.F. Computer-aided design of 1,4-naphthoquinone-based inhibitors targeting cruzain and rhodesain cysteine proteases. *Bioorg. Med. Chem.* **2021**, *41*, 116213. [CrossRef] [PubMed]
15. Ramos, E.I.; Garza, K.M.; Krauth-Siegel, R.L.; Bader, J.; Martinez, L.E.; Maldonado, R.A. 2,3-Diphenyl-1,4-Naphthoquinone: A potential chemotherapeutic agent against trypanosoma cruzi. *J. Parasitol.* **2009**, *95*, 461–466. [CrossRef]
16. Becerra, N.A.; Espinosa-Bustos, C.; Vázquez, K.; Rivera, G.; Paulino, M.; Cantero, J.; Nogueda, B.; Chacón-Vargas, F.; Castillo-Velazquez, U.; Rodríguez, A.F.E.; et al. Expanding the chemical space of aryloxy-naphthoquinones as potential anti-Chagasic agents: Synthesis and trypanosomicidal activity. *Med. Chem. Res.* **2021**, *30*, 2256–2265. [CrossRef]
17. Da Cunha-Júnior, E.F.; Pacienza-Lima, W.; Alves Ribeiro, G.; Daher Netto, C.; Do Canto-Cavalheiro, M.M.; Monteiro da Silva, A.J.; Ribeiro Costa, P.R.; Rossi-Bergamann, B.; Torres-Santo, E.C. Effectiveness of the local or oral delivery of the novel naphthopterocarpanquinone LQB-118 against cutaneous leishmaniasis. *J. Antimicrob. Chemother.* **2011**, *66*, 1555–1559. [CrossRef]
18. De Araújo, M.V.; De Souza, P.S.O.; De Queiroz, A.C.; Da Matta, B.; Brandao Leite, A.; Da Silva, A.E.; de Franca, J.A.A.; Silva, T.M.S.; Camara, C.A.; Alexandre-Moreira, M.S. Synthesis, leishmanicidal activity and theoretical evaluations of a series of substituted bis-2-Hydroxy-1,4-Naphthoquinones. *Molecules* **2014**, *19*, 15180–15195. [CrossRef]
19. Guimarães, T.T.; Pinto, M.C.F.R.; Lanza, J.S.; Melo, M.N.; Do Monte-Neto, R.L.; De Melo, I.M.M.; Diogo, E.B.T.; Ferreira, V.F.; Camara, C.A.; Valenca, W.O.; et al. Potent naphthoquinones against antimony-sensitive and -resistant Leishmania parasites: Synthesis of novel α- And nor-α-lapachone-based 1,2,3-triazoles by copper-catalyzed azide-alkyne cycloaddition. *Eur. J. Med. Chem.* **2013**, *63*, 523–530. [CrossRef]
20. Teixeira, M.J.; De Almeida, Y.M.; Viana, J.R.; Holanda Filha, J.G.; Rodrigues, T.P.; Prata, J.R., Jr.; Coelho, I.C.B.; Rao, V.S.; Pompeu, M.M.L. In vitro and in vivo leishmanicidal activity of 2-hydroxy-3-(3-methyl-2-butenyl)-1,4-naphthoquinone (lapachol). *Phytother. Res.* **2001**, *15*, 44–48. [CrossRef]
21. Lima, N.M.F.; Corraia, C.S.; Leon, L.L.; Machado, G.M.C.; De Fátima Madeir, A.M.; Santana, G.A.E.; Goulart, M.O.F. Antileishmanial activity of lapachol analogues. *Mem. Inst. Oswaldo Cruz* **2004**, *99*, 757–761. [CrossRef]
22. Pandey, R.K.; Kumbhar, B.V.; Sundar, S.; Kunwar, A.; Prajapati, V.K. Structure-based virtual screening, molecular docking, ADMET and molecular simulations to develop benzoxaborole analogs as potential inhibitor against Leishmania donovani trypanothione reductase. *J. Recept. Signal Transduct.* **2017**, *37*, 60–70. [CrossRef] [PubMed]

23. Kim, Y.S.; Park, S.Y.; Lee, H.J.; Suh, M.E.; Schollmeyer, D.; Lee, C.O. Synthesis and cytotoxicity of 6,11-Dihydro-pyrido- and 6,11-Dihydro-benzo [2,3-b]phenazine-6,11-dione derivatives. *Bioorg. Med. Chem.* **2003**, *11*, 1709–1714. [CrossRef]
24. Da Silva Júnior, E.N.; Diogo, E.B.T.; Dias, G.G.; Rodrigues, B.L.; Guimarães, T.T.; Valenca, W.O.; Camara, C.A.; De Oliveira, M.R.N.; Camara, C.A.; De Oliveira, R.A.; et al. Synthesis and anti-Trypanosoma cruzi activity of Naphthoquinone-containing Triazoles: Electrochemical studies on the effects of the quinoidal moiety. *Bioorg. Med. Chem.* **2013**, *21*, 6337–6348. [CrossRef]
25. Bahia, S.B.B.B.; Reis, W.J.; Jardim, G.A.M.; Souto, F.T.; De Simone, C.A.; Gatto, C.C.; Menna-Barreto, R.F.S.; De Castro, S.L.; Cavalvanti, B.C.; Pessoa, C.; et al. Molecular hybridization as a powerful tool towards multitarget quinoidal systems: Synthesis, trypanocidal and antitumor activities of naphthoquinone-based 5-iodo-1,4-disubstituted-, 1,4- and 1,5-disubstituted-1,2,3-triazoles. *Med. Chem. Comm.* **2016**, *7*, 1555–1563. [CrossRef]
26. Pinto, A.V.; Pinto, C.N.; Pinto, M.D.C.F.R.; Rita, R.S.; Pezzella, C.A.C. Trypanocidal Activity of Synthetic Heterocyclic Derivatives of Active Quinones from *Tabebuia* sp. *Arzneimittelforschung* **1997**, *47*, 21045. [CrossRef]
27. Jardim, G.A.M.; Silva, T.L.; Goulart, M.O.F.; De Simone, C.A.; Barbosa, J.M.C.; Salomão, K.; De Castro, S.L.; Bower, J.F.; Da Silva Júnio, R.E.N. Rhodium-catalyzed C-H bond activation for the synthesis of quinonoid compounds: Significant Anti-Trypanosoma cruzi activities and electrochemical studies of functionalized quinones. *Eur. J. Med. Chem.* **2017**, *136*, 406–419. [CrossRef]
28. Ferreira, S.B.; Salomão, K.; De Carvalho da Silva, F.; Ventura Pinto, A.; Kaiser, C.R.; Pinto, A.C.; Ferreira, V.F.; De Castro, S.L. Synthesis and anti-Trypanosoma cruzi activity of β-lapachone analogues. *Eur. J. Med. Chem.* **2011**, *46*, 3071–3077. [CrossRef]
29. Da Silva Júnior, E.N.; De Mel, I.M.M.; Diogo, E.B.T.; Costa, V.A.; De Souza Felho, J.D.; Valencia, W.O.; Camara, C.A.; De Oliveira, R.N.; De Araujo, A.S.; Emery, F.S.; et al. On the search for potential anti-Trypanosoma cruzi drugs: Synthesis and biological evaluation of 2-hydroxy-3-methylamino and 1, 2, 3-triazolic naphthoquinoidal compounds obtained by click chemistry reactions. *Eur. J. Med. Chem.* **2012**, *52*, 304–312. [CrossRef]
30. Da Silva, E.N.; Menna-Barreto, R.F.S.; Pinto, M.C.F.R.; Silva, R.S.F.; Teixeira, D.V.; De Souza, C.B.V.; De Simone, C.A.; De Castro, S.L.; Ferreira, V.L.; Pinto, A.V. Naphthoquinoidal [1,2,3]-triazole, a new structural moiety active against Trypanosoma cruzi. *Eur. J. Med. Chem.* **2008**, *43*, 1774–1780. [CrossRef]
31. Da Silva Júnior, E.N.; De Souza, M.C.; Fernandes, M.C.; Menna-Barreto, R.F.S.; Pinto, M.C.F.R.; De Assis Lopes, F.; de Simone, C.A.; Andrade, C.K.; Pinto, A.V.; Ferreira, V.F.; et al. Synthesis and anti-Trypanosoma cruzi activity of derivatives from nor-lapachones and lapachones. *Bioorg. Med. Chem.* **2008**, *16*, 5030–5038. [CrossRef]
32. Ryu, C.K.; Kim, D.H. The antimicrobial activities of some 1,4-naphthalenediones (III). *Arch. Pharmacal Res.* **1993**, *16*, 161–163. [CrossRef]
33. Salomão, K.; De Santana, N.A.; Molina, M.T.; De Castro, S.L.; Menna-Barreto, R.F.S. Trypanosoma cruzi mitochondrial swelling and membrane potential collapse as primary evidence of the mode of action of naphthoquinone analogues. *BMC Microbiol.* **2013**, *13*, 196. [CrossRef] [PubMed]
34. Valderrama, J.A.; Benites, J.; Cortés, M.; Pessoa-Mahana, H.; Prina, E.; Fournet, A. Studies on quinones. Part 38: Synthesis and leishmanicidal activity of sesquiterpene 1,4-quinones. *Bioorg. Med. Chem.* **2003**, *13*, 4713–4718. [CrossRef] [PubMed]
35. Valderrama, J.A.; Zamorano, C.; González, M.F.; Prina, E.; Fournet, A. Studies on quinones. Part 39: Synthesis and leishmanicidal activity of acylchloroquinones and hydroquinones. *Bioorg. Med. Chem.* **2005**, *13*, 4153–4159. [CrossRef]
36. Da Silva, A.J.M.; Netto, C.D.; Pacienza-Lima, W.; Torres-Santo, E.C.; Rosii-Bergmann, B.; Maurel, S.; Valentin, A.; Costa, P.R.R. Antitumoral, Antileishmanial and Antimalarial Activity of Pentacyclic 1,4-Naphthoquinone Derivatives. *J. Braz. Chem. Soc.* **2009**, *20*, 176–182. [CrossRef]
37. De Araújo, M.V.; David, C.C.; Netto, J.C.; De Oliveira, L.A.P.L.; Da Silva, K.C.J.; Dos Santos, J.M.; Da Silva, J.K.S.; De A Brandão, V.B.C.; Silva, T.M.S.; Camara, C.A.; et al. Evaluation on the leishmanicidal activity of 2-N,N′-dialkylamino-1,4-naphthoquinone derivatives. *Exp. Parasitol.* **2017**, *176*, 46–51. [CrossRef]
38. Da Silva, P.R.; De Oliveira, J.F.; Da Silva, A.L.; Marques Queiroz, C.; de Lima, M.D.C.A.; Sampaio Feitosa, A.P.; Araújo Duarte, D.M.; Da Silva, A.C.; Brelaz de Castro, M.C.A.; Alves Pereira, V.R.; et al. Novel indol-3-yl-thiosemicarbazone derivatives: Obtaining, evaluation of in vitro leishmanicidal activity and ultrastructural studies. *Chem.-Biol. Interact.* **2020**, *315*, 108899. [CrossRef]
39. Scarim, C.B.; Jornada, D.H.; Machado, M.G.M.; Ferreira, C.M.R.; Dos Santos, J.L.; Chung, M.C. Thiazole, thio and semicarbazone derivatives against tropical infective diseases: Chagas disease, human African trypanosomiasis (HAT), leishmaniasis, and malaria. *Eur. J. Med. Chem.* **2019**, *162*, 378–395. [CrossRef]
40. Pinto, E.G.; Santo, I.O.; Schmidt, T.J.; Borborema, S.E.T.; Ferreira, V.F.; Rocha, D.R.; Templone, A.G. Potential of 2-hydroxy-3-phenylsulfanylmethyl-[1,4]-naphthoquinones against *Leishmania* (L.) infantum: Biological activity and structure-activity relationships. *PLoS ONE* **2014**, *9*, e105127. [CrossRef]
41. Tapia, R.A.; Tapia, R.A.; Prieto, Y.; Pautet, M.; Domard, M.; Domard, M.; Sarciron, M.E.; Walchshofer, N.; Walchshofer, N.; Fillion, H. Synthesis and Antileishmanial Activity of Indoloquinones Containing a Fused Benzothiazole Ring. *Eur. J. Org. Chem* **2002**, *2002*, 4005–4010. [CrossRef]
42. Di Giorgio, C.; Delmas, F.; Filloux, N.; Robin, M.; Seferian, L.; Azas, N.; Gasquet, M.; Costa, M.; Timon-David, P.M.; Galy, J.P. In vitro activities of 7-substituted 9-chloro and 9-amino-2-methoxyacridines and their bis- and tetra-acridine complexes against Leishmania infantum. *Antimicrob. Agents Chemother.* **2003**, *47*, 174–180. [CrossRef] [PubMed]

43. Cunha Araújo, I.A.; De Paula, R.C.; Alves, C.L.; Ferraz Faria, K.; De Oliveira, M.M.; Gonçalves Mendes, G.; Ferreira Abdia Dias, E.M.; Ribeiro, R.R.; De Oliveira, A.B.; Da Silva, S.M. Efficacy of lapachol on treatment of cutaneous and visceral leishmaniasis. *Exp. Parasitol.* **2019**, *199*, 67–73. [CrossRef] [PubMed]
44. Dos Santos Faiões, V.; Da Frota, L.C.R.; Cunha-Junior, E.F.; Barcellos, J.C.F.; Da Silva, T.; Netto, C.D.; Gonçalves Da Silva, S.A.; Da Silva, A.J.M.; Costa, P.R.R.; Torres-Santos, E.C. Second-generation pterocarpanquinones: Synthesis and antileishmanial activity. *J. Venom. Anim. Toxins Incl. Trop. Dis.* **2018**, *24*, 35. [CrossRef] [PubMed]
45. Jentzsch, J.; Koto, W.S.; Al Nasr, I.S.; Schobert, R.; Ersfeld, K.; Biersack, B. New Antiparasitic Bis-Naphthoquinone Derivatives. *Chem. Biodivers.* **2020**, *17*, e1900597. [CrossRef]
46. Ramírez-Macías, I.; Marín, C.; Es-Samti, H.; Fernandéz, A.; Guardia, J.J.; Zentar, H.; Agil, a.; Chamboun, R.; Alvarez-Manzaneda, E.; Sánchez-Moreno, M. Taiwaniaquinoid and abietane quinone derivatives with trypanocidal activity against *T. cruzi* and *Leishmania* spp. *Parasitol. Int.* **2012**, *61*, 405–413. [CrossRef]
47. Da Cruz, E.H.G.; Hussene, C.M.B.; Diasa, G.G.; Diogo, E.B.T.; De Melo, I.M.M.; Rodrigues, B.L.; Da Silva Júnior, E.N.; Da Silva, M.G.; Valencia, W.O.; Camara, C.A. 1,2,3-Triazole-, arylamino- and thio-substituted 1,4-naphthoquinones: Potent antitumor activity, electrochemical aspects, and bioisosteric replacement of C-ring-modified lapachones. *Bioorg. Med. Chem.* **2014**, *22*, 1608–1619. [CrossRef]
48. Ramirez, O.; Motta-Mena, L.B.; Cordova, A.; Garza, K.M. A small library of synthetic Di-substituted 1, 4-naphthoquinones induces ROS-mediated cell death in murine fibroblasts. *PLoS ONE* **2014**, *9*, e106828. [CrossRef]
49. Liu, Z.; Zhang, Z.; Zhang, W.; Yan, D. 2-Substituted-1-(2-morpholinoethyl)-1H-naphtho [2,3-d]imidazole-4,9-diones: Design, synthesis and antiproliferative activity. *Bioorg. Med. Chem. Lett.* **2018**, *28*, 2454–2458. [CrossRef]
50. Baiju, T.V.; Almeida, R.G.; Sivanandam, S.T.; De Simone, C.A.; Brito, L.M.; Cavalcanti, B.C.; Pessoa, C.; Namboothiti, I.N.N.; Da Silva Júnior, E.N. Quinonoid compounds via reactions of lawsone and 2-aminonaphthoquinone with α-bromonitroalkenes and nitroallylic acetates: Structural diversity by C-ring modification and cytotoxic evaluation against cancer cells. *Eur. J. Med. Chem.* **2018**, *151*, 686–704. [CrossRef]
51. Da Silva Júnior, E.N.; De Souza, M.C.B.V.; Pinto, A.V.; Pinto, C.C.; Goulart, M.O.F.; Barros, F.W.A.; Pessoa, C.; Costa-Lotufo, L.V.; Montenegro, R.C.; de Moraes, M.O.; et al. Synthesis and potent antitumor activity of new arylamino derivatives of nor-β-lapachone and nor-α-lapachone. *Bioorg. Med. Chem.* **2007**, *15*, 7035–7041. [CrossRef]
52. Hoffmann, R.; Minkin, V.I.; Carpenter, B.K. Ockham's Razor and chemistry. *Int. J. Philos. Chem.* **1997**, *3*, 3–28. [CrossRef]
53. Laboratoire de Chemoinformatique. Available online: http://infochim.u-strasbg.fr/spip.php?rubrique41 (accessed on 29 August 2021).
54. Wei Yap, C. PaDEL-Descriptor: An Open Source Software to Calculate Molecular Descriptors and Fingerprints. *J. Comput. Chem.* **2010**, *31*, 671–690. [CrossRef]
55. Durant, J.L.; Leland, B.A.; Henry, D.R.; Nourse, J.G. Reoptimization of MDL keys for use in drug discovery. *J. Chem. Inf. Model.* **2002**, *42*, 1273–1280. [CrossRef] [PubMed]
56. Martiní, J.R.V.; Ponce, Y.M.; Jacas, C.R.G.; Mayorga, K.M. QuBiLS—MAS, open source multi—platform software for atom-and bond-based topological descriptors computations. *J. Cheminform.* **2017**, *9*, 35. [CrossRef] [PubMed]
57. Ghose, A.K.; Crippen, G.M. Atomic Physicochemical Parameters for Three-Dimensional-Structure-Directed Quantitative Structure-Activity Relationships. 2. Modeling Dispersive and Hydrophobic Interactions. *J. Chem. Inf. Comput. Sci.* **1987**, *27*, 21–35. [CrossRef] [PubMed]
58. Klekota, J.; Roth, F.P. Chemical substructures that enrich for biological activity. *Bioinformatics* **2008**, *24*, 2518–2525. [CrossRef]
59. Martínez, M.J.; Ponzoni, I.; Díaz, M.F.; Vazquez, G.E.; Soto, A.J. Visual analytics in cheminformatics: User—supervised descriptor selection for QSAR methods. *J. Cheminform.* **2015**, *7*, 39. [CrossRef]
60. Garro Martinez, J.C.; Andrada, M.F.; Vega-Hissi, E.G.; Garibotto, F.M.; Nogueras, M.; Rodríguez, R.; Cobo, J.; Enriz, R.D.; Estrada, M.R. Dihydrofolate reductase inhibitors: A quantitative structure—activity relationship study using 2D-QSAR and 3D-QSAR methods. *Med. Chem. Res.* **2016**, *26*, 247–261. [CrossRef]
61. Insubria QSAR PaDEL-Descriptor Model for Prediction of Endocrine Disruptors Chemicals (EDC) Estrogen Receptor (ER)-Binding Affinity. Available online: http://padel.nus.edu.sg/software/padeldescriptor/index.html (accessed on 5 October 2021).
62. Samuelson, J. Why Metronidazole Is Active against both Bacteria and Parasites. *ASM* **1999**, *43*, 1533–1541. [CrossRef]
63. Cardoso-Silva, J.; Papadatos, G.; Papageorgiou, L.G.; Tsoka, S. Optimal Piecewise Linear Regression Algorithm for QSAR Modelling. *Mol. Inform.* **2019**, *38*, 1800028. [CrossRef]
64. Thurston, B.A.; Ferguson, A.L. Machine learning and molecular design of self-assembling-conjugated oligopeptides. *Mol. Simul.* **2018**, *44*, 930–945. [CrossRef]
65. Ibrahum, Z.Y.; Uzairu, A.; Shallangwa, G.; Abechi, S. Theoretical design of novel antimalarial agents against P. falciparum strain, Dd2 through the QSAR modeling of synthesized 2′-substituted triclosan derivatives. *Heliyon* **2020**, *6*, e05032. [CrossRef] [PubMed]
66. García-Jacas, C.R.; Barigye, S.J.; Marrero-Ponce, Y.; Acevedo-Martínez, L.; Valdés-Martiní, J.R.; Contreras-Torres, E. QuBiLS-MIDAS: A Parallel Free-Software for Molecular Descriptors Computation Based on Multilinear Algebraic Maps. *J. Comput. Chem.* **2014**, *35*, 1395–1409. [CrossRef] [PubMed]
67. Ghose, A.K.; Viswanadhan, V.N.; Wendoloski, J.J. Prediction of Hydrophobic (Lipophilic) Properties of Small Organic Molecules Using Fragmental Methods: An Analysis of ALOGP and CLOGP Methods. *J. Phys. Chem.* **1998**, *5639*, 3762–3772. [CrossRef]

68. Lanez, T.; Ahmedi, R. AlogP calculation of octanol-water partition coefficient of ferrocene derivatives. *Int. J. Pharm.Tech. Res.* **2015**, *8*, 408–414. [CrossRef]
69. Prasanna, S.; Doerksen, R.J. Topological Polar Surface Area: A Useful Descriptor in 2D-QSAR. *Curr. Med. Chem.* **2009**, *16*, 21–41. [CrossRef]
70. Organisation de Coopération et de Développement Economiques. *Guidance Document on the Validation of (Quantitative)Structure-Activity Relationships [(Q)SAR] Models*; OECD: Paris, France, 2007.
71. Ciubotariu, D.; Medeleanu, M.; Vlaia, V.; Olariu, T.; Ciubotariu, C.; Dragos, D.; Corina, S. Molecular van der Waals Space and Topological Indices from the Distance Matrix. *Molecules* **2004**, *9*, 1053–1078. [CrossRef]
72. Andrew, G.; Pablo, R. *Chemometrics Applocations and Research QSAR in Medicinal Chemistry*, 1st ed.; Appe Academic Press: Burlington, ON, Canada; Cambridge, MA, USA, 2016; pp. 366–381.
73. Fernandes, J.; Gattass, C.R. Topological polar surface area defines substrate transport by multidrug resistance associated protein 1 (MRP1/ABCC1). *J. Med. Chem* **2009**, *52*, 1214–1218. [CrossRef]
74. Gozalbes, R.; Doucet, J.P.; Derouin, F. Application of Topological Descriptors in QSAR and Drug Design: History and New Trends. *Curr. Drug Targets Infect. Disord.* **2002**, *2*, 93–102. [CrossRef]
75. Tandon, H.; Ranjan, P.; Chakraborty, T.; Suhag, V. Polarizability: A promising descriptor to study chemical–biological interactions. *Mol. Divers.* **2021**, *25*, 249–262. [CrossRef]
76. Putz, M.V.; Ionaşcu, C.; Putz, A.M.; Ostafe, V. Alert-QSAR. Implications for electrophilic theory of chemical carcinogenesis. *Int. J. Mol. Sci.* **2011**, *12*, 5098–5134. [CrossRef] [PubMed]
77. Bhal, S.K.; Kassam, K.; Peirson, I.G.; Pearl, G.M. The rule of five revisited: Applying log D in place of log P in drug-likeness filters. *Mol. Pharm.* **2007**, *4*, 556–560. [CrossRef] [PubMed]
78. Golbraikh, A.; Tropsha, A. Beware of q 2! *J. Mol. Graph. Model.* **2002**, *20*, 269–276. [CrossRef]
79. Nossa, D.L.; Rozo Núñez, W.E.; Gómez Castaño, J.A.; Duchowicz, P.R. Antiprotozoal QSAR modelling for trypanosomiasis (Chagas disease) based on thiosemicarbazone and thiazole derivatives. *J. Mol. Graph. Model.* **2021**, *103*, 107821. [CrossRef] [PubMed]
80. Roy, K. On some aspects of validation of predictive quantitative structure—Activity relationship models. *Drug Discov.* **2007**, *2*, 1567–1578. [CrossRef] [PubMed]
81. López López, L.I.; Nery Flores, S.D.; Silva Belmares, S.Y.; Sáenz Galindo, A. Naphthoquinones: Biological properties and synthesis of lawsone and derivatives—A structured review. *Vitae* **2014**, *21*, 248–258.
82. Rodrigues Coura, J.; De Castro, S.L. A critical review on chagas disease chemotherapy. *Mem. Inst. Oswaldo Cruz* **2002**, *97*, 3–24. [CrossRef]
83. Silva, R.S.F.; De Amorim, M.B.C.; Pinto, F.R.; Emery, F.S.; Goulart, M.O.F.; Pinto, A.V. Chemoselective Oxidation of Benzophenazines by m-CPBA: N-Oxidation vs. Oxidative Cleavage. *J. Braz. Chem. Soc.* **2007**, *18*, 759–764. [CrossRef]
84. Pacheco, P.A.F.; Galvão, R.M.S.; Faria, A.F.M.; Von Ranke, N.I.; Rangel, M.S.; Ribeiro, T.M.; Bello, M.I.; Rodrigues, C.R.; Ferreira, V.F.; Da Rocha, D.R.; et al. 8-Hydroxy-2-(1H-1,2,3-triazol-1-yl)-1,4-naphtoquinone derivatives inhibited P2X7 Receptor-Induced dye uptake into murine Macrophages. *Bioorg. Med. Chem.* **2019**, *27*, 1449–1455. [CrossRef]
85. Chacón-Vargas, K.F.; Nogueda-Torres, B.; Sánchez-Torres, L.E.; Suarez-Contreras, E.; Villalobos-Rocha, J.C.; Torres-Martinez, Y.; Lara-Ramirez, E.E.; Fiorani, G.; Krauth-Siegel, R.L.; Bolognesi, M.L.; et al. Trypanocidal activity of quinoxaline 1,4 Di-N-oxide derivatives as trypanothione reductase inhibitors. *Molecules* **2017**, *22*, 220. [CrossRef]
86. Bond, C.S.; Zhang, Y.; Berriman, M.; Cunningham, M.L.; Fairlamb, A.H.; Hunter, W.N. Crystal structure of Trypanosoma cruzi trypanothione reductase in complex with trypanothione, and the structure-based discovery of new natural product inhibitors. *Structure* **1999**, *7*, 81–89. [CrossRef]
87. Chen, C.K.; Leung, S.F.; Guilbert, C.; Jacobson, M.P.; Mckerrow, J.H.; Podust, L.M. Structural characterization of CYP51 from Trypanosoma cruzi and Trypanosoma brucei bound to the antifungal drugs posaconazole and fluconazole. *PLoS Negl. Trop. Dis.* **2010**, *4*, e651. [CrossRef] [PubMed]
88. Cardoso, M.F.C.; Forezi, L.S.M.; De Souza, A.S.; Faria, A.F.M.; Galvão, R.M.S.; Bello, M.L.; Da Silva, F.C.; Faria, R.X.; Ferreira, V.F. Tandem Synthesis of Furanaphthoquinones via Enamines and Evaluation of Their Antiparasitic Effects against Trypanosoma cruzi. *J. Braz. Chem. Soc.* **2022**, *33*, 238–250. [CrossRef]
89. Inacio Filho, J.D. Estudo do Efeito da EGCG In Vitro e In Vivo, Suas Associações e Mecanismo Molecular de Ação em Leishmania Infantum. Ph.D. Thesis, Fundação Oswaldo Cruz, Rios de Janeiro, Brazil, 2018.
90. Reynolds, K.A. Design and Synthesis of Quinoline, Cinchona Alkaloids and Other Potential Inhibitors or Leishmaniasis. Ph.D. Thesis, Griffith University, Brisbane, Australia, 2012.
91. Braga, S.S. Multi-target drugs active against leishmaniasis: A paradigm of drug repurposing. *Eur. J. Med. Chem.* **2019**, *183*, 111660. [CrossRef] [PubMed]
92. Ilari, A.; Baiocco, P.; Messori, L.; Fiorillo, A.; Boffi, A.; Gramiccia, M.; Di Muccio, T.; Colotti, G. A gold-containing drug against parasitic polyamine metabolism:The X-ray structure of trypanothione reductase from Leishmania infantum in complex with auranofin reveals a dual mechanism of enzyme inhibition. *Amino Acids* **2012**, *42*, 803–811. [CrossRef]
93. Venkatesan, S.K.; Shukla, A.K.; Dubey, V.K. Molecular Docking Studies of Selected Tricyclic and Quinone Derivatives on Trypanothione Reductase of Leishmania infantum. *J. Comp. Chem.* **2010**, *32*, 174–182. [CrossRef]

94. Manjolin, L.C.; Dos Reis, M.B.G.; Do Carmo Maquiaveli, C.; Santos-Filho, O.A.; Da Silva, E.R. Dietary flavonoids fisetin, luteolin and their derived compounds inhibit arginase, a central enzyme in Leishmania (Leishmania) amazonensis infection. *Food Chem.* **2013**, *141*, 2253–2262. [CrossRef]
95. De Lima, E.C.; Castelo-Branco, F.S.; Maquiaveli, C.C.; Farias, A.B.; Rennó, M.N.; Boechat, N.; Silva, E.R. Phenylhydrazides as inhibitors of Leishmania amazonensis arginase and antileishmanial activity. *Bioorg. Med. Chem.* **2019**, *27*, 3853–3859. [CrossRef]
96. Kanyo, Z.F.; Scolnick, L.R.; Ash, D.E.; Christianson, D.W. Structure of unique binuclear manganese cluster in arginase. *Lett. Nat.* **1996**, *383*, 554–557. [CrossRef]
97. Estrada, E.; Molina, E. Novel local (fragment-based) topological molecular descriptors for QSPR / QSAR and molecular design. *J. Mol. Graph. Model.* **2001**, *20*, 54–64. [CrossRef]
98. Daina, A.; Michielin, O.; Zoete, V. SwissADME: A free web tool to evaluate pharmacokinetics, drug-likeness and medicinal chemistry friendliness of small molecules. *Sci. Rep.* **2017**, *7*, 42717. [CrossRef] [PubMed]
99. Zafar, F.; Gupta, A.; Thangavel, K.; Khayana, K.; Sani, A.A.; Ghosal, A.; Tandon, P.; Nishat, N. Physicochemical and Pharmacokinetic Analysis of Anacardic Acid Derivatives. *ACS Omega* **2020**, *5*, 6021–6030. [CrossRef] [PubMed]
100. Bhal, S.K. *Advanced Chemistry Development (ACD/LABS). Log P—Making Sense of the Value*; Advanced Chemistry Development: Toronto, ON, Canada, 2007.
101. Lipinski, C.A.; Lombardo, F.; Dominy, B.W.; Feeney, P.J. Experimental and computational approaches to estimate solubility and permeability in drug discovery and development settings. *Adv. Drug Deliv. Rev.* **2012**, *64*, 4–17. [CrossRef]
102. Mahanthesh, M.T.; Ranjith, D.; Raghavendra, Y.; Jyothi, R.; Narappa, G.; Ravi, M.V. Swiss ADME prediction of phytochemicals present in *Butea monosperma* (Lam.) Taub. *J. Pharmacogn. Phytochem.* **2020**, *9*, 1799–1809.
103. Delaney, J.S. ESOL: Estimating aqueous solubility directly from molecular structure. *J. Chem. Inf. Comput. Sci.* **2004**, *44*, 1000–1005. [CrossRef]
104. Ali, P.; Camilleri, P.; Brown, M.B.; Hutt, A.J.; Kirton, S.B. Revisiting the general solubility equation: In silico prediction of aqueous solubility incorporating the effect of topographical polar surface area. *J. Chem. Inf. Model.* **2012**, *52*, 420–428. [CrossRef]
105. Löbenberg, R.; Amidon, G.L.; Ferraz, H.G.; Bou-Chacra, N. Mechanism of gastrointestinal drug absorption and application in therapeutic drug delivery. In *Therapeutic Delivery Methods: A Concise Overview of Emerging Areas*; Future Science Ltd.: London, UK, 2013; pp. 8–22. [CrossRef]
106. Osorio, E.J.; Robledo, S.M.; Arango, G.J.; Muskus, C.E. Leishmania: Papel de la glicoproteína P en la mediación de resistencia a medicamentos y estrategias de reversión. *Biomédica* **2005**, *25*, 242. [CrossRef]
107. Finch, A.; Pillans, P. P-glycoprotein and its role in drug-drug interactions. *Aust. Prescr.* **2014**, *37*, 137–139. [CrossRef]
108. Daina, A.; Zoete, V. A BOILED-Egg To Predict Gastrointestinal Absorption and Brain Penetration of Small Molecules. *Chem. Pub. Soc. Eur.* **2016**, *11*, 1117–1121. [CrossRef]
109. Potts, R.O.; Guy, R.H. Predicting Skin Permeability. *Pharm. Res.* **1992**, *9*, 663–669. [CrossRef]
110. Ranjith, D.; Ravikumar, C. SwissADME predictions of pharmacokinetics and drug-likeness properties of small molecules present in Ipomoea mauritiana Jacq. *J. Pharmacogn. Phytochem.* **2019**, *8*, 2063–2073. Available online: http://www.swissadme.ch/index.php (accessed on 30 April 2022).
111. Jaimes-Santoyo, J.; De Montesinos-Sampedro, A.; Barbosa-Cobos, R.E.; Moreno-Mutio, S.G.; Rodriguez-Ballesteros, D.; Ramos-Cervantes, T.; Ocharán-Hernández, M.E.; Toscano-Garibay, J.; Beltrán-Ramírez, O. El Citocromo P-450. *Rev. Hosp. Juárez Mex.* **2014**, *81*, 250–256.
112. Deodhar, M.; Al Rihani, S.B.; Arwood, M.J.; Drakjian, L.; Dow, P.; Turgeon, J.; Michaud, V. Mechanisms of cyp450 inhibition: Understanding drug-drug interactions due to mechanism-based inhibition in clinical practice. *Pharmaceutics* **2020**, *12*, 846. [CrossRef] [PubMed]
113. Ogu, C.C.; Maxa, J.L. Drug Interactions Due to Cytochrome P450. *Bayl. Univ. Med. Cent.* **2017**, *8280*, 11–14. [CrossRef]
114. Ghose, A.K.; Viswanadhan, V.N.; Wendoloski, J.J. A Knowledge-Based Approach in Designing Combinatorial or Medicinal Chemistry Libraries for Drug Discovery. 1. A Qualitative and Quantitative Characterization of Known Drug Databases. *J. Comb. Chem.* **1999**, *1*, 55–68. [CrossRef]
115. Veber, D.F.; Johnson, S.R.; Cheng, H.J.; Smith, B.R.; Ward, K.W.; Kopple, K.D. Molecular Properties That Influence the Oral Bioavailability of Drug Candidates. *J. Med. Chem.* **2002**, *45*, 2615–2623. [CrossRef]
116. Egan, W.J.; Merz, K.M.; Baldwin, J.J. Prediction of Drug Absorption Using Multivariate Statistics. *J. Med. Chem.* **2000**, *43*, 3867–3877. [CrossRef]
117. Muegge, I.; Heald, S.L.; Brittelli, D. Simple Selection Criteria for Drug-like Chemical Matter. *J. Med. Chem.* **2001**, *44*, 1841–1846. [CrossRef]
118. Martin, Y.C. A Bioavailability Score. *J. Med. Chem.* **2005**, *48*, 3164–3170. [CrossRef]
119. *ACD/ChemSketch*; Versión 2021.1.3; Advanced Chemistry Development, Inc.: Toronto, ON, Canada, 2021. Available online: www.acdlabs.com (accessed on 30 April 2022).
120. Mold2_FDA. Available online: https://www.fda.gov/science-research/bioinformatics-tools/mold2 (accessed on 29 August 2021).
121. Laboratory of Chemoinformatique. 2013. Available online: http://infochim.u-strasbg.fr/ (accessed on 30 April 2022).
122. Mercader, A.G.; Duchowicz, P.; Ferna, F. Replacement Method and Enhanced Replacement Method Versus the Genetic Algorithm Approach for the Selection of Molecular Descriptors in QSPR/QSAR Theories. *J. Chem. Inf. Model.* **2010**, *50*, 1542–1548. [CrossRef]

123. Mathworks, MATLAB—Mathworks—MATLAB & Simulink. 2016. Available online: https://nl.mathworks.com/products/matlab.html%0Ahttp://www.mathworks.com/products/matlab/ (accessed on 29 August 2021).
124. Gramatica, P. Principles of QSAR models validation: Internal and external. *QSAR Comb. Sci.* **2007**, *26*, 694–701. [CrossRef]
125. Veerasamy, R.; Rajak, H.; Jain, A.; Sivadasan, S.; Varghese, C.P.; Agrawal, R.K. Validation of QSAR Models—Strategies and Importance. *Int. J. Drug Des. Discov.* **2011**, *2*, 511–519.
126. Singh, B.K.; Sarkar, N.; Jagannadham, M.V.; Dubey, V.K. Modeled structure of trypanothione reductase of Leishmania infantum. *BMB Rep.* **2008**, *41*, 444–447. [CrossRef] [PubMed]
127. Baiocco, P.; Colotti, G.; Franceschini, S.; Ilari, A. Molecular Basis of Antimony Treatment in Leishmaniasis. *J. Med. Chem.* **2009**, *52*, 2603–2612. [CrossRef]
128. Antonio, E.L.D.; Ullman, B.; Roberts, S.C.; Dixit, U.P.; Wilson, M.E.; Hai, Y.; Christianson, D.W. Crystal structure of arginase from Leishmania mexicana and implications for the inhibition of polyamine biosynthesis in parasitic infections. *Arch. Biochem. Biophys.* **2013**, *535*, 163–176. [CrossRef]
129. Moreno, M.A.; Abramov, A.; Abendroth, J.; Alonso, A.; Zhang, S.; Alcolea, P.J.; Edwards, T.; Lorimer, D.; Myley, P.J.; Larraga, V. Structure of tyrosine aminotransferase from Leishmania infantum. *Acta Crystallogr.* **2014**, *70*, 583–587. [CrossRef]
130. Molexus, Molegro Virtual Docker-Manual, Copyrigh, M. 2019. Available online: http://molexus.io/molegro-virtual-docker/ (accessed on 30 April 2022).
131. Filgueira De Azevedo, W. *Docking Screens for Drug Discovery*; Humana Press: Ria Grande Do Sul, Brazil, 2019.
132. Frisch, J.P.M.J.; Trucks, G.W.; Schlegel, H.B.; Scuseria, G.E.; Robb, M.A.; Cheeseman, J.R.; Zakrzewski, V.G.; Montgomery, J.A., Jr.; Stratmann, R.E.; Burant, J.C.; et al. *Gaussian 98, Revision A. 7*; Gaussian Inc.: Pittsburgh, PA, USA, 1998; p. 49.
133. Thomsen, R.; Christensen, M.H. MolDock: A New Technique for High-Accuracy Molecular Docking. *J. Med. Chem.* **2006**, *49*, 3315–3321. [CrossRef]
134. De Azevedo, W.F., Jr. MolDock Applied to Structure-Based Virtual Screening. *Curr. Drug Targets* **2010**, *11*, 327–334. [CrossRef]
135. Da Cunha, E.F.F.; Azevedo Martins, R.C.; Girão Albuquerque, M.; de Alencastro, R.B. LIV-3D-QSAR model for estrogen receptor ligands. *J. Mol. Model.* **2004**, *10*, 297–304. [CrossRef]

pharmaceuticals

MDPI

Article

QSAR, ADMET In Silico Pharmacokinetics, Molecular Docking and Molecular Dynamics Studies of Novel Bicyclo (Aryl Methyl) Benzamides as Potent GlyT1 Inhibitors for the Treatment of Schizophrenia

Mohamed El fadili [1,*], Mohammed Er-Rajy [1], Mohammed Kara [2,*], Amine Assouguem [3], Assia Belhassan [4], Amal Alotaibi [5], Nidal Naceiri Mrabti [1], Hafize Fidan [6], Riaz Ullah [7], Sezai Ercisli [8], Sara Zarougui [1] and Menana Elhallaoui [1]

1 Engineering Materials, Modeling and Environmental Laboratory, Faculty of Sciences Dhar El Mehraz, Sidi Mohammed Ben Abdellah University, Fez 30000, Morocco; mohamed.errajy@usmba.ac.ma (M.E.-R.); nidal_chimie@yahoo.fr (N.N.M.); sara.zerougui@gmail.com (S.Z.); menana.elhallaoui@usmba.ac.ma (M.E.)
2 Laboratory of Biotechnology, Conservation and Valorisation of Naturals Resources, Faculty of Sciences Dhar El Mehraz, Sidi Mohamed Ben Abdellah University, Fez 30000, Morocco
3 Laboratory of Functional Ecology and Environment, Faculty of Sciences and Technology, Sidi Mohamed Ben Abdellah University, Imouzzer Street, Fez 30000, Morocco; assougam@gmail.com
4 Molecular Chemistry and Natural Substances Laboratory, Department of Chemistry, Faculty of Sciences, University Moulay Ismail, Meknes 50000, Morocco; assiabelhassan2013@gmail.com
5 Department of Basic Science, College of Medicine, Princess Nourah Bint Abdulrahman University, Riyadh 11671, Saudi Arabia; amaalotaibi@pnu.edu.sa
6 Department of Tourism and Culinary Management, Faculty of Economics, University of Food Technologies, 4000 Plovdiv, Bulgaria; hfidan@abv.bg
7 Department of Pharmacognosy (MAPPRC), College of Pharmacy, King Saud University, Riyadh 11451, Saudi Arabia; rullah@ksu.edu.sa
8 Department of Horticulture, Agricultural Faculty, Ataturk University, Erzurum TR-25240, Turkey; sercisli@gmail.com
* Correspondence: mohamed.elfadili@usmba.ac.ma (M.E.f.); mohammed.kara@usmba.ac.ma (M.K.)

Citation: El fadili, M.; Er-Rajy, M.; Kara, M.; Assouguem, A.; Belhassan, A.; Alotaibi, A.; Mrabti, N.N.; Fidan, H.; Ullah, R.; Ercisli, S.; et al. QSAR, ADMET In Silico Pharmacokinetics, Molecular Docking and Molecular Dynamics Studies of Novel Bicyclo (Aryl Methyl) Benzamides as Potent GlyT1 Inhibitors for the Treatment of Schizophrenia. *Pharmaceuticals* **2022**, *15*, 670. https://doi.org/10.3390/ph15060670

Academic Editor: Osvaldo Andrade Santos-Filho

Received: 5 May 2022
Accepted: 21 May 2022
Published: 27 May 2022

Abstract: Forty-four bicyclo ((aryl) methyl) benzamides, acting as glycine transporter type 1 (GlyT1) inhibitors, are developed using molecular modeling techniques. QSAR models generated by multiple linear and non-linear regressions affirm that the biological inhibitory activity against the schizophrenia disease is strongly and significantly correlated with physicochemical, geometrical and topological descriptors, in particular: Hydrogen bond donor, polarizability, surface tension, stretch and torsion energies and topological diameter. According to in silico ADMET properties, the most active ligands (L6, L9, L30, L31 and L37) are the molecules having the highest probability of penetrating the central nervous system (CNS), but the molecule 32 has the highest probability of being absorbed by the gastrointestinal tract. Molecular docking results indicate that Tyr124, Phe43, Phe325, Asp46, Phe319 and Val120 amino acids are the active sites of the dopamine transporter (DAT) membrane protein, in which the most active ligands can inhibit the glycine transporter type 1 (GlyT1). The results of molecular dynamics (MD) simulation revealed that all five inhibitors remained stable in the active sites of the DAT protein during 100 ns, demonstrating their promising role as candidate drugs for the treatment of schizophrenia.

Keywords: GlyT1; QSAR; schizophrenia; ADMET; molecular docking; DAT; MD

1. Introduction

About 1% of the worldwide population is affected by schizophrenia as a serious neuropsychiatric disease [1]. Despite the current regimens with favorable levels of efficacy and the great advancement in the treatment of schizophrenia, no antipsychotic medication can completely treat the cognitive dysfunction associated with this disorder, because its present treatments are accompanied by undesirable secondary effects. Therefore, the discovery of more clinically effective antipsychotic drugs are still necessary [2]. For this goal, the glycine transporter type 1 (GlyT1) inhibitors approved by the Food and Drug Administration (FDA) are a key therapeutic development strategy to treat a variety of central nervous system (CNS) disorders, in particular schizophrenia and cognitive disorders [3,4]. In this regard, type 1 glycine transporters regulate N-methyl-D-Aspartate (NMDA) receptor function via modulation of glycine concentration at the glutamatergic synapses, but their deficiency may affect the higher central nervous system functions [5,6]. In this paper, a systematic in silico study was performed on 44 GlyT1 inhibitors, which were tested in a locomotor activity assay (LMA) of the MK801 mouse to model the treatment of positive and negative symptoms of schizophrenia [4], by means of the following molecular modeling techniques: first of all, the quantitative structure activity relationships (QSAR) as a technology widely used in drug discovery, indicating ligands with a high affinity for a given macromolecular target and optimizing the quantitative linear and non-linear relationship established between structure and inhibitory activity [7,8]; secondly, in silico ADMET prediction of newly engineered drugs [9]; and third, the molecular docking study as an approach designed in computational chemistry to accelerate drug discovery at the early stages through the detection of typical intermolecular interactions, established between the potent ligands and the responsible protein target [10]. The last step concerns the molecular dynamics (MD) simulation as an efficient technique to investigate the dynamic conformational changes of the selected complexes (active ligands-protein target) [11,12]. In this context, we started our study with a molecular descriptors calculation for each GlyT1 inhibitor, using a quantum chemistry computation with the assistance of the molecular modeling method of MM2 type and the density functional theory (DFT) based on B3LYP/6-31 + G(d,p) level, in order to optimize the molecular configurations of all inhibitors [13]. Then, we reduced the dimension of the molecular descriptors using a principal component analysis (PCA) based on the correlation matrix. Next, two QSAR models were developed using multiple linear regression (MLR) and multiple nonlinear regression (MNLR). The robustness and reliability of the established QSAR models were examined using the external validation technique, followed by Y-randomization test, an applicability domain and a cross-validation technique with the Leave-One-Out process, as one of the decisive steps to assess the confidence of the developed model's predictions for a new data set [14,15]. Moreover, we predicted the molecules having the highest inhibitory activity, based on their adsorption, distribution, metabolism, excretion and toxicity (ADMET) properties and the conditions mentioned in the rules of Lipinski, Ghose, Veber and Egan [16]. Additionally, we studied the intermolecular interactions established between the more active ligands and the dopamine transporter (DAT) membrane protein, encoded 4M48 as a crucial target for schizophrenia, with the assistance of the molecular docking approach [2,17], which was validated using docking validation protocol [18]. Lastly, we performed the molecular dynamics simulations to analyze and elaborate the details of interaction and stability of the potent ligands in the protein targets [19].

2. Results and Discussion

2.1. Pricipal Component Analysis

Principal component analysis (PCA) is one of the most widely applied multivariate techniques. It is used to reduce the size of the variables into a limited number of principal components (linear combinations of the original variables) [20]. In this paper, we calculated 40 different descriptors, which were later reduced to 27 descriptors based on the correlation matrix, since descriptors that are strongly correlated with each other (r *pearson* > 0.9) were removed. From this reduced number of variables, we were able to visualize the projection of the new database on the first two principal components (factorial axes), as shown in Figure 1, which clearly indicates that molecules 1 and 32 are poorly explained. Consequently, they are considered as outliers.

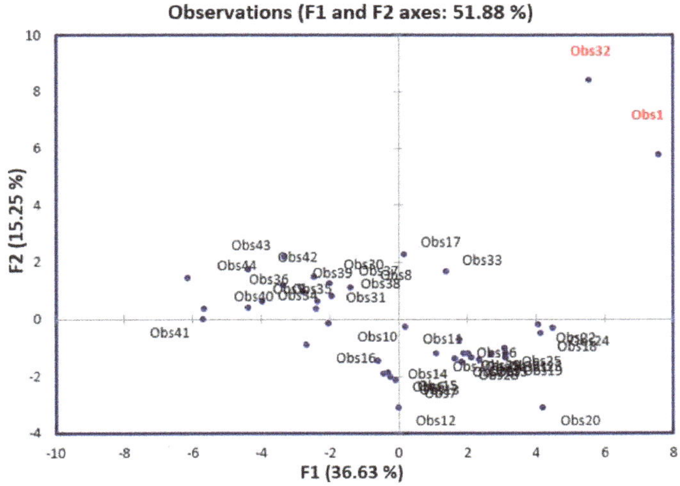

Figure 1. Data visualization on the first two principal components.

2.2. Statistical Database

Although observations 1 and 32 are considered as outliers, the new database will be represented by a matrix of 27 descriptors and 42 molecules. Using the k-means method, we randomly divided the database into training and test sets. The first one includes 80% of the total data (35 molecules) and was taken to develop the QSAR models, while the second one contains 20% of the total data (7 molecules) and was used to assess the validity of the developed models [21].

2.3. Multiple Linear Regression

The Quantitative structure-activity relationships (QSAR) have the potential to reduce the time and effort of molecular screening using mathematical predictive models [22]. One of these models is obtained by the multiple linear regression (MLR) technique, as a statistical tool for estimating the linear relationship between more than two variables which have cause-effect relations [23]. Thus, the first QSAR model was applied using the MLR technique with stepwise selection, on a training set of thirty-five molecules ($N = 35$), where the process was repeated more than a thousand times based on statistical criteria: in particular, the determination and correlation coefficients, provided that they will be validated in the next stage. Accordingly, the best QSAR model is given by the following equation:

$$\text{Log}_{10}\text{IC}_{50} = -10{,}407 - 0.279 \times \alpha e + 0.069 \times \gamma + 0.156 \times \text{TE} + 1.83 \times \text{HBD} + 1.716 \times \text{SE} + 1.029 \times \text{TD}. \quad (1)$$

This constructed model shows that the biological activity at the log scale is a quantitative variable affected by the following six descriptors: polarizability (αe), surface tension (γ), torsion energy (TE), Hydrogen bond donor (HBD), stretch energy (SE) and topological diameter (TD), which have been calculated and presented in Table 1. Moreover, the significance test demonstrates that the slope of each variable has a probability inferior to 5% as shown in Table 2, and so the selected descriptors have a significant weight on the biological inhibitory activity at a 95% confidence interval. Except the polarizability, all five molecular descriptors affect positively the biological activity as shown in Figure 2, where a molecule can be more active if it is less polar and has higher values of surface tension, torsion and stretch energies, hydrogen bond donor and topological diameter.

Table 1. The values of selected descriptors for 44 molecules.

N°	*ae*	γ	TE	HBD	SE	TD	$Log_{10}IC_{50}$
2	41.05	40.3	12.9136	1	2.609	11	0.47712126
3	43.9	43.9	12.833	1	3.43	11	1.61278386
4	43.9	43.9	12.2837	1	3.7251	11	0.77815125
5	41.96	44.6	10.5041	1	3.3398	11	1.96378783
6	43.87	50.9	5.8562	1	3.5148	10	0
7	43.11	54.3	10.9678	1	3.5012	10	0.77815125
8	44.29	57.7	10.6827	1	3.31	10	0.47712126
10	43.05	49.2	13.6092	1	3.581	10	2.69372695
11	43.82	51.6	16.8366	1	3.7574	10	2.67577834
12	42.28	53.7	12.0135	1	3.2349	10	1.87506126
13	43.11	54.3	15.9864	1	3.5181	10	2.90794852
14	43.87	50.9	12.0765	1	3.6081	10	1.36172784
15	43.11	54.3	15.211	1	3.5393	10	1.65321251
17	45.28	46.3	11.4242	1	4.1245	10	0.77815125
18	46.55	43.3	11.1295	1	4.5556	11	2.53147892
19	45.81	43.2	11.5098	1	4.5198	11	2.71096312
20	46.95	45.7	12.3354	1	3.7527	11	0.95424251
21	45.81	43.2	11.5767	1	3.7965	11	1.462398
22	46.55	43.3	12.3649	1	4.0183	12	2.24797327
23	45.81	43.2	11.5647	1	3.7752	12	3.23121465
24	46.55	43.3	12.3272	1	3.9781	13	3.24526584
25	41.5	38.4	18.5378	1	3.5883	11	3.52659771
26	40.85	43.8	14.1068	1	3.3294	11	1.8920946
29	43.14	46.6	17.5352	1	3.5318	11	2.95616843
30	42.67	45.3	11.6496	1	3.2701	10	0
31	43.05	49.2	15.9695	1	3.5677	10	0
33	52.92	45	13.4879	1	3.9397	14	2.97589114
34	41.86	48.5	7.3285	2	2.3774	10	0.47712126
37	45.11	46	10.9824	1	3.3677	10	0
38	44.35	48.9	16.6401	1	3.3293	10	1
40	39.53	51.1	7.6774	2	2.2337	10	1.76342799
41	38.77	54.5	13.3491	2	2.2124	10	1.65321251
42	40.15	49.3	8.3209	1	3.3316	10	0.84509804
43	41.98	47.7	10.8208	1	3.622	10	0.47712126
44	38.2	52.2	5.2114	2	2.8062	10	2.22530928
1 *	45.25	41.3	39.2347	1	2.6809	13	1.56820172
9 *	43.81	46.2	10.3084	1	3.6309	10	0
16 *	43.6	55.2	8.802	2	3.3159	10	0.90308999
27 *	43.14	46.6	18.0072	1	3.6639	11	1.25527251
28 *	43.14	46.6	18.0105	1	3.682	11	2.32428246
32 *	53.84	50.1	58.0893	1	5.1759	14	0
35 *	41.48	47.3	9.0526	1	2.9116	10	0.47712126
36 *	43.31	45.9	9.4978	1	3.0768	10	0.60205999
39 *	44.32	54.8	9.9783	1	2.9	10	0.30103

* indicates test set molecules.

Table 2. Significance test of the slopes.

Source	Value	Standard Deviation	t	Pr > |t|	Lower Terminal (95%)	Higher Terminal (95%)
Constante	−10.408	3.172	−3.281	0.003	−16.905	−3.910
αe	−0.279	0.079	−3.550	0.001	−0.441	−0.118
γ	0.070	0.033	2.101	0.045	0.002	0.138
TE	0.156	0.042	3.731	0.001	0.071	0.242
HBD	1.830	0.571	3.208	0.003	0.661	2.999
SE	1.716	0.387	4.429	0.000	0.922	2.510
TD	1.030	0.208	4.956	<0.0001	0.604	1.455

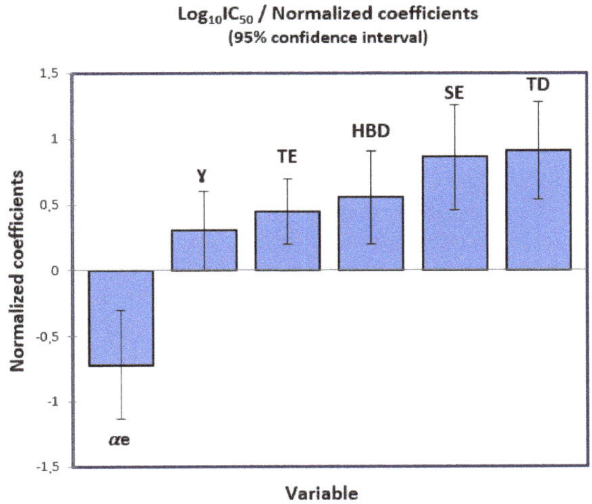

Figure 2. Influence degree of the descriptors on the biological activity.

Additionally, the null hypothesis (H0) postulated by the Fisher statistical test is rejected, because the calculated Fisher value ($F = 10.325$) is so much higher than its critical value: [F (35,6) = 2.37, $p < 0.0001$], as presented in the one Anova test (Table 3). Therefore, the variance between the response ($Log_{10}IC_{50}$) and the six predictor variables is homogeneous. Moreover, the correlation and determination coefficients of $R = 0.83$ and $R^2 = 0.69$, respectively, confirm that there is a strong relationship between the descriptors and the inhibitory activity. Thus, the first QSAR model generated via MLR technique has a good predictive performance, with a low standard error ($RMSE = 0.66$).

Table 3. Variance analysis.

Source	DDL	Total Square	Mean Square	*F*	*Pr > F*
Model	6	26.753	4.459	10.325	<0.0001
Error	28	12.092	0.432		
Adjusted total	34	38.846			

2.4. Multiple Non-Linear Regression

The multiple non-linear regression (MNLR) technique is applied using a set of adapted algorithms to generate the quantitative predictive models [24]. In the present study, we relied on the programmed function of the type:

$$Y = a0 + \sum_{i=1}^{n} \left(ai \times Xi + bi \times Xi^2 \right) \quad (2)$$

As:
Y: is the predicted biological activity ($Log_{10}IC_{50}$)
Xi: is the explicative variable
a0: is the constant of the QSAR model
ai and bi: are the slopes of each descriptor to one and two degrees, respectively.
Finally, we arrived at the second QSAR model given by the following equation:

$$Log_{10}IC_{50} = -19.699 - 0.009 \times \alpha e - 0.056 \times \gamma - 0.161 \times TE + 1.466 \times HBD + 0.5 \times SE + 2.693 \times TD - 0.002 \times \alpha e^{\wedge 2} + 0.001 \times \gamma^{\wedge 2} + 0.013 \times TE^{\wedge 2} + 0.148 \times SE^{\wedge 2} - 0.07 \times TD^{\wedge 2}. \quad (3)$$

This mathematical model has a good predictive capacity, justified by a strong non-linear relationship between the biological activity and the six descriptors, as it is defined by a good correlation coefficient ($R = 0.84$) and a good coefficient of determination ($R^2 = 0.71$), in addition to its minimal mean square error ($RMSE = 0.72$).

2.5. QSAR Model Validation

2.5.1. Applicability Domain

The applicability domain (AD) of a quantitative structure-activity relationship (QSAR) model is necessary to verify its reliability on new compounds (test set) that were not considered during its development [25]. This technique has been evaluated by an analysis expressed as a Williams diagram (Figure 3), which confirms that the molecules (1 and 32) belonging to the test set are really outliers, because they exceed the warning leverage ($h^* = 0.6$), where: $h^* = 3 \times K/n$ and $K = p + 1$, ($p = 6$, $K = 7$, $n = 35$) as, n: is the number of training set, and p: is the number of predictor descriptors [26,27]. Next, we noted that the compound 33 from training test is not an outlier because it does not exceed the critical leverage (h^*). Therefore, except for molecules (1 and 32), all the others are well explained because they have in addition a normalized residual included in the 3 times standard deviation interval. Consequently, the 42 remaining molecules are tested in the applicability domain and the QSAR model was predicted correctly.

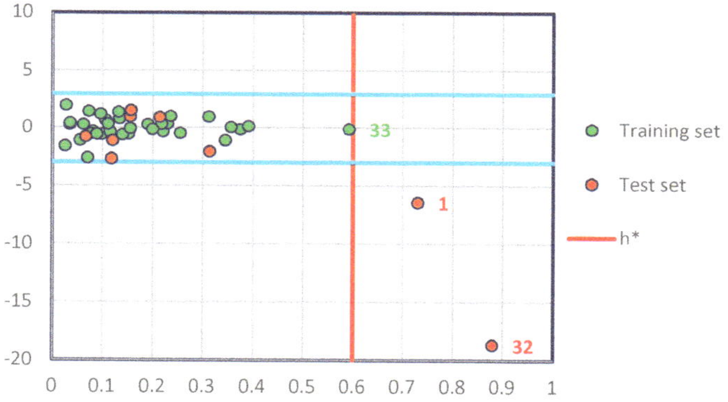

Figure 3. William's diagram of the MLR model established by Equation (1). 1 and 32 are outliers in the test set and 33 is a non-aberrant molecule in the training test.

2.5.2. External Validation

To assess the accuracy of the QSAR predictive model and guarantee its generalizability, it is absolutely needed to validate it on new molecules included in the test set, before its application in clinical practice [28]. Based on a training test (35 molecules), we tested the seven new molecules from the test set and got the results presented in Table 4.

Table 4. External validation results of the MLR and MNLR models.

Molecule Number	Observed $Log_{10}IC_{50}$	Predicted $Log_{10}IC_{50}$(MLR)	Predicted $Log_{10}IC_{50}$(MNLR)
9 *	0.000	0.545	0.380
16 *	0.903	2.285	2.134
27 *	1.255	3.051	3.342
28 *	2.324	3.083	3.372
35 *	0.477	−0.158	−0.164
36 *	0.602	−0.414	−0.429
39 *	0.301	−0.304	−0.046

* Indicates test set molecules.

The results mentioned in Figure 4 indicate that the MLR QSAR model is given by an external validation correlation coefficient (R^2ext = 0.63), and the results noted in Figure 5 indicate that the MNLR QSAR model is characterized by an external validation correlation coefficient of R^2ext = 0.68. According to the Alexander Golbraikh and Alexander Tropsha theory, a QSAR model is externally validated if the correlation coefficient of its external validation is greater than 0.6. Therefore, the mathematical models developed with the help of MLR and MNLR techniques are externally validated.

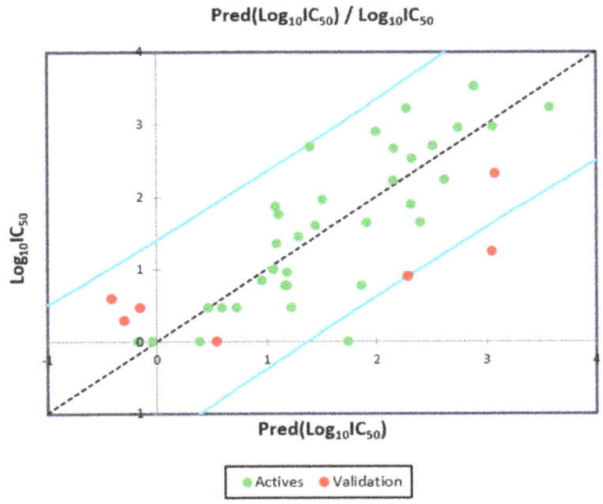

Figure 4. Correlation between the observed and predicted activities using MLR technique.

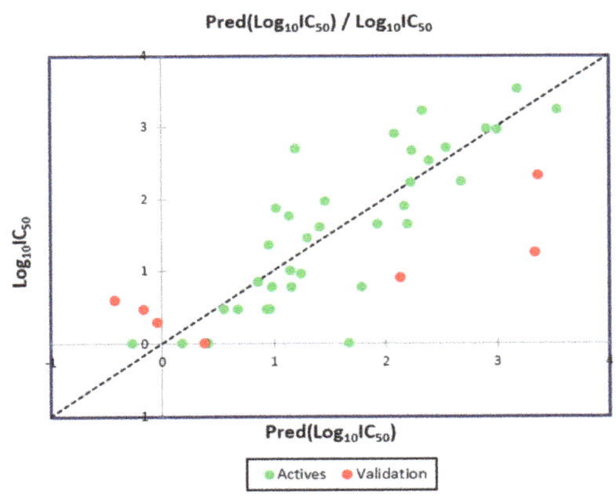

Figure 5. Correlation between the observed and predicted activities using MNLR technique.

2.5.3. Internal Validation

To validate internally the QSAR model, we applied the cross-validation technique with the leave-one-out procedure (CVLOO), so that each observation is tested exactly once, by executing a new model each run on thirty-four compounds (N-1 = 34) and predicting the biological activity of the removed sample, as shown in Table 5. This technique is based on the calculation of the quadratic coefficient of cross validation (Q^2cv), which is expressed in the following equation [29,30]: $Q^2cv = 1 - \frac{\sum_i^n (Ypred - Yobs)^2}{\sum_i^n (Yobs - Ymean)^2}$ (4) AS: *Ypred*: is the predicted activity value, *Yobs*: is the observed activity value, *Ymean*: is the mean of the observed activity values. A high value of Q^2cv = 0.57 (superior than 0.5) signifies that the established model is reliable, robust and has better internal predictivity.

Table 5. Observed and predicted activity values from the QSAR models.

Molecules Number	Observed $Log_{10}IC_{50}$	Predicted $Log_{10}IC_{50}$ (MLR)	Predicted $Log_{10}IC_{50}$ (MNLR)	Predicted $Log_{10}IC_{50}$ (CV)
2	0.47712126	0.588	0.679	0.664
3	1.61278386	1.439	1.415	1.428
4	0.77815125	1.860	1.790	1.922
5	1.96378783	1.511	1.464	1.441
6	0	−0.040	0.405	−0.053
7	0.77815125	1.186	1.157	1.245
8	0.47712126	0.721	0.933	0.801
10	2.69372695	1.397	1.195	1.321
11	2.67577834	2.157	2.240	2.057
12	1.87506126	1.083	1.018	0.970
13	2.90794852	2.000	2.081	1.827
14	1.36172784	1.093	0.954	1.075
15	1.65321251	1.915	1.933	1.959
17	0.77815125	1.163	0.982	1.247
18	2.53147892	2.322	2.392	2.250
19	2.71096312	2.520	2.548	2.458
20	0.95424251	1.189	1.245	1.217
21	1.462398	1.289	1.302	1.272
22	2.24797327	2.623	2.680	2.667
23	3.23121465	2.281	2.338	2.174
24	3.24526584	3.578	3.538	3.710
25	3.52659771	2.891	3.183	2.562
26	1.8920946	2.311	2.171	2.396
29	2.95616843	2.751	3.000	2.717
30	0	0.391	0.176	0.443
31	0	1.744	1.675	1.934
33	2.97589114	3.062	2.907	3.204
34	0.47712126	0.463	0.555	0.454
37	0	−0.178	−0.276	−0.228
38	1	1.056	1.151	1.068
40	1.76342799	1.104	1.136	0.867
41	1.65321251	2.404	2.199	2.852
42	0.84509804	0.959	0.855	0.993
43	0.47712126	1.226	0.961	1.294

2.5.4. Validation Using Y-Randomisation Test

The statistical study of Alexander Golbraikh and Alexander Tropsha confirms that the cross-validation technique is necessary but not sufficient, as the internal predictive accuracy of the cross-validation procedure tends to be overestimated and the high value of the quadratic coefficient may be the result of chance correlation. For this reason, the Y-randomisation test is necessary [31]. Using java Platform SE binary, we tested the QSAR model quality by running one hundred randomizations, as presented in Table 6. The results of the Y-randomisation test demonstrate that the (cR^2p = 0.602) criteria is superior than 0.5; moreover, the R, R^2 and R^2cv values of the original model are much better than the values obtained by 100 randomizations. Consequently, the biological activity values predicted by the original model are not due to chance.

Table 6. Y-randomization test results.

Model	*R*	*R*^2	*Q*^2	Model	*R*	*R*^2	*Q*^2
Original	**0.829884**	**0.688707**	**0.572045**	Random 51	0.206983	0.042842	−0.46272
Random 1	0.252331	0.063671	−0.50878	Random 52	0.537396	0.288794	−0.15592
Random 2	0.457615	0.209411	−0.17702	Random 53	0.379861	0.144294	−0.43774
Random 3	0.47795	0.228436	−0.41001	Random 54	0.367538	0.135084	−0.29876
Random 4	0.375518	0.141014	−0.34708	Random 55	0.179251	0.032131	−0.54121
Random 5	0.422447	0.178462	−0.39625	Random 56	0.663141	0.439756	0.029755
Random 6	0.480602	0.230979	−0.17775	Random 57	0.36146	0.130653	−0.41471
Random 7	0.306791	0.09412	−0.47744	Random 58	0.445943	0.198865	−0.22915
Random 8	0.354955	0.125993	−0.40713	Random 59	0.417956	0.174687	−0.19669
Random 9	0.209847	0.044036	−0.71484	Random 60	0.204369	0.041767	−0.88175

Table 6. *Cont.*

Model	R	R^2	Q^2	Model	R	R^2	Q^2
Random 10	0.395267	0.156236	−0.36218	Random 61	0.557804	0.311145	0.016035
Random 11	0.520928	0.271366	−0.1806	Random 62	0.50639	0.256431	−0.3063
Random 12	0.510412	0.260521	−0.21009	Random 63	0.37293	0.139077	−0.46899
Random 13	0.427634	0.182871	−0.23082	Random 64	0.383643	0.147182	−0.41262
Random 14	0.445148	0.198156	−0.41414	Random 65	0.414428	0.171751	−0.30301
Random 15	0.21278	0.045275	−0.4451	Random 66	0.292763	0.08571	−0.36258
Random 16	0.516892	0.267178	−0.45198	Random 67	0.526141	0.276824	−0.1287
Random 17	0.37686	0.142024	−0.55449	Random 68	0.284657	0.08103	−0.54548
Random 18	0.154692	0.023929	−0.85659	Random 69	0.456042	0.207974	−0.2171
Random 19	0.491084	0.241163	−0.24676	Random 70	0.451139	0.203526	−0.15451
Random 20	0.424795	0.180451	−0.30099	Random 71	0.402163	0.161735	−0.15347
Random 21	0.513699	0.263886	−0.1961	Random 72	0.480122	0.230517	−0.17729
Random 22	0.316251	0.100015	−0.30938	Random 73	0.426294	0.181727	−0.22948
Random 23	0.301949	0.091173	−0.63655	Random 74	0.475859	0.226442	−0.23411
Random 24	0.332628	0.110641	−0.8224	Random 75	0.462608	0.214006	−0.12839
Random 25	0.633727	0.401609	0.166923	Random 76	0.53816	0.289616	−0.33075
Random 26	0.328704	0.108046	−0.48201	Random 77	0.383709	0.147233	−0.30145
Random 27	0.46585	0.217016	−0.16011	Random 78	0.38822	0.150715	−0.41903
Random 28	0.441731	0.195126	−0.25279	Random 79	0.528782	0.279611	−0.29561
Random 29	0.355019	0.126039	−0.31878	Random 80	0.330001	0.1089	−0.41611
Random 30	0.329982	0.108888	−0.42698	Random 81	0.413654	0.171109	−0.22613
Random 31	0.378435	0.143213	−0.25482	Random 82	0.493491	0.243533	−0.12853
Random 32	0.462326	0.213746	−0.13151	Random 83	0.381202	0.145315	−0.49761
Random 33	0.343488	0.117984	−0.53921	Random 84	0.323593	0.104712	−0.30559
Random 34	0.462673	0.214066	−0.27221	Random 85	0.32106	0.103079	−0.33856
Random 35	0.35063	0.122941	−0.3394	Random 86	0.30071	0.090427	−0.55488
Random 36	0.522964	0.273491	−0.09258	Random 87	0.518334	0.26867	−0.1494
Random 37	0.222631	0.049564	−0.75169	Random 88	0.387695	0.150307	−0.45639
Random 38	0.241784	0.058459	−0.47485	Random 89	0.36652	0.134337	−0.30196
Random 39	0.339537	0.115286	−0.4132	Random 90	0.279562	0.078155	−0.47573
Random 40	0.448316	0.200987	−0.47037	Random 91	0.575806	0.331552	−0.03852
Random 41	0.487561	0.237716	−0.34662	Random 92	0.5706	0.325585	0.021398
Random 42	0.369003	0.136164	−0.33599	Random 93	0.381837	0.1458	−0.44739
Random 43	0.400756	0.160605	−0.30621	Random 94	0.385236	0.148406	−0.6547
Random 44	0.343595	0.118058	−0.42487	Random 95	0.251773	0.06339	−0.49809
Random 45	0.390289	0.152325	−0.27962	Random 96	0.446548	0.199405	−0.47359
Random 46	0.350185	0.12263	−0.22911	Random 97	0.316743	0.100326	−0.95316
Random 47	0.463947	0.215247	−0.27397	Random 98	0.367366	0.134958	−0.3352
Random 48	0.37435	0.140138	−0.27999	Random 99	0.631342	0.398592	0.090509
Random 49	0.452168	0.204456	−0.40118	Random 100	0.56162	0.315417	0.016006
Random 50	0.266881	0.071225	−0.47945				

2.5.5. Golbreikh and Tropsha Criteria

The quantitative structure-activity relationship (QSAR) model, defined by the first Equation (1), satisfies the threshold criteria postulated by Golbraikh and Tropsha theory, as shown in Table 7.

Table 7. Golbraikh and Tropsha statistical criteria to validate the designed QSAR model.

Parameter	Equation	Model Score	Threshold	Comment
R^2	$R^2 = 1 - \frac{\sum (Yobs - Y\,cal)^2}{\sum (Yobs - \overline{Yobs})^2}$	0.69	>0.6	Accepted
R^2adj	$R^2adj = \frac{(N-1)R^2 - p}{N-p-1}$	0.62	>0.6	Accepted
R^2test	$R^2test = 1 - \frac{\sum (Ycal(test) - Y\,obs(test))^2}{\sum (Yobs(test) - \overline{Yobs}(train))^2}$	0.63	>0.6	Accepted
Q^2cv	$Q^2cv = 1 - \frac{\sum (Ycal - Y\,obs)^2}{\sum (Yobs - \overline{Yobs})^2}$	0.57	>0.5	Accepted

Table 7. *Cont.*

Parameter	Equation	Model Score	Threshold	Comment
R^2 rand	Average of the 100 R^2 rand (i)	0.17	$<R^2$	Accepted
Q^2cv 'LOO' rand	Average of the 100 Q^2cv 'LOO' rand (i)	−0.34	$<Q^2cv$	Accepted
cR^2p	cR2p = $R^* \sqrt[2]{(R^2 - (\,Average\ R_{rand}\,)^2)}$	0.60	>0.5	Accepted

Yobs and *Ycalc*: refer to the observed and calculated/predicted response values. $\overline{Yobs}$ and $\overline{Ycal}$ refer to the mean of the observed and calculated/predicted response values. *N* and *p* refer to the number of data points (compounds) and descriptors.

2.6. In Silico Pharmacokinetics ADMET Prediction

The most active ligands (L6, L9, L30, L31, L32 and L37), acting as inhibitors of type 1 glycine transporters, were tested based on the rules of Lipinski, Veber, Egan, and Ghose, and the pharmacokinetic properties (ADMET) [32], which were compared to the obtained results for nortriptyline as a co-crystallized ligand bound to the dopamine transporter (DAT) membrane protein encoded 4M48. The results presented in Table 8 indicate that all molecules respect the rules of Lipinski, Veber, Egan and Ghose except the ligand 32, because its molar refractivity index exceeds 130 and its Ghose violation number is equal to 2 (exceed 1). Additionally, the exact predictive model (BOILED-Egg), highly practical in the context of drug discovery and medicinal chemistry, and based on the calculation of lipophilicity given by the logarithm of the partition coefficient between n-octanol and water (Log $P_{O/W}$) and polarity signaled by the topological polar surface area (TPSA) of small molecules, clearly shows that the molecule (L32) is the only one that does not belong to the yellow Egan-egg, as presented in Figure 6. Therefore, the five ligands (L6, L9, L30, L31 and L37) are the molecules having the highest probability to penetrate the brain. In comparison, the molecule 32 belonging to the white region of the egg has the highest probability of being absorbed by the gastrointestinal tract [33], which is why it was an outlier in the previous QSAR study.

Table 8. Prediction of the physicochemical properties of nortriptyline and more active ligands, based on Lipinski, Veber, Egan and Ghose violations.

Ligands Number	Physico-Chemical Propities						Lipinski Violations	Veber Violations	Egan Violations	Ghose Violations	Synthetic Accessiblity
	Molecular Weight (g/mol)	Molar Refractive Index	Rotatable Bonds	Log *p* (Octanol/Water)	H-BA	H-BD					
Rule	≤500	40 ≤ MR ≤ 130	<10	<5	≤10	<5	≤1	Yes/No	Yes/No	Yes/No	0 < S.A < 10
(1) L6	403.34	115.02	5	3.60	2	1	1	Yes	Yes	Yes	4.24
(2) L9	362.51	114.93	5	3.58	2	1	0	Yes	Yes	Yes	4.21
(3) L30	366.50	112.17	5	3.75	3	1	0	Yes	Yes	Yes	4.97
(4) L31	363.50	112.73	5	3.15	3	1	0	Yes	Yes	Yes	4.28
(5) L32	480.66	140.34	8	3.61	4	1	0	Yes	Yes	No	5.19
(6) L37	377.52	121.65	6	3.23	3	2	0	Yes	Yes	Yes	4.47
(7) nortriptyline	265.39	85.74	4	3.24	1	1	1	Yes	Yes	Yes	3.28

The pharmacokinetic parameters of adsorption, distribution, metabolism, excretion and toxicity (ADMET) of the most active ligands as presented in Table 9 indicate that the ligands have a good absorption in the human intestine (IAH so higher than 70%), and a good distribution, since their human distribution volumes are estimated to be greater than −0.44 Log L/kg. Their permeability to the blood-brain barrier (BBB) is greater than −1 Log BB, and their permeability to the central nervous system (CNS) outside the interval (of −2 to −3) Log PS. Thus, they all penetrate the central nervous system (CNS) with the exception of ligands L32 and L30. In addition, the molecules are all predicted as inhibitors of cytochrome 2D6 except ligand 32. Consequently, the ligands (L6, L9, L30, L31 and L37) are designed to be agents of the central nervous system due to the highest probability of penetrating the blood-brain barrier (BBB).

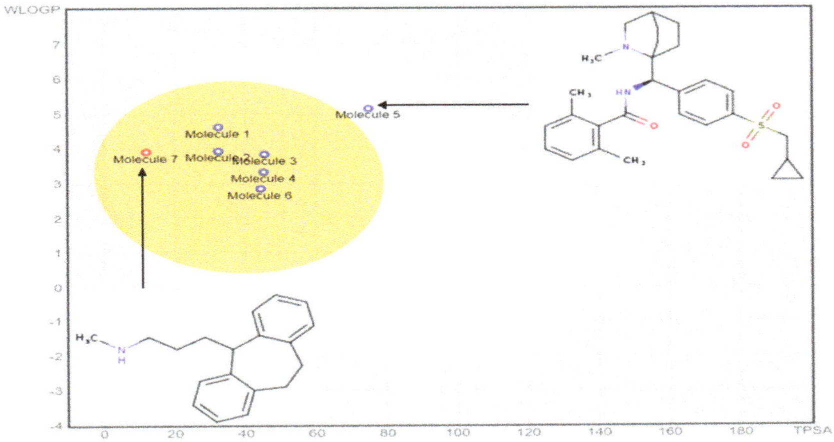

Figure 6. BOILED-egg predictive model of the most active ligands.

Table 9. Prediction of ADMET pharmacokinetic properties of nortriptyline and more active ligands.

Ligands Number	Absorption	Distribution			Metabolism							Excretion	Toxicity
					Substrate		Inhibitor						
	Intestinal Absorption (Human)	VDss (Human)	BBB Permeability	CNS Permeability	CYP							Total Clearance	AMES Toxicity
					2D6	3A4	1A2	2C19	2C9	2D6	3A4		
	Numeric (% Absorbed)	Numeric (Log L/kg)	Numeric (Log BB)	Numeric (Log PS)	Categorical (Yes/No)							Numeric (Log ml/min/kg)	Categorical (Yes/No)
(1) L6	91.194	1.431	0.199	−1.06	Yes	Yes	Yes	Yes	No	Yes	Yes	1.058	Not toxic
(2) L9	93.373	1.477	0.223	−1.072	Yes	Yes	Yes	No	No	Yes	No	0.978	Not toxic
(3) L30	93.344	1.242	0.176	−2.055	Yes	Yes	No	No	No	Yes	No	0.883	Not toxic
(4) L31	95.105	1.187	0.048	−1.976	Yes	Yes	No	No	No	Yes	Yes	0.948	Not toxic
(5) L32	94.331	1.038	−0.378	−2.005	No	Yes	Yes	No	No	No	Yes	0.85	Not toxic
(6) L37	92.765	1.814	0.044	−0.657	Yes	Yes	No	No	No	Yes	No	0.905	Not toxic
(7) nortriptyline	98.519	1.688	0.854	−1.287	No	Yes	Yes	No	No	Yes	No	1.077	Not toxic

2.7. Molecular Docking

Molecular docking results are focused on the dopamine transporter (DAT) bound to the tricyclic antidepressant nortriptyline, as a transmembrane protein that removes the neurotransmitter dopamine from the synaptic cleft and transports it into the cytosol of surrounding cells. The crystal structure of this receptor is extracted using the X-ray diffraction method at a resolution of 2.96 Å taken from the protein data base (PDB) [34–36]. In this part of the research, the molecular docking process is started for the following most active molecules (L6, L9, L30, L31 and L37) to predict the type of Intermolecular interactions established with the protein encoded 4M48, compared to the established interactions with the co-crystallized ligand (nortriptyline) pictured in Figure 7, which indicate that Phe43A, Phe325A and Tyr124A amino acids, are the active sites of the target protein, as sourced using the ProteinsPlus online server [37].

The results of molecular docking applied on the more active ligands, presented in Figure 8, show that the ligands L6 and L9 share common molecular interactions as the chemical bonds of type pi-sigma and Pi-Pi T-shaped established between the benzenic cycle and (Val120 and Tyr124) amino acids respectively, in addition to two bonds of alkyl type with Phe325 and Phe43 amino acids. L30 and L31 ligands also form common bonds, like the hydrogen bond linked to the nitrogen atom, with the amino acid Asp46 at the same nuclear distance (5.5 Å), in addition to the alkyl bond with bicyclo group and Tyr124 amino acid. The same type of bond was established between the methyl group and the amino acid Phe325 at a nuclear distance of 5.5 Å, more than Pi-Pi bonds with Phe43 and Phe319 amino acids. Even the ligand L37 formed an alkyl bond with Tyr124 amino acid, and two Pi-Pi chemical bonds with Phe325 and Phe319 amino acids. Therefore, we can conclude that Tyr124, Phe43, Phe325, Asp46, Phe319 and Val120 amino acids are the active sites of the dopamine transporter (DAT) membrane protein, in which the most active ligands can inhibit the glycine transporter type 1 (GlyT1).

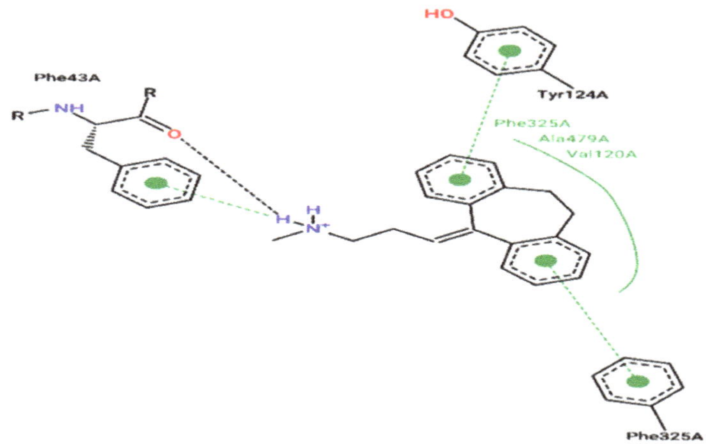

Figure 7. Experimental pose view of Nortriptyline with the protein's active sites.

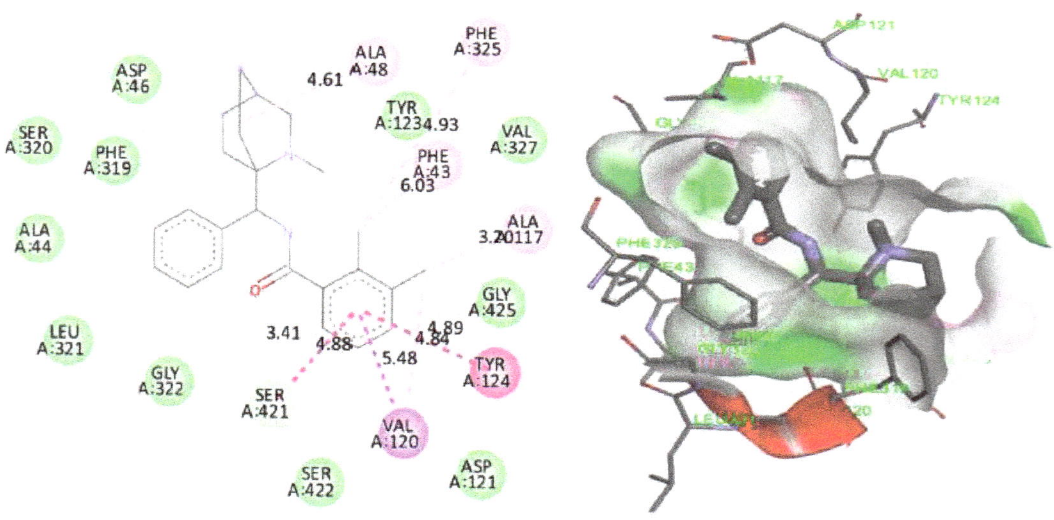

L6

Figure 8. *Cont.*

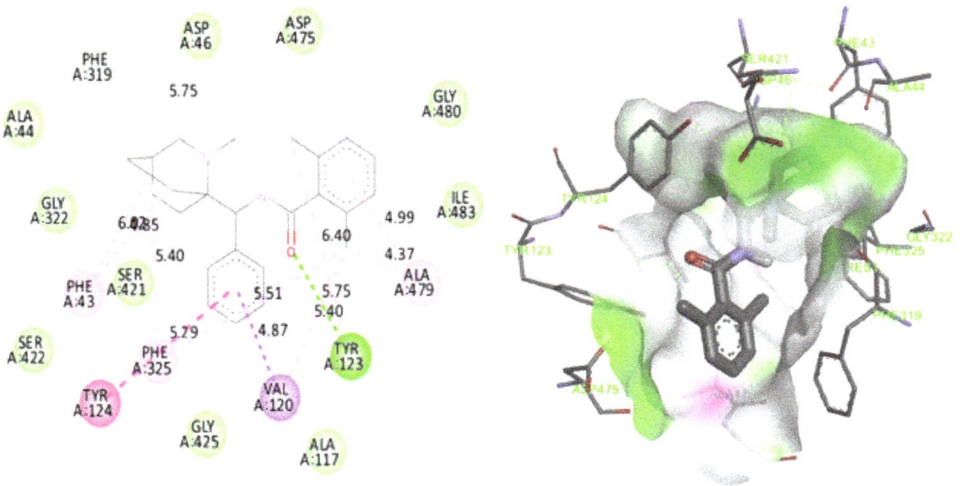

L9

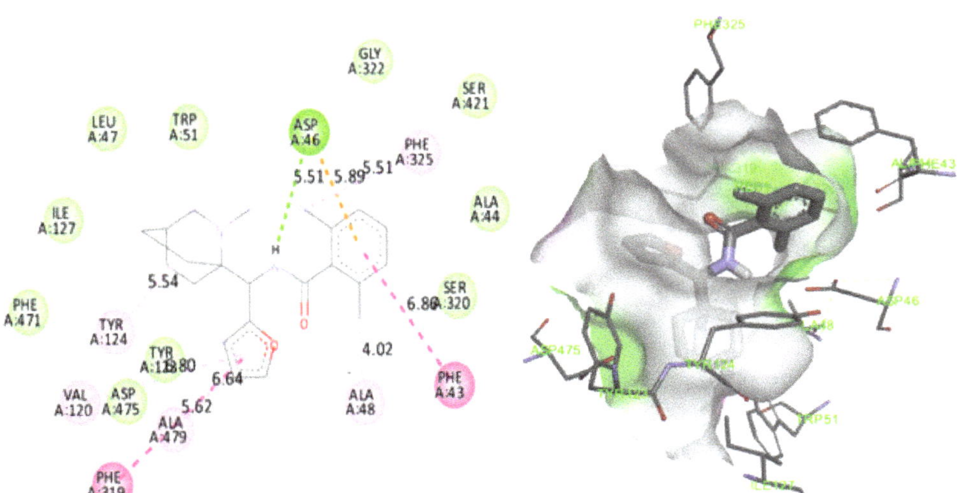

L30

Figure 8. *Cont.*

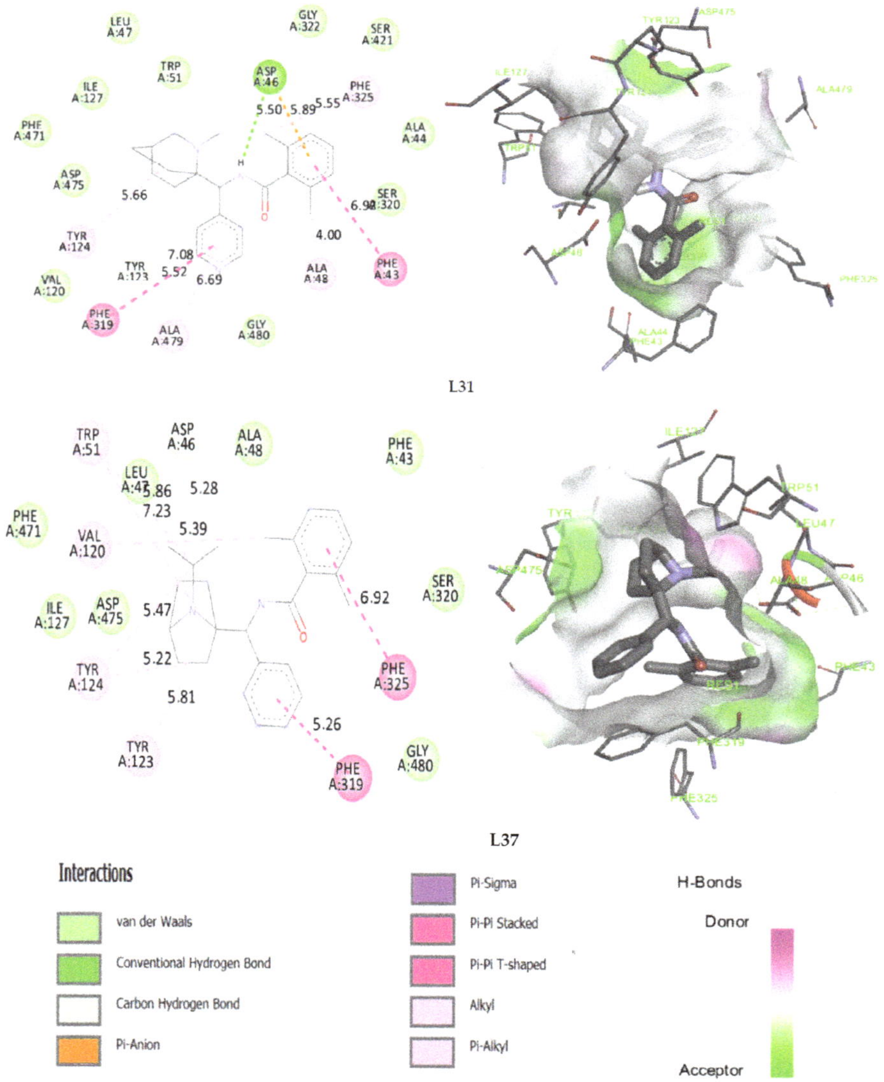

Figure 8. 2D and 3D visualization of intermolecular interactions between DAT (PDB code: 4M48) and the more active ligands (L6, L9, L30, L31 and L37), with binding energies of −10.74 kcal/mol, −10.22 kcal/mol, −8.46 kcal/mol, −8.78 kcal/mol and −8.59 kcal/mol, respectively.

2.8. Docking Validation Protocol

The efficiency of the molecular docking algorithms was tested using the re-docking methodology, which is based on the superposition of the docked ligand on the protein-bound ligand, as shown in Figure 9. The superposition result indicates a root mean square deviation smaller than 2 (*RMSD* = 0.022 Å), which explains an exact pose prediction. Additionally, 2D and 3D visualization (Figure 10) of the intermolecular interaction between the docked nortriptyline and the protein target indicates that the chemical bonds formed with Phe43A and Tyr124A amino acids are the same as those observed experimentally. Thus, the molecular docking protocol is successfully validated [18].

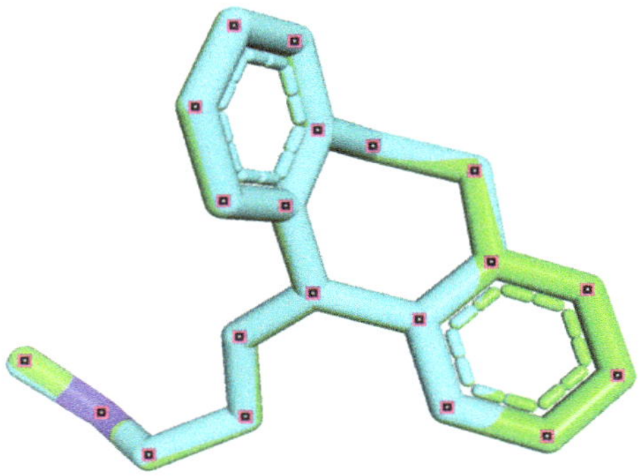

Figure 9. Re-docking pose with RMSD equal to 0.022 Å (original nortriptyline of cyan color, and docked nortriptyline of green color).

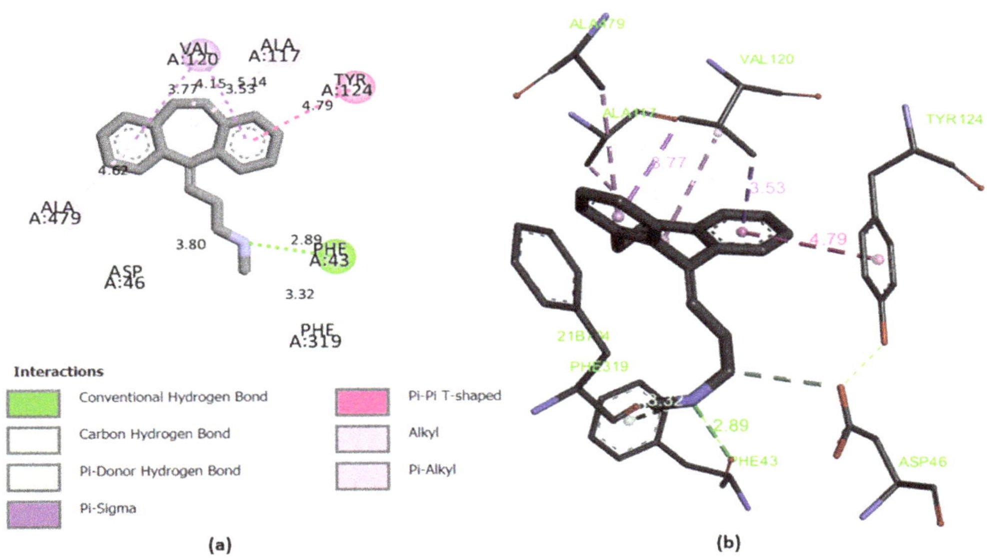

Figure 10. 2D (**a**) and 3D (**b**) visualization of intermolecular interaction between the docked nortriptyline and the protein target (binding energy of −9.11 kcal/mol).

2.9. Molecular Dynamics Simulations

The most active ligands (L6, L9, L30, L31 and L37) were chosen for the molecular dynamic's simulation during 100 ns, to examine their stability toward DAT protein, where the conformational changes of one of these ligands are presented in Figure 11, and the others were presented in Figure S1.

The dynamic changes of conformation for (L9-protein) complex shown in Figure 11, indicate that the simulation is well-equilibrated, as the fluctuations of the root mean square deviation (RMSD) of the protein (left *Y*-axis) are around the thermal mean structure throughout the simulation time (100 ns), because the changes of the order of 1–3 Å are perfectly acceptable for small globular proteins. Moreover, the RMSD evolution of the heavy atoms of the ligand (right *Y*-axis) shows its stability with respect to the protein, when the protein-ligand complex is first aligned on the protein backbone of the reference, because the observed values are significantly smaller than the RMSD of the protein, and so the ligand did not diffuse away from its initial binding site.

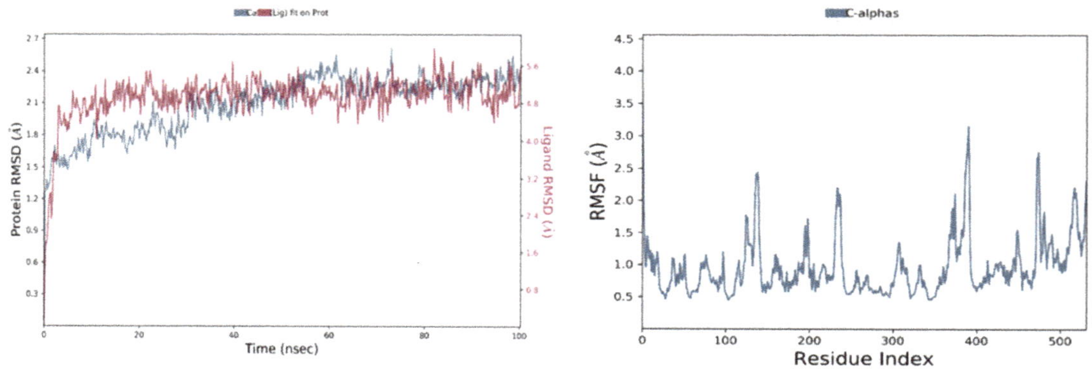

Figure 11. RMSD and RMSF graphs for the ligand 9 complexed with the dopamine transporter membrane protein during 100 ns.

The root mean square fluctuation (RMSF) values are also computed to examine the impact of the ligand binding on the internal dynamics of the target protein during 100 ns, where the tails (N- and C-terminal) fluctuate more than any other part of the protein and the secondary structure elements like alpha helices and beta strands are usually more rigid than the unstructured part of the protein; for this reason, they fluctuate less than the loop regions. Except for a single fluctuation of 3.2 Å, detected in the loop region of residue 390, all fluctuations were less than 3 Å, indicating the binding strength between the ligand 9 and the DAT protein, and no significant change in the protein conformation resulting from ligand binding.

Additionally, the radius of gyration (r Gyr) values fluctuated in a small interval from 3.45 to 3.76 Å until the end of the simulation, as shown in Figure 12, indicating that there are just some changes in the compactness of the ligand; thus, the protein has a good flexibility after its binding with the ligand 9. Moreover, the solvent accessibility of the protein-ligand 9 complex was evaluated by the solvent accessible surface area (SASA) analysis, which fluctuated between 0 and 15 Å^2 for 100 ns; this graph revealed that the structure of compound 9 was relatively stable during the simulation time. The polar surface area (PSA) is a solvent accessible surface area in a molecule contributed only by oxygen and nitrogen atoms; this parameter varies between 8 and 32 Å^2, accompanied by some maximal and minimal fluctuations during the simulation time. The contributions of this type of atoms make the ligand relatively unstable. However, the molecular surface area (MolSA) illustrates the molecular surface calculation with a probe radius of 1.4 Å, equivalent to a Van der Waals surface, showing only minimal fluctuations.

Lastly, the graph of the total energy presented in Figure 12 shows a minimal variation about the average -53.8682 kcal.mol^{-1}, which means that the energy of the L9- DAT protein complex remained in equilibrium throughout the MD simulation.

The dynamic changes of conformation for other complexes are available in the supplementary material (Figure S1). The protein-ligands interactions fluctuate with a root mean square deviation (RMSD) of 1 to 3 Å along the simulation time (100 ns), except for the L31-protein complex, which oscillates for the first 20 nanoseconds from 1 to 3 Å, then destabilizes until 50 ns, and stabilizes again with a deviation 4 Å of about until the end of the simulation time.

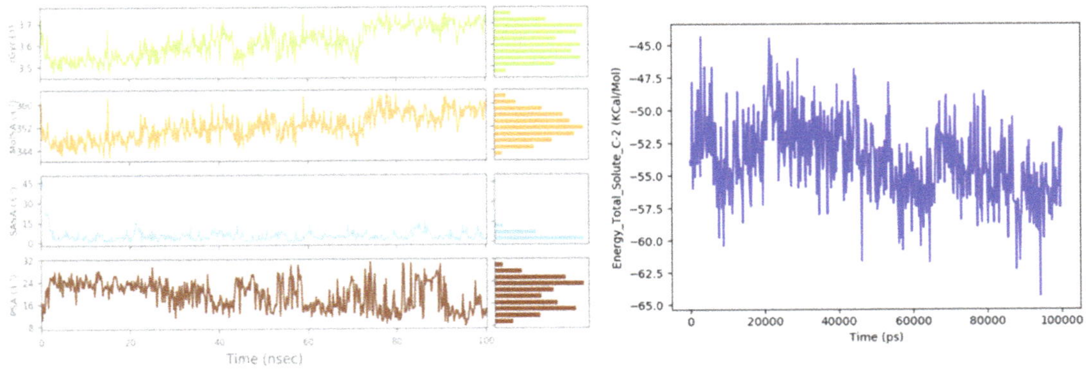

Figure 12. Rg, MolSA, SASA and PSA during 100 ns of MD simulation, and the variation of total free energy for the ligand 9 complexed with DAT protein.

Minimal fluctuations have been observed during the established interactions between the protein and the ligand 6, such as the observed root mean square fluctuations (RMSF) of 3.4 Å, 4.4 Å and 3.9 Å detected in the loop region of 10, 240 and 480 residues, respectively, in addition to a maximal fluctuation of 5.5 Å recorded in the loop area of residue 380. No fluctuation was noticed greater than 3 Å for L30-protein and L37-protein complexes. Three fluctuations have been recorded for L31-protein complex of 3.6 Å, 3.5 Å and 7 Å reported in the loop zone of 10, 480 and 520 residues, respectively.

Overall, we note that the protein has a good flexibility of binding with L6, L30, L31 and L37 inhibitors, as there are just a few changes in the compactness of the ligand, since the r Gyr, SASA, MolSA and PSA parameters are varied with minimal fluctuations about the mean along 100 ns.

Finally, the total energy plots presented in Figure S2 show a minimal variance around the average energy of the total system, which was in Kcal/mol of −47.7003, −48.8821 −49.5236 and −62.5749 for L30, L31, L37 and L6 inhibitors, respectively, indicating that the energies of the ligands-protein complexes have remained in equilibrium over the course of the MD simulation.

We conclude that the molecular dynamics simulations reinforce the previous results obtained by QSAR and docking studies, since the ligands L6, L9, L30, L31 and L37 are the most active inhibitors, forming typical static interactions with some amino acids of the target protein. These interactions form dynamically stable complexes during the 100 ns of the simulation time, as there is no change in their properties, except for the minimal fluctuations that were observed.

3. Materials and Methods

3.1. Database

The present study is performed on 44 bicyclo ((aryl) methyl) benzamides as glycine transporter type 1 (GlyT1) inhibitors, whose biological activities are expressed on a logarithmic decimal scale ($\log_{10}IC_{50}$), as illustrated in Table S1.

3.2. Molecular Descriptors Calculation

To build the quantitative structure-activity relationship (QSAR) models that provide information on the correlation between activities and structure-based molecular descriptors, we calculated various types of molecular descriptors [38], as shown in Table S2. Initially, the constitutional descriptors were calculated using the ACD/chemsketch software [39]. Subsequently, the thermodynamic and physicochemical descriptors were extracted using the MM2 technique via the ChemBio3D software [40]. Lastly, the quantum descriptors are calculated through Gaussian 09 software [41], using the density function theory (DFT)/B3LYP [42], combined with the 6-31 + G(d,p) basis set, in order to ensure the molecules stability and optimize their three-dimensional geometries.

3.3. Statistical Methods

The Quantitative structure-activity relationships (QSARs) are developed with the help of XLSTAT 2014 software [43], using different statistical methods such as: the principal component analysis (PCA), multiple linear regression (MLR) and multiple non-linear regression (MNLR). The principal component analysis method is a very important step that serves to minimize the molecular descriptor dimension so as to identify the most predictive variables [44]. This limited number of descriptors is mathematically modeled by the multiple linear regression (MLR) and multiple non-linear regression (MNLR) techniques. Therefore, the two obtained QSAR models were generated to predict the linear and non-linear relationships established between the biological activity of glycine transporter type 1 (GlyT1) inhibitors and their relevant descriptors. For their applicability, these two models have been evaluated by external and internal validation, as well as the molecules, which have been tested in the applicability domain [45]. Additionally, the Golbreikh and Tropsha criteria and the Y-randomization test were used to verify the robustness and predictive potential of the established QSAR model [31,46].

3.4. Drug Likeness and In Silico Pharmacokinetics ADMET Prediction

To make the drugs applicable in clinical trials, it is necessary to study their absorption, distribution, metabolism, excretion and toxicity (ADMET) in the human body before starting the investigation protocols [21,47], respecting some important rules such as those of Lipinski [48], Veber [49], Ghose [50] and Egan [51,52]. This technique is also applied to eliminate the compounds with potentially undesirable physiological qualities, taking into account toxicity and pharmacokinetic properties [53]. For this task, we estimated the drug similarity and in silico pharmacokinetic properties of the newly selected molecules as GluT1 inhibitory agents, using the online SwissADMET [54] and pkCSM [55] servers, respectively.

3.5. Molecular Docking Modeling

The computational technique of molecular docking is an efficient, fast and powerful tool for drug discovery [56]. For this project, we uploaded the three-dimensional coordinates of the target protein from the protein data bank (pdb) using the Discovery Studio 2021 (BIOVIA) software package [57]. To improve the performance of the cavity method, water molecules and suspended ligands bound to the protein were removed and polar hydrogens were added. Accordingly, the prepared protein was docked with the most active ligands, previously optimized by the density functional theory (DFT), with the assistance of AutoDock 4.2 [58]. Moreover, the grid box was centralized on (−42.562 Å, −0.46 Å, −55.066 Å) with the help of AUTOGRID algorithm, by putting the sizes (80, 80, 80) in their three-dimensional structure, and running 10 genetic algorithms with a total of 25 million trials. Finally, the molecular interactions of the protein-ligand were visualized using discovery studio 2021 [59].

3.6. Molecular Dynamics

Based on QSAR and molecular docking results, the five best-docked ligands, having the highest activity, were chosen for the molecular dynamics simulations in order to identify the molecular recognition between the ligand and the dopamine transporter (DAT) membrane protein. The MD simulations were performed for 100 nanoseconds using Desmond software, a package of Schrödinger LLC [60]. The first stage in the molecular dynamic's simulation of protein-ligand complexes was obtained by docking studies, and preprocessed using Protein Preparation Maestro, which performs optimization and minimization of complexes that have been prepared by the System Builder tool using a solvent model with an orthorhombic box that was chosen as TIP3P (transferable intermolecular interaction potential 3 points), using the OPLS force field [61]. At 300 K temperature and 1 atm pressure, the models were made neutral with the addition of water molecules, and counter ions, such as 0.15 M salt (Na^+, Cl^-) were added to mimic the physiological conditions. Finally, the trajectories were saved after every 10 ps for analysis, and the stability of simulations was evaluated by calculating the root mean square deviation (RMSD) of the protein and ligand over time. In addition, the root-mean-square fluctuation (RMSF), gyration radius (Rg), solvent accessible surface area (SASA), molecular surface area (MolSA) and polar surface area (PSA) were recorded for 100 ns, and the free energies of the inhibitors-protein interactions were evaluated using MM-GBSA approach [62].

4. Conclusions

A systematic in silico study was applied on 44 bicyclo((aryl)methyl)benzamide derivatives as glycine transporter type 1 (GlyT1) inhibitors to discover effective antipsychotic candidates for the treatment of schizophrenia. Initially, two QSAR models were developed using MLR and MNLR techniques and were examined through external and internal validation, applicability domain (AD), Y-randomization test and Golbreikh and tropsha criteria, indicating a significant effect of hydrogen bond donor, polarizability, surface tension, stretch and torsion energies and topological diameter on the locomotor activity (LMA). Subsequently, ADMET in silico pharmacokinetics prediction revealed a favorable profile of the most active ligands, where L6, L9, L30, L31 and L37 were predicted as non-toxic inhibitors for 2D6 cytochrome, which respect the rules of Lipinski, Veber, Egan and Ghose, with an excellent absorption exceeded 91% and highest probability to penetrate the central nervous system (CNS). In contrast, the ligand L32 as an outlier in the QSAR study has an unfavorable ADMET profile with the highest probability of being absorbed by the gastrointestinal tract. Lastly, the obtained results were further strengthened and qualified using molecular docking and molecular dynamics studies, which confirm that L6, L9, L30, L31 and L37 react specifically with Tyr124, Phe43, Phe325, Asp46, Phe319 and Val120 amino acids of the dopamine transporter (DAT) membrane protein in a way that blocks glycine transporter type 1 (GlyT1) forming dynamically stable complexes during 100 ns of MD simulation time. Therefore, they could be used as therapeutics in medicine to treat schizophrenia. However, they must be subjected to in vitro and in vivo investigations to evaluate their efficacy and safety as anti-schizophrenia drugs.

Supplementary Materials: The following are available online at https://www.mdpi.com/article/10.3390/ph15060670/s1, Table S1: The 44 molecules and their biological activities. Figure S1: RMSD and RMSF graphs for L6, L30, L31, L37 ligands complexed with the dopamine transporter membrane protein during 100 ns. Figure S2: Rg, MolSA, SASA and PSA during 100 ns of MD simulation, and the variation of total free energy for L6, L30, L31 and L37 ligands complexed with DAT protein. Table S2: The calculated molecular descriptors.

Author Contributions: Conceptualization, M.E.f., M.E. and M.K.; methodology, M.E.f., A.A. (Amine Assouguem) and M.E.-R.; software, M.E.f. and A.A. (Amal Alotaibi); validation, A.B., N.N.M. and H.F. data curation, R.U., S.E. and S.Z.; writing—original draft preparation, M.E.f. and M.E.-R.; writing—review and editing, M.K. and M.E.; supervision, M.E. All authors have read and agreed to the published version of the manuscript.

Funding: This research was funded by Princess Nourah bint Abdulrahman University Researchers Supporting Project number (PNURSP2022R33), Princess Nourah bint Abdulrahman University, Riyadh, Saudi Arabia.

Institutional Review Board Statement: Not applicable.

Informed Consent Statement: Not applicable.

Data Availability Statement: Data is contained within the article and Supplementary Materials.

Acknowledgments: Authors wish to thank Princess Nourah bint Abdulrahman University Researchers Supporting Project number (PNURSP2022R33), Princess Nourah bint Abdulrahman University, Riyadh, Saudi Arabia, for financial support.

Conflicts of Interest: The authors declare no conflict of interest.

References

1. Zheng, X.; Wang, C.; Zhai, N.; Luo, X.; Liu, G.; Ju, X. In Silico Screening of Novel A1-GABAA Receptor PAMs towards Schizophrenia Based on Combined Modeling Studies of Imidazo [1,2-a]-Pyridines. *Int. J. Mol. Sci.* **2021**, *22*, 9645. [CrossRef] [PubMed]
2. Gao, L.; Hao, C.; Chen, J.; Ma, R.; Zheng, L.; Wu, Q.; Liu, X.; Liu, B.-F.; Zhang, G.; Chen, Y.; et al. Discovery of a New Class of Multi-Target Heterocycle Piperidine Derivatives as Potential Antipsychotics with pro-Cognitive Effect. *Bioorg. Med. Chem. Lett.* **2021**, *40*, 127909. [CrossRef] [PubMed]
3. Shahsavar, A.; Stohler, P.; Bourenkov, G.; Zimmermann, I.; Siegrist, M.; Guba, W.; Pinard, E.; Seeger, M.A.; Schneider, T.R.; Dawson, R.J.P.; et al. *Structural Insights into Glycine Reuptake Inhibition*; 2020; BioRxiv. Available online: https://www.biorxiv.org/content/10.1101/2020.12.20.110478v1 (accessed on 14 April 2022).
4. Varnes, J.G.; Xiong, H.; Forst, J.M.; Holmquist, C.R.; Ernst, G.E.; Frietze, W.; Dembofsky, B.; Andisik, D.W.; Palmer, W.E.; Hinkley, L.; et al. Bicyclo((Aryl)Methyl)Benzamides as Inhibitors of GlyT1. *Bioorg. Med. Chem. Lett.* **2018**, *28*, 1043–1049. [CrossRef] [PubMed]
5. Cubelos, B.; Giménez, C.; Zafra, F. The Glycine Transporter GLYT1 Interacts with Sec3, a Component of the Exocyst Complex. *Neuropharmacology* **2005**, *49*, 935–944. [CrossRef] [PubMed]
6. Marques, B.L.; Oliveira-Lima, O.C.; Carvalho, G.A.; de Almeida Chiarelli, R.; Ribeiro, R.I.; Parreira, R.C.; da Madeira Freitas, E.M.; Resende, R.R.; Klempin, F.; Ulrich, H.; et al. Neurobiology of Glycine Transporters: From Molecules to Behavior. *Neurosci. Biobehav. Rev.* **2020**, *118*, 97–110. [CrossRef] [PubMed]
7. Lill, M.A. Multi-Dimensional QSAR in Drug Discovery. *Drug Discov. Today* **2007**, *12*, 1013–1017. [CrossRef]
8. Vilar, S.; Cozza, G.; Moro, S. Medicinal Chemistry and the Molecular Operating Environment (MOE): Application of QSAR and Molecular Docking to Drug Discovery. *Curr. Top. Med. Chem.* **2008**, *8*, 1555–1572. [CrossRef]
9. Tian, S.; Wang, J.; Li, Y.; Li, D.; Xu, L.; Hou, T. The Application of in Silico Drug-Likeness Predictions in Pharmaceutical Research. *Adv. Drug Deliv. Rev.* **2015**, *86*, 2–10. [CrossRef]
10. Serrano, A.; Imbernón, B.; Pérez-Sánchez, H.; Cecilia, J.M.; Bueno-Crespo, A.; Abellán, J.L. QN-Docking: An Innovative Molecular Docking Methodology Based on Q-Networks. *Appl. Soft Comput.* **2020**, *96*, 106678. [CrossRef]
11. El Khatabi, K.; El-mernissi, R.; Aanouz, I.; Ajana, M.A.; Lakhlifi, T.; Shahinozzaman, M.; Bouachrine, M. Benzimidazole Derivatives in Identifying Novel Acetylcholinesterase Inhibitors: A Combination of 3D-QSAR, Docking and Molecular Dynamics Simulation. *Phys. Chem. Res.* **2022**, *10*, 237–249. [CrossRef]
12. de Oliveira, T.A.; Medaglia, L.R.; Maia, E.H.B.; Assis, L.C.; de Carvalho, P.B.; da Silva, A.M.; Taranto, A.G. Evaluation of Docking Machine Learning and Molecular Dynamics Methodologies for DNA-Ligand Systems. *Pharmaceuticals* **2022**, *15*, 132. [CrossRef] [PubMed]
13. Wang, H.; Jia, Y.; Jing, G.; Wu, X. A Novel Toxicity Prediction Model for Hydrazine Compounds Based on 1D–3D Molecular Descriptors. *Comput. Toxicol.* **2021**, *18*, 100169. [CrossRef]
14. Halder, A.K.; Jha, T. Validated Predictive QSAR Modeling of N-Aryl-Oxazolidinone-5-Carboxamides for Anti-HIV Protease Activity. *Bioorg. Med. Chem. Lett.* **2010**, *20*, 6082–6087. [CrossRef] [PubMed]
15. Roy, K.; Kar, S.; Das, R.N. Validation of QSAR Models. In *Understanding the Basics of QSAR for Applications in Pharmaceutical Sciences and Risk Assessment*; Elsevier: Amsterdam, The Netherlands, 2015; pp. 231–289. ISSN 978-0-12-801505-6.
16. El Mchichi, L.; El Aissouq, A.; Kasmi, R.; Belhassan, A.; El-Mernissi, R.; Ouammou, A.; Lakhlifi, T.; Bouachrine, M. In Silico Design of Novel Pyrazole Derivatives Containing Thiourea Skeleton as Anti-Cancer Agents Using: 3D QSAR, Drug-Likeness Studies, ADMET Prediction and Molecular Docking. *Mater. Today Proc.* **2021**, *45*, 7661–7674. [CrossRef]
17. Mazigh, M.; El'mbarki, C.; Hadni, H.; Elhallaoui, M. QSAR Studies Combined with DFT-Calculations and Molecular Docking of Polyamine-Sensitive Inhibitors of the NMDA Receptor. *Mediterr. J. Chem.* **2019**, *9*, 164–174. [CrossRef]
18. Abdullahi, M.; Shallangwa, G.A.; Uzairu, A. In Silico QSAR and Molecular Docking Simulation of Some Novel Aryl Sulfonamide Derivatives as Inhibitors of H5N1 Influenza A Virus Subtype. *Beni-Suef Univ. J. Basic Appl. Sci.* **2020**, *9*, 2. [CrossRef]
19. Krieger, E.; Darden, T.; Nabuurs, S.B.; Finkelstein, A.; Vriend, G. Making Optimal Use of Empirical Energy Functions: Force-Field Parameterization in Crystal Space. *Proteins Struct. Funct. Bioinforma.* **2004**, *57*, 678–683. [CrossRef]
20. Bastianoni, A.; Guastaldi, E.; Barbagli, A.; Bernardinetti, S.; Zirulia, A.; Brancale, M.; Colonna, T. Multivariate Analysis Applied to Aquifer Hydrogeochemical Evaluation: A Case Study in the Coastal Significant Subterranean Water Body between "Cecina River and San Vincenzo", Tuscany (Italy). *Appl. Sci.* **2021**, *11*, 7595. [CrossRef]
21. Daoui, O.; Elkhattabi, S.; Chtita, S.; Elkhalabi, R.; Zgou, H.; Benjelloun, A.T. QSAR, Molecular Docking and ADMET Properties in Silico Studies of Novel 4,5,6,7-Tetrahydrobenzo[D]-Thiazol-2-Yl Derivatives Derived from Dimedone as Potent Anti-Tumor Agents through Inhibition of C-Met Receptor Tyrosine Kinase. *Heliyon* **2021**, *7*, e07463. [CrossRef]
22. Matsuzaka, Y.; Uesawa, Y. A Deep Learning-Based Quantitative Structure–Activity Relationship System Construct Prediction Model of Agonist and Antagonist with High Performance. *Int. J. Mol. Sci.* **2022**, *23*, 2141. [CrossRef]
23. Uyanık, G.K.; Güler, N. A Study on Multiple Linear Regression Analysis. *Procedia Soc. Behav. Sci.* **2013**, *106*, 234–240. [CrossRef]

24. Kravić, N.; Savosina, J.; Agafonova-Moroz, M.; Babain, V.; Legin, A.; Kirsanov, D. Nonlinear Multivariate Regression Algorithms for Improving Precision of Multisensor Potentiometry in Analysis of Spent Nuclear Fuel Reprocessing Solutions. *Chemosensors* **2022**, *10*, 90. [CrossRef]
25. Ruiz, I.L.; Gómez-Nieto, M.Á. Study of the Applicability Domain of the QSAR Classification Models by Means of the Rivality and Modelability Indexes. *Molecules* **2018**, *23*, 2756. [CrossRef] [PubMed]
26. Pourbasheer, E.; Riahi, S.; Ganjali, M.R.; Norouzi, P. Quantitative Structure–Activity Relationship (QSAR) Study of Interleukin-1 Receptor Associated Kinase 4 (IRAK-4) Inhibitor Activity by the Genetic Algorithm and Multiple Linear Regression (GA-MLR) Method. *J. Enzyme Inhib. Med. Chem.* **2010**, *25*, 844–853. [CrossRef]
27. Chtita, S.; Belhassan, A.; Bakhouch, M.; Taourati, A.I.; Aouidate, A.; Belaidi, S.; Moutaabbid, M.; Belaaouad, S.; Bouachrine, M.; Lakhlifi, T. QSAR Study of Unsymmetrical Aromatic Disulfides as Potent Avian SARS-CoV Main Protease Inhibitors Using Quantum Chemical Descriptors and Statistical Methods. *Chemom. Intell. Lab. Syst.* **2021**, *210*, 104266. [CrossRef]
28. de Castro Rezende, K.B.; da Cunha, A.J.L.; Amim Junior, J.; Bornia, R.G. External Validation of the Fetal Medicine Foundation Algorithm for the Prediction of Preeclampsia in a Brazilian Population. *Pregnancy Hypertens.* **2019**, *17*, 64–68. [CrossRef]
29. Rafało, M. Cross Validation Methods: Analysis Based on Diagnostics of Thyroid Cancer Metastasis. *ICT Express* **2021**, S2405959521000552. [CrossRef]
30. Chtita, S.; Ghamali, M.; Ousaa, A.; Aouidate, A.; Belhassan, A.; Taourati, A.I.; Masand, V.H.; Bouachrine, M.; Lakhlifi, T. QSAR Study of Anti-Human African Trypanosomiasis Activity for 2-Phenylimidazopyridines Derivatives Using DFT and Lipinski's Descriptors. *Heliyon* **2019**, *5*, e01304. [CrossRef]
31. Golbraikh, A.; Tropsha, A. Beware of Q2! *J. Mol. Graph. Model.* **2002**, *20*, 269–276. [CrossRef]
32. Daina, A.; Michielin, O.; Zoete, V. ILOGP: A Simple, Robust, and Efficient Description of *n* -Octanol/Water Partition Coefficient for Drug Design Using the GB/SA Approach. *J. Chem. Inf. Model.* **2014**, *54*, 3284–3301. [CrossRef]
33. Daina, A.; Zoete, V. A BOILED-Egg To Predict Gastrointestinal Absorption and Brain Penetration of Small Molecules. *ChemMedChem* **2016**, *11*, 1117–1121. [CrossRef] [PubMed]
34. Belhassan, A.; Zaki, H.; Benlyas, M.; Lakhlifi, T.; Bouachrine, M. Study of Novel Triazolo-Benzodiazepine Analogues as Antidepressants Targeting by Molecular Docking and ADMET Properties Prediction. *Heliyon* **2019**, *5*, e02446. [CrossRef] [PubMed]
35. Adamski, A.; Kruszka, D.; Dutkiewicz, Z.; Kubicki, M.; Gorczyński, A.; Patroniak, V. Novel Family of Fused Tricyclic [1,4]Diazepines: Design, Synthesis, Crystal Structures and Molecular Docking Studies. *Tetrahedron* **2017**, *73*, 3377–3386. [CrossRef]
36. Penmatsa, A.; Wang, K.H.; Gouaux, E. X-Ray Structure of Dopamine Transporter Elucidates Antidepressant Mechanism. *Nature* **2013**, *503*, 85–90. [CrossRef] [PubMed]
37. Zentrum Für Bioinformatik: Universität Hamburg-Proteins Plus Server. Available online: https://proteins.plus/ (accessed on 8 March 2022).
38. Spiegel, J.; Senderowitz, H. Evaluation of QSAR Equations for Virtual Screening. *Int. J. Mol. Sci.* **2020**, *21*, 7828. [CrossRef] [PubMed]
39. Österberg, T.; Norinder, U. Prediction of Drug Transport Processes Using Simple Parameters and PLS Statistics The Use of ACD/LogP and ACD/ChemSketch Descriptors. *Eur. J. Pharm. Sci.* **2001**, *12*, 327–337. [CrossRef]
40. Milne, G.W.A. Software Review of ChemBioDraw 12.0. *J. Chem. Inf. Model.* **2010**, *50*, 2053. [CrossRef]
41. Citation Gaussienne 09 | Gaussian.Com. Available online: https://gaussian.com/g09citation/ (accessed on 8 March 2022).
42. Parr, R.G.; Weitao, Y. *Density-Functional Theory of Atoms and Molecules*; International Series of Monographs on Chemistry; Oxford University Press: New York, NY, USA, 1995; ISBN 978-0-19-509276-9.
43. Introducing the XLSTAT Free Edition. Available online: https://www.xlstat.com/en/news/introducing-the-xlstat-free-edition (accessed on 8 March 2022).
44. Guerra Tort, C.; Aguiar Pulido, V.; Suárez Ulloa, V.; Docampo Boedo, F.; López Gestal, J.M.; Pereira Loureiro, J. Electronic Health Records Exploitation Using Artificial Intelligence Techniques. *Proceedings* **2020**, *54*, 60. [CrossRef]
45. Hadni, H.; Elhallaoui, M. 3D-QSAR, Docking and ADMET Properties of Aurone Analogues as Antimalarial Agents. *Heliyon* **2020**, *6*, e03580. [CrossRef]
46. van der Voet, H. Comparing the Predictive Accuracy of Models Using a Simple Randomization Test. *Chemom. Intell. Lab. Syst.* **1994**, *25*, 313–323. [CrossRef]
47. Ebenezer, O.; Damoyi, N.; Jordaan, M.A.; Shapi, M. Unveiling of Pyrimidindinones as Potential Anti-Norovirus Agents—A Pharmacoinformatic-Based Approach. *Molecules* **2022**, *27*, 380. [CrossRef] [PubMed]
48. Lipinski, C.A.; Lombardo, F.; Dominy, B.W.; Feeney, P.J. Experimental and Computational Approaches to Estimate Solubility and Permeability in Drug Discovery and Development Settings. *Adv. Drug Deliv. Rev.* **1997**, *23*, 3–25. [CrossRef]
49. Veber, D.F.; Johnson, S.R.; Cheng, H.-Y.; Smith, B.R.; Ward, K.W.; Kopple, K.D. Molecular Properties That Influence the Oral Bioavailability of Drug Candidates. *J. Med. Chem.* **2002**, *45*, 2615–2623. [CrossRef] [PubMed]
50. Yalcin, S. Molecular Docking, Drug Likeness, and ADMET Analyses of Passiflora Compounds as P-Glycoprotein (P-Gp) Inhibitor for the Treatment of Cancer. *Curr. Pharmacol. Rep.* **2020**, *6*, 429–440. [CrossRef]
51. Egan, W.J.; Merz, K.M.; Baldwin, J.J. Prediction of Drug Absorption Using Multivariate Statistics. *J. Med. Chem.* **2000**, *43*, 3867–3877. [CrossRef]
52. Egan, W.J.; Lauri, G. Prediction of Intestinal Permeability. *Adv. Drug Deliv. Rev.* **2002**, *54*, 273–289. [CrossRef]

53. Gomes, D.; Silvestre, S.; Duarte, A.P.; Venuti, A.; Soares, C.P.; Passarinha, L.; Sousa, Â. In Silico Approaches: A Way to Unveil Novel Therapeutic Drugs for Cervical Cancer Management. *Pharmaceuticals* **2021**, *14*, 741. [CrossRef]
54. Daina, A.; Michielin, O.; Zoete, V. SwissADME: A Free Web Tool to Evaluate Pharmacokinetics, Drug-Likeness and Medicinal Chemistry Friendliness of Small Molecules. *Sci. Rep.* **2017**, *7*, 42717. [CrossRef]
55. PkCSM. Available online: http://biosig.unimelb.edu.au/pkcsm/run_example? (accessed on 8 March 2022).
56. Bassani, D.; Pavan, M.; Bolcato, G.; Sturlese, M.; Moro, S. Re-Exploring the Ability of Common Docking Programs to Correctly Reproduce the Binding Modes of Non-Covalent Inhibitors of SARS-CoV-2 Protease Mpro. *Pharmaceuticals* **2022**, *15*, 180. [CrossRef]
57. Iqbal, D.; Rehman, M.T.; Bin Dukhyil, A.; Rizvi, S.M.D.; Al Ajmi, M.F.; Alshehri, B.M.; Banawas, S.; Khan, M.S.; Alturaiki, W.; Alsaweed, M. High-Throughput Screening and Molecular Dynamics Simulation of Natural Product-like Compounds against Alzheimer's Disease through Multitarget Approach. *Pharmaceuticals* **2021**, *14*, 937. [CrossRef]
58. Norgan, A.P.; Coffman, P.K.; Kocher, J.-P.A.; Katzmann, D.J.; Sosa, C.P. Multilevel Parallelization of AutoDock 4.2. *J. Cheminformatics* **2011**, *3*, 12. [CrossRef] [PubMed]
59. BIOVIA Discovery Studio - BIOVIA - Dassault Systèmes®. Available online: https://www.3ds.com/products-services/biovia/products/molecular-modeling-simulation/biovia-discovery-studio/ (accessed on 8 March 2022).
60. Desmond | Schrodinger. Available online: https://www.schrodinger.com/products/desmond (accessed on 28 April 2022).
61. Kaminski, G.A.; Friesner, R.A.; Tirado-Rives, J.; Jorgensen, W.L. Evaluation and Reparametrization of the OPLS-AA Force Field for Proteins via Comparison with Accurate Quantum Chemical Calculations on Peptides. *J. Phys. Chem. B* **2001**, *105*, 6474–6487. [CrossRef]
62. Wang, E.; Sun, H.; Wang, J.; Wang, Z.; Liu, H.; Zhang, J.Z.H.; Hou, T. End-Point Binding Free Energy Calculation with MM/PBSA and MM/GBSA: Strategies and Applications in Drug Design. *Chem. Rev.* **2019**, *119*, 9478–9508. [CrossRef] [PubMed]

pharmaceuticals

MDPI

Article

Structural Elucidation of Rift Valley Fever Virus L Protein towards the Discovery of Its Potential Inhibitors

Mubarak A. Alamri [1,†], Muhammad Usman Mirza [2,†], Muhammad Muzammal Adeel [3,†], Usman Ali Ashfaq [4], Muhammad Tahir ul Qamar [4,*], Farah Shahid [4], Sajjad Ahmad [5], Eid A. Alatawi [6], Ghadah M. Albalawi [7,8], Khaled S. Allemailem [7,*] and Ahmad Almatroudi [7]

1 Department of Pharmaceutical Chemistry, College of Pharmacy, Prince Sattam Bin Abdulaziz University, Al-Kharj 16273, Saudi Arabia; m.alamri@psau.edu.sa
2 Department of Chemistry and Biochemistry, University of Windsor, Windsor, ON N9B 3P4, Canada; mumirza@uwindsor.ca
3 3D Genomics Research Center, College of Informatics, Huazhong Agricultural University, Wuhan 430070, China; m.muzammal.adeel@outlook.com
4 Department of Bioinformatics and Biotechnology, Government College University Faisalabad, Faisalabad 38000, Pakistan; usmancemb@gmail.com (U.A.A.); farahshahid24@gcuf.edu.pk (F.S.)
5 Department of Health and Biological Sciences, Abasyn University, Peshawar 25000, Pakistan; sajjad.ahmad@abasyn.edu.pk
6 Department of Medical Laboratory Technology, Faculty of Applied Medical Sciences, University of Tabuk, Tabuk 71491, Saudi Arabia; eid.alatawi@ut.edu.sa
7 Department of Medical Laboratories, College of Applied Medical Sciences, Qassim University, Buraydah 51452, Saudi Arabia; galbalawi080@gmail.com (G.M.A.); aamtrody@qu.edu.sa (A.A.)
8 Department of Laboratory and Blood Bank, King Fahd Specialist Hospital, Tabuk 47717, Saudi Arabia
* Correspondence: tahirulqamar@gcuf.edu.pk (M.T.u.Q.); k.allemailem@qu.edu.sa (K.S.A.)
† These authors contributed equally to this work.

Citation: Alamri, M.A.; Mirza, M.U.; Adeel, M.M.; Ashfaq, U.A.; Tahir ul Qamar, M.; Shahid, F.; Ahmad, S.; Alatawi, E.A.; Albalawi, G.M.; Allemailem, K.S.; et al. Structural Elucidation of Rift Valley Fever Virus L Protein towards the Discovery of Its Potential Inhibitors. *Pharmaceuticals* **2022**, *15*, 659. https://doi.org/10.3390/ph15060659

Academic Editor: Marialuigia Fantacuzzi

Received: 23 April 2022
Accepted: 20 May 2022
Published: 25 May 2022

Publisher's Note: MDPI stays neutral with regard to jurisdictional claims in published maps and institutional affiliations.

Abstract: Rift valley fever virus (RVFV) is the causative agent of a viral zoonosis that causes a significant clinical burden in domestic and wild ruminants. Major outbreaks of the virus occur in livestock, and contaminated animal products or arthropod vectors can transmit the virus to humans. The viral RNA-dependent RNA polymerase (RdRp; L protein) of the RVFV is responsible for viral replication and is thus an appealing drug target because no effective and specific vaccine against this virus is available. The current study reported the structural elucidation of the RVFV-L protein by in-depth homology modeling since no crystal structure is available yet. The inhibitory binding modes of known potent L protein inhibitors were analyzed. Based on the results, further molecular docking-based virtual screening of Selleckchem Nucleoside Analogue Library (156 compounds) was performed to find potential new inhibitors against the RVFV L protein. ADME (Absorption, Distribution, Metabolism, and Excretion) and toxicity analysis of these compounds was also performed. Besides, the binding mechanism and stability of identified compounds were confirmed by a 50 ns molecular dynamic (MD) simulation followed by MM/PBSA binding free energy calculations. Homology modeling determined a stable multi-domain structure of L protein. An analysis of known L protein inhibitors, including Monensin, Mycophenolic acid, and Ribavirin, provide insights into the binding mechanism and reveals key residues of the L protein binding pocket. The screening results revealed that the top three compounds, A-317491, Khasianine, and VER155008, exhibited a high affinity at the L protein binding pocket. ADME analysis revealed good pharmacodynamics and pharmacokinetic profiles of these compounds. Furthermore, MD simulation and binding free energy analysis endorsed the binding stability of potential compounds with L protein. In a nutshell, the present study determined potential compounds that may aid in the rational design of novel inhibitors of the RVFV L protein as anti-RVFV drugs.

Keywords: RVFV; RdRp; structural modeling; virtual screening; docking; MD simulation

1. Introduction

Rift Valley fever is a hemorrhagic ailment caused by the Rift Valley Viral Infection (RVVI), affecting humans and livestock. Mosquitos are the vectors for this disease. The first case of RVVI was reported in East Africa's Rift Valley in Kenya, which made it known as RVF. In its first instance, a significant population of farmed sheep was killed from 1930 to 1931. *Aedex* and *cules* are the two common vectors (mosquitoes) transmitting this virus [1]. Post RVVI, flu-like common symptoms have lasted up to seven days. Although most human infections are mild, approximately four percent of the cases have been severe and show symptoms such as Hemorrhagic fever, meningoencephalitis, and ocular type [2].

The virus responsible for this disease is Rift Valley Fever Virus (RVFV), a single-stranded RNA virus belonging to the Phenuviridae Family and the genus Phlebovirus. Rift Valley fever (RVF) is caused by RVFV and has a wide range of clinical symptoms. A mild febrile illness is common in humans and can lead to more severe illnesses such as encephalitis, hemorrhagic fever, and liver disease. Neurological issues including dizziness, paralysis, headaches, hallucinations, vertigo, and delirium are also observed [3]. Up to 10% of RVFV-infected humans experience ophthalmologic complications, including retinal hemorrhaging and photophobia. Sheep, cattle, and goats are more susceptible to RVFV, with a 20–30% mortality rate in adult ruminants and 70% in young animals. Spontaneous abortion in infected pregnant animals is alarmingly high, ranging from 40–100 percent [4].

RVF outbreaks are sporadic and linked to meteorological, hydrological, and socioeconomic factors. RVF outbreaks have been reported to produce considerable numbers of infected human cases, which have substantially impacted the healthcare system [5]. According to an analysis by the Center for Disease Control and Prevention (CDC), several RVF outbreaks have occurred in various countries, resulting in hundreds of thousands of human illnesses and human casualties [6]. This disease has spread from the African region to the Arabian to the USA, making it a grave concern to affected regions and the whole world [7]. Epizootics that occur in livestock frequently precede human epidemics. In other words, reducing RVVI in animals is expected to break the transmission cycle and help avoid human sickness [8]. The CDC and the U.S Department of Agriculture (USDA) both classify RVFV as a select agent because of its ability to cause morbidity and mortality and its potential use as a bioterrorism agent [4,9]. Unfortunately, there are no FDA-approved vaccines for humans, but some approved vaccines are available for veterinary use. Similarly, there are no therapeutics available to treat RVFV, requiring additional research in this area.

As per the structure of RVF, it is a high-molecular-weight, single-stranded, linear virion (2–2.5 nm in diameter, 200–300 nm in length, and displaying helical symmetry) enclosed within the ribonucleo-capsid [10]. Three segments of the RVFV genome (S, M, and L-segments) have previously been described as having three separate open reading frames (ORFs) coding for three distinct proteins (viral polymerase, L-protein, and S-protein) [11,12]. The L segment, which encodes only one protein, RNA-dependent RNA polymerase (RdRp), commonly referred to as L protein, is particularly important to our research. The L protein is involved in genomic replication and viral mRNA transcription. The middle region of the L protein contains an RdRp domain, which is found in all RNA viral polymerases and is required for viral RNA production. The RdRp domain retains the six characteristic conserved structural motifs, including PreA/F, A, B, C, D, and E in the central core region [12–15]. Most of these motifs are located in the palm subdomain and characterize the active site chamber formation [14]. These host mRNAs are employed as primers for viral transcription and suppress viral-RNA-induced immune responses [16]. L protein has an endonuclease domain at its N-terminus that is necessary for cap-snatching, in which it cleaves 50 m7G caps from host mRNAs [17,18]. Viruses translate and reproduce their genome in the cell cytoplasm for survival and growth. During the replication, the virus uses a technique termed cap-snatching, which means taking advantage of two known viral L protein functions: the capability to bind cap structures and cut off the cellular mRNA attached to [19].

The rational drug design process is greatly accelerated by using different computer-aided drug designing applications for in silico drug screening [20–27]. A virtual screening-based drug discovery strategy has been identified as one of the most effective ways to discover and develop new drugs [28]. RVFV L protein was selected for the current study as a potential target for which no drug has been reported so far. Besides evolutionarily conserved motifs in the core region, RdRp has channels/tunnels that link the active site chamber with the exterior and therefore emerge as a potential target for developing antiviral inhibitors [29–32], which is evident from the inhibitor design against many deadly viruses such as *Zika virus* (ZIKV) [33–36], *Japanese encephalitis virus* (JEV) [37], *West Nile virus* (WNV) [38], *Dengue virus* (DENV) [39–41], HCV [24,42–44], HIV [45], SARS-CoV-2 [25], and most of the drugs have been reported against *Ebola* polymerase L (EBOV) [26]. The current study aimed to use the virtual screening approach to identify potential RVFV L protein inhibitors and inhibitory binding modes of known potent inhibitors, followed by molecular docking analysis to discover novel inhibitors that could be used as potential leads for *RVVI* treatment.

2. Results and Discussion

2.1. Protein Structural Analysis

Homology modeling is a well-established technique in modern drug discovery, and with more advancement in machine learning approaches, it is now possible to build a homology model with high accuracy even from a template with a low identity. Recent advances in homology modeling have proven their effectiveness as an alternative [46,47] and retrospective analysis, and validate the usefulness of homology modeling in SBVS. [48–51]. In the current study, the 3D structure of RVFV L protein was predicted by using the homology modeling approach via Modeller.v9.11. It was observed that the crystal structure and cryo-EM structure of severe fever with thrombocytopenia syndrome virus L (SFTSV L) protein (PDB IDs: 6L42 and 6Y6K) were the best hits based on query coverage and percentage identity. 6L42 showed a 34.41% sequence identity and a 91% query coverage during the sequence to structure alignment, while 6Y6K showed a 34.28% sequence identity and a 91% query coverage against the target sequence (Figure S1). Hence, these models were considered the best templates for homology modeling. Chain "A" of both templates were used for downstream structure prediction steps. Studies have suggested that more than 90% confidence indicates that the core model is precise and correct, deviating 2–4 Å in RMSD from the native protein structure [52]. Moreover, a good percentage of identity with maximum coverage between the template and the query sequence indicates a high level of accuracy in the model. The structural superposition/RMSD of the model with the templates is depicted in (Figure S2).

Overall, the newly predicted structure showed a pretty stable arrangement of amino-acid residues; apparently, no structural distortion was observed, and a total of 82 helices, 40 sheets, and 118 coils were detected (Figure 1A). Deep structural analysis suggested that the computational model of RVFV protein contains seven domains, i.e., the endoN domain (amino acids 25–205), separated by a linker of span 206–295; the PA-C-like domain from 296 to 762 amino acid; the RdRp core from 763 to 1345 amino acid; the PB2-N-like domain with residues 1346–1571 span; the arm domain contains two spans 1615–1696 and 1811–1932 that are separated by a blocker motif of 1811–1852 residues; the next domain was CBD with the residues 1697–1810, and on the C-terminal, a lariat domain (1933–2049 amino acid) was observed as previously reported [53] (Figure 1B). Some of the RVFV protein model domains were reported as structurally similar to SFTSV-L (severe fever with thrombocytopaenia syndrome virus –L protein) [54], which seems evident because these proteins shared the same values as the *Phenuiviridae* protein family. The orientation of each domain determines the functional specificity of protein and facilitates inter-molecular interactions for domain organization [19,53].

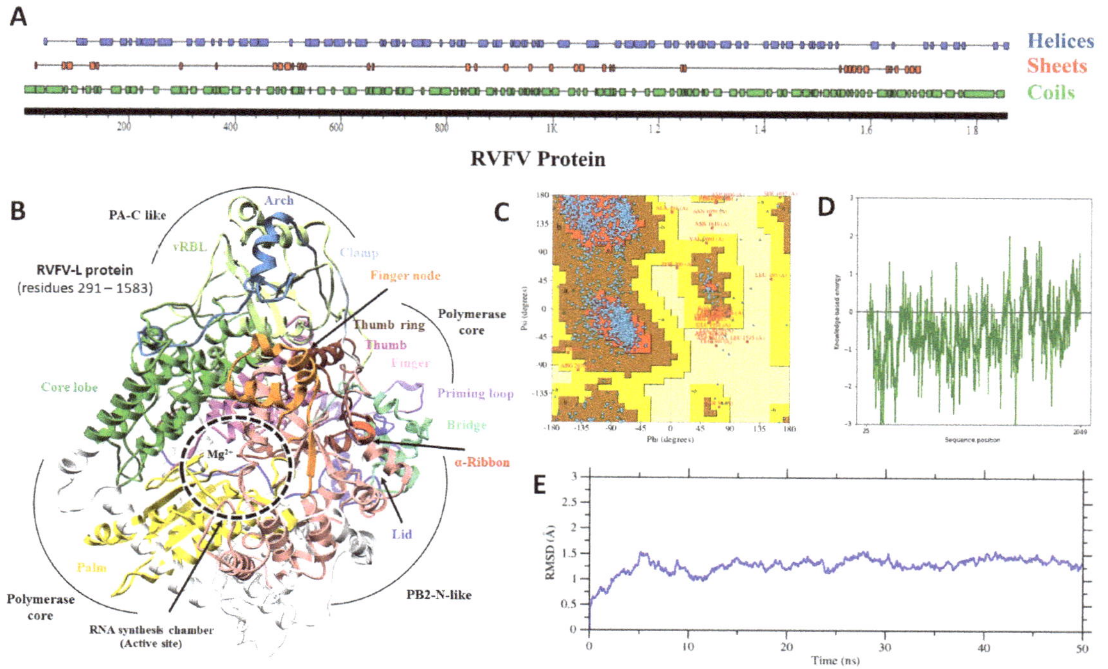

Figure 1. RVFV L protein structural analysis: (**A**) Two-dimensional representation of RVFV L protein showing the helices (blue), sheets (red), and coils (green) information (top to bottom). The horizontal black bar is representing the length of a protein. (**B**) Ribbon representation of 3D-model of RVFV L Protein (residues from 291–1583 are highlighted) with divalent cation, presumed to be a magnesium ion (circle Mg^{2+}). Each structural component is highlighted with a different color. (**C**) Ramachandran plot contains four quadrants. The 1st and 3rd quadrant indicate the allowed region, while 2nd and 4th show the disallowed region. Blue dots are showing the density of amino acid residues. (**D**) Model energy calculation graph showing the local energy estimation of a model. The *X*-axis indicates the sequence length, while *Y*-axis shows the energy values. (**E**) RMSD of $C\alpha$ atoms of the RVFV L protein over a period of 50 ns.

Multiple methods were employed for the validation of the 3D model. The Ramachandran plot indicates that 82.8% of residues were present in the favored region, 15.4% were present in additional allowed regions, and 0.7% were present in disallowed regions (Figure 1C). The presence of 82% of residues in the favored region indicates the high quality of the model. The functional properties of a protein depend mainly on its 3D structure and these properties were analyzed based on secondary structures. It is beneficial to identify secondary structure elements and structural motifs when studying the protein 3D structure [55]. Structural components of L protein were analyzed by PDBsum [56]; results showed the presence of multiple structural components such as 18 Beta-hairpins, 84 helices, 1Psi-loops, 40 strands, 155 Beta-turns, 44 Gamma-turns, 1 Beta-alpha-beta-unit, and 111 helix–helix interactions. Since we detected the 84 helices and 111 helix–helix interactions, such a high number of helices content determines the high chirality of proteins and thus provides structural compactness [57]. The distribution of structural components suggested the potential stability of the newly designed model, which was cross-validated by MD-simulations in subsequent steps. The lowest energy of a model also determines its quality, here we have applied the ProsaWeb server [58] to determine the overall local energy of the RVFV protein model at the amino acid level, results showed that most of the amino acids were showing the lowest energy below the threshold (Figure 1D). A 50 ns MD simulation further evaluated the generated model, and less than a 1.5 Å average RMSD was found that endorsed the reliability of the predicted RVFV-L protein model. An RMSD trajectory plot depicted the overall backbone structure stability of RVFV's core L protein subdomains (Figure 1E). The backbone Cα-RMSD of RVFV-L fluctuated in the start and converged afterwards. Protein expansion during the start of the simulation probably led to a somewhat larger RMSD of model structure to achieve a more stable conformation. Additionally, the RVFV-L protein homology model was compared with the corresponding template using TM align [59] to identify the likelihood of a similar structural fold (RdRp polymerase chamber) as categorized in SCP/CATH. The TM-algin is the protein structural alignment program for comparing proteins. The TM-align ranked the RVFV-RdRp with up to an 88% similar fold. Reverse template selection by the profunc server [60] (which scans auto-generated templates from the query structure against the most representative structures in PDB using Jess, a fast and accurate 3D-structure search algorithm) also determined SFTSV L (6L42) as the best hits with an E-value of 0.00E+00 and structural similarity of 99.9% (Table S1).

2.2. Binding Site Determination

The identification and characterization of binding sites of target proteins using various in silico methods are of main consideration for structure-based drug design. For binding site analysis, careful consideration was given to the biological suggestive templates. As RdRps are encoded by a wide range of viruses and play an important role in the replication and transcription of viral RNA [61] and have a conserved RdRp core region including the characteristic conserved finger, palm, and thumb subdomains with conserved 6 structural motifs (motifs A–F), which are essential for polymerase function [31]. Therefore, more in-depth information was extracted from other templates (with low identity) that showed sequence identity in the core region. The overall predicted binding site is diagrammatically illustrated in Figure 2.

Despite the low sequence identity (<35% identity), the RVFV-L RdRp core (residues 769–1358) displayed characteristic features of the polymerase core domain, which included the RNA synthesis chamber configured by representative RdRp conserved structural motifs connected to the exterior by four channels (for template entry and exit, NTP entry, and product exit) (Figure 2). The active site chamber of the RVFV-L RdRp core is formed by conserved RdRp motifs A-F located in the palm domain as reported in other RNA polymerases, notably in *orthobunyavirus* polymerases [14,62]. For molecular docking, the active site residues were further predicted using COACH and 3DLigandSite, and both servers predicted Arg926, Ile928, Asp991, Lys994, Trp995, Asn996, Gln1084, Ser1132, Asp1133, Asp1134 and Ser1175, and Phe1191 and Phe1194 as common binding site residues. Interestingly, the structural superimposition of RdRp core regions of RVFV-L and SFTSV-L demonstrated these residues to be entirely inside the functionally conserved structural motifs A-F. These include premotif A (motif F) (919-QQHGGL**R**E**I**-928), motif A (991-**D**AR**KWN**-996) with a conserved divalent cation binding residue Asp991, motif B (1084-**Q**GILHYTSSLLH-1095), catalytic signature motif C (1132-**SDD**-1134) located between two β-strands, motif D (1173-YP**S**EKST-1179), and motif E (1186-MEYNS**EFYF**-1194). To further evaluate the binding site for docking simulations, poliovirus elongation complex structure (PDB ID: 3OL8) [63] and foot-and-mouth disease virus in complex with RTP (PDB ID: 2E9R) [64] were superimposed and positions of catalytic divalent cations and conformation of RTP were analyzed. The superimposition revealed that the position of divalent cations was in close connection with functionally conserved aspartates of motif C (Asp1133) and motif A (Asp991) [65,66]. The importance of these aspartates is apparent from a number of mutational studies that uncovered altered polymerase activity in several RdRp viruses [63,67–73]. The conservation of core residues in these motifs suggests a conserved evolutionary link between RNA polymerase viruses and pinpoints the potential of exploiting the core architecture with other related segmented (−) ssRNA viruses in order to predict their structural/functional features even with a low sequence homology [32,74–76]. The docking grid was generated to cover these structural motifs for molecular docking.

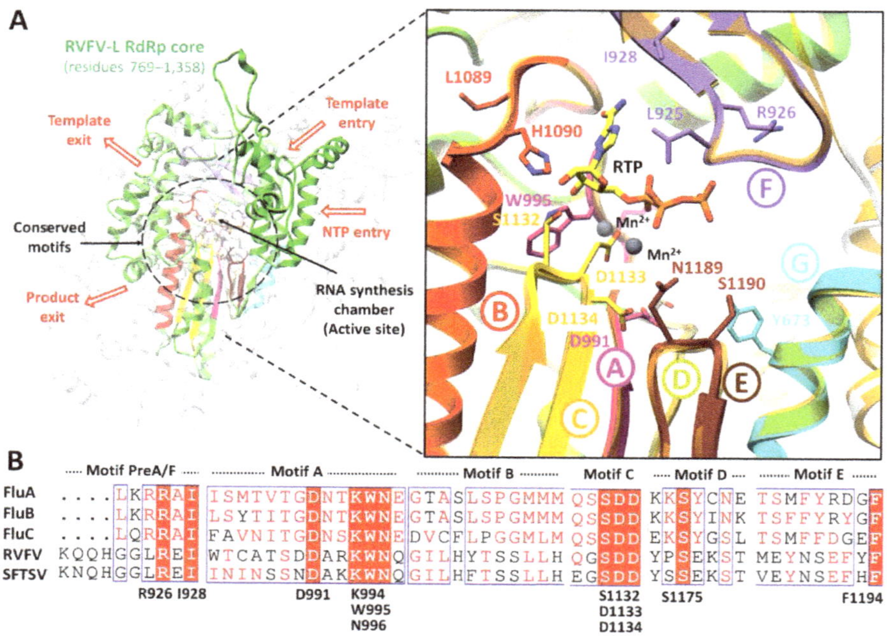

Figure 2. The predicted RVFV-L RdRp active site. (**A**) The RVFV-L RdRp core (residues 769–1358) is highlighted in green with conserved RNA synthesis chamber (active site), organized by conserved structural motifs in distinct colors. The four predicted tunnels are marked with arrows as an entrance (template and NTP entry) into the active site chamber and exit tunnels (template and product exit). The arrangement of structurally conserved RdRp motifs are colored magenta, red, golden, khaki, brown, purple, and cyan for motifs A–F, respectively, and superimposed on SFTSV-L RdRp core (light orange). (**B**) The predicted binding site residues are aligned and highlighted through multiple structure alignment (MSA) in representative motifs. These conserved residues are highlighted in stick representation accordingly. Superposition of the poliovirus elongation complex structure (PDB ID: 3OL8) and foot-and-mouth disease virus in complex with RTP (PDB ID: 2E9R) displays the conformation of RTP (yellow) and positions of the catalytic divalent cations (black spheres). Viral names in MSA are abbreviated as follows: Influenza A (FluA), B (FluB), and C (FluC) virus polymerase, Rift valley fever virus (RVFV), and Severe fever with thrombocytopenia syndrome virus (SFTSV).

2.3. Molecular Docking

Molecular docking is a modeling technique that examines how ligands and receptors fit together and how enzymes interact with ligands [77,78]. The docking computations were done three times, and the compound conformations were sorted by binding energy in kcal/mol. Initially, three known potent inhibitors with distinct chemical structures, namely, Monensin, Mycophenolic acid, and Ribavirin were docked [79]. Monensin inhibits host cell entry by blocking endocytic organelles' acidification [80]. Mycophenolic acid and Ribavirin act directly by inhibiting the RdRp enzyme or indirectly via the inhibition of cellular enzymes necessary for the biosynthesis of guanine-nucleotide [81,82]. The docking grid-box in Autodock Vina was set up to cover the predicted active site residues within the conserved structural RdRp motifs. As shown in Figure 3, the docked complexes obtained a similar binding orientation within the active chamber RdRp core. For Monensin, it forms hydrogen bonds with the side chains of Arg 672, Asp 990, Asp 1133 (belong to motif C), and Ala 992 (belong to motif A) residues with a binding energy score of −8.5 kcal/mol (Figure 3B). Mycophenolic acid forms hydrogen bonds with residues Arg 1197 and Asn 984 having a binding score of −7.0 kcal/mol (Figure 3D), while Ribavirin forms hydrogen bonds with residues Asp 1134 (belong to motif C), Tyr 757, Ser 1190 (belong to motif E), Arg 672, Asp 991 (a conserved divalent cation binding residue), and Asp 1133 (functionally conserved aspartates of motif C) having a binding score of −6.7 kcal/mol (Figure 3F).

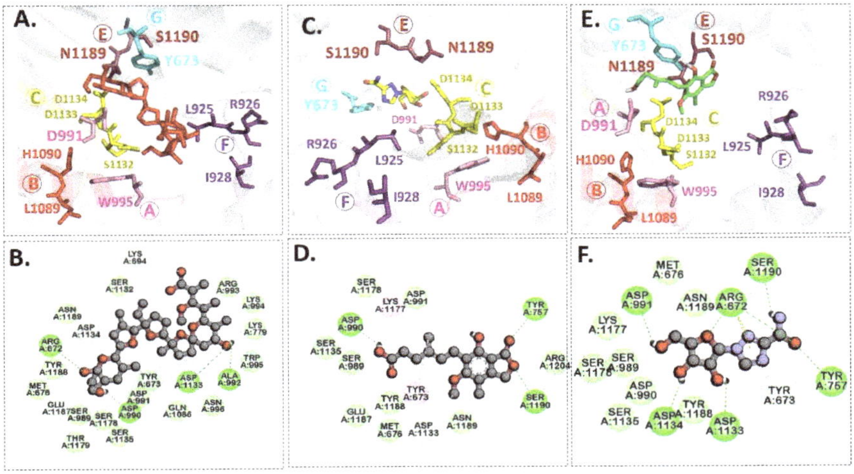

Figure 3. Binding modes and interaction mechanisms of known L protein inhibitors. Close-up view into 3D binding mode of (**A**) Monensin, (**C**) Mycophenolic acid, and (**E**) Ribavirin. The main residues that involve in the formation of the active site within the structurally conserved RdRp motifs that are show in in stickes. 2D interaction analysis of (**B**) Monensin, (**D**) Mycophenolic acid, and (**F**) Ribavirin.

Subsequently, the structure-based virtual screening of the Selleckchem Nucleoside Analogue Library containing 156 diverse compounds against the L protein was performed. Nucleoside or nucleotide analogue is an important class of antiviral therapeutics [83]. It is a powerful tool for dissecting the mechanisms and functions of viral DNA and RNA polymerases [84,85]. This screening selected top-ranking compounds with better binding scores than control compounds for further analysis. The virtual screening results for the top compounds with a binding affinity > −1.5 kcal/mol are shown in Table S2. Table 1 depicts a general overview of the binding energies and residues of control drugs. The docking analysis revealed that A-317491, followed by VER155008, and Khasianine were the best binders among the docked compounds used in this study. The selected compounds exhibited their binding energies in −8.7 kcal/mol to −6.7 kcal/mol.

Figure 4 shows the binding modes and 2D interaction mechanisms of top docked compounds. The 2D plot shows that A-317491 is involved in hydrogen bonding with several residues, such as His1090 and Gln1086 within motif E, Asp991, Ala992, Trp995, and Asn996 within motif A, and Lys 1177 within motif D, with a binding energy score of −8.7 kcal/mol (Figure 4B). Khasianine formed hydrogen bonding with a Gln997 side chain with a binding score of −7.1 kcal/mol (Figure 4C), while VER155008 was involved in making hydrogen bonds with residues Arg672, Lys779, Asp991, Lys1177, Tyr1188, and Ser1190 with a binding score of −7.8 kcal/mol (Figure 4D).

Table 1. Binding energy and binding residues of docked complexes.

Docked Complex	Chemical Structure	Binding Energy kcal/mol	Binding Residues (Amino Acid ID)	
			Van der Waals	Hydrogen Bonds
A-317491	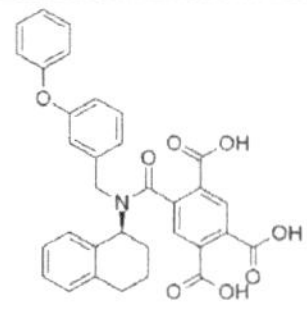	−8.7	673, 1132, 1133	1090, 995, 1134, 925, 1086, 924, 996, 779, 992, 1177, 993, 991, 676, 672, 1188, 1189
Monensin	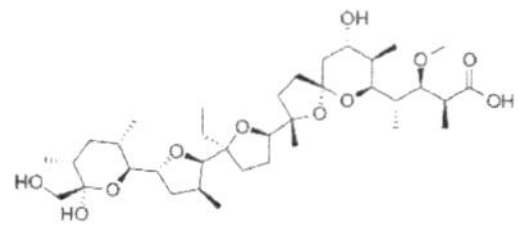	−8.5	676, 1187, 989, 1179, 1135, 991, 673, 995, 694, 1134, 1189	672, 990, 1133, 992
VER155008	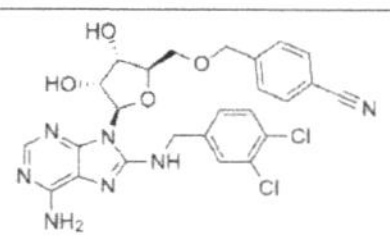	−7.8	925, 1189, 1187, 676, 989, 1179, 1178, 673, 1133, 1086	779, 1190, 1188, 672, 991, 1177
Khasianine	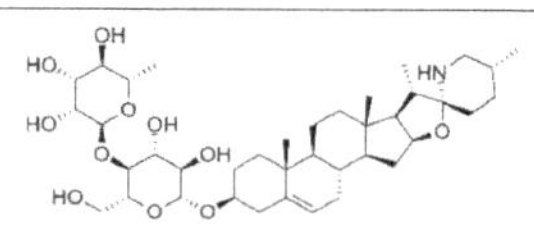	−7.1	1189, 1204, 924, 1133, 925, 993, 995, 996, 994, 779, 694, 1177, 670, 669, 673, 1134	997
Mycophenolic acid	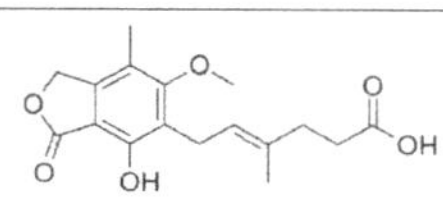	−7.0	1181, 1180, 1127, 1126, 1183, 751, 667, 985, 1171, 1128, 668, 1170	1197, 984
Ribavirin	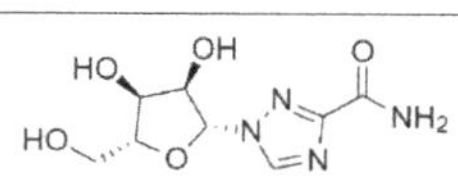	−6.7	1135, 1188, 990, 989, 1178, 1177, 676, 1189	1134, 757, 1190, 672, 991, 1133

Notably, both known inhibitors and the identified compounds occupied the binding site pockets within the RdRp core with a similar interaction pattern (Figure 5). Both control drugs and selected compounds formed hydrogen bonds with functionally conserved aspartates of motif C, namely, Asp 1133 and the conserved divalent cation binding residue, Asp991 [24]. Our screened nucleoside compounds displayed higher binding energies and interacting profiles than Monensin, mycophenolic acid, and Ribavirin. Most ligands tended to bind the residues belonging to the PA-C-Like domain and the RdRp core domain. Since both these domains are actively involved in forming active site chamber and vRNA binding. Previously published data have proposed that RdRp and PA-C-Like domains facilitate the template-directed RNA synthesis in SFTSV-L protein by providing the NTP entry into the catalytic chamber [62]. Overall, both these domains and endo N domain are critical for product synthesis and the safest release in the cell [53]. These findings suggested that the compounds identified in our study could be more useful candidates for RVFV drug therapy. Previously, a number of studies on RdRp have identified several leads using various computational and experimental techniques. The compounds revealed to interact with RdRp binding pocket residues reported herein [86,87]. However, RVFV RdRp has not been explored much, and the current study is a pioneer work in this regard.

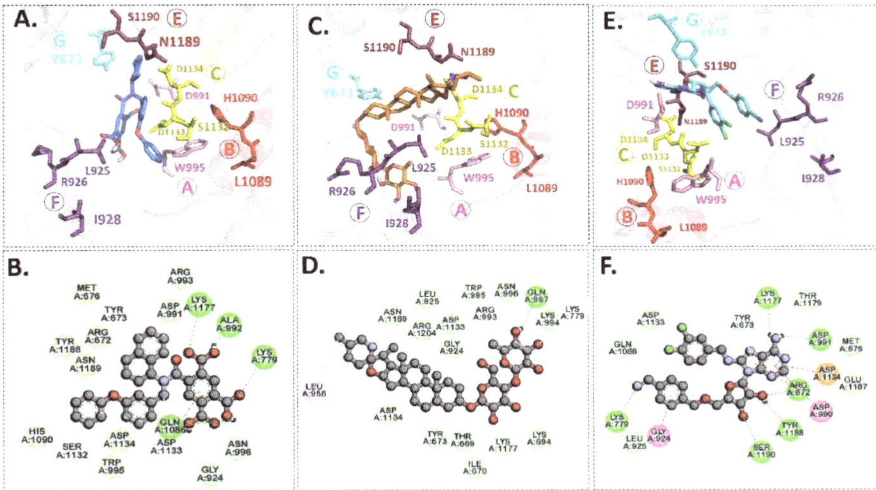

Figure 4. Binding modes and interaction mechanisms of novel L protein inhibitors. (**A**) Close-up view into binding mode of (**A**) A-317491, (**C**) Khasianine, and (**E**) VER155008. The main residues involved in the formation of the active site within the structurally conserved RdRp motifs shown in stickes. 2D interaction analysis of (**B**) A-317491, (**D**) Khasianine, and (**F**) VER155008.

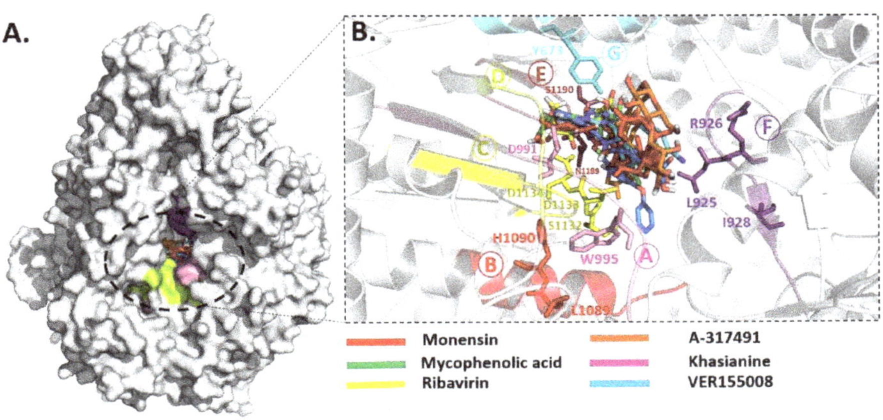

Figure 5. Binding modes of compounds. (**A**) Molecular surface representation for the inhibitory binding pattern of all ligands. (**B**) Close-up view into the binding mode of all compounds within the active site of RdRp core. The main residues involved in the formation of the active site within the structurally conserved RdRp motifs that are shown in stickes.

2.4. ADME and Toxicity Prediction Analysis

Predicting ADME profiles using an in silico approach has long been proven to be a reliable method of determining a compound's pharmacokinetic properties. Evaluating lead compounds' ADME properties is a major challenge in the drug development [88]. Because of poor toxicity and pharmacokinetic properties, most drugs fail to pass the drug development process. The development of high-throughput and fast ADMET profiling assays has aided the detection of active lead compounds during early drug discovery [89]. Swiss ADMET and ADMETlab 2.0 were used to predict the absorption, distribution, metabolism, excretion, and toxicity (ADME) studies of the top three compounds, and their results are presented in Table 2. Gastro-intestinal absorption (GI) and blood-brain barrier (BBB) permeation indicate drug absorption and distribution of drug molecules [71]. One of the primary factors optimising drug discovery is information about drug distribution via BBB [90]. According to Table 2 results, all compounds show low gastro-intestinal absorption and no BBB permeation. The compounds cannot cross the blood-brain barrier (blood-brain barrier negative), so their consumption is not linked to the onset of neurological disorders. The absorption of the compounds was further revealed by caco-2 permeability values ranging from −6.019 to −5.727 log unit. A permeability of >−5.15 log unit in the ADMETlab 2.0 server indicates optimal caco-2 absorption. Oral bioavailability is frequently viewed as crucial in determining the drug-likeness of active compounds as therapeutic agents [91]. Furthermore, a variety of cytochromes (CYPs) regulate drug metabolism, with CYP2C19, CYP1A2, CYP2C9, CYP3A4, and CYP2D6 being critical for the biotransformation of drug molecules. The ability of a drug to inhibit or act as a substrate of the cytochrome P450 (CYP450) subfamily determines its therapeutic action [92]. A-317491 is an inhibitor of CYP2C9 while being a non-inhibitor and a non-substrate of other isoforms, while Khasianine is a non-inhibitor and a non-substrate of all isoforms, and VER155008 is an inhibitor of CYP3A4 and a non-inhibitor and non-substrates of other isoforms. Besides, p-glycoprotein inhibitors reduce the bioavailability of drugs that are known to be transported by it [93]. Except for Khasianine, all of the compounds in our analysis are inhibitors and negative substrates of p-glycoprotein, which explains the good absorption profile of the compounds. All of the compounds studied were nontoxic in terms of AMES toxicity. Following that, the safety profile of the three compounds was assessed by conducting toxicity prediction studies with an online tool: ProTox-II. This server classified substances into six toxicity classes (1–6), with class one being the most lethal and toxic, with an estimated lethal dose (LD50) of $\leq$5, and class six designating non-toxicity of the compound with an LD50 > 5000. A-317491 falls in class five with an LD50 value of 2500 mg/kg, while Khasianine falls in class four with an LD50 value of 500 mg/kg, and VER155008 falls in class six with an LD50 value of 7000 mg/kg. The findings strongly support the ability of the compounds studied to act as drugs against RVFV.

Table 2. Predicted ADME and Toxicity properties of identified nucleoside analogs. The probability of each parameter is depicted. **BBB**: blood–brain barrier; **CYP450**: cytochrome P450.

Parameters	Compounds		
	A-317491	**Khasianine**	**VER155008**
	Absorption		
BBB	No	No	No
GI absorption	Low	Low	Low
Caco-2 permeability	−6.019	−5.356	−5.727
Human oral bioavailability	0.56	0.17	0.17
Log P	5.296	2.723	2.136
TPSA (Å^2)	141.44	179.56	166.21
	Metabolism		
P-glycoprotein substrate	No	Yes	No
P-glycoprotein inhibitor	No	No	No
CYP450 2C9 substrate	No	No	No
CYP450 2D6 substrate	No	No	No
CYP450 3A4 substrate	No	No	No
CYP450 1A2 inhibitor	No	No	No
CYP450 2C9 inhibitor	Yes	No	No
CYP450 2D6 inhibitor	No	No	No
CYP450 2C19 inhibitor	No	No	No
CYP450 3A4 inhibitor	No	No	Yes

Table 2. *Cont.*

Parameters	Compounds		
	A-317491	**Khasianine**	**VER155008**
	Toxicity		
AMES Toxicity	Non-toxic	Non-toxic	Non-toxic
Carcinogens	Non-carcinogenic	Non-carcinogenic	Non-carcinogenic
Acute oral toxicity	2500 mg/kg	500 mg/kg	7000 mg/kg

2.5. MD Simulation

To understand the structural–functionality relationship of the target protein, MD simulations are essential in computer-aided drug design (CADD) [21]. MD simulations provide detailed biomolecule dynamical structural information and surface wealth of protein-ligand interactions and energetic data. MD simulations have been very successful in recent years for optimizing the docked hits [24,25,45,94,95] and related studies [23,52,95–97]. This data set can guide novel drug design, making MD simulation a valuable tool in modern drug discovery.

2.5.1. Root Mean Square Deviation (RMSD)

MD simulations of 50 ns were performed for the top three complexes and controls to elucidate compound binding stability and extract receptors/compound structural information that is important in the binding, and that may be altered to improve binding conformation and, ultimately, a compound affinity for the target biomolecule [95]. The RMSD is a frequently applied analysis to measure the structural similarity between superimposed proteins; smaller RMSD corresponds to similar structures and vice versa. The RMSD of each complex was calculated as carbon alpha deviations by superimposing 50,000 snapshots over the initial reference structure versus time. The RMSDs of the top three compounds were: A-317491-L (maximum, 6.76 Å; mean, 5.64 Å), VER155008-L (maximum, 7.82 Å; mean, 6.20 Å), and Khasianine-L (maximum, 7.67 Å; mean, 6.20 Å), while the RMSDs of the control drugs were: Monensin-L (maximum, 7.02 Å; mean, 5.95 Å), Mycophenolic acid-L (maximum, 7.24 Å; mean, 5.80 Å), and Ribavirin-L (maximum, 6.92 Å; mean, 6.0 Å) (Figure 6A). All the systems depicted uniform RMSD patterns, and no prominent peak was observed throughout the length of simulation time. The RMSD from the initial simulation time can be seen continuously for all complexes and converged at 10–15 ns. This is rightly possible because of the sudden exposure of the systems to a dynamic environment. This forces the receptor enzyme loops to acquire a more stable conformation. After 10 ns the systems can be witnessed in a more stable behavior until the end of the simulation time. The RdRp has been explored in SARS-CoV-2 for dynamics in the presence of a variety of drug molecules. The studies have found several leads that experience stable conformational dynamics and showed significant intermolecular stability with enzyme's active pockets [98–100]. However, RdRp from RVFV is not investigated so far, making the findings of the current study interesting for experimentalists to test them in in vivo and in vitro validation.

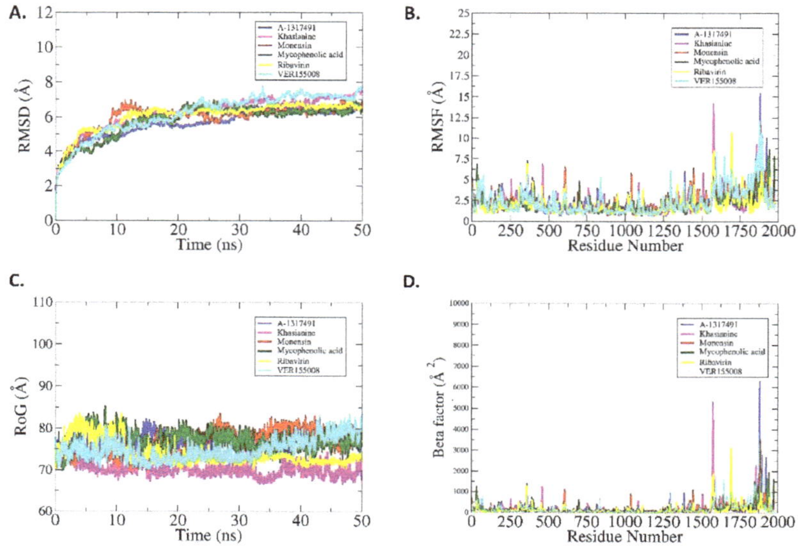

Figure 6. MD-Simulation studies of ligand bounded complexes. (**A**) Root mean square deviation. (**B**) Root mean square fluctuations (endoN domain 25–205 aa; PA-C-like domain 296–762 aa; RdRp core 763–1345 aa; PB2-N-like domain 1346–1571 aa; arm domain two spans 1615–1696 and 1811 aa; CBD domain 1697–1810 aa; and C-terminal domain 1933–2049 aa). (**C**) Radius of Gyrations. (**D**) Beta-factor analysis, each ligand is represented with different color such as A-1317491 (blue), Khasianane (pink), Monensin (Red), Mycophenolic acid (dark green), Ribavirin (Yellow), and Ver155008 (Cyan).

2.5.2. Root Mean Square Fluctuation (RMSF) Analysis

The residual flexibility and stability of complexes were further computed. The mean RMSF for A-317491-L is 2.38 Å, VER155008-L is 2.37 Å, Khasianine-L is 2.23 Å, Monensin-L is 2.31 Å, mycophenolic acid-L is 2.16 Å, and Ribavirin-L is 1.98 Å. These values indicate a high level of agreement on intermolecular stability. Overall, a high rate of fluctuations was observed starting from residue 1250 to onward, and Khasianine-L and A-317491-L were among the ligands showing a high tendency to fluctuate (Figure 6B). It was observed that part of the RdRp core, PB2-N-like domain, CBD domain, and the C-terminal domain comprise a large percentage of flexible loops, forcing these segments to behave more dynamically. This may be a natural mechanism of the protein to confer some flexibility for mediating the proper accommodation of the substrate/ligand molecule inside the pocket and accomplish the catalytic mechanism. Moreover, the predicted binding site residues and their corresponding structural motifs were stable within a ~2 Å fluctuation in the presence of ligands. The less flexibility in the RdRp core region indicated that the ligands adopted a more stable conformation and established consistent interactions with the important surrounding residues.

2.5.3. Radius of Gyration (Rg)

Furthermore, Rg analysis was used to assess structural equilibrium and protein compactness over the simulation time. Rg is employed to investigate whether the binding of the compounds affects the overall structural stability of the receptor enzyme. Lower Rg indicates the tight packing of the enzyme atoms and less effect of the compounds on the enzyme structure upon binding, thus presenting the stable nature of the subject complex. The Rg of the complexes follows; A-317491-L (maximum, 82.41 Å; mean, 76.76 Å), Khasianine-L (maximum, 76.76 Å; mean,70.16 Å), VER155008-L (maximum, 83.67 Å; mean, 75.05 Å), Monensin-L (maximum, 83.64 Å; mean, 76.43 Å), Mycophenolic acid-L (maximum,

85.40 Å; mean, 77.29 Å), and Ribavirin-L (maximum, 83.76 Å; mean, 74.09 Å) (Figure 6C). All six complexes are quite stable and remain compact. These Rg results complement the RMSD result in interpreting the docked complex stability.

2.5.4. B-Factor Analysis

B-factors were also derived from simulation trajectories to probe highly mobile regions of the complexes. The B-factor monitors the thermal motion of protein atoms, side chains, and whole regions. The B-factor is commonly used to identify internal protein motions, probing rigid and flexible regions important in proteins/enzyme functionality. The average values of the B-factor for the top three complexes A-317491-L, VER155008-L Khasianine-L, and control drugs Monensin-L, Mycophenolic acid-L, and Ribavirin-L were: 201.68 Å^2, 210.62 Å^2,187.20 Å^2, 183.67 Å^2, 155.86 Å^2, and 139.35 Å^2, respectively (Figure 6D). It demonstrates that these complexes have good stability throughout the 50 ns simulation period. From the simulation results, it can be concluded that all the studied systems are structurally stable, and the intermolecular interactions remained strong throughout the simulation time.

2.6. MMGBA/PBSA Analysis

Binding free energies were estimated using MMPBSA and MMGBSA techniques to understand better the compounds' binding potential with the L protein. Table 3 shows the detailed binding energies of the complexes [101,102]. As all binding interactions are energetically favorable, stable complexes are formed. Gas-phase energy dominates the system energy in all complexes, with van der Waals playing a significant role, while electrostatic energy plays a minor role. This reflects that both van der Waals and electrostatic interactions are key in intermolecular stability. The polar solvation energy is unfavorable in binding, whereas the nonpolar energy appears to be favourable in complex equilibration. The complexes' MMGBSA net binding-energy rankings were as follows: A-317491-L > VER155008-L > Khasianine-L > Mycophenolic acid-L > Monensin-L > Ribavirin-L. The complexes' MMPBSA net binding-energy rankings were as follows: A-317491-L > Khasianine-L > VER155008-L > Monensin-L > Mycophenolic acid-L > Ribavirin-L. These results indicate that our compounds have high binding free energies than control drugs.

Table 3. Binding free energy of docked complexes. The energy values are given in kcal/mol units.

Energy Component	Average	Standard Error of Mean	Average	Standard Error of Mean	Average	Standard Error of Mean	Average	Standard Error of Mean	Average	Standard Error of Mean	Average	Standard Error of Mean
	A-1317491		Khasianine		Monensin		Mycophenolic Acid		Ribavirin		VER155008	
						MM-GBSA						
ΔE_{vdw}	−65.37	2.72	−54.45	4.89	−53.83	3.23	−48.81	5.00	−26.20	3.57	−51.64	3.87
ΔE_{ele}	−56.86	6.92	−257.10	17.11	−80.72	5.55	−30.21	4.83	−155.72	7.14	−87.45	11.03
ΔG_p	74.46	6.80	275.40	16.39	100.29	4.76	42.30	4.30	158.69	5.83	98.08	8.68
ΔG_{np}	−7.10	0.19	−6.51	0.31	−6.92	0.39	−5.04	0.18	−3.75	0.26	−5.72	0.29
ΔE_{MM}	−122.23	7.68	−311.55	18.54	−134.56	6.12	−79.03	8.37	−181.93	7.33	−139.09	9.68
ΔG_{sol}	67.36	6.68	268.88	16.23	93.36	4.68	37.26	4.21	154.93	5.86	92.35	8.74
ΔG_{total}	−54.87	2.75	−42.66	4.16	−41.19	2.89	−41.76	4.96	−26.99	4.216	−46.73	3.41
						MM-PBSA						
ΔE_{vdw}	−65.37	2.72	−54.45	4.89	−53.83	3.23	−48.81	5.00	−26.20	3.57	−51.64	3.87
ΔE_{ele}	−56.86	6.92	−257.10	17.1	−80.72	5.55	−30.21	4.83	−155.72	7.14	−87.45	11.03

Table 3. *Cont.*

Energy Component	Average	Standard Error of Mean	Average	Standard Error of Mean	Average	Standard Error of Mean	Average	Standard Error of Mean	Average	Standard Error of Mean	Average	Standard Error of Mean
	A-1317491		Khasianine		Monensin		Mycophenolic Acid		Ribavirin		VER155008	
ΔG_p	95.85	7.89	288.12	16.80	114.98	8.24	57.57	5.53	166.11	6.22	118.11	7.49
ΔG_{np}	−4.73	0.10	−4.99	0.13	−5.52	0.16	−3.18	0.08	−2.34	0.07	−4.44	0.12
ΔE_{MM}	−122.2	7.68	−311.55	18.54	−134.56	6.12	−79.03	8.37	−181.93	7.33	−139.09	9.68
ΔG_{sol}	91.12	7.84	283.12	16.76	109.45	8.19	54.39	5.53	163.77	6.20	113.66	7.49
ΔG_{total}	−31.11	4.89	−28.42	4.30	−25.10	5.39	−24.64	6.16	−18.16	5.23	−25.42	5.87

3. Materials and Methods

3.1. Homology Modeling

Drug discovery relies heavily on homology modeling, with current efforts resulting in unprecedented accuracy models, even with low sequence identity [32,103–107]. Because L protein lacked a crystal structure, homology modeling was required to determine target structure elucidation. The L protein sequence was obtained from the UniProt database (P27316 (L_RVFVZ)) to perform homology modeling [108]. Sequence to Structure alignment was performed using PSI-BLAST against Protein Data Bank (PDB) to find suitable templates for the three-dimensional (3D) structure prediction [109,110]. The initial alignment between the target and the template was generated using the ALIGN2D module. The final model was built using a restrained-based approach in Modeller.v9.11 with the most-fitted template and secondary structural information obtained by manual curation after superimposition between all generated models and the template [111]. Modeller's secondary structure module was used to model the final structure using the extracted spatial secondary structure restraints.

3.2. Structure Validation

Accurate evaluation of the 3D model is considered one of the core elements of computational structure prediction. The emergence of rapidly endorsed and highly efficient approaches for structure evaluation has paved new ways to assess the quality of newly designed models [112,113]. Ramachandran plots are a quick and easy way to evaluate the quality of a 3D structure. The Ramachandran plot was used to determine the energetically permissible and prohibited phi (ϕ) and psi (ψ) dihedral angles of amino acid residues [114]. The 3D structure was further analyzed by PDBsum [56]. PDBsum is a database that summarises the contents of 3D macromolecular structures. In addition, the predicted 3D structure was refined and validated by using 50 ns MD simulations.

3.3. Target Protein Preparation

3D structure of L protein predicted from Modeller and validated with 50 ns MD simulations were prepared using the AMBER 18 program [115]. The ff14SB force field [116] was utilized to parameterize amino acids. AMBER18's tleap module was used to add complementary hydrogen atoms missed by crystallography. Energy minimization of the target protein was performed first for 1000 steepest descent steps and then for 500 conjugate gradient steps, allowing the step size to be 0.02 Å. After MD clustering, the most stable conformation was selected from the cluster (with RMSD < 1 Å) for further processing.

3.4. Compound Preparation

The Selleckchem Nucleoside Analogue Library (https://www.selleckchem.com/screening/Nucleoside-Analogue-Library.html, accessed on 15 February 2021) was used to identify molecules with the highest binding affinity to the L-protein. The library composed of 156 natural compounds was downloaded in 3D SDF format. A recent study reported

Monensin, Mycophenolic acid, and Ribavirin as potent inhibitors of RVFV-L protein [79]. To get an insight into the mechanism of the binding of known inhibitors, these three potent inhibitors were docked as controls in the present study. These drugs were retrieved from the PubChem database (https://pubchem.ncbi.nlm.nih.gov, accessed on 15 February 2021) in 3D SDF format [117].

3.5. Structure-Based Virtual Screening

The AutoDock Vina implicated in the PyRx (version 0.8) was used to perform the virtual screening of the compounds against the target protein [118,119]. The control drugs and chemical library of 156 compounds in SDF format were imported in the Open-babel program of PyRx for further energy minimization, followed by conversion of all the ligands into AutoDock PDBQT format. Further, the top three ligands were subjected to docking against the L protein of RVFV using AutoDock Vina. The grid box was set to cover the entire binding site within the core chamber of RdRp with box_size of (x = 20, y = 20, z = 20 Å) and dimensions of (x = 122.005, y = 105.326, and z = 137.824). Dockings were run in triplicates to ensure absolute consistency of the results. The docked solutions were clustered using an RMSD of 1 Å. The 3D structural alignment, visualization and analysis, and docking figures production were carried out using Discovery Studio 2019 software [120], PyMOL [121], and UCSF Chimera 1.14 [122].

3.6. ADME and Toxicity Prediction Analysis

The analysis of the pharmacological activity of drug candidates is a critical step in drug discovery [93]. Therefore, in silico prediction of pharmacophore properties of active compounds is critical for accelerating the drug development process. Absorption, distribution, metabolism, excretion, and toxicity (ADMET) are the most plausible drug-like properties to evaluate virtual hits. ADME analysis was carried out by submitting the compounds' canonical simplified molecular-input line-entry system (SMILES) to online servers; ADMETlab 2.0 [123] and Swiss ADME [124]. Acute oral toxicity was predicted by the Protox II web server [125].

3.7. MD Simulations

AMBER18 was used to perform MD simulations of the docked solutions [115]. The same MD simulation protocol was adopted in the current study as described in previous studies [22,94,126–128]. The Antechamber package of AmberTools was employed to generate the general AMBER force field (GAFF) parameters for the studied ligands using AM1–BCC charge definitions. Each top complex was explicitly solvated with water molecules, and then counter ions were added to create a neutral system. A water box with a thickness of 12 Å was created using the TIP3P solvent model to encircle the complex [129,130]. The complex was simulated using periodic boundary conditions, with electrostatic interactions modeled using the particle mesh Ewald procedure [131]. For nonbounded interactions, a threshold value of 8 Å was defined during the procedure. Water molecules were minimized for 500 cycles, and then the entire system was minimized for 1000 rounds. The temperature of each system was then steadily increased to 300 K. Solutes in the first phase were restrained for 50 ps during equilibration of counterions and water molecules, while protein side chains were relaxed afterwards. At 300 K and 1 atm, a 50 ns MD simulation was performed, and coordinate trajectories were collected every 2 ps during the simulation under the NPT ensemble. While the SHAKE algorithm [132] constrained covalent and hydrogen bonds, Langevin dynamics [133] was used to control the system temperature. The original structure was used as a reference, and AMBER's CPPTRAJ [134,135] was used to generate an RMSD (root mean square deviation) plot to assess the system's MD simulation convergence [136]. The structural flexibility of ligands was calculated using ligand RMSD. The radius of gyration (RoG) was analyzed to determine the complex's compactness and three-dimensional packing. RMSF reflects the root mean square averaged distance between an atom and its average geometric position [137]. The Term β–factor, which is closely related to the RMSF, measures the spatial displacement of atoms around their mean positions, as well as a thermal and local vibrational movement [138].

3.8. MMGBA/PBSA Analysis

AMBER18 MM/PBSA and MM/PBSA methods were used to estimate the binding free energy (G binding) of the complexes [101,139]. The method has been well-documented in our previous studies, implemented in AMBER 18. The free energy difference was calculated using 100 snapshots from simulated trajectories at regular intervals. The total binding free energy is calculated as a sum of the molecular mechanics binding energy (ΔE_{MM}) and solvation free energy (ΔG_{sol}) as follows:

$$\Delta E_{MM} = \Delta E_{int} + \Delta E_{ele} + \Delta E_{vdw}$$

$$\Delta G_{sol} = \Delta G_{p} + \Delta G_{np}$$

$$\Delta G_{total} = \Delta E_{MM} + \Delta G_{sol}$$

$$\Delta G_{bind} = \Delta E_{MM} + \Delta G_{sol} - T\Delta S$$

In these equations, ΔE_{MM} is further divided into internal energy (ΔE_{int}), electrostatic energy (ΔE_{ele}), and van der Waals energy (ΔE_{vdw}), and the total solvation free energy (ΔG_{sol}) is contributed by the sum of polar (ΔG_{p}) and non-polar (ΔG_{np}) components. ΔG_{bind} is the free energy of binding of the ligand evaluated after entropic calculations ($T\Delta S$). We excluded entropic term, $T\Delta S$, from the calculation due to its intensive computational cost [101,102,140,141]. These methods have been well documented [101,128,140] and considered reliable end-point binding free energy estimations [102,141].

4. Conclusions

A combination of virtual screening and molecular docking analysis was used to identify inhibitors of RVFV L protein in the present study. The 3D structure of the RVFV-L enzyme was predicted, and the findings could aid researchers working on RVFV drug development. The Selleckchem Nucleoside Analogue Library (156 compounds) was screened, and the top three compounds, A-317491, VER155008, and Khasianine exhibit a high binding affinity compared to the control drugs chosen that may inhibit RVFV-L enzyme activity and hence virus replication. Compounds also show good pharmacodynamic and pharmacokinetic profiles based on toxicity and ADME studies. Overall, the results reveal that all of the compounds fit into the same binding pocket of the protein, suggesting that they could be good therapeutic candidates for RVFV. However, further in-vivo and in-vitro experiments are required to convert these potential inhibitors into clinical drugs. We anticipate that the findings of this study will be useful in the future for developing and exploring novel natural anti-RVFV therapeutic agents.

Supplementary Materials: The following supporting information can be downloaded at: https://www.mdpi.com/article/10.3390/ph15060659/s1, Figure S1. Sequence alignment of RVFV L protein with the templates (Structure of the alpha-Synuclein (PDB ID: 6I42 and severe fever with thrombocytopenia syndrome virus L protein (PDB ID: 6Y6K). Figure S2. Structural superposition of the RVFV L protein model with the templates. The RMSD values between the model and 6I42 and 6Y6K are 0.179 and 1.165 Å, respectively. Table S1. Reverse template comparison of RVFV L protein model with the representative structures in PDB using ProFunc reverse template search program. Table S2. Virtual Screening result of Selleckchem Nucleoside Analogue Library (compounds with binding affinity > −1.5 kcal/mol) against model of RVFV-L RdRp core.

Author Contributions: Conceptualization, U.A.A., M.T.u.Q., S.A. and K.S.A.; data curation, M.T.u.Q., F.S., S.A., E.A.A., G.M.A. and A.A.; formal analysis, M.A.A., M.U.M., M.M.A., U.A.A. and S.A.; funding acquisition, K.S.A.; investigation, M.A.A., M.U.M., M.M.A., F.S., E.A.A. and G.M.A.; methodology, M.A.A., M.U.M., M.M.A., U.A.A., M.T.u.Q., S.A., E.A.A., G.M.A., K.S.A. and A.A.; project administration, M.T.u.Q. and K.S.A.; resources, K.S.A.; software, M.A.A., M.U.M., M.M.A. and S.A.;

supervision, U.A.A. and K.S.A.; validation, U.A.A., M.T.u.Q., F.S., S.A., E.A.A., G.M.A., K.S.A. and A.A.; visualization, M.A.A., M.U.M. and M.M.A.; writing—original draft, M.A.A., M.U.M., M.M.A. and F.S.; writing—review and editing, U.A.A., M.T.u.Q., S.A., E.A.A., G.M.A., K.S.A. and A.A. All authors have read and agreed to the published version of the manuscript.

Funding: This research received no external funding.

Institutional Review Board Statement: Not applicable.

Informed Consent Statement: Not applicable.

Data Availability Statement: The data presented in this study are available within the article and Supplementary Material.

Acknowledgments: The researchers would like to thank the Deanship of Scientific Research, Qassim University for funding the publication of this project.

Conflicts of Interest: The author declares no conflict of interest.

References

1. Pepin, M.; Bouloy, M.; Bird, B.H.; Kemp, A.; Paweska, J. Rift Valley fever virus (Bunyaviridae: Phlebovirus): An update on pathogenesis, molecular epidemiology, vectors, diagnostics and prevention. *Vet. Res.* **2010**, *41*, 61. [CrossRef] [PubMed]
2. Bird, B.H.; Ksiazek, T.G.; Nichol, S.T.; MacLachlan, N.J. Rift Valley fever virus. *J. Am. Vet. Med. Assoc.* **2009**, *234*, 883–893. [CrossRef] [PubMed]
3. Hartman, A. Rift valley fever. *Clin. Lab. Med.* **2017**, *37*, 285–301. [CrossRef] [PubMed]
4. Ikegami, T.; Makino, S. The pathogenesis of Rift Valley fever. *Viruses* **2011**, *3*, 493–519. [CrossRef]
5. Drake, J.M.; Hassan, A.N.; Beier, J.C. A statistical model of Rift Valley fever activity in Egypt. *J. Vector Ecol.* **2013**, *38*, 251–259. [CrossRef]
6. Helmy, Y.A.; El-Adawy, H.; Abdelwhab, E.M. A comprehensive review of common bacterial, parasitic and viral zoonoses at the human-animal interface in Egypt. *Pathogens* **2017**, *6*, 33. [CrossRef]
7. Gaudreault, N.N.; Indran, S.V.; Bryant, P.; Richt, J.A.; Wilson, W.C. Comparison of Rift Valley fever virus replication in North American livestock and wildlife cell lines. *Front. Microbiol.* **2015**, *6*, 664. [CrossRef]
8. McElroy, A.K.; Albariño, C.G.; Nichol, S.T. Development of a RVFV ELISA that can distinguish infected from vaccinated animals. *Virol. J.* **2009**, *6*, 1–11. [CrossRef]
9. Lumley, S.; Horton, D.L.; Hernandez-Triana, L.L.; Johnson, N.; Fooks, A.R.; Hewson, R. Rift Valley fever virus: Strategies for maintenance, survival and vertical transmission in mosquitoes. *J. Gen. Virol.* **2017**, *98*, 875–887. [CrossRef]
10. Ikegami, T. Molecular biology and genetic diversity of Rift Valley fever virus. *Antiviral Res.* **2012**, *95*, 293–310. [CrossRef]
11. Gerrard, S.R.; Nichol, S.T. Synthesis, proteolytic processing and complex formation of N-terminally nested precursor proteins of the Rift Valley fever virus glycoproteins. *Virology* **2007**, *357*, 124–133. [CrossRef] [PubMed]
12. Müller, R.; Poch, O.; Delarue, M.; Bishop, D.; Bouloy, M. Rift Valley fever virus L segment: Correction of the sequence and possible functional role of newly identified regions conserved in RNA-dependent polymerases. *J. Gen. Virol.* **1994**, *75*, 1345–1352. [CrossRef] [PubMed]
13. Poch, O.; Sauvaget, I.; Delarue, M.; Tordo, N. Identification of four conserved motifs among the RNA-dependent polymerase encoding elements. *EMBO J.* **1989**, *8*, 3867–3874. [CrossRef] [PubMed]
14. Gerlach, P.; Malet, H.; Cusack, S.; Reguera, J. Structural insights into bunyavirus replication and its regulation by the vRNA promoter. *Cell* **2015**, *161*, 1267–1279. [CrossRef] [PubMed]
15. Kinsella, E.; Martin, S.G.; Grolla, A.; Czub, M.; Feldmann, H.; Flick, R. Sequence determination of the Crimean–Congo hemorrhagic fever virus L segment. *Virology* **2004**, *321*, 23–28. [CrossRef]
16. Bouloy, M.; Weber, F. Molecular biology of Rift Valley fever virus. *Open Virol. J.* **2010**, *4*, 8. [CrossRef]
17. Morin, B.; Coutard, B.; Lelke, M.; Ferron, F.; Kerber, R.; Jamal, S.; Frangeul, A.; Baronti, C.; Charrel, R.; De Lamballerie, X. The N-terminal domain of the arenavirus L protein is an RNA endonuclease essential in mRNA transcription. *PLoS Pathog.* **2010**, *6*, e1001038. [CrossRef]
18. Patterson, J.; Holloway, B.; Kolakofsky, D. La Crosse virions contain a primer-stimulated RNA polymerase and a methylated cap-dependent endonuclease. *J. Virol.* **1984**, *52*, 215–222. [CrossRef]
19. Gogrefe, N.; Reindl, S.; Günther, S.; Rosenthal, M. Structure of a functional cap-binding domain in Rift Valley fever virus L protein. *PLoS Pathog.* **2019**, *15*, e1007829. [CrossRef]
20. Sarwar, S.; Abdul Qadir, M.; Alharthy, R.D.; Ahmed, M.; Ahmad, S.; Vanmeert, M.; Mirza, M.U.; Hameed, A. Folate Conjugated Polyethylene Glycol Probe for Tumor-Targeted Drug Delivery of 5-Fluorouracil. *Molecules* **2022**, *27*, 1780. [CrossRef]
21. Salo-Ahen, O.M.H.; Alanko, I.; Bhadane, R.; Bonvin, A.M.J.J.; Honorato, R.V.; Hossain, S.; Juffer, A.H.; Kabedev, A.; Lahtela-Kakkonen, M.; Larsen, A.S. Molecular Dynamics Simulations in Drug Discovery and Pharmaceutical Development. *Processes* **2021**, *9*, 71. [CrossRef]

22. Ahmad, S.; Lee, Y.K.; Nazir, M.; Abdul Rahman, N.; Trant, J.F.; Abdullah, I. Fragment-based in silico design of SARS CoV-2 main protease inhibitors. *Chem. Biol. Drug Des.* **2021**, *98*, 604–619. [CrossRef] [PubMed]
23. Durrani, F.G.; Gul, R.; Mirza, M.U.; Kaderbhai, N.N.; Froeyen, M.; Saleem, M. Mutagenesis of DsbAss is Crucial for the Signal Recognition Particle Mechanism in Escherichia coli: Insights from Molecular Dynamics Simulations. *Biomolecules* **2019**, *9*, 133. [CrossRef] [PubMed]
24. Khalid, H.; Landry, K.B.; Ijaz, B.; Ashfaq, U.A.; Ahmed, M.; Kanwal, A.; Froeyen, M.; Mirza, M.U. Discovery of novel Hepatitis C virus inhibitor targeting multiple allosteric sites of NS5B polymerase. *Infect. Genet. Evol.* **2020**, *84*, 104371. [CrossRef] [PubMed]
25. Mirza, M.U.; Ahmad, S.; Abdullah, I.; Froeyen, M. Identification of novel human USP2 inhibitor and its putative role in treatment of COVID-19 by inhibiting SARS-CoV-2 papain-like (PLpro) protease. *Comput. Biol. Chem.* **2020**, *89*, 107376. [CrossRef]
26. Mirza, M.U.; Vanmeert, M.; Ali, A.; Iman, K.; Froeyen, M.; Idrees, M. Perspectives towards antiviral drug discovery against Ebola virus. *J. Med. Virol.* **2019**, *91*, 2029–2048. [CrossRef]
27. ul Qamar, M.T.; Ahmad, S.; Khan, A.; Mirza, M.U.; Ahmad, S.; Abro, A.; Chen, L.-L.; Almatroudi, A.; Wei, D.-Q. Structural probing of HapR to identify potent phytochemicals to control Vibrio cholera through integrated computational approaches. *Comput. Biol. Med.* **2021**, *138*, 104929. [CrossRef]
28. Sliwoski, G.; Kothiwale, S.; Meiler, J.; Lowe, E.W. Computational methods in drug discovery. *Pharmacol. Rev.* **2014**, *66*, 334–395. [CrossRef]
29. Jácome, R.; Becerra, A.; de León, S.P.; Lazcano, A. Structural analysis of monomeric RNA-dependent polymerases: Evolutionary and therapeutic implications. *PLoS ONE* **2015**, *10*, e0139001. [CrossRef]
30. Van Der Linden, L.; Vives-Adrián, L.; Selisko, B.; Ferrer-Orta, C.; Liu, X.; Lanke, K.; Ulferts, R.; De Palma, A.M.; Tanchis, F.; Goris, N. The RNA template channel of the RNA-dependent RNA polymerase as a target for development of antiviral therapy of multiple genera within a virus family. *PLoS Pathog.* **2015**, *11*, e1004733. [CrossRef]
31. Ferrer-Orta, C.; Arias, A.; Escarmís, C.; Verdaguer, N. A comparison of viral RNA-dependent RNA polymerases. *Curr. Opin. Struct. Biol.* **2006**, *16*, 27–34. [CrossRef] [PubMed]
32. Mirza, M.U.; Vanmeert, M.; Froeyen, M.; Ali, A.; Rafique, S.; Idrees, M. In silico structural elucidation of RNA-dependent RNA polymerase towards the identification of potential Crimean-Congo Hemorrhagic Fever Virus inhibitors. *Sci. Rep.* **2019**, *9*, 6809. [CrossRef] [PubMed]
33. Godoy, A.S.; Lima, G.M.; Oliveira, K.I.; Torres, N.U.; Maluf, F.V.; Guido, R.V.; Oliva, G. Crystal structure of Zika virus NS5 RNA-dependent RNA polymerase. *Nat. Commun.* **2017**, *8*, 14764. [CrossRef] [PubMed]
34. Zhang, C.; Feng, T.; Cheng, J.; Li, Y.; Yin, X.; Zeng, W.; Jin, X.; Li, Y.; Guo, F.; Jin, T. Structure of the NS5 methyltransferase from Zika virus and implications in inhibitor design. *Biochem. Biophys. Res. Commun.* **2017**, *492*, 624–630. [CrossRef] [PubMed]
35. Hercík, K.; Kozak, J.; Šála, M.; Dejmek, M.; Hřebabecký, H.; Zborníková, E.; Smola, M.; Ruzek, D.; Nencka, R.; Boura, E. Adenosine triphosphate analogs can efficiently inhibit the Zika virus RNA-dependent RNA polymerase. *Antivir. Res.* **2017**, *137*, 131–133. [CrossRef]
36. Pattnaik, A.; Palermo, N.; Sahoo, B.R.; Yuan, Z.; Hu, D.; Annamalai, A.S.; Vu, H.L.; Correas, I.; Prathipati, P.K.; Destache, C.J. Discovery of a non-nucleoside RNA polymerase inhibitor for blocking Zika virus replication through in silico screening. *Antivir. Res.* **2018**, *151*, 78–86. [CrossRef]
37. Lu, G.; Gong, P. Crystal structure of the full-length Japanese encephalitis virus NS5 reveals a conserved methyltransferase-polymerase interface. *PLoS Pathog.* **2013**, *9*, e1003549. [CrossRef] [PubMed]
38. Malet, H.; Egloff, M.-P.; Selisko, B.; Butcher, R.E.; Wright, P.J.; Roberts, M.; Gruez, A.; Sulzenbacher, G.; Vonrhein, C.; Bricogne, G. Crystal structure of the RNA polymerase domain of the West Nile virus non-structural protein 5. *J. Biol. Chem.* **2007**, *282*, 10678–10689. [CrossRef]
39. Noble, C.G.; Lim, S.P.; Chen, Y.-L.; Liew, C.W.; Yap, L.; Lescar, J.; Shi, P.-Y. Conformational flexibility of the Dengue virus RNA-dependent RNA polymerase revealed by a complex with an inhibitor. *J. Virol.* **2013**, *87*, 5291–5295. [CrossRef]
40. Noble, C.G.; Chen, Y.-L.; Dong, H.; Gu, F.; Lim, S.P.; Schul, W.; Wang, Q.-Y.; Shi, P.-Y. Strategies for development of dengue virus inhibitors. *Antivir. Res.* **2010**, *85*, 450–462. [CrossRef] [PubMed]
41. El Sahili, A.; Lescar, J. Dengue virus non-structural protein 5. *Viruses* **2017**, *9*, 91. [CrossRef] [PubMed]
42. De Francesco, R.; Tomei, L.; Altamura, S.; Summa, V.; Migliaccio, G. Approaching a new era for hepatitis C virus therapy: Inhibitors of the NS3-4A serine protease and the NS5B RNA-dependent RNA polymerase. *Antivir. Res.* **2003**, *58*, 1–16. [CrossRef]
43. Dhanak, D.; Duffy, K.J.; Johnston, V.K.; Lin-Goerke, J.; Darcy, M.; Shaw, A.N.; Gu, B.; Silverman, C.; Gates, A.T.; Nonnemacher, M.R. Identification and biological characterization of heterocyclic inhibitors of the hepatitis C virus RNA-dependent RNA polymerase. *J. Biol. Chem.* **2002**, *277*, 38322–38327. [CrossRef]
44. Gemma, S.; Brogi, S.; Novellino, E.; Campiani, G.; Maga, G.; Brindisi, M.; Butini, S. HCV-targeted antivirals: Current status and future challenges. *Curr. Pharm. Des.* **2014**, *20*, 3445–3464. [CrossRef] [PubMed]
45. Mirza, M.U.; Saadabadi, A.; Vanmeert, M.; Salo-Ahen, O.M.H.; Abdullah, I.; Claes, S.; De Jonghe, S.; Schols, D.; Ahmad, S.; Froeyen, M. Discovery of HIV entry inhibitors via a hybrid CXCR4 and CCR5 receptor pharmacophore-based virtual screening approach. *Eur. J. Pharm. Sci.* **2020**, *155*, 105537. [CrossRef] [PubMed]
46. Cavasotto, C.N.; Phatak, S.S. Homology modeling in drug discovery: Current trends and applications. *Drug Discov. Today* **2009**, *14*, 676–683. [CrossRef]

47. Hillisch, A.; Pineda, L.F.; Hilgenfeld, R. Utility of homology models in the drug discovery process. *Drug Discov. Today* **2004**, *9*, 659–669. [CrossRef]
48. Oshiro, C.; Bradley, E.K.; Eksterowicz, J.; Evensen, E.; Lamb, M.L.; Lanctot, J.K.; Putta, S.; Stanton, R.; Grootenhuis, P.D.J. Performance of 3D-database molecular docking studies into homology models. *J. Med. Chem.* **2004**, *47*, 764–767. [CrossRef]
49. Kairys, V.; Fernandes, M.X.; Gilson, M.K. Screening drug-like compounds by docking to homology models: A systematic study. *J. Chem. Inf. Model* **2006**, *46*, 365–379. [CrossRef]
50. Fernandes, M.X.; Kairys, V.; Gilson, M.K. Comparing ligand interactions with multiple receptors via serial docking. *J. Chem. Inf. Comput. Sci.* **2004**, *44*, 1961–1970. [CrossRef]
51. McGovern, S.L.; Shoichet, B.K. Information decay in molecular docking screens against holo, apo, and modeled conformations of enzymes. *J. Med. Chem.* **2003**, *46*, 2895–2907. [CrossRef] [PubMed]
52. Mirza, M.U.; Rafique, S.; Ali, A.; Munir, M.; Ikram, N.; Manan, A.; Salo-Ahen, O.M.; Idrees, M. Towards peptide vaccines against Zika virus: Immunoinformatics combined with molecular dynamics simulations to predict antigenic epitopes of Zika viral proteins. *Sci. Rep.* **2016**, *6*, 1–17. [CrossRef] [PubMed]
53. Wang, P.; Liu, L.; Liu, A.; Yan, L.; He, Y.; Shen, S.; Hu, M.; Guo, Y.; Liu, H.; Liu, C. Structure of severe fever with thrombocytopenia syndrome virus L protein elucidates the mechanisms of viral transcription initiation. *Nat. Microbiol.* **2020**, *5*, 864–871. [CrossRef] [PubMed]
54. Vogel, D.; Thorkelsson, S.R.; Quemin, E.R.; Meier, K.; Kouba, T.; Gogrefe, N.; Busch, C.; Reindl, S.; Günther, S.; Cusack, S. Structural and functional characterization of the severe fever with thrombocytopenia syndrome virus L protein. *Nucleic Acids Res.* **2020**, *48*, 5749–5765. [CrossRef] [PubMed]
55. Eisenberg, D. The discovery of the α-helix and β-sheet, the principal structural features of proteins. *Proc. Natl. Acad. Sci. USA* **2003**, *100*, 11207–11210. [CrossRef] [PubMed]
56. Laskowski, R.A.; Jabłońska, J.; Pravda, L.; Vařeková, R.S.; Thornton, J.M. PDBsum: Structural summaries of PDB entries. *Protein Sci.* **2018**, *27*, 129–134. [CrossRef]
57. Sidorova, A.E.; Malyshko, E.V.; Lutsenko, A.O.; Shpigun, D.K.; Bagrova, O.E. Protein Helical Structures: Defining Handedness and Localization Features. *Symmetry* **2021**, *13*, 879. [CrossRef]
58. Wiederstein, M.; Sippl, M.J. ProSA-web: Interactive web service for the recognition of errors in three-dimensional structures of proteins. *Nucleic Acids Res.* **2007**, *35*, W407–W410. [CrossRef]
59. Zhang, Y.; Skolnick, J. TM-align: A protein structure alignment algorithm based on the TM-score. *Nucleic Acids Res.* **2005**, *33*, 2302–2309. [CrossRef]
60. Laskowski, R.A.; Watson, J.D.; Thornton, J.M. ProFunc: A server for predicting protein function from 3D structure. *Nucleic Acids Res.* **2005**, *33*, W89–W93. [CrossRef]
61. Sun, Y.; Li, J.; Gao, G.F.; Tien, P.; Liu, W. Bunyavirales ribonucleoproteins: The viral replication and transcription machinery. *Crit. Rev. Microbiol.* **2018**, *44*, 522–540. [CrossRef] [PubMed]
62. Pflug, A.; Guilligay, D.; Reich, S.; Cusack, S. Structure of influenza A polymerase bound to the viral RNA promoter. *Nature* **2014**, *516*, 355. [CrossRef] [PubMed]
63. Arnold, J.J.; Ghosh, S.K.B.; Cameron, C.E. Poliovirus RNA-dependent RNA polymerase (3Dpol): Divalent cation modulation of primer, template, and nucleotide selection. *J. Biol. Chem.* **1999**, *274*, 37060–37069. [CrossRef]
64. Ferrer-Orta, C.; Arias, A.; Pérez-Luque, R.; Escarmís, C.; Domingo, E.; Verdaguer, N. Sequential structures provide insights into the fidelity of RNA replication. *Proc. Natl. Acad. Sci. USA* **2007**, *104*, 9463–9468. [CrossRef] [PubMed]
65. Amroun, A.; Priet, S.; de Lamballerie, X.; Quérat, G. Bunyaviridae RdRps: Structure, motifs, and RNA synthesis machinery. *Crit. Rev. Microbiol.* **2017**, *43*, 753–778. [CrossRef]
66. Rothwell, P.J.; Waksman, G. Structure and mechanism of DNA polymerases. *Adv. Protein Chem.* **2005**, *71*, 401–440.
67. Biswas, S.K.; Nayak, D.P. Mutational analysis of the conserved motifs of influenza A virus polymerase basic protein 1. *J. Virol.* **1994**, *68*, 1819–1826. [CrossRef]
68. Sánchez, A.B.; de la Torre, J.C. Genetic and biochemical evidence for an oligomeric structure of the functional L polymerase of the prototypic arenavirus lymphocytic choriomeningitis virus. *J. Virol.* **2005**, *79*, 7262–7268. [CrossRef]
69. Vázquez, A.L.; Alonso, J.M.M.; Parra, F. Mutation analysis of the GDD sequence motif of a calicivirus RNA-dependent RNA polymerase. *J. Virol.* **2000**, *74*, 3888–3891. [CrossRef]
70. Zhou, Y.; Zheng, H.; Gao, F.; Tian, D.; Yuan, S. Mutational analysis of the SDD sequence motif of a PRRSV RNA-dependent RNA polymerase. *Sci. China Life Sci.* **2011**, *54*, 870–879. [CrossRef]
71. Abdelrheem, D.A.; Rahman, A.A.; Elsayed, K.N.; Abd El-Mageed, H.; Mohamed, H.S.; Ahmed, S.A. Isolation, characterization, in vitro anticancer activity, dft calculations, molecular docking, bioactivity score, drug-likeness and admet studies of eight phytoconstituents from brown alga sargassum platycarpum. *J. Mol. Struct.* **2021**, *1225*, 129245. [CrossRef]
72. Bergeron, É.; Albariño, C.G.; Khristova, M.L.; Nichol, S.T. Crimean-Congo hemorrhagic fever virus-encoded ovarian tumor protease activity is dispensable for virus RNA polymerase function. *J. Virol.* **2010**, *84*, 216–226. [CrossRef]
73. Dunn, E.F.; Pritlove, D.C.; Jin, H.; Elliott, R.M. Transcription of a recombinant bunyavirus RNA template by transiently expressed bunyavirus proteins. *Virology* **1995**, *211*, 133–143. [CrossRef] [PubMed]
74. Beerens, N.; Selisko, B.; Ricagno, S.; Imbert, I.; Van Der Zanden, L.; Snijder, E.J.; Canard, B. De novo initiation of RNA synthesis by the arterivirus RNA-dependent RNA polymerase. *J. Virol.* **2007**, *81*, 8384–8395. [CrossRef]

75. Boonrod, K.; Chotewutmontri, S.; Galetzka, D.; Krczal, G. Analysis of tombusvirus revertants to identify essential amino acid residues within RNA-dependent RNA polymerase motifs. *J. Gen. Virol.* **2005**, *86*, 823–826. [CrossRef] [PubMed]
76. Pasternak, A.O.; Spaan, W.J.M.; Snijder, E.J. Nidovirus transcription: How to make sense? *J. Gen. Virol.* **2006**, *87*, 1403–1421. [CrossRef] [PubMed]
77. Qamar, M.T.; Ashfaq, U.A.; Tusleem, K.; Mumtaz, A.; Tariq, Q.; Goheer, A.; Ahmed, B. In-silico identification and evaluation of plant flavonoids as dengue NS2B/NS3 protease inhibitors using molecular docking and simulation approach. *Pak. J. Pharm. Sci.* **2017**, *30*, 2119–2137. [PubMed]
78. Muhseen, Z.T.; Hameed, A.R.; Al-Hasani, H.M.; Ahmad, S.; Li, G. Computational Determination of Potential Multiprotein Targeting Natural Compounds for Rational Drug Design Against SARS-COV-2. *Molecules* **2021**, *26*, 674. [CrossRef]
79. Piper, M.E.; Gerrard, S.R. A novel system for identification of inhibitors of Rift Valley fever virus replication. *Viruses* **2010**, *2*, 731–747. [CrossRef]
80. Ausubel, F.M. *Current Protocols in Molecular Biology*; Greene Pub. Associates and Wiley-Interscience: New York, NY, USA, 1987; Volume 1.
81. Graci, J.D.; Cameron, C.E. Mechanisms of action of ribavirin against distinct viruses. *Rev. Med. Virol.* **2006**, *16*, 37–48. [CrossRef]
82. Allison, A.C.; Eugui, E.M. Mycophenolate mofetil and its mechanisms of action. *Immunopharmacology* **2000**, *47*, 85–118. [CrossRef]
83. Seley-Radtke, K.L.; Yates, M.K. The evolution of nucleoside analogue antivirals: A review for chemists and non-chemists. Part 1: Early structural modifications to the nucleoside scaffold. *Antivir. Res.* **2018**, *154*, 66–86. [CrossRef] [PubMed]
84. Kuchta, R.D. Nucleotide Analogues as Probes for DNA and RNA Polymerases. *Curr. Protoc. Chem.* **2010**, *2*, 111–124. [CrossRef] [PubMed]
85. Ju, J.; Kumar, S.; Li, X.; Jockusch, S.; Russo, J.J. Nucleotide analogues as inhibitors of viral polymerases. *BioRxiv* **2020**.
86. Ghazwani, M.Y.; Bakheit, A.H.; Hakami, A.R.; Alkahtani, H.M.; Almehizia, A.A. Virtual Screening and Molecular Docking Studies for Discovery of Potential RNA-Dependent RNA Polymerase Inhibitors. *Crystals* **2021**, *11*, 471. [CrossRef]
87. Gajjar, N.D.; Dhameliya, T.M.; Shah, G.B. In search of RdRp and Mpro inhibitors against SARS CoV-2: Molecular docking, molecular dynamic simulations and ADMET analysis. *J. Mol. Struct.* **2021**, *1239*, 130488. [CrossRef]
88. Lin, J.H.; Lu, A.Y. Role of pharmacokinetics and metabolism in drug discovery and development. *Pharmacol. Rev.* **1997**, *49*, 403–449.
89. Tsaioun, K.; Bottlaender, M.; Mabondzo, A. ADDME–Avoiding Drug Development Mistakes Early: Central nervous system drug discovery perspective. *BMC Neurol.* **2009**, *9*, 1–11. [CrossRef]
90. Alavijeh, M.S.; Chishty, M.; Qaiser, M.Z.; Palmer, A.M. Drug metabolism and pharmacokinetics, the blood-brain barrier, and central nervous system drug discovery. *NeuroRx* **2005**, *2*, 554–571. [CrossRef]
91. Thomas, V.H.; Bhattachar, S.; Hitchingham, L.; Zocharski, P.; Naath, M.; Surendran, N.; Stoner, C.L.; El-Kattan, A. The road map to oral bioavailability: An industrial perspective. *Expert Opin. Drug Metab. Toxicol.* **2006**, *2*, 591–608. [CrossRef]
92. Das, P.; Majumder, R.; Mandal, M.; Basak, P. In-Silico approach for identification of effective and stable inhibitors for COVID-19 main protease (Mpro) from flavonoid based phytochemical constituents of Calendula officinalis. *J. Biomol. Struct. Dyn.* **2020**, *39*, 6265–6280. [CrossRef] [PubMed]
93. Mohammed, I. Virtual screening of Microalgal compounds as potential inhibitors of Type 2 Human Transmembrane serine protease (TMPRSS2). *arXiv* **2021**, arXiv:2108.13764.
94. Anwar, F.; Saleem, U.; Ahmad, B.; Ashraf, M.; Rehman, A.U.; Froeyen, M.; Kee, L.Y.; Abdullah, I.; Mirza, M.U.; Ahmad, S. New naphthalene derivative for cost-effective AChE inhibitors for Alzheimer's treatment: In silico identification, in vitro and in vivo validation. *Comput. Biol. Chem.* **2020**, *89*, 107378. [CrossRef] [PubMed]
95. Guterres, H.; Im, W. Improving protein-ligand docking results with high-throughput molecular dynamics simulations. *J. Chem. Inf. Model* **2020**, *60*, 2189–2198. [CrossRef]
96. Vanmeert, M.; Razzokov, J.; Mirza, M.U.; Weeks, S.D.; Schepers, G.; Bogaerts, A.; Rozenski, J.; Froeyen, M.; Herdewijn, P.; Pinheiro, V.B. Rational design of an XNA ligase through docking of unbound nucleic acids to toroidal proteins. *Nucleic Acids Res.* **2019**, *47*, 7130–7142. [CrossRef]
97. Rehman, H.M.; Mirza, M.U.; Ahmad, M.A.; Saleem, M.; Froeyen, M.; Ahmad, S.; Gul, R.; Alghamdi, H.A.; Aslam, M.S.; Sajjad, M. A putative prophylactic solution for COVID-19: Development of novel multiepitope vaccine candidate against SARS-COV-2 by comprehensive immunoinformatic and molecular modelling approach. *Biology* **2020**, *9*, 296. [CrossRef]
98. Koulgi, S.; Jani, V.; Uppuladinne, M.V.; Sonavane, U.; Joshi, R. Remdesivir-bound and ligand-free simulations reveal the probable mechanism of inhibiting the RNA dependent RNA polymerase of severe acute respiratory syndrome coronavirus 2. *RSC Adv.* **2020**, *10*, 26792–26803. [CrossRef]
99. Hosseini, M.; Chen, W.; Xiao, D.; Wang, C. Computational molecular docking and virtual screening revealed promising SARS-CoV-2 drugs. *Precis. Clin. Med.* **2021**, *4*, 1–16. [CrossRef]
100. Rudrapal, M.; Gogoi, N.; Chetia, D.; Khan, J.; Banwas, S.; Alshehri, B.; Alaidarous, M.A.; Laddha, U.D.; Khairnar, S.J.; Walode, S.G. Repurposing of phytomedicine-derived bioactive compounds with promising anti-SARS-CoV-2 potential: Molecular docking, MD simulation and drug-likeness/ADMET studies. *Saudi J. Biol. Sci.* **2021**, *29*, 2432–2446. [CrossRef]
101. Genheden, S.; Ryde, U. The MM/PBSA and MM/GBSA methods to estimate ligand-binding affinities. *Expert Opin. Drug Discov.* **2015**, *10*, 449–461. [CrossRef]

102. Wang, E.; Sun, H.; Wang, J.; Wang, Z.; Liu, H.; Zhang, J.Z.H.; Hou, T. End-point binding free energy calculation with MM/PBSA and MM/GBSA: Strategies and applications in drug design. *Chem. Rev.* **2019**, *119*, 9478–9508. [CrossRef] [PubMed]
103. Fiser, A.; Sali, A. Modeller: Generation and refinement of homology-based protein structure models. *Methods Enzym.* **2003**, *374*, 461–491. [CrossRef]
104. Fan, H.; Irwin, J.J.; Webb, B.M.; Klebe, G.; Shoichet, B.K.; Sali, A. Molecular Docking Screens Using Comparative Models of Proteins. *J. Chem. Inf. Model* **2009**, *49*, 2512–2527. [CrossRef] [PubMed]
105. Mariani, V.; Kiefer, F.; Schmidt, T.; Haas, J.; Schwede, T. Assessment of template based protein structure predictions in CASP9. *Proteins* **2011**, *79* (Suppl. 10), 37–58. [CrossRef] [PubMed]
106. Huang, Y.J.; Mao, B.; Aramini, J.M.; Montelione, G.T. Assessment of template-based protein structure predictions in CASP10. *Proteins* **2014**, *82* (Suppl. 2), 43–56. [CrossRef]
107. Webb, B.; Sali, A. Protein Structure Modeling with MODELLER. *Methods Mol. Biol.* **2014**, *1137*, 1–15. [CrossRef]
108. Consortium, U. UniProt: A worldwide hub of protein knowledge. *Nucleic Acids Res.* **2019**, *47*, D506–D515. [CrossRef]
109. Sussman, J.L.; Lin, D.; Jiang, J.; Manning, N.O.; Prilusky, J.; Ritter, O.; Abola, E.E. Protein Data Bank (PDB): Database of three-dimensional structural information of biological macromolecules. *Acta Crystallogr. Sect. D Biol. Crystallogr.* **1998**, *54*, 1078–1084. [CrossRef]
110. Altschul, S.F.; Madden, T.L.; Schäffer, A.A.; Zhang, J.; Zhang, Z.; Miller, W.; Lipman, D.J. Gapped BLAST and PSI-BLAST: A new generation of protein database search programs. *Nucleic Acids Res.* **1997**, *25*, 3389–3402. [CrossRef]
111. Eswar, N.; Eramian, D.; Webb, B.; Shen, M.-Y.; Sali, A. Protein structure modeling with MODELLER. In *Structural Proteomics*; Springer: Berlin/Heidelberg, Germany, 2008; pp. 145–159.
112. Querin, O.; Young, V.; Steven, G.; Xie, Y. Computational efficiency and validation of bi-directional evolutionary structural optimisation. *Comput. Methods Appl. Mech. Eng.* **2000**, *189*, 559–573. [CrossRef]
113. Tahir ul Qamar, M.; Mirza, M.U.; Song, J.-M.; Rao, M.J.; Zhu, X.; Chen, L.-L. Probing the structural basis of Citrus phytochrome B using computational modelling and molecular dynamics simulation approaches. *J. Mol. Liq.* **2021**, *340*, 116895. [CrossRef]
114. Gopalakrishnan, K.; Sowmiya, G.; Sheik, S.; Sekar, K. Ramachandran plot on the web (2.0). *Protein Pept. Lett.* **2007**, *14*, 669–671. [CrossRef] [PubMed]
115. Case, D.; Darden, T.; Cheatham, T., III; Simmerling, C.; Wang, J.; Duke, R.; Luo, R.; Crowley, M.; Walker, R.; Zhang, W. *AMBER 10*; University of California: San Francisco, CA, USA, 2008.
116. Maier, J.A.; Martinez, C.; Kasavajhala, K.; Wickstrom, L.; Hauser, K.E.; Simmerling, C. ff14SB: Improving the accuracy of protein side chain and backbone parameters from ff99SB. *J. Chem. Theory Comput.* **2015**, *11*, 3696–3713. [CrossRef]
117. Kim, S.; Thiessen, P.A.; Bolton, E.E.; Chen, J.; Fu, G.; Gindulyte, A.; Han, L.; He, J.; He, S.; Shoemaker, B.A. PubChem substance and compound databases. *Nucleic Acids Res.* **2016**, *44*, D1202–D1213. [CrossRef] [PubMed]
118. Dallakyan, S.; Olson, A.J. Small-Molecule Library Screening by Docking with PyRx. In *Chemical Biology*; Springer: Berlin/Heidelberg, Germany, 2015; pp. 243–250.
119. Trott, O.; Olson, A.J. AutoDock Vina: Improving the speed and accuracy of docking with a new scoring function, efficient optimization, and multithreading. *J. Comput. Chem.* **2010**, *31*, 455–461. [CrossRef]
120. Jejurikar, B.L.; Rohane, S.H. Drug Designing in Discovery Studio. *Asian J. Res. Chem.* **2021**, *14*, 135–138.
121. DeLano, W.L. Pymol: An open-source molecular graphics tool. *CCP4 Newsl. Protein Crystallogr.* **2002**, *40*, 82–92.
122. Pettersen, E.F.; Goddard, T.D.; Huang, C.C.; Couch, G.S.; Greenblatt, D.M.; Meng, E.C.; Ferrin, T.E. UCSF Chimera—A visualization system for exploratory research and analysis. *J. Comput. Chem.* **2004**, *25*, 1605–1612. [CrossRef]
123. Xiong, G.; Wu, Z.; Yi, J.; Fu, L.; Yang, Z.; Hsieh, C.; Yin, M.; Zeng, X.; Wu, C.; Lu, A. ADMETlab 2.0: An integrated online platform for accurate and comprehensive predictions of ADMET properties. *Nucleic Acids Res.* **2021**, *49*, W5–W14. [CrossRef]
124. Daina, A.; Michielin, O.; Zoete, V. SwissADME: A free web tool to evaluate pharmacokinetics, drug-likeness and medicinal chemistry friendliness of small molecules. *Sci. Rep.* **2017**, *7*, 1–13. [CrossRef]
125. Banerjee, P.; Eckert, A.O.; Schrey, A.K.; Preissner, R. ProTox-II: A webserver for the prediction of toxicity of chemicals. *Nucleic Acids Res.* **2018**, *46*, W257–W263. [CrossRef] [PubMed]
126. Malik, A.; Arooj, M.; Butt, T.T.; Zahid, S.; Zahid, F.; Jafar, T.H.; Waquar, S.; Gan, S.H.; Ahmad, S.; Mirza, M.U. In silico and in vivo characterization of cabralealactone, solasodin and salvadorin in a rat model: Potential anti-inflammatory agents. *Drug Des. Dev. Ther.* **2018**, *12*, 1431. [CrossRef] [PubMed]
127. Naheed, N.; Maher, S.; Saleem, F.; Khan, A.; Wadood, A.; Rasheed, S.; Choudhary, M.I.; Froeyen, M.; Abdullah, I.; Mirza, M.U. New isolate from Salvinia molesta with antioxidant and urease inhibitory activity. *Drug Dev. Res.* **2021**, *82*, 1169–1181. [CrossRef] [PubMed]
128. Alamri, M.A.; Tahir ul Qamar, M.; Mirza, M.U.; Bhadane, R.; Alqahtani, S.M.; Muneer, I.; Froeyen, M.; Salo-Ahen, O.M.H. Pharmacoinformatics and molecular dynamics simulation studies reveal potential covalent and FDA-approved inhibitors of SARS-CoV-2 main protease 3CLpro. *J. Biomol. Struct. Dyn.* **2020**, *39*, 4936–4948. [CrossRef] [PubMed]
129. Man, V.H.; Wu, X.; He, X.; Xie, X.-Q.; Brooks, B.R.; Wang, J. Determination of van der Waals Parameters Using a Double Exponential Potential for Nonbonded Divalent Metal Cations in TIP3P Solvent. *J. Chem. Theory Comput.* **2021**, *17*, 1086–1097. [CrossRef]

130. Amin, S.A.; Ghosh, K.; Gayen, S.; Jha, T. Chemical-informatics approach to COVID-19 drug discovery: Monte Carlo based QSAR, virtual screening and molecular docking study of some in-house molecules as papain-like protease (PLpro) inhibitors. *J. Biomol. Struct. Dyn.* **2021**, *39*, 4764–4773. [CrossRef]
131. Ngo, S.T.; Quynh Anh Pham, N.; Thi Le, L.; Pham, D.-H.; Vu, V.V. Computational determination of potential inhibitors of SARS-CoV-2 main protease. *J. Chem. Inf. Model* **2020**, *60*, 5771–5780. [CrossRef]
132. Kräutler, V.; Van Gunsteren, W.F.; Hünenberger, P.H. A fast SHAKE algorithm to solve distance constraint equations for small molecules in molecular dynamics simulations. *J. Comput. Chem.* **2001**, *22*, 501–508. [CrossRef]
133. Bussi, G.; Parrinello, M. Accurate sampling using Langevin dynamics. *Phys. Rev. E* **2007**, *75*, 056707. [CrossRef]
134. Bhowmik, D.; Nandi, R.; Jagadeesan, R.; Kumar, N.; Prakash, A.; Kumar, D. Identification of potential inhibitors against SARS-CoV-2 by targeting proteins responsible for envelope formation and virion assembly using docking based virtual screening, and pharmacokinetics approaches. *Infect. Genet. Evol.* **2020**, *84*, 104451. [CrossRef]
135. Roe, D.R.; Cheatham III, T.E. PTRAJ and CPPTRAJ: Software for processing and analysis of molecular dynamics trajectory data. *J. Chem. Theory Comput.* **2013**, *9*, 3084–3095. [CrossRef] [PubMed]
136. Kouznetsova, V.L.; Zhang, A.; Tatineni, M.; Miller, M.A.; Tsigelny, I.F. Potential COVID-19 papain-like protease PLpro inhibitors: Repurposing FDA-approved drugs. *PeerJ* **2020**, *8*, e9965. [CrossRef] [PubMed]
137. Alamri, M.A.; ul Qamar, M.T.; Afzal, O.; Alabbas, A.B.; Riadi, Y.; Alqahtani, S.M. Discovery of anti-MERS-CoV small covalent inhibitors through pharmacophore modeling, covalent docking and molecular dynamics simulation. *J. Mol. Liq.* **2021**, *330*, 115699. [CrossRef]
138. Kuzmanic, A.; Zagrovic, B. Determination of ensemble-average pairwise root mean-square deviation from experimental B-factors. *Biophys. J.* **2010**, *98*, 861–871. [CrossRef]
139. Homeyer, N.; Gohlke, H. Free energy calculations by the molecular mechanics Poisson— Boltzmann surface area method. *Mol. Inform.* **2012**, *31*, 114–122. [CrossRef] [PubMed]
140. Sun, H.; Duan, L.; Chen, F.; Liu, H.; Wang, Z.; Pan, P.; Zhu, F.; Zhang, J.Z.H.; Hou, T. Assessing the performance of MM/PBSA and MM/GBSA methods. 7. Entropy effects on the performance of end-point binding free energy calculation approaches. *Phys. Chem. Chem. Phys.* **2018**, *20*, 14450–14460. [CrossRef] [PubMed]
141. Tuccinardi, T. What is the current value of MM/PBSA and MM/GBSA methods in drug discovery? *Expert Opin. Drug Discov.* **2021**, *16*, 1233–1237. [CrossRef] [PubMed]

pharmaceuticals

Review

Drug Design by Pharmacophore and Virtual Screening Approach

Deborah Giordano [1], Carmen Biancaniello [2], Maria Antonia Argenio [1] and Angelo Facchiano [1,*]

1 National Research Council, Institute of Food Science, Via Roma 64, 83110 Avellino, Italy; deborah.giordano@isa.cnr.it (D.G.); maria.antonia.argenio@gmail.com (M.A.A.)
2 Doctorate School in Computational and Quantitative Biology, University of Naples "Federico II", 80100 Naples, Italy; carmenbnl93@gmail.com
* Correspondence: angelo.facchiano@isa.cnr.it

Abstract: Computer-aided drug discovery techniques reduce the time and the costs needed to develop novel drugs. Their relevance becomes more and more evident with the needs due to health emergencies as well as to the diffusion of personalized medicine. Pharmacophore approaches represent one of the most interesting tools developed, by defining the molecular functional features needed for the binding of a molecule to a given receptor, and then directing the virtual screening of large collections of compounds for the selection of optimal candidates. Computational tools to create the pharmacophore model and to perform virtual screening are available and generated successful studies. This article describes the procedure of pharmacophore modelling followed by virtual screening, the most used software, possible limitations of the approach, and some applications reported in the literature.

Keywords: structure-based pharmacophore modeling; ligand-based pharmacophore modeling; virtual screening; drug discovery; bioinformatics; computational biology

Citation: Giordano, D.; Biancaniello, C.; Argenio, M.A.; Facchiano, A. Drug Design by Pharmacophore and Virtual Screening Approach. *Pharmaceuticals* **2022**, *15*, 646. https://doi.org/10.3390/ph15050646

Academic Editor: Osvaldo Andrade Santos-Filho

Received: 30 April 2022
Accepted: 21 May 2022
Published: 23 May 2022

1. Introduction

Computer-Aided Drug Discovery (CADD) investigates molecular properties to develop novel therapeutic solutions by way of computational tools and data resources. In its broadest meaning, it includes computational approaches for designing or selecting compounds as potential candidates before they are synthesized and tested for their biological activity [1]. Bioinformatics and computational tools offer an in silico approach to reducing costs and times, i.e., the factors that influence the progress of the research and, in the specific field of drug development, limit the possibilities of fighting more pathologies. To date, in vitro screening is expensive and time-consuming, and alternatives are highly desirable. Virtual Screening (VS) is a CADD method that involves in silico screening of a library of chemical compounds, to identify those that are most likely to bind to a specific target [2]. In this way, it is possible to reduce the impact of these limiting factors on drug discovery, meeting the needs due to health emergencies, as well as the spread of personalized medicine. This process can be speeded up using pharmacophore models used as the query with which compound libraries can be searched to pull out molecules of interest with desired properties. Indeed, pharmacophore-based methods are widely used tools in CADD and are of great interest in the chemo-informatics field [2], since they find many applications in drug discovery projects including not only the virtual screening but also scaffold hopping, lead optimization, ligand profiling, target identification, multi-target drug or de novo drug design.

The concept of a pharmacophore was coined in the 19th century when Langley first suggested that certain drug molecules might act on particular receptors. Only later, with the discovery of Salvarsan by Paul Elrich, the selectivity of drug–target interactions was recognized. Several years of experimentation confirmed its therapeutic effect. This discovery had found support in the statement of Emil Fisher who, following his research, had defined the concept "Lock & Key" in 1894, according to which a ligand and its receptor fits like a key with its lock to interact with the on top of each other through a chemical bond [3].

Hence, historically the term "pharmacophore" was used to indicate the functional or structural capacity of a compound with specific characteristics towards a biological target [4].

Schueler provided the basis for our modern understanding of a pharmacophore, defined by the International Union of Pure and Applied Chemistry (IUPAC) as "the ensemble of steric and electronic features that is necessary to ensure the optimal supra-molecular interactions with a specific biological target structure and to trigger (or to block) its biological response" [3,5,6].

Pharmacophoric modelling is based on the theory that having common chemical functionalities, and maintaining a similar spatial arrangement, leads to biological activity on the same target. The chemical characteristics of a molecule capable of creating interactions with its ligand are represented in the pharmacophoric model as geometric entities such as spheres, planes and vectors. The most important pharmacophoric feature types are: hydrogen bond acceptors (HBAs); hydrogen bond donors (HBDs); hydrophobic areas (H); positively and negatively ionizable groups (PI/NI); aromatic groups (AR); and metal coordinating areas (Figure 1). Additional size restrictions in the form of a shape or exclusion volumes (XVOL)—forbidden areas—can be added to represent the size and the shape of the binding pocket [7].

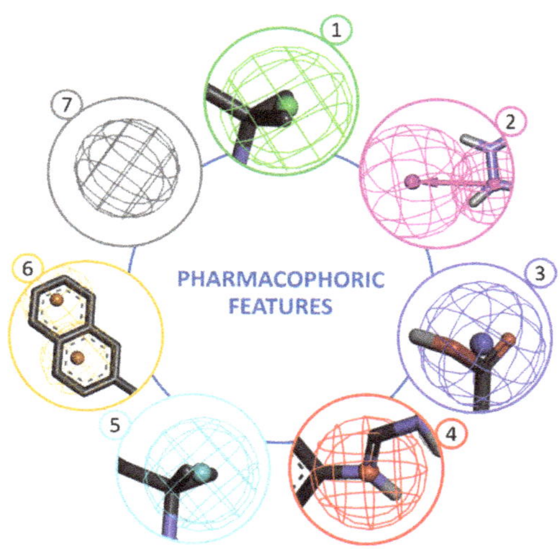

Figure 1. Pharmacophoric features. Main pharmacophoric feature types are represented by geometric entities and include: 1—hydrogen bond acceptor (HBA), 2—hydrogen bond donor (HBD), 3—negative ionizable (NI), 4—positive ionizable (PI), 5—hydrophobic (H), 6—aromatic (AR), 7—exclusion volume (XVOL).

Since the models themselves do not focus on actual atoms, but on chemical functionalities, they are good tools in recognizing similarities between molecules. Pharmacophore activity is independent of the scaffold, and this explains why similar biological events can be triggered by chemically divergent molecules. The use of these models as a query allows performing searches in the large libraries of compounds made available on the computational platform in order to select molecules of interest for the next vs. or in the chemo-informatics field [7].

Pharmacophore models can be generated using two different approaches depending on the input data employed for model construction, which are, namely, "structure-based" and "ligand-based" pharmacophore modelling. The structure-based approach uses the structural information of the target proteins like enzymes or receptors, to identify compounds that can potentially be used as a drug. On the other hand, the ligand-based approach consists of the development of 3D pharmacophore models and modelling quantitative structure-activity relationship (QSAR) or quantitative structure-property relationship (QSPR), using only the physicochemical properties of known ligand molecules for drug development. The choice of the best approach to use depends on several factors such as data availability, data quality, computational resources and also the intended use of the generated pharmacophore models. In the following paragraphs, we describe both strategies and their implementation in virtual screening is provided below to guide the non-experts on this topic in their application by explaining the basic concepts these methods are based on.

2. Structure-Based Pharmacophore Modelling

The structure-based approach owns its name to the fact that the three-dimensional structure of a macromolecule target is the essential prerequisite to obtaining a structure-based pharmacophore. The 3D structure of a protein provides significant details at the atomic level that can be very useful for the design or discovery of new drugs. As previously outlined, a pharmacophore is an abstract picture showing the stereo-electronic features, which make a ligand bioactive toward a specific target, and this type of information can be extracted from the 3D structure of the protein target in its holo or apo form. Typically, the workflow of the structure-based approach (Figure 2, left side of the flow) consists of different steps: protein preparation, identification or prediction of ligand binding site, pharmacophore features generation, and the selection of relevant features for ligand activity [8,9].

The 3D structure of the target or the ligand–target complex is the required starting point of this methodology. The RCSB Protein Data Bank (PDB) [www.rcsb.org] (accessed on 20 May 2022) includes thousands of protein structures at high resolution alone or in the presence of a bound ligand, mainly solved by X-ray crystallography or NMR spectroscopy. In case experimental structural data are lacking, computational techniques such as homology modelling [10] may be an alternative strategy to retrieve a 3D model and machine learning-based methods are successfully applied to retrieve protein structures, a powerful example is ALPHAFOLD2 [11]. Molecular docking is another method to study in silico the interaction of a known active compound towards a specific receptor and derive protein-ligand complexes from the most favorable binding poses [12].

A practical tip for those who want to use this approach is to perform a deep analysis of the quality of input data before using the target structure since it directly influences the quality of the pharmacophore model. For this reason, the protein structure preparation is the first step to carry out by evaluating, for instance, the residues' protonation states, the position of hydrogen atoms (that are absent in X-ray solved structures), the presence of non-protein groups which may have or not some functional roles, eventual missing residues or atoms, the stereochemical and energetic parameters accounting for the general quality and biological-chemical sense of the investigated target, also in the case of experimentally solved structures that may contain errors [8].

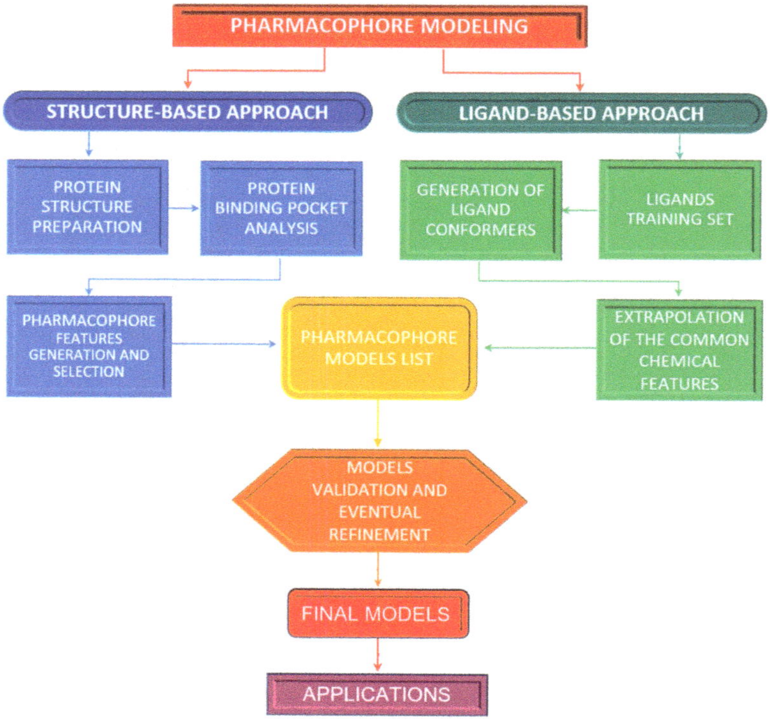

Figure 2. Pharmacophore modeling workflow. A pharmacophore model can be generated using two approaches. In the structure-based approach (on the left side), the structural information of the macromolecular target, alone or bounded to a ligand, is evaluated for its correctness and used to analyze the ligand binding sites in order to derive and select ligand complementary characteristics composing the pharmacophore models. In the ligand-based approach (on the right side), the first step is the construction of a training set made up of known active ligands structures. From each of them, conformers are generated and then used to extrapolate common features that are combined in different pharmacophore models. The resultant models undergo a validation and refinement procedure to obtain the final models exploitable for practical applications.

Once the target structure is identified and critically evaluated, ligand-binding site detection is the next crucial step. This can be manually inferred by analyzing the area including residues suggested to have a key role from experimental data such as site-directed mutagenesis or X-ray structures of the protein co-crystallized with ligands, but it also requires time and expert knowledge of the target and ligands. Nowadays this purpose can be easily and quickly achieved using bioinformatics tools based on different methods which inspect the protein surface to search for potential ligand-binding sites according to various properties (evolutionary, geometric, energetic, statistical, or a combination of them), and which are particularly useful if the ligand information is not available [13]. Examples of computer programs developed for this purpose are GRID [14] and LUDI [15]. The first one, as suggested by the name, is a grid-based method that uses different molecules or functional groups to sample a specific protein region defined with a regular grid to identify grid points with which they make energetically favorable interactions, thus generating molecular interaction fields [14]. The second one predicts potential interaction sites using the knowledge from distributions of non-bonded contacts in experimental structures or geometric rules [15].

Since the goal of the structure-based method is to generate a pharmacophore model from the interactions between an active molecule (the ligand) and its protein target (enzyme or receptor), the characterization of the ligand-binding site can be used to derive a map of interaction and to build accordingly one or more pharmacophore hypotheses describing the type and the spatial arrangement of the chemical features required for a ligand to interact with the residues of the binding region. Initially, many features are detected with this approach and therefore only those that are essential for ligand bioactivity should be selected and incorporated into the final model to have a more reliable and selective pharmacophore hypothesis [9,16]. This operation can be accomplished in different ways, such as removing features that do not strongly contribute to the energy binding, identifying the most conserved interaction if multiple protein–ligands structures exist, preserving residue with key functions from sequence alignments or variation analysis, and incorporating spatial constraints from the receptor information [8].

If the structure of a protein–ligand complex is available, the pharmacophore features generation and selection can be achieved more accurately. The 3D information of the ligand in its bioactive conformation directs the identification and the spatial disposition of the pharmacophore features in correspondence with its functional groups directly involved in the interactions with the target. Moreover, the presence of the receptor allows accounting for spatial restrictions from the binding site shape through the addition of the exclusion volumes. In this ideal situation, pharmacophore models of high quality can be obtained. In case the available structural data do not include a bound ligand, the pharmacophore modelling depends only on the target structure which can be analyzed to detect all possible ligands interaction points in the binding sites and, therefore, to compute the complementary features that a ligand should match to potentially bind the receptor. However, in the absence of a ligand counterpart, several pharmacophoric features are calculated and approximately positioned resulting in less accurate models that should be manually refined [3,16,17].

3. Ligand-Based Pharmacophore Modelling

So far, we have mentioned the importance of the availability of the structure for modelling pharmacophores suitable to accommodate the best interaction features. However, even if this still represents one of the best strategies for modelling a pharmacophore, often the target molecule is not available. To overcome this problem, an alternative approach to structural-based modelling is represented by ligand-based pharmacophore modelling.

The starting point of this strategy is the knowledge of active compounds, which bind the same protein target with a similar orientation [4] that could allow the extraction of chemical features in common and, therefore, the pharmacophore construction. Due to the unknown bioactive conformations of the input compounds, a critical step, before the extraction of the shared features, is the generation of ligand conformers, so that, from each set of conformers, at list one should correspond to the bioactive conformation of the ligand [3].

In more detail, two datasets are necessary to generate a ligand-based pharmacophore, i.e., a training set and a test set. The training set composition differs according to the algorithm employed and the data availability, varying from the simplest, composed of at least two active compounds, to the most complex, for which it is possible to set multiple compounds with a different activity. The test set, instead, should contain as many active and inactive structurally different compounds as possible, preferring the inclusion of experimentally confirmed inactive compounds and compounds judged as active by experimentally proven direct interaction and with suitable activity cutoffs (i.e., low EC50/IC50 and high binding affinity values). In the case of unknown inactive ligands, decoy molecules could be used [6], which are available from a specific repository such as DUD (Directory of Useful Decoys) [18] or by generating them by service as DUD-E [19]. In addition to what could be extrapolated from pertinent literature, the source of molecules to be employed in the construction of the dataset could be chemical databases such as OpenPHACTS [20], ChEMBL [21] or Drugbank [22], for compounds with a target-based activity, ChEMBL,

PubChem Bioassay [23] and Tox21 [24] for research on the inactive molecules. In principle, all the algorithms appointed to the ligand-based pharmacophore modelling, starting from the active compounds of the training set, extrapolate from them common chemical functionalities, related for instance to the presence of hydrogen bond donors or acceptors, of a positively or negatively charged ionizable group, of aromatic ring systems or hydrophobic areas, and use these features for model design. This step is followed by an improvement of the pharmacophore model including shape features and spatial constrains which take care of specific regions occupied by inactive molecules [25]. The pharmacophore models obtained are ranked by the best ability to fit the active molecules but not the inactive ones. The best models obtained from this first phase are chosen for the validation and refinement using the test set. The purpose of this second phase is to evaluate if the generated models can fit most of the active molecules rejecting the inactive ones, to select only models which show the major sensitivity and specificity. A summary of the described process is described in Figure 2 (right side of the flow).

Despite the accuracy of the pharmacophore construction being highly dependent on the quality of the training set, its final composition is conditioned by the algorithm used for modelling [7]. In general, ligand-based pharmacophore modelling could be performed following two main strategies: the common feature pharmacophore and the QSAR based pharmacophore.

In the common feature approach, generally, an algorithm of alignment is involved, its purpose is basically to extrapolate and align specific and common features: starting from a defined feature for each active element the algorithm combines it with the corresponding features of the other molecules, from this alignment a novel feature, combination of the previous, is generated; reiterating this procedure for each set of overlapping features a pharmacophore of shared feature is built. This is for example the case of the espresso algorithm implemented in LigandScout [26,27], which achieved the pharmacophore modelling by dividing the procedure previously described into six steps exploiting various algorithms and two alignment methods: the first, based on a combination of shared pharmacophore feature and the second, based on a merged pharmacophore feature. Finally, the common features present in all training compounds are included in the common features models and all features of the aligned compounds are summated in a merged feature pharmacophore [28]. Another example of similar functionality is given by the HipHop algorithm provided by DiscoveryStudio [29], which builds several pharmacophore models starting from identifying the common chemical features arrangement of the training set structures. Beginning with a few groups of features, which are extended until no more shared configuration features are found, several models are obtained and ranked based on the fitness of the training compounds. Models are refined by the HipHop Refinement algorithm, which adds space restrains imposed by the structures of inactive compounds.

QSAR (Quantitative structure-activity relationships) based pharmacophore is a mathematical model that tries to find statistical correlations between structures and functions, quantifying the impacts in a biological activity of specific structural modifications in existing or predicted molecules [30]. Based on the idea that molecules with similar physico-chemical properties show a similar binding affinity for a protein target, nowadays the QSAR approach is used in drug discovery to build statistical models derived from these correlations exploiting for the prediction of the bioavailability, the ADMET profile (toxicity), adsorption, distribution, metabolism, binding affinity, biological activity and elimination of novel compounds [31].

There are six classifications of the QSAR approaches, from the 1D to the 6D-QSAR, according to the different dimensions of the method (Figure 3).

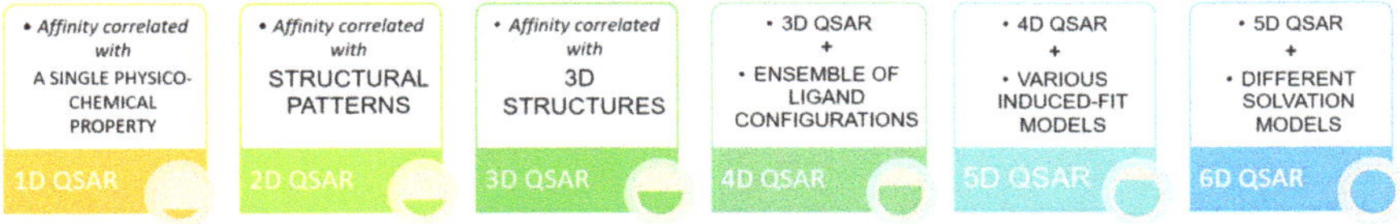

Figure 3. QSAR classifications. The QSAR approaches are classified from the 1D to the 6D-QSAR according to the different dimensions of the descriptors implemented in the method.

1D-QSAR takes into account a single physico-chemical property of the ligand, for an example the pKa value. In the 2D-QSAR, instead, affinity is correlated with structural patterns, while in the 3D-QSAR with the 3D structure of the ligand and its interactions. The concept extends as dimension rises: 4D-QSAR incorporates an ensemble of ligand configurations in 3D-QSAR, 5D-QSAR adds to 4D-QSAR various induced-fit models, 6D-QSAR implements 5D-QSAR with different solvation models [25].

Pharmacophore Models Validation

Once one or more pharmacophore models have been computed, a validation step is crucial before their implementation for practical purposes. Pharmacophore validation could be performed by exploiting several methods, such as the goodness of hit list (GH), receiver operating characteristic (ROC) curves construction, Fischer's method, or other statistical analysis, which relies on screening a test set and decoy set (if needed) to evaluate the model ability to distinguish active and inactive molecules and provide an estimation of its quality [9].

Mainly, the quality of a model can be described by four parameters: the sensitivity (capacity to detect active compounds), the specificity (capacity to exclude the inactive molecules), the yield of actives (the ratio between true positives and the number of hits) and the enrichment factor (which relates the yield of actives to the composition of the screening dataset) [7].

The GH scoring method consists of calculating the percentage of sensitivity, the percentage of the yield of actives the enrichment factor and the Güner–Henry score, which gives an evaluation of the efficiency of the screening dataset search and can vary from 0 to 1 where 1 is the value for the ideal model [32]. The ROC curve shows the enrichment power of a model plotting the sensitivity against 1—specificity (the false positive rate). The area under this curve (AUC) gives a measure of the pharmacophore's performance and it is useful for multiple models evaluation. AUC can vary from 0 to 1, where 1 corresponds to an ideal case in which all the active compounds are detected at first, 0 to the collection of the inactive ones at first and 0.5 to random results [33]. Fisher's randomization test validation method is instead used to analyze the significance of the statistical correlation between structure and biological activity [34]. Regression analysis can also be applied to check for the correlation between the compounds predicted as active and those whose bioactivity is experimentally confirmed.

In case the validation process reveals low-quality results, manual refinement could be a way to improve its performance by applying some changes in chemical features' selection or definition settings, training or test sets composition or in the pharmacophore building procedure, but a new model generation with a different approach and algorithm should not be excluded.

4. Pharmacophore-Based Virtual Screening

Among the strategies for the identification of new bioactive substances, VS techniques play a prominent role. VS tools are important in drug discovery as they increase the speed of the bioactive molecule discovery process through computational simulations by selecting from large libraries the compounds that are most likely to interact with the identified target. In addition, VS identifies compounds that may be toxic or have unfavorable pharmacodynamic (for example, potency, affinity, selectivity) and pharmacokinetic (for example, absorption, metabolism, bioavailability) properties [35].

In this context, pharmacophore models can be successfully applied to filter large collections of compounds to find the so-called hits, i.e., novel molecules matching the pharmacophoric features required to be potentially active against a specific target. Since a pharmacophore does not represent exact chemical groups but chemical functionalities and their spatial relationships, the retrieved hits usually include structurally different compounds, making pharmacophores useful tools for scaffold hopping [7].

The pharmacophore-based screening can be performed directly using some of the software already mentioned for the pharmacophore generation, which allows doing this on a manually created dataset. Other useful open-access platforms for virtual screening are Pharmit (http://pharmit.csb.pitt.edu) (accessed on 20 May 2022) and ZINCPharmer (http://zincpharmer.csb.pitt.edu/) (accessed on 20 May 2022). The first one allows the user to import a predefined pharmacophore query or elucidate pharmacophore and shape queries from the receptor and/or ligand structures, and to use it to screen a desired dataset among a set of provided compounds libraries or a personal one. The results are quickly computed and classified according to different criteria such as energy minimization [36]. ZINCPharmer is a user-friendly online web server, which, exploiting the Pharmer research technology, allows screening of the purchasable molecules present only in the ZINC database using a pharmacophore model imported from other tools or directly derived from ligands or structures [37].

In general, once the model to use has been defined, the first step in virtual screening is to consult a database that contains a large number of compounds annotated with information about the 3D structure, known target, and in some cases the purchasability. Some of the free databases include the Protein Data Bank (PDB) [38], PubChem [39], ChEMBL [21], Zinc [40], and Drugbank [22]. Moreover, there are some commercially available databases such as the MDL Drug Data Report. Usually, due to the presence of a multitude of compounds in these repositories, the strategy adopted by many researchers is to filter the data by applying different parameters to reduce the computational cost of the pharmacophore searching. This may be obtained through the exclusion of compounds that are too big for the ligand pocket, the use of Lipinski's Rule of Five or standard metrics for lead-likeness, and removing compounds deemed to be pan-assay interference compounds (PAINS) [35,41]. In addition, a combination of filtering for desired pharmacological and adsorption, distribution, metabolism, excretion, and toxicological (ADMET) properties is advisable to be applied early in the virtual screening process [42]. These filters should be considered suggestions, not mandatory, and they can be applied depending on the specific case. As an example, the Rule of Five is not an absolute rule, as many drugs go under the "beyond the rule of five" [43]. To efficiently filter a library of compounds against such criteria, several online tools have been developed. For example, the commercial software ACD/LogD Suite (https://www.acdlabs.com/products/percepta-platform/physchem-suite/logd/) (accessed on 20 May 2022) by Advanced Chemistry Development (ACD/Labs) can be used to predict ADME-related properties including hydrophobicity, lipophilicity and pKa, while Pharma Algorithms provided a suite of products via ADME Boxes (the company joined ACD/Labs and the ADME Suite is now available at https://www.acdlabs.com/products/percepta-platform/adme-suite/) (accessed on 20 May 2022) that addresses issues such as solubility, oral bioavailability, absorption and distribution [1]. It is necessary to underline that in some protocols reported in the literature, the evaluation of toxicity and of the ADME profile is made only after molecular docking. Therefore, it is in the choice of the researcher the use of a protocol that adds a preliminary filter, thus reducing the number of molecules on which to apply further analysis or proceed on a larger number of molecules to identify potential ligands that, if not usable directly because of their toxicity, could serve as the basis for the synthesis of new molecules. If the structure information of the target is available, the retrieved pool of compounds can be further selected by molecular docking with programs such as DOCK [44] or Autodock (http://autodock.scripps.edu/) (accessed on 20 May 2022) [45], to have a preliminary evaluation of binding affinities and exclude molecules with very low values, as well as to obtain preliminary protein-ligand complexes. Molecular docking is a computational process where ligands are moved in 3D space to find a configuration of the target and ligand that maximizes the scoring function [1]. With docking, therefore, ligand–target complexes are obtained and can be evaluated more in depth, by specific methods, to verify if these compounds can be used subsequently for in vitro experimentation. One of these evaluation methods is the molecular dynamics (MD) approach. It is the pivotal theoretical approach, which can be utilized to gain molecular insight into the stability of the binding pose of the screened molecules in the active site [46], giving a more accurate evaluation of their binding affinity. At the end of the virtual screening, the selected compounds matching the desired properties and giving the best results must undergo an in vitro validation process to verify if indeed the results obtained in silico are reliable. Everything said up to now represents a typical workflow followed in a virtual screening analysis and it is graphically depicted in Figure 4.

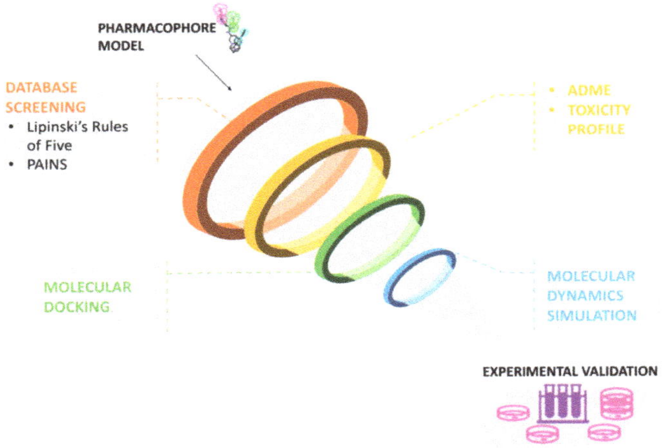

Figure 4. Virtual screening workflow. Basic filters and methods applicable for a virtual screening process. Scheme of the multistage vs. approach. The application of vs. follows a typical sequence of processes with a cascade of filters able to narrow down and choose a set of hits with potential biological activities.

Recently, MD simulations have been used to perform a thorough conformational search without any help of traditional docking procedures, with accurate all-atom force field and enhanced sampling techniques, obtaining accurate results for both binding modes and binding affinities [47,48].

Finally, it is necessary to also mention the free energy calculations used to obtain protein–ligand binding affinity by MD simulations in conjunction with molecular docking [49–52].

5. Limitations and Possible Solutions

As shown, pharmacophore modelling is a very useful tool for many applications in drug discovery or drug design. However, despite its strength, this method is not free of limitations that have implications in virtual screening increasing the rate of false positives and/or false negatives, and that should be in mind to find proper solutions, when possible, and to have a critical view of the results.

As explained in the previous paragraphs the quality of a pharmacophore model is strictly related to that of the input dataset and the algorithm used for the modelling. Indeed, the quality of the structures used for pharmacophore building, refinement, and validation greatly affect its reliability, and to overcome this limit many authors suggest a manual inspection of the structures used and of the annotations regarding the biological data associated with them. For what concerns the choice of the algorithm, it is important to underline that different algorithms can give different results with no overlap starting from the same macromolecular target. This could be attributed to the different screening methodology of the algorithm, but also to the specific screening dataset used among the several publicly available screening platforms [7]. Therefore, an integration of different tools is recommended to cover a larger chemical space and obtain different chemotypes.

Moreover, whether the structure-based or the ligand-based approach is used, both present some intrinsic limitations. In particular, flexibility is the main drawback of the structure-based strategy. As already explained, a structure-based pharmacophore derives from the 3D structure of a macromolecule target, ideally complexed with an active compound. A single structure represents a static image reproducing a single binding mode of a ligand towards its target without taking into account the dynamic nature of the system due to receptor and ligand conformational flexibility [53]. This lacking information results in pharmacophore models that may be defective in some features that could be relevant for the binding of different ligands and, therefore, in retrieving new potential hits. If experimental structures of the same protein target complexed with different ligands exist, it is possible to reduce this limit by using them to extract and merge features responsible for ligands interactions into a more refined model. However, this does not often happen and an alternative way to handle the flexibility consists in employing computational techniques such as flexible docking and/or MD simulations of the investigated system. Dynamic pharmacophores can be computed from protein-ligand MD trajectories and have been successfully applied in recent studies showing a better performance in the virtual screening of bioactive compounds compared to the classic rigid approach [54–56]. Nevertheless, this methodology needs higher computational resources (a problem that is less relevant due to the increasing availability of computing resources, and in case of application to a small set of selected ligands) and expert knowledge since it produces many models that should be averaged or clustered to derive more representative pharmacophores [57].

Another common problem affecting the structure-based approach is the detection of a high number of unprioritized pharmacophoric features, especially when apo-structures are the only available starting point. In this case, the derived pharmacophore model is too restrictive for virtual screening making the identification of structurally different compounds with similar characteristics difficult [17]. Given this, the reduction of chemical features is crucial to obtaining a reasonable and usable model. Some strategies to apply for this purpose have already been discussed, but they depend on available data and an expert manual intervention is often required.

Regarding the ligand-based method, the major limitation is the absence of receptor complementary information related to the interaction pattern with the binding pocket or even just about its shape. By its nature, the ligand-based approach is founded on all possible chemical features and geometric information inferable from the input compounds and their flexible alignment. However, more are the chemical features to be taken into account by the algorithm, more is the time cost of it. Therefore, this approach is limited to small compounds and simple chemical features by computational/time costs, generating a less tailored pharmacophore model [27].

A further complication for the ligand-based modelling is the low availability of inactive compounds, due to the lack in the literature of negative results. The use of a not enough number of molecules known as inactive for a specific protein target has an impact on the selectivity and sensitivity of the pharmacophore model obtained [6].

Above the individual deficiencies, another key point to place is that the pharmacophore represents a model of the chemical features but other variables that can influence the binding of active compounds to a specific target, such as chemical solubility, cell metabolism, membrane permeability, the particular toxicologic effect could not be considered or well-integrated on it; this could have a strong impact on the real capacity of the selected compounds to have a suitable biological effect on the target [7].

In general, even if some of these issues could be addressed by the use of accurate structures, training and test sets, the validity of the model obtained should be always compared to the statistical robustness of the input dataset, because no matter how complete the dataset employed could be, no model can be judged as universal [58].

Because of the things reviewed above, the simultaneous use of both strategies, when it is allowed, is advantageous since the weaknesses of one can be balanced by the strengths of the other. Moreover, their combination with multiple approaches at different stages, such as MD simulation, docking studies and machine learning approaches, could be a valuable resource to overcome the inherent limitations of the pharmacophore modelling, improving the chance to have more complete and reliable results.

6. Software for Pharmacophore Modelling

Several articles reported lists of software, databases and online tools for CADD applications [1,25,59]. Moreover, online services and catalogues provide links to many resources (see https://www.click2drug.org/ or https://bio.tools/) (accessed on 20 May 2022). In this paragraph, we report the most used and reliable, in our opinion, and findable at the time of the writing of this review. Several programs have been developed to perform the pharmacophore modeling in an automated way using different algorithms, such as LigandScout, Schrodinger-Maestro, MOE, and Discovery Studio. Among them, LigandScout [60] is widely used for pharmacophores generation from a protein–ligand complex and performs a step-by-step ligand topology interpretation including aromatic ring detection, the assignment of functional group patterns, the determination of hybridization state and bond types, followed by ligand and binding site analysis to automatically detect and classify protein–ligand interactions into hydrogen bonding, ionic, aromatic and lipophilic contacts according to geometric constraints. The ligand features composing this set of paired interactions define a pharmacophore model which can be also modified by removing specific features [60]. The Schrodinger–Maestro suite allows the generation of e-pharmacophores, energetically-optimized pharmacophores using the Glide XP scoring function to prioritize protein-ligands interaction sites and shows good speed and performance in virtual screening [61]. MOE is an integrated computer-aided molecular design platform that offers many different services, from drug design to virtual screening and molecular simulations. Drug design by MOE allows exploiting different methods such as the structure-based design, the ligand-based design and the fragment-based discovery (www.chemcomp.com/MOE-Molecular_Operating_Environment.htm/) (accessed on 20 May 2022). Another commonly used software is Discovery Studio (BIOVIA, Dassault Systèmes), which allows deriving structure-based and/or ligand-based pharmacophores. In the first case, it offers three methods to build pharmacophores: structure-based, fragment-based or receptor-ligand pharmacophores according to the available structural data. In absence of a bound ligand, this program implements the Interaction Generation protocol to create LUDI interaction maps for hydrogen and hydrophobic contacts with the binding site that can be manually selected or computationally computed. The interaction map is then converted into pharmacophore models consisting of different combinations of at least three features complementary to those of residue in the binding pocket in terms of chemical nature and location, and the resultant models are scored and ranked according to their target selectivity [62]. For ligand-based pharmacophore generation, besides the use of the HipHop algorithm, DiscoveryStudio gives also the opportunity to explore the QSAR approach by the HypoGen algorithm [63]. The purpose of this algorithm is to find a spatial 3D arrangement of the features shared by the training molecules whose activity on a specific target has been measured. To do so, it needs as input at least 16 compounds covering four orders of magnitudes: H-bond donors, H-bond acceptor, aromatic ring, hydrophobicity. The algorithm works in three phases: the constructive, the subtractive and the optimization. In the first phase, all the pharmacophoric conformations, which preserve at most five default features, are collected and pharmacophores preserving features shared by all the bioactive training compounds are generated; only pharmacophores fitting other active molecules are kept. In the second phase, pharmacophores fitting inactive molecules are removed; in the last, pharmacophore collection is optimized by simulating annealing algorithm. Only the pharmacophore models showing the highest score are given as output [7]. Other examples of 3D QSAR programs, which generate predictive models include PHASE [64], comparative molecular field analysis (CoMFA) [65] and comparative similarity indices analysis (CoMSIA) [66]. For a more exhaustive list, we remand to Gurung et colleagues' review of 2021 [26].

The software tools mentioned above are commercial but there are also academic programs freely accessible. For instance, Pocket v.2 is a structure-based pharmacophore program available either on the web (http://www.pkumdl.cn:8080/pocketv2.html) (accessed on 20 May 2022) or a stand-alone version that uses the Pocket module of LigBuilder (for de novo structure-based ligand design) to analyze the binding site of the target receptor by scored grids. The basic required input is the protein 3D structure in PDB format that is employed to generate pharmacophore models from receptor structures with or without a bound compound [67].

A user-friendly and freely-available web server, which exploited the common feature approach for ligand-based modelling, is represented by PharmaGist [68]. The main window of PharmaGist requires only the uploading of up to 32 input molecules in mol2 format (uploadable in single or in a unique zip file), with bonds angles and length already corrected and hydrogens atoms explicitly specified, the selection of the number of output of pharmacophores that will be showed, and an e-mail address where the link to the results, stored at least for a month, will be sent. Besides this standard research PharmaGist gives also the possibility to choose some advanced options as: i. the selection of a key molecule, by this option all the other molecules will be aligned to the compound selected, otherwise all compounds are selected as key compounds; ii. the minimum number of features in pharmacophore iii. the feature weighting options, by which it is possible to modify the weight of some features (aromatic ring, hydrogen bond donor/acceptor, anion/cation and hydrophobic properties) in the scoring function; iv. User-defined features, by which additional feature types can be defined by a supported feature file format created by the user. The output consists of several tables: the first gives a summary of the input molecules' features and the following summarized the results starting always with the highest scoring pharmacophore.

For those who are researching an easy to use and free available tool which exploits the QSAR method without requiring particular informatics skills, or who simply want to start learning about pharmacophore construction, the web portal 3d-qsar.com (accessed on 20 May 2022) represents a valid opportunity, being a platform hosting several applications which guide the user along the correct workflow necessary to build a pharmacophore model. The first is represented by Py-MolEdit which allows the correct compilation and uploading of the training and the test dataset in any format, giving also the possibility to draw your molecules. After using that tool, the platform gives the discretionary option to align your dataset by exploiting the Py-Align tool. At this point is possible to perform the building of a pharmacophore model with Py-CoMFA, obtained which, can be easily analyzed by Py-ConfSearch tool that performs a conformational analysis. Py-CoMFA allows the building and validation of the 3-D QSAR model with the same style as the original CoMFA software, which seems to reproduce published results with a very good agreement. The platform also provides the opportunity to make docking simulations (by Py-Docking), or to use a different QSAR algorithm (Py-ComBinE). An interface to the Protein Data Bank is also provided (by Py-PDB) [69].

7. Examples and Case Studies

Many examples in the literature present pharmacophore models obtained by QSAR and common feature pharmacophore approaches. In addition to articles and reviews published in the past that report on successful applications in pharmacophore modeling and virtual screening [70–74], we highlight some specific example of studies.

Schuster and colleagues performed the ligand-based pharmacophore modelling for selective and nonselective 11β-HSD1 inhibitors. Their pharmacophore models, after a virtual screening procedure, led to the in vitro validation of 30 compounds among which seven were found to inhibit more than 70% of the activity of 11β -HSD1 when measured in cell lysates with IC50 values below 10 μM and without cytotoxicity at concentrations up to 40 μM [75]. Pal and colleagues exploited the 3D-QSAR pharmacophore hypothesis and found relevant binding features of novel topoisomerase inhibitors [46].

In a recent study, a pharmacophore model based on the experimental structure of AKT1 protein complexed with an inhibitor has been used for virtual screening on a database of natural compounds. The most promising compounds obtained by the screening have been further investigated by toxicity profile and ADMET analyses, together with molecular docking for better prediction of the potential binding [76]. Experimental studies confirmed the potential inhibitory role of at least one of the selected compounds [76] and, in addition, its synergic effect with quercetin to inhibition of cell growth and induce apoptosis [77].

Due to the pandemic, many research teams explored the opportunity to find novel drugs through time-saving CADD approaches. This is the case of a study oriented to finding novel inhibitors of TMPRSS2, or type II transmembrane serine protease, a human protein involved in the activating processes of SARS-CoV-2 [78]. TMPRSS2 is of particular interest for its involvement also in cancer pathologies. The in silico screening has been performed by a pharmacophore-based approach, starting from camostat mesylate, a known inhibitor of serine protease 2, also approved for drug. The authors selected 10 pharmacophoric features of camostat mesylate and selected 2140 compounds from a public database containing more than 30,000 natural compounds. After a molecular docking analysis, the 2140 compounds were filtered to 85 candidates with docking scores similar to or better than the known inhibitor. The computational study has been further extended to analyze the list of filtered compounds for matching with Lipinski's rule of five and for ADMET properties. The study has been cited many times in literature, due to the interest in the results and the need to verify by experimental approaches the real potential inhibitory activity of filtered compounds.

8. Future Perspectives

CADD approaches have been successfully developed to improve the ability to discover new drugs. The increasing computational power of hardware opens the perspective of many more applications, also by increasing the availability of protein target structures through deep learning and AI-based prediction tools [79]. The deep learning approaches have been also recently applied to drug-target interaction [80]. However, the experimental steps needed to validate the compound activity and safety remain time-consuming and will always slow down the whole drug discovery process. From this point of view, the pharmacophore modelling followed by the virtual screening of databases of approved drugs, in the drug repurposing perspective, represents the most advanced rational approach, and the most promising way to find novel therapies.

Author Contributions: All authors contributed to conceptualization, writing—review and editing. All authors have read and agreed to the published version of the manuscript.

Funding: This research received no external funding. DG is supported by a post-doc fellowship under the project framework "CIR01_00017-"CNRBiOmics–Centro Nazionale di Ricerca in Bioinformatica per le Scienze "Omiche"–Rafforzamento del capitale umano" funded by MUR, CUP B56J20000960001.

Institutional Review Board Statement: Not applicable.

Informed Consent Statement: Not applicable.

Data Availability Statement: No new data were created or analyzed in this study. Data sharing is not applicable to this article.

Conflicts of Interest: The authors declare no conflict of interest.

References

1. Song, C.M.; Lim, S.J.; Tong, J.C. Recent Advances in Computer-Aided Drug Design. *Brief. Bioinform.* **2009**, *10*, 579–591. [CrossRef] [PubMed]
2. Voet, A.; Banwell, E.F.; Sahu, K.K.; Heddle, J.G.; Zhang, K.Y.J. Protein Interface Pharmacophore Mapping Tools for Small Molecule Protein: Protein Interaction Inhibitor Discovery. *Curr. Top. Med. Chem.* **2013**, *3*, 989–1001. [CrossRef] [PubMed]
3. Seidel, T.; Schuetz, D.A.; Garon, A.; Langer, T. The Pharmacophore Concept and Its Applications in Computer-Aided Drug Design. *Prog. Chem. Org. Nat. Prod.* **2019**, *110*, 99–141. [PubMed]
4. Seidel, T.; Wieder, O.; Garon, A.; Langer, T. Applications of the Pharmacophore Concept in Natural Product Inspired Drug Design. *Mol. Inform.* **2020**, *39*, 1–11. [CrossRef]
5. Wermuth, C.G.; Ganellin, C.R.; Lindberg, P.; Mitscher, L.A. Glossary of terms used in medicinal chemistry. *Pure Appl. Chem.* **1998**, *70*, 1129–1142. [CrossRef]
6. Kaserer, T.; Beck, K.R.; Akram, M.; Odermatt, A.; Schuster, D.; Willett, P. Pharmacophore Models and Pharmacophore-Based Virtual Screening: Concepts and Applications Exemplified on Hydroxysteroid Dehydrogenases. *Molecules* **2015**, *20*, 22799–22832. [CrossRef]
7. Vuorinen, A.; Schuster, D. Methods for generating and applying pharmacophore models as virtual screening filters and for bioactivity profiling. *Methods* **2015**, *71*, 113–134. [CrossRef]
8. Sanders, M.P.A.; McGuire, R.; Roumen, L.; de Esch, I.J.P.; de Vlieg, J.; Klomp, J.P.G.; de Graaf, C. From the Protein's Perspective: The Benefits and Challenges of Protein Structure-Based Pharmacophore Modeling. *MedChemComm* **2012**, *3*, 28–38. [CrossRef]
9. Chandrasekaran, B.; Agrawal, N.; Kaushik, S. Pharmacophore Development. In *Encyclopedia of Bioinformatics and Computational Biology: ABC of Bioinformatics*; Elsevier: Amsterdam, The Netherlands, 2018; Volume 1–3, pp. 677–687. [CrossRef]
10. Muhammed, M.T.; Aki-Yalcin, E. Homology modeling in drug discovery: Overview, current applications, and future perspectives. *Chem. Biol. Drug Des.* **2019**, *93*, 12–20. [CrossRef]
11. Jumper, J.; Evans, R.; Pritzel, A.; Green, T.; Figurnov, M.; Ronneberger, O.; Tunyasuvunakool, K.; Bates, R.; Žídek, A.; Potapenko, A.; et al. Highly accurate protein structure prediction with AlphaFold. *Nature* **2021**, *596*, 583–589. [CrossRef]
12. Sousa, S.F.; Fernandes, P.A.; Ramos, M.J. Protein-ligand docking: Current status and future challenges. *Proteins* **2006**, *65*, 15–26. [CrossRef]
13. Xie, Z.R.; Hwang, M.J. Methods for predicting protein-ligand binding sites. *Methods Mol. Biol.* **2015**, *1215*, 383–398.
14. Goodford, P.J. A computational procedure for determining energetically favorable binding sites on biologically important macromolecules. *J. Med. Chem.* **1985**, *28*, 849–857. [CrossRef]
15. Böhm, H.J. The computer program LUDI: A new method for the de novo design of enzyme inhibitors. *J. Comput. Aided Mol. Des.* **1992**, *6*, 61–78. [CrossRef]
16. Choudhury, C.; Narahari Sastry, G. Pharmacophore Modelling and Screening: Concepts, Recent Developments and Applications in Rational Drug Design. *Chall. Adv. Comput. Chem. Phys.* **2019**, *27*, 25–53.
17. Yang, S.Y. Pharmacophore modeling and applications in drug discovery: Challenges and recent advances. *Drug Discov. Today* **2010**, *15*, 444–450. [CrossRef]
18. Huang, N.; Shoichet, B.K.; Irwin, J.J. Benchmarking Sets for Molecular Docking. *J. Med. Chem.* **2006**, *49*, 6789–6801. [CrossRef]
19. Mysinger, M.M.; Carchia, M.; Irwin, J.J.; Shoichet, B.K. Directory of Useful Decoys, Enhanced (DUD-E): Better Ligands and Decoys for Better Benchmarking. *J. Med. Chem.* **2012**, *55*, 6582–6594. [CrossRef]
20. Chichester, C.; Digles, D.; Siebes, R.; Loizou, A.; Groth, P.; Harland, L. Drug discovery FAQs: Workflows for answering multidomain drug discovery questions. *Drug Discov. Today* **2015**, *20*, 399–405. [CrossRef]
21. Gaulton, A.; Hersey, A.; Nowotka, M.; Bento, A.P.; Chambers, J.; Mendez, D.; Mutowo, P.; Atkinson, F.; Bellis, L.J.; Cibrián-Uhalte, E.; et al. The ChEMBL Database in 2017. *Nucleic Acids Res.* **2017**, *45*, D945–D954. [CrossRef]
22. Wishart, D.S.; Knox, C.; Guo, A.C.; Cheng, D.; Shrivastava, S.; Tzur, D.; Gautam, B.; Hassanali, M. DrugBank: A knowledgebase for drugs, drug actions and drug targets. *Nucleic Acids Res.* **2008**, *36*, D901–D906. [CrossRef] [PubMed]
23. Wang, Y.; Bryant, S.H.; Cheng, T.; Wang, J.; Gindulyte, A.; Shoemaker, B.A.; Thiessen, P.A.; He, S.; Zhang, J. PubChem BioAssay: 2017 update. *Nucleic Acids Res.* **2017**, *45*, D955–D963. [CrossRef] [PubMed]
24. Thomas, R.S.; Paules, R.S.; Simeonov, A.; Fitzpatrick, S.C.; Crofton, K.M.; Casey, W.M.; Mendrick, D.L. The US Federal Tox21 Program: A strategic and operational plan for continued leadership. *ALTEX* **2018**, *35*, 163–168. [CrossRef] [PubMed]
25. Gurung, A.B.; Ali, M.A.; Lee, J.; Farah, M.A.; Al-Anazi, K.M. An Updated Review of Computer-Aided Drug Design and Its Application to COVID-19. *Biomed. Res. Int.* **2021**, *2021*, 8853056. [CrossRef]
26. Seidel, T.; Ibis, G.; Bendix, F.; Wolber, G. Strategies for 3D pharmacophore-based virtual screening. *Drug Discov. Today Technol.* **2010**, *7*, e221–e228. [CrossRef]
27. Wolber, G.; Dornhofer, A.A.; Langer, T. Efficient overlay of small organic molecules using 3D pharmacophores. *J. Comput. Aided Mol. Des.* **2006**, *20*, 773–788. [CrossRef]
28. Tyagi, R.; Singh, A.; Chaudhary, K.K. Pharmacophore modeling and its application. In *Bioinformatics: Methods and Applications*; Singh, D.B., Pathak, R.K., Eds.; Academic Press: Cambridge, MA, USA, 2021.

29. Barnum, D.; Greene, J.; Smellie, A.; Sprague, P. Identification of common functional configurations among molecules. *J. Chem. Inf. Comput. Sci.* **1996**, *36*, 563–571. [CrossRef]
30. Prieto-Martínez, F.D.; Norinder, U.; Medina-Franco, J.L. Cheminformatics Explorations of Natural Products. In *Progress in the Chemistry of Organic Natural Products*; Kinghorn, A.D., Gibbons, H.F.S., Kobayashi, J., Asakawa, Y., Liu, J.K., Eds.; Springer: Cham, Switzerland, 2019.
31. Lill, M.A. Multi-dimensional QSAR in drug discovery. *Drug Discov. Today* **2007**, *12*, 1013–1017. [CrossRef]
32. Lu, S.-H.; Wu, J.W.; Liu, H.-L.; Zhao, J.-H.; Liu, K.-T.; Chuang, C.-K.; Lin, H.-Y.; Tsai, W.-B.; Ho, Y. The discovery of potential acetylcholinesterase inhibitors: A combination of pharmacophore modeling, virtual screening, and molecular docking studies. *J. Biomed. Sci.* **2011**, *18*, 8. [CrossRef]
33. Triballeau, N.; Acher, F.; Brabet, I. Virtual Screening Workflow Development Guided by the "Receiver Operating Characteristic" Curve Approach. Application to High-Throughput Docking on Metabotropic Glutamate Receptor Subtype 4. *J. Med. Chem.* **2005**, *48*, 2534–2547. [CrossRef]
34. Mitra, I.; Saha, A.; Roy, K. Pharmacophore mapping of arylamino-substituted benzo[b]thiophenes as free radical scavengers. *J. Mol. Model.* **2010**, *16*, 1585–1596. [CrossRef]
35. Maia, E.H.B.; Assis, L.C.; de Oliveira, T.A.; da Silva, A.M.; Taranto, A.G. Structure-Based Virtual Screening: From Classical to Artificial Intelligence. *Front. Chem.* **2020**, *8*, 343. [CrossRef]
36. Sunseri, J.; Koes, D.R. Pharmit: Interactive exploration of chemical space. *Nucleic Acids Res.* **2016**, *44*, W442–W448. [CrossRef]
37. Koes, D.R.; Camacho, C.J. ZINCPharmer: Pharmacophore search of the ZINC database. *Nucleic Acids Res.* **2012**, *40*, W409–W414. [CrossRef]
38. Burley, S.K.; Bhikadiya, C.; Bi, C.; Bittrich, S.; Chen, L.; Crichlow, G.V.; Christie, C.H.; Dalenberg, K.; Di Costanzo, L.; Duarte, J.M.; et al. RCSB Protein Data Bank: Powerful new tools for exploring 3D structures of biological macromolecules for basic and applied research and education in fundamental biology, biomedicine, biotechnology, bioengineering and energy sciences. *Nucleic Acids Res.* **2021**, *49*, D437–D451. [CrossRef]
39. Kim, S.; Chen, J.; Cheng, T.; Gindulyte, A.; He, J.; He, S.; Li, Q.; Shoemaker, B.A.; Thiessen, P.A.; Yu, B.; et al. PubChem in 2021: New data content and improved web interfaces. *Nucleic Acids Res.* **2021**, *49*, D1388–D1395. [CrossRef]
40. Irwin, J.J.; Shoichet, B.K. ZINC—A Free Database of Commercially Available Compounds for Virtual Screening. *J. Chem. Inf. Model.* **2005**, *45*, 177–182. [CrossRef]
41. Carpenter, K.A.; Huang, X. Machine Learning-Based Virtual Screening and Its Applications to Alzheimer's Drug Discovery: A Review. *Curr. Pharm. Des.* **2018**, *24*, 3347–3358. [CrossRef]
42. Lionta, E.; Spyrou, G.; Vassilatis, D.K.; Cournia, Z. Structure-based virtual screening for drug discovery: Principles, applications and recent advances. *Curr. Top. Med. Chem.* **2014**, *14*, 1923–1938. [CrossRef]
43. Tyagi, M.; Begnini, F.; Poongavanam, V.; Doak, B.C.; Kihlberg, J. Drug Syntheses Beyond the Rule of 5. *Chemistry* **2020**, *26*, 49–88. [CrossRef]
44. Allen, W.J.; Balius, T.E.; Mukherjee, S.; Brozell, S.R.; Moustakas, D.T.; Lang, P.T.; Case, D.A.; Kuntz, I.D.; Rizzo, R.C. DOCK 6: Impact of new features and current docking performance. *J. Comput. Chem.* **2015**, *36*, 1132–1156. [CrossRef] [PubMed]
45. Morris, G.M.; Huey, R.; Olson, A.J. Using AutoDock for ligand-receptor docking. In *Current Protocols in Bioinformatics*; John Wiley & Sons, Inc.: Hoboken, NJ, USA, 2008; Chapter 8, Unit 8.14.
46. Pal, S.; Kumar, V.; Kundu, B.; Bhattacharya, D.; Preethy, N.; Reddy, M.P.; Talukdar, A. Ligand-based Pharmacophore Modeling, Virtual Screening and Molecular Docking Studies for Discovery of Potential Topoisomerase I Inhibitors. *Comput. Struct. Biotechnol. J.* **2019**, *17*, 291–310. [CrossRef] [PubMed]
47. Boz, E.; Stein, M. Accurate Receptor-Ligand Binding Free Energies from Fast QM Conformational Chemical Space Sampling. *Int. J. Mol. Sci.* **2021**, *22*, 3078. [CrossRef] [PubMed]
48. Sun, Z.; Huai, Z.; He, Q.; Liu, Z. A General Picture of Cucurbit[8]uril Host-Guest Binding. *J. Chem. Inf. Model.* **2021**, *61*, 6107–6134. [CrossRef]
49. Case, D.A. Normal mode analysis of protein dynamics. *Curr. Opin. Struct. Biol.* **1994**, *4*, 285–290. [CrossRef]
50. Gallicchio, E.; Levy, R.M. Recent theoretical and computational advances for modeling pro-tein-ligand binding affinities. *Adv. Protein Chem. Struct Biol.* **2011**, *85*, 27–80.
51. Genheden, S.; Ryde, U. The MM/PBSA and MM/GBSA methods to estimate ligand-binding affinities. *Expert Opin. Drug Discov.* **2015**, *10*, 449–461. [CrossRef]
52. Qiu, L.; Yan, Y.; Sun, Z.; Song, J.; Zhang, J.Z.H. Interaction entropy for computational alanine scanning in protein-protein binding. *Wires Comput. Mol. Sci.* **2018**, *8*, e1342. [CrossRef]
53. Whitesides, G.M.; Krishnamurthy, V.M. Designing ligands to bind proteins. *Q. Rev. Biophys.* **2005**, *38*, 385–395. [CrossRef]
54. Polishchuk, P.; Kutlushina, A.; Bashirova, D.; Mokshyna, O.; Madzhidov, T. Virtual Screening Using Pharmacophore Models Retrieved from Molecular Dynamic Simulations. *Int. J. Mol. Sci.* **2019**, *20*, 5834. [CrossRef]
55. Wieder, M.; Garon, A.; Perricone, U.; Boresch, S.; Seidel, T.; Almerico, A.M.; Langer, T. Common Hits Approach: Combining Pharmacophore Modeling and Molecular Dynamics Simulations. *J. Chem. Inf. Model.* **2017**, *57*, 365–385. [CrossRef]
56. Lombino, J.; Gulotta, M.R.; De Simone, G.; Mekni, N.; De Rosa, M.; Carbone, D.; Parrino, B.; Cascioferro, S.M.; Diana, P.; Padova, A.; et al. Dynamic-shared Pharmacophore Approach as Tool to Design New Allosteric PRC2 Inhibitors, Targeting EED Binding Pocket. *Mol. Inform.* **2021**, *40*, e2000148. [CrossRef]

57. Caporuscio, F.; Tafi, A. Pharmacophore modelling: A forty year old approach and its modern synergies. *Curr. Med. Chem.* **2011**, *18*, 2543–2553. [CrossRef]
58. Prathipati, P.; Dixit, A.; Saxena, A.K. Computer-aided drug design: Integration of structure-based and ligand-based approaches in drug design. *Curr. Comput. Aided Drug Des.* **2007**, *3*, 133–148. [CrossRef]
59. Ferreira, L.G.; Dos Santos, R.N.; Oliva, G.; Andricopulo, A.D. Molecular docking and structure-based drug design strategies. *Molecules* **2015**, *20*, 13384–13421. [CrossRef]
60. Wolber, G.; Langer, T. LigandScout: 3-D Pharmacophores Derived from Protein-Bound Ligands and Their Use as Virtual Screening Filters. *J. Chem. Inf. Model.* **2005**, *45*, 160–169. [CrossRef]
61. Salam, N.K.; Nuti, R.; Sherman, W. Novel method for generating structure-based pharmacophores using energetic analysis. *J. Chem. Inf. Model.* **2009**, *49*, 2356–2368. [CrossRef]
62. Sutter, J.; Li, J.; Maynard, A.J.; Goupil, A.; Luu, T.; Nadassy, K. New features that improve the pharmacophore tools from Accelrys. *Curr. Comput. Aided Drug Des.* **2011**, *7*, 173–180. [CrossRef]
63. Li, H.; Sutter, J.; Hoffmann, R. HypoGen: An Automated System for Generating Predictive 3D Pharmacophore Models. In *Pharmacophore Perception, Development, and Use in Drug Design*; Güner, O.F., Ed.; International University Line: La Jolla, CA, USA, 2000.
64. Dixon, S.L.; Smondyrev, A.M.; Knoll, E.H.; Rao, S.N.; Shaw, D.E.; Friesner, R.A. PHASE: A new engine for pharmacophore perception, 3D QSAR model development, and 3D database screening: 1. Methodology and preliminary results. *J. Comput. Aided Mol. Des.* **2006**, *20*, 647–671. [CrossRef]
65. Cramer, R.D.; Patterson, D.E.; Bunce, J.D. Comparative molecular field analysis (CoMFA). 1. Effect of shape on binding of steroids to carrier proteins. *J. Am. Chem. Soc.* **1988**, *10*, 5959–5967. [CrossRef]
66. Klebe, G.; Abraham, U.; Mietzner, T. Molecular similarity indices in a comparative analysis (CoMSIA) of drug molecules to correlate and predict their biological activity. *J. Med. Chem.* **1994**, *37*, 4130–4146. [CrossRef] [PubMed]
67. Chen, J.; Lai, L. Pocket v.2: Further Developments on Receptor-Based Pharmacophore Modeling. *J. Chem. Inf. Model.* **2006**, *46*, 2684–2691. [CrossRef] [PubMed]
68. Schneidman-Duhovny, D.; Dror, O.; Inbar, Y.; Nussinov, R.; Wolfson, H.J. PharmaGist: A webserver for ligand-based pharmacophore detection. *Nucleic Acids Res.* **2008**, *36*, W223–W228. [CrossRef] [PubMed]
69. Ragno, R. www.3d-qsar.com: A web portal that brings 3-D QSAR to all electronic devices-the Py-CoMFA web application as tool to build models from pre-aligned datasets. *J. Comput. Aided Mol. Des.* **2019**, *33*, 855–864. [CrossRef]
70. Reddy, A.S.; Pati, S.P.; Kumar, P.P.; Pradeep, H.N.; Sastry, G.N. Virtual screening in drug discovery—A computational perspective. *Curr. Protein Pept. Sci.* **2007**, *8*, 329–351. [CrossRef]
71. Kar, S.; Roy, K. How far can virtual screening take us in drug discovery? *Expert Opin. Drug Discov.* **2013**, *8*, 245–261. [CrossRef]
72. Danishuddin, M.; Khan, A.U. Structure based virtual screening to discover putative drug candidates: Necessary considerations and successful case studies. *Methods* **2015**, *71*, 135–145. [CrossRef]
73. Damm-Ganamet, K.L.; Arora, N.; Becart, S.; Edwards, J.P.; Lebsack, A.D.; McAllister, H.M.; Nelen, M.I.; Rao, N.L.; Westover, L.; Wiener, J.J.M.; et al. Accelerating Lead Identification by High Throughput Virtual Screening: Prospective Case Studies from the Pharmaceutical Industry. *J. Chem. Inf. Model.* **2019**, *59*, 2046–2062. [CrossRef]
74. Temml, V.; Kutil, Z. Structure-based molecular modeling in SAR analysis and lead optimization. *Comput. Struct. Biotechnol. J.* **2021**, *19*, 1431–1444. [CrossRef]
75. Schuster, D.; Maurer, E.M.; Laggner, C.; Nashev, L.G.; Wilckens, T.; Langer, T.; Odermatt, A. The Discovery of New 11β-Hydroxysteroid Dehydrogenase Type 1 Inhibitors by Common Feature Pharmacophore Modeling and Virtual Screening. *J. Med. Chem.* **2006**, *49*, 3454–3466. [CrossRef]
76. Dotolo, S.; Cervellera, C.; Russo, M.; Russo, G.L.; Facchiano, A. Virtual Screening of Natural Compounds as Potential PI3K-AKT1 Signaling Pathway Inhibitors and Experimental Validation. *Molecules* **2021**, *26*, 492. [CrossRef]
77. Cervellera, C.; Russo, M.; Dotolo, S.; Facchiano, A.; Russo, G.L. STL1, a New AKT Inhibitor, Synergizes with Flavonoid Quercetin in Enhancing Cell Death in A Chronic Lymphocytic Leukemia Cell Line. *Molecules* **2021**, *26*, 5810. [CrossRef]
78. Rahman, N.; Basharat, Z.; Yousuf, M.; Castaldo, G.; Rastrelli, L.; Khan, H. Virtual Screening of Natural Products against Type II Transmembrane Serine Protease (TMPRSS2), the Priming Agent of Coronavirus 2 (SARS-CoV-2). *Molecules* **2020**, *25*, 2271. [CrossRef]
79. Rossi Sebastiano, M.; Ermondi, G.; Hadano, S.; Caron, G. AI-based protein structure databases have the potential to accelerate rare diseases research: AlphaFoldDB and the case of IAHSP/Alsin. *Drug Discov. Today* **2021**, *27*, 1652–1660. [CrossRef]
80. Song, T.; Zhang, X.; Ding, M.; Rodriguez-Paton, A.; Wang, S.; Wang, G. DeepFusion: A Deep Learning Based Multi-Scale Feature Fusion Method for Predicting Drug-Target Interactions. *Methods* **2022**, in press. [CrossRef]

pharmaceuticals

Article

Virtual Screening Based on Machine Learning Explores Mangrove Natural Products as $KRAS^{G12C}$ Inhibitors

Lianxiang Luo [1,2,*], Tongyu Zheng [3], Qu Wang [3], Yingling Liao [3], Xiaoqi Zheng [3], Ai Zhong [3], Zunnan Huang [4,5,*] and Hui Luo [1,2,*]

1 The Marine Biomedical Research Institute, Guangdong Medical University, Zhanjiang 524023, China
2 The Marine Biomedical Research Institute of Guangdong Zhanjiang, Zhanjiang 524023, China
3 The First Clinical College, Guangdong Medical University, Zhanjiang 524023, China; dzheng@gdmu.edu.com (T.Z.); wang15728276376@hotmail.com (Q.W.); lyl212608@gdmu.edu.cn (Y.L.); zxqzxq@gdmu.edu.cn (X.Z.); zhongai@gdmu.edu.cn (A.Z.)
4 School of Pharmacy, Guangdong Medical University, Dongguan 523808, China
5 Key Laboratory of Big Data Mining and Precision Drug Design of Guangdong Medical University, Dongguan 523808, China
* Correspondence: luolianxiang321@gdmu.edu.cn (L.L.); zn_huang@gdmu.edu.cn (Z.H.); luohui@gdmu.edu.cn (H.L.)

Citation: Luo, L.; Zheng, T.; Wang, Q.; Liao, Y.; Zheng, X.; Zhong, A.; Huang, Z.; Luo, H. Virtual Screening Based on Machine Learning Explores Mangrove Natural Products as $KRAS^{G12C}$ Inhibitors. *Pharmaceuticals* **2022**, *15*, 584. https://doi.org/10.3390/ph15050584

Academic Editor: Osvaldo Andrade Santos-Filho

Received: 11 April 2022
Accepted: 5 May 2022
Published: 8 May 2022

Abstract: Mangrove secondary metabolites have many unique biological activities. We identified lead compounds among them that might target $KRAS^{G12C}$. KRAS is considered to be closely related to various cancers. A variety of novel small molecules that directly target KRAS are being developed, including covalent allosteric inhibitors for $KRAS^{G12C}$ mutant, protein–protein interaction inhibitors that bind in the switch I/II pocket or the A59 site, and GTP-competitive inhibitors targeting the nucleotide-binding site. To identify a candidate pool of mangrove secondary metabolic natural products, we tested various machine learning algorithms and selected random forest as a model for predicting the targeting activity of compounds. Lead compounds were then subjected to virtual screening and covalent docking, integrated absorption, distribution, metabolism and excretion (ADME) testing, and structure-based pharmacophore model validation to select the most suitable compounds. Finally, we performed molecular dynamics simulations to verify the binding mode of the lead compound to $KRAS^{G12C}$. The lazypredict function package was initially used, and the Accuracy score and F1 score of the random forest algorithm exceeded 60%, which can be considered to carry a strong ability to distinguish the data. Four marine natural products were obtained through machine learning identification and covalent docking screening. Compound **44** and compound **14** were selected for further validation after ADME and toxicity studies, and pharmacophore analysis indicated that they had a favorable pharmacodynamic profile. Comparison with the positive control showed that they stabilized switch I and switch II, and like MRTX849, retained a novel binding mechanism at the molecular level. Molecular dynamics analysis showed that they maintained a stable conformation with the target protein, so compound **44** and compound **14** may be effective inhibitors of the G12C mutant. These findings reveal that the mangrove-derived secondary metabolite compound **44** and compound **14** might be potential therapeutic agents for $KRAS^{G12C}$.

Keywords: mangrove natural products; $KRAS^{G12C}$; machine learning; molecular docking; drug discovery; virtual screening; molecular dynamics

1. Introduction

Plants are an important source of drugs and many compounds extracted from plants have been shown to have excellent medicinal properties [1]. In China and India, drugs extracted from plants have been widely put into use. For example, ethyl acetate compounds obtained from the flowers of Cassia fistula [2]. Mangroves are widely distributed in tropical and subtropical beach areas and grow a variety of plants with rich medicinal value, such as Scyphiphora and Clerodendruminerme [3]. Additionally, mangroves have unique biochemical properties that produce a large number of novel natural products and complex skeletons, and various extracts of mangrove plants have been used to treat tumors and bacterial infections [4]. Mangrove secondary metabolite extracts contain a large number of medicinal compounds similar to tannins, steroids, triterpenes, saponins, etc. [5]. These medicinal compounds play a unique role in the fight against human and animal pathogens.

KRAS targets have long been considered typically non-targetable targets in drug discovery, circulating in active and inactive GTPase [6–8]. RAS is a GTPase that cycles between GTP-bound (active) state and GDP-bound (inactive) forms through the actions of guanine nucleotide exchange factors (GEFs) and GTPase-activating proteins (GAPs). In the active state, KRAS can maintain affinity with many proteins, among which RAF and PI3K pathways may be the most typical [9–11]. Although the KRAS protein is closely associated with cancer, recent studies have shown that the KRAS protein can cause oncogenic mutations around activation sites (e.g., G12C, G12D, etc.), leading to downstream RAFs and overexpression of PI3K proteins. This leads to a range of cancerous lesions and over-proliferation of cancer cells [12]. In KRAS mutations, mutations in Cys12 cause the $KRAS^{G12C}$ protein to lose its inherent catalytic activity and at the same time to lose the GTPase-activated protein (GAP). The enhanced catalytic effect leads to the activation of its structure and disrupts the inactive state of KRAS, causing cancer cells to promote proliferation. Lung cancer is the leading cause of cancer deaths in Western countries. In the course of the current study, although we have made substantial progress in treating genetic subtypes (e.g., patients with EGFR mutations or ALK-translocated lung cancer), the most common (30% genetically defined subtypes) and effective treatment strategies are still lacking. Cys12 mutations caused by codon 12 mutations account for nearly 50% of patients with KRAS mutations [13–15]. Therefore, drugs that target $KRAS^{G12C}$ may have important therapeutic effects. Although KRAS is one of the first oncogenes to be discovered, it has two features that make it nearly impossible to be suppressed. 1. KRAS binds to GTP and GDP with a dermo maline affinity, which makes it difficult to develop nucleotide-based inhibitors [16]. 2. The hydrophobic pocket of KRAS is shallow, resulting in the insufficient affinity of the compound with the KRAS protein, resulting in off-target effects and increasing the difficulty of finding high-affinity allosteric inhibitors [17].

In 2013, Shokat and his colleagues used a new strategy for Cys12 for $KRAS^{G12C}$ [18]. They suggested that covalent bonds formed with Cys12 residue could interfere with the activity of $KRAS^{G12C}$, thereby locking it into an inactive state bound to GTP, thereby downregulating the downstream signaling pathway. After that, the researchers developed a series of covalent inhibitors (ARS1620, AMG510, MRTX849) [19–22], that passed with Cys12 and switch II (amino acids 60–68) binds and occupies an allogeneic pocket on KRAS, and in these findings, the hydrophobic fraction of the new inhibitor penetrates switch II. In the allogeneic pockets below the ring area (residue His95, Tyr96, Gln99), these inhibitors are highly selective for the state in which $KRAS^{G12C}$ binds to GTP and can maintain the inactivity of the $KRAS^{G12C}$ protein in the formation of its covalent complex.

To begin with, we performed preliminary virtual filtering based on ligand structures. Then, we constructed training and test sets based on a selection of $KRAS^{G12C}$ inhibitors from the ChEMBL library and trained a random forest classifier to prospectively predict a library of candidate compounds that were then predicted to be active by covalent screening. More effective chemical structures than positive compounds were screened by comprehensive evaluation of docking score and MM-GBSA score, and lead compounds were selected by ADME toxicity analysis. A compound adapted to $KRAS^{G12C}$ was selected and it can be considered that it may be an inhibitor of $KRAS^{G12C}$. Under this process, we can predict the lead components that may target $KRAS^{G12C}$ in the mangrove natural product library under the algorithm that is most suitable for the training set and then select the compounds with better docking effects than the positive control for ADME property analysis to reduce false positives in ADME screening as much as possible. Pharmacophore validation demonstrated that the lead compound and the positive control had more common features, and kinetics further validated the binding activity of the selected compounds (Figure 1).

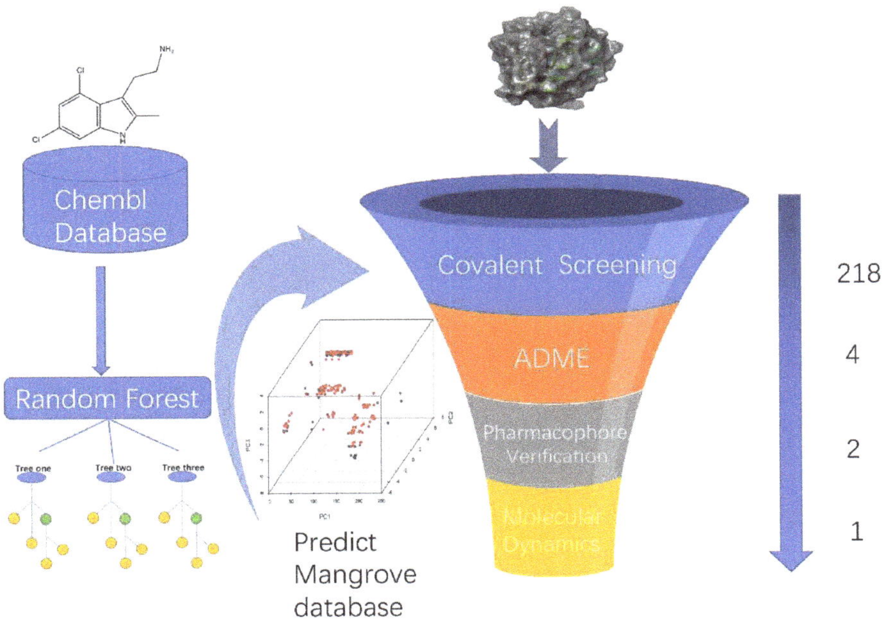

Figure 1. A virtual screening workflow (VSW) was used to identify molecules that hit KRAS^{G12C}. A workflow overview of machine learning, covalent screening, elimination, and toxicity (ADMET) approaches for pharmacophore validation and MD simulations.

2. Result

2.1. Candidate Compound Library Data

The dataset for external use was from the ChEMBL database, and all data excluded compounds that did not have semi-concentration inhibition activity. To obtain the distribution of compound species in the mangrove secondary metabolite library, we calculated the structural similarity score (volume score) between each compound in the dataset. The volume score is between 0 and 1, and a higher value indicates higher structural similarity. The following figure reports the volume score between the two compounds. The two-volume score was obtained by fractional normalization based on the backbone of the first or second compound. Additionally, the result demonstrates the cluster analysis of the corresponding volume score sizes for different compounds in the mangrove natural product library, where most compounds have a similarity score of less than 0.4. Figure 2A reveals three sets, compounds **0–50**, compounds **50–100**, the high similarity of compounds **125–200** may be due to the presence of co-backbone structures in the mangrove secondary metabolite pool (Figure 2B–D).

2.2. Machine Learning Models

To screen the mangroves in the laboratory to find inhibitors that can better target KRAS^{G12C}, we used machine learning technology to better predict the activity of these compounds on the target protein. Machine learning models were developed using the random forest model and the various algorithms included in the lazypredict package. All data were cross-validated by 10x, and from our result, it is clear that different predictive statistics for all machine learning algorithms were implemented using training data alone. At a threshold of 6.5um, the random forest algorithm performed best among all candidate classification algorithms, with the highest Accuracy and F1 score, indicating that the random forest algorithm had the best-fit value. (Figure 3) Therefore, we chose the random forest classification algorithm in Weka (version 3.8) to train the pubchem molecular fingerprint and analyze its 882 features. However, in real-world analysis, many features are complex and have noise implications for the analysis. Therefore, with the Rank and CfsSubsetEval modules, we removed features that were not related to structure–activity effects and finally analyzed the remaining 404 features, improving the performance of the random forest algorithm. Consequently, from a variety of classifiers, we screened and applied the random forest classifier that best fit the dataset, showing its good discriminative power.

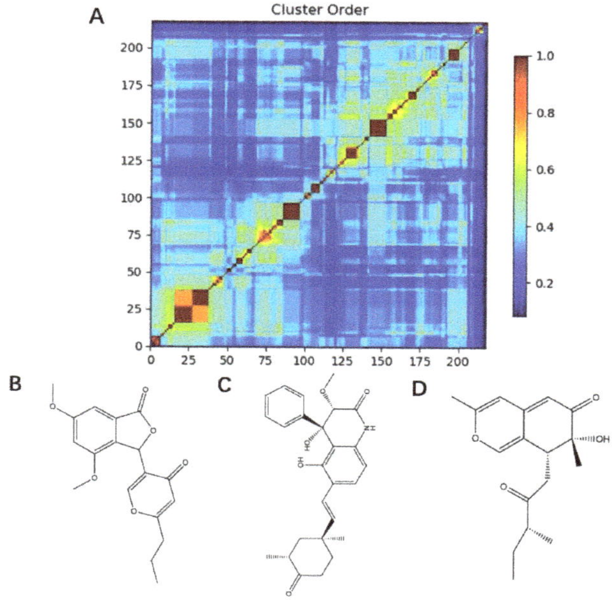

Figure 2. Clustering and typical frameworks of clusters in mangrove secondary metabolite library. (**A**) Clustering of clusters in the mangrove secondary metabolite library; (**B–D**) typical frameworks in the candidate compound library.

2.3. Random Forest Classification Model

After identifying the machine learning classifier likely to best fit the ChEMBL dataset, we performed a new round of parameter tuning for the random forest algorithm, which helped to better identify new molecules with similar properties that bind to the target protein. The descriptor set obtained by the feature selection method was used to establish a classification model, and the machine learning algorithm of random forest classification was used to evaluate the molecular descriptor set to be selected in detail. Confusion matrices are visualization tools used in machine learning to show accuracy assessments in supervised learning. The records in the dataset were summarized in matrix form based on the two criteria for the actual category and the classification judgments made by the classification model. The random forest model was suitable for both true positives and true negatives (Figure 4A,B), with a false positive number of 9 and a false negative number of 24 in the training set. The number of false positives in the test set is 3 and the number of false negatives is 8. Compared with true positives and true negatives in the matrix, good classification effects can be shown. A good binary classification model usually has good sensitivity and resolution, accuracy, and a larger area under ROC. If both sensitivity and resolution are high, the accuracy will be biased towards the highest value. Figure 4D shows the area under the ROC curve of the machine learning algorithm. It can be seen that it has a high ROC value (ROC = 0.965), which partly indicates that it has a strong ability to distinguish between molecular descriptors. Additionally, it is sufficient for the activity differentiation of mangrove natural product libraries. In Tables 1 and 2, the predicted values, recall values, F-scores, and MCC scores of the active and inactive compound classifiers are given, and the values of the average model after the mixture of the two are given. The predicted, recall values, and F-scores of the active and inactive compounds in the training set were all close to 1, showing excellent sensitivity, with an average model MCC value of 0.825. While the average model in the test set has better overall statistics, a better balance is achieved between recall and specificity.

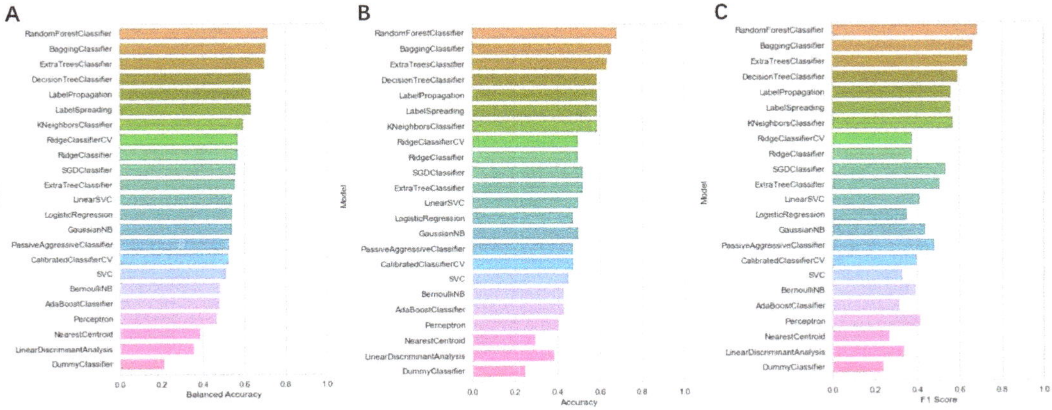

Figure 3. The accuracy of each machine learning algorithm trained using the lazypredict package. (**A**) Balanced Accuracy value of each machine learning classifier; (**B**) Accuracy value of each machine learning classifier; (**C**) F1 score value of each machine learning classifier.

Table 1. Prediction values for the training set for the random forest classifier.

Class	Precision	Recall	F-Measure	MCC
Active	0.946	0.993	0.969	0.825
Inactive	0.962	0.758	0.847	0.825
Weighted Avg	0.949	0.949	0.946	0.825

Table 2. Predicted values for the test set of a random forest classifier.

Class	Precision	Recall	F-Measure	MCC
Active	0.795	0.939	0.861	0.289
Inactive	0.600	0.273	0.375	0.289
Weighted Avg	0.746	0.773	0.740	0.289

2.4. Chemical Space

The chemical space of the mangrove secondary metabolite library is highly diverse, consisting of aldehydes, alcohols, and esters. The data set for this study was established using compounds extracted from secondary metabolites of mangroves collected in published papers. The data set was constructed with Schrodinger software, and a total of 281 molecules from different bacterial groups were collected. Principal component analysis was performed on secondary metabolic natural products in mangrove forests (Figure 4C). When analyzed using molecular fingerprint descriptors, it can be seen that $KRAS^{G12C}$ is spatially well-arranged, active and inactive molecules are well-arranged and are located in large clusters with wider distributions. Splitting the test data in the compound library into the 80% training dataset and 20% test dataset shows the considerable overlap between the two sets (Figure 4C), which shows that the classifier is validated based on COM with similar intervals.

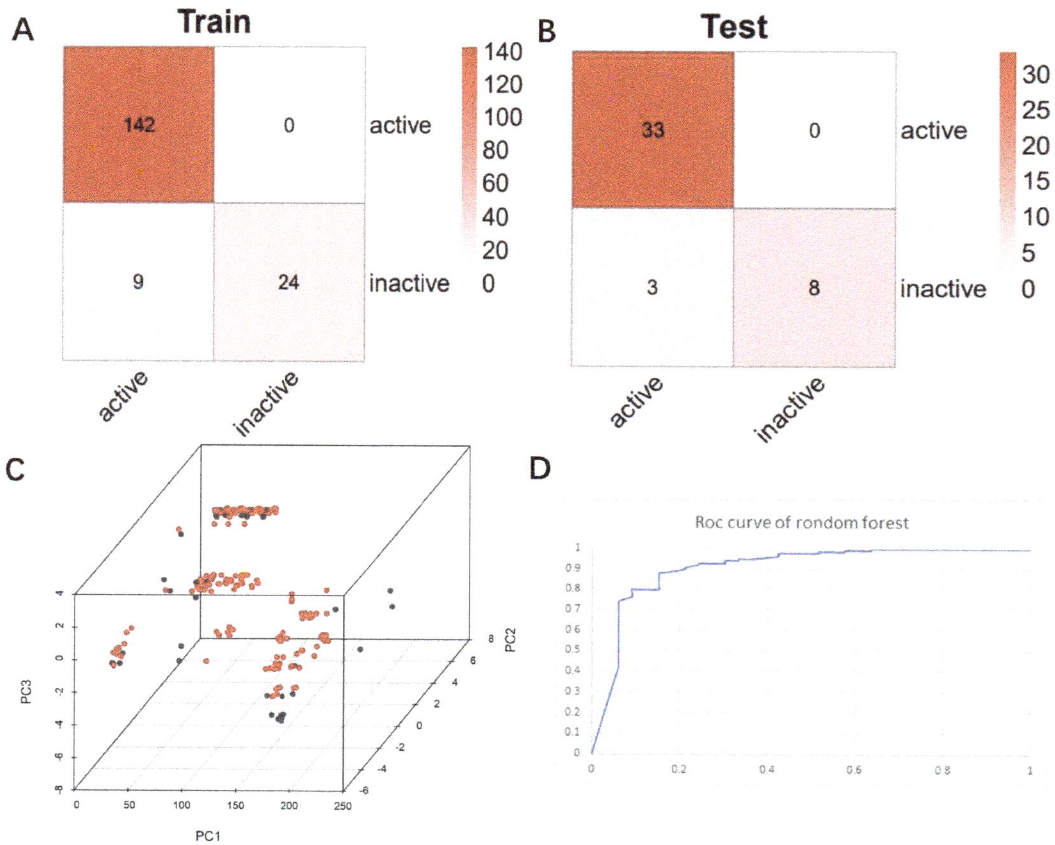

Figure 4. Chaos matrix and roc curve of the constructed random forest classifier and the chemical space of the candidate mangrove compound library. (**A**) Confusion matrix of random forest classifier to distinguish the training set; (**B**) confusion matrix of random forest classifier to distinguish the test set; (**C**) chemical space of the candidate compound library; (**D**) ROC curve of the random forest classifier.

2.5. Prediction of Prospects

Candidate compounds were scored by a random forest model and compounds labeled as active were selected for subsequent docking experiments. From this point of view, compounds are docked based on reliability, which may provide a degree of confidence for these predictions.

2.6. Docking

Molecular docking can better reveal how compounds bind to targets. The selected lead compounds were covalently docked in the Schrödinger Suite 18.4. After the ligand minimization step, the interaction energy of each compound at each docking position was calculated. The compounds with better performance than the positive control MRTX849 score were selected to show the most favorable conformation. It can be seen that the final selected compound is better combined in the preset binding pocket and wrapped tightly, so it is judged that its off-target possibility is not high. Figure 5 shows 2D and 3D interaction patterns of compounds **44** and **14** docking. Among them, the 2D interaction diagram of compound **44** can be seen in Figure 5A and the 3D docking mode diagram in Figure 5C. For compound **14**, its two-dimensional interaction diagram and three-dimensional docking model diagram are shown in Figure 5B,D. It can be seen that both compounds are linked to the H95 cryptocodon of KRAS^{G12C} and form an irreversible covalent bond with Cys12. Both compounds are connected to the switch II region, where the KRAS^{G12C} protein can be inactivated by regulation. Compound **14** had a solid docking conformation by interacting with Gly60 to form a hydrogen bond, forming a hydrogen bond with Gly10. Compound **44** is firmly present by forming the ΠΠ interaction with Arg68 and a hydrogen bond interaction and forming hydrogen bonds with Peo34, surrounded by hydrophobic bonds in the pocket. The results of validation and docking are consistent, which is qualitatively expected for an inhibitor of KRAS^{G12C}. The RMSD values of compound **44** and compound **14** with the best docking effect are 7.9196 and 9.1083, respectively, which are in line with the docking agreement among all the compounds with better docking effects, showing that the overlap with MRTX849 fluctuates less (Table 3).

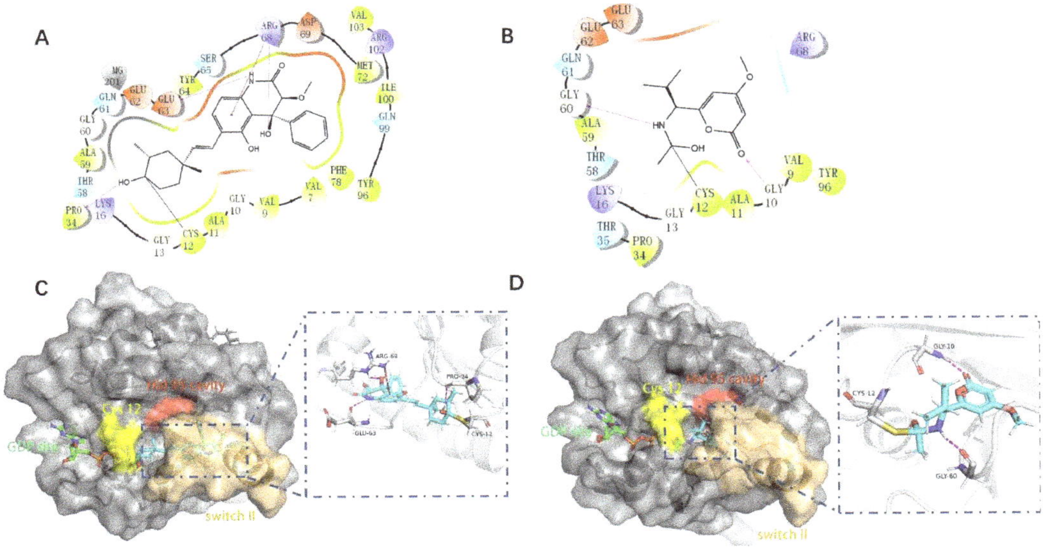

Figure 5. The most pharmaceutically available compound **44** with compound **14** and the KRAS^{G12C} docking structure diagram. (**A**) Two-dimensional binding mode of compound **44** and protein complex; (**B**) two-dimensional binding mode of compound **14** and protein complex; (**C**) three-dimensional binding mode of compound **44** and protein complex; (**D**) three-dimensional binding modes of compound and protein complexes. The purple sticks are hydrogen bonds and the red sticks are ΠΠ cation interactions.

Table 3. Docking RMSD between ligand pose and crystal coordinates for compounds with better docking results than positive controls.

Name	2D Structure	RMSD	Docking Score
8	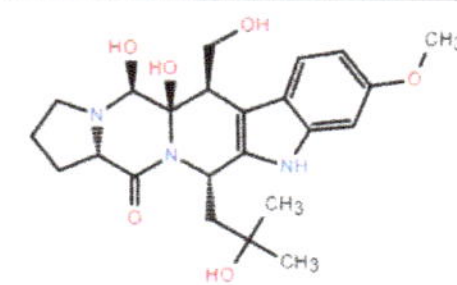	8.7699	−6.518
14	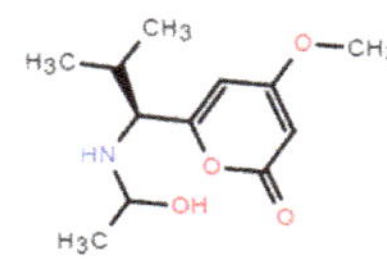	9.1083	−6.707
15	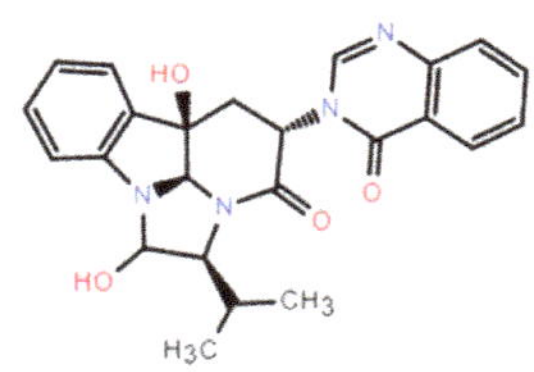	8.3822	−6.432
31	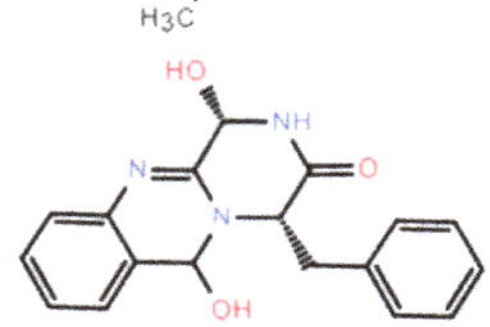	10.9337	−6.52
44	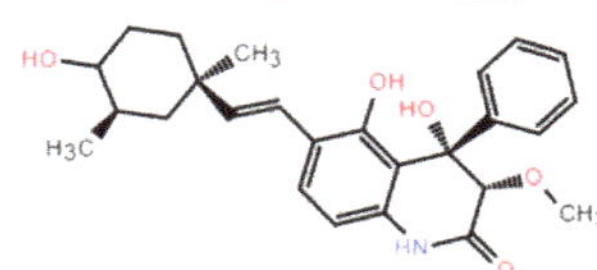	7.9196	−6.916
75	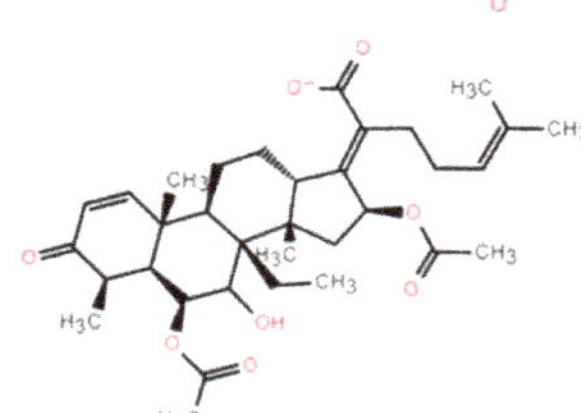	8.4722	−6.65
102	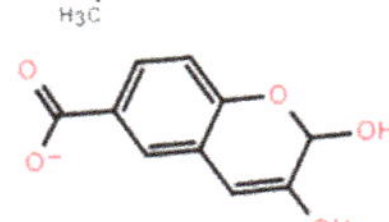	12.8430	−7.618
127	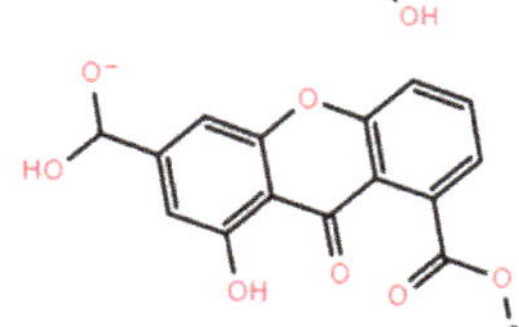	12.7782	−7.701

2.7. MM-GBSA

Binding free energies calculated by molecular mechanics generalized born surface area (MM-GBSA) indicate that the compensation between binding enthalpy and entropy plays a crucial role in drug–protein binding. For the alternative lead compound, calculations were also performed in the MM-GBSA module in the Schrödinger Suite 18.4. The values of MM-GBSA for each compound were obtained, and the compound superior to the positive control MRTX849 was selected (Figure 6). We describe the surrounding kinetic environment by analyzing the conformation of protein ligands, but the calculations are too complex to be easily controlled. We selected conformation by analyzing intermolecular MM-GBSA scores and binding fractions, which not only focus on binding but also visualize it by a fraction. The MRTX849 compound has an MM-GBSA score of −3.58, and compound **127** (score = −55.97), compound **44** (score = −6.35), compound **14** (score = −32.68), compound **31** (score = −25.13), and compound **15** (score = −4.43) are higher than the MRTX849, indicating that these compounds may have a better conformation than the positive control.

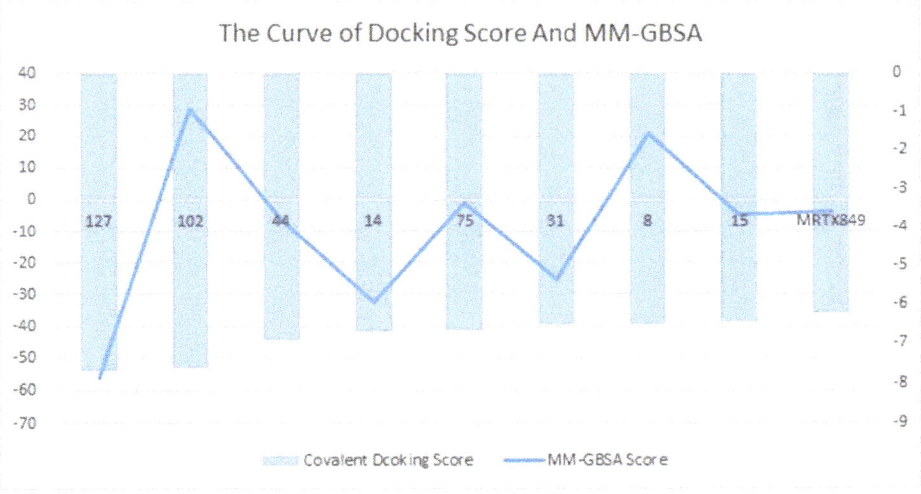

Figure 6. Compounds that were identified as active by random forest classifiers and were superior to positive controls in covalent screening with KRAS^{G12C} protein docking results and MM-GBSA results.

2.8. ADME

ADME (Absorption, Distribution, Metabolism, and Excretion) is a key aspect for predicting the pharmacodynamics of the molecule under study which could be used as a future lead molecule for drug development. Swiss-ADME is a website (https://www.swissadme.ch, accessed on 17 December 2021) that allows users to draw individual ligands or drug molecules or contains molecules from pubchem smiles data and provides information such as fat solubility (iLOGP, XLOGP3, WLOGP, MLOGP, SILICOS-IT, Log Po/w), Water Soluble Log S (ESOL, ALI, SILICOS-IT), drug-like rules (Lipinski, Ghose, Veber), and other parameters. ADME prediction studies for design compounds are shown in Table 4. Swiss-ADME is based in part on Lipinski, Ghose, Veber, Egan, and the five different rules identified by Muegge give the physicochemical properties of a possible oral drug candidate [23–26]. The logarithmic S reference values for medium soluble and highly soluble molecules are −4 to −6 and −2~−4, respectively. Based on the results, all molecules are classified as medium soluble and highly soluble. ADME drug capability assessment was performed on four selected compounds, where compounds **127** and **31** violated Lipinsky's rule of five, but compound **44** and compound **14** exhibited good ADME properties (Figure 7) and were reserved for the next evaluation and submitted for bone toxicity analysis, where the benzene backbone of compound **31** showed stronger toxicity (Figure 8) (https://mcule.com/apps/toxicity-checker/, accessed on 19 January 2022). The next evaluation was skipped. All of these parameters infer that compounds **44** and **14** are close to a drug-like molecule.

Table 4. ADME properties of ligands selected from the Marine Natural Products Library.

Molecule	MW	Rotatable Bonds	H-Bond Acceptors	H-Bond Donors	ESOL Log S	TPSA	WLOGP	GI Absorption	log Kp (cm/s)
14	241.28	5	5	2	−1.93	71.7	0.95	High	−7.02
31	323.35	2	4	3	−2.69	85.16	−0.38	High	−7.58
44	437.53	4	5	4	−4.66	99.02	3.01	High	−6.6
127	315.25	3	7	2	−3.04	120.03	1.54	High	−7.11

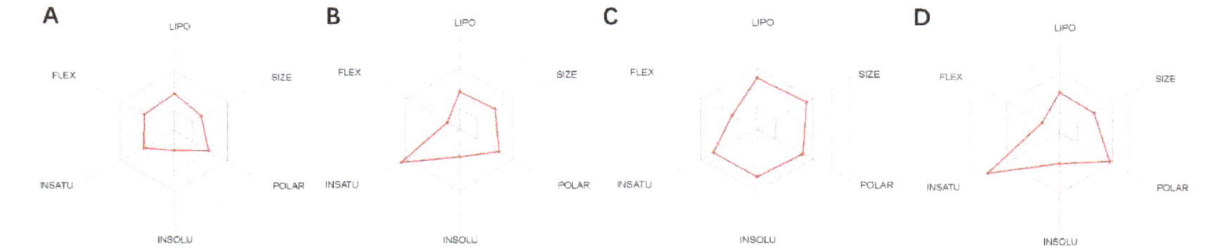

Figure 7. ADME properties of compounds obtained after the covalent screening. (**A**) ADME properties of compound **14**; (**B**) ADME properties of compound **31**; (**C**) ADME properties of compound **44**; (**D**) ADME properties of compound **127**.

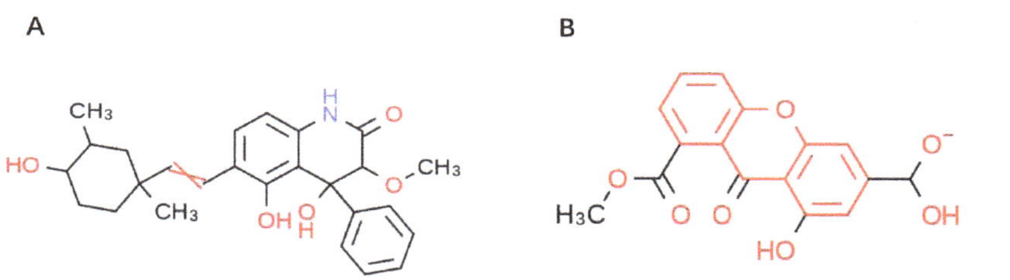

Figure 8. Toxicity alerts for compounds **44** and **31** are displayed in red font. Toxicity alerts for compounds **44** and **31** are displayed in red font. (**A**) Toxicity alert for compound **44**; (**B**) toxicity alert for compound **31**.

2.9. Pharmacophore Analysis

During the process of virtual screening, the pharmacophore model can be used to characterize the active conformation of the ligand molecule by conformational search and molecular superposition, and the possible mode of action between the receptor and the ligand molecule can be deduced and explained accordingly. Based on the ranking and scoring results of the pharmacophores given by the platform (Table 5), the best pharmacophores we selected (rank score = 52.937) have four hydrophobic characteristics and three hydrogen bond receptors. The results confirm that both drug candidates match the selected model, with compound **44** being the best match to the pharmacophore, matching the three hydrophobic interaction features and one hydrogen bond acceptor feature (green) of the model (Figure 9). It can be assumed that both compounds are more similar to the known inhibitors in terms of distribution of spatial pharmacodynamic curves.

Table 5. Feature composition and ranking score of 10 pharmacophore hypothesis models generated based on common features of positive compounds.

ID	Features	Rank	Direct Hit	Partial Hit	Max Fit
1	HHHHAAA	52.937	111	000	7
2	HHHHAAA	52.338	111	000	7
3	HHHHAAA	51.858	111	000	7
4	HHHHHAA	51.669	111	000	7
5	HHHHHAA	51.530	111	000	7
6	HHHHAAA	51.409	111	000	7
7	HHHHHAA	51.359	111	000	7
8	HHHHHAA	51.352	111	000	7
9	HHHHAAA	51.242	111	000	7
10	HHHHAAA	51.236	111	000	7

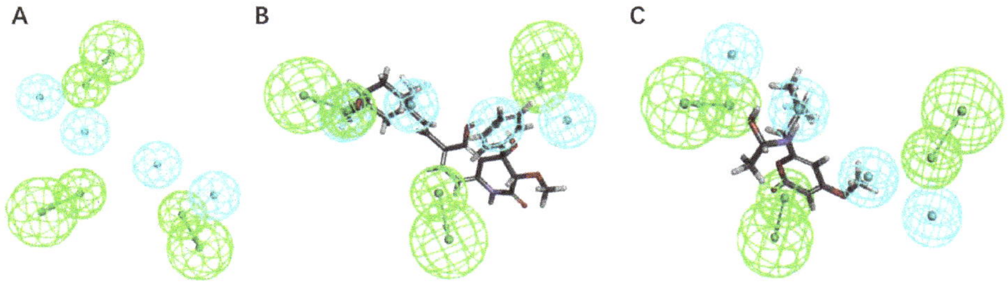

Figure 9. The pharmacophore model was generated based on the common features of the positive compounds and the matching status of the two candidate molecules with the model. (**A**) The common feature pharmacophore model; (**B**) the matching status of compound **44** and the model; (**C**) the matching status of compound **14** with the model.

2.10. Root Mean Square Deviation (RMSD) Analysis

To obtain the equilibration time for each simulated protein–ligand complex during the MD simulation, the RMSD of the skeleton was calculated. RMSD plots are typically used to evaluate the time it takes for a system to reach structural balance and to estimate the duration of running a simulation. RMSD is an important parameter for estimating changes or changes in molecular conformation. Due to sudden changes in structural conditions, the RMSD value of analog complexes, including references, increases suddenly, which is related to protein crystallization. The latter effect is to be expected since, in the crystal structure, the protein is rigid, and when it dissolves in the tank it resumes its dynamic movement.

A complex system with a time frame x should have an *RMSD* that can be calculated from the following equation [27,28].

$$RMSD_x = \sqrt{\frac{1}{N}\sum_{i=1}^{N}(r'_i(t_x)) - r_i\left(t_{ref}\right))^2} \quad (1)$$

Here, the $RMSD_x$ is the calculation of *RMSD* for the specific number of frames, *N* is the number of selected atoms; t_{ref} is the reference or mentioned time, r' is the selected atom in the frame x after super imposing on the reference frame, and t_x is the recording intervals.

2.11. Root Mean Square Volatility (RMSF) Analysis

As shown in Figure 10A, the entire $KRAS^{G12C}$ system is in equilibrium in the first 62 ns of the simulated 100 ns (RMSD value is 0.52 nm), and then fluctuates to the RMSD of 0.50 nm after 62 ns and in equilibrium in the remaining 38 ns; the entire system can eventually be in equilibrium in this 100 ns without much fluctuation in the process. For the system of compound **14**, the RMSD of the system is finally stable at 0.23 nm and the RMSD of its ligand is stable at around 0.16 nm. However, in the 100 ns simulation process, it can be seen that there are four relatively long-term fluctuations. Interestingly, the system finally stabilizes and is 0.27 nm lower than the RMSD value of compound **44** (Figure 11A). To determine the deviation of the ligand from the initial posture and the degree of movement of the protein residues, the RMSF values of all sampled conformations during the 30 ns simulation were also calculated. RMSF fluctuates greatly, indicating that the residue is unstable; otherwise, the residue is stable. The RMSF of the residue is *i* ccalculated from the following equation [29].

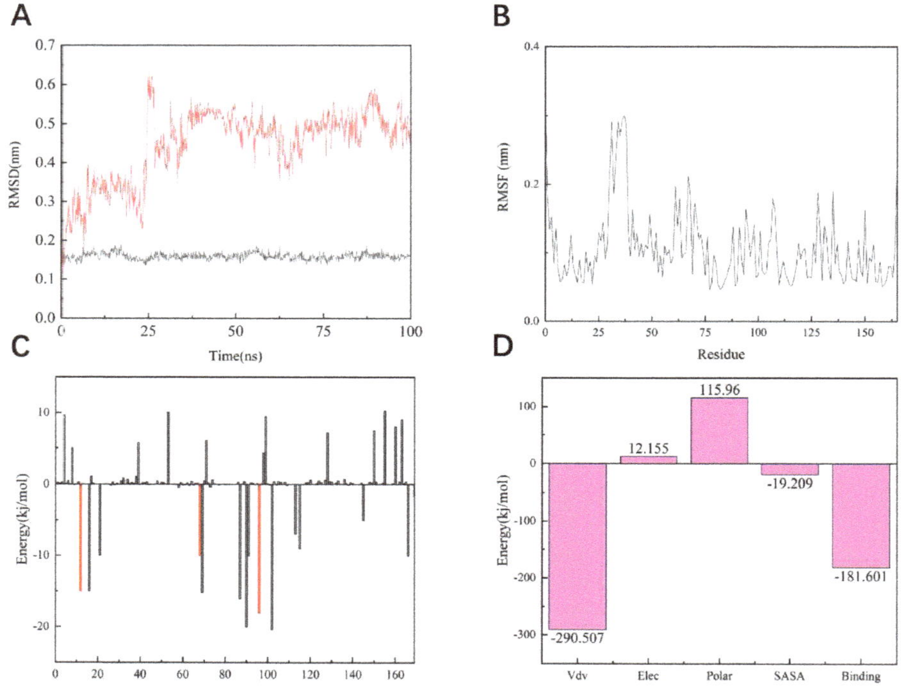

Figure 10. Dynamic simulation results. (**A**) RMSD values extracted from protein fit ligand of the protein-ligand docked complexes and ligand. RMSD plot of KRAS^{G12C} complex (red) and ligand 44 (black). (**B**) The RMSF graph of all complexes along with the protein during 100 ns MD simulation. RMSF plot of the KRAS^{G12C} complex (black). (**C**) Residue-wise decomposition of binding free energies obtained from the MM-PBSA analyses. Red bars indicate CYS-12, ARG-68, and TYR-96. (**D**) Binding energy of binding for the protein complexed with ligand 44.

As shown in Figure 10B, the RMSF range of the entire system is between 0.05 and 0.3 nm. From this numerical range, the flexibility of the entire complex system is relatively low, and each residue does not fluctuate too much. The RMSF value of the residue ranged from 0.05 to 0.15 nm, indicating that the binding site of compound **44** with the target fluctuated significantly and the binding was stable. The RMSF of another system is basically consistent with the overall surface line of RMSF of compound **44**. After visualization, the RMSF of compound **14** is significantly larger on the key residues Cys12, Arg68, and Tyr96. The flexibility of these residues shows that compound **14** is not as effective as compound **44** (Figure 11B).

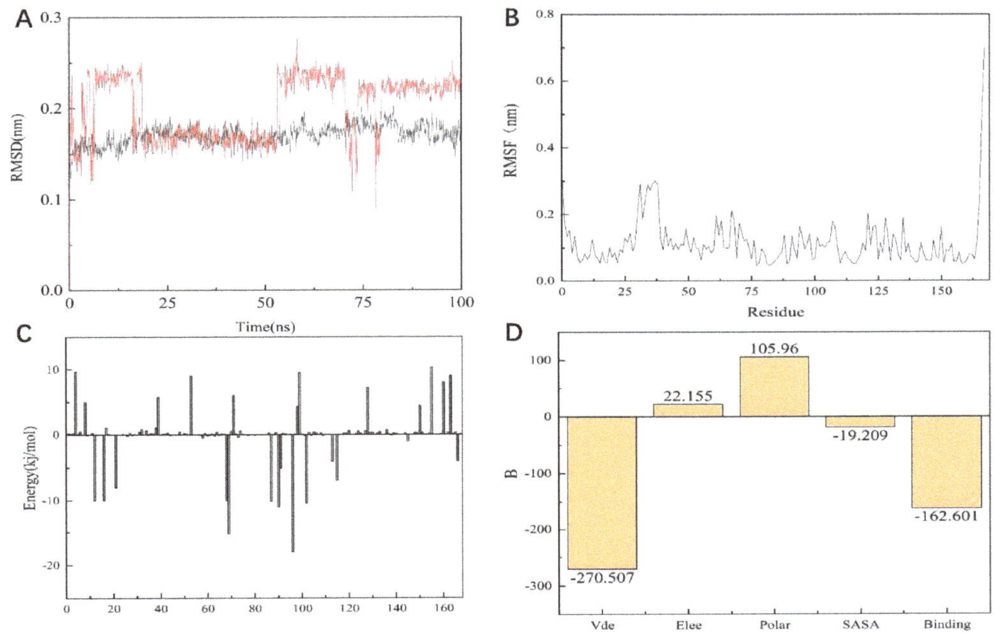

Figure 11. Dynamic simulation results. (**A**) RMSD values extracted from protein fit ligand of the protein-ligand docked complexes and ligand. RMSD plot of the KRAS^{G12C} complex (red) and ligand 14 (black). (**B**) The RMSF graph of all complexes along with protein during 100 ns MD simulation. RMSF plot of the KRAS^{G12C} complex (black). (**C**) Residue-wise decomposition of binding free energies obtained from the MM-PBSA analyses. (**D**) Binding energy of binding for the protein complexed with ligand 14.

2.12. MM/PBSA Analysis

For molecular mechanics, Poisson–Boltzmann surface area (MM/PBSA) is an efficient and reliable method for calculating the free energy of small inhibitors bound to their protein targets. In general, low binding energy values indicate that the binding between the ligand and the target is good, and the results of the g_mmpbsa are shown in Figure 10C,D. In Figure 10C we can see that for the key residues Cys12, Arg68, and Tyr96, the energy contribution of Cys12, Arg68, and Tyr96 is −15.05, −15.21, and −18.02 kj/mol, which also corresponds to the interaction forces shown in the molecular docking section results. It is shown that the interaction force acts in this system. In terms of the specific energy contribution of key residues Cys12, Arg68, and Tyr96, the energy value of compound 14 is not very good. These values are −10.03, −11.21, and −12.02 kj/mol, respectively (Figure 11C). In addition, in the energy decomposition of compound 44 and the target (Figure 10B), the total binding energy is −181.601 kj/mol, the energy of van der Waals is −290.5 kj/mol, the energy of electrostatic energy is 12.155 kj/mol, the energy of polarization is 115.96 kj/mol, and the final energy of SASA is −19.209 kj/mol. Overall, compound **44** binds very well to KRAS^{G12C}. The total combined energy of compound **14** is −162.601 kj/mol, van der Waals energy is −290.5 kj/mol, electrostatic energy is 22.155 kj/mol, polarization energy is 105.96kj/mol, and the final energy of Sasa is −19.209 kj/mol (Figure 11D).

3. Discussion

KRAS is the cancer gene with the most mutations in a single place and is the first to be identified to have a causal relationship with human cancer [30]. Mutations in KRAS are common among the three deadliest cancers: pancreatic, colorectal, and lung cancers [31].

Frequent mutations in the KRAS gene lead to increased demand for drug development, but due to its strong affinity with GTP and lack of deep hydrophobic pockets, the hydrogen bond formed by molecular docking has difficultly accurately anchoring its active pocket, which makes the development of corresponding small molecule inhibitors very difficult. However, recently, after the single mutation KRAS^{G12C} was identified as an inhibitor that could be used in clinical trials. There have been an increasing number of studies on KRAS^{G12C}, the most common KRAS mutation in lung cancer individuals.

In recent years, due to the low affinity of the binding form formed by the hydrogen bond and the limited binding efficiency of the active pocket, people have gradually begun to focus on covalent docking. Covalent bonds are directly connected to the target residues; thus, providing a more stable and higher affinity than hydrogen bonds. Therefore, in this paper, due to the special form of KRAS^{G12C} protein, we chose covalent screening as a way to find lead compounds, hoping to find new inhibitors from the mangrove natural product library through machine learning high-throughput screening.

In this study, 281 published small molecules targeting KRAS^{G12C} were selected from the ChEMBL database and all of them were converted into pubchem molecular fingerprints. Molecular descriptors were evaluated with the lazypredict package in Python. The random forest classifier had higher AUC values among all the classifiers used. This means that compared to other machine learning methods, random forest outperforms all methods on the KRAS^{G12C} dataset, so the random forest classifier chosen in this study seems suitable for prospective prediction. Therefore, we characterized the data in Weka (version 3.8) to make the algorithm fit the data better, the AUC area under the ROC curve of the random forest classifier indicates that the model has a good degree of discrimination, and the real number of filters in the confusion matrix with positive numbers for the training and test sets also indicate that the model has moderate to high reliability for forward-looking predictions. The mangrove secondary metabolite library in the laboratory contained a large number of molecules with different frames, which showed the diversity of candidate compounds. PCA results showed that the mangrove natural product library had a broader space of chemical properties. After the compounds screened by the random forest classifier were introduced into the covalent screening module of Schrödinger Suite 18.4, the control compounds with higher scores were selected for further analysis by comparison with the positive control MRTX849. From the docking results, it seems that the carbon–carbon double bond and the imine group can form a covalent bond with the Csy12 group of KRAS^{G12C} through Michael addition reaction, and these warheads were proved to be feasible in this study. Binding modes and molecular interactions reveal the mode of action of the selected ligands for KRAS^{G12C}. The comparison with the positive control showed that the warhead of compound **14** covalently bound to the receptor was similar, which may instruct us to modify it for better effect in the following experiments. Interestingly, the skeleton of compound **44** is similar to that of the positive control MRTX849, which allows compound **44** to have more favorable interactions and better probe itself into the shallow hydrophobic pocket of KRAS^{G12C} to interact with the better receptor combination. Toxicity testing shows that the structure of compound **14** has no components that are toxic to humans, but compound **44** has groups that may be harmful to humans, which is very important for future research. We may be able to optimize the functional groups of the lead compounds to provide them with better performance when targeting KRAS^{G12C}. In addition, quantum/molecular mechanics (QM/MM) calculations can be performed on the complexes, and finally, the conformation is selected from the docking simulations [32].

After years of development and calibration, the QM/MM hybrid method has become an indispensable tool for studying the kinetics of various chemical and biochemical processes. QM/MM is mainly used to characterize and study the transition states and activation energies of enzymatic reactions. Conformations computed in this way describe the surrounding environment in more detail. However, the calculations become more complex and not easy to control. We chose the conformation by analyzing the interaction between the molecule and the binding moiety, which focuses not only on the binding mode but also the moiety to be referenced. However, some compounds change mating conformations due to changes in the environment, regardless of environmental influences. Machine learning to resolve inhibitors is an emerging technology that is an important branch of artificial intelligence to extract useful and thematically relevant data when analyzing large samples. In this study, we focused on the classification analysis and principal component analysis of machine learning, allowing the compounds in the data set to pass activity prediction, so that the virtual screening can obtain more drug-like results. At the same time, in the machine learning analysis, if the docking score is more balanced by improving the docking score, it can also accurately filter out potential lead compounds from the virtual screening [33]. Compared with the QSAR analysis under the traditional algorithm [34], the active structure–activity relationship model constructed by machine learning can better fit the data and can have better performance in terms of robustness and prediction accuracy [35]. We, therefore, identified compounds in the mangrove secondary metabolite pool that might target $KRAS^{G12C}$, which exhibited favorable pharmacokinetic properties and docking effects and also received high scores in machine learning models. In the following research, its inhibitory activity can be verified experimentally to better obtain its inhibitory effect in animals and humans.

All in all, in terms of statistical machine learning methods, docking scores, and in silico ADMET studies, the results are satisfactory, indicating that virtual screening strategies combined with machine learning as well as structure-based molecular docking can improve the efficiency and accuracy of screening of target compounds.

4. Materials and Methods

4.1. Protein Pretreatment

We used the PDB website (https://www.rcsb.org/, accessed on 1 May 2021) to select and download $KRAS^{G12C}$'s structure (PDB id:5F2E) [36], and then imported it into the Schrödinger Suite 18.4 to perform protein processing preparation. Pre-processing took place in the prepwizard module (Schrödinger Inc., New York, NY, USA), flipping pairs of Asn, Gln, and His by 180°. The terminal X angle of the residue was sampled to optimize the hydrogen bond network, and the hydrogen on the hydroxyl and thiols was sampled to optimize the hydrogen bond network. After hydrogen bond optimization, we used impact's imperf module and OPLS-2005. It also minimizes the structure of the protein; thus allowing the entire structural system to relax. In a protein minimization protocol, including all atoms and pure hydrogen atoms, the conditional criterion for termination was based on the root mean square deviation of the heavy atoms from their initial positions. At the same time, all water molecules were removed under the premise of optimizing hydrogen bonds and retaining the necessary water molecules at the minimum stage.

4.2. Machine Learning

4.2.1. Data

The dataset constructed to train the machine learning classifier was extracted and queried separately in the ChEMBL database, and the reference protein we chose was ChEMBL2189121. The activity set was defined as compounds with a molecular weight < 1000, and the activity type (Standard type = "IC50") that detected inhibition had a STANDARD_UNITS value of "NM". After removal of duplicate structures and no experimentally determined definitive IC50 values, the active set included 98 structures. Standard Relation =">" for the inactive compound set, which means that the construct did not show any activity at the concentrations used for screening. The inhibitory activity type of the resulting structure was also IC50, and its STANDARD_UNITS was also "NM". After deduplication, the inactive set contained 72 structures. The electrical properties of the compounds were restored to electrical neutrality for both test and training sets. All machine learning classifiers use L1 regularization to weed out unimportant descriptors. The area under the curve (AUC) of the receiver operator characteristic (ROC) and the number of true positives (TP), true negatives (TN), false positives (FP), and false negatives (FN) were used as metrics for the classification model.

4.2.2. Machine Learning Models

Some of the molecular descriptors in the sample were noisy and irrelevant. We needed to remove them without missing too much information to reduce the likelihood of overfitting. From here, a condition was introduced to remove the unwanted descriptor, which measures the correlation between the descriptor and the sample output by the classifier [37]. For this purpose, we used a feature selection project, which selected the appropriate descriptor in a sample that contains a small amount of information without losing a lot of information. This study used the Rank method in the Select Attributes module in Weka [38] to rank each feature in descending order and then delete the lower-ranked feature. At the same time, the CfsSubsetEval method was used to predict the degree of complexity between each feature and the predicted feature for classification.

4.2.3. QSAR Modeling

The QSAR classification model can reflect the molecular descriptor as a correspondence between the independent and dependent variables, each representing the category of the corresponding sample (KRAS^{G12C} inhibitory activity). Machine learning algorithms can group observations or instances into classes. In structure–activity relationships, it tended to be complex and nonlinear, in which case QSAR modeling had shown excellent performance [39]. Lazypredict Pack (https://github.com/shankarpandala/lazypredict/tree/master, accessed on 12 January 2022) uses a variety of machine learning algorithms to verify which algorithm is better suited for a dataset in Python. The machine learning software Weka (Waikato Knowledge Analysis Environment) [38] version 3.8 was used to perform a random forest algorithm selected by lazy prediction. Weka implemented 10 cross-validations to get the best fit on the training set.

4.2.4. Principal Component Analysis

Principal component analysis (PCA) was performed on the mangrove secondary metabolite library data set to assess its chemical space. We used the Scikit-Learn 40 (0.22.2) for the PCA algorithm. The pubchem fingerprint reduces the feature dimension to 3. Molecular descriptors and fingerprints were from the Cheminformatics Library Rdkit (1 March 2020).

4.3. *Covalent Docking*

To further screen candidate compounds, the resulting candidate compounds were subjected to covalent docking virtual screening (CovDock-VS) based on the KRAS^{G12C} structure (PDB ID:5F2E). Molecular docking studies were conducted using the Maestro program. The ray structure of the KRAS^{G12C} protein (PDB ID:5F2E) with a resolution of 1.40 Å was selected for covalent docking. The ligands were prepared in Schrödinger's LigPrep module (Schrödinger Inc., New York, NY, USA). Protonation and ionization states of various stereoisomers, tautomers, and ligands were generated at pH 7.4 using an ionizer. Finally, the energy of the ligand was minimized using the OPLS2005 force field. The LigPrep-generated ligands were docked into the receptor grid in a covalent docking manner and the Michael addition reaction was selected as the reaction equation. The active functional group of the ligand was limited to 5 Å of the active amino acid residue, according to the previously obtained binding sites. A receptor grid with X = 14.9, Y = 10.5, and Z = 14.3 was prepared. The energy was minimized after docking, and each ligand outputs up to three optimal poses. Unless otherwise noted, all docking results were visually screened and conformations with the best docking scores were retained. CovDock used Cys12 as a covalently mated nucleophilic residue that conjugates to CovDock's preset alkyne hydrocarbons (carbonyl activation). Ligands with reactive functional groups in the range of 5 Å form covalent bonds specified by the reaction. Ligands were selected and ranked based on the Glide score of the reaction complex binding pattern [40]. To ensure the accuracy of the docking protocol, we chose the superposition module in maestro to calculate the docking RMSD between the ligand's pose and crystal coordinates, while using MRTX849 as a control.

4.4. ADME

ADME's analysis of the pharmacodynamics of this pharmaceutically acceptable small molecule was of great significance. The Swiss ADME Server (http://www.swissadme.ch/, accessed on 17 December 2021) evaluates lead compounds retained after machine learning and covalent docking screening. This was described based on the specification SMILES [41]. The ADME properties of the selected compound were calculated by the website. The main relevant parameters such as pharmacokinetic properties and drug solubility were taken into account. The observed attribute values are shown in Table 3.

4.5. Pharmacophore Modeling and Matching Validation

By using the Discovery Studio platform (Discovery Studio 4.5, Accelrys, Co., Ltd., 175 Wyman Street, 02451 WALTHAM, MA, USA), we spatially aligned three known positive compounds and generated 10 hypothetical pharmacophore models based on molecular common characteristics. We selected hydrogen bond receptors, hydrogen bond donors, and hydrophobicity features as model pharmacodynamic features. The minimum distance was set between pharmacodynamic features within the model to 2.97 Å and the best conformation method was applied to generate the potential conformation of the positive compound. According to the pharmacophore ranking score given by the platform, the optimal pharmacophore was selected to match the two candidate molecules to assess whether the candidate molecules were consistent with the common pharmacodynamic characteristics of known inhibitor molecules.

4.6. Molecular Dynamics (MD) Simulation

After docking, an MD simulation of the compounds **14** and **44** with $KRAS^{G12C}$ was used to check the stability of the compound in the binding bag. Then, the GROMACS 2019.1 package [42], amber 99sb-ildn force field (https://www.gromcs.org/About_Gromacs, accessed on 26 December 2021), and single point charge (SPC216) model were used for molecular dynamics simulations of 100 ns. To guarantee the total charge neutrality of the simulated system, a corresponding number of sodium ions are added to replace the water molecules in the system to produce a solvent cartridge of appropriate size. Then, the periodic boundary condition (PBC) was applied in the three directions of the system [43]. Using the amber99sb-ildn force field, the force field parameters obtained for the entire atom can be found on the Acpype website [44] (https://www.bio2byte.be/acpype/, accessed on 29 December 2021). The first pass (EM) minimizes the energy of the entire system at 50,000 steps below 300 K. Then, through MD simulations with position constraints, collected by NVT (constant particle count, volume, and temperature), and finally by NPT (constant particle number, pressure, and temperature) [45]. In addition, we balanced enzymes, ligand molecules, and solvents. Among them, we carried out non-standardized residual treatment of covalent bonds in the system.

4.7. MM-PBSA

Poisson Boltzmann Surface Area is open-source software, and g_mmpbsa was primarily used to calculate the free energy of binding between the receptor and the inhibitor after MD [46]. As a scoring function, MM-PBSA has been used in computational methods for drug design. In this study, MM-PBSA was used to determine the binding free energy of $KRAS^{G12C}$ with molecules 44 and 14, respectively.

The following Equation (2) describes the binding free energy:

$$G_{binding} = G_{complex} - \left(G_{protein} + G_{ligand}\right) \tag{2}$$

The free energy of the protein–inhibitor complex was represented by the $G_{\_complex}$, the free energy of the protein in the solvent is represented by the $G_{\_protein}$, and the free energy of the inhibitor in the solvent is represented by the $G_{\_ligand}$.

5. Conclusions

In summary, marine natural products are an important source of lead compounds, especially mangroves and their secondary metabolites have many potential antitumor lead compounds. In the present study, we constructed a random forest classifier with excellent discriminatory power and sensitivity and used it to predict mangrove-derived compounds with potential $KRAS^{G12C}$ inhibitory activity. Subsequently, further covalent docking and MM-GBSA analysis results confirmed the stable binding ability of two mangrove-derived compounds **14** and **44**. To investigate the commonalities in the potency of our two selected mangrove compounds and previously reported $KRAS^{G12C}$ inhibitors, a pharmacophore model based on molecular common features was also used to further extend our study and corroborate the potential of both compounds to inhibit $KRAS^{G12C}$. Next, our work is focused on improving the biochemical and pharmacological profiles of mangrove secondary metabolite compounds **14** and **44** through further medicinal chemistry work and structural studies. Although the development of $KRAS^{G12C}$ inhibitors is still considered a challenging task in the field of drug discovery and development, our work expands new horizons for this field.

Author Contributions: L.L. conceived and designed the study. X.Z., T.Z., A.Z., Q.W. and Y.L. performed data mining and analysis. X.Z. and L.L. wrote the manuscript. Z.H., H.L. and L.L. reviewed the paper and provided comments. All authors contributed to the article and approved the submitted version. All authors have read and agreed to the published version of the manuscript.

Funding: This project was supported by Basic and Applied Basic Research Program of Guangdong Province (2019A1515110201); Discipline Construction Project of Guangdong Medical University (4SG21004G). Science and technology program of Guangdong Province (2019B090905011).

Institutional Review Board Statement: Not applicable.

Informed Consent Statement: Not applicable.

Data Availability Statement: The data used to support the findings of this study are included within the article.

Acknowledgments: We thank the Public Service Platform of South China Sea for R&D Marine Biomedicine Resources for support.

Conflicts of Interest: The authors declare that they have no competing interest.

References

1. Ruhil, S.; Balhara, M.; Dhankhar, S.; Chhillar, A.K. Aegle marmelos (Linn.) Correa: A potential source of Phytomedicine. *J. Med. Plants Res.* **2011**, *5*, 1497–1507.
2. Duraipandiyan, V.; Ignacimuthu, S. Antibacterial and antifungal activity of Cassia fistula L.: An ethnomedicinal plant. *J. Ethnopharmacol.* **2007**, *112*, 590–594. [CrossRef]
3. Bunyapraphatsara, N.; Jutiviboonsuk, A.; Sornlek, P.; Therathanathorn, W.; Aksornkaew, S.; Fong, H.H.; Pezzuto, J.M.; Kosmeder, J. Pharmacological studies of plants in the mangrove forest. *Thai J. Phytopharm.* **2003**, *10*, 1–12.
4. Bobbarala, V.; Vadlapudi, V.R.; Naidu, C.K. Antimicrobial potentialities of mangrove plant Avicennia marina. *J. Pharm. Res.* **2009**, *2*, 1019–1021.
5. Chen, S.; Cai, R.; Liu, Z.; Cui, H.; She, Z. Secondary metabolites from mangrove-associated fungi: Source, chemistry and bioactivities. *Nat. Prod. Rep.* **2022**. [CrossRef] [PubMed]
6. Uprety, D.; Adjei, A.A. KRAS: From undruggable to a druggable Cancer Target. *Cancer Treat. Rev.* **2020**, *89*, 102070. [CrossRef] [PubMed]
7. Kano, Y.; Gebregiworgis, T.; Marshall, C.B.; Radulovich, N.; Poon, B.P.K.; St-Germain, J.; Cook, J.D.; Valencia-Sama, I.; Grant, B.M.M.; Herrera, S.G.; et al. Tyrosyl phosphorylation of KRAS stalls GTPase cycle via alteration of switch I and II conformation. *Nat. Commun.* **2019**, *10*, 224. [CrossRef] [PubMed]

8. Yang, L.; Zhou, Y.; Li, Y.; Zhou, J.; Wu, Y.; Cui, Y.; Yang, G.; Hong, Y. Mutations of p53 and KRAS activate NF-κB to promote chemoresistance and tumorigenesis via dysregulation of cell cycle and suppression of apoptosis in lung cancer cells. *Cancer Lett.* **2015**, *357*, 520–526. [CrossRef]
9. Drosten, M.; Barbacid, M. Targeting the MAPK Pathway in KRAS-Driven Tumors. *Cancer Cell* **2020**, *37*, 543–550. [CrossRef] [PubMed]
10. Zeitouni, D.; Pylayeva-Gupta, Y.; Der, C.; Bryant, K. KRAS Mutant Pancreatic Cancer: No Lone Path to an Effective Treatment. *Cancers* **2016**, *8*, 45. [CrossRef]
11. Fakih, M. Targeting mechanisms of resistance to anti-EGF receptor therapy in KRAS wild-type colorectal cancer: The path to more personalized medicine. *Future Oncol.* **2013**, *9*, 551–560. [CrossRef] [PubMed]
12. Haigis, K.M. KRAS Alleles: The Devil Is in the Detail. *Trends Cancer* **2017**, *3*, 686–697. [CrossRef] [PubMed]
13. Seashore-Ludlow, B.; Rees, M.G.; Cheah, J.H.; Cokol, M.; Price, E.V.; Coletti, M.E.; Jones, V.; Bodycombe, N.E.; Soule, C.K.; Gould, J.; et al. Harnessing Connectivity in a Large-Scale Small-Molecule Sensitivity Dataset. *Cancer Discov.* **2015**, *5*, 1210–1223. [CrossRef]
14. Wang, X.; Meng, Q.; Wang, C.; Li, F.; Zhu, Z.; Liu, S.; Shi, Y.; Huang, J.; Chen, S.; Li, C. Investigation of transrenal KRAS mutation in late stage NSCLC patients correlates to disease progression. *Biomarkers* **2016**, *22*, 654–660. [CrossRef]
15. Takagi, M.; Shinoda, K.; Piao, J.; Mitsuiki, N.; Takagi, M.; Matsuda, K.; Muramatsu, H.; Doisaki, S.; Nagasawa, M.; Morio, T.J.B. Autoimmune lymphoproliferative syndrome–like disease with somatic KRAS mutation. *J. Am. Soc. Hematol.* **2011**, *117*, 2887–2890. [CrossRef]
16. Christensen, J.G.; Olson, P.; Briere, T.; Wiel, C.; Bergo, M.O. Targeting Kras g12c-mutant cancer with a mutation-specific inhibitor. *J. Intern. Med.* **2020**, *288*, 183–191. [CrossRef] [PubMed]
17. Wang, Y.; Kaiser, C.E.; Frett, B.; Li, H.-Y. Targeting Mutant KRAS for Anticancer Therapeutics: A Review of Novel Small Molecule Modulators. *J. Med. Chem.* **2013**, *56*, 5219–5230. [CrossRef] [PubMed]
18. Ostrem, J.M.; Peters, U.; Sos, M.L.; Wells, J.A.; Shokat, K.M. K-Ras(G12C) inhibitors allosterically control GTP affinity and effector interactions. *Nature* **2013**, *503*, 548–551. [CrossRef] [PubMed]
19. Lim, S.M.; Westover, K.D.; Ficarro, S.B.; Harrison, R.A.; Choi, H.G.; Pacold, M.E.; Carrasco, M.; Hunter, J.; Kim, N.D.; Xie, T.; et al. Therapeutic Targeting of Oncogenic K-Ras by a Covalent Catalytic Site Inhibitor. *Angew. Chem. Int. Ed.* **2014**, *53*, 199–204. [CrossRef]
20. Janes, M.R.; Zhang, J.; Li, L.-S.; Hansen, R.; Peters, U.; Guo, X.; Chen, Y.; Babbar, A.; Firdaus, S.J.; Darjania, L.; et al. Targeting KRAS Mutant Cancers with a Covalent G12C-Specific Inhibitor. *Cell* **2018**, *172*, 578–589.e517. [CrossRef] [PubMed]
21. Canon, J.; Rex, K.; Saiki, A.Y.; Mohr, C.; Cooke, K.; Bagal, D.; Gaida, K.; Holt, T.; Knutson, C.G.; Koppada, N.; et al. The clinical KRAS(G12C) inhibitor AMG 510 drives anti-tumour immunity. *Nature* **2019**, *575*, 217–223. [CrossRef] [PubMed]
22. Hallin, J.; Engstrom, L.D.; Hargis, L.; Calinisan, A.; Aranda, R.; Briere, D.M.; Sudhakar, N.; Bowcut, V.; Baer, B.R.; Ballard, J.A.; et al. The KRASG12C Inhibitor MRTX849 Provides Insight toward Therapeutic Susceptibility of KRAS-Mutant Cancers in Mouse Models and Patients. *Cancer Discov.* **2020**, *10*, 54–71. [CrossRef]
23. Egan, W.J.; Merz, K.M.; Baldwin, J.J. Prediction of Drug Absorption Using Multivariate Statistics. *J. Med. Chem.* **2000**, *43*, 3867–3877. [CrossRef]
24. Ghose, A.K.; Viswanadhan, V.N.; Wendoloski, J.J. A Knowledge-Based Approach in Designing Combinatorial or Medicinal Chemistry Libraries for Drug Discovery. 1. A Qualitative and Quantitative Characterization of Known Drug Databases. *J. Comb. Chem.* **1998**, *1*, 55–68. [CrossRef]
25. Lipinski, C.A.; Lombardo, F.; Dominy, B.W.; Feeney, P.J. Experimental and computational approaches to estimate solubility and permeability in drug discovery and development settings. *Adv. Drug Deliv. Rev.* **2001**, *46*, 3–26, reprinted in *Adv. Drug Deliv. Rev.* **2001**, *46*, 3–26. [CrossRef]
26. Muegge, I.; Heald, S.L.; Brittelli, D. Simple Selection Criteria for Drug-like Chemical Matter. *J. Med. Chem.* **2001**, *44*, 1841–1846. [CrossRef]
27. Coutsias, E.A.; Wester, M.J. RMSD and Symmetry. *J. Comput. Chem.* **2019**, *40*, 1496–1508. [CrossRef]
28. Anuar, N.F.S.K.; Wahab, R.A.; Huyop, F.; Halim, K.B.A.; Hamid, A.A.A. In silico mutation on a mutant lipase from Acinetobacter haemolyticus towards enhancing alkaline stability. *J. Biomol. Struct. Dyn.* **2019**, *38*, 4493–4507. [CrossRef]
29. Oyewusi, H.A.; Huyop, F.; Wahab, R.A. Molecular docking and molecular dynamics simulation of Bacillus thuringiensis dehalogenase against haloacids, haloacetates and chlorpyrifos. *J. Biomol. Struct. Dyn.* **2020**, *40*, 1979–1994. [CrossRef]
30. Simanshu, D.K.; Nissley, D.V.; McCormick, F. RAS Proteins and Their Regulators in Human Disease. *Cell* **2017**, *170*, 17–33. [CrossRef]
31. Hobbs, G.A.; Der, C.J.; Rossman, K.L. RAS isoforms and mutations in cancer at a glance. *J. Cell Sci.* **2016**, *129*, 1287–1292. [CrossRef] [PubMed]
32. Ryde, U. QM/MM Calculations on Proteins. In *Computational Approaches for Studying Enzyme Mechanism Part A*; Methods in Enzymology; Elsevier: Amsterdam, The Netherlands, 2016; pp. 119–158.
33. Choi, J.; Tark, D.; Lim, Y.-S.; Hwang, S.B. Identification of African Swine Fever Virus Inhibitors through High Performance Virtual Screening Using Machine Learning. *Int. J. Mol. Sci.* **2021**, *22*, 13414. [CrossRef] [PubMed]
34. Lonsdale, R.; Burgess, J.; Colclough, N.; Davies, N.L.; Lenz, E.M.; Orton, A.L.; Ward, R.A. Expanding the Armory: Predicting and Tuning Covalent Warhead Reactivity. *J. Chem. Inf. Modeling* **2017**, *57*, 3124–3137. [CrossRef] [PubMed]

35. King, R.D.; Hirst, J.D.; Sternberg, M. New approaches to QSAR: Neural networks and machine learning. *Perspect. Drug Discov. Des.* **1993**, *1*, 279–290. [CrossRef]
36. Patricelli, M.P.; Janes, M.R.; Li, L.-S.; Hansen, R.; Peters, U.; Kessler, L.V.; Chen, Y.; Kucharski, J.M.; Feng, J.; Ely, T.; et al. Selective Inhibition of Oncogenic KRAS Output with Small Molecules Targeting the Inactive State. *Cancer Discov.* **2016**, *6*, 316–329. [CrossRef]
37. Jovic, A.; Brkic, K.; Bogunovic, N. A review of feature selection methods with applications. In Proceedings of the 2015 38th International Convention on Information and Communication Technology, Electronics and Microelectronics (MIPRO), Opatija, Croatia, 25–29 May 2015; pp. 1200–1205.
38. Frank, E.; Hall, M.A.; Witten, I.H. *The WEKA Workbench*; Morgan Kaufmann: Burlington, MA, USA, 2016.
39. Lavecchia, A. Machine-learning approaches in drug discovery: Methods and applications. *Drug Discov. Today* **2015**, *20*, 318–331. [CrossRef]
40. Toledo Warshaviak, D.; Golan, G.; Borrelli, K.W.; Zhu, K.; Kalid, O. Structure-Based Virtual Screening Approach for Discovery of Covalently Bound Ligands. *J. Chem. Inf. Modeling* **2014**, *54*, 1941–1950. [CrossRef]
41. Daina, A.; Michielin, O.; Zoete, V. SwissADME: A free web tool to evaluate pharmacokinetics, drug-likeness and medicinal chemistry friendliness of small molecules. *Sci. Rep.* **2017**, *7*, 42717. [CrossRef]
42. Abraham, M.J.; Murtola, T.; Schulz, R.; Páll, S.; Smith, J.C.; Hess, B.; Lindahl, E. GROMACS: High performance molecular simulations through multi-level parallelism from laptops to supercomputers. *SoftwareX* **2015**, *1*, 19–25. [CrossRef]
43. Mark, P.; Nilsson, L. Structure and Dynamics of the TIP3P, SPC, and SPC/E Water Models at 298 K. *J. Phys. Chem. A* **2001**, *105*, 9954–9960. [CrossRef]
44. Sousa da Silva, A.W.; Vranken, W.F. ACPYPEAnte-Chamber PYthon Parser interfacE. *BMC Res. Notes* **2012**, *5*, 367. [CrossRef] [PubMed]
45. Miller, A.; Carchman, R.; Long, R.; Denslow, S.A. La Crosse Viral Infection in Hospitalized Pediatric Patients in Western North Carolina. *Hosp. Pediatrics* **2012**, *2*, 235–242. [CrossRef] [PubMed]
46. Kumari, R.; Kumar, R.; Lynn, A. g_mmpbsa—A GROMACS Tool for High-Throughput MM-PBSA Calculations. *J. Chem. Inf. Modeling* **2014**, *54*, 1951–1962. [CrossRef] [PubMed]

pharmaceuticals MDPI

Article

Chromene Derivatives as Selective TERRA G-Quadruplex RNA Binders with Antiproliferative Properties

Roberta Rocca [1,2,†], Francesca Scionti [3,†], Matteo Nadai [4], Federica Moraca [2,5], Annalisa Maruca [2,6], Giosuè Costa [2,6], Raffaella Catalano [2,6], Giada Juli [1], Maria Teresa Di Martino [1], Francesco Ortuso [2,6], Stefano Alcaro [2,6], Pierosandro Tagliaferri [1], Pierfrancesco Tassone [1], Sara N. Richter [4,*] and Anna Artese [2,6,*]

1 Department of Experimental and Clinical Medicine, Magna Graecia University of Catanzaro, Campus "Salvatore Venuta", Viale Europa, 88100 Catanzaro, Italy; rocca@unicz.it (R.R.); giadajuli@libero.it (G.J.); teresadm@unicz.it (M.T.D.M.); tagliaferri@unicz.it (P.T.); tassone@unicz.it (P.T.)
2 Net4science Srl, Magna Graecia University of Catanzaro, 88100 Catanzaro, Italy; federica.moraca@unina.it (F.M.); maruca@unicz.it (A.M.); gscosta@unicz.it (G.C.); catalano@unicz.it (R.C.); ortuso@unicz.it (F.O.); alcaro@unicz.it (S.A.)
3 Institute for Biomedical Research and Innovation (IRIB), National Research Council of Italy (CNR), 98164 Messina, Italy; francesca.scionti@irib.cnr.it
4 Department of Molecular Medicine, University of Padua, Via A. Gabelli 63, 35121 Padua, Italy; matteo.nadai@unipd.it
5 Department of Pharmacy, University of Napoli Federico II, Via D. Montesano 49, 80131 Napoli, Italy
6 Department of Health Sciences, Magna Graecia University of Catanzaro, Campus "Salvatore Venuta", Viale Europa, 88100 Catanzaro, Italy
* Correspondence: sara.richter@unipd.it (S.N.R.); artese@unicz.it (A.A.)
† These authors contributed equally to this work.

Citation: Rocca, R.; Scionti, F.; Nadai, M.; Moraca, F.; Maruca, A.; Costa, G.; Catalano, R.; Juli, G.; Di Martino, M.T.; Ortuso, F.; et al. Chromene Derivatives as Selective TERRA G-Quadruplex RNA Binders with Antiproliferative Properties. *Pharmaceuticals* **2022**, *15*, 548. https://doi.org/10.3390/ph15050548

Academic Editor: Osvaldo Andrade Santos-Filho

Received: 18 January 2022
Accepted: 22 April 2022
Published: 28 April 2022

Abstract: In mammalian cells, telomerase transcribes telomeres in large G-rich non-coding RNA, known as telomeric repeat-containing RNA (TERRA), which folds into noncanonical nucleic acid secondary structures called G-quadruplexes (G4s). Since TERRA G4 has been shown to be involved in telomere length and translation regulation, it could provide valuable insight into fundamental biological processes, such as cancer growth, and TERRA G4 binders could represent an innovative strategy for cancer treatment. In this work, the three best candidates identified in our previous virtual screening campaign on bimolecular DNA/RNA G4s were investigated on the monomolecular Tel DNA and TERRA G4s by means of molecular modelling simulations and in vitro and in cell analysis. The results obtained in this work highlighted the stabilizing power of all the three candidates on TERRA G4. In particular, the two compounds characterized by a chromene scaffold were selective TERRA G4 binders, while the compound with a naphthyridine core acted as a dual Tel/TERRA G4-binder. A biophysical investigation by circular dichroism confirmed the relative stabilization efficiency of the compounds towards TERRA and Tel G4s. The TERRA G4 stabilizing *hits* showed good antiproliferative activity against colorectal and lung adenocarcinoma cell lines. Lead optimization to increase TERRA G4 stabilization may provide new powerful tools against cancer.

Keywords: G-quadruplex DNA; TERRA; docking; circular dichroism; mass spectrometry; biological assays

1. Introduction

The dynamic nucleoprotein telomerase plays a central role in cellular senescence by maintaining chromosomal integrity. In particular, it adds TTAGGG sequences to the end of the chromosomes, known as telomeres, preventing chromosomal degradation or end-to-end fusion events that may cause genomic instability [1]. Telomeres are guanine-rich (G-rich) sequences, characterized by non-canonical higher-order structures called G-quadruplexes (G4s). These are characterized by two or more stacked G-tetrads that are constituted by four guanines held in a planar arrangement through a network of Hoogsteen hydrogen bonds. Moreover, further stabilization is provided by a monovalent cation coordinating the O6-lone pairs of each guanine [2]. Based on the environmental conditions, G4 can assume multiple folding topologies influenced by the number and orientation of the strands (parallel, antiparallel, and hybrid 1 and 2 types), the loop size, the groove width, and the *syn*/*anti* glycosidic bond orientation of the guanines [2,3]. For the human telomeric sequence (HTS), several G4 DNA topologies have been observed in the presence of K^+ ions. Specifically, the parallel-stranded conformation is the only one found for the wild-type Tel_{22} $AG_3[T_2AG_3]_3$ crystallographic structure [4], while hybrid 1 and hybrid 2 topologies are prevalent in NMR solutions [5,6]. Conversely, antiparallel folding was revealed by NMR studies in the presence of Na^+ [7]. Furthermore, several bimolecular and tetramolecular G4 structures can be obtained in vitro by nucleic acid sequences that include groups of contiguous guanine residues [8–10]. At first, telomeres were considered as transcriptionally silent regions of mammalian chromosomes, but Azzalin et al. pointed out their transcription by detecting non-coding telomeric repeat-containing RNAs (TERRA) into mammalian cells [11]. TERRA can play significant a significant role in different biological processes, such as end protection, telomeric replication, and telomerase recruitment [12,13]. Interestingly, Xu et al. demonstrated that human TERRA molecules folded in G4s similarly to the telomeric DNA and provided direct evidence about the presence of the parallel-stranded TERRA G4s in living cells, through a light-switching pyrene probe [14]. Moreover, several TERRA-binding proteins have been discovered, including telomeric duplex DNA binding proteins TRF1 and TRF2, which are Shelterin key components able to protect telomeres [15]. Balasubramanian and co-workers also demonstrated that TRF2 interacts with the G4 conformation of TERRA for binding more tightly to telomeric DNA (Tel) [16]. TRF2 promotes telomere folding by hiding the 3′-end overhang, which is not recognized as damaged DNA, thus preventing DNA damage response (DDR) activation [17]. Because the maintenance of telomeres is a key tract of cancer cells, compounds that target telomeres and their transcripts have been investigated as anticancer strategies. The therapeutic evaluation of TERRA-mediated telomerase regulation in cancer cells showed promising results. Indeed, previous studies demonstrated TERRA downregulation in advanced stages of various human cancers compared to normal tissues, suggesting that telomeric transcription is downregulated in advanced tumors [18]. Moreover, recent studies demonstrated that the identification of TERRA G4-targeting drugs induced a cytotoxic effect on high TERRA-expressing cells, where they induce a DDR at telomeres, probably by displacing TERRA from telomeres [19]. In light of this, TERRA provides a promising antitumor target as it is necessary for the formation of telomeric heterochromatin in all tumor cells, even those not expressing telomerase (ALT-positive tumors) [20]. The availability of TERRA experimental (NMR or X-ray) structures, together with a deep understanding of their topologies, is extremely helpful for the rational design of their selective ligands. Interestingly, CD, NMR, and X-ray crystallographic studies pointed out the parallel "propeller" topology as the most predominant for TERRA [21], if compared to the wide variety of G4 conformations observed for Tel [4–6,22,23]. Unfortunately, only the bimolecular sequence of TERRA was solved [21,24], while its unimolecular counterpart is still unavailable. While several Tel ligands have been identified and studied [25–30], few compounds have yet been proposed as TERRA binders. Among them, Collie et al. described a naphthalene diimide able to bind bimolecular TERRA with higher selectivity than BRACO-19, a ligand more selective towards Tel. This observation is suggested to be related to the presence of the 2′-OH groups in the RNA sugars, which reduce groove and loop widths, making important changes in the portion interacting with the ligand sidechains as well [31]. Therefore, the hydrogen bonds (H-bonds) network, involving the O2′ hydroxyl groups of the ribonucleotide sugars in TERRA, can be considered an important structural feature for the drug-design of selective TERRA-ligands [32]. In particular, this H-bond network tunes down the negative electrostatic surface of the target, partially explaining the observed selectivity of carboxypyridostatin (*c*PDS) [33]. A previous computational study by us pointed out that the *c*PDS high electrostatic surface, coupled to a conformational profile able to maximize the solvation contribution, is an important feature to make it selective against TERRA [34]. Starting from our previous virtual screening (VS) campaign on bimolecular telomeric DNA and RNA G4 structures (named Tel_2 and $TERRA_2$ G4, respectively) [35], in this work, the three best candidates (Figure 1) were submitted to molecular recognition studies on the 3D coordinates of monomolecular Tel and TERRA. A computational approach, based on molecular dynamics (MD) and docking simulations, was applied to target the monomolecular Tel of the 22-nt telomeric sequence 5′-AGGGTTAGGGTTAGGGTTAGGG-3′ (PDB code: 1KF1) [31] and its TERRA counterpart sequence 22-nt 5′-AGGGUUAGGGUUAGGGUUAGGG-3′. In particular, we investigated the binding affinity of the three best candidates **7**, **15**, and **17** previously discovered as dual Tel_2 and $TERRA_2$ binders [35], towards their Tel and TERRA monomolecular counterparts. With this aim, the homology model of the monomolecular TERRA was built and submitted to MD simulations to assess its geometric stability with respect to the corresponding Tel conformation. Subsequently, our docking simulations allowed us to predict the putative binding mode of all three candidates on TERRA. Furthermore, biophysical assays confirmed their stabilizing power.

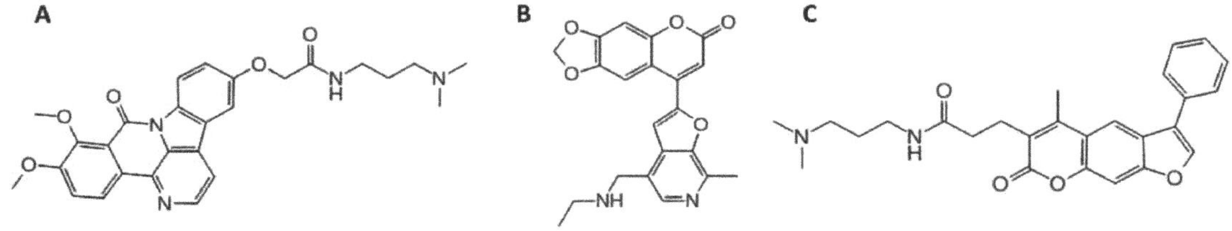

Figure 1. **The** 2D chemical structures of the three best *hits* found in our previous VS campaign on bimolecular $Tel_2/TERRA_2$ G4s: (**A**) *hit* **7**, characterized by a naphthyridine scaffold with a ((dimethylamino)propyl)acetamide side chain; (**B**) *hit* **15**, exhibiting a furo-chromene structure; and (**C**) *hit* **17**, distinguished by a benzofuran ring [35].

2. Results and Discussion

2.1. Computational Studies

The binding capability of the three best *hits*, discovered in a previous VS on bimolecular $Tel_2/TERRA_2$ G4s [35], was computationally investigated on the corresponding monomolecular structures. The G4 crystallographic model of Tel (PDB ID: 1KF1) was used as template to build the corresponding TERRA G4 structure through the *"homology modelling"* approach and was submitted to MD simulations to verify the geometrical stability. MD simulations agree with the experimental data [36,37], showing higher structural stability for TERRA with respect to Tel (Supplementary Figure S1), as demonstrated by the average of the Root Mean Square deviation (RMSd) on all the heavy atoms, which is equal to 0.26 nm and 0.34 nm, respectively, for TERRA and Tel. This observation is further confirmed by the RMSd matrix (Supplementary Figure S2) calculated on the heavy atoms among all MDs conformations, from which it turns out that Tel exhibited a more significant heterogeneity than TERRA, as highlighted by the wider orange and red areas (Supplementary Figure S2A), associated with the higher RMSd values. A cluster analysis performed on all the nucleic acid heavy atoms allowed us to select the most representative conformations of both G4 targets. Specifically, to perform the subsequent docking studies, four and three conformations for Tel and TERRA, respectively, were selected, thus considering the flexibility of both targets. A visual inspection analysis of all the most representative conformations (cluster 1, 2, 3, and 4 of Tel and cluster 1, 2, and 3 of TERRA) (Supplementary Figure S3) retrieved a well-structured G-core with partial coverage of the G-tetrad at the top of the residue DA1 (Deoxyribonucleotide Adenine 1) and RA1 (Ribonucleotide Adenine 1) in Tel and TERRA, respectively. Moreover, the structure of the Tel cluster 4 was exhibited in the top position in the presence of an additional residue, DA7 (Supplementary Figure S3B). Interestingly, TERRA and Tel showed two different behaviors in the bottom position. While all TERRA representative conformations showed that the G-tetrad at the bottom position is free to interact with any end-stacking ligands, in three Tel structures (cluster 1, cluster 3, and cluster 4), we observed residue DT17 (Deoxyribonucleotide Thymine 17) interacting through stacking interactions with DG16 (Deoxyribonucleotide Guanine 16), partially preventing ligands access (Supplementary Figure S3B). The greatest structural difference between the target-selected conformations of both Tel and TERRA was instead found in the loops, where the highest heterogeneity was observed. In order to investigate the differences in the recognition of the unimolecular telomeric G4s for the three ligands, we clusterized all generated docking poses obtained against all clusters by using the angle descriptor defined by three dummy atoms, as reported in a previous work [38]. As shown in Supplementary Figure S4, *hits* **15** and **17** bound to loop in both targets, while *hit* **7** exhibited a greater number of poses positioned at the bottom of the TERRA molecule. The second favorite binding site for all compounds was the bottom position. The top position was not a favorite binding site for these compounds: we hypothesize that the presence of DA1 and RA1 in Tel and TERRA, respectively, blocks the access to the G-tetrad. In Supplementary Figure S5, we report a deeper analysis for the distribution of the binding poses to the most representative conformations of both targets. Regarding TERRA clusters, we observed heterogeneous behaviour. In fact, although all 3D structures showed that the G-tetrad in the bottom position is free to interact with the three studied compounds, as previously described, only cluster 1 and cluster 2 for *hit* **7**, and cluster 2 and cluster 1 for *hits* **15** and **17**, respectively, seem to favour this binding mode. Conversely, the lateral position appeared to be preferred in the rest of the clusters, with a higher prevalence for *hits* **15** and **17**, suggesting the conformation of the loops more favourable to accommodate a ligand. Interestingly, for cluster 4 of the Tel target, a single binding mode could be observed for all generated docking poses since all compounds bind the nucleic acid in a lateral position. In addition, Tel cluster 2 showed a preference to bind the ligands in a lateral position, especially for *hits* **7** and **17**. Finally, despite the presence at the bottom of residue DT17 that partially covers the G-tetrad, clusters 1 and 3 of all *hits* seemed to slightly prefer this binding site. Then, for each compound, we selected and deeply analyzed the energetically most stable complex with both targets (Supplementary Table S1). All three compounds showed better binding free energies when they were docked against TERRA, with ΔG_{bind} values ranging from −58.86 to −88.77 kcal/mol. Conversely, Tel complexes were characterized by ΔG_{bind} values higher than −57.96 kcal/mol. Thus, *hit* **7** potentially maintained its dual Tel/TERRA ligand profile, as previously also observed on the respective bimolecular Tel_2/$TERRA_2$ G4s [35]. Surprisingly, *hit* **15** and *hit* **17**, previously characterized as selective Tel_2 ligands [35], turned out to have a better theoretical affinity towards the monomolecular TERRA G4. An analysis of the related single contributions of ΔG_{bind} highlighted the better contribution of Van der Waals (ΔG_{bind_vdW}), lipophilic (ΔG_{bind_Lipo}), and packing energy ($\Delta G_{bind\_Packing}$), that is, the π–π packing correction, in TERRA complexes compared to Tel ones [39]. We next analyzed the interaction pattern of the best thermodynamic complexes (Figure 2). Specifically, *hit* **7** recognized the bottom of TERRA, confirming this binding site as the most geometrically and energetically favored (Figure 2A). The complex was stabilized by four π–π interactions, established between the naphthyridine moiety of the ligand and the nitrogenous base of the nucleobase RG10 (Ribonucleotide Guanine 10), and a π–cation between *hit* **7** pyridine ring and the potassium coordinating the last G-tetrad. This ligand also engaged three H-bonds with nucleobases RG10, RG4, and RA7 by means of the carbonyl group on the naphtyridine ring, the linear amide, and the quaternary ammonium, respectively. Its positive charge was also involved in three salt bridges with nucleobases RU5 (Ribonucleotide Uracil 5), RA7, and RG9. Conversely, in the Tel complex, *hit* **7** behaved as a loop binder by preventing the formation of the stacking interactions that stabilize its bond with TERRA (Figure 2D). This ligand interacted with Tel through three H-bonds with nucleobases DA14 and DA19 by employing its quaternary ammonium, its amide group, and its pyridinium ring, respectively. Two salt bridges were also engaged between the quaternary ammonium and the pyridinium ring of the ligand and nucleobases DA19 and DA14, respectively. *Hit* **15** (Figure 2B) appeared to form the most energetically stable complex for both G4 structures by acting as a loop binder, in agreement with the geometrical analysis of the docking binding sites. In the complex between *hit* **15** and TERRA, electrostatic contributions were the driving interactions (Supplementary Table S1). Specifically, a salt bridge, involving the quaternary ammonium of the ligand and the phosphoric group of the RG16 nucleobase, and four H-bonds were established. These latter interactions were engaged between the 1,3-dioxole portion; the furan ring; and the quaternary ammonium of the ligand and nucleobases RU17, RA19, and RG15, respectively. Conversely, in the Tel complex (Figure 2E), *hit* **15** engaged only two H-bonds between the carbonyl group of the chromene moiety and the quaternary ammonium of the ligand with nucleobases DT11 and DG10, respectively. In the complex between *hit* **15** and Tel, we observed four π–π interactions between the chromene ring and the furopyridine moiety with the nucleobases DG8 and DA13, respectively. Although only two π–π interactions were observed in the TERRA complex between the 1,3 dioxole portion and the pyridine ring of *hit* **15** with nucleobases RA19 and RU18, respectively, the ligand was able to establish several hydrophobic interactions, as highlighted by the lipophilic energetic terms in Supplementary Table S1 (ΔG_{bind_Lipo} and $\Delta G_{bind\_Packing}$). Finally, the energetic analysis confirmed the behavior of loop binders for *hit* **17** when complexed to TERRA (Figure 2C). At the same time, the bottom position was disclosed as the best binding site on Tel G4 for the same compound (Figure 2F). Moreover, the best energy evaluation for the complex between *hit* **17** and TERRA G4 was related to the higher number of established favorable interactions compared to Tel. Specifically, *hit* **17** was involved in three π–π interactions and two H-bonds with TERRA G4, while in the Tel complex only one π–π interaction and one H-bond were observed. In detail, the TERRA complex showed the phenyl ring and the chromene moiety of the ligand interacting with nucleobases RG8 and RG14, respectively, through π–π interactions. Instead, the amide moiety and the quaternary ammonium engaged two H-bonds with nucleobases RA13 and RU12, respectively. Regarding the Tel complex, we observed π–π interactions between the ligand furan ring and DT17 nucleobase, while the amide portion interacted through an H-bond with DG22. Both complexes of *hit* **17** shared a salt bridge, involving its quaternary ammonium and nucleobases RU12 and DG22 for TERRA and Tel, respectively.

In a second step, we evaluated the ability of the three compounds to stabilize both TERRA and Tel. We performed 200 ns long MDs starting with thermodynamically best complexes and compared the results with respect to the stability of the related cluster conformation for each target. As shown in Supplementary Figure S6, the analysis of the RMSd trend, calculated on the heavy atoms of both targets, showed a better ability to stabilize TERRA for all compounds, compared to Tel complexes. Interestingly, *hit* **7** exhibited the best stabilizing profile on TERRA, with an average RMSd value of 0.17 nm. Moreover, it is the only compound able to form a complex with Tel showing an RMSd trend (with an average RMSd value of 0.26 nm) similar to that of the related unbound target structure (with an average RMSd value of 0.24 nm). Conversely, *hit* **17** exhibited the worst trend of RMSd on Tel (with an average RMSd value of 0.35 nm) since we observed for the entire duration of the MDs higher RMSd values compared to the unbound target, with a further increase in the last 50 ns. Regarding *hit* **15**, although in the first 100 ns of MDs it seemed to stabilize both G4 structures, in the last part of the simulation it showed a gradual increase in the RMSd trend of Tel. Finally, for each complex, the most populated structure during the MDs was selected and deeply analyzed (Supplementary Table S2 and Supplementary Figure S6). As observed in docking simulation, all the three compounds confirmed a better binding free energy if complexed with TERRA, with ΔG_{bind} values ranging from −38.36 to −85.93 kcal/mol. Conversely, Tel complexes were characterized by ΔG_{bind} values higher than −35.01 kcal/mol, except for the complex of *hit* **7**, which exhibited ΔG_{bind} value of −45.85 kcal/mol. Regarding the binding mode and the interaction pattern of the most populated structure during MDs, we observed the maintenance of the binding site only in the TERRA complexes

(Supplementary Figure S7A–C). In particular, *hit* **7** always bonded the bottom portion of TERRA, as in the docking pose, and it established excellent π–π interactions between its naphthyridine moiety and nucleobases RG10 and RG16, as well as a π–cation interaction and an H-bond with RG22 and RG16, respectively. On the other hand, when comparing this structure with the initial docking pose (Figure 2A), we observed the rotation of the ligand with good interactions between its lateral chain and the first loop of TERRA. Specifically, two salt bridges were established between the quaternary ammonium of *hit* **7** and the phosphoric groups of nucleobases RA7 and RU5, while two H-bonds were observed with the sugar and the base of the RG4 (Supplementary Figure S7A). As noted in the docking pose (Figure 2B), *hit* **15** kept its lateral binding mode by establishing two π–π and a π–cation interaction with the RA19 nucleobase (Supplementary Figure S7B). Regarding *hit* **17**, the comparison of the most populated structure during MDs with the docking pose (Figure 2C) highlighted the absence of interactions between the ligand side-chain and the TERRA loop. Conversely, *hit* **17** strengthened π–π interactions between its psoralen portion and nucleobases RG8 and RG14, and it also established an additional H-bond between its carbonyl amide and RA (Supplementary Figure S7C). Interestingly, the most populated structures of MDs for Tel complexes showed a complete change in the binding site (Supplementary Figure S7D–E), except for *hit* **17**. During MDs, *hits* **7** and **15** changed their binding sites, moving from the lateral (Figure 2D–E) to the top position. The new binding mode of *hit* **7** was characterized by a strong interaction between the ligand naphthyridine moiety and nucleobase DG8, thanks to formation of six π–π, two π–cations, and one H-bond (Supplementary Figure S7D). Moreover, we also observed a π–π interaction with nucleobase DA1 and an H-bond between the ammonium group of the ligand and the sugar portion of DG14. Additionally, for *hit* **15**, we beheld several π–π interactions between its furo-chromen ring and nucleobases DG14 and DG8, but, as shown in Supplementary Figure S7E, these events caused the alteration and destabilization of the G-tetrad formed by nucleobases DG2, DG8, DG14, and DG20. Moreover, the ammonium group of the ligand was involved in two H-bonds with nucleobase DG8. Finally, the most populated structure of MDs for *hit* **17** exhibited two salt bridges between its ammonium group and the DG21 and DG22 nucleobases, an H-bond between the amide group and the DT17 and four π–π interactions with DG16 and DG10 (Supplementary Figure S7F). As noted for *hit* **15**, in this case the ligand also appeared able to induce the alteration and destabilization of the interacting G-tetrad.

2.2. In Vitro Analysis

Hits **7**, **15**, and **17** were tested for their ability to stabilize the target Tel and TERRA G4s by means of circular dichroism (CD) melting experiments. This technique is used to obtain information about the G4 topology and stability (melting temperature, T_m) of the G4 structured oligonucleotides. Tel G4 displayed the well-known hybrid 3 + 1 topology and a T_m of 67.2 ± 0.2 °C: when incubated with *hit* **7**, we observed a topological change with the appearance of a peak around 260 nm that could be ascribed to the contribution of the parallel structure, and stabilization by 5.8 °C. No significant topological changes and stabilization were observed when the target Tel G4 was incubated with *hits* **15** and **17** (Figures 3 and S8).

TERRA G4 showed a prevalently parallel topology, with a maximum peak of around 260 nm and a shoulder of around 300 nm, and T_m of 75.2 ± 0.7 °C. Incubation with *hits* **7**, **15**, and **17** did not alter its topology but led to great stabilization of the structure, with *hit* **7** being the best stabilizer (ΔT_m 11.2 °C), followed by *hit* **15** (ΔT_m 9.5 °C) and *hit* **17** (ΔT_m 7.7 °C) (Figures 4 and S9). These in vitro data are in perfect agreement with our MD simulations.

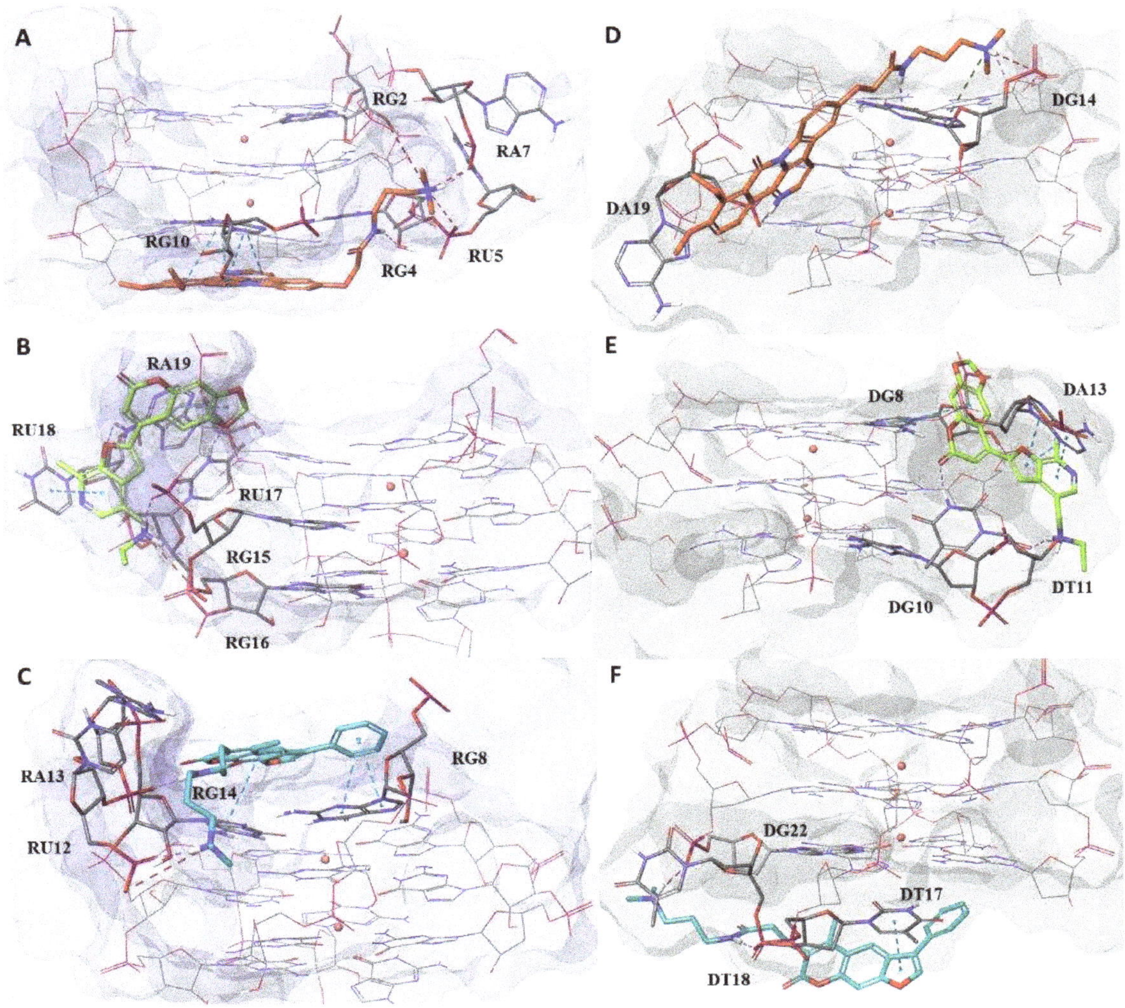

Figure 2. A docking pose analysis of the best thermodynamic complexes of *hits* **7** (panels (**A**,**D**)), **15** (panels (**B**,**E**)), and **17** (panels(**C**,**F**)) in complex with TERRA and Tel, respectively. For *hits* **7**, **15**, and **17**, the ligand is depicted as orange, green, and cyan carbon sticks, respectively. The nucleic acids are shown as faded blue and grey surfaces for TERRA and Tel, respectively, while the guanine residues, forming the G-tetrads, are shown as lines. Moreover, the residues interacting with the ligands are depicted as faded blue and grey carbon sticks for TERRA and Tel, respectively. K^+ ions are represented as pink spheres. Hydrogen bonds, salt bridges, and π–π and π–cation interactions are shown as dashed violet, red, cyan, and green lines, respectively.

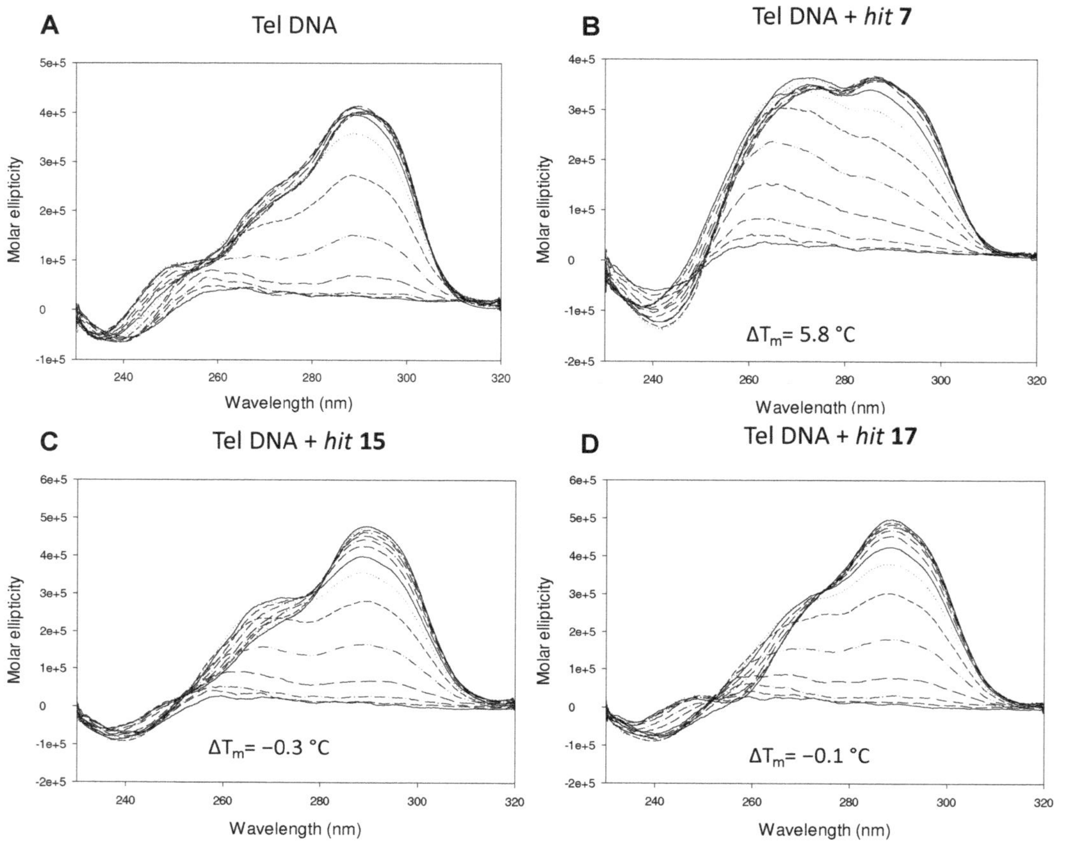

Figure 3. The CD thermal unfolding spectra of the nucleic acid Tel G4 4 µM in 100 mM K^+ alone (**A**) and in the presence of the *hit* **7** 16 µM (**B**), *hit* **15** 16 µM (**C**), and *hit* **17** 16 µM (**D**).

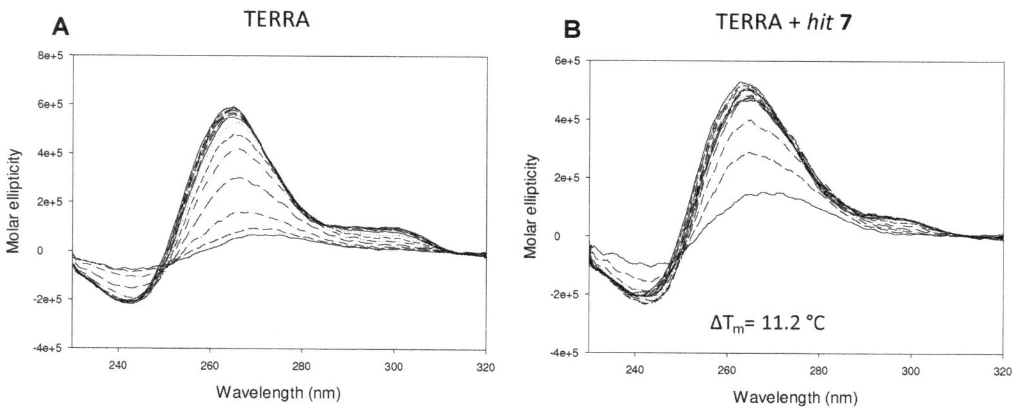

Figure 4. *Cont.*

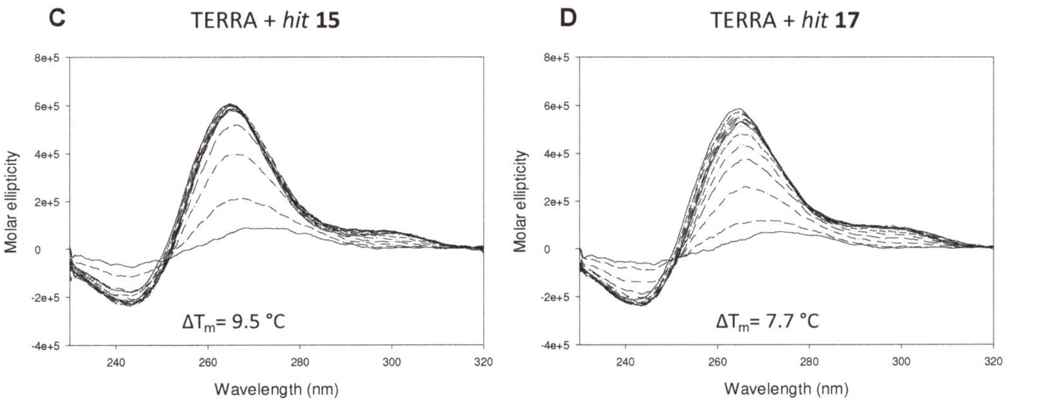

Figure 4. The CD thermal unfolding spectra of the nucleic acid TERRA G4 4 μM in 100 mM K^+ alone (**A**) and in the presence of *hit* **7** 16 μM (**B**), *hit* **15** 16 μM (**C**), and *hit* **17** 16 μM (**D**).

To measure the binding affinity of the hits to the G4-folded oligonucleotides with unmodified 5′- and 3′-ends (i.e., lacking fluorophores or biotin), we employed ESI-MS analysis, as previously described [40,41]. All *hits* displayed both a 1:1 and 1:2 binding ratio, albeit adducts with 2 bound *hit* molecules were 2–3 times less abundant than those with 1 bound *hit* molecule. For each *hit*, the binding affinity (K_D) of the 1:1 complex with Tel and TERRA G4s was measured at three compound concentrations, corresponding to 1:1, 1:2, and 1:4 G4:compound ratios. K_D values were 3.4 ± 0.2 μM, 7.1 ± 1.2 μM, and 6.1 ± 0.2 μM for binding of *hits* **7**, **15,** and **17**, respectively, to TERRA G4 (Figures 5 and S11). Binding affinity to Tel G4 was in general lower, with K_D values of 11.0 ± 0.7 μM, 18.0 ± 4.2 μM, and 22.9 ± 6.4 μM for binding of *hits* **7**, **15,** and **17**, respectively (Figure S10).

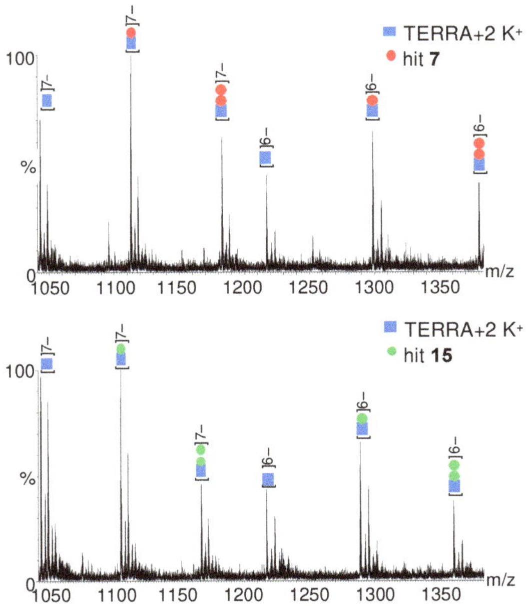

Figure 5. *Cont.*

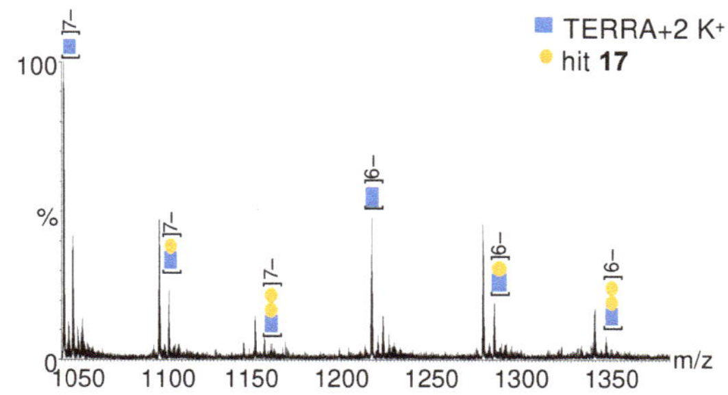

Figure 5. The MS spectra of TERRA (blue squares) incubated with the indicated *hits*. Samples containing TERRA oligonucleotide (5 μM) and *hit* molecule (10 μM) were incubated in MS buffer (HFIP 120 mM/TEA pH 7.4, KCl 0.8 mM, isopropanol 20%) overnight before MS analysis. A zoom on the most significant m/z range is shown. The larger m/z range is provided in Figure S11.

2.3. In Cell Assays

The cytotoxic activity of the tested compounds was evaluated on a panel of cultured human tumor cell lines: MCF7 (mammary gland adenocarcinoma), HT-29 (colorectal adenocarcinoma), and A549 (lung adenocarcinoma) cells. After 48 h treatment with the compounds, cytotoxicity was assessed by the MTT test and indicated as the concentration able to kill 50% of the cell population (CC_{50}). As reported in Table 1, the colorectal adenocarcinoma HT-29 cell line was the most sensitive to compound treatment, with CC_{50} in the low micromolar range for *hits* **7** and **17** and in the nanomolar range for *hit* **15**. A549 cells had intermediate sensitivity to the *hits*, while MCF7 cells were the least affected by compounds' treatment. In these cells, it was not possible to obtain a discrete CC_{50} value for of *hit* **7** as it exceeded the compound limit of solubility. *Hit* **15** was the most effective compound against HT-29 and A549 cells.

Table 1. Cytotoxicity CC_{50} (μM) in human tumor cell lines measured 48 h post administration of *hits* **7**, **15**, and **17**.

	MCF7	HT-29	A549
hit **7**	>50	1.9 ± 0.2	20.3 ± 0.4
hit **15**	62.0 ± 4.1	0.3 ± 0.1	1.1 ± 0.2
hit **17**	28.9 ± 2.0	1.0 ± 0.1	7.9 ± 0.3

The sensitivity of a particular cell line to a given compound is influenced not only by the intrinsic nature of the drug but also by the characteristics of cancer, including mutations, gene expression, and copy number variation. Thus, the different response of the three cell lines observed in this study is probably due to that distinct oncogenic drivers and drug resistance mechanisms that operate in each cell line and create perturbations of the downstream pathways triggered by the compounds.

3. Materials and Methods

3.1. Target Preparation for In Silico Analysis

The crystal structure with PDB code 1KF1 and 2.1 Å resolution was selected as a tridimensional model of the parallel stranded Tel G4, featured by the 22-nt human telomeric sequence *d*[$AG_3(T_2AG_3)_3$] [7]. The same structure was used as a template to generate TERRA homology modeling by adding hydroxyl groups to the sugar ring. The TERRA G4 is known to be characterized by a monomorphic nature since only the parallel topology was experimentally observed [36]. K^+ ions, coordinating the G-tetrad O6 atoms and vertically aligned in the internal G-delimited channel, were retained at their respective crystallographic positions, while all the crystallized water molecules were removed. Both

Tel and TERRA structures were submitted to MD simulations, using GROMACS code ver. 4.5.1 [42]. Both nucleic acids were treated with standard *parm99* Amber force field with modified parmbsc0 [43,44] and combined with corrections ε/ζOL1 and χOL4, to improve the description of ε/ζ and χ G4 torsions, respectively [45–47]. For each system, the tleap module of the AmberTools program was employed to generate a topology file, which was converted into a suitable GROMACS file format using the Acpype script [48]. A truncated dodecahedron box with the TIP3P water solvent model [49] was built using periodic boundary conditions, and the global negative charge was neutralized by adding K^+ counter-ions. To resolve bad steric contacts, both systems were energy-minimized, using 5000 steps with the steepest descent algorithm; equilibrated at 300 K through 5 ns MD under NVT conditions; and then equilibrated in the isothermal–isobaric (NPT) ensemble at 1 atm. An MD production run (200 ns) was performed in NPT, using a time step of 2 fs. The V-rescale algorithm [50] and Parrinello–Rahman barostat [51] were used to control and monitor temperature and pressure, respectively. Finally, for both targets, all conformations found during MD runs were submitted to cluster analysis with the GROMOS algorithm [52], by the g-cluster tool implemented in the GROMACS package [42]. A cut-off of 2.5 Å was used in the cluster process, with the aim to select different representative structures for the two G4 targets.

3.2. Molecular Docking Protocol

The most representative structures of the two G4 targets, obtained during MD runs, were used to generate grids by applying default parameters. Each energy grid was built centering the docking box on the G-tetrads centroid and setting its outer box size to 48 × 48 × 48 Å. For each docking run, 10 poses per ligand were generated and the scaling factor for the target Van der Waals radii was set to 1.0. We used the Standard Precision (SP) scoring function of Glide ver. 7.8 software of the Schrödinger suite [53] to perform docking calculations of the most promising compounds found in our previous screening on the bimolecular target [35]. The molecular structures of *hits* **7**, **15**, and **17** were previously built using the Maestro graphical user interface (*Schrödinger Release 2019: Maestro, Schrödinger, LLC., New York, NY, 2019*) [54], while their most probable protonation state at physiological pH 7.4 was computed using LigPrep (LigPrep version 2.5, *Schrödinger, LLC., New York, NY, 2012*) tool [55]. All complexes generated with the docking procedure were further submitted to the Molecular Mechanics Generalized Born/Surface Area (MM-GBSA) method [56], applying molecular mechanics and continuum solvation models, to compute their binding free energies (ΔG_{bind}) [57]. The docking pose of each compound with the best ΔG_{bind} was selected and further analyzed.

3.3. Molecular Dynamics of the Thermodynamically Best Complexes

For each compound, the best thermodynamics complex was submitted to MD simulations, using the same MD protocol applied for both targets. To consider a comparable starting point, also the TERRA and Tel clusters that provided the best complex thermodynamics were submitted to MDs to investigate the stabilizing power of each compound. For each ligand, we calculated the electrostatic potential (ESP) by Jaguar ver. 9.3 software [58], using the 6-31G* basis set at the Hartree–Fock theory level. The restrained electrostatic potential (RESP) [59] was computed using Antechamber [60] and parameterized with General Amber Force Field (GAFF) [61]. Finally, all conformations found during MD runs were submitted to cluster analysis with the GROMOS algorithm [52], by the g-cluster tool implemented in the GROMACS package [42]. MD frames were aligned on the nucleic acid targets, and RMSd values were computed on the heavy atoms of both the target and ligand. In this case, 1.5 Å cut-off was used in the cluster process to select different representative structures of the complex for all ligands.

3.4. Circular Dichroism

Circular dichroism spectra were recorded on a Chirascan-Plus (Applied Photophysics, Leatherhead, UK) equipped with a Peltier temperature controller using a quartz cell of 5-mm optical path length and a scanning speed of 50 nm/min, with a response time of 4 sec over a wavelength range of 230–320 nm. The reported spectrum of each sample represents the average of 2 scans. Observed ellipticities were converted to the mean residue ellipticity (θ) = deg × cm^2 × $dmol^{-1}$ (molar ellipticity). Oligonucleotides were diluted from stock to the final concentration (4 μM) in the Li cacodylate buffer (10 mM, pH 7.4) with 100 mM KCl, annealed by heating at 95 °C for 5 min, and gradually cooled to room temperature. Compounds were added at 4 × G4 final concentration (16 μM). CD spectra were recorded after 24 h from 20 °C to 95 °C, with a temperature increase of 5 °C. T_m values were calculated according to the van't Hoff equation, applied for a two-state transition from a folded to an unfolded state, assuming that the heat capacity of the folded and unfolded states are equal [62].

3.5. Binding Affinity

To determine the K_D of *hit* ligands to Tel and TERRA G4s, mass spectrometry (MS) analysis was performed on mixtures of oligonucleotide (5 μM) + *hit* compound (5, 10, and 20 μM). A mixture of 2 μM reference dT6 + 5 μM oligonucleotide + 5 or 10 μM *hits* was also used to check for unspecific *hit* binding. Oligonucleotides were heat denatured on MS buffer (HFIP 120 mM/TEA pH 7.4, KCl 0.8 mM, isopropanol 20%) for 5 min at 95 °C and gradually cooled to room temperature to allow the correct folding. After 4 h, *hits* were added, and samples were incubated over night at room temperature. Samples were analyzed by direct infusion electrospray ionization (ESI)-MS on a Xevo G2-XS QTOF mass spectrometer (Waters, Manchester, UK). This is a high-resolution instrument that allowed us to visualize the isotopic pattern, identify the charge state, and therefore unambiguously calculate the neutral mass of the detected species. The injection was automatically performed by an Agilent 1290 Infinity HPLC (Agilent Technologies, Santa Clara, CA, USA) equipped with an autosampler; the carrying buffer was HFIP 120 mM/TEA pH 7.4 with 20% isopropanol. A volume of 5 μL of each sample was typically injected. In all experiments, ESI source settings were electrospray capillary voltage, 1.8 kV; source and desolvation temperatures, 45 °C and 65 °C, respectively; and sampling cone voltage, 65 V. All these parameters ensured minimal DNA complex fragmentation. The instrument was calibrated using a 2 mg/mL solution of sodium iodide in 50% isopropanol. The additional use of the LockSpray during analysis provided typical <5 ppm mass accuracy. The internal standard LockSpray consisted of a solution of leu-enkephalin (1 μg/mL) in acetonitrile/water (50:50, *v*/*v*) containing 0.1% formic acid. Peak areas were used to calculate the concentration ratios, as previously reported [40,41], using the formulas:

$$[\text{oligo}]_{\text{free}} = C_0 \times A(\text{oligo})^{n-} / (A(\text{oligo})^{n-} + A(\text{oligo} + hit)^{n-})$$

$$[\text{oligo} + hit] = C_0 \times A(\text{oligo} + hit)^{n-} / (A(\text{oligo})^{n-} + A(\text{oligo} + hit)^{n-})$$

$$[hit]_{\text{free}} = [hit]_{\text{tot}} - [\text{oligo} + hit]$$

$$K_d = [hit]_{\text{free}} \times [\text{oligo}]_{\text{free}} / [\text{oligo} + hit]$$

where $[\text{oligo}]_{\text{free}}$ and $[hit]_{\text{free}}$ are the concentrations of the unbound oligonucleotide and *hit*, respectively; $[hit]_{\text{tot}}$ is the total concentration of *hit*; [oligo + *hit*] is the concentration of *hit* bound to oligonucleotide; C_0 is the starting oligo (Tel or TERRA G4) concentration; $A(\text{oligo})^{n-}$ is the peak area of the oligonucleotide alone at charge state n^-; and $A(\text{oligo} + hit)^{n-}$ is the peak area of *hit* bound to oligo at charge state n^-. Peak areas were calculated using MassLynx 4.1 software (Waters), after processing steps consisting of smoothing, background subtraction, and conversion to centroid.

3.6. Compounds' Cytotoxicity

Cytotoxic effects were determined by MTT assay. Compounds were dissolved and diluted into working concentrations with DMSO. All cell lines were obtained from ATCC (MCF7, human breast adenocarcinoma, cat. # HTB-22, HT-29, human colorectal adenocarcinoma, cat # HTB-38, A549, human lung carcinoma, cat # CCL-185), grown and maintained according to the manufacturer's instructions (https://www.lgcstandards-atcc.org (accessed on 8 June 2020)). Cells were plated into 96-microwell plates to a final volume of 100 μL and allowed to attach overnight. The following day, the tested compounds were added to each well with a 0.5% final concentration of DMSO per well; each concentration was tested in triplicate. Compounds were incubated for 48 h, and control cells (without any compound but with 0.5% DMSO) were treated in the exact same conditions. Cell survival was evaluated by MTT assay: 10 μL of freshly dissolved solution of MTT (5 mg/mL in PBS) was added to each well, and after 4 h of incubation, MTT crystals were solubilized in solubilization solution (10% sodium dodecyl sulphate (SDS) and 0.01 M HCl). After overnight incubation at 37 °C, absorbance was read at 540 nm. Data were expressed as mean values of at least three experiments conducted in triplicate. The percentage of cell survival was calculated as follows: cell survival = $(A_{well} - A_{blank})/(A_{control} - A_{blank}) \times 100$, where blank denotes the medium without cells. Each experiment was repeated at least three times.

4. Conclusions

In this study, three compounds (*hit* **7**, *hit* **15**, and *hit* **17**), previously identified by means of a virtual screening campaign on bimolecular DNA/RNA G4s, were investigated on the monomolecular Tel DNA and TERRA G4s. Molecular docking calculations indicated all ligands were able to better recognize TERRA with respect to Tel. As previously observed on the bimolecular Tel_2/$TERRA_2$ G4s, *hit* **7** maintained its behavior as a dual Tel/TERRA ligand. Conversely, *hit* **15** and *hit* **17**, previously characterized as selective Tel_2 ligands [35], showed better theoretical affinity towards the monomolecular TERRA G4. Moreover, MDs results highlighted that all the analyzed *hits* better stabilized TERRA G4 folding if compared to Tel, while the naphthyridine *hit* **7** confirmed its dual profile. The in vitro data corroborated our MDs since the relative *hit* stabilization efficiency on TERRA and Tel corresponded to that calculated by MDs. Analysis in cells showed that these compounds have anticancer activity. *Hit* **15**, i.e., the compound that displayed the highest selective stabilization towards TERRA, was the most active compound. Our data indicate that the tested *hits* have enhanced activity towards HT-29 cell, a model line for colorectal adenocarcinoma [63]. In particular, *hit* **15**, being over 200 times more efficient on HT-29 cell that MCF7 cells, could be a promising compound to be further optimized against colorectal cancer.

Supplementary Materials: The following supporting information can be downloaded at: https://www.mdpi.com/article/10.3390/ph15050548/s1, Figure S1: the plot of the RMSd values calculated on all heavy atoms during 200 ns of MDs, performed on both the parallel telomeric (Tel) DNA (black line) and TERRA (red line) G-quadruplex (G4) structures; Figure S2: the RMSd matrices calculated on the heavy atoms of all the saved structures throughout all the MDs of the parallel telomeric Tel (A) and TERRA (B) G4 structures; Figure S3: the 3D structure of all the most representative conformations of (A) TERRA and (B) Tel G4. All clusters have been superimposed, while the single cluster and the most interesting residues are shown as surface and carbon sticks, respectively. Cluster 1, cluster 2, cluster 3, and cluster 4 are reported as red, faded-blue, green, and faded-plum surface, respectively; Figure S4: a pie chart showing the distribution of all the generated docking poses of hits 7, 15, and 17, obtained against all clusters, by considering the site analysis towards both TERRA and Tel G4 targets; Figure S5: an analysis of the binding modes of hits 7, 15, and 17 on each single cluster of both G4 targets, according to the geometrical descriptors reported in a previous work [38]; Figure S6: a plot of the RMSd values calculated on all heavy atoms during 200 ns of MDs, performed on the best thermodynamic complexes of the three hits with both Tel and TERRA G4 and on the related cluster structures of both receptors. (A) An RMSd plot of TERRA cluster 2 (red line) and its related complex with hit 7 (orange line). (B) An RMSd plot of TERRA cluster 3 (red line) and its related complexes with hit 15 and hit 17 (green and cyan lines, respectively). (C) An RMSd plot of Tel cluster 4 (black line) and its related complexes with hit 7 and hit 17 (orange and cyan lines, respectively). (D) An RMSd plot of Tel cluster 1 (black line) and its related complex with hit 15 (green line); Figure S7: a binding pose analysis of the MD-generated, most populated structure of hit 7 (panels (A,D)), hit 15 (panels (B,E)), and hit 17 (panels (C,F)) in complex with TERRA and Tel, respectively. Hit 7, hit 15, and hit 17 are depicted as orange, green, and cyan carbon sticks, respectively. The nucleic acids are shown as faded blue and grey surface for TERRA and Tel, respectively, while the guanine residues, forming the G-tetrads, are shown as lines. Moreover, the residues interacting with the ligands are depicted as faded blue and grey carbon sticks for TERRA and Tel, respectively. K+ ions are represented as pink spheres. Hydrogen bonds, salt bridges, and π–π and π–cation interactions are shown as dashed violet, red, cyan, and green lines, respectively; Figure S8: the CD thermal unfolding analysis of Tel DNA G4 in complex with hits 7, 15, and 17. The melting curves of Tel G4 (4 μM) in the absence and presence of each hit (16 μM), plotted at the wavelength corresponding to the maximum CD signal; Figure S9: the CD thermal unfolding analysis of TERRA G4 in complex with hits 7, 15, and 17. The melting curves of TERRA G4 (4 μM) in the absence and presence of each hit (16 μM), plotted at the wavelength corresponding to the maximum CD signal; and Figure S10: the MS spectra of Tel (grey squares) incubated with the indicated hits. Samples containing Tel DNA oligonucleotide (5 μM) and hit molecule (10 μM) were incubated in MS buffer (HFIP 120 mM/TEA pH 7.4, KCl 0.8 mM, isopropanol 20%) overnight before MS analysis. The relevant m/z range is shown, Figure S11: the MS spectra of TERRA (blue squares) were incubated with the indicated hits. Samples containing TERRA oligonucleotide (5 μM) and hit molecule (10 μM) were incubated in MS buffer (HFIP 120 mM/TEA pH 7.4, KCl 0.8 mM, isopropanol 20%) overnight before MS analysis. The relevant m/z range is shown; Table S1: ΔGbind and related single contributions of the binding free energy for the best thermodynamic complex of hits 7, 15, and 17 with both Tel and TERRA G4. All thermodynamic values are reported in kcal/mol. In Table S1, we also reported the related cluster for each hit-target most stable complex, Table S2: ΔGbind and related single contributions of the binding free energy of the most populated cluster structure of hits 7, 15, and 17 complexed with both Tel and TERRA G4. All thermodynamic values are reported in kcal/mol.

Author Contributions: Conceptualization, A.A. and R.R.; methodology, G.C.; software, F.O.; validation, R.R., A.M. and R.C.; formal analysis, R.R., F.M. and F.S.; investigation, F.S., G.J., M.T.D.M. and M.N.; resources, S.A., P.T. (Pierosandro Tagliaferri) and P.T. (Pierfrancesco Tassone); data curation, R.R., F.S., and M.N.; writing—original draft preparation, R.R., M.N. and F.M.; writing—review and editing, A.A. and S.N.R.; visualization, all; supervision, S.A., P.T. (Pierosandro Tagliaferri) and P.T. (Pierfrancesco Tassone); project administration, S.A., A.A., P.T. (Pierfrancesco Tassone) and S.N.R.; funding acquisition, S.A., P.T. (Pierfrancesco Tassone) and S.N.R. All authors have read and agreed to the published version of the manuscript.

Funding: This research was funded by the PRIN 2017 research project "Novel anticancer agents endowed with multi-targeting mechanism of action", grant number 201744BN5T to A.M., Italian Association for Cancer Research (AIRC) Investigator Grant "Small molecule-based targeting of lncRNAs 3D structure: a translational platform for treatment of multiple myeloma" Project N. 21588 to R.R. and the Investigator Grant "Characterization and targeting of G-quadruplexes in the MDM2 P2 promoter for the treatment of liposarcomas" Project N. 21850 to S.N.R.

Institutional Review Board Statement: Not applicable.

Informed Consent Statement: Not applicable.

Data Availability Statement: Data is contained in the article and Supplementary Material.

Acknowledgments: The authors acknowledge Mu.Ta.Lig. COST ACTION CA15135.

Conflicts of Interest: The authors declare no conflict of interest.

References

1. Gordon, K.E.; Parkinson, E.K. Analysis of telomerase activity and telomere function in cancer. *Methods Mol. Biol.* **2004**, *281*, 333–348. [CrossRef] [PubMed]
2. Parrotta, L.; Ortuso, F.; Moraca, F.; Rocca, R.; Costa, G.; Alcaro, S.; Artese, A. Targeting unimolecular G-quadruplex nucleic acids: A new paradigm for the drug discovery? *Expert Opin. Drug Discov.* **2014**, *9*, 1167–1187. [CrossRef] [PubMed]

3. Dai, J.; Carver, M.; Yang, D. Polymorphism of human telomeric quadruplex structures. *Biochimie* **2008**, *90*, 1172–1183. [CrossRef] [PubMed]
4. Parkinson, G.N.; Lee, M.P.; Neidle, S. Crystal structure of parallel quadruplexes from human telomeric DNA. *Nature* **2002**, *417*, 876–880. [CrossRef] [PubMed]
5. Dai, J.; Punchihewa, C.; Ambrus, A.; Chen, D.; Jones, R.A.; Yang, D. Structure of the intramolecular human telomeric G-quadruplex in potassium solution: A novel adenine triple formation. *Nucleic Acids Res.* **2007**, *35*, 2440–2450. [CrossRef] [PubMed]
6. Dai, J.; Carver, M.; Punchihewa, C.; Jones, R.A.; Yang, D. Structure of the Hybrid-2 type intramolecular human telomeric G-quadruplex in K+ solution: Insights into structure polymorphism of the human telomeric sequence. *Nucleic Acids Res.* **2007**, *35*, 4927–4940. [CrossRef] [PubMed]
7. Wang, Y.; Patel, D.J. Solution structure of the human telomeric repeat d [AG3 (T2AG3) 3] G-tetraplex. *Structure* **1993**, *1*, 263–282. [CrossRef]
8. Campbell, N.H.; Parkinson, G.N.; Reszka, A.P.; Neidle, S. Structural basis of DNA quadruplex recognition by an acridine drug. *J. Am. Chem. Soc.* **2008**, *130*, 6722–6724. [CrossRef]
9. Hounsou, C.; Guittat, L.; Monchaud, D.; Jourdan, M.; Saettel, N.; Mergny, J.L.; Teulade-Fichou, M.P. G-quadruplex recognition by quinacridines: A SAR, NMR, and biological study. *ChemMedChem* **2007**, *2*, 655–666. [CrossRef]
10. Phan, A.T.; Patel, D.J. Two-repeat human telomeric d(TAGGGTTAGGGT) sequence forms interconverting parallel and antiparallel G-quadruplexes in solution: Distinct topologies, thermodynamic properties, and folding/unfolding kinetics. *J. Am. Chem. Soc.* **2003**, *125*, 15021–15027. [CrossRef]
11. Azzalin, C.M.; Reichenbach, P.; Khoriauli, L.; Giulotto, E.; Lingner, J. Telomeric repeat containing RNA and RNA surveillance factors at mammalian chromosome ends. *Science* **2007**, *318*, 798–801. [CrossRef] [PubMed]
12. Feuerhahn, S.; Iglesias, N.; Panza, A.; Porro, A.; Lingner, J. TERRA biogenesis, turnover and implications for function. *FEBS Lett.* **2010**, *584*, 3812–3818. [CrossRef]
13. Porro, A.; Feuerhahn, S.; Delafontaine, J.; Riethman, H.; Rougemont, J.; Lingner, J. Functional characterization of the TERRA transcriptome at damaged telomeres. *Nat. Commun.* **2014**, *5*, 5379. [CrossRef] [PubMed]
14. Xu, Y.; Kaminaga, K.; Komiyama, M. G-quadruplex formation by human telomeric repeats-containing RNA in Na+ solution. *J. Am. Chem. Soc.* **2008**, *130*, 11179–11184. [CrossRef] [PubMed]
15. Deng, Z.; Norseen, J.; Wiedmer, A.; Riethman, H.; Lieberman, P.M. TERRA RNA binding to TRF2 facilitates heterochromatin formation and ORC recruitment at telomeres. *Mol. Cell* **2009**, *35*, 403–413. [CrossRef]
16. Biffi, G.; Tannahill, D.; Balasubramanian, S. An intramolecular G-quadruplex structure is required for binding of telomeric repeat-containing RNA to the telomeric protein TRF2. *J. Am. Chem. Soc.* **2012**, *134*, 11974–11976. [CrossRef] [PubMed]
17. Baker, A.M.; Fu, Q.; Hayward, W.; Victoria, S.; Pedroso, I.M.; Lindsay, S.M.; Fletcher, T.M. The telomere binding protein TRF2 induces chromatin compaction. *PLoS ONE* **2011**, *6*, e19124. [CrossRef] [PubMed]
18. Bae, S.U.; Park, W.J.; Jeong, W.K.; Baek, S.K.; Lee, H.W.; Lee, J.H. Prognostic impact of telomeric repeat-containing RNA expression on long-term oncologic outcomes in colorectal cancer. *Medicine* **2019**, *98*, e14932. [CrossRef] [PubMed]
19. Marzano, S.; Pagano, B.; Iaccarino, N.; Di Porzio, A.; De Tito, S.; Vertecchi, E.; Salvati, E.; Randazzo, A.; Amato, J. Targeting of Telomeric Repeat-Containing RNA G-Quadruplexes: From Screening to Biophysical and Biological Characterization of a New Hit Compound. *Int. J. Mol. Sci.* **2021**, *22*, 10315. [CrossRef] [PubMed]
20. Bryan, T.M.; Englezou, A.; Gupta, J.; Bacchetti, S.; Reddel, R.R. Telomere elongation in immortal human cells without detectable telomerase activity. *EMBO J.* **1995**, *14*, 4240–4248. [CrossRef]
21. Collie, G.W.; Haider, S.M.; Neidle, S.; Parkinson, G.N. A crystallographic and modelling study of a human telomeric RNA (TERRA) quadruplex. *Nucleic Acids Res.* **2010**, *38*, 5569–5580. [CrossRef]
22. Lim, K.W.; Amrane, S.; Bouaziz, S.; Xu, W.; Mu, Y.; Patel, D.J.; Luu, K.N.; Phan, A.T. Structure of the human telomere in K+ solution: A stable basket-type G-quadruplex with only two G-tetrad layers. *J. Am. Chem. Soc.* **2009**, *131*, 4301–4309. [CrossRef]
23. Phan, A.T.; Kuryavyi, V.; Luu, K.N.; Patel, D.J. Structure of two intramolecular G-quadruplexes formed by natural human telomere sequences in K+ solution. *Nucleic Acids Res.* **2007**, *35*, 6517–6525. [CrossRef]
24. Martadinata, H.; Phan, A.T. Structure of human telomeric RNA (TERRA): Stacking of two G-quadruplex blocks in K(+) solution. *Biochemistry* **2013**, *52*, 2176–2183. [CrossRef] [PubMed]
25. Yan, Y.; Tan, J.; Ou, T.; Huang, Z.; Gu, L. DNA G-quadruplex binders: A patent review. *Expert Opin. Ther. Pat.* **2013**, *23*, 1495–1509. [CrossRef] [PubMed]
26. Rocca, R.; Moraca, F.; Costa, G.; Alcaro, S.; Distinto, S.; Maccioni, E.; Ortuso, F.; Artese, A.; Parrotta, L. Structure-based virtual screening of novel natural alkaloid derivatives as potential binders of h-telo and c-myc DNA G-quadruplex conformations. *Molecules* **2014**, *20*, 206–223. [CrossRef] [PubMed]
27. Rocca, R.; Costa, G.; Artese, A.; Parrotta, L.; Ortuso, F.; Maccioni, E.; Pinato, O.; Greco, M.L.; Sissi, C.; Alcaro, S. Hit Identification of a Novel Dual Binder for h-telo/c-myc G-Quadruplex by a Combination of Pharmacophore Structure-Based Virtual Screening and Docking Refinement. *ChemMedChem* **2016**, *11*, 1721–1733. [CrossRef] [PubMed]
28. Alcaro, S.; Musetti, C.; Distinto, S.; Casatti, M.; Zagotto, G.; Artese, A.; Parrotta, L.; Moraca, F.; Costa, G.; Ortuso, F.; et al. Identification and characterization of new DNA G-quadruplex binders selected by a combination of ligand and structure-based virtual screening approaches. *J. Med. Chem.* **2013**, *56*, 843–855. [CrossRef]

29. Costa, G.; Rocca, R.; Moraca, F.; Talarico, C.; Romeo, I.; Ortuso, F.; Alcaro, S.; Artese, A. A Comparative Docking Strategy to Identify Polyphenolic Derivatives as Promising Antineoplastic Binders of G-quadruplex DNA c-myc and bcl-2 Sequences. *Mol. Inf.* **2016**, *35*, 391–402. [CrossRef] [PubMed]
30. Catalano, R.; Moraca, F.; Amato, J.; Cristofari, C.; Rigo, R.; Via, L.D.; Rocca, R.; Lupia, A.; Maruca, A.; Costa, G.; et al. Targeting multiple G-quadruplex-forming DNA sequences: Design, biophysical and biological evaluations of indolo-naphthyridine scaffold derivatives. *Eur. J. Med. Chem.* **2019**, *182*, 111627. [CrossRef] [PubMed]
31. Collie, G.; Reszka, A.P.; Haider, S.M.; Gabelica, V.; Parkinson, G.N.; Neidle, S. Selectivity in small molecule binding to human telomeric RNA and DNA quadruplexes. *Chem. Commun.* **2009**, 7482–7484. [CrossRef] [PubMed]
32. Xu, Y.; Komiyama, M. Structure, function and targeting of human telomere RNA. *Methods* **2012**, *57*, 100–105. [CrossRef] [PubMed]
33. Di Antonio, M.; Biffi, G.; Mariani, A.; Raiber, E.A.; Rodriguez, R.; Balasubramanian, S. Selective RNA versus DNA G-quadruplex targeting by in situ click chemistry. *Angew. Chem. Int. Ed. Engl.* **2012**, *51*, 11073–11078. [CrossRef] [PubMed]
34. Rocca, R.; Talarico, C.; Moraca, F.; Costa, G.; Romeo, I.; Ortuso, F.; Alcaro, S.; Artese, A. Molecular recognition of a carboxy pyridostatin toward G-quadruplex structures: Why does it prefer RNA? *Chem. Biol. Drug Des.* **2017**, *90*, 919–925. [CrossRef] [PubMed]
35. Rocca, R.; Moraca, F.; Costa, G.; Nadai, M.; Scalabrin, M.; Talarico, C.; Distinto, S.; Maccioni, E.; Ortuso, F.; Artese, A.; et al. Identification of G-quadruplex DNA/RNA binders: Structure-based virtual screening and biophysical characterization. *Biochim. Biophys. Acta Gen. Subj.* **2017**, *1861*, 1329–1340. [CrossRef]
36. Xu, Y. Chemistry in human telomere biology: Structure, function and targeting of telomere DNA/RNA. *Chem. Soc. Rev.* **2011**, *40*, 2719–2740. [CrossRef]
37. Xu, Y.; Ishizuka, T.; Kimura, T.; Komiyama, M. A U-tetrad stabilizes human telomeric RNA G-quadruplex structure. *J. Am. Chem. Soc.* **2010**, *132*, 7231–7233. [CrossRef] [PubMed]
38. Alcaro, S.; Costa, G.; Distinto, S.; Moraca, F.; Ortuso, F.; Parrotta, L.; Artese, A. The polymorphisms of DNA G-quadruplex investigated by docking experiments with telomestatin enantiomers. *Curr. Pharm. Des.* **2012**, *18*, 1873–1879. [CrossRef]
39. Li, J.; Abel, R.; Zhu, K.; Cao, Y.; Zhao, S.; Friesner, R.A. The VSGB 2.0 model: A next generation energy model for high resolution protein structure modeling. *Proteins* **2011**, *79*, 2794–2812. [CrossRef] [PubMed]
40. Lombardo, C.M.; Sánchez Martínez, I.; Haider, S.; Gabelica, V.; De Pauw, E.; Moses, J.E.; Neidle, S. Structure-based design of selective high-affinity telomeric quadruplex-binding ligands. *Chem. Commun.* **2010**, *46*, 9116–9118. [CrossRef]
41. Scalabrin, M.; Nadai, M.; Tassinari, M.; Lago, S.; Doria, F.; Frasson, I.; Freccero, M.; Richter, S.N. Selective Recognition of a Single HIV-1 G-Quadruplex by Ultrafast Small-Molecule Screening. *Anal. Chem.* **2021**, *93*, 15243–15252. [CrossRef]
42. Hess, B.; Kutzner, C.; van der Spoel, D.; Lindahl, E. GROMACS 4: Algorithms for Highly Efficient, Load-Balanced, and Scalable Molecular Simulation. *J. Chem. Theory Comput.* **2008**, *4*, 435–447. [CrossRef]
43. Weiner, S.J.; Kollman, P.A.; Case, D.A.; Singh, U.C.; Ghio, C.; Alagona, G.; Profeta, S.; Weiner, P. A new force field for molecular mechanical simulation of nucleic acids and proteins. *J. Am. Chem. Soc.* **1984**, *106*, 765–784.
44. Cheatham, T.E.; Cieplak, P.; Kollman, P.A. A modified version of the Cornell et al. force field with improved sugar pucker phases and helical repeat. *J. Biomol. Struct. Dyn.* **1999**, *16*, 845–862. [CrossRef]
45. Pérez, A.; Marchán, I.; Svozil, D.; Sponer, J.; Cheatham, T.E.; Laughton, C.A.; Orozco, M. Refinement of the AMBER force field for nucleic acids: Improving the description of alpha/gamma conformers. *Biophys. J.* **2007**, *92*, 3817–3829. [CrossRef]
46. Zgarbová, M.; Luque, F.J.; Sponer, J.; Cheatham, T.E.; Otyepka, M.; Jurečka, P. Toward Improved Description of DNA Backbone: Revisiting Epsilon and Zeta Torsion Force Field Parameters. *J. Chem. Theory Comput.* **2013**, *9*, 2339–2354. [CrossRef]
47. Krepl, M.; Zgarbová, M.; Stadlbauer, P.; Otyepka, M.; Banáš, P.; Koča, J.; Cheatham, T.E.; Jurečka, P.; Sponer, J. Reference simulations of noncanonical nucleic acids with different χ variants of the AMBER force field: Quadruplex DNA, quadruplex RNA and Z-DNA. *J. Chem. Theory Comput.* **2012**, *8*, 2506–2520. [CrossRef]
48. Sousa da Silva, A.W.; Vranken, W.F. ACPYPE—AnteChamber PYthon Parser interfacE. *BMC Res. Notes* **2012**, *5*, 367. [CrossRef]
49. Jorgensen, W.L.; Madura, J.D. Quantum and statistical mechanical studies of liquids. 25. Solvation and conformation of methanol in water. *J. Am. Chem. Soc.* **1983**, *105*, 1407–1413.
50. Bussi, G.; Donadio, D.; Parrinello, M. Canonical sampling through velocity rescaling. *J. Chem. Phys.* **2007**, *126*, 014101. [CrossRef]
51. Parrinello, M.; Rahman, A. Polymorphic transitions in single crystals: A new molecular dynamics method. *J. Appl. Phys.* **1981**, *52*, 7182–7190.
52. Daura, X.; Gademann, K.; Jaun, B.; Seebach, D.; Van Gunsteren, W.F.; Mark, A.E. Peptide folding: When simulation meets experiment. *Angew. Chem. Int. Ed.* **1999**, *38*, 236–240.
53. Schrödinger. *Glide*; Schrödinger, LLC.: New York, NY, USA, 2018.
54. Schrödinger. *Maestro*; Schrödinger, LLC.: New York, NY, USA, 2019.
55. Schrödinger. *LigPrep*; Schrödinger, LLC.: New York, NY, USA, 2018.
56. Kollman, P.A.; Massova, I.; Reyes, C.; Kuhn, B.; Huo, S.; Chong, L.; Lee, M.; Lee, T.; Duan, Y.; Wang, W.; et al. Calculating Structures and Free Energies of Complex Molecules: Combining Molecular Mechanics and Continuum Models. *Acc. Chem. Res.* **2000**, *33*, 889–897. [CrossRef]
57. *Prime*; Schrodinger, LLC.: New York, NY, USA, 2018.

58. Bochevarov, A.D.; Harder, E.; Hughes, T.F.; Greenwood, J.R.; Braden, D.A.; Philipp, D.M.; Rinaldo, D.; Halls, M.D.; Zhang, J.; Friesner, R.A. Jaguar: A high-performance quantum chemistry software program with strengths in life and materials sciences. *Int. J. Quantum Chem.* **2013**, *113*, 2110–2142. [CrossRef]
59. Cornell, W.D.; Cieplak, P.; Bayly, C.I.; Kollman, P.A. Application of RESP charges to calculate conformational energies, hydrogen bond energies, and free energies of solvation. *J. Am. Chem. Soc.* **2002**, *115*, 9620–9631. [CrossRef]
60. Wang, J.; Wang, W.; Kollman, P.A.; Case, D.A. Automatic atom type and bond type perception in molecular mechanical calculations. *J. Mol. Graph. Model.* **2006**, *25*, 247–260. [CrossRef]
61. Wang, J.; Wolf, R.M.; Caldwell, J.W.; Kollman, P.A.; Case, D.A. Development and testing of a general amber force field. *J. Comput. Chem.* **2004**, *25*, 1157–1174. [CrossRef]
62. Greenfield, N.J. Using circular dichroism collected as a function of temperature to determine the thermodynamics of protein unfolding and binding interactions. *Nat. Protoc.* **2006**, *1*, 2527–2535. [CrossRef]
63. Fogh, J.; Trempe, G. New human tumor cell lines. In *Human Tumor Cells in Vitro*; Springer: Boston, MA, USA, 1975; pp. 115–159.

pharmaceuticals

MDPI

Article

Improved Database Filtering Technology Enables More Efficient Ab Initio Design of Potent Peptides against Ebola Viruses

Thomas Ripperda †, Yangsheng Yu †, Atul Verma, Elizabeth Klug, Michellie Thurman, St Patrick Reid * and Guangshun Wang *

Department of Pathology and Microbiology, College of Medicine, University of Nebraska Medical Center, 985900 Nebraska Medical Center, Omaha, NE 68198-5900, USA; ripperdatj@gmail.com (T.R.); yangshengyu@unmc.edu (Y.Y.); atul.k.verma@hotmail.com (A.V.); liz.klug@unmc.edu (E.K.); michelliethurman19@gmail.com (M.T.)

* Correspondence: patrick.reid@unmc.edu (S.P.R.); gwang@unmc.edu (G.W.); Tel.: +1-(402)-559-3644 (S.P.R.); +1-(402)-559-4176 (G.W.)

† These authors contributed equally to this work.

Abstract: The rapid mutations of viruses such as SARS-CoV-2 require vaccine updates and the development of novel antiviral drugs. This article presents an improved database filtering technology for a more effective design of novel antiviral agents. Different from the previous approach, where the most probable parameters were obtained stepwise from the antimicrobial peptide database, we found it possible to accelerate the design process by deriving multiple parameters in a single step during the peptide amino acid analysis. The resulting peptide DFTavP1 displays the ability to inhibit Ebola virus. A deviation from the most probable peptide parameters reduces antiviral activity. The designed peptides appear to block viral entry. In addition, the amino acid signature provides a clue to peptide engineering to gain cell selectivity. Like human cathelicidin LL-37, our engineered peptide DDIP1 inhibits both Ebola and SARS-CoV-2 viruses. These peptides, with broad antiviral activity, may selectively disrupt viral envelopes and offer the lasting efficacy required to treat various RNA viruses, including their emerging mutants.

Keywords: antimicrobial peptide database; antiviral peptides; database filtering technology; SARS-CoV-2; Ebola virus; peptide design

Citation: Ripperda, T.; Yu, Y.; Verma, A.; Klug, E.; Thurman, M.; Reid, S.P.; Wang, G. Improved Database Filtering Technology Enables More Efficient Ab Initio Design of Potent Peptides against Ebola Viruses. *Pharmaceuticals* **2022**, *15*, 521. https://doi.org/10.3390/ph15050521

Academic Editor: Osvaldo Andrade Santos-Filho

Received: 29 March 2022
Accepted: 22 April 2022
Published: 24 April 2022

1. Introduction

Emerging viral infections can cause harm to our society. This was made crystal clear in the previous Spanish flu and the current severe acute respiratory syndrome coronavirus 2 (SARS-CoV-2) pandemic. According to the World Health Organization, COVID-19 has caused 464 million infections and 6.06 million cumulative deaths globally as of March 21, 2022 [1]. SARS-CoV-2 has also added a burden to our economic, educational, and health care systems around the world. Similarly, Ebola viruses have a major impact on our society, causing a significant number of mortalities. Ebola viruses are highly lethal and have an average mortality rate of 50% [2,3]. Fortunately, vaccines have proven to be effective to protect humans from SARS-CoV-2 and Ebola virus (EBOV) infections [4–6]. However, viruses mutate rapidly and have evolved into numerous mutants that could compromise vaccine protection and cause breakthrough coronavirus infections [7]. Hence, there is a need to develop alternatives such as antiviral drugs to better manage viral infections.

Antimicrobial peptides (AMPs) are an important factor of the innate immune defense for both invertebrates and vertebrates, including humans [8–14]. Recently, human defensins have been shown to inhibit SARS-CoV-2 infection [15]. Likewise, human cathelicidin LL-37, another key AMP, also demonstrated antiviral activity against SARS-CoV-2 [16]. These antiviral peptides can work through different mechanisms, ranging from immune regulation to direct inactivation via membrane disruption [17–20]. Hence, natural AMPs may be engineered into new therapeutics to help control these viruses [11,12,21–23]. As a proof of concept, we previously demonstrated that LL-37 could be engineered to inhibit Ebola virus entry [24].

As an alternative approach, we found it useful to discover novel antimicrobials based on the antimicrobial peptide database (APD) [25]. This was made possible due to our systematic classification of AMPs based on the sequence length, net charge, hydrophobic ratio, post-translational modification, structure, activity, and source organism. In the APD, most of the AMPs had a peptide length of less than 60 amino acids. The net charge of a peptide was calculated at pH 7 and chemical modification was considered. The majority of the peptides in the APD have a net charge in the range of +1 to +7. The hydrophobic amino acids were defined based on the Kyte–Doolittle hydrophobic scale [26], where residues of leucine (L), isoleucine (I), valine (V), alanine (A), methionine (M), cysteine (C), and phenylalanine (F) are hydrophobic. In addition, the APD included tryptophan (W) in the hydrophobic group. The hydrophobic ratio of a peptide was calculated based on the sum of all the hydrophobic amino acids mentioned above divided by the peptide length. The dominant hydrophobic ratios for AMPs are located between 20 and 70%. Peptide structures are separated into four classes based on the presence or absence of the α-helix and β-sheet (i.e., α, β, αβ, and non-αβ). In the current APD, 478 peptides are found to have an α-helical structure based on nuclear magnetic resonance (NMR) spectroscopy and/or circular dichroism (CD). Only 88 peptides are determined to have a β-sheet structure, while 116 entries are known to adopt an αβ fold. Finally, the structures of 22 peptides are found to belong to the non-αβ class (i.e., no α-helix nor β-sheet). Both the peptide sequence and post-translational modification play an important role in determining 3D structure and biological activity (e.g., antibacterial, antiviral, antiparasitic, antifungal, and anticancer) [27].

This study reports the design of novel antiviral peptides by developing an improved version of the database filtering technology [28], making peptide design more efficient. Following up on our initial observation of Ebola virus entry inhibition, we validate the utility of the database filtering approach in designing new antiviral peptides using an Ebola virus pseudo-type system. In addition, we also evaluate the antiviral effects of DDIP1, a database-designed inhibitory peptide 1 [27], using both Ebola virus and SARS-CoV-2.

2. Results and Discussion

2.1. Peptide Design via an Improved Database Filtering Technology

The APD, originally established in 2003, was expanded and described in 2009 and 2016 [25,27]. To learn the wisdom of nature, the APD currently focuses on natural peptides with determined antimicrobial activity, known amino acid sequences, and less than 100 amino acids, leading to a widely used core data set. Our careful annotation of peptide activity data (e.g., antibacterial, antiviral, antifungal, antiparasitic, spermicidal, and anticancer) laid a solid foundation for designing peptides with the desired activity. In addition, peptide properties, such as the length, net charge, hydrophobicity, and structure, can be searched for in a systematic manner. Each parameter can be arrayed to identify the optimum. These database features enabled the development of database technology for peptide design. The database filtering technology (DFT) is one such approach that designs new peptides based on the most probable parameters within a set of peptides with common activity [28]. The DFT is an ab initio approach to designing peptides because, unlike de novo approaches, it makes no prior assumptions. The first proposed version of the DFT designed a peptide with activity against methicillin-resistant *Staphylococcus aureus* (MRSA), but did not inhibit Gram-negative bacteria. To design antiviral peptides, the first database filter selected all 190 antiviral peptides in the database (Summer 2021) as templates. These peptides were analyzed to determine the AMP length with the highest abundance. The search was conducted in 10 amino acid increments. The 21–30 residue range had the highest peptide count (Figure 1). This range would be the most probable length for our peptide design. Considering the cost of making longer peptides, however, we selected a peptide length of 20, which was closest to the lower optimal boundary. We then derived the rest of the peptide parameters based on the antiviral peptides with 11–20 amino acids. To study the impact of the AMP length on antiviral activity, we also designed two shorter peptides with 12 and 16 amino acids. In the original DFT design method, a series of filtering steps were involved in deriving numerous parameters. For example, three separate filters were used to determine the frequency of amino acids, net charge, and the hydrophobicity of the anti-MRSA peptide. Here, we found it possible to derive these three parameters in one step by analyzing the amino acid frequency plot for the 11–20-peptide length group. In this plot (Figure 2A), the 20 standard amino acids were separated into four groups based on their common features: (1) hydrophobic (I, V, L, F, C, M, A, and W), (2) special glycine/proline (G and P), (3) polar and hydrophilic (T, S, Y, Q, and N), and (4) charged (E, D, H, K, and R) [25]. We then selected the most abundant amino acid in each group as a representative. In this manner, 20 amino acids were reduced to four for our peptide design (solid columns in Figure 2A, top panel). In this plot, the four representative amino acids were leucine (L), glycine (G), serine (S), and arginine (R). Interestingly, we were not alone in utilizing this reductionist approach, since nature also uses a small set of amino acids to design peptides such as θ-defensins. While the hydrophobic group contained I, V, F, L, and C, the other three groups consisted of a single amino acid (glycine, threonine, and arginine, respectively) (Figure 2B) [29]. This plot indicated that other amino acids in the special GP, polar, and charged groups were not preferred in the known θ-defensins. Next, in our improved design, the amino acid percentages within each amino acid group were summed (Figure 2A bottom panel) to represent the percentage for each of the four selected amino acids (L, G, S, or R) in the designed peptides. To design a 20-mer peptide, we calculated the numbers of the four amino acids L, G, S, and R for this peptide by multiplying the percentage for each amino acid with the targeted peptide length. Thus, this procedure enabled us to determine the types and contents of the four representative amino acids (including hydrophobic and cationic) in one step, increasing the efficiency of this ab initio method. Next, the most probable structure of the peptide was determined to be α-helical, because this structure had the highest occurrence in the 11–20 residue range (Figure 3). This allowed us to place charged and hydrophobic amino acids in a classic amphipathic pattern, where every two leucines were dispersed with two hydrophilic amino acids. To determine the potential combinations of these amino acids in the sequence, a statistical analysis was performed on the possible sequence motifs (four amino acids) that could be formed. The motifs with the highest abundance in the database were selected to connect the leucine pairs. The amino acid sequence of the first peptide (DFTavP1) designed to inhibit viral replication is given in Table 1. For antiviral assays, we utilized a pseudotyped Ebola virus as described previously [24]. In this study, the designed peptides displayed different degrees of inhibitory effects on pseudo-EBOV VSV-eGP (vesicular stomatitis virus-Ebola glycoprotein) infection. DFTavP1, the 20mer, showed an 18% higher inhibition than LL-37 at 2.5 μM (Figure 4). Also, the inhibition increased as the peptide dosage increased.

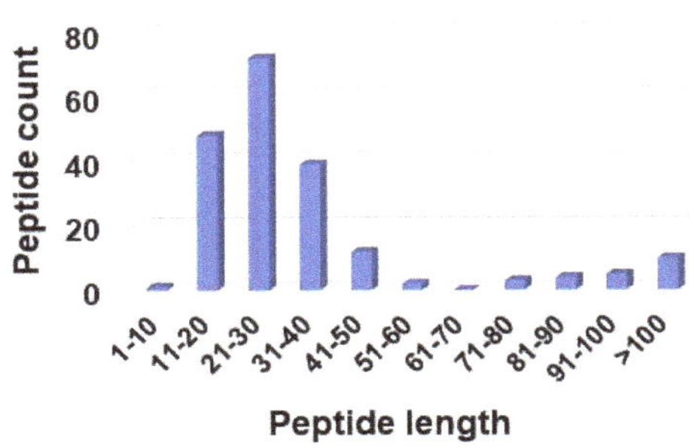

Figure 1. Antiviral peptide count in the antimicrobial peptide database at various peptide length ranges [25]. Peptides in the range of 21–30 amino acids were dominant. This length range would be

the most probable length based on our previous design idea [28]. To reduce peptide cost, we selected a peptide length of 20 in this study and two even shorter peptides were also designed based on the peptide parameters with 11–20 amino acids.

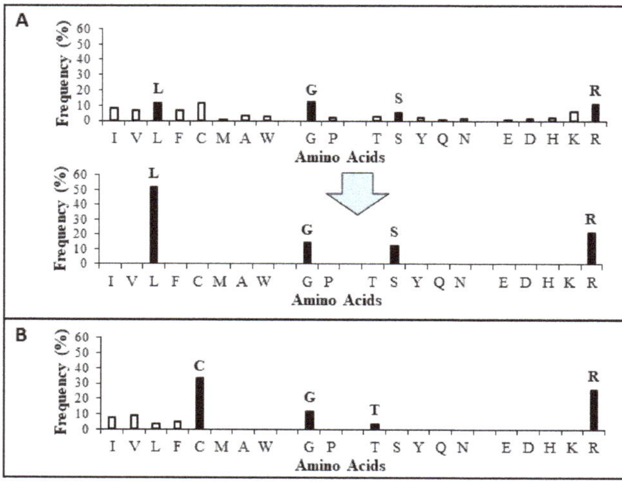

Figure 2. A single-step amino acid analysis of antiviral peptides with 11–20 amino acids to derive multiple most probable parameters for peptide design. (**A**) Four frequent amino acids (L, G, S, and R, solid column) were identified from the four groups of amino acids. The percentages of amino acids for each group were then merged into L, G, S, and R. (**B**) The amino acid analysis of 19 θ-defensins registered in the APD. It is remarkable that in nature, θ-defensins are designed in a similar way by mainly using C, G, T, and R dotted with a few other hydrophobic amino acids.

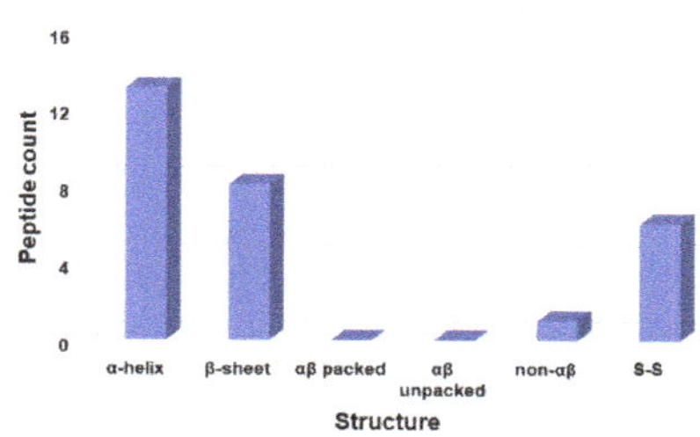

Figure 3. Count of antiviral peptides with different structures. Data were obtained from the antimicrobial peptide database [25] for antiviral peptides with 11–20 amino acids. Antiviral peptides with an α-helical structure were dominant with 13 counts. In addition, there were eight antiviral peptides in the selected length group with β-sheet structures. No antiviral peptides in this length group had a determined αβ structure (packed or unpacked). Only one antiviral peptide in this group had a non-αβ structure. In addition, six antiviral peptides in this group were disulfide-linked (S-S), although their 3D structures are unknown. Note that a similar plot was obtained for antiviral peptides with 21–30 amino acids (not shown). Therefore, α-helical structure was decided as the most probable structure for this design.

Table 1. Database-designed antiviral peptides and their properties.

Peptide	Amino Acid Sequence [a]	Length	Net Charge	Pho [b]	Boman Index [c]	GRAVY
DFTavP1	RWLRGLLSGLLRRLLSGLLL	20	+5	55	0.6	0.815
DFTavP2	RWLRGLLSGLLRRLLS	16	+5	50	1.73	0.331
DFTavP3	RWLRGLLSGLLR	12	+4	50	1.61	0.25
DFTavP4	RWVRGVVSGVVRRVVS	16	+5	50	2.12	0.506
DDIP1 [d]	GLRCRLGRLLRRLGRCLLR	19	+7	47	3.4	−0.0579

[a] All the peptides were C-terminally amidated except for DDIP1. A tryptophan was introduced into the DFT peptides to facilitate peptide quantification (see Methods section). [b] Hydrophobic content. [c] Boman index (originally called protein binding potential in kcal/mol) [8] was renamed by the APD in 2003 [25]. [d] All were D-amino acids. In addition, a disulfide bond exists between the two cysteines C4 and C16 of DDIP1.

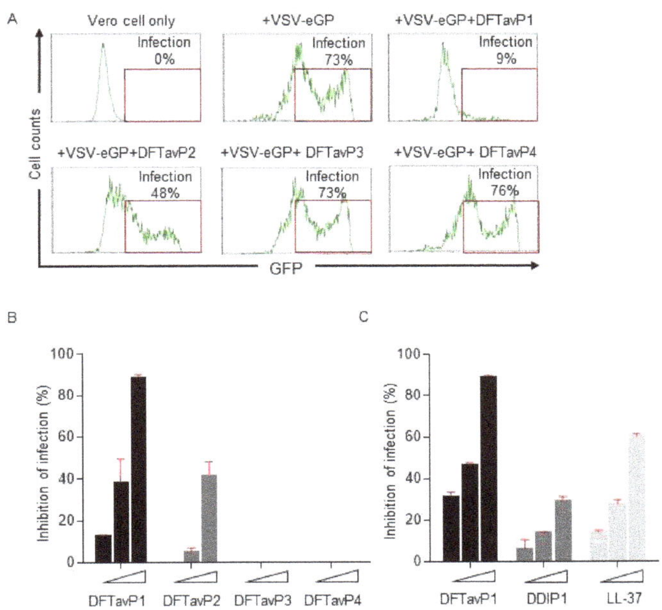

Figure 4. Designed AMPs inhibited the infection of pseudo-EBOV virion in Vero cells. (**A**) AMPs inhibited pseudo-EBOV (VSV-eGP) infection in Vero cells. Vero cells were pretreated with individual AMPs at 10 μM for 2 h before VSV-eGP viruses were added. After 24 h of culture, Vero cells were harvested for flow cytometry analysis to measure viral infection. Percentages of GFP-positive cells represent percentages of cells infected with VSV-eGP. (**B**) DFTavP1 and its derivatives inhibited pseudo-EBOV (VSV-eGP) infection in Vero cells in a dose-dependent manner. Since AMPs usually inhibit microbes at micromolar, Vero cells were pretreated with individual AMPs (at 2.5, 5, or 10 μM) for 2 h before VSV-eGP viruses were added. After 24 h of culture, Vero cells were harvested for flow cytometry analysis to measure viral infection. (**C**) DFTavP1, DDIP1, and LL37 inhibited pseudo-EBOV (VSV-eGP) infection in Vero cells in a dose-dependent manner. Vero cells were pretreated with individual AMPs (at 2.5, 5, or 10 μM) for 2 h before VSV-eGP viruses were added. After 24 h of culture, Vero cells were harvested for flow cytometry analysis to measure viral infection.

2.2. Validation of the Most Probable Parameters

Next, we validated the improved methodology by designing additional peptides with parameters deviated from the optima. A 16 mer (DFTavP2) was designed in the same manner as DFTavP1 (sequence in Table 1). This peptide length decrease caused a 33% decrease in the viral inhibition of DFTavP2 at 5 μM compared to DFTavP1. A further deviation from the most probable length led to DFTavP3 (a 12 mer in Table 1), which did not inhibit the VSV–eGP (Figure 4B). Hence, the peptide close to the most probable peptide length range was more potent than the sequence-shortened counterparts.

To further validate the most probable amino acids, leucine in DFTavP2 was converted to valine, leading to DFTavP4 (sequence in Table 1). The flow cytometry results suggested that DFTavP4 entirely lost the ability to inhibit the Ebola pseudo-virus (Figure 4B). This observation indicated the significance of the most probable hydrophobic leucine in conferring antiviral activity to the peptide. The reason for this might be twofold. First, leucine is more hydrophobic than valine, enabling a better binding to viruses. Second, leucine has a higher potential than valine in forming the helical structure required for target binding [25]. To fully validate this, leucine may be converted to other hydrophobic amino acids (I, F, A, M, C, and W) as well. A previous study revealed the peptide became less soluble when substituted by isoleucine [28]. Thus, we did not make the same change. As alanine is even less hydrophobic than valine, we predicted that alanine substitution would also lead to an inactive peptide. We did not test methionine, since this residue is not favorable for peptide design due to its readiness of being oxidized. While phenylalanine and tryptophan substitutions may be of interest for future studies, we included one, W, here for UV quantification. In a different design below, two leucines were transformed to cysteines.

Additional proof of the most probable principle in peptide design came from our previous database-guided design. The GLK-19 peptide (a 19-residue peptide containing G, L, and K) designed based on the frequently occurring amino acids from amphibian peptides [25] became active to human immunodeficiency virus type 1 (HIV-1) when all lysines were replaced with arginines. These changes were determined based on the arginine/lysine ratios in antibacterial, antifungal, antiviral, and anticancer peptides in the APD, where only in the antiviral peptides was the arginine/lysine ratio greater than one [30]. Since cysteine is also abundant in the hydrophobic group of the antiviral peptide amino acid signature (e.g., see Figure 2A), we changed two leucines in GLR-19 to two cysteines at positions 4 and 16. These changes led to DDIP1 with a disulfide bond. For this study, we created a new version of DDIP1, where all L-amino acids were converted to D-amino acids to gain stability to proteases. Our previous study suggested the importance of peptide stability for inhibiting Ebola viruses [24]. In the inhibition experiment, DDIP1 displayed 7% inhibition at 2.5 μM and 14% inhibition at 5 μM against the virus. Human LL-37, a known antiviral peptide [16,24,30], showed a higher viral inhibition than DDIP1 (Figure 4C).

2.3. *Antiviral Efficacy of Peptides Treated before or after Viral Infection*

We then compared the treatment efficacy of DDIP1 and DFTavP1 postinfection. Human LL-37 was included as a positive control. At 0, 2, and 4 h postinfection, a dose-responsive viral inhibition was observed for all the peptides, indicating the effect results from the peptide treatment (Figure 5A). When treated immediately after infection (delay 0 h), DDIP1, DFTavP1, and LL-37 displayed ~15%, 69%, and 9% inhibitions at 2.5 μM, respectively. Hence, DDIP1 and DFTavP1 demonstrated a higher inhibition than LL-37. DFTavP1, in the 4 h postinfection treatment study, showed a major decrease of 54% inhibition at 5 μM. The inhibition of the Ebola pseudovirus was reduced with a longer delay after infection for both DDIP1 and DFTavP1, implying an action on viral entry. The decrease in inhibition was caused by the decrease in viral load in the extracellular fluid because the intracellular viral load was increasing. Interestingly, the effect of human LL-37 was relatively constant. More experiments are required to determine the precise mechanism of DFTavP1 or DDIP1.

We also tested the antiviral activity of DDIP1 against SARS-CoV-2. Like LL-37, DDIP1 showed an inhibitory effect on SARS-CoV-2 in a dose-dependent manner (Figure 5B). At 5 μM, LL-37 inhibited 18% of the virus, while DDIP1 suppressed 42%. At 10 μM, DDIP1 (~55% inhibition) was more potent than LL-37 (~27% inhibition) as well. These results reinforced the antiviral potency of the database-designed antiviral peptides.

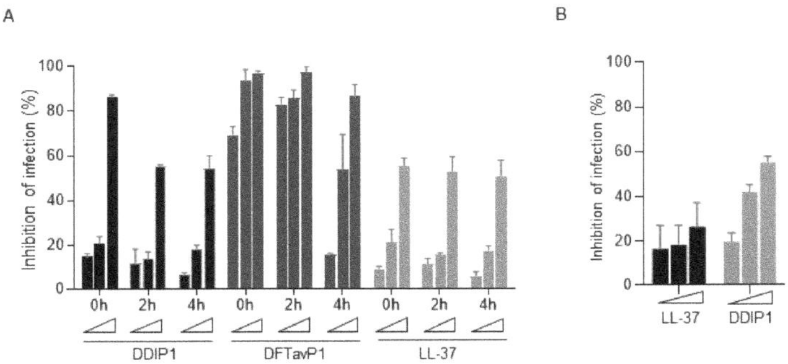

Figure 5. Designed AMPs inhibited EBOV cell entry and SARS-CoV-2 infection. (**A**) AMPs targeted pseudo-EBOV (VSV-eGP) at the early stage of infection. Vero cells were treated with individual AMPs (at 2.5, 5, or 10 μM) at the same time with VSV-eGP (0 h), or at 2 or 4 h after VSV-eGP infection. Vero cells were harvested for flow cytometry analysis of GFP levels at 24 h post infection. (**B**) DDIP1 inhibited SARS-CoV-2 infection. Vero cells were pretreated with individual AMPs (at 2.5, 5, or 10 μM) for 2 h before SARS-CoV-2 viruses were added. After 24 h of culture, Vero cells were harvested for immunofluorescence staining to access infection activity.

2.4. Different Requirements for Antiviral and Antibacterial Properties

As our antiviral peptides were designed based on the antimicrobial peptide database [25], one may wonder whether they are active against bacteria. To obtain a more complete picture, we used two Gram-positive and four Gram-negative bacterial strains and the minimum inhibitory concentrations (MIC) of the peptides are provided in Table 2. In contrast to the antiviral case, DFTavP1 was less active against bacteria than the two shortened peptides DFTavP2 and DFTavP3 (low MIC values). Interestingly, DDIP1 displayed excellent MIC values against all the tested antibiotic-resistant pathogens (e.g., MRSA, *Escherichia coli*, *Pseudomonas aeruginosa*, and *Klebsiella pneumoniae*) in the range of 2–8 μM, comparable to the two shorter DFT peptides (Table 2). These results unveiled different parameter requirements for designing antibacterial and antiviral peptides. We speculate that such a difference primarily resulted from the potential differences in pathogenic targets. It is likely that our designed peptides (e.g., DDIP1) targeted the viral envelope since many AMPs act on bacterial membranes [8–10]. Another in silico study screened antiviral peptides by docking known antiviral peptides to the major protease (M^{Pro}) of SARS-CoV-2 without experimental validation [31]. Future studies on both viruses and bacteria could validate such mechanisms of action. Our speculation was supported by our previous knowledge on human cathelicidin LL-37 peptides (e.g., GF-17 and GI-20), which inhibit both bacteria and viruses [32]. However, the peptide lost its antiviral effects when the helical structure was disrupted by partially incorporating D-amino acids. In terms of the mechanism, the helical structure of LL-37 peptides was not a must for targeting bacterial membranes, but essential to inhibit HIV-1 reverse transcriptase [33]. In the case of Ebola viruses, only the engineered peptides such as 17BIPHE2 were effective at the endosomal cell entry step by impairing the cathepsin-B-mediated processing of the Ebola viral glycoprotein [34].

Table 2. Minimum inhibitory concentration (μM) of database-designed antiviral peptides.

Peptide	*S. aureus* USA300	*Staphylococcus epidermidis* 1457	*Escherichia coli* E416-7	*Pseudomonas aeruginosa* #2	*Klebsiella pneumoniae* E406-17	*Acinetobacter baumannii* B28-16
DFTavP1	8–16	8–16	16	32	16–32	8
DFTavP2	4	2	4	8	4	2
DFTavP3	4	8	2–4	4–8	8	4
DFTavP4	>64	NA	16	NA	NA	NA
DDIP1	4	4–8	2	4	4	2–4

2.5. Cytotoxicity of Antiviral Peptides

For therapeutic use, it is important that the designed peptides had minimal toxic effects on mammalian cells. To evaluate the cytotoxicity of the new peptides, we utilized several cell lines. Vero cells are a model cell for viral infection, derived from the kidney epithelia of the African green monkey. It appeared that Vero cells were highly sensitive to DFTavP1 (TC_{50} 2.4 μM), but became less sensitive to DDIP1 (TC_{50} 13.0 μM in Table 3). Because SARS-CoV-2 infects lung cells, we also tested their cytotoxicity to Calu3 cells. Both DFTavP1 and DDIP1 showed a TC_{50} in the range of 12–14 μM, comparable to the human host defense cathelicidin peptide LL-37 (TC_{50} 19.1 μM). These results indicated a direct antiviral effect of our peptides at a low peptide concentration (e.g., 2.5 μM), where its secondary toxic effect on host cells might play a role. The toxic effect of the designed peptides depended on cell types. The 50% hemolytic concentration (HC_{50}) for DDIP1 was greater than 160 μM, the highest concentration we tested (Table 3). However, both DFTavP1 and DFTavP2 were highly hemolytic, with an HC_{50} below 12.5 μM, while DFTavP3, the shortest 12-mer peptide, had an HC_{50} of 50 μM. Likewise, DDIP1 was poorly hemolytic to murine red blood cells as well (HC_{50} > 160 μM), while DFTavP1 was highly hemolytic (Table 3). In the case of skin HaCaT cells, the HC_{50} was 25 μM for DFTavP1, but greater than 100 μM for DDIP1. These results confirmed the toxicity of DFT peptides. However, the engineered peptide DDIP1 was much more selective and showed cell-dependent toxicity (Table 3).

Table 3. Cytotoxicity comparison of antiviral peptides to different cells.

Peptide	hRBC HC_{50} [a]	mRBC HC_{50} [b]	HaCaT TC_{50} [c]	Vero Cell TC_{50}	Calu3 Cell TC_{50}
DFTavP1	<12.5 μM	<10 μM	25 μM	2.39	11.88
DDIP1	>160 μM	>160 μM	>100 μM	13	14.25

[a] hRBC, human red blood cells; [b] mRBC, BALB/c mouse red blood cells; [c] TC_{50}, the peptide concentration that killed 50% of human keratinocytes.

3. Materials and Methods

3.1. The Antimicrobial Peptide Database

The APD was originally established in 2003. Since then, it has been updated regularly and expanded substantially [25,27]. For scientific rigor, the APD applied a set of criteria for peptide registration (natural peptides, known sequences, known activity, and a size of less than 100 amino acids). Thus, this database currently focuses on natural peptides from six life kingdoms, including bacteria, archaea, protists, fungi, plants, and animals [25]. After over 18 years, 26 types of peptide activities (e.g., antibacterial, antiviral, antifungal, antiparasitic, spermicidal, and anticancer) have been annotated. Such a well-annotated peptide sequence–activity database provides a unique platform for peptide prediction and design. The APD enables a thorough statistical analysis of natural AMPs through a variety of search functions and database filters. Such an analysis identifies key parameters for peptide design [27].

3.2. Database Filtering Technology (DFT) vs. Improved DFT

The rigorous registration of the data in the APD set the stage for us to develop database-guided approaches for peptide discovery, ranging from database screening to database filtering technology [27]. The original database filtering technology [28] consisted of multiple database filters that allowed us to derive a family of peptides with desired biological activity, followed by deriving key peptide parameters step by step. In the original DFT, the first filter selected a set of peptides with activity against Gram-positive bacteria, whereas the improved DFT used here selected a group of peptides annotated with antiviral activity. The second filter is common and was used to identify the most probable peptide length. This was achieved by statistically analyzing the peptides in the APD in bins (every 10 s), so that the peptide length with the highest count was found. Subsequently, the original DFT identified the most probable amino acid frequency, net charge, and hydrophobic amino acid in three steps. In contrast, the improved DFT derived frequency, net charge, and hydrophobic content in one step. The rest of the steps in identifying the most probable structure and motifs are shared by both methods and were detailed elsewhere [28].

3.3. Chemicals and Peptides

All the chemicals were purchased from established vendors such as Fisher and Sigma. Peptides were created by Genemed Synthesis, Inc. (San Antonio, TX, USA). All the peptides were highly purified and reached over 95% purity based on HPLC. The correct mass of each peptide was validated by mass spectrometry (Shimadzu MALDI-8020, Kyoto, Japan or Thermo Fisher Scientific SALDI-TOF-MS, Waltham, MA, USA). The incorporation of a tryptophan (W) for each peptide at position 2 (in replacement of a leucine in Table 1) facilitated peptide quantification on a UV spectrometer (Ultraspec 1100 pro, Amersham Biosciences) at 280 nm.

3.4. SARS-CoV-2 Safety Statement

All experiments involving SARS-CoV-2 were conducted in an approved BSL-3 facility of the University of Nebraska Medical Center (UNMC) by dedicated trained personnel.

3.5. Antiviral Assays

Peptide activity against Ebola pseudo-virus was tested using established lab protocols as described [24]. Inhibitory effects on SARS-CoV-2 were tested as below. Live virus experiments were performed in the BSL3 laboratory at the UNMC (Omaha, NE, USA). Briefly, Vero cells (~10,000 cells/well) were seeded in a 96-well plate and cultured in complete medium overnight. In the prevention experiments, cells were pretreated with compounds for 2 h at 37 °C. Treatments were washed off and cells were infected with SARS-CoV-2 WI at a multiplicity of infection (MOI) of 0.1 in complete media. After 24 h, cells were fixed with 4% buffered paraformaldehyde for 30 min at room temperature. The fixed cells were washed with phosphate-buffered saline (PBS), permeabilized with 0.1% (v/v) Triton X-100 solution for 10 min, then blocked with 3% bovine serum albumin–PBS solution. The cells were incubated with anti-SARS-CoV-2 spike protein rabbit monoclonal antibody (Sino Biological, Beijing, China) at 1:1000 overnight at 4 °C, followed by incubation with 1:2000 diluted Alexa Fluor 488 conjugated secondary antibody (Jackson ImmunoResearch) for 1 h at room temperature. Cell nuclei were counterstained using Hoechst 33,342 (Invitrogen, #H3570), and cytoplasmic membranes were stained with CellMask (Invitrogen, #C10046). Noninfected cells and untreated virus-infected cells were included as internal controls. Cells were imaged using a high-content analysis system, Operetta CLS (PerkinElmer Inc., Waltham, MA, USA). Percentage inhibition of viral infection was calculated using Harmony 4.9 software (PerkinElmer Inc.).

3.6. Antibacterial Assays

Peptide activity against bacteria was tested using established lab protocols as described previously [28]. In brief, a peptide concentration gradient with two-fold dilution was created in the 96-well polystyrene microplates at 10 μL per well. From overnight cultures, six bacteria (Table 2) were grown to the logarithmic phase (i.e., optical density at 600 nm $\approx$ 0.5), diluted to ~10^5 CFU/mL, and partitioned into the 96-well microplates at 90 μL per well. The microplates were incubated at 37 °C overnight and read on a ChroMate 4300 Microplate Reader at 600 nm (GMI, Ramsey, MN, USA).

3.7. Cytotoxicity

Peptide toxicity was evaluated by using human red blood cells (hRBCs) and other host cells. Hemolysis was conducted as described elsewhere [28]. Briefly, hRBCs, obtained from the UNMC Blood Bank, were washed three times with phosphate-buffered saline (PBS) and diluted to a 2% solution (v/v). After peptide treatment, incubation at 37 °C for one hour, and centrifugation at 13,000 rpm, aliquots of the supernatant were carefully transferred to a fresh 96-well microplate. The amount of hemoglobin released was measured at 545 nm. The percent lysis was calculated by assuming 100% release when human blood cells were treated with 2% Triton X-100, and 0% release when incubated with PBS buffer. The peptide concentration that caused 50% lysis of hRBCs was defined as HC_{50}.

Vero cells (ATCC, CCL-81) or Calu-3 (ATCC, HTB-55) cells were seeded into 96-well tissue culture plates (Greiner Bio-One, Monroe, NC) and treated with different concentrations of peptides for 24/48 h at 37 °C. Cell viability was examined by Vybrant® MTT Cell Proliferation Assay Kit (Thermo Fisher Scientific, Grand Island, NY) following the manufacturer's instructions. Toxicity assays using HaCaT cells were conducted similarly as described elsewhere [34].

4. Conclusions

It is useful to identify antiviral peptides that can eliminate all kinds of SARS-CoV-2 variants: alpha, beta, delta, omicron, etc. Based on the antimicrobial peptide database [25], we previously developed a database filtering technology [28], which was recently proved to be useful for us in the design of anti-MRSA peptides with systemic efficacy in mice [34]. Here, we improved the original stepwise database filtering method by deriving multiple most probable parameters in a single amino acid composition analysis for designing antiviral peptides, thereby accelerating this peptide design process based on the antimicrobial peptide database. Our designed peptides were indeed inhibitory to the Ebola pseudo-virus. In addition, both human cathelicidin LL-37 and DDIP1 could inhibit SARS-CoV-2. The decrease in or loss of activity of peptides created with deviated most probable parameters further validated the improved method. Our study demonstrated that the designed peptides were inhibitory to the Ebola pseudo-virus in either prevention or treatment experiments. The reduced antiviral effect of the designed peptides after additional delay postinfection implied the blockage of viral entry. Our engineered disulfide-containing peptide DDIP1 with numerous desired properties could be further optimized to remove toxicity and developed into a novel treatment for viral infections such as COVID-19. This should require the study of pharmacokinetics and pharmacodynamics of the optimized peptide in animal models. It is predicted that DDIP1 is effective against a variety of mutated viral strains, since it may damage viral envelopes to prevent infection in a similar manner to disrupt bacterial membranes. Our discovery of novel antiviral peptides may be further accelerated by applying the machine learning/artificial intelligence algorithms [35–43] that enable the prediction of both the antiviral activity and toxicity of peptides with the accumulation of experimental data of AMPs.

Author Contributions: G.W. conceived the study; Y.Y., T.R., S.P.R. and G.W. designed the study; T.R., Y.Y., A.V., E.K. and M.T. conducted the experiments; T.R., Y.Y., S.P.R. and G.W. wrote the manuscript. All authors have read and agreed to the published version of the manuscript.

Funding: This study was supported in part by the NIGMS, NIH grant number GM138552 and the state grant to GW.

Institutional Review Board Statement: Not applicable.

Informed Consent Statement: Not applicable.

Data Availability Statement: Publicly available datasets were analyzed in this study. This data can be found here: https://aps.unmc.edu (accessed on 1 June 2021) [44].

Acknowledgments: T.R. is a summer student who gratefully appreciates the support of the Summer Undergraduate Research Fellowship provided by the Department of Pathology and Microbiology, University of Nebraska Medical Center.

Conflicts of Interest: The authors declare no conflict of interest.

References

1. WHO Website. Available online: https://covid19.who.int/ (accessed on 21 March 2022).
2. Da Costa, S.M. The impact of the Ebola crisis on mortality and welfare in Liberia. *Health Econ.* **2020**, *29*, 1517–1532. [CrossRef]
3. Shimizu, K.; Checchi, F.; Warsame, A. Disparities in Health Financing Allocation among Infectious Diseases in Ebola Virus Disease (EVD)-Affected Countries, 2005–2017. *Healthcare* **2022**, *10*, 179. [CrossRef]
4. El-Masry, E.A. Immunization against severe acute respiratory syndrome Coronavirus 2: An overview. *Afr. Health Sci.* **2021**, *21*, 1574–1583. [CrossRef]
5. Diakou, K.I.; Mitsis, T.; Pierouli, K.; Papakonstantinou, E.; Bongcam-Rudloff, E.; Wayengera, M.; Vlachakis, D. Ebola Virus Disease and Current Therapeutic Strategies: A Review. *Adv. Exp. Med. Biol.* **2021**, *1339*, 131–137.
6. Chen, W.H.; Strych, U.; Hotez, P.J.; Bottazzi, M.E. The SARS-CoV-2 Vaccine Pipeline: An Overview. *Curr. Trop. Med. Rep.* **2020**, *7*, 61–64. [CrossRef]
7. Lechmere, T.; Snell, L.B.; Graham, C.; Seow, J.; Shalim, Z.A.; Charalampous, T.; Alcolea-Medina, A.; Batra, R.; Nebbia, G.; Edgeworth, J.D.; et al. Broad Neutralization of SARS-CoV-2 Variants, Including Omicron, following Breakthrough Infection with Delta in COVID-19-Vaccinated Individuals. *Mbio* **2022**, e0379821. [CrossRef]
8. Boman, H.G. Antibacterial peptides: Basic facts and emerging concepts. *J. Intern. Med.* **2003**, *254*, 197–215. [CrossRef]
9. Etayash, H.; Hancock, R.E.W. Host Defense Peptide-Mimicking Polymers and Polymeric-Brush-Tethered Host Defense Peptides: Recent Developments, Limitations, and Potential Success. *Pharmaceutics* **2021**, *13*, 1820. [CrossRef]
10. Bevins, C.L. Innate immune functions of α-defensins in the small intestine. *Dig. Dis.* **2013**, *31*, 299–304. [CrossRef]
11. Mammari, N.; Krier, Y.; Albert, Q.; Devocelle, M.; Varbanov, M. On Behalf of the Oemonom. Plant-Derived Antimicrobial Peptides as Potential Antiviral Agents in Systemic Viral Infections. *Pharmaceuticals* **2021**, *14*, 774. [CrossRef]
12. Brice, D.C.; Diamond, G. Antiviral Activities of Human Host Defense Peptides. *Curr. Med. Chem.* **2020**, *27*, 1420–1443. [CrossRef]
13. Bhopale, G.M. Antimicrobial Peptides: A Promising Avenue for Human Healthcare. *Curr. Pharm. Biotechnol.* **2020**, *21*, 90–96. [CrossRef]
14. Ferrera, L.; Cappiello, F.; Loffredo, M.R.; Puglisi, E.; Casciaro, B.; Botta, B.; Galietta, L.J.V.; Mori, M.; Mangoni, M.L. Esc peptides as novel potentiators of defective cystic fibrosis transmembrane conductance regulator: An unprecedented property of antimicrobial peptides. *Cell. Mol. Life Sci.* **2021**, *79*, 67. [CrossRef]
15. Xu, C.; Wang, A.; Marin, M.; Honnen, W.; Ramasamy, S.; Porter, E.; Subbian, S.; Pinter, A.; Melikyan, G.B.; Lu, W.; et al. Human Defensins Inhibit SARS-CoV-2 Infection by Blocking Viral Entry. *Viruses* **2021**, *13*, 1246. [CrossRef]
16. Wang, C.; Wang, S.; Li, D.; Chen, P.; Han, S.; Zhao, G.; Chen, Y.; Zhao, J.; Xiong, J.; Qiu, J.; et al. Human Cathelicidin Inhibits SARS-CoV-2 Infection: Killing Two Birds with One Stone. *ACS Infect. Dis.* **2021**, *7*, 1545–1554. [CrossRef]
17. Solanki, S.S.; Singh, P.; Kashyap, P.; Sansi, M.S.; Ali, S.A. Promising role of defensins peptides as therapeutics to combat against viral infection. *Microb. Pathog.* **2021**, *155*, 104930. [CrossRef]
18. Fu, Y.; Jaarsma, A.H.; Kuipers, O.P. Antiviral activities and applications of ribosomally synthesized and post-translationally modified peptides (RiPPs). *Cell. Mol. Life Sci.* **2021**, *78*, 3921–3940. [CrossRef]
19. Chessa, C.; Bodet, C.; Jousselin, C.; Wehbe, M.; Lévêque, N.; Garcia, M. Antiviral and Immunomodulatory Properties of Antimicrobial Peptides Produced by Human Keratinocytes. *Front. Microbiol.* **2020**, *11*, 1155. [CrossRef]
20. Hartshorn, K.L. Role of surfactant protein A and D (SP-A and SP-D) in human antiviral host defense. *Front. Biosci (Schol. Ed.)* **2010**, *2*, 527–546. [CrossRef]
21. Laneri, S.; Brancaccio, M.; Mennitti, C.; De Biasi, M.G.; Pero, M.E.; Pisanelli, G.; Scudiero, O.; Pero, R. Antimicrobial Peptides and Physical Activity: A Great Hope against COVID 19. *Microorganisms* **2021**, *9*, 1415. [CrossRef]
22. Rani, P.; Kapoor, B.; Gulati, M.; Atanasov, A.G.; Alzahrani, Q.; Gupta, R. Antimicrobial peptides: A plausible approach for COVID-19 treatment. *Expert Opin. Drug Discov.* **2022**, *in press*. [CrossRef]
23. Enayathullah, M.G.; Parekh, Y.; Banu, S.; Ram, S.; Nagaraj, R.; Kumar, B.K.; Idris, M.M. Gramicidin S and melittin: Potential anti-viral therapeutic peptides to treat SARS-CoV-2 infection. *Sci. Rep.* **2022**, *12*, 3446. [CrossRef] [PubMed]
24. Yu, Y.; Cooper, C.L.; Wang, G.; Morwitzer, M.J.; Kota, K.; Tran, J.P.; Bradfute, S.B.; Liu, Y.; Shao, J.; Zhang, A.K.; et al. Engineered Human Cathelicidin Antimicrobial Peptides Inhibit Ebola Virus Infection. *Iscience* **2020**, *23*, 100999. [CrossRef]
25. Wang, G.; Li, X.; Wang, Z. APD2: The updated antimicrobial peptide database and its application in peptide design. *Nucleic Acids Res.* **2009**, *37*, D933-7. [CrossRef]
26. Kyte, J.; Doolittle, R.F. A simple method for displaying the hydropathic character of a protein. *J. Mol. Biol.* **1982**, *157*, 105–132. [CrossRef]
27. Wang, G. Database-Guided Discovery of Potent Peptides to Combat HIV-1 or Superbugs. *Pharmaceuticals* **2013**, *6*, 728–758. [CrossRef]
28. Mishra, B.; Wang, G. *Ab initio* design of potent anti-MRSA peptides based on database filtering technology. *J. Am. Chem. Soc.* **2012**, *134*, 12426–12429. [CrossRef] [PubMed]
29. Tang, Y.Q.; Yuan, J.; Osapay, G.; Osapay, K.; Tran, D.; Miller, C.J.; Ouellette, A.J.; Selsted, M.E. A cyclic antimicrobial peptide produced in primate leukocytes by the ligation of two truncated alpha-defensins. *Science* **1999**, *286*, 498–502. [CrossRef]
30. Wang, G.; Watson, K.M.; Peterkofsky, A.; Buckheit, R.W., Jr. Identification of novel human immunodeficiency virus type 1-inhibitory peptides based on the antimicrobial peptide database. *Antimicrob. Agents Chemother.* **2010**, *54*, 1343–1346. [CrossRef] [PubMed]

31. Mahmud, S.; Paul, G.K.; Biswas, S.; Afrose, S.; Mita, M.A.; Hasan, M.R.; Shimu, M.S.S.; Hossain, A.; Promi, M.M.; Ema, F.K.; et al. Prospective Role of Peptide-Based Antiviral Therapy Against the Main Protease of SARS-CoV-2. *Front. Mol. Biosci.* **2021**, *8*, 628585. [CrossRef]
32. Wang, G.; Watson, K.M.; Buckheit, R.W., Jr. Anti-human immunodeficiency virus type 1 activities of antimicrobial peptides derived from human and bovine cathelicidins. *Antimicrob. Agents Chemother.* **2008**, *52*, 3438–3440. [CrossRef]
33. Wong, J.H.; Legowska, A.; Rolka, K.; Ng, T.B.; Hui, M.; Cho, C.H.; Lam, W.W.; Au, S.W.; Gu, O.W.; Wan, D.C. Effects of cathelicidin and its fragments on three key enzymes of HIV-1. *Peptides* **2011**, *2*, 1117–1122. [CrossRef] [PubMed]
34. Lakshmaiah Narayana, J.; Mishra, B.; Lushnikova, T.; Wu, Q.; Chhonker, Y.S.; Zhang, Y.; Zarena, D.; Salnikov, E.S.; Dang, X.; Wang, F.; et al. Two distinct amphipathic peptide antibiotics with systemic efficacy. *Proc. Natl Acad. Sci. USA* **2020**, *117*, 19446–19454. [CrossRef] [PubMed]
35. Chowdhury, A.S.; Reehl, S.M.; Kehn-Hall, K.; Bishop, B.; Webb-Robertson, B.M. Better understanding and prediction of antiviral peptides through primary and secondary structure feature importance. *Sci. Rep.* **2020**, *10*, 19260. [CrossRef] [PubMed]
36. Li, C.; Sutherland, D.; Hammond, S.A.; Yang, C.; Taho, F.; Bergman, L.; Houston, S.; Warren, R.L.; Wong, T.; Hoang, L.M.N.; et al. AMPlify: Attentive deep learning model for discovery of novel antimicrobial peptides effective against WHO priority pathogens. *BMC Genom.* **2022**, *23*, 77. [CrossRef]
37. Ma, Y.; Guo, Z.; Xia, B.; Zhang, Y.; Liu, X.; Yu, Y.; Tang, N.; Tong, X.; Wang, M.; Ye, X.; et al. Identification of antimicrobial peptides from the human gut microbiome using deep learning. *Nat. Biotechnol.* **2022**. [CrossRef]
38. Wang, G.; Vaisman, I.I.; van Hoek, M.L. Machine Learning Prediction of Antimicrobial Peptides. *Methods Mol Biol.* **2022**, *2405*, 1–37. [PubMed]
39. Khabbaz, H.; Karimi-Jafari, M.H.; Saboury, A.A.; BabaAli, B. Prediction of antimicrobial peptides toxicity based on their physico-chemical properties using machine learning techniques. *BMC Bioinform.* **2021**, *22*, 549. [CrossRef] [PubMed]
40. Yaseen, A.; Gull, S.; Akhtar, N.; Amin, I.; Minhas, F. HemoNet: Predicting hemolytic activity of peptides with integrated feature learning. *J. Bioinform. Comput. Biol.* **2021**, *19*, 2150021. [CrossRef] [PubMed]
41. Timmons, P.B.; Hewage, C.M. HAPPENN is a novel tool for hemolytic activity prediction for therapeutic peptides which employs neural networks. *Sci. Rep.* **2020**, *10*, 10869. [CrossRef]
42. Plisson, F.; Ramírez-Sánchez, O.; Martínez-Hernández, C. Machine learning-guided discovery and design of non-hemolytic peptides. *Sci. Rep.* **2020**, *10*, 16581. [CrossRef] [PubMed]
43. Porto, W.F.; Ferreira, K.C.V.; Ribeiro, S.M.; Franco, O.L. Sense the moment: A highly sensitive antimicrobial activity predictor based on hydrophobic moment. *Biochim. Biophys. Acta Gen. Subj.* **2022**, *1866*, 130070. [CrossRef] [PubMed]
44. The Antimicrobial Peptide Database. Available online: https://aps.unmc.edu (accessed on 1 June 2021).

Pharmaceuticals **2022**, *15*, 501
pharmaceuticals
MDPI

Article

Toward the Identification of Natural Antiviral Drug Candidates against Merkel Cell Polyomavirus: Computational Drug Design Approaches

Amer H. Asseri [1,2,†], Md. Jahidul Alam [3,†], Faisal Alzahrani [1,4,†], Ahmed Khames [5,†], Mohammad Turhan Pathan [6,†], Mohammed A. S. Abourehab [7], Salman Hosawi [1,2], Rubaiat Ahmed [8,†], Sifat Ara Sultana [9], Nazia Fairooz Alam [8], Nafee-Ul Alam [10], Rahat Alam [11,12,†], Abdus Samad [11,12,†], Sushil Pokhrel [13], Jin Kyu Kim [14], Foysal Ahammad [12,15,*], Bonglee Kim [14,*] and Shing Cheng Tan [16,*]

1 Biochemistry Department, Faculty of Science, King Abdul-Aziz University, Jeddah 21589, Saudi Arabia; ahasseri@kau.edu.sa (A.H.A.); faahalzahrani@kau.edu.sa (F.A.); shosawi@kau.edu.sa (S.H.)
2 Centre for Artificial Intelligence in Precision Medicines, King Abdul-Aziz University, Jeddah 21589, Saudi Arabia
3 Department of Applied Chemistry and Chemical Engineering, Noakhali Science and Technology University, Noakhali 3814, Bangladesh; mdjahidulalam.nstu.bd@gmail.com
4 King Fahd Medical Research Center, Embryonic Stem Cells Unit, Department of Biochemistry, Faculty of Science, King Abdul-Aziz University, Jeddah 21589, Saudi Arabia
5 Department of Pharmaceutics and Industrial Pharmacy, College of Pharmacy, Taif University, P.O. Box 11099, Taif 21944, Saudi Arabia; dr.akhamies@gmail.com
6 Department of Biochemistry and Microbiology, North South University, Dhaka 1229, Bangladesh; turhan.pathan@hotmail.com
7 Department of Pharmaceutics, Faculty of Pharmacy, Umm Al-Qura University, Makkah 21955, Saudi Arabia; maabourehab@uqu.edu.sa
8 Department of Biochemistry and Molecular Biology, University of Dhaka, Dhaka 1000, Bangladesh; rubaiat1ahmed@gmail.com (R.A.); nazia.fairooz@gmail.com (N.F.A.)
9 Department of Pharmacy, Faculty of Pharmacy, University of Dhaka, Dhaka 1000, Bangladesh; sifatarasultana@gmail.com
10 Department of Biotechnology, College of Life Science and Medicine, Zhejiang Sci-Tech University, Hangzhou 310018, China; nafee.alam@hotmail.com
11 Department of Genetic Engineering and Biotechnology, Faculty of Biological Science and Technology, Jashore University of Science and Technology, Jashore 7408, Bangladesh; rahatalam1643@gmail.com (R.A.); kazisamad50@gmail.com (A.S.)
12 Laboratory of Computational Biology, Biological Solution Centre (BioSol Centre), Jashore 7408, Bangladesh
13 Department of Biomedical Engineering, State University of New York (SUNY), Binghamton, NY 13902, USA; sushilpokhrel@binghamton.edu
14 College of Korean Medicine, Kyung Hee University, Kyungheedae-ro 26, Dongdaemun-gu, Seoul 05254, Korea; wlsrb7330@khu.ac.kr
15 Department of Biological Sciences, Faculty of Science, King Abdul-Aziz University (KAU), Jeddah 21589, Saudi Arabia
16 UKM Medical Molecular Biology Institute, Universiti Kebangsaan Malaysia, Kuala Lumpur 56000, Malaysia
* Correspondence: foysalgebt@gmail.com (F.A.); bongleekim@khu.ac.kr (B.K.); sctan@ukm.edu.my (S.C.T.)
† These authors contributed equally to this work.

Citation: Asseri, A.H.; Alam, M.J.; Alzahrani, F.; Khames, A.; Pathan, M.T.; Abourehab, M.A.S.; Hosawi, S.; Ahmed, R.; Sultana, S.A.; Alam, N.F.; et al. Toward the Identification of Natural Antiviral Drug Candidates against Merkel Cell Polyomavirus: Computational Drug Design Approaches. *Pharmaceuticals* **2022**, *15*, 501. https://doi.org/10.3390/ph15050501

Academic Editor: Osvaldo Andrade Santos-Filho

Received: 7 March 2022
Accepted: 12 April 2022
Published: 20 April 2022

Abstract: Merkel cell carcinoma (MCC) is a rare form of aggressive skin cancer mainly caused by Merkel cell polyomavirus (MCPyV). Most MCC tumors express MCPyV large T (LT) antigens and play an important role in the growth-promoting activities of oncoproteins. Truncated LT promotes tumorigenicity as well as host cell proliferation by activating the viral replication machinery, and inhibition of this protein in humans drastically lowers cellular growth linked to the corresponding cancer. Our study was designed with the aim of identifying small molecular-like natural antiviral candidates that are able to inhibit the proliferation of malignant tumors, especially those that are aggressive, by blocking the activity of viral LT protein. To identify potential compounds against the target protein, a computational drug design including molecular docking, ADME (absorption, distribution, metabolism, and excretion), toxicity, molecular dynamics (MD) simulation, and molecular mechanics generalized Born surface area (MM-GBSA) approaches were applied in this study.

Initially, a total of 2190 phytochemicals isolated from 104 medicinal plants were screened using the molecular docking simulation method, resulting in the identification of the top five compounds having the highest binding energy, ranging between −6.5 and −7.6 kcal/mol. The effectiveness and safety of the selected compounds were evaluated based on ADME and toxicity features. A 250 ns MD simulation confirmed the stability of the selected compounds bind to the active site (AS) of the target protein. Additionally, MM-GBSA analysis was used to determine the high values of binding free energy (ΔG bind) of the compounds binding to the target protein. The five compounds identified by computational approaches, Paulownin (CID: 3084131), Actaealactone (CID: 11537736), Epigallocatechin 3-O-cinnamate (CID: 21629801), Cirsilineol (CID: 162464), and Lycoricidine (CID: 73065), can be used in therapy as lead compounds to combat MCPyV-related cancer. However, further wet laboratory investigations are required to evaluate the activity of the drugs against the virus.

Keywords: Merkel cell polyomavirus; Merkel cell carcinomas; drug design; molecular docking; ADMET; MD simulation

---

1. Introduction

Human polyomaviruses are a broad community of human pathogens that normally induce asymptomatic infection in healthy people [1]. The polyomavirus family, which includes the Trichodysplasia spinulosa polyomavirus (TSPyV), John cunningham polyomavirus (JCPyV), BK polyomavirus (BKPyV), and MCPyV, are linked to the growth of various malignant tumors. However, of these, current research only supports the involvement of MCPyV in human carcinogenicity [2,3]. MCPyV is a tiny, non-enveloped, circular double-strand DNA virus that has gained the most attention due to its link with a rare human cancer [4]. The virus is a member of the *Polyomaviridae* family that was first isolated from MCC in 2008 by a group of researchers from the University of Pittsburgh [4–6]. Research from diverse geographic regions indicates that approximately 80% of MCC cases occur through MCPyV [6]. MCC is an aggressive neuroendocrine skin cancer linked with immunosuppression induced by MCPyV DNA [6], which has a five-year average survival rate of 40% [7]. The disease is more prevalent in those suffering from leukemia [8] or HIV infection [9] as well as in immunocompromised persons that have undergone organ transplantation [10]. The disease has a mortality rate of 30%, making it more lethal than other cancers, and the incidence of MCC has increased almost four-fold over the past 20 years in the USA [2]. To date, there are no specific therapeutics or vaccines available against the disease.

MCPyV can replicate its own DNA by using the host cell replication machinery [11]. The 5000 base pairs (bp) of the MCPyV closed-circular viral genome can be split up into three regions, namely the viral regulatory, early coding, and late coding regions [6]. The early coding region expresses four unique gene products known as the large T (LT), small T (ST), and 57kT antigens as well as the overprinting gene known as the Alternate frame of the Large T Open reading frame (ALTO), shown in Figure 1 [4,12]. These genes are transcribed before viral DNA replication and express the tumor (T) antigen in the host cell [6]. MCPyV LT antigen is a multifunctional protein that contains several common motifs and domains important for facilitating the viral life cycle [4]. The N-terminal end of MCPyV LT (1–70) amino acids (AA) contains a DnaJ domain comprising conserved region 1 (CR1) followed by the HPDKGG hexapeptide sequence responsible for Hsc70 binding. LT encodes a MCPyV unique region (MUR) binding motif that interacts with vacuolar sorting protein Vam6p in regulating LT stability via multiple E3 ligase interactions (Figure 1). It also contains a LXCXE motif between the first exon and the OBD (~100–300 aa), a stretch of sequences that interferes with retinoblastoma protein (RB) and promotes host cell proliferation [13]. The LT C-terminal region includes an Ori-binding domain (OBD), required for LT to bind to viral Ori, and a helicase domain that stimulates viral genome replication [4]. The majority of MCPyV LT is truncated at 258 aa and thus loses its C-terminal domain responsible for viral replication, whereas the N-terminal contains the RB-interacting domain and promotes cancer development [4,11]. Thus, the integrated virus LT amino terminus plays an important role in virus replication and cancer progression. Therefore, inhibition of the virus LT protein will hinder the replication process as well as the development of MCC.

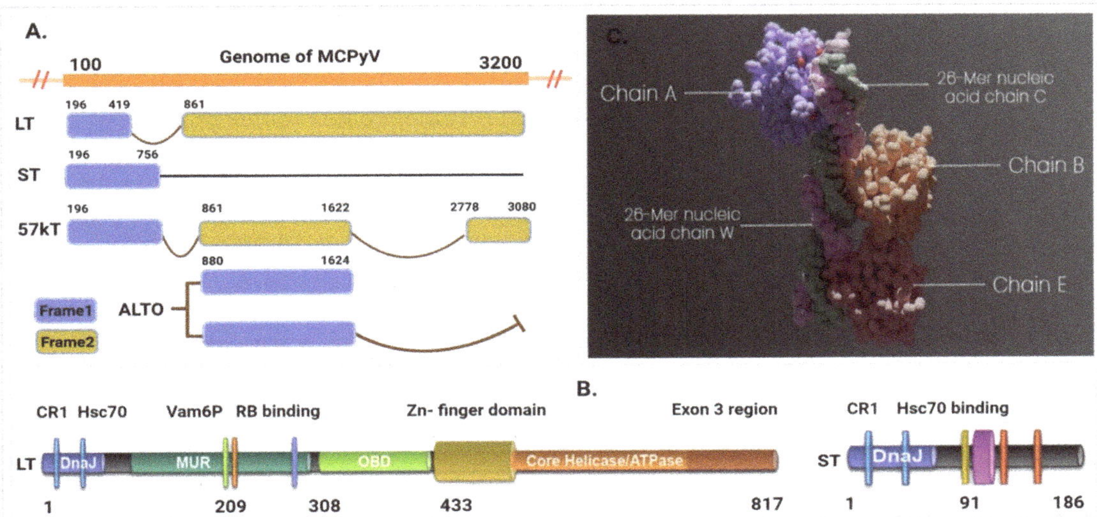

Figure 1. Representing the early region of MCPyV that contains the T (tumor) antigen genome structure. (**A**) The four unique gene products known as the large T (LT), small T (ST), 57kT, and ALTO expressed in the early coding region. (**B**) The large T antigens (left) and small T antigens (right). (**C**) Asymmetric assembly of MCPyV LT antigen origin-binding domains in complex with viral origin DNA retrieved from PDB ID: 3QFQ, adapted from ref. [14].

Plant secondary metabolites and derivatives have gained an abundance of new therapeutic applications in the last century, particularly when applied against cancer [15–17]. For instance, plants have aided in the discovery or development of over 60% of anticancer products, either directly or indirectly [18,19]. Previously, numerous plant species and their active components functioning against different diseases have been assessed and shown enhanced activity against different viral and cancer-related diseases [20–22]. Natural compounds and their derivatives account for more than half of all FDA-approved medications [18]. However, the identification of molecules that could be promising candidates for drug development is not an easy task because various screening paradigms are required to identify hit molecules [23,24]. For example, high-throughput screening (HTS) involves the screening of an entire compound library directly against the drug target or in a more complex assay system, which is costly and time consuming. In this regard, in silico approaches can be beneficial for discovering new plant-based drugs since they allow the faster completion of a variety of complex tasks, including library screening, drug target prediction, and binding site prediction [21,25]. Computer-aided drug design (CADD) approaches increase the probabilities of recognizing molecules with desirable properties and hastened hit-to-lead development [26,27]. Moreover, new methodology incorporating structure-based drug design with the assistance of informatics tools and analytical approaches has significantly accelerated the drug development process [28,29]. Regarding traditional drug discovery, large-scale in vitro and in vivo trials are needed to calculate a compound's binding efficacy and toxicity [30]. In this regard, CADD approaches comprise a molecular docking method that can initially screen many compounds with higher binding efficacy. The approaches can also be used to evaluate pharmacokinetic (PK) properties, bioavailability, toxicity, and efficacy of a compound within short periods [31,32]. Additionally, CADD approaches can predict the binding stability of a ligand to its receptor through molecular dynamics (MD) simulation approaches, which is more appropriate [33,34]. Therefore, the goal of this research was to utilize CADD approaches, including molecular docking, pharmacoinformatic, MD simulation, and MM-GBSA methods, to identify bioactive natural compounds that can be used against MCPyV and thereby help in the fight against MCC.

2. Results

2.1. Protein Preparation

The structure determined for the large T-antigen protein (PDB ID: 3QFQ) with a resolution of 2.90 Å consists of 440 amino acids with a standardized weight of 62.91 kDa, represented in Figure 1C [14]. The asymmetric assembly of MCPyV LT antigen origin-binding domains have three (A, B, and E) identical LT antigen chain in complex with viral origin DNA (C and W) (Figure S1). As the A, B, and E chain are functionally similar proteins that have a similar and identical amino acid (AA) sequence, therefore the B, C, E, and W chains were removed, and A chain was kept for molecular docking simulation. The structure was further modified through two steps in the protein preparation process. In the first step, the metal ions, cofactors, and water beyond 5 Å from the groups were removed, nonpolar hydrogen (H) was merged, and polar H atoms were assigned and saved in PDB file format for further use (Figure S1A). In the second step, the protein was prepared without removing the water and metal ion because water and metal ions sometimes play an important role in the accuracy of ligand–protein docking predictions. As the selected protein crystal structures (3QFQ) contain metal ions and water molecules in their binding sites, the protein was therefore saved with water molecules to determine their role in protein–ligand binding activity (Figure S1B).

2.2. Phytochemical Retrieval and Preparation

The IMPPAT database was used to select the readily accessible compounds of the desired medicinal plants [24]. A total of 2190 phytochemicals were identified from 104 medicinal plants. The medicinal plants and their corresponding compounds used in this study are listed in Supplementary Tables S1 and S7 (Excel), respectively. The compounds were retrieved from the IMPPAT database and saved in 3D SDF format. Medicinal plants were selected based on a literature review, and their corresponding compounds were retrieved to observe their binding activity toward the MCPyV LT proteins.

2.3. Active Site Identification and Receptor Grid Generation

The CASTp server was used to predict the location of the active pocket as well as the binding sites of the MCPyV LT protein [35]. The CASTp web-based tool identified 19 different surface pockets while the probe radius was set to 1.4 Å (Figure S2 and Table S2). Predicted surface pockets were sorted according to area and volume. Among the 19 active pockets, the first 4 active pockets and their corresponding aa residues were chosen based on the surface area and volume listed in Table S3. The first four pockets have a significant area coverage ranging from 103.342 to 4.777 A^2, where volumes of $\geq$1 (SA) are shown in Figure 2. The AS residues identified through this evaluation process were utilized for molecular docking purposes. Maximization of receptor active pocket was confirmed through receptor grid box selection process. The prepared protein was imported in PyRx to assign a grid box that generated a box having a center of X = 38.74, Y = −56.48, and Z = −35.11 along with dimensions of X = 30.90, Y = 26.5, and Z = 26.46 Å.

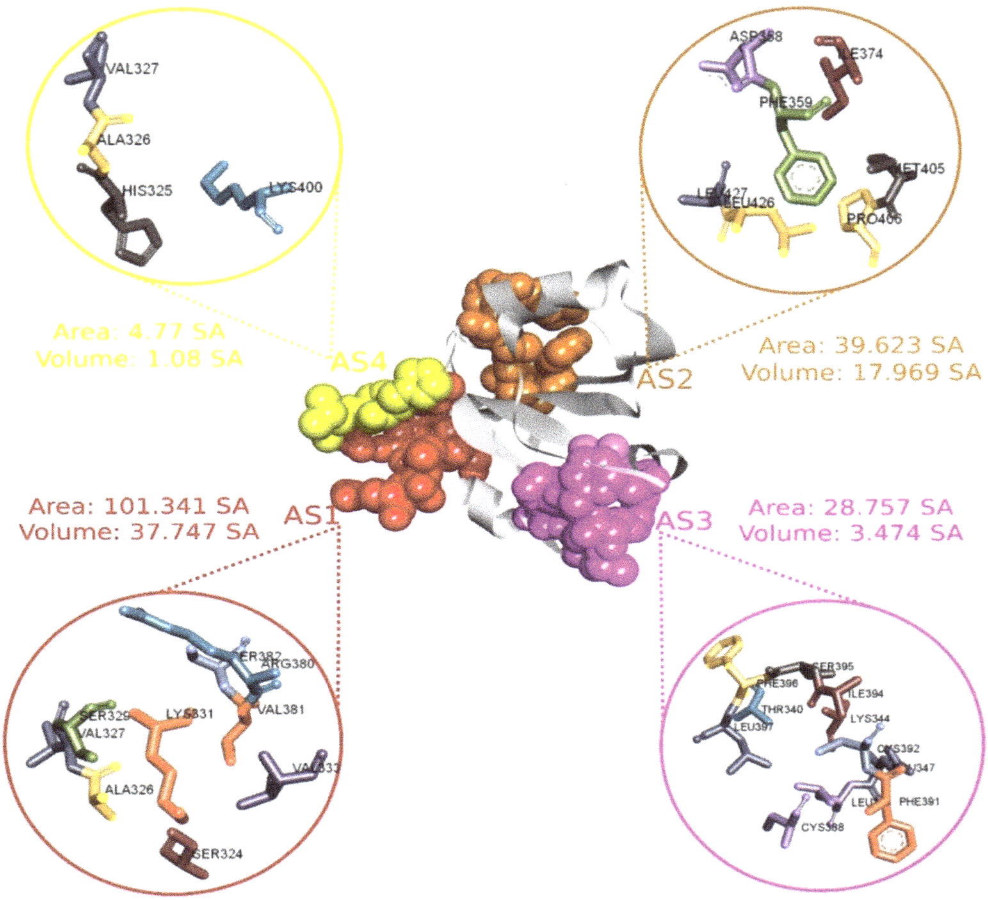

Figure 2. The four selected active pockets of MCPyV LT (PDB: 3QFQ) with the surface area calculated by the CASTp server, adapted from ref. [14]. The first active site (AS1) and its corresponding aa are represented in red, AS2 in orange, AS3 in purple, and AS4 in yellow.

2.4. Molecular Docking Analysis

PyRx tools, specifically the AutoDock Vina wizard, were used to perform molecular docking between 2190 phytochemicals and the target protein [36]. Initially, the compounds were docked with protein that does not contain any water molecules in its structure. The docking study found that the binding affinity of compounds ranged between −3.1 and −7.6 kcal/mol. Based on the binding affinity of the five compounds with the highest values, as listed in Table 1, a threshold energy value of ≥−6.50 kcal/mol was chosen for further evaluation. The five selected compounds were subsequently docked with the same protein chain now containing water molecules in the crystal structure. The docking was performed to see how water affected the compound's binding affinity. Analysis of the docking results show that the presence of water molecules did not substantially alter the binding affinities of the compounds (Table S4).

Table 1. List of compounds, CAS ID, PubChem CID, chemical formula, and two-dimensional (2D) structure of the five selected compounds with the highest binding affinity.

No.	CAS ID	PubChem CID	Chemical Name	Chemical Formula	2D Structure	Docking Score (kcal/mol)
1	13040-46-5	CID: 3084131	Paulownin	$C_{20}H_{18}O_7$	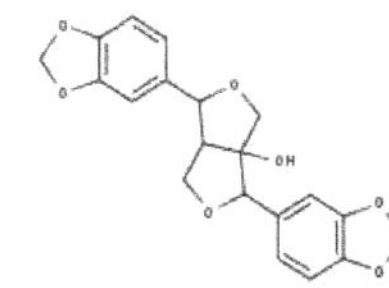	−7.6
2	108907-46-6	CID: 21629801	Epigallocatechin 3-O-cinnamate	$C_{24}H_{20}O_8$	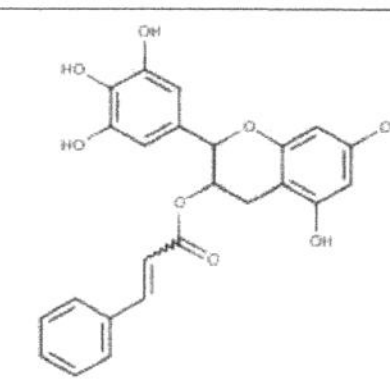	−7.1
3	874359-26-9	CID: 11537736	Actaealactone	$C_{18}H_{14}O_8$	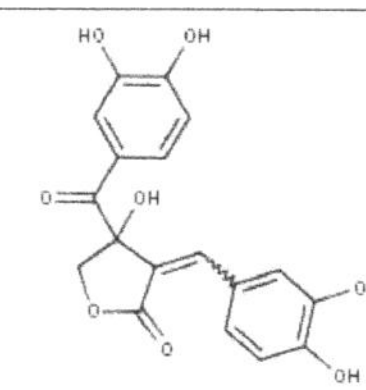	−6.7
4	19622-83-4	CID: 73065	Lycoricidine	$C_{14}H_{13}NO_6$	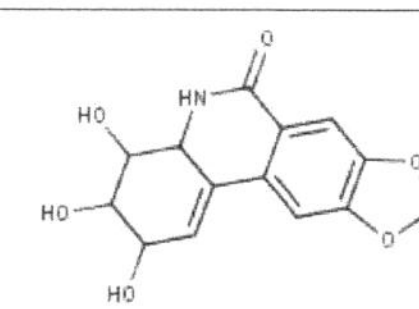	−6.6
5	41365-32-6	CID: 162464	Cirsilineol	$C_{18}H_{16}O_7$	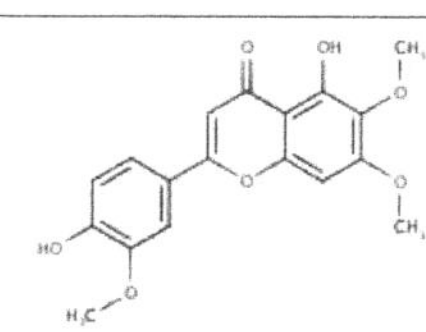	−6.5

2.5. Interpretations of Protein–Ligand Interactions

Protein–ligand interaction studies are important for understanding the mechanisms of biological regulation, and they provide a theoretical basis for the design and discovery of new drug. They can be categorized into four types: hydrogen bonds, hydrophobic, ionic, and water Bridges. Each interaction type contains more specific subtypes. The interactions are essential to developing novel drug leads, predicting side-effects of approved drugs and candidates, and de-orphaning phenotypic hits [37]. Therefore, the interaction between the five ligands and the target protein was visualized using the BIOVIA Discovery Studio Visualizer software [30]. Interactions between the selected compounds and target protein (with and without water) were also analyzed to observe the different interactions formed in the presence and absence of water and represented in Figure S3.

It has been observed that the compound CID: 162464 forms numerous conventional and carbon–hydrogen bonds with the target MCPyV LT protein. It was also found that three conventional hydrogen bonds form at the residue positions SER329 (1.95 Å), LYS400 (2.74 Å), and CYS399 (2.47 Å). Two carbon–hydrogen bonds with LYS331 (3.37 Å) and

LEU397 (3.55 Å) were also observed during the interaction of the compound CID: 162464 with the protein. Alkyl and pi-Alkyl bonds were found to form at positions LYS385 (3.72 Å) and VAL381 (4.08 Å) and positions LYS385 (4.72 Å) and VAL381 (5.28 Å), respectively, as shown in Figure 3A and Table S5.

In the case of compound CID: 73065, it was discovered that five conventional hydrogen bonds form at residue positions VAL327 (1.87 Å), SER329 (2.21 Å), SER329 (2.93 Å), SER382 (2.27 Å), and VAL381 (2.67 Å). One pi-alkyl bond was found to form at position VAL381 (4.96 Å) shown in Figure 3B and Table S5. The compound CID: 3084131 generated two conventional hydrogen bonds and one pi-donor hydrogen bond. Two conventional hydrogen bonds were formed at residue positions SER329 (2.15 Å) and SER324 (2.97Å), whereas one pi-donor hydrogen bond was observed at VAL381 (3.81 Å). One pi-sigma bond formed at VAL381 (3.52 Å), and two pi-alkyl bonds formed at ALA326 (4.93 Å) and ARG380 (5.17 Å), as shown in Figure 3C and Table S5. The compound CID: 11537736 was found to form six conventional hydrogen bonds with the target molecule, at positions SER324 (1.82 Å), ALA326 (2.43 Å), SER329 (2.44 Å), ARG380 (2.74 Å), SER382 (2.04 Å), and CYS399 (2.48 Å). One pi-sigma bond formed at VAL381 (3.53 Å), and two pi-alkyl bonds were generated at ALA326 (4.11 Å) and VAL381 (5.10 Å), as shown in Figure 3D and Table S5. For the compound CID: 21629801, five conventional hydrogen bonds and two carbon–hydrogen bonds, and a pi-donor hydrogen bond with the target protein were identified. Five conventional hydrogen bonds at the positions of ARG380 (2.35 Å), VAL381 (2.95 Å), SER382 (2.07 Å), ASN330 (2.05 Å), and CYS399 (2.84 Å) were observed, while two carbon–hydrogen bonds formed at the positions of SER382 (3.21 Å) and SER382 (3.22 Å). One pi-donor hydrogen bond was established at SER324 (2.94 Å), as shown in Figure 3E and Table S5.

2.6. Pharmacokinetics (PK) Properties Analysis

PK is a field of pharmacology that employs statistical models to explain and forecast the time course of drug concentrations in body fluids [38]. PK analysis in drug development helps to optimize the absorption, distribution, metabolism, and excretion (ADME) properties of lead compounds. Early PK analysis also helps to develop a therapeutic candidate with an appropriate concentration–time profile in the body for the optimal effectiveness and protection profile [39]. The SwissADME server generates a set of parameters that characterize the drug's kinetic activity in the body after administration [40]. The tool allows researchers to save time when making informed decisions about the nature and course of studying a molecule's PK [38]. Therefore, the tool was used to predict the PK properties of the selected molecular candidates. Pharmacological, physicochemical, and PK properties including lipophilicity, solubility, gastrointestinal (GI) absorption, blood–brain barrier (BBB) penetration, and synthesis accessibility of the selected molecules were evaluated and are listed in Table 2 and depicted in Figures S4 and S5.

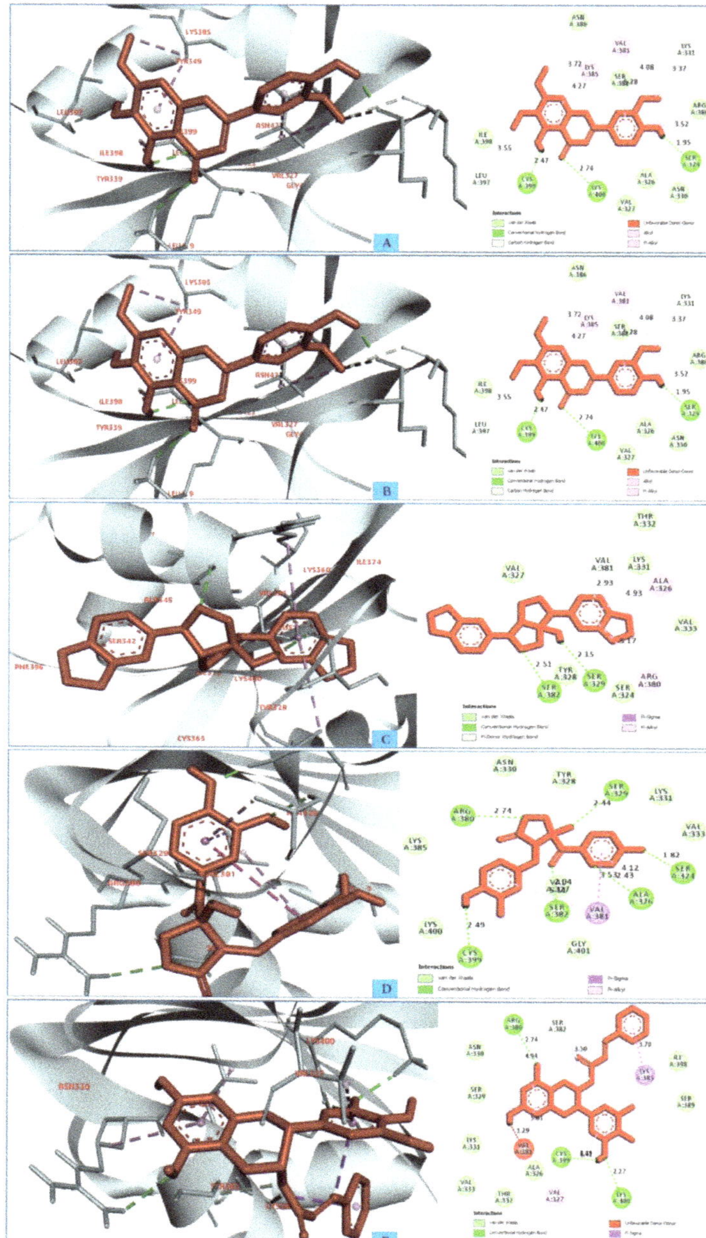

Figure 3. The interactions between the MCPyV large T antigen and five selected natural compounds. The protein–ligand interactions are represented in 3D on the left side of the figure and in 2D on the right side of the figure. The represented interactions are between the MCPyV LT protein and the compounds (**A**) CID: 162464, (**B**) CID: 73065, (**C**) CID: 3084131, (**D**) CID: 11537736, and (**E**) CID: 21629801.

Table 2. List of pharmacokinetic properties, including ADME properties, of the five selected natural compounds. The list also includes the different physicochemical properties of the compounds.

Properties		CID: 73065	CID: 11537736	CID: 3084131	CID: 21629801	CID: 162464
Physicochemical Properties	Formula	$C_{14}H_{13}NO_6$	$C_{18}H_{14}O_8$	$C_{20}H_{18}O_7$	$C_{24}H_{20}O_8$	$C_{18}H_{16}O_7$
	MW (g/mol)	291.26	358.30	370.35	436.41	344.32
	Heavy atoms	21	26	27	32	25
	Arom. atoms	6	12	12	18	16
	Rotatable bonds	0	3	2	5	4
	H-bond acceptors	6	8	7	8	7
	H-bond donors	4	5	1	5	2
Lipophilicity	C Log Po/w	−0.42	0.78	2.10	2.45	2.53
Water Solubility	Log S (ESOL)	−1.01	−2.9	−3.35	−4.31	−4.33
Pharmacokinetics	GI absorption	High	Moderate	High	Moderate	High
	BBB permeant	No	No	No	No	No
Drug Likeness	RO5 Violation	0	0	0	0	0
Medi. Chemistry	Synth. ability	4.01	3.61	4.22	4.38	3.43

2.7. Toxicity Prediction

An in silico toxicity analysis was performed using the pkCSM web portal to identify the toxic effects of the selected compounds [32]. Oral rat chronic toxicity (LOAEL), oral rat acute toxicity (LD50), AMES toxicity, hepatotoxicity, and skin sensitization of drug candidates were evaluated by the pkCSM server and are listed in Table 3.

Table 3. A list of the drug-induced toxicity profile for the five selected natural compounds.

Target	CID: 73065	CID: 11537736	CID: 3084131	CID: 21629801	CID: 162464
AMES toxicity	No	No	No	No	No
LD_{50}	1.981	2.154	2.241	2.769	2.258
LOAEL	2.907	3.172	1.684	3.834	0.953
Hepatotoxicity	No	No	No	No	No
Skin Sensitization	No	No	No	No	No

2.8. MD Simulation Analysis

The binding stability of protein–ligand complexes was investigated and validated by using molecular dynamics (MD) simulations. Data focusing on intermolecular interaction were recorded by the MD simulation throughout the orientation time. The study utilized a 250 ns MD simulation to determine the stability of the protein–ligand complexes. The MD simulation findings are reported based on the root mean square deviation (RMSD), root mean square fluctuation (RMSF), intramolecular hydrogen bonding (Intra HB), and protein–ligand contact analysis (P–L contact).

2.8.1. RMSD Analysis

The RMSD is used to quantify the average change in position of a chosen set of atoms relative to a reference atom [41]. The RMSD analysis is used to describe the system equilibration in terms of stability and reliability.

The smaller range of RMSD and constant fluctuation throughout the simulation imply that the protein backbone is stable. On the other hand, a larger RMSD and/or significant variation from the native structure suggest that the protein–ligand combination is more unstable [42]. The mean or average value change between a specific frame and a reference frame with a range order of 1–3 Å is entirely permissible, where a value larger than the required range indicates that the protein has undergone a significant conformational shift. The MD simulation with a time step of 250 ns was used to provide the RMSD that was calculated from Equation (1) and described below.

Initially, the MCPyV LT protein frames were aligned on the reference frame backbone (blue), and the RMSD of the selected compounds CID: 73065 (red), CID: 3084131 (yellow), and CID: 11537736 (light blue), CID: 21629801 (green), and CID: 162464 (purple) were calculated and are depicted in Figure 4 and Figure S6. The RMSD was computed for the Cα atoms of apoprotein, and the selected compounds increase somewhat but then re-equilibrate toward the conclusion of the 250 ns MD simulation. The RMSD values for the ligand–protein complex was computed and compared with the apoprotein, and the optimal variation was seen for all five molecules. The compound CID: 73065 showed a slight fluctuation between 125 and 175 ns and showed a state of equilibration with the apo structure the rest of the time (Figure 4A). The fluctuations increased for the compound CID: 11537736 from the start of the 25–125 ns MD simulation time and then stabilized with a slight fluctuation between the 166 and 187 ns intervals (Figure 4B). The average RMSD of the compound was 2.067, indicating good stability of the compound with the target protein. The compound CID: 3084131 demonstrates confirmational stability most of the time, having an average RMSD value of 1.25 Å, indicating good stability of the compound with the AS of the protein (Figure 4C). The compound CID: 21629801 exhibits the optimum conformational stability of around 1.2 Å between 200 and 250 ns of the MDS. The highest fluctuation (<2.0 Å) found for the compound is from 50 to 125 ns simulation time, followed by gradual stabilization, indicating that the compound has undergone minor conformational change during the simulation (Figure 4D). In the case of the compound CID: 162464, very low fluctuation was observed during the 250 ns simulation time, although some variations were seen between 25 and 75 ns simulation time, with an average RMSD of 2.5 Å (Figure 4E). Conformational stability was achieved later, from 100 ns and toward the conclusion of the simulation. The measured values for the ligands were less than for the apoprotein RMSD, indicating that the ligand would not dissociate from its original binding site.

2.8.2. RMSF Analysis

The root mean square fluctuation (RMSF) can be used to predict the occurrence of local variations in protein chain residues as well as changes in the location of ligand atoms at a given temperature and pressure [43]. Additionally, the RMSF assists in evaluating the flexibility of each atom to get a better understanding of how ligand binding impacts protein flexibility [44]. Low RMSF values of the AA residues suggest that the complex has achieved more stability, while higher values indicate that the complex has achieved less stability [42]. Thus, the RMSF values of the chosen natural compounds CID: 73065 (red), CID: 3084131 (yellow), CID: 11537736 (light blue), (D) CID: 21629801 (green), and CID: 162464 (purple) in combination with the MCPyV LT protein have been analyzed using Equation (2) and are illustrated in Figure 5. In Figure 5, peaks represent the areas of the aa residues that fluctuate the most during the 250 simulations. There was higher fluctuation from the starting to endpoint aa residues of the complex systems than for any other part of the protein due to the location of the N- and C-terminal domains.

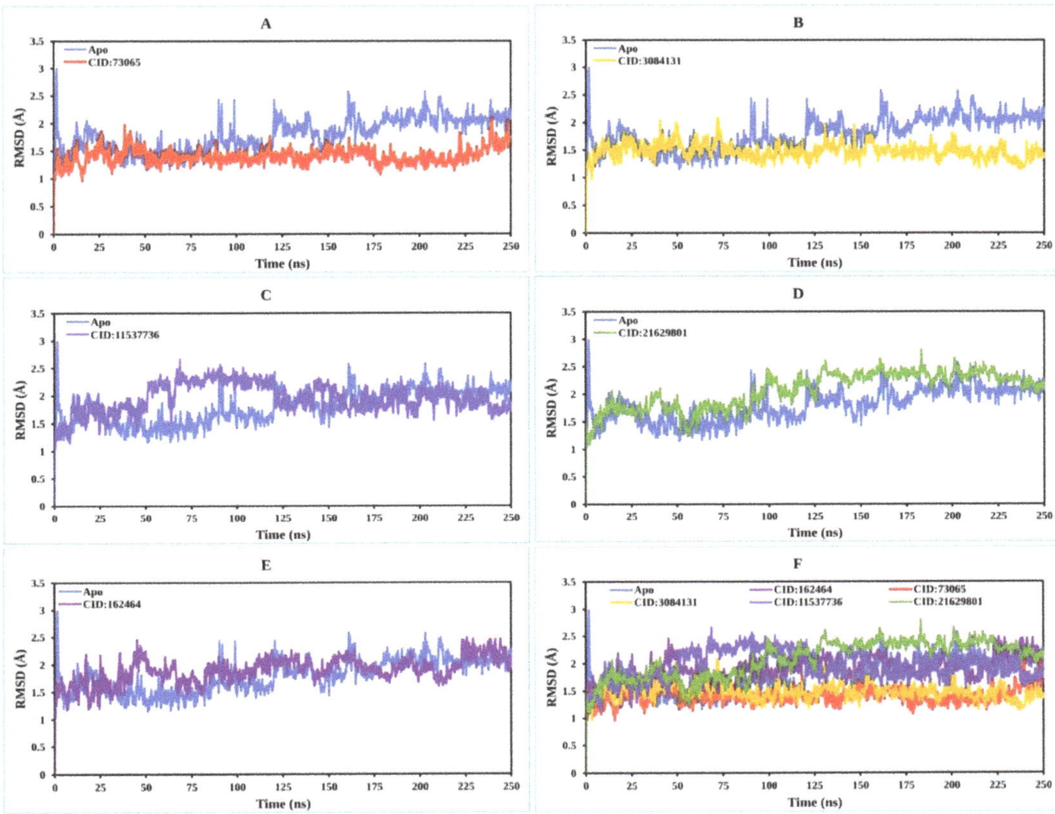

Figure 4. The RMSD values extracted for the Cα atoms of the five selected compounds in complex with the MCPyV LT protein (blue) for the compounds (**A**) CID: 73065 (red), (**B**) CID: 3084131 (yellow), (**C**) CID: 11537736 (light blue), (**D**) CID: 21629801 (green), and (**E**) CID: 162464 (purple), and (**F**) shows all the RMSD for all compounds and the protein together.

In the case of the apoprotein, the maximum fluctuation was observed between residue positions 325 and 330 aa, with a fluctuation of 2.35 Å at VAL327. The apo structure also showed a low level of fluctuation at residue positions LEU367 and THR 393. The apo structure was then compared with the compound CID: 73065 in complex with the protein, in which low fluctuation at residue positions VAL327, LEU367, and THR393 was found (Figure 5A). CID:3084131 seems to have the lowest average RMSF range between 1.0 and 1.3 Å, and the fluctuation of VAL327, LEU367, and THR393 was also low compared to that of the apoprotein structure (Figure 5B). However, the RMSF graph demonstrated average low and significant values of the MCPyV LT protein in complex with CID: 11537736 (0.98 to 1.01 Å), CID: 21629801 (1–1.3 Å), and CID: 162464 (1–1.4 Å) compared to the reference apo structure, as shown in Figure 5C–F. As previously stated, a low RMSF value indicates higher protein stability, whereas the RMSF values found for each protein–ligand system in this study were lower than those for apoprotein. Therefore, the compounds are expected to retain stable contact with the protein without altering its structure.

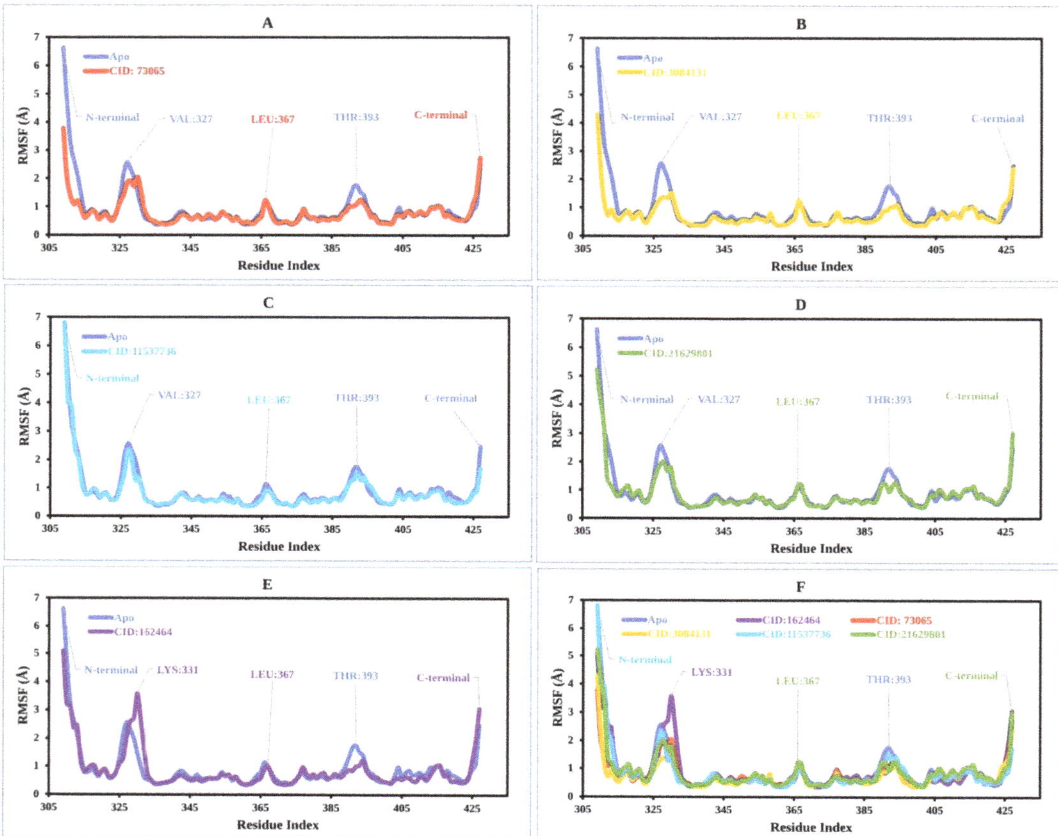

Figure 5. The RMSF values extracted for the Cα atoms of the five selected compounds in complex with the MCPyV LT protein (blue) in complex with the compounds (**A**) CID: 73065 (red), (**B**) CID: 3084131 (yellow), (**C**) CID: 11537736 (light blue), (**D**) CID: 21629801 (green), and (**E**) CID: 162464 (purple), and (**F**) shows the RMSF for all compounds and the protein together.

2.8.3. Protein–Ligand Contacts

The bonding interaction between the molecules and the target protein plays an important role in the stability as well as PK properties. For example, hydrogen bonds of molecules affect drug selectivity, adsorption, and metabolism. Therefore, the protein complex with the selected ligands and their intermolecular interactions were studied using a simulation interactions diagram (SID). The interactions that occur for more than 30.0% of the simulation time between the natural compound (CID: 73065, CID: 3084131, CID: 11537736, CID: 21629801, and CID: 162464) atoms and the MCPyV LT protein residues were characterized based on hydrogen, hydrophobic, ionic, and water bridge bonds and are represented in Figure 6. Additionally, a stacked bar chart representation of the protein–ligand interactions found during the 250 ns simulation run is also provided in Figure S7. The interaction between the protein and ligands can be described based on an interaction fraction value (IFV), such as that an IFV value of 0.7 suggests that the specific interaction is maintained for 70% of the simulation time. Values over 1.0 (>100%) are possible, as some protein residues may make multiple contacts of the same subtype with the ligand. For example, the ARG side chain has four H-bond donors that can produce four hydrogen bond interactions with a single H-bond acceptor.

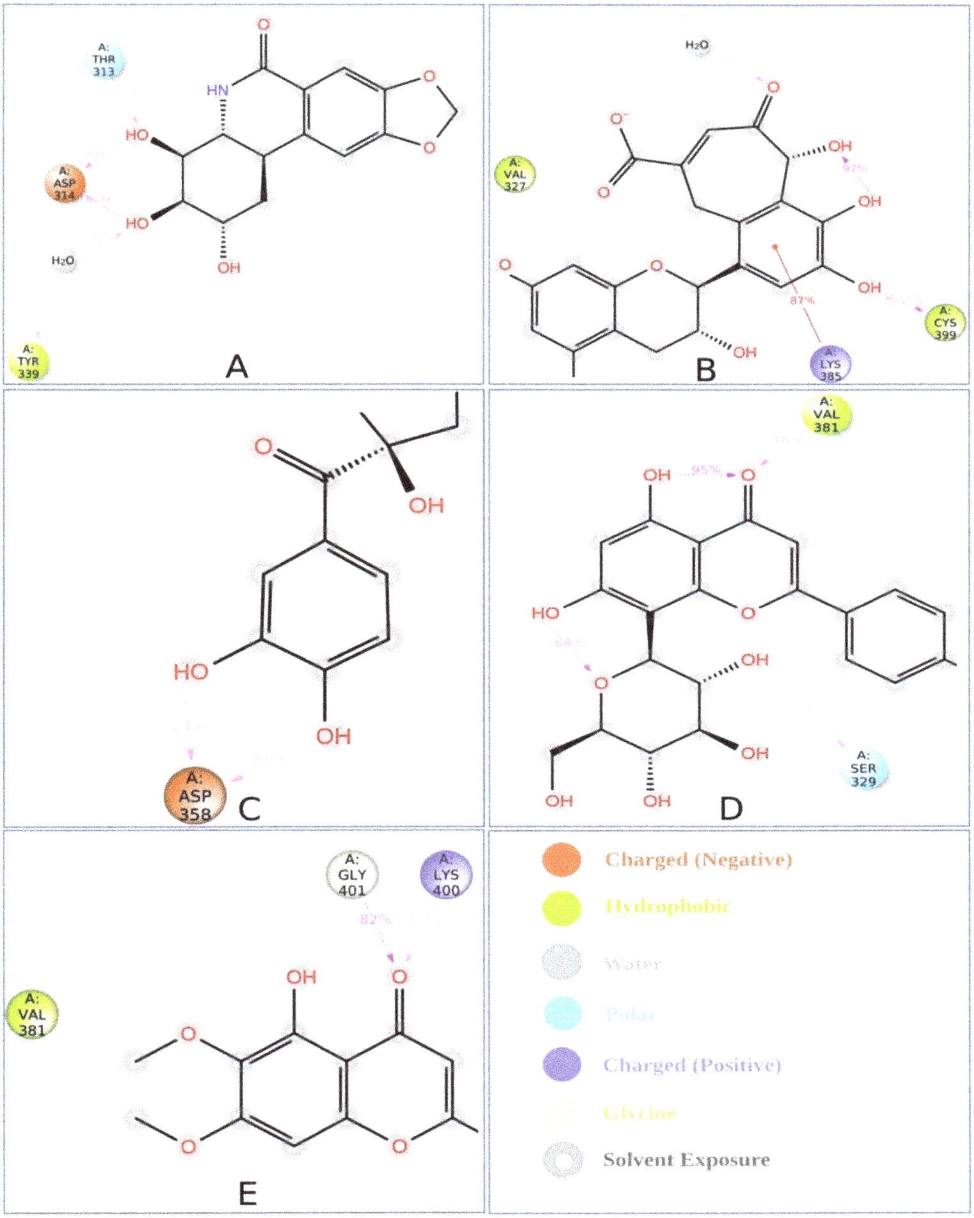

Figure 6. Schematic representation of interactions of selected ligand atoms with MCPyV LT protein residues shown for interactions that occur more than 30.0% of the simulation time between the protein and the compounds (**A**) P CID: 73065, (**B**) CID: 3084131, (**C**) CID: 11537736, (**D**) CID: 21629801, and (**E**) CID: 162464 in the selected trajectory (0.00 through 250.00 ns).

In this study, atoms of the compound CID: 73065 formed interactions at ASP314 and TYR339 protein residues for more than 30.0% of the simulation time with an IFV of 1.4 and 0.6, respectively, indicating that the specific interaction was maintained for 140% and 60%

of simulation time via multiple contacts of the same subtype in the ligand (Figure 6A and Figure S6A). The compound CID: 3084131 produced multiple contacts at LYS385, ASN386, and CYS399 aa residues with 2.0, 0.75, and 1.2 IFV, respectively (Figure 6B and Figure S6B), where the compound CID: 11537736 formed multiple contacts with ASP358 residue with an IFV of 1.2 (Figure 6C and Figure S6C). In the case of the compound CID: 21629801, contact occurred at SER329 and VAL381 residues for more than 30.0% of the simulation time with IFVs of 0.78 and 0.65, respectively (Figure 6D and Figure S6D). Finally, the compound CID: 162464 was found to form multiple interactions for more than 30.0% of the simulation time at the residue positions LYS400 and GLY401 with an IFV of 0.88 and 0.8, respectively, suggesting that the specific interaction will be maintained by multiple contacts for 88% and 80% of the simulation time, respectively, and help to ensure stable binding with the target protein (Figure 6E and Figure S6E).

2.9. MM-GBSA Analysis

The MM-GBSA approach helps to determine the binding free energy of a molecule to the target protein. The binding free energy of the selected molecules to the target protein were evaluated based on the MD simulation trajectory and are represented in Figure 7. The MM-GBSA of the complex structure was computed for every single frame generated for the 250 ns MD simulation trajectory. The analysis of the complex structure identified higher net negative binding free energy values of −47.91 ± 3.92, −29.67 ± 9.53, −39.98 ± 7.20, −28.34 ± 10.05, and −36.67 ± 11.0 kcal/mol for the five selected molecules CID: 162464, CID: 73065, CID: 3084131, CID: 11537736, and CID: 21629801, respectively, with the target protein (Figure 7).

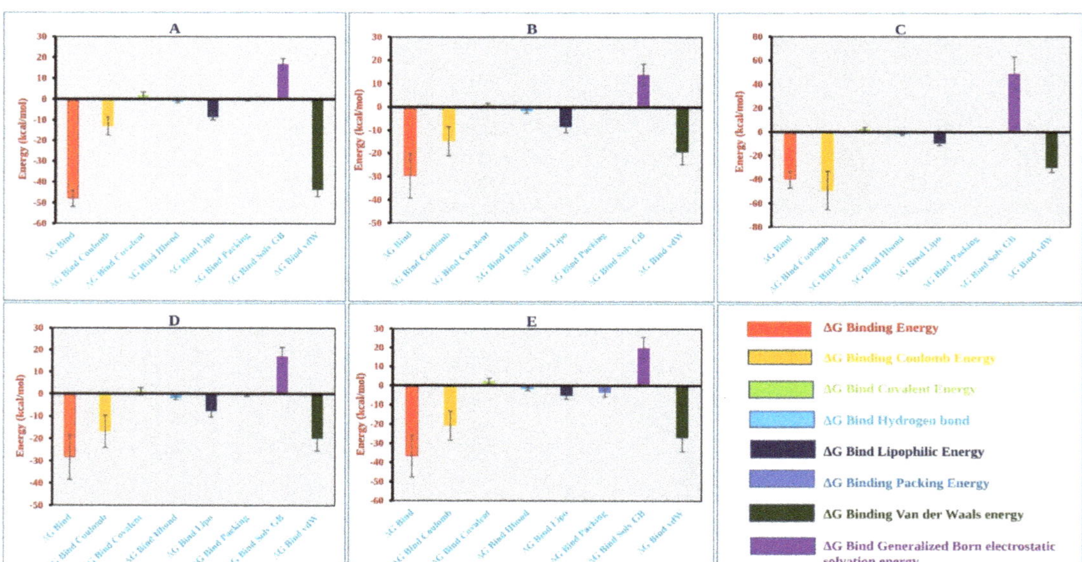

Figure 7. Different energy components and net MM-GBSA binding free energy (kcal/mol) along with the standard deviation values calculated from 250 ns MD simulation trajectory of MCPyV LT protein in complex with the selected compounds (**A**) CID: 162464, (**B**) CID: 73065, (**C**) CID: 3084131, (**D**) CID: 11537736, and (**E**) CID: 21629801.

In addition, the physicochemical contributions to total energy from the analysis of different components found a significant contribution of coulomb, covalent, van der Waals, lipophilic, and generalized Born electrostatic solvation energy shown in Figure 7 and listed in Table S6. Therefore, it can be said that the five selected molecules will maintain a stable interaction with the target protein.

3. Discussion

MCC is a very rare disease in which malignant (cancer) cells form on the top layer of the skin. MCPyV is responsible for at least 80% of all cases of MCC, which has a high risk of returning (recurring) and spreading (metastasizing) [4,45–47]. MCC has a mortality rate of 30%, and to date, no specific drugs are available against the disease [11]. Therefore, the study aimed to identify effective drug candidates against the disease using CADD approaches. CADD approaches have proven efficient and successful in the field of drug design and development, as they enable researchers to rapidly identify the most successful drug candidates. It has been found that CADD approaches can reduce the cost of the drug development process by up to 50% [48]. These approaches can be used to search for new compounds based on specific targets and, in the screening process, increase the possible number of compounds evaluated in a short time. CADD approaches include virtual scanning, molecular docking, ADMET, and MD simulation and are commonly used to find, produce, and study drugs and related bioactive molecules [30].

Molecular docking is a popular method used in the rational design of a drug that involves the analysis and prediction of binding behaviors and interaction affinities between ligands and receptors [49,50]. To identify the interaction between the desired target with different natural compounds in this study, a molecular docking-based screening process was initially applied. This study conducted the simulated screening of a vast library of natural phytochemicals that could target the MCPyV LT protein. The docking technique efficiently screened and ranked 2190 phytochemicals based on a scoring function, whereby the top five phytochemicals were selected based on having the highest binding affinity. The five selected compounds CID: 73065, CID: 11537736, CID: 21629801, CID: 162464, and CID: 3084131 had the highest binding scores of −6.6, −6.7, −7.1, −6.5, and −7.6 kcal/mol, respectively. The selected compounds were further evaluated based on their PK properties.

PK is the study of how small drug-like molecules are absorbed, distributed, metabolized, and excreted (ADME) by the body [39]. Since ADME processes influence the intensity and duration of a drug's operation, their interpretation is critical for supervising the drug development phase and clinical decision-making. Understanding a drug's absorption and distribution properties helps us to estimate how much of an administered dosage can penetrate the bloodstream and hit the target site of action. Furthermore, knowledge of drug metabolism and elimination accounts for the prediction of concentrations for drugs that are provided regularly [51]. Therefore, the study also evaluated a drug's effectiveness by determining its ADME properties [52]. As a result of pharmacokinetic analysis, the optimal GI absorption of the selected compounds with no BBB permeation was identified. The consensus log Po/w value of candidate molecule <5 indicates that it is lipophilic and, therefore, capable of crossing lipid membranes found within the body. Lipinski's rule of five (LR5) assesses the drug-like properties of chosen compounds to determine if they are orally bioavailable for humans, and the selected compounds were found to have good drug-likeness properties.

In the human body system, biological regulators control a variety of cellular processes, including biosynthesis, signal transduction, transport, storage, and metabolism. The undesired activity of a drug candidate with a bioregulator, excluding the primary target, can show toxic effects [53]. One of the most prominent causes of late-stage drug development failure is drug toxicity [54]. It has been found that 20% of late-stage drug discovery failures are due to molecule toxicity [32]. Recently, high toxicity estimation approaches for the early stages of drug production have evolved, which maximize the success ratio of corresponding drug development phases [54]. Early-stage toxicity of drug candidates can be evaluated through in silico toxicology techniques that utilize both quantitative and qualitative methods. In silico methods have many advantages, including the potential to analyze hypothetical substances, their low expense, and the fact that such simulated studies are usually focused on human results, which eliminate the issue of interspecies transferability [53]. Therefore, the study evaluated the toxicity of the selected drug candidates through computational approaches. The top five phytochemicals were evaluated based on mutagenicity, organ toxicity, and animal-based toxicity analysis. The Ames analysis is a bacterial mutation assay that was used in this study to determine whether the medications may trigger such gene mutations that cause genetic disruptions to a cell that can eventually lead to cancer [55], and showed that all tested compounds were negative. Besides this, they were not found to chemically alter the skin, which may result in a prolonged T-cell-induced allergic reaction [56], nor to trigger hepatic dysfunction [57]. LD50 estimates the short-term toxicity efficiency of compounds over a specific time [54], and all compounds were found to have optimum acute toxicity. Moreover, the chosen phytochemicals exhibited favorable results in chronic toxicity tests that were repeated over a longer duration on the living organism.

The compounds that have been chosen based on docking, PK, and toxicity properties were further evaluated through MD simulation methods. MD simulation was used to identify the binding stability of the selected compounds to the AS of the target protein. MD simulations help to determine the physical motions of molecules inside a desirable macromolecule and have become an integral part of the CADD process [58]. MD simulations enable analyzing an intended drug candidate's stability in the presence of a certain macromolecule. Therefore, the LT protein in complex with the five selected small molecules was evaluated based on the RMSD, RMSF, and ligand–protein interactions generated from the 250 ns simulation trajectories. Optimal RMSD and RMSF values for all five compounds were obtained, and the protein–ligand interactions indicated the stability of the five selected molecules to the AS of the protein. Additionally, in the MM-GBSA calculated from the simulation trajectory, a high ΔGbind value was found, as well as coulomb, covalent, vdw, lipophilic, and solv gb energy, indicating the stability of the selected compounds to the target protein for long-term simulation.

The comprehensive CADD approaches successfully identified five compounds, namely Lycoricidine (CID: 73065), Actaealactone (CID: 11537736), Epigallocatechin 3-O-cinnamate (CID: 21629801), Cirsilineol (CID: 162464), and Paulownin (CID: 3084131), which have previously shown activity against different diseases. For example, Lycoricidine, a type of amaryllidaceae alkaloid and constituent of the medicinal plant *Lycoris radiata*, which has shown anti-HCV activity by downregulating the expression of host heat-stress cognate 70 (Hsc70) [59]. Paulownin, found in *Gmelina arborea*, has recently been reported to have a potential inhibitory effect against key receptors of estrogen-positive breast cancer, including FGFR2, ESR1, PIK3CA, PIK3CB, and PIK3CD [60]. The compound has also been reported to have anti-inflammatory and analgesic properties and boost immunity as well as lower blood glucose levels [61]. Actaealactone, a type of neolignan found in the extracts of *Actaea racemose*, is reported to have antioxidant activity [62]. On the other hand, Cirsilineol, a flavone from *Artemisia capillaris*, has many medicinal properties such as anti-neoplastic activity [63], induction of ROS-mediated apoptosis [64], and inhibition of IFN-g signaling in a murine model [65]. The role of the compound Epigallocatechin 3-O-cinnamatein in different diseases, however, has not yet been studied. The study here identified potential inhibitory compounds that may act against the MCPyV LT protein. Previously, most studies were designed to find a potential lead compound by analyzing a plethora of similar compounds. In this study, however, we have analyzed various compounds that cover a wide array of natural compounds, enhancing the chance of discovering a promising drug candidate against MCPyV LT antigen.

4. Materials and Methods

4.1. Protein Preparation

The three-dimensional (3D) structure of the MCPyV large T antigen protein was obtained from the Protein Data Bank (www.rcsb.org//pdb, accessed on 9 December 2021) and has previously been generated via X-ray diffraction. PyMOL v2.4.1 was chosen to view the PDB configuration of the receptor, which was prepared for further analysis using Schrödinger's Protein Preparation Wizard [66].

4.2. Compound Retrieval and Preparation

Indian Medicinal Plants, Phytochemistry, And Therapeutics (IMPPAT) (https://cb.imsc.res.in/imppat/home) (accessed on 9 December 2021) is a manually compiled database of 1742 Indian Medicinal Plants and 9596 stereochemically diverse bioactive compounds [24]. Phytochemicals from a variety of medicinal plants were retrieved from the database and prepared by applying OPLS_2005 as a force field. The Epik ionization tool of Schrödinger Suite was utilized to obtain the ionization state of the compound, where the pH was set within the range of 7 ± 2 [67]. All possible deprotonated and ionization states along with their tautomers, stereochemistry, and ring conformations of the compound were also determined during the ligand preparation process.

4.3. Active Site Identification and Receptor Grid Generation

The active site (AS) of a protein or enzyme is a complex structure of different aa residues in a particular region that aid in the formation of a temporary attachment with the substrate [68]. The active sites forming aa residues are also known as the binding site, which enable the enzyme to bind to a chemical substrate and catalyze the reaction. Additionally, it aids in the stabilization of reaction intermediates and helps recognizing the ligand and forming a tight binding relationship with the protein [32]. Identification of the AS position in a protein can help to generate enough contact points with the ligands and significantly increase the docking efficiency. Therefore, the Computed Atlas of Protein Surface Topography (CASTp) 3.0, a web-based tool (http://sts.bioe.uic.edu/castp/) (accessed on 9 December 2021) was used to classify all surface pockets, internal cavities, and cross-channels in our refined protein structured model [35]. The refined 3D protein structure was uploaded to the website to analyze the binding pocket of the MCPyV LT protein. Additionally, the area and volume of the binding pocket as well as the aa residues required for binding interaction were estimated.

4.4. Molecular Docking

PyRx software was used to upload the refined 3D structure of target proteins and small phytochemical molecules for structure-based virtual screening [36]. Before beginning the simulated screening process, the referenced 3D protein was transformed into a macromolecule, and all phytochemicals were subjected to an energy minimization phase [69]. PyRx virtual scanning tools convert the PDB format of a macromolecule and SDF format of small molecules to Autodock's Pdbqt format using the Open Babel widget according to default configuration parameters. Afterward, all aa residues were selected for the following process using the CASTp server. The grid box was adjusted using Vina Wizard to guarantee that all chosen amino acid residues are contained inside the grid box for running Vina Wizard. Finally, it analyzes the protein binding free energy, which is associated with the scoring mechanism for deciding which phytochemicals are more likely to attach to the target [49], and the phytochemicals containing the highest binding energy (kcal/mol) with a negative sign were selected for further analysis. Finally, the binding interaction between the protein and ligand complex was visualized using BIOVIA Discovery Studio Visualizer v 20.1.0.19295 (BIOVIA) [70].

4.5. Pharmacokinetic (PK) Properties Analysis

Pharmacokinetics is the analysis of how drug concentrations change with time in various body fluids in consideration of the drug absorption, distribution, metabolism, and excretion (ADME) properties. Lipinski's rule specifies the following criteria for an orally active drug: MW (200~500), HBAs (0~10), HBDs (0~5), ClogP $\leq$ 5, and ROTBs (0~10) [71]. The PK properties of the compounds were evaluated using the SwissADME (http://www.swissadme.ch/index.php) server (accessed on 12 December 2021) [40]. The

SwissADME tool predicts the pharmacokinetic, pharmacological, and physicochemical properties, including gastrointestinal (GI) absorption, lipophilicity (consensus Log Po/w), blood–brain barrier (BBB) penetration, solubility (ESOL), drug likeness, and medicinal chemistry friendliness [72].

4.6. Toxicity Prediction

The pkCSM (http://biosig.unimelb.edu.au/pkcsm/) server (accessed on 13 December 2021) is a freely available web server for developing statistical models of drug discovery using a graph-based signature that assesses the toxicity of a variety of substances to guarantee the clinical effectiveness of drug candidates [73]. The pkCSM web server was used here to predict the toxicity parameters, including AMES toxicity, oral rat acute toxicity, oral rat chronic toxicity, hepatotoxicity, and skin sensitization of the compounds.

4.7. MD Simulations

MD simulations were conducted using the Desmond v3.6 program in Schrödinger to determine the stable interactions of the ligands to the binding pockets of the receptors [67]. The stability of the selected compounds in binding the target protein was determined through 250 ns MD simulations. For the prediction of the equation of state (EOS), this software allowed automated simulation and free energy perturbation (FEP) computation, which was combined with various temperatures. The system was solvated using a predefined TIP3P water model, in which an orthorhombic periodic boundary box shape with 10 Å was employed to assign both sides to retain a certain volume. The system was electronically neutralized using suitable ions such as Na^+ and Cl^- with salt concentration of 0.15 M. After creating the solvated system that included the protein in complex with the ligand, the system was optimized by employing the OPLS-2005 force field. Ensembles of NPT (constant number of particles, pressure, and temperature) particles were maintained at 300 K and 1.0 atmospheric (1.01325 bar) pressure, followed by 250 PS recording intervals with an energy of 1.2, in which the solvent and ions were evenly distributed around the protein–ligand complex.

4.8. Simulation Trajectory Analysis

The quality of the MD simulation was verified, and the simulation event was analyzed using simulation interaction diagram (SID) available in the Schrödinger package [68]. The stability of the complex structure was assessed based on the RMSD, RMSF, protein–ligand interactions (P–L contacts), and hydrogen bond interactions found from the trajectory.

4.8.1. RMSD Analysis

The RMSD of a protein–ligand complex system enables the average distance produced by the dislocation of a chosen atom over a certain period to be determined and indicates the stability of a protein [45,74]. When initializing the simulation, the protein structures and the reference frame backbone were aligned, and after that, the RMSD of the whole system was computed for about the duration that the MD simulations ran (in our instance, 250 ns). The RMSD of a complicated system with a time of x may be computed using the below equation.

$$\text{RMSD}_x = \sqrt{\frac{1}{N}\sum_{\text{i}=1}^{\text{N}}(r'_i(\text{t}_x)) - r_i(\text{t}_{\text{ref}}))^2} \quad (1)$$

where N is the atom selection number, t_{ref} is the reference time (usually the first frame is a reference and time t = 0), and x is the location of the chosen atoms when superimposed with the reference frame. Every simulation frame undergoes the process.

4.8.2. RMSF Analysis

The generated RMSF information plays an important role in identifying the local conformational change of a protein coupled with ligands by calculating the average observed atomic changes compared to the number of atoms [30,32]. The following equation may be used to determine the RMSF value of a protein, where the number of residues is denoted by i.

$$\mathrm{RMSF}_i = \sqrt{\frac{1}{\mathrm{T}} \sum_{\mathrm{t}=1}^{\mathrm{T}} < (r_i'(\mathrm{t})) - r_i(\mathrm{t_{ref}}))^2 >} \quad (2)$$

where T denotes the trajectory time interval used to calculate the RMSF, $\mathrm{t_{ref}}$ denotes the reference time interval, r_i denotes the location of residue i, r_i' denotes the location of the atoms in residue i after their overlap upon that reference, and the angle brackets (< >) denote that the square distance is averaged across the residue's atoms.

4.9. MM-GBSA Analysis

MM-GBSA is a popular method to calculate the binding free energy of a complex of molecules with a protein or a free ligand [70]. The MM-GBSA of a complex system can be calculated based on MD simulation trajectory, which is more accurate than most scoring functions. Therefore, to determine the binding free energy (ΔGbind) of the selected molecules in complex with MCPyV LT protein, the MM-GBSA methods were utilized through the Prime MM-GBSA module in the Schrödinger Maestro package [67].

5. Conclusions

Premature stop codon mutations in the truncated MCPyV LT protein are primarily responsible for the proliferation of cutaneous malignant cells that lead to MCC through Merkel cell transformation [7,11]. However, no effective drugs have been identified that target the protein and may thus help to combat against MCC-related human cancers. Therefore, this study aimed to finding natural and effective chemicals that might restrict the function of protein and, hence, impede cancer growth. To achieve this, the research applied a broad range of computational methods, including molecular docking, ADMET, MD simulation, and MM-GBSA approaches, and identified five promising therapeutic candidates, namely Lycoricidine (CID:73065), Actaealactone (CID:11537736), Epigallocatechin 3-O-cinnamate (CID:21629801), Cirsilineol (CID:162464), and Paulownin (CID:3084131), which can inhibit the MCPyV LT protein activity and subsequently block cancer formation. However, these phytochemicals must be subjected to in vitro and in vivo investigations to evaluate their effectiveness and safety as anti-MCPyV medicines in humans. Developing the selected phytochemicals as drug candidates against MCPyV is both therapeutically and commercially feasible.

Supplementary Materials: The following are available online at https://www.mdpi.com/article/10.3390/ph15050501/s1. Figure S1: Representing the MCPyV LT protein retrieved from the protein data bank (PDB ID: 3QFQ-A). Herein, (A). Asymmetric assembly of MCPyV LT antigen origin-binding domains in complex with viral origin DNA. (B) The prepared protein chain without the water molecules, and (C) the prepared protein chain with the water molecules. Figure S2: The active pocket of MCPYV LT (PDB: 3QFQ) with surface area and volume calculated by the CASTp server indicated in the red circle. The server generated a total of 19 pockets, but one was excluded from the figure due to the active pocket being nonvisible due to low surface area and volume. Figure S3: The interaction between the MCPyV LT protein and five selected natural compounds. Interaction of the ligands and protein with water are represented in the left side of the figure, and the interaction of ligands and protein without water are depicted in right side of the figure. The interaction is shown between MCPyV LT protein and the compounds (A) CID: 162464, (B) CID: 73065, (C) CID: 3084131, (D) CID: 11537736, and (E) CID: 21629801. Figure S4: Data visualization of amino acid interaction for (A) comparative bond length, (B) bond category, and (C) bond distance. Figure S5: Data visualization of (A) molecular weight, (B) number of heavy atoms, (C) aromatic heavy atoms, (D) rotatable bonds, (E) hydrogen bond acceptors, (F) hydrogen bond donors, (G) lipophilicity, and (H) water solubility of selected molecules. Figure S6: Representing multiple repetition of RMSD value for each 50 ns interval obtained from 250 ns Simulation time. Herein, A. 1–50 ns, B. 50–100 ns, C. 100–150 ns, D. 150–200 ns, and E. 200–250 ns RMSD of the selected protein–ligand's complex structure. Figure S7: Stacked bar charts representing the protein–ligand interactions found during the 250 ns simulation run for (A) CID: 73065, (B) CID: 3084131, (C) CID: 11537736, (D) CID: 21629801, and (E) CID: 162464 compounds in complex with the MCPyV LT protein. Table S1: List of plants and their antiviral activity against different viruses, and the compounds derived from them are retrieved from the IMPPAT database for this study. Table S2: Active pocket of the MCPyV LT protein (PDB ID: 3QFQ; Chain: A) with surface area and volume. Table S3: First four active pockets and their corresponding aa residues retrieved from the MCPyV LT protein (PDB ID: 3QFQ; Chain: A). Table S4: Comparative docking score of compounds for docking of the protein with water and without water. Table S5: List of bonding interactions between five selected phytochemicals with MCPyV large T antigen. Table S6: The contributions to the total energy from the analysis of different components through MM-GBSA energy calculation method. Analysis of MM-GBSA for five selected compounds found a significant contribution in the binding, coulomb, covalent, van der Waals, lipophilic, and generalized Born electrostatic solvation energy. Table S7: Corresponding compounds of medicinal plants used in this study.

Author Contributions: Conceptualization, A.H.A., F.A. (Faisal Alzahra), A.K., M.A.S.A., R.A. (Rahat Alam), A.S., F.A. (Foysal Ahammad), B.K. and S.C.T.; data curation, M.J.A., M.T.P., R.A. (Rubaiat Ahmed), S.A.S., N.F.A., N.-U.A., S.P. and J.K.K.; formal analysis, M.J.A., M.T.P., R.A. (Rubaiat Ahmed), S.A.S., N.F.A., N.-U.A. and S.P.; funding acquisition, A.H.A., F.A. (Faisal Alzahra), A.K., M.A.S.A., S.H., J.K.K., F.A. (Foysal Ahammad), B.K. and S.C.T.; investigation, A.H.A., F.A. (Faisal Alzahra), A.K., M.A.S.A., S.H., R.A. (Rahat Alam), A.S., J.K.K., F.A. (Foysal Ahammad), B.K. and S.C.T.; project administration, A.H.A., F.A. (Faisal Alzahra), A.K., M.A.S.A., S.H., R.A. (Rahat Alam), A.S., J.K.K., F.A. (Foysal Ahammad), B.K. and S.C.T.; methodology, M.J.A., M.T.P., R.A. (Rubaiat Ahmed), S.A.S., N.F.A., N.-U.A., R.A. (Rahat Alam), F.A. (Foysal Ahammad), and A.S.; resources, M.J.A., M.T.P., R.A. (Rubaiat Ahmed), S.A.S., N.F.A., S.H., N.-U.A., R.A. (Rahat Alam), F.A. (Foysal Ahammad), and A.S.; software, M.J.A., M.T.P., R.A. (Rubaiat Ahmed), S.A.S., N.F.A., N.-U.A., R.A. (Rahat Alam), F.A. (Foysal Ahammad), and A.S.; supervision, A.H.A., F.A. (Faisal Alzahra), A.K., M.A.S.A., S.H., J.K.K., F.A. (Foysal Ahammad), B.K. and S.C.T.; visualization, M.J.A., M.T.P., R.A. (Rubaiat Ahmed), S.A.S., N.F.A., N.-U.A., R.A. (Rahat Alam), and A.S.; writing—original draft, M.J.A., M.T.P., R.A. (Rubaiat Ahmed), S.A.S., N.F.A. and N.-U.A.; writing—review and editing, A.H.A., R.A. (Rahat Alam), A.S. and F.A. (Foysal Ahammad) All authors have read and agreed to the published version of the manuscript.

Funding: This research was funded by the Deanship of Scientific Research (DSR) at King Abdul-Aziz University, Jeddah, Saudi Arabia, grant number FP-54-42. The Taif University Researchers Supporting Project number (TURSP-2020/68), Taif University, Taif, Saudi Arabia. The Deanship of Scientific Research at Umm Al-Qura University Grant Code: (22UQU4290565DSR18). Basic Science Research Program through the National Research Foundation of Korea (NRF) funded by the Ministry of Education (NRF-2020R1I1A2066868), the National Research Foundation of Korea (NRF) grant funded by the Korea government (MSIT) (No. 2020R1A5A2019413), a grant of the Korea Health Technology R&D Project through the Korea Health Industry Development Institute (KHIDI), funded by the Ministry of Health & Welfare, Republic of Korea (grant number: HF20C0116), and a grant of the Korea Health Technology R&D Project through the Korea Health Industry Development Institute (KHIDI), funded by the Ministry of Health & Welfare, Republic of Korea (grant number: HF20C0038).

Institutional Review Board Statement: Not applicable.

Informed Consent Statement: Not applicable.

Data Availability Statement: Data is contained within the article and Supplementary Material.

Acknowledgments: We extend our gratitude to the Deanship of Scientific Research (DSR) at King Abdul-Aziz University, Jeddah, Saudi Arabia for supporting the study through grant FP-54-42. The authors would like to thank the Taif University Researchers Supporting Project number (TURSP-2020/68), Taif University, Taif, Saudi Arabia. The authors also would like to thank the Deanship of Scientific Research at Umm Al-Qura University for supporting this work by Grant Code: (22UQU4290565DSR18). We thank the Biological Solution Centre (https://biosolcentre.org/, accessed on 15 December 2021) for providing technical support. We also thank the authority of King Abdul-Aziz University High-Performance Computing Center (Aziz Supercomputer) (http://hpc.kau.edu.sa, accessed on 15 December 2021) for providing facilities for different computational work.

Conflicts of Interest: The authors declare no conflict of interest.

References

1. Maginnis, M.S. *Human Polyomaviruses (Papillomaviridae)*; Elsevier: Amsterdam, The Netherlands, 2021; pp. 518–527. [CrossRef]
2. Prado, J.C.M.; Monezi, T.A.; Amorim, A.T.; Lino, V.; Paladino, A.; Boccardo, E. Human polyomaviruses and cancer: An overview. *Clinics* **2018**, *73*, e558s. [CrossRef] [PubMed]
3. Ahammad, F.; Abd Rashid, T.R.; Mohamed, M.; Tanbin, S.; Fuad, F.A. Contemporary strategies and current trends in designing antiviral drugs against dengue fever via targeting host-based approaches. *Microorganisms* **2019**, *7*, 296. [CrossRef] [PubMed]
4. MacDonald, M.; You, J. Merkel cell polyomavirus: A new DNA virus associated with human cancer. *Adv. Exp. Med. Biol.* **2017**, *1018*, 35–56. [CrossRef] [PubMed]
5. Feng, H.; Shuda, M.; Chang, Y.; Moore, P.S. Clonal integration of a polyomavirus in human Merkel cell carcinoma. *Science* **2008**, *319*, 1096–1100. [CrossRef]
6. Shuda, M. *Polyomaviruses in Human Cancer*, 3rd ed.; Elsevier: Amsterdam, The Netherlands, 2018; Volume 3, ISBN 9780128124857.
7. Kervarrec, T.; Aljundi, M.; Appenzeller, S.; Samimi, M.; Maubec, E.; Cribier, B.; Deschamps, L.; Sarma, B.; Sarosi, E.M.; Berthon, P.; et al. Polyomavirus-Positive Merkel Cell Carcinoma Derived from a Trichoblastoma Suggests an Epithelial Origin of this Merkel Cell Carcinoma. *J. Investig. Dermatol.* **2020**, *140*, 976–985. [CrossRef]
8. Giudicessi, J.R.; Ackerman, B.M. NIH Public Access. *Bone* **2008**, *23*, 179–196.
9. Engels, E.A.; Frisch, M.; Goedert, J.J.; Biggar, R.J.; Miller, R.W. Merkel cell carcinoma and HIV infection. *Lancet* **2002**, *359*, 497–498. [CrossRef]
10. Clarke, C.A.; Robbins, H.A.; Tatalovich, Z.; Lynch, C.F.; Pawlish, K.S.; Finch, J.L.; Hernandez, B.Y.; Fraumeni, J.F.; Madeleine, M.M.; Engels, E.A. Risk of Merkel cell carcinoma after solid organ transplantation. *J. Natl. Cancer Inst.* **2015**, *107*, dju382. [CrossRef]
11. Liu, W.; You, J. Molecular Mechanisms of Merkel Cell Polyomavirus Transformation and Replication. *Annu. Rev. Virol.* **2020**, *7*, 289–307. [CrossRef]
12. IARC Working Group on the Evaluation of Carcinogenic Risks to Humans. Malaria and Some Polyomaviruses (Sv40, Bk, Jc, and Merkel Cell Viruses). *IARC Monogr. Eval. Carcinog. Risks Hum.* **2014**, *104*, 9–350.
13. Shuda, M.; Feng, H.; Kwun, H.J.; Rosen, S.T.; Gjoerup, O.; Moore, P.S.; Chang, Y. T antigen mutations are a human tumor-specific signature for Merkel cell polyomavirus. *Proc. Natl. Acad. Sci. USA* **2008**, *105*, 16272–16277. [CrossRef] [PubMed]
14. Harrison, C.J.; Meinke, G.; Kwun, H.J.; Rogalin, H.; Phelan, P.J.; Bullock, P.A.; Chang, Y.; Moore, P.S.; Bohm, A. Asymmetric assembly of merkel cell polyomavirus large T-antigen origin binding domains at the viral origin. *J. Mol. Biol.* **2011**, *409*, 529–542. [CrossRef] [PubMed]
15. Mustafa, G.; Arif, R.; Atta, A.; Sharif, S.; Jamil, A. Bioactive Compounds from Medicinal Plants and Their Importance in Drug Discovery in Pakistan. *Matrix Sci. Pharma* **2017**, *1*, 17–26. [CrossRef]
16. Rahman, S.M.M.; Atikullah, M.; Islam, M.N.S.; Mohaimenul, M.; Ahammad, F.; Islam, M.N.S.; Saha, B.; Rahman, M.H. Anti-inflammatory, antinociceptive and antidiarrhoeal activities of methanol and ethyl acetate extract of Hemigraphis alternata leaves in mice. *Clin. Phytosci.* **2019**, *5*, 16. [CrossRef]
17. Mou, M.A.; Keya, N.A.; Islam, M.; Hossain, M.J.; Al Habib, M.S.; Alam, R.; Rana, S.; Samad, A.; Ahammad, F. Validation of CSN1S1 transcriptional expression, promoter methylation, and prognostic power in breast cancer using independent datasets. *Biochem. Biophys. Rep.* **2020**, *24*, 100867. [CrossRef]
18. Anand, U.; Jacobo-Herrera, N.; Altemimi, A.; Lakhssassi, N. A comprehensive review on medicinal plants as antimicrobial therapeutics: Potential avenues of biocompatible drug discovery. *Metabolites* **2019**, *9*, 258. [CrossRef]
19. Raphela-Choma, P.P.; Simelane, M.B.C.; Choene, M.S. Evaluation of the antiproliferative effect of Iso-mukaadial acetate on breast and ovarian cancer cells. *Adv. Tradit. Med.* **2022**, 1–10. [CrossRef]
20. Akram, M. Herbal treatment of viral cancer. *Pak. J. Med. Biol. Sci.* **2018**, *2*. Available online: https://www.researchgate.net/publication/329512172_Herbal_treatment_of_viral_cancer (accessed on 15 December 2021).
21. Alam, R.; Rahman Imon, R.; Enamul, M.; Talukder, K.; Akhter, S.; Hossain, M.A.; Ahammad, F.; Rahman, M.M. GC-MS analysis of phytoconstituents from Ruellia prostrata and Senna tora and identification of potential anti-viral activity against SARS-CoV-2. *RSC Adv.* **2021**, *11*, 40120–40135. [CrossRef]
22. Islam, M.A.; Zilani, M.N.H.; Biswas, P.; Khan, D.A.; Rahman, M.H.; Nahid, R.; Nahar, N.; Samad, A.; Ahammad, F.; Hasan, M.N. Evaluation of in vitro and in silico anti-inflammatory potential of some selected medicinal plants of Bangladesh against cyclooxygenase-II enzyme. *J. Ethnopharmacol.* **2022**, *285*, 114900. [CrossRef]
23. Fang, J.; Liu, C.; Wang, Q.; Lin, P.; Cheng, F. In silico polypharmacology of natural products. *Brief. Bioinform.* **2017**, *19*, 1153–1171. [CrossRef] [PubMed]
24. Mohanraj, K.; Karthikeyan, B.S.; Vivek-Ananth, R.P.; Chand, R.P.B.; Aparna, S.R.; Mangalapandi, P.; Samal, A. IMPPAT: A curated database of Indian Medicinal Plants, Phytochemistry and Therapeutics. *Sci. Rep.* **2018**, *8*, 4329. [CrossRef] [PubMed]
25. Lee Ventola, C. Cancer immunotherapy, part 3: Challenges and future trends. *Pharm. Ther.* **2017**, *42*, 514–521. [CrossRef]
26. Prada-Gracia, D.; Huerta-Yépez, S.; Moreno-Vargas, L.M. Aplicación de métodos computacionales para el descubrimiento, diseño y optimización de fármacos contra el cáncer. *Bol. Med. Hosp. Infant. Mex.* **2016**, *73*, 411–423. [CrossRef]
27. Aljahdali, M.O.; Habibur, M.; Molla, R.; Ahammad, F. Immunoinformatics and Computer-Aided Drug Design as New Approaches against Emerging and Re-Emerging Infectious Diseases. In *Antiviral Drugs [Working Title]*; Intechopen: London, UK, 2022. [CrossRef]

28. Baldi, A. Computational approaches for drug design and discovery: An overview. *Syst. Rev. Pharm.* **2010**, *1*, 99–105. [CrossRef]
29. Rafi, J.H.; Jafar, T.; Pathan, M.T.; Reza, R.; Islam, S.; Sourna, I.J.; Alam, R.; Samad, A.; Ahammad, F. High expression of bone morphogenetic protein 1 (BMP1) is associated with a poor survival rate in human gastric cancer, a dataset approaches. *Genomics* **2021**, *113*, 1141–1154. [CrossRef]
30. Opo, F.A.D.M.; Rahman, M.M.; Ahammad, F.; Ahmed, I.; Bhuiyan, M.A.; Asiri, A.M. Structure based pharmacophore modeling, virtual screening, molecular docking and ADMET approaches for identification of natural anti-cancer agents targeting XIAP protein. *Sci. Rep.* **2021**, *11*, 4049. [CrossRef]
31. Zhou, S.F.; Zhong, W.Z. Drug design and discovery: Principles and applications. *Molecules* **2017**, *22*, 279. [CrossRef]
32. Ahammad, F.; Alam, R.; Mahmud, R.; Akhter, S.; Talukder, E.K.; Tonmoy, A.M.; Fahim, S.; Al-Ghamdi, K.; Samad, A.; Qadri, I. Pharmacoinformatics and molecular dynamics simulation-based phytochemical screening of neem plant (*Azadiractha indica*) against human cancer by targeting MCM7 protein. *Brief. Bioinform.* **2021**, *22*, bbab098. [CrossRef]
33. Duru, I.A. Natural Product Chemistry and Computer Aided Drug Design an Approach to Natural Product Chemistry and Computer Aided Drug Design an Approach to Drug Discovery: A Review Article. *Int. J. Pharmacogn. Chin. Med.* **2020**, *4*, 000207. [CrossRef]
34. Islam, M.R.; Awal, M.A.; Khames, A.; Abourehab, M.A.S.; Samad, A.; Hassan, W.M.I.; Alam, R.; Osman, O.I.; Nur, S.M.; Molla, M.H.R.; et al. Computational Identification of Druggable Bioactive Compounds from Catharanthus roseus and Avicennia marina against Colorectal Cancer by Targeting Thymidylate Synthase. *Molecules* **2022**, *27*, 2089. [CrossRef] [PubMed]
35. Tian, W.; Chen, C.; Lei, X.; Zhao, J.; Liang, J. CASTp 3.0: Computed atlas of surface topography of proteins. *Nucleic Acids Res.* **2018**, *46*, W363–W367. [CrossRef] [PubMed]
36. Dallakyan, S.; Olson, A.J. Small-molecule library screening by docking with PyRx. *Methods Mol. Biol.* **2015**, *1263*, 243–250. [CrossRef] [PubMed]
37. Li, L.; Koh, C.C.; Reker, D.; Brown, J.B.; Wang, H.; Lee, N.K.; Liow, H.H.; Dai, H.; Fan, H.M.; Chen, L.; et al. Predicting protein-ligand interactions based on bow-pharmacological space and Bayesian additive regression trees. *Sci. Rep.* **2019**, *9*, 7703. [CrossRef]
38. Ruiz-Garcia, A.; Bermejo, M.; Moss, A.; Casabo, V.G. Pharmacokinetics in drug discovery. *J. Pharm. Sci.* **2008**, *97*, 654–690. [CrossRef]
39. Reichel, A.; Lienau, P. Pharmacokinetics in drug discovery: An exposure-centred approach to optimising and predicting drug efficacy and safety. In *Handbook of Experimental Pharmacology*; Springer: New York, NY, USA, 2016; Volume 232, pp. 235–260.
40. Palleria, C.; Di Paolo, A.; Giofrè, C.; Caglioti, C.; Leuzzi, G.; Siniscalchi, A.; De Sarro, G.; Gallelli, L. Pharmacokinetic drug-drug interaction and their implication in clinical management. *J. Res. Med. Sci.* **2013**, *18*, 600–609.
41. Samad, A.; Ahammad, F.; Nain, Z.; Alam, R.; Imon, R.R.; Hasan, M.; Rahman, M.S. Designing a multi-epitope vaccine against SARS-CoV-2: An immunoinformatics approach. *J. Biomol. Struct. Dyn.* **2020**, *40*, 14–30. [CrossRef]
42. Sinha, S.K.; Prasad, S.K.; Islam, M.A.; Gurav, S.S.; Patil, R.B.; AlFaris, N.A.; Aldayel, T.S.; AlKehayez, N.M.; Wabaidur, S.M.; Shakya, A. Identification of bioactive compounds from Glycyrrhiza glabra as possible inhibitor of SARS-CoV-2 spike glycoprotein and non-structural protein-15: A pharmacoinformatics study. *J. Biomol. Struct. Dyn.* **2020**, *39*, 4686–4700. [CrossRef]
43. Sharma, P.; Joshi, T.; Joshi, T.; Chandra, S.; Tamta, S. Molecular dynamics simulation for screening phytochemicals as α-amylase inhibitors from medicinal plants. *J. Biomol. Struct. Dyn.* **2020**, *39*, 6524–6538. [CrossRef]
44. Islam, R.; Parves, M.R.; Paul, A.S.; Uddin, N.; Rahman, M.S.; Al Mamun, A.; Hossain, M.N.; Ali, M.A.; Halim, M.A. A molecular modeling approach to identify effective antiviral phytochemicals against the main protease of SARS-CoV-2. *J. Biomol. Struct. Dyn.* **2021**, *39*, 3213–3224. [CrossRef]
45. Samad, A.; Haque, F.; Nain, Z.; Alam, R.; Al Noman, M.A.; Rahman Molla, M.H.; Hossen, M.S.; Islam, M.R.; Khan, M.I.; Ahammad, F. Computational assessment of MCM2 transcriptional expression and identification of the prognostic biomarker for human breast cancer. *Heliyon* **2020**, *6*, e05087. [CrossRef] [PubMed]
46. Tabassum, A.; Nazmus Samdani, M.; Chandra Dhali, T.; Alam, R.; Samad, A.; Karpiński, T.M.; Arabia, S. Transporter Associated with Antigen Processing 1 (TAP1) as a Potential Biomarker for Breast, Lung, Liver and Ovarian Cancer using Health Informatics. *Preprints* **2020**, 2020080322. [CrossRef]
47. Alam, R.; Biswas, S.; Haque, F.; Pathan, M.T.; Imon, R.R.; Talukder, M.E.K.; Samad, A.; Asseri, A.H.; Ahammad, F. A systematic analysis of ATPase Cation transporting 13A2 (ATP13A2) transcriptional expression and prognostic value in human brain cancer. *Biomed. Signal Process. Control* **2022**, *71*, 103183. [CrossRef]
48. Baig, M.H.; Ahmad, K.; Rabbani, G.; Danishuddin, M.; Choi, I. Computer Aided Drug Design and its Application to the Development of Potential Drugs for Neurodegenerative Disorders. *Curr. Neuropharmacol.* **2017**, *16*, 740–748. [CrossRef] [PubMed]
49. Cui, W.; Aouidate, A.; Wang, S.; Yu, Q.; Li, Y.; Yuan, S. Discovering Anti-Cancer Drugs via Computational Methods. *Front. Pharmacol.* **2020**, *11*, 733. [CrossRef]
50. Bhuiyan, M.A.; Quayum, S.T.; Ahammad, F.; Alam, R.; Samad, A.; Nain, Z. Discovery of potential immune epitopes and peptide vaccine design—A prophylactic strategy against Rift Valley fever virus. *F1000Research* **2020**, *9*, 999. [CrossRef]
51. Luer, M.S.; Penzak, S.R. Pharmacokinetic properties. In *Applied Clinical Pharmacokinetics and Pharmacodynamics of Psychopharmacological Agents*; Springer International Publishing: Berlin/Heidelberg, Germany, 2016; pp. 3–27. ISBN 9783319278834.
52. Abdulrahman, H.L.; Uzairu, A.; Uba, S. Computational pharmacokinetic analysis on some newly designed 2-anilinopyrimidine derivative compounds as anti-triple-negative breast cancer drug compounds. *Bull. Natl. Res. Cent.* **2020**, *44*, 63. [CrossRef]

53. Vedani, A.; Smiesko, M. In silico toxicology in drug discovery—Concepts based on three-dimensional models. *Altern. Lab. Anim.* **2009**, *37*, 477–496. [CrossRef]
54. Wang, Y.; Xing, J.; Xu, Y.; Zhou, N.; Peng, J.; Xiong, Z.; Liu, X.; Luo, X.; Luo, C.; Chen, K.; et al. In silico ADME/T modelling for rational drug design. *Q. Rev. Biophys.* **2015**, *48*, 488–515. [CrossRef]
55. Mortelmans, K.; Mortelmans, K.; Zeiger, E. The Ames Salmonella/microsome mutagenicity assay. *Mutat. Res./Fundam. Mol. Mech. Mutagenesis* **2000**, *455*, 29–60. [CrossRef]
56. Basketter, D.; Darlenski, R.; Fluhr, J.W. Skin irritation and sensitization: Mechanisms and new approaches for risk assessment—2. Skin sensitization. *Skin Pharmacol. Physiol.* **2008**, *21*, 191–202. [CrossRef] [PubMed]
57. Björnsson, E.S. Hepatotoxicity by drugs: The most common implicated agents. *Int. J. Mol. Sci.* **2016**, *17*, 20224. [CrossRef] [PubMed]
58. Zhou, W.; Wang, Y.; Lu, A.; Zhang, G. Systems pharmacology in small molecular drug discovery. *Int. J. Mol. Sci.* **2016**, *17*, 20246. [CrossRef] [PubMed]
59. Chen, D.Z.; Jiang, J.D.; Zhang, K.Q.; He, H.P.; Di, Y.T.; Zhang, Y.; Cai, J.Y.; Wang, L.; Li, S.L.; Yi, P.; et al. Evaluation of anti-HCV activity and SAR study of (+)-lycoricidine through targeting of host heat-stress cognate 70 (Hsc70). *Bioorg. Med. Chem. Lett.* **2013**, *23*, 2679–2682. [CrossRef] [PubMed]
60. Jain, S.; Das, A. Virtual screening of natural compounds as combinatorial agents from indian medicinal plants against estrogen positive breast cancer. *Int. J. Integr. Educ.* **2020**, *3*, 266–275. [CrossRef]
61. He, T.; Vaidya, B.; Perry, Z.; Parajuli, P.; Joshee, N. Paulownia as a Medicinal Tree: Traditional Uses and Current Advances. *Eur. J. Med. Plants* **2016**, *14*, 1–15. [CrossRef]
62. Pan, J.Y.; Chen, S.L.; Yang, M.H.; Wu, J.; Sinkkonen, J.; Zou, K. An update on lignans: Natural products and synthesis. *Nat. Prod. Rep.* **2009**, *26*, 1251–1292. [CrossRef]
63. Sheng, X.; Sun, Y.; Yin, Y.; Chen, T.; Xu, Q. Cirsilineol inhibits proliferation of cancer cells by inducing apoptosis via mitochondrial pathway. *J. Pharm. Pharmacol.* **2008**, *60*, 1523–1529. [CrossRef]
64. Pathak, G.; Singh, S.; Kumari, P.; Hussain, Y.; Raza, W.; Luqman, S.; Meena, A. Cirsilineol inhibits proliferation of lung squamous cell carcinoma by inducing ROS mediated apoptosis. *Food Chem. Toxicol.* **2020**, *143*, 111550. [CrossRef]
65. Sun, Y.; Wu, X.X.; Yin, Y.; Gong, F.Y.; Shen, Y.; Cai, T.T.; Zhou, X.B.; Wu, X.F.; Xu, Q. Novel immunomodulatory properties of cirsilineol through selective inhibition of IFN-γ signaling in a murine model of inflammatory bowel disease. *Biochem. Pharmacol.* **2010**, *79*, 229–238. [CrossRef]
66. Lill, M.A.; Danielson, M.L. Computer-aided drug design platform using PyMOL. *J. Comput. Aided. Mol. Des.* **2011**, *25*, 13–19. [CrossRef] [PubMed]
67. Pokhrel, S.; Bouback, T.A.; Samad, A.; Nur, S.M.; Alam, R.; Abdullah-Al-Mamun, M.; Nain, Z.; Imon, R.R.; Talukder, M.E.K.; Tareq, M.M.I.; et al. Spike protein recognizer receptor ACE2 targeted identification of potential natural antiviral drug candidates against SARS-CoV-2. *Int. J. Biol. Macromol.* **2021**, *191*, 1114–1125. [CrossRef] [PubMed]
68. Ahmed Bhuiyan, M.; Atia Keya, N.; Susan Mou, F.; Rahman Imon, R.; Alam, R.; Ahammad, F. Discovery of Potential Compounds Against Nipah Virus: A Molecular Docking and Dynamics Simulation Approaches. *Res. Sq.* **2022**. [CrossRef]
69. Ahammad, F.; Fuad, F.A.A. The in silico identification of potent natural bioactive anti-dengue agents by targeting the human hexokinase 2 enzyme. In Proceedings of the 5th International Electronic Conference on Medicinal Chemistry, Basel, Switzerland, 1–30 November; MDPI: Basel, Switzerland, 2020; p. 6342.
70. Bouback, T.A.; Pokhrel, S.; Albeshri, A.; Aljohani, A.M.; Samad, A.; Alam, R.; Hossen, M.S.; Al-Ghamdi, K.; Talukder, M.E.K.; Ahammad, F.; et al. Pharmacophore-Based Virtual Screening, Quantum Mechanics Calculations, and Molecular Dynamics Simulation Approaches Identified Potential Natural Antiviral Drug Candidates against MERS-CoV S1-NTD. *Molecules* **2021**, *26*, 4961. [CrossRef]
71. Lipinski, C.A.; Lombardo, F.; Dominy, B.W.; Feeney, P.J. Experimental and computational approaches to estimate solubility and permeability in drug discovery and development settings. *Adv. Drug Deliv. Rev.* **2012**, *64*, 4–17. [CrossRef]
72. Daina, A.; Michielin, O.; Zoete, V. SwissADME: A free web tool to evaluate pharmacokinetics, drug-likeness and medicinal chemistry friendliness of small molecules. *Sci. Rep.* **2017**, *7*, 42717. [CrossRef]
73. Pires, D.E.V.; Blundell, T.L.; Ascher, D.B. pkCSM: Predicting small-molecule pharmacokinetic and toxicity properties using graph-based signatures. *J. Med. Chem.* **2015**, *58*, 4066–4072. [CrossRef]
74. Aljahdali, M.O.; Molla, M.H.R.; Ahammad, F. Compounds Identified from Marine Mangrove Plant (*Avicennia alba*) as Potential Antiviral Drug Candidates against WDSV, an In-Silico Approach. *Mar. Drugs* **2021**, *19*, 253. [CrossRef]

pharmaceuticals

Article

Rethinking Protein Drug Design with Highly Accurate Structure Prediction of Anti-CRISPR Proteins

Ho-Min Park [1,2], Yunseol Park [1], Joris Vankerschaver [1,3], Arnout Van Messem [4], Wesley De Neve [1,2] and Hyunjin Shim [1,*]

1 Center for Biosystems and Biotech Data Science, Ghent University Global Campus, Incheon 21985, Korea; homin.park@ghent.ac.kr (H.-M.P.); yunseol.park@ghent.ac.kr (Y.P.); joris.vankerschaver@ghent.ac.kr (J.V.); wesley.deneve@ghent.ac.kr (W.D.N.)
2 Department of Electronics and Information Systems, Ghent University, 9000 Ghent, Belgium
3 Department of Applied Mathematics, Computer Science and Statistics, Ghent University, 9000 Ghent, Belgium
4 Department of Mathematics, University of Liège, 4000 Liège, Belgium; arnout.vanmessem@uliege.be
* Correspondence: hyunjin.shim@ghent.ac.kr

Abstract: Protein therapeutics play an important role in controlling the functions and activities of disease-causing proteins in modern medicine. Despite protein therapeutics having several advantages over traditional small-molecule therapeutics, further development has been hindered by drug complexity and delivery issues. However, recent progress in deep learning-based protein structure prediction approaches, such as AlphaFold2, opens new opportunities to exploit the complexity of these macro-biomolecules for highly specialised design to inhibit, regulate or even manipulate specific disease-causing proteins. Anti-CRISPR proteins are small proteins from bacteriophages that counter-defend against the prokaryotic adaptive immunity of CRISPR-Cas systems. They are unique examples of natural protein therapeutics that have been optimized by the host-parasite evolutionary arms race to inhibit a wide variety of host proteins. Here, we show that these anti-CRISPR proteins display diverse inhibition mechanisms through accurate structural prediction and functional analysis. We find that these phage-derived proteins are extremely distinct in structure, some of which have no homologues in the current protein structure domain. Furthermore, we find a novel family of anti-CRISPR proteins which are structurally similar to the recently discovered mechanism of manipulating host proteins through enzymatic activity, rather than through direct inference. Using highly accurate structure prediction, we present a wide variety of protein-manipulating strategies of anti-CRISPR proteins for future protein drug design.

Keywords: in-silico drug design; AlphaFold; anti-CRISPR proteins; prokaryotic defence mechanisms; bacteriophages; structural biology; protein drug

Citation: Park, H.-M.; Park, Y.; Vankerschaver, J.; Van Messem, A.; De Neve, W.; Shim, H. Rethinking Protein Drug Design with Highly Accurate Structure Prediction of Anti-CRISPR Proteins. *Pharmaceuticals* **2022**, *15*, 310. https://doi.org/10.3390/ph15030310

Academic Editor: Osvaldo Andrade Santos-Filho

Received: 27 January 2022
Accepted: 1 March 2022
Published: 4 March 2022

1. Introduction

Proteins are macromolecules composed of amino-acid residues that perform diverse roles in biological entities, including catalysing biochemical reactions, providing cell/capsid structure, transporting molecules, replicating genetic material, and responding to stimuli. It is estimated there are over 25,000 functionally distinct proteins in the human body [1,2], and mutations or abnormalities in these proteins may result in diseases. Thus, modern medicine has focused on targeting such proteins to alleviate diseases, mostly through small-molecule therapeutic agents acting as competitive or non-competitive inhibitors [3]. However, it is estimated that only ~10% of the human proteome can be targeted with small-molecule drugs [3]. Since the introduction of human insulin as the first recombinant protein therapeutic in the 1980s [4,5], protein-based therapeutics have expanded the scope of "druggable proteins". Compared to small-molecule drugs, the major advantage of protein therapeutics is improved target specificity and reduced immunogenicity due to their proteinaceous nature [5]. Protein therapeutics can also serve complex functions that simple chemical compounds cannot achieve, such as replacing a deficient protein or providing a protein of novel function (Figure 1a). Furthermore, protein therapeutics can inhibit disease-related proteins that small-molecule drugs cannot target due to the lack of a cavity to bind. Currently, there are over 130 protein therapeutics commercially available and intense research efforts are ongoing to better design protein therapeutics [5].

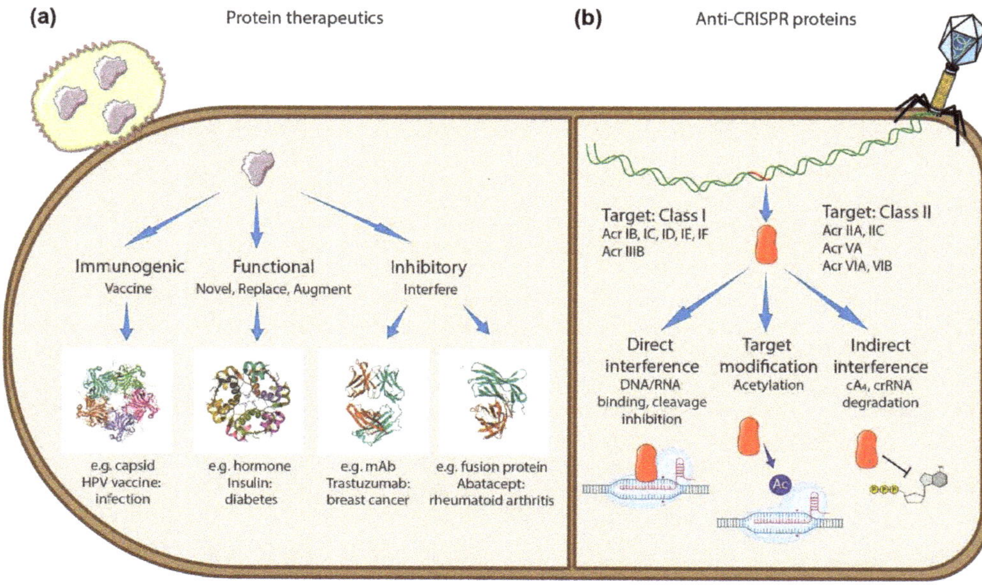

Figure 1. Mechanisms of protein therapeutics and anti-CRISPR proteins. (**a**) Mechanism of protein therapeutics. The first group consists of prophylactic or therapeutic vaccines that induce immunity against foreign or cancer cells. A highly successful protein vaccine against human papillomavirus (HPV) combining the capsids from four pathogenic HPV strains is given as an example (PDB: 2R5K [6]). The second group consists of protein therapeutics that provide novel functions, replace deficient or abnormal proteins, or augment existing activities. The approval of recombinant insulin in the 1980s to treat diabetes as the first abundant, inexpensive and low immunogenic therapeutic protein is given as an example (PDB: 4F8F [7]). The third group consists of proteins that interfere with target proteins through high binding specificity. Some monoclonal antibodies use antigen recognition sites or receptor-binding domains like Trastuzumab against breast cancer cells (PDB: 6MH2 [8,9]). Some fusion proteins inhibit target proteins by blocking interaction sites like Abatacept against rheumatoid arthritis (PDB: 1DQT [8,9]). (**b**) Mechanisms of anti-CRISPR proteins. Upon successful infection, phage genomes express anti-CRISPR proteins that neutralize host CRISPR-Cas immunity. Anti-CRISPR proteins target various types of both Class I and Class II CRISPR-Cas systems and the inhibitory mechanisms are highly diverse, including direct interference of DNA/RNA binding and cleavage of Cas complexes, enzymatic inhibition of the active site by acetylation, and nuclease activity of degrading the signalling molecule (cyclic nucleotide cA_4).

In this study, we present a group of naturally-occurring protein therapeutics, called anti-CRISPR (Acr) proteins, as a good example of how small proteins are used by invading bacteriophages (phages) in nature to control host proteins. Phages are the most abundant and diverse biological entities in the biosphere (estimated 10^{31} existing phages) that infect and replicate within host prokaryotes (such as bacteria or archaea) [10]. High selective pressures between these parasites and hosts drive dynamic coevolution of genomic and proteomic mechanisms and systems [11–13]. In particular, the evolutionary arms race between phages and prokaryotes has resulted in a vast arsenal of immune systems, including the prokaryotic adaptive immune system known as CRISPR-Cas [14,15]. CRISPR-Cas systems are defence mechanisms against phages (and other mobilomes) through a complex of RNA-guided Cas proteins (Figure 1b). Remarkably, prokaryotic genomes with CRISPR-Cas systems can acquire short fragments of foreign genetic sequences in their CRISPR arrays, which serve as RNA templates to recognize and cleave invading phages through the nuclease complex of Cas proteins [16]. Since the successful application of CRISPR-Cas systems as genome-editing tools [17,18], there has been a burst in the discovery of diverse CRISPR-Cas systems [19], followed by the discovery of Acr proteins that neutralize the activity of this prokaryotic adaptive immune system [20] (Figure 1b). A family of Acr proteins was first identified in the CRISPR-Cas-inactivating prophages of *Pseudomonas* genomes that disable Type I-F and Type I-E CRISPR-Cas systems [20,21]. A number of Acr proteins inhibiting type II CRISPR-Cas systems have since been applied as regulators of gene-editing activities [22]. The Acr protein families are known to have short sequences (<100 amino acids) with no common genetic features, and interact directly with Cas proteins to inhibit target DNA binding, DNA cleavage, CRISPR RNA loading and protein-complex formation [22,23]. A recent study reveals that AcrVA5 proteins inactivate Cas12a of Type V CRISPR-Cas systems enzymatically by acetylation of the active site, with structural similarity to an acetyltransferase protein [24].

In this study, we conducted a comprehensive analysis on the key characteristics of Acr proteins viewed from the perspective of naturally-occurring protein therapeutics that effectively inhibit host protein functions. Motivated by the observation that these Acr proteins are genetically diverse, we examined the protein structure of these diverse proteins using AlphaFold2 [25]. AlphaFold is a state-of-the-art deep learning-based approach that performs protein structure prediction, which takes a protein sequence as an input to predict its 3-D protein structure through an iterative exchange of information between its genetic representation and its structural representation. The recent release of AlphaFold2, the winner of CASP14, which achieves highly accurate protein structure predictions [25,26], is revolutionary for the field of life sciences and medicine, and is expected to accelerate critical research in a large number of fields ranging from structural biology to drug discovery. In this study, we first assessed the performance of AlphaFold2 in predicting the 3-D structures of Acr proteins based on similarity metrics against their experimentally reconstructed 3-D macromolecular structures. Using this performance as a basis, we further examined the Acr proteins without experimental structures with AlphaFold2, to predict the structural diversity of these genetically distinct proteins that are natural inhibitory proteins against prokaryotic CRISPR-Cas systems. We used AlphaFold-predicted structures of Acr proteins to infer a range of inhibition mechanisms through homology search and functional analysis, to demonstrate how bacteriophages exploit diverse strategies to manipulate host immune systems, with the long-term goal of providing a unique opportunity to learn from the evolution-optimized inhibitor proteins for future protein drug design.

2. Results

2.1. AlphaFold2 Prediction of Anti-CRISPR Protein Structures

The Acr protein datasets were acquired from various viral and prokaryotic genomes, including *Pseudomonas phage*, *Pseudomonas aeruginosa* and *Escherichia coli* [27], which were categorised into three sets: verified Acr proteins with experimental structure (Set A), verified Acr proteins without experimental structure (Set B), and putative Acr proteins with experimental structure (Set C) (Supplementary Table S1). From the AlphaFold-predicted structures of each set (Figure 2a), we compared the prediction performance between CASP14 (52 AlphaFold2 evaluation results from the CASP14 competition), Set A and Set C (Figure 2b,c), based on TM-scores, relative Z-errors (see Section 4 for details) and root mean square deviation (RMSD) (Supplementary Figure S1) against the true experimental structures (Supplementary Table S2), where Set B without experimental structures was excluded. According to the TM-score, CASP14 had a higher median than Set A and Set C

(0.925 vs. 0.895; 0.843, respectively), but Set A had the highest mean as compared to Set C and CASP14 (0.896 vs. 0.868; 0.882, respectively). Furthermore, Set A and Set C had significantly smaller standard deviations than CASP14 (0.095; 0.092, respectively, vs. 0.120), indicating that, according to the TM-score, their predictions are more accurate. According to the relative Z-error, CASP14 recorded a lower median than Set A and Set C (0.201 vs. 0.217; 0.230, respectively), but Set A recorded the lowest mean as compared to CASP14 and Set C (0.211 vs. 0.237; 0.259, respectively). Like the TM-score, Set A and Set C recorded smaller standard deviations than CASP14 (0.128; 0.129 vs. 0.141, respectively). For RMSD, Set A and Set C have more outliers and higher mean values than CASP 14 (2.206; 2.271 vs. 1.106, respectively). As can be seen in the boxplots (Figure 2b,c and Figure S1), there was no significant difference in prediction performance, validating that AlphaFold2 predicts 3-D structures of Acr proteins as accurately as the CASP14 dataset. Previous studies demonstrated that structures of identical proteins obtained from different experimental techniques had RMSD values of around 2.3 Å [28]. Thus, the average result of 2.271 Å in the RMSD distribution in Set C further validates the prediction performance of AlphaFold2 on Acr proteins.

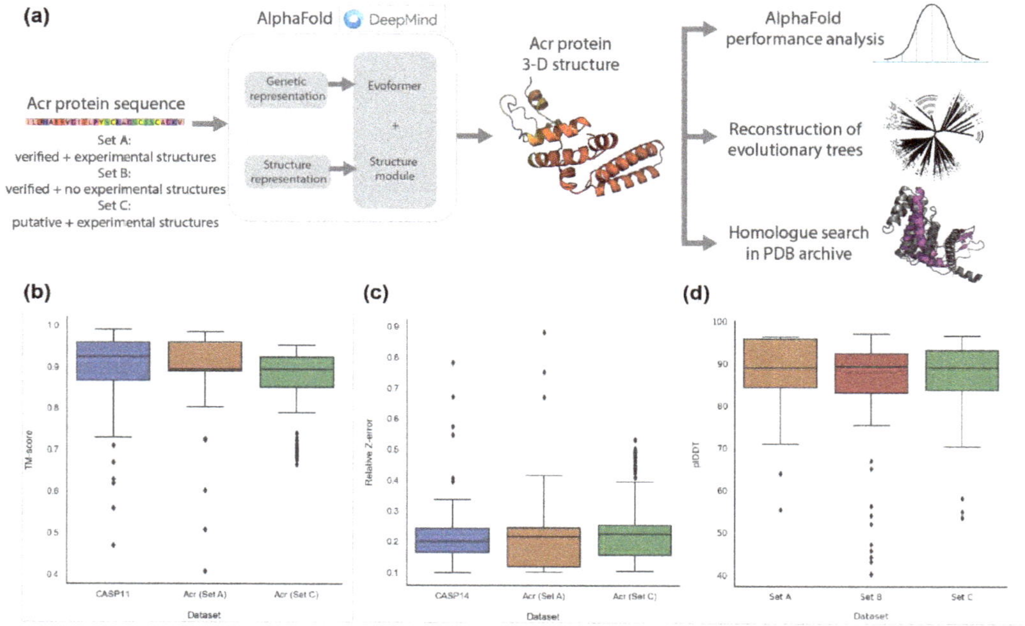

Figure 2. Performance analysis of AlphaFold2 on anti-CRISPR proteins in comparison to the CASP14 dataset. (**a**) Overall workflow to analyse the 3-D macromolecular structures of Acr protein sequences predicted with AlphaFold2. (**b**) The performance of AlphaFold2 on the Acr protein datasets in comparison to the CASP14 dataset using TM-scores. The closer the TM-score is to 1, the more similar the predicted structure is to its true experimental structure. (**c**) The performance of AlphaFold2 on the Acr protein datasets in comparison to the CASP14 dataset using relative Z-errors. The closer the relative Z-error is to 0, the more similar the predicted structure is to its true experimental structure. (**d**) The performance of AlphaFold2 on the Acr protein datasets using plDDT. The closer the plDDT is to 100, the higher the confidence level of prediction by AlphaFold2. (Set A: Verified Acr proteins with experimental structures, Set B: Verified Acr proteins without experimental structures, Set C: Putative Acr proteins with experimental structures).

For Set B without experimental structures, we calculated the predicted local distance difference test (plDDT) to check the confidence level of AlphaFold2 (Figure 2d). The median plDDT of Set B was almost identical to that of Set A and Set C (89.4 vs. 89.2; 89.1, respectively), but Set B had a slightly higher standard deviation (13.48 vs. 8.4; 7.84, respectively). However, as all the plDDT values of Set A, Set B and Set C (excluding a few outliers) were above the lower cut-off value of AlphaFold2 given as 70 [29], we concluded that the prediction quality of Set B was not significantly different from that of Set A and Set C.

2.2. Evolutionary Trees of Anti-CRISPR Proteins

The Acr proteins are known to be genetically diverse; this raises an intriguing question about the origin and evolution of Acr proteins. We reconstructed evolutionary trees of the verified Acr proteins (Set A + Set B; $n = 207$), using sequence-based and structure-based methods (see Section 4 for details). As expected, the phylogenetic tree built using genetic sequences (Figure 3a) shows high levels of variation, while forming consistent clades with the high bootstrap support. Analysis of the clades reveals some degree of clustering by the Acr family at the shallower nodes; however, this clustering is mostly due to the near-identical protein sequences. For instance, many of the AcrIIA proteins were derived from AcrIIA1 and AcrIIA2, driven by the technological interest to regulate CRISPR-Cas gene-editing activities in different cell types [22]. Otherwise, the phylogenetic tree shows absence of clustering by other biological features such as taxonomy and inhibition mechanism.

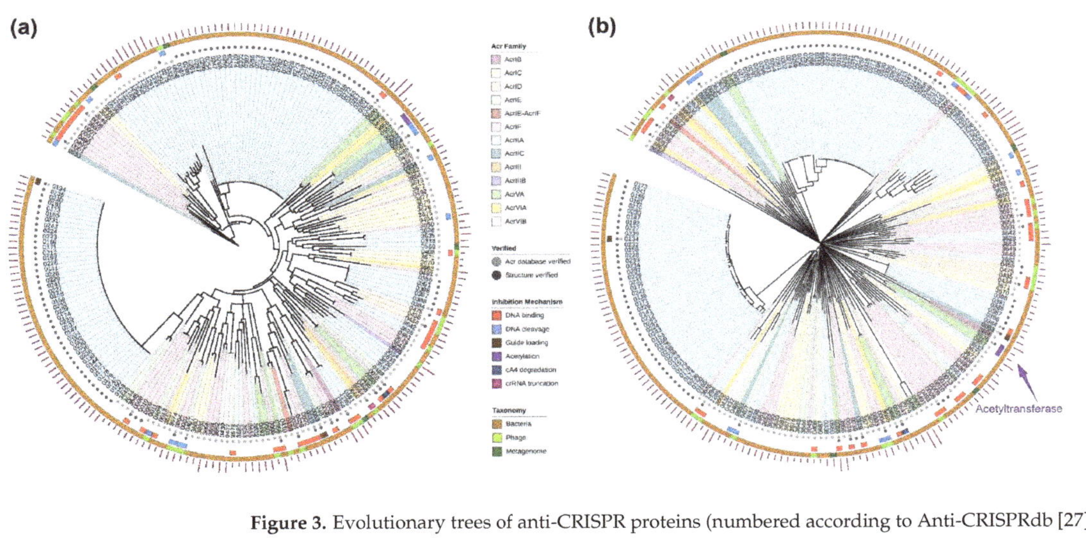

Figure 3. Evolutionary trees of anti-CRISPR proteins (numbered according to Anti-CRISPRdb [27]). (**a**) The phylogenetic tree of anti-CRISPR proteins reconstructed using sequence-based methods (Set A + Set B; $n = 207$). (**b**) The structural tree of anti-CRISPR proteins reconstructed using structure-based methods (Set A + Set B; $n = 207$). The clades of the two evolutionary trees were coloured by the Acr Family. The inner to outer rings display the Acr verification status, structural verification status, inhibition mechanism and source organism taxonomy. The outer magenta bars represent the genetic sequence length of each protein.

Given the low sequence similarity among the Acr proteins, we built a structure-based tree using AlphaFold-predicted structures, which included 98 Acr proteins without experimental structures (Figure 3b). The structural tree showed an even higher level of diversity in the Acr proteins than the phylogenetic tree. In the structural tree, the Acr proteins share no common ancestor and display deep branches, consistent with earlier observations of how evolutionary pressure drives immunity-related mechanisms of hosts and parasites to coevolve rapidly [12,13]. The structural tree also shows some degrees of clustering by the Acr family, but the clusters do not always coincide between the two evolutionary trees. The visual analysis of the protein structures show that the branches of the structural tree are placed randomly in terms of representative structural forms and the functions are only related at the clade level (Supplementary Figure S2).

It is evident that the sequence-based and structure-based trees capture different evolutionary relationships between the Acr proteins. The 3-D structures of homologous proteins were previously shown to be better conserved than their corresponding genetic sequences, particularly when the sequence similarity was below 30% [30]. From the multiple sequence alignment, no site of the Acr proteins was conserved at 30% and only very few sites were conserved at 15% (Supplementary Figures S3 and S4). We calculated the congruence among distance matrices of the sequence-based and structure-based trees to be very low according to the measure of congruence (Kendall's coefficient of concordance, $W = 6.58 \times 10^{-1}$), confirming the correlation between these two types of evolutionary trees is poor among highly divergent proteins [30].

2.3. Structural Homology to Predicted Anti-CRISPR Structures

The characterised Acr proteins use diverse strategies to interfere directly with CRISPR-Cas systems, including inhibiting DNA binding, DNA cleavage, guide loading and ribonuclease activity [22]. To investigate the relation between the 3-D protein structures and their inhibitory functions, we identified homologous structures to the AlphaFold-predicted Acr proteins using structure-based distance measures [31] (see Section 4 for details).

First, we used a subset of the Acr dataset with experimental structures (Set A) to successfully validate the closest structural homologue to each AlphaFold-predicted Acr protein matched with its true experimental structure (Supplementary Table S3).

Second, we analysed the Acr proteins without experimental structures (Set B) by matching the AlphaFold-predicted structures to the closest homologues from the Protein Data Bank archive [31] (Supplementary Table S4). We first validated that Acr proteins retrieved their neighbours in the same clade as the closest homologue, for those cases where their neighbouring proteins had experimental structures in the Protein Data Bank. For example, the Acr proteins labelled '0434' and '0435' are in the same clade, and the closest homologue of the Acr protein '0435' matched with the experimental structure of the Acr protein '0434'. Functional analysis of the closest homologue to each Acr protein revealed a wide variety of protein functions, including polymerase, ligase, nuclease, regulation, and transport (Figure 4c). We acknowledge that some of the closest homologues have low structural similarity (Z-score below 4); however, it is intriguing that these Acr proteins have no close structural homologues in the Protein Data Bank. Some Acr proteins from the families AcrIC6, AcrVIA2, AcrIIA19, and AcrIF8 (Figure 4a) have no structural homologues (significance threshold for similarity: Z-score = 2).

Third, we cross-examined the Acr proteins whose inhibitory mechanism was experimentally characterised to verify that the homologues retrieved were functionally related (indicated as the middle ring in Figure 3b). The homologue functions of this subset were related to a wide variety of functional domains (Supplementary Table S4). For instance, the two Acr proteins in the same clade (labelled '3628' and '3642') were characterised to inhibit the DNA-binding of Cas proteins [32] and their structural homologues have functional domains of ligase. A few closest homologues with functions related to acetyltransferase drew particular attention, as a recent biochemical study revealed an unprecedented mechanism of inhibiting CRISPR-Cas systems through enzymatic activity rather than through direct interaction [24]. According to this study, the closest structural homologue to this Acr protein (labelled '3625') was found to be N-Alpha-Acetyltransferase from *Homo sapiens* (4U9W-C) (Figure 4b), despite their low sequence similarity. We found another homologue (1Y9W-A) with a better similarity score to the AlphaFold-predicted structure of this Acr protein, that had the functional annotation of acetyltransferase from *Bacillus cereus* (Table 1).

In addition, we found several uncharacterised Acr proteins in the same clade of the structural tree (between '0430' and '3681') related to Acetylglucosaminidase from various Acr families, including AcrIC, AcrIE, AcrIF, AcrIIA, and AcrVIB. Intriguingly, several proteins have homologues with the functional annotations of nuclease activity, which is reminiscent of the newly-discovered mechanism of nuclease activity against crRNAs and CRISPR-Cas signalling molecules [33,34].

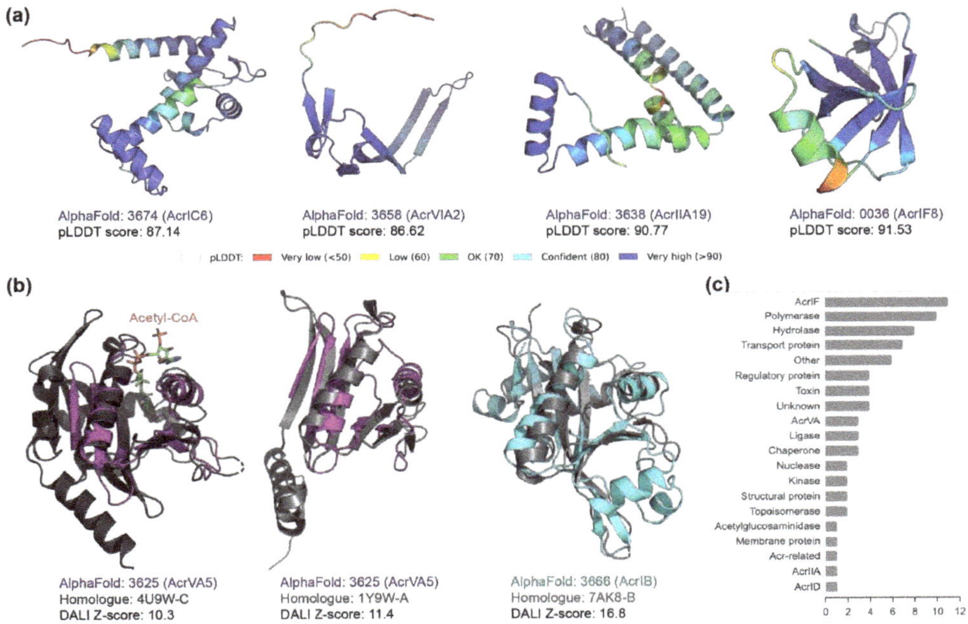

Figure 4. AlphaFold-predicted 3-D structures of outlier anti-CRISPR proteins. (**a**) The AlphaFold-predicted structures of the Acr proteins without homologues in the Protein Data Bank archive (Dali Z-score < 2). The 3-D protein structures are coloured according to the b-factor spectrum in PyMol, with a per-residue estimate of the AlphaFold2 confidence on a scale from 0–100 (high pLDDT accuracy in blue, low pLDDT accuracy in red). (**b**) Superimposition of the AlphaFold-predicted structures of Acr proteins and their closest structural homologues retrieved from the Protein Data Bank archive. All the closest structural homologues in grey have functional annotations related to acetyltransferase. The homologue to the Acr protein labelled '3625' has a cofactor (acetyl-CoA) bound, revealing the functionally critical site of the enzyme. (**c**) Functional analysis of the closest homologues to the AlphaFold-predicted Acr proteins without experimental structures (Set B). Only the functional annotations above the significance threshold of Dali Z-score (>4) were included.

Table 1. Closest homologue to the AlphaFold-predicted structure of Acr proteins with acetyltransferase annotations.

Acr ID	Family	Type	Length	Homologue	Dali Z-Score	Annotation	%ID Structure	%ID Sequence
3625	AcrVA5	V-A	92	4U9W-C	10.3	N-Alpha-Acetyltransferase	14	6.8
3625	AcrVA5	V-A	92	1Y9W-A	11.3	Acetyltransferase	22	16.8
3666	AcrIB	I-B	193	7AK8-B	16.8	Acetyltransferase	21	17.6

%ID structure: percentage identity in structure. %ID sequence: percentage identity in sequence.

2.4. New Anti-CRISPR Family of Acetylation Inhibition

Previously described Acr proteins of the Acr family VA5 disable Type V Cas12a by acetylation, which leads to a complete loss of the DNA-cleavage activity [24]. We found that this AcrVA5 protein (labelled '3625') structurally aligned closer to *Bacillus cereus* acetyltransferase than the previous structural homology of *Homo sapiens* acetyltransferase (Figure 4b). We further identified other Acr proteins that are related to this AcrVA5 protein on the evolutionary trees of the Acr proteins (Figure 3b). Notably, there are two Acr proteins in the same clade as the AcrVA5 protein on the structural tree, one of which was lacking experimentally validated structure or function. Analysis of its function using the structural homologues reveals that this Acr protein (labelled '3666') is related to acetyltransferase. Interestingly, this Acr protein belongs to a different Acr family (AcrIB) than the previously identified AcrVA5. Its superimposition with the closest structural homologue reveals a similar structural alignment at the functionally critical site of the acetyltransferase where acetyl-CoA binds (Figure 4b). The sequence identity of the AcrIB protein to its closest homologue was found to be 17.6% (Supplementary Table S4), while the structural identity between these two proteins in 3-D was found to be higher at 21% (Table 1 and Supplementary Figure S5). On the phylogenetic tree, this AcrIB protein was not placed close to the other two Acr proteins of acetyltransferase function (labelled '3625' and '0557') (Figure 3a), demonstrating that these two types of Acr proteins have close structural similarity but not genetic similarity. This finding suggests that for proteins with low sequence similarity, structure-based trees cluster proteins with most similar biochemical functional properties perform better than sequence-based trees [30]. Using the structural tree, we discovered a new family of Acr proteins belonging to AcrIB that was structurally similar to acetyltransferase from a different organism (gram-negative bacteria *Salmonella enterica*), whereas the previously characterised AcrVA5 matched to acetyltransferase from gram-positive bacteria *Bacillus cereus*.

3. Discussion

We show that the 3-D structures of Acr proteins predicted with AlphaFold2 achieve high accuracy. The structural tree reconstructed from these AlphaFold-predicted structures display more diversity of Acr proteins with no common evolutionary origin as compared to the phylogenetic tree. On the structural tree, the Acr proteins form small clades by their unique structural similarity, which are also related by the inhibition mechanism. The functional annotations of the Acr protein homologues are extremely diverse, relating to a wide range of enzymatic and regulatory activities from different organisms. Most characterised Acr proteins inhibit host CRISPR-Cas systems by direct interference; we show that this category of Acr proteins displays various functional annotations and unique structural forms in the multiple branches of the structural tree.

Specifically, we found a number of Acr proteins with homologue annotations related to acetylation. A recent discovery of Acr proteins that manipulate CRISPR-Cas systems through enzymatic activities demonstrates extensive phage defence mechanisms driven by the intense host-parasite arms race [24,33]. Through the AlphaFold-predicted structural analysis, we found a novel family of Acr proteins (AcrIB) from the genome of a human pathogen (*Leptotrichia buccalis* C-1013-b) that shows more structural similarity to acetyltransferase than the previously characterised AcrVA protein. Intriguingly, other Acr proteins on the multiple branches of the structural tree have homologues related to different types of acetyltransferase enzymes from heterologous species. As Acr proteins with acetyltransferase activities permanently disable Cas proteins by covalent modification [24], other Acr proteins with enzymatic activities such as acetylglucosaminidase are expected to have similar inactivation functions of biochemically modifying CRISPR-Cas systems. The Acr proteins could evolve independently from various host genomes and mobile genetic elements, exploiting a vast inventory of protein structures as the basis for their counter-defence advantage [10,13,35].

More broadly, Acr proteins are exceptional examples of coevolution dynamics optimizing the phage genomes to manipulate host systems and maximize survival. As phages can only replicate within host cells and are void of metabolic capacity to synthesize small molecules, their counter-defence machinery against the sophisticated and extensive prokaryotic anti-phage systems is protein-based. Nonetheless, phages are the most abundant biological entities in the biosphere [36], and their successful protein-based viral arsenals such as Acr proteins provide an important insight on how to expand the potential of protein therapeutics. Specifically, we could get inspiration from these phage-derived protein structures that resemble segments of related target proteins, to design highly-specialised protein inhibitors with diverse protein-manipulating strategies [37]. In future, utilizing the ability of small proteins to engage in indirect interference through enzymatic activities is to be explored against disease-causing proteins (such as in cancer) and disease-causing organisms (such as drug-resistant bacteria) [36].

4. Materials and Methods

4.1. Curation of Anti-CRISPR Datasets

The anti-CRISPR dataset contained 443 Acr proteins (207 verified, 236 putative) that inhibit a wide range of CRISPR-Cas systems including I, II, III and VI from the Anti-CRISPRdb [27]. The term 'verified' indicates that the protein was validated as CRISPR-Cas-inactivating Acr (either by the database or other published papers), while 'putative' indicates the protein was predicted to be Acr without sufficient experimental support. The anti-CRISPR dataset was further curated into Set A, Set B, and Set C for AlphaFold2, according to the availability of experimentally reconstructed 3-D macromolecular structures (hereby referred to as "experimental structures") (Supplementary Table S1). Each protein was annotated with the Acr family, type of inhibited CRISPR-Cas systems, NCBI accession, genetic sequence, source organism, taxonomy, and inhibitory mechanism when available (Supplementary Tables S3 and S4).

4.2. Prediction of Anti-CRISPR Protein Structure with AlphaFold2

We predicted the 3-D protein structures of each set with AlphaFold2, using the Acr protein sequence as the input to AlphaFold2 (Figure 2a). AlphaFold2 creates genetic and structural representations by comparing the protein sequence with several pre-installed databases. Those representations are used as input to five prediction models to generate five candidate 3-D structures. The result with the highest per-residue confidence score (pLDDT: per residue estimate of confidence on a scale from 0 to 100 [29]) among the five results was determined as the final structure and saved in a protein data bank (PDB) format (Supplementary Figure S6). For the Acr datasets, we used the PDB archive until 31 December 2012 as templates in AlphaFold2 to exclude the true experimental structures of the Acr proteins. The details of the experiments related to the hardware specification and to the processor performance are given in the Supplementary Material (Supplementary Table S5 and Supplementary Table S6, respectively).

4.3. Comparison of AlphaFold2 Performance on Anti-CRISPR against CASP14

To validate the performance of AlphaFold2 for predicting Acr structures, we benchmarked the CASP14 dataset against Set A and Set C of Acr proteins with the corresponding true experimental structures available. We excluded predicted structure and experimental structure pairs for which the TM-score and/or the Z-score were too low. Finally, 52 pairs of CASP14, 99 pairs of Set A, and 207 pairs of Set C were used for the comparison study. We used the TM-score [38,39] and Dali Z-score [40] as similarity measures between the predicted and the experimental structures. Unlike traditional metrics (e.g., root-mean-square deviation), the TM-score is length-independent and more sensitive to the global similarity than to the local variation. The Dali Z-score is the sum of the equivalent residue-wise intermolecular distances among two proteins, and does not have a fixed upper bound [40]. We then used the following relative Z-error to calculate the relative difference:

$$Z_{error} = \frac{Z_{gt} - Z_{pd}}{Z_{gt}} \tag{1}$$

where Z_{gt} is the self Dali Z-score between experimental structure and itself, and Z_{pd} is the Dali Z-score between experimental structure and predicted structure. We obtained the Z_{pd} and TM-score for the CASP14 set of AlphaFold2 from the CASP14 assessment scores [41], whereas Z_{gt} of CASP14 and Z_{gt} and Z_{pd} of Set A and Set C were calculated using DaliLite.v5 [40]. Finally, a protein structure comparison and clustering tool called MaxCluster [42] was used to calculate the TM-scores of Set A and Set C. Both distance metrics have values between 0 and 1, with 1 as the best score for TM-scores and 0 as the best score for relative Z-errors.

4.4. Reconstruction of Evolutionary Trees of Anti-CRISPR Proteins

We reconstructed the evolutionary trees of the anti-CRISPR dataset (Set A and Set B) using sequence-based and structure-based inference. Set C was excluded from the evolutionary analysis due to the absence of functional verification and due to sequence variation (Supplementary Figure S3). The sequence-based tree of the Acr proteins was built by aligning the amino acid sequences using a multiple alignment program, MAFFT (version 7.471, -auto option) [43]. The multiple sequence alignment of the Acr proteins was then visualized using Jalview (version 2.11.1.3) with a conservation visibility of 15% (Supplementary Figure S2) [44]. Subsequently, a phylogenetic tree of the Acr proteins was built with IQ-Tree using ModelFinder (-auto option) to find the best-fit model among the supported range of protein substitution models [45,46] (Supplementary Table S7). Using the best-fit substitution model, 1000 ultrafast bootstrap replicates were run to check bootstrap support of the reconstructed tree topology [47].

The structure-based tree of the Acr proteins was built by calculating the similarity matrix between the Dali Z-scores of the AlphaFold-predicted structures and its corresponding experimental structures. We used the Dali server [40] for generating structural trees from hierarchical clustering of the similarity matrix. The structural tree of the Acr proteins was generated from distance matrices, where the pseudo-distance between two structures Q and T was defined as [48]:

$$D_{QT} = Z_{QQ} + Z_{TT} - 2Z_{QT} \tag{2}$$

The hierarchical clustering of the similarity matrix was outputted as a Newick formatted dendrogram. The phylogenetic tree and the structural tree of the Acr proteins were visualized with iTOL (version 4) and iTOL annotation editor [49,50] with the following labels: Acr Family, Taxonomy, and Inhibition Mechanism.

4.5. Congruence among Distance Matrices of Sequence-Based and Structure-Based Trees

We measured the congruence among distance matrices of the reconstructed trees from the sequence-based and structure-based methods using Kendall's coefficient of concordance, W, which ranges from 0 (no congruence) to 1 (complete congruence) [51]. First, we computed the cophenetic value of pairwise distances between the terminals from a phylogenetic tree using its branch lengths with the function cophenetic.phylo from ape-package (version 5.0) [52]. Then, we used the function CADM.global to calculate the coefficient of concordance among the distance matrices of the sequence-based and structure-based trees of the Acr proteins through a permutation test.

4.6. Visualization of Protein Structure Superimposition

For functional analysis, the AlphaFold-predicted structures with functional annotations of interest were superimposed with their structural homologues using PyMol (version 2.5.2) to visualize the overlap in structure of the functionally active sites. The inhibitory mechanism of the Acr proteins without experimental structure was inferred through examining functional annotations of the structural homologues to the AlphaFold-predicted structure, with the significance threshold of Z-score > 4.

4.7. Code Availability

Protein structures were predicted with AlphaFold2, available under an open-source license at https://github.com/deepmind/alphafold, accessed on 27 September 2021. For protein structure similarity metrics, we used MaxCluster (http://www.sbg.bio.ic.ac.uk/~maxcluster/index.html, accessed on 13 October 2021) for TM-score and DaliLite.v5 (http://ekhidna2.biocenter.helsinki.fi/dali/README.v5.html, accessed on 24 October 2021) for the Dali Z-score. For MSA, we used MAFFT.v7 (https://mafft.cbrc.jp/alignment/server, accessed on 29 October 2021) and Jalview.v2 (https://www.jalview.org, accessed on 29 October 2021) for visualization. For phylogenetic tree reconstruction, we used IQ-Tree (http://www.iqtree.org, accessed on 14 November 2021) with ModelFinder and UFBoot options. For structural tree reconstruction, we used the Dali server (http://ekhidna2.biocenter.helsinki.fi/dali, accessed on 16 November 2021) for building dendrograms. The 3-D Structure visualizations were created in Pymol v.2.5.2 (https://pymol.org, accessed on 4 November 2021) and Py3DMol v.1.7.0 (https://pypi.org/project/py3Dmol, accessed on 26 October 2021) with Jupyter v.1.0.0 (https://jupyter.org, accessed on 26 October 2021). For data analysis, Python v.3.6.4 (https://www.python.org, accessed on 27 November 2021), NumPy v.1.17.5 (https://github.com/numpy/numpy, accessed on 27 November 2021), SciPy v.1.1.0 (https://www.scipy.org, accessed on 27 November 2021), seaborn v.0.9.0 (https://github.com/mwaskom/seaborn, accessed on 25 November 2021), Matplotlib v.3.3.4 (https://github.com/matplotlib/matplotlib, accessed on 24 November 2021), pandas v.0.22.0 (https://github.com/pandas-dev/pandas, accessed on 24 November 2021) were used.

5. Conclusions

The high biodegradability issue of protein therapeutics has partially been solved by the recent success of mRNA vaccine delivery using lipid nanoparticles [53], making low risk protein therapeutics ever more attractive to the industry. From the AlphaFold-predicted structures, we accelerated the structural and functional analysis of the Acr proteins whose experimental 3-D structures remain to be resolved. In conclusion, we wonder whether there is a vast repertoire of unexplored protein structural configurations that can be exploited for protein drug design, given the number of Acr proteins without homologues in the current protein structure domain.

Supplementary Materials: The following supporting information can be downloaded at: https://www.mdpi.com/article/10.3390/ph15030310/s1. Figure S1. The performance of AlphaFold2 on the Acr protein datasets in comparison to the CASP14 dataset using RMSD; Figure S2. The structural tree of anti-CRISPR proteins reconstructed using structure-based methods; Figure S3. Multiple sequence alignment of anti-CRISPR proteins using MAFFT, visualized with Jalview; Figure S4. The structural tree of anti-CRISPR proteins reconstructed using structure-based methods; Figure S5. A scatter plot of percentage identity in structure against percentage identity in sequence of the closest homologue to each protein; Figure S6. Outlier AlphaFold structures with bad scores; Table S1. Acr protein types in Anti-CRISPRdb; Table S2. Detailed statistics and scores on AlphaFold prediction performance; Table S3. Closest homologue (highest TM score) to the AlphaFold-predicted structure of Acr proteins with experimentally reconstructed 3-D macromolecular structures (Set A) from the Protein Data Bank archive; Table S4. Closest homologue (highest DALI Z-score) to the AlphaFold-predicted structure of Acr proteins without experimentally reconstructed 3-D macromolecular structures (Set B) from the Protein Data Bank archive; Table S5. Hardware specification for AlphaFold experiments; Table S6. Time to create a 3-D structure from one protein sequence (in seconds); Table S7. The best-fit-model of the phylogenetic tree of each Acr set using IQ-TREE ModelFinder.

Author Contributions: Conceptualization, H.S.; methodology, H.-M.P. and H.S.; software, H.-M.P. and H.S.; validation, H.-M.P., Y.P. and H.S.; formal analysis, H.-M.P., Y.P. and H.S.; investigation,

H.-M.P., Y.P. and H.S.; resources, J.V. and W.D.N.; data curation, H.-M.P. and H.S.; writing, H.-M.P., Y.P., J.V., A.V.M., W.D.N. and H.S.; visualization, H.-M.P. and H.S. All authors have read and agreed to the published version of the manuscript.

Funding: This research was funded by Ghent University Global Campus grant number [RC4].

Institutional Review Board Statement: Not applicable.

Informed Consent Statement: Not applicable.

Data Availability Statement: Publicly available datasets were analyzed in this study. All the input protein sequences analysed in this study are available in Anti-CRISPRdb at https://doi.org/10.1093/nar/gkx835 (accessed on 13 November 2021). As well as our project GitHub page which can be found here: https://github.com/powersimmani/ACR_alphafold, accessed on 28 November 2021. All the 3-D structures used as ground truth for calculating Dali Z-scores and TM-scores; and superimposing structures in this study are available in Protein Data Bank at https://www.rcsb.org/ accessed on 13 November 2021. CASP (Critical Assessment of Structure Prediction) competition datasets were used for measuring AlphaFold performance. This data can be found here: https://predictioncenter.org/casp14/, accessed on 29 September 2021.

Acknowledgments: We thank members of the Center for Biosystems and Biotech Data Science at GUGC for helpful discussions.

Conflicts of Interest: The authors declare no conflict of interest.

References

1. Lander, E.S.; Linton, L.M.; Birren, B.; Nusbaum, C.; Zody, M.C.; Baldwin, J.; Devon, K.; Dewar, K.; Doyle, M.; FitzHugh, W.; et al. Initial sequencing and analysis of the human genome. *Nature* **2001**, *409*, 860–921. [PubMed]
2. Venter, J.C.; Adams, M.D.; Myers, E.W.; Li, P.W.; Mural, R.J.; Sutton, G.G.; Smith, H.O.; Yandell, M.; Evans, C.A.; Holt, R.A.; et al. The sequence of the human genome. *Science* **2001**, *291*, 1304–1351. [CrossRef]
3. Hopkins, A.L.; Groom, C.R. The druggable genome. *Nat. Rev. Drug Discov.* **2002**, *1*, 727–730. [CrossRef]
4. Goeddel, D.V.; Kleid, D.G.; Bolivar, F.; Heyneker, H.L.; Yansura, D.G.; Crea, R.; Hirose, T.; Kraszewski, A.; Itakura, K.; Riggs, A.D. Expression in Escherichia coli of chemically synthesized genes for human insulin. *Proc. Natl. Acad. Sci. USA* **1979**, *76*, 106–110. [CrossRef] [PubMed]
5. Leader, B.; Baca, Q.J.; Golan, D.E. Protein therapeutics: A summary and pharmacological classification. *Nat. Rev. Drug Discov.* **2008**, *7*, 21–39. [CrossRef] [PubMed]
6. Bishop, B.; Dasgupta, J.; Klein, M.; Garcea, R.L.; Christensen, N.D.; Zhao, R.; Chen, X.S. Crystal structures of four types of human papillomavirus L1 capsid proteins: Understanding the specificity of neutralizing monoclonal antibodies. *J. Biol. Chem.* **2007**, *282*, 31803–31811. [CrossRef]
7. Fávero-Retto, M.P.; Palmieri, L.C.; Souza, T.A.C.B.; Almeida, F.C.L.; Lima, L.M.T.R. Structural meta-analysis of regular human insulin in pharmaceutical formulations. *Eur. J. Pharm. Biopharm.* **2013**, *85*, 1112–1121. [CrossRef]
8. Luthra, A.; Langley, D.B.; Schofield, P.; Jackson, J.; Abdelatti, M.; Rouet, R.; Nevoltris, D.; Mazigi, O.; Crossett, B.; Christie, M.; et al. Human antibody bispecifics through phage display selection. *Biochemistry* **2019**, *58*, 1701–1704. [CrossRef]
9. Ostrov, D.A.; Shi, W.; Schwartz, J.C.; Almo, S.C.; Nathenson, S.G. Structure of murine CTLA-4 and its role in modulating T cell responsiveness. *Science* **2000**, *290*, 816–819. [CrossRef] [PubMed]
10. Dion, M.B.; Oechslin, F.; Moineau, S. Phage diversity, genomics and phylogeny. *Nat. Rev. Microbiol.* **2020**, *18*, 125–138. [CrossRef] [PubMed]
11. Koonin, E.V.; Dolja, V.V.; Krupovic, M. Origins and evolution of viruses of eukaryotes: The ultimate modularity. *Virology* **2015**, *479–480*, 2–25. [CrossRef] [PubMed]
12. Watson, B.N.J.; Steens, J.A.; Staals, R.H.J.; Westra, E.R.; van Houte, S. Coevolution between bacterial CRISPR-Cas systems and their bacteriophages. *Cell Host Microbe* **2021**, *29*, 715–725. [CrossRef]
13. Hampton, H.G.; Watson, B.N.J.; Fineran, P.C. The arms race between bacteria and their phage foes. *Nature* **2020**, *577*, 327–336. [CrossRef] [PubMed]
14. Jansen, R.; van Embden, J.D.A.; Gaastra, W.; Schouls, L.M. Identification of genes that are associated with DNA repeats in prokaryotes. *Mol. Microbiol.* **2002**, *43*, 1565–1575. [CrossRef] [PubMed]
15. Mojica, F.J.M.; Díez-Villaseñor, C.; García-Martínez, J.; Soria, E. Intervening sequences of regularly spaced prokaryotic repeats derive from foreign genetic elements. *J. Mol. Evol.* **2005**, *60*, 174–182. [CrossRef] [PubMed]
16. Barrangou, R.; Fremaux, C.; Deveau, H.; Richards, M.; Boyaval, P.; Moineau, S.; Romero, D.A.; Horvath, P. CRISPR provides acquired resistance against viruses in prokaryotes. *Science* **2007**, *315*, 1709–1712. [CrossRef]
17. Deltcheva, E.; Chylinski, K.; Sharma, C.M.; Gonzales, K.; Chao, Y.; Pirzada, Z.A.; Eckert, M.R.; Vogel, J.; Charpentier, E. CRISPR RNA maturation by trans-encoded small RNA and host factor RNase III. *Nature* **2011**, *471*, 602–607. [CrossRef]

18. Jinek, M.; Chylinski, K.; Fonfara, I.; Hauer, M.; Doudna, J.A.; Charpentier, E. A programmable dual-RNA-guided DNA endonuclease in adaptive bacterial immunity. *Science* **2012**, *337*, 816–821. [CrossRef] [PubMed]
19. Makarova, K.S.; Wolf, Y.I.; Iranzo, J.; Shmakov, S.A.; Alkhnbashi, O.S.; Brouns, S.J.J.; Charpentier, E.; Cheng, D.; Haft, D.H.; Horvath, P.; et al. Evolutionary classification of CRISPR-Cas systems: A burst of class 2 and derived variants. *Nat. Rev. Microbiol.* **2020**, *18*, 67–83. [CrossRef] [PubMed]
20. Bondy-Denomy, J.; Pawluk, A.; Maxwell, K.L.; Davidson, A.R. Bacteriophage genes that inactivate the CRISPR/Cas bacterial immune system. *Nature* **2013**, *493*, 429–432. [CrossRef] [PubMed]
21. Pawluk, A.; Bondy-Denomy, J.; Cheung, V.H.W.; Maxwell, K.L.; Davidson, A.R. A new group of phage anti-CRISPR genes inhibits the type I-E CRISPR-Cas system of *Pseudomonas aeruginosa*. *MBio* **2014**, *5*, e00896:1–e00896:7. [CrossRef] [PubMed]
22. Marino, N.D.; Pinilla-Redondo, R.; Csörgő, B.; Bondy-Denomy, J. Anti-CRISPR protein applications: Natural brakes for CRISPR-Cas technologies. *Nat. Methods* **2020**, *17*, 471–479. [CrossRef]
23. Pawluk, A.; Staals, R.H.J.; Taylor, C.; Watson, B.N.J.; Saha, S.; Fineran, P.C.; Maxwell, K.L.; Davidson, A.R. Inactivation of CRISPR-Cas systems by anti-CRISPR proteins in diverse bacterial species. *Nat. Microbiol.* **2016**, *1*, 16085:1–16085:6. [CrossRef] [PubMed]
24. Dong, L.; Guan, X.; Li, N.; Zhang, F.; Zhu, Y.; Ren, K.; Yu, L.; Zhou, F.; Han, Z.; Gao, N.; et al. An anti-CRISPR protein disables type V Cas12a by acetylation. *Nat. Struct. Mol. Biol.* **2019**, *26*, 308–314. [CrossRef] [PubMed]
25. Jumper, J.; Evans, R.; Pritzel, A.; Green, T.; Figurnov, M.; Ronneberger, O.; Tunyasuvunakool, K.; Bates, R.; Žídek, A.; Potapenko, A.; et al. Highly accurate protein structure prediction with AlphaFold. *Nature* **2021**, *596*, 583–589. [CrossRef]
26. Callaway, E. 'It will change everything': DeepMind's AI makes gigantic leap in solving protein structures. *Nature* **2020**, *588*, 203–204. [CrossRef] [PubMed]
27. Dong, C.; Hao, G.F.; Hua, H.L.; Liu, S.; Labena, A.A.; Chai, G.; Huang, J.; Rao, N.; Guo, F.B. Anti-CRISPRdb: A comprehensive online resource for anti-CRISPR proteins. *Nucleic Acids Res.* **2018**, *46*, D393–D398. [CrossRef] [PubMed]
28. Kufareva, I.; Abagyan, R. Methods of protein structure comparison. *Methods Mol. Biol.* **2012**, *857*, 231–257. [PubMed]
29. Tunyasuvunakool, K.; Adler, J.; Wu, Z.; Green, T.; Zielinski, M.; Žídek, A.; Bridgland, A.; Cowie, A.; Meyer, C.; Laydon, A.; et al. Highly accurate protein structure prediction for the human proteome. *Nature* **2021**, *596*, 590–596. [CrossRef] [PubMed]
30. Balaji, S.; Srinivasan, N. Comparison of sequence-based and structure-based phylogenetic trees of ho-mologous proteins: Inferences on protein evolution. *J. Biosci.* **2007**, *32*, 83–96. [CrossRef]
31. Berman, H.M.; Westbrook, J.; Feng, Z.; Gilliland, G.; Bhat, T.N.; Weissig, H.; Shindyalov, I.N.; Bourne, P.E. The protein data bank. *Nucleic Acids Res.* **2000**, *28*, 235–242. [CrossRef] [PubMed]
32. Watters, K.E.; Shivram, H.; Fellmann, C.; Lew, R.J.; McMahon, B.; Doudna, J.A. Potent CRISPR-Cas9 inhibitors from Staphylococcus genomes. *Proc. Natl. Acad. Sci. USA* **2020**, *117*, 6531–6539. [CrossRef] [PubMed]
33. Athukoralage, J.S.; McMahon, S.A.; Zhang, C.; Grüschow, S.; Graham, S.; Krupovic, M.; Whitaker, R.J.; Gloster, T.M.; White, M.F. An anti-CRISPR viral ring nuclease subverts type III CRISPR immunity. *Nature* **2020**, *577*, 572–575. [CrossRef] [PubMed]
34. Knott, G.J.; Thornton, B.W.; Lobba, M.J.; Liu, J.J.; Al-Shayeb, B.; Watters, K.E.; Doudna, J.A. Broad-spectrum enzymatic inhibition of CRISPR-Cas12a. *Nat. Struct. Mol. Biol.* **2019**, *26*, 315–321. [CrossRef] [PubMed]
35. Shim, H. Feature learning of virus genome evolution with the nucleotide skip-gram neural network. *Evol. Bioinform.* **2019**, *15*, 1176934318821072:1–1176934318821072:10. [CrossRef] [PubMed]
36. Frost, L.S.; Leplae, R.; Summers, A.O.; Toussaint, A. Mobile genetic elements: The agents of open source evolution. *Nat. Rev. Microbiol.* **2005**, *3*, 722–732. [CrossRef] [PubMed]
37. Shim, H.; Shivram, H.; Lei, S.; Doudna, J.A.; Banfield, J.F. Diverse ATPase proteins in mobilomes constitute a large potential sink for prokaryotic host ATP. *Front. Microbiol.* **2021**, *12*, 691847:1–691847:11. [CrossRef] [PubMed]
38. Xu, J.; Zhang, Y. How significant is a protein structure similarity with TM-score = 0.5? *Bioinformatics* **2010**, *26*, 889–895. [CrossRef]
39. Zhang, Y.; Skolnick, J. Scoring function for automated assessment of protein structure template quality. *Proteins* **2004**, *57*, 702–710. [CrossRef]
40. Holm, L. Using Dali for protein structure comparison. *Methods Mol. Biol.* **2020**, *2112*, 29–42. [PubMed]
41. Kryshtafovych, A.; Schwede, T.; Topf, M.; Fidelis, K.; Moult, J. Critical assessment of methods of pro-tein structure prediction (CASP)-Round XIV. *Proteins* **2021**, *89*, 1607–1617. [CrossRef] [PubMed]
42. Siew, N.; Elofsson, A.; Rychlewski, L.; Fischer, D. MaxSub: An automated measure for the assessment of protein structure prediction quality. *Bioinformatics* **2000**, *16*, 776–785. [CrossRef] [PubMed]
43. Katoh, K.; Rozewicki, J.; Yamada, K.D. MAFFT online service: Multiple sequence alignment, interactive sequence choice and visualization. *Brief. Bioinform.* **2019**, *20*, 1160–1166. [CrossRef]
44. Taylor, W.R. Residual colours: A proposal for aminochromography. *Protein Eng.* **1997**, *10*, 743–746. [CrossRef]
45. Nguyen, L.T.; Schmidt, H.A.; von Haeseler, A.; Minh, B.Q. IQ-TREE: A Fast and Effective Stochastic Algorithm for Estimating Maximum-Likelihood Phylogenies. *Mol. Biol. Evol.* **2015**, *32*, 268–274. [CrossRef]
46. Kalyaanamoorthy, S.; Minh, B.Q.; Wong, T.K.F.; von Haeseler, A.; Jermiin, L.S. ModelFinder: Fast model selection for accurate phylogenetic estimates. *Nat. Methods* **2017**, *14*, 587–589. [CrossRef]
47. Hoang, D.T.; Chernomor, O.; von Haeseler, A.; Minh, B.Q.; Vinh, L.S. UFBoot2: Improving the Ultra-fast Bootstrap Approximation. *Mol. Biol. Evol.* **2018**, *35*, 518–522. [CrossRef]
48. Holm, L. DALI and the persistence of protein shape. *Protein Sci.* **2019**, *29*, 128–140. [CrossRef] [PubMed]

49. Letunic, I.; Bork, P. Interactive Tree Of Life (iTOL) v4: Recent updates and new developments. *Nucleic Acids Res.* **2019**, *47*, W256–W259. [CrossRef] [PubMed]
50. Letunic, I.; Bork, P. Interactive Tree Of Life (iTOL): An online tool for phylogenetic tree display and annotation. *Bioinformatics* **2007**, *23*, 127–128. [CrossRef] [PubMed]
51. Legendre, P. Species associations: The Kendall coefficient of concordance revisited. *JABES* **2005**, *10*, 226–245. [CrossRef]
52. Paradis, E.; Schliep, K. ape 5.0: An environment for modern phylogenetics and evolutionary analyses in R. *Bioinformatics* **2019**, *35*, 526–528. [CrossRef]
53. Jackson, N.A.C.; Kester, K.E.; Casimiro, D.; Gurunathan, S.; Derosa, F. The promise of mRNA vaccines: A biotech and industrial perspective. *npj Vaccines* **2020**, *5*, 11:1–11:6. [CrossRef] [PubMed]

pharmaceuticals MDPI

Article

Exploring the Prominent and Concealed Inhibitory Features for Cytoplasmic Isoforms of Hsp90 Using QSAR Analysis

Magdi E. A. Zaki [1,*], Sami A. Al-Hussain [1], Syed Nasir Abbas Bukhari [2], Vijay H. Masand [3,*], Mithilesh M. Rathore [3], Sumer D. Thakur [4] and Vaishali M. Patil [5]

1 Department of Chemistry, Faculty of Science, Imam Mohammad Ibn Saud Islamic University, Riyadh 13318, Saudi Arabia; sahussain@imamu.edu.sa
2 Department of Pharmaceutical Chemistry, College of Pharmacy, Jouf University, Al Jouf 72388, Saudi Arabia; sbukhari@ju.edu.sa
3 Department of Chemistry, Vidya Bharati Mahavidyalaya, Amravati 444 602, Maharashtra, India; mithsrathore@gmail.com
4 Department of Chemistry, RDIK and NKD College, Badnera-Amravati 444 701, Maharashtra, India; sdthakur11@gmail.com
5 Department of Pharmaceutical Chemistry, KIET School of Pharmacy, KIET Group of Institutions, Delhi-NCR, Ghaziabad 201206, Uttar Pradesh, India; vaishuwise@gmail.com
* Correspondence: mezaki@imamu.edu.sa (M.E.A.Z.); vijaymasand@gmail.com (V.H.M.)

Citation: Zaki, M.E.A.; Al-Hussain, S.A.; Bukhari, S.N.A.; Masand, V.H.; Rathore, M.M.; Thakur, S.D.; Patil, V.M. Exploring the Prominent and Concealed Inhibitory Features for Cytoplasmic Isoforms of Hsp90 Using QSAR Analysis. *Pharmaceuticals* **2022**, *15*, 303. https://doi.org/10.3390/ph15030303

Academic Editor: Osvaldo Andrade Santos-Filho

Received: 21 January 2022
Accepted: 23 February 2022
Published: 1 March 2022

Abstract: Cancer is a major life-threatening disease with a high mortality rate in many countries. Even though different therapies and options are available, patients generally prefer chemotherapy. However, serious side effects of anti-cancer drugs compel us to search for a safer drug. To achieve this target, Hsp90 (heat shock protein 90), which is responsible for stabilization of many oncoproteins in cancer cells, is a promising target for developing an anti-cancer drug. The QSAR (Quantitative Structure–Activity Relationship) could be useful to identify crucial pharmacophoric features to develop a Hsp90 inhibitor. Therefore, in the present work, a larger dataset encompassing 1141 diverse compounds was used to develop a multi-linear QSAR model with a balance of acceptable predictive ability (Predictive QSAR) and mechanistic interpretation (Mechanistic QSAR). The new developed six-parameter model satisfies the recommended values for a good number of validation parameters such as R2tr = 0.78, Q2LMO = 0.77, R2ex = 0.78, and CCCex = 0.88. The present analysis reveals that the Hsp90 inhibitory activity is correlated with different types of nitrogen atoms and other hidden structural features such as the presence of hydrophobic ring/aromatic carbon atoms within a specific distance from the center of mass of the molecule, etc. Thus, the model successfully identified a variety of reported as well as novel pharmacophoric features. The results of QSAR analysis are further vindicated by reported crystal structures of compounds with Hsp90.

Keywords: Hsp90; cancer; QSAR; machine learning; pharmacophores

1. Introduction

Cancer kills; therefore, medicinal chemists are continuously trying to develop therapeutic agents that could retard the growth of cancer cells. In cancer cells, a protein Hsp90 (heat shock protein 90, also known as HSPC) is overexpressed [1]. It is a highly conserved, non-fibrous, and chaperone protein with a key role in many cellular processes like proper folding of other proteins, apoptosis, cell cycle control, cell viability, and degradation and signaling events [1–6]. As the name indicates, Hsp (heat shock proteins) shield cells when stressed by higher temperatures. The number "90" comes from the fact that it weighs about 90 kDa. There are two isoforms of Hsp90: Hsp90α (the inducible form) and Hsp90β (the constitutive form), which are found in cytoplasm and share 85% sequence identity [1–6]. These two isoforms are like flexible biological catalysts and interact with a good number of newly synthesized proteins, such as Akt2, CDKs, PKC, MAP kinases, steroid receptors,

BCL-6, CAR, p53, Oct4, etc., to avoid their aggregation or mistakes in their folding [6]. Despite a crucial role, in cancer cells, these are responsible for the stabilization of a number of oncoproteins required for tumor growth, leading to their overexpression [1–6]. Consequently, Hsp90 is an attractive target for developing a drug for cancer.

The majority of Hsp90 inhibitors occupy the ATP (adenosine tri-phosphate) pocket in the N-terminal domain of Hsp90, leading to limited ATPase activity [1–6]. At present, several natural and semi-synthetic Hsp90 inhibitors (see Figure 1) are in different stages of clinical trials for a variety of cancers [2,3,7–9].

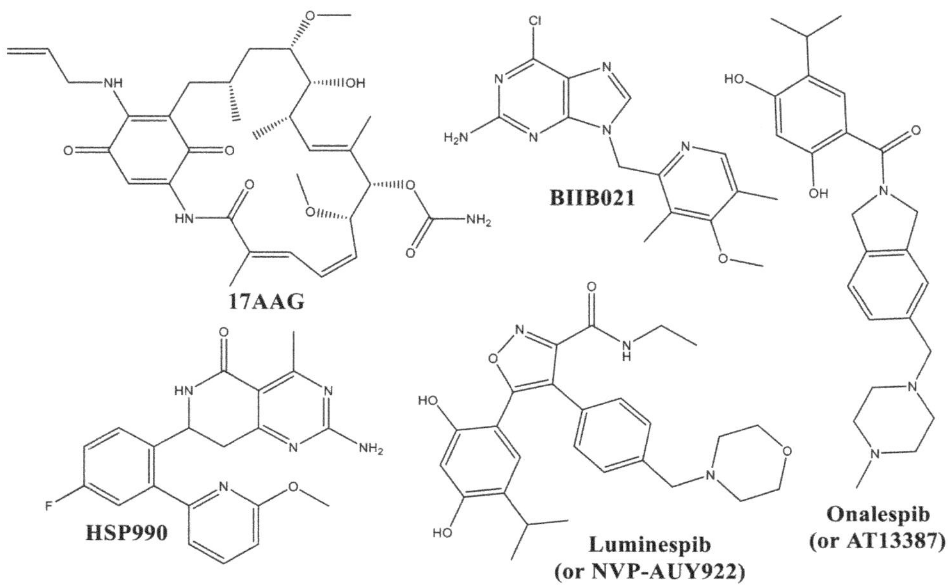

Figure 1. Different clinical trial candidates as inhibitors of Hsp90.

Unfortunately, several inhibitors have shown hepatotoxicity and ocular toxicity [2,10]; consequently, there is a need to modify them with retention of activity against Hsp90, which could be achieved on knowing the structural features responsible for their Hsp90 inhibitory activity. A simple, cost-effective, and faster yet effective strategy to know crucial pharmacophoric features is to use QSAR (Quantitative Structure–Activity Relationships), a successful, contemporary, and widely used branch of computer assisted-drug designing [11–16].

In QSAR analysis, generally, a good number of inhibitors are analyzed using a suitable technique like machine learning, deep learning, etc. There are two main advantages of using the QSAR approach [11,17,18]: (a) the analysis helps to identify the prominent structural features or patterns that influence the bioactivity profile of molecules (Mechanistic interpretation or Qualitative QSAR), and (b) the analysis could be used to predict the desired bioactivity of a molecule prior to its synthesis and lab testing (Predictive ability or Predictive QSAR). Therefore, many researchers prefer QSAR as a method of choice for drug/lead optimization. Nowadays, a QSAR analysis with a balance of mechanistic interpretation with predictive ability is highly preferred.

The literature survey reveals that QSAR analyses have been reported for Hsp90, but they are either based on a small dataset, lack general applicability, have poor predictive ability, are deficient of a mechanistic interpretation, or a combination of these factors, which limit their use [9,19–22]. Therefore, in the present work, we accomplished QSAR analysis for a larger and diverse dataset of Hsp90 inhibitors, and followed the OECD

(Organization for Economic Cooperation and Development) guidelines while developing a QSAR model to have a balance of mechanistic interpretation with predictive ability.

2. Results

The exhaustive and heuristic search resulted in the development of a six-descriptor-based QSAR model (see model-A), which was subjected to thorough statistical validation for internal and external validations.

Model-A: pIC_{50} (M) = 3.903 (± 0.134) + 0.101 (± 0.013) × **com_ringChyd_4A** + 0.433 (± 0.058) × **faroCN2B** + 0.714 (± 0.214) × **aroCminus_sumpc** + 0.065 (± 0.005) × **aroC_aroN_5B** + 0.266 (± 0.048) × **fringNsp3C5B** + 0.59 (± 0.082) × **da_amdN_6B**

Statistical validation of model-A:

$N_{tr} = 915$, $N_{ext} = 226$, $R^2_{tr} = 0.779$, $R^2_{adj.} = 0.777$, $R^2_{tr} - R^2_{adj.} = 0.002$, LOF = 0.244, Kxx = 0.219, $\Delta K = 0.122$, $RMSE_{tr} = 0.487$, $MAE_{tr} = 0.404$, $RSS_{tr} = 217.321$, $CCC_{tr} = 0.876$, s = 0.489, F = 533.134, R^2_{cv} (Q^2loo) = 0.775, $R^2\text{-}R^2_{cv} = 0.004$, $RMSE_{cv} = 0.491$, $MAE_{cv} = 0.407$, $PRESS_{cv} = 220.839$, $CCC_{cv} = 0.874$, $Q^2_{LMO} = 0.775$, $R^2_{Yscr} = 0.007$, $Q^2_{Yscr} = -0.009$, $RMSE_{ex} = 0.474$, $MAE_{ex} = 0.383$, $PRESS_{ext} = 50.675$, $R^2_{ex} = 0.779$, $Q^2\text{-}F^1 = 0.778$, $Q^2\text{-}F^2 = 0.778$, $Q^2\text{-}F^3 = 0.791$, $CCC_{ex} = 0.876$, R^2-ExPy = 0.779, $R'^2_o = 0.727$, k' = 0.989, $1-(R^2/R'^2_o) = 0.066$, $r'^2m = 0.602$, $R_o^2 = 0.779$, k = 1.005, $1 - (R^2 - ExPy/R_o^2) = 0$, $r^2m = 0.766$

Different researchers have recommended the above statistical parameters to judge the robustness and external predictive ability of a QSAR model [11–16,23–31]. The formula to calculate them is available in the Supplementary Materials. It is clear that model-A fulfils the recommended threshold for many validation parameters and other criteria. A high value of different parameters like R^2_{tr} (coefficient of determination), $R^2_{adj.}$ (adjusted coefficient of determination), and R^2_{cv} (Q^2loo, cross-validated coefficient of determination for leave-one-out), R^2_{ex} (external coefficient of determination), Q^2-F^n, and CCC_{ex} (Concordance Correlation Coefficient), etc., and a low value of LOF (lack-of-fit), $RMSE_{tr}$ (root mean square error), MAE_{tr} (mean absolute error), R^2_{Yscr} (R^2 for Y-scrambling), etc. along with the different graphs (see Figure 2) associated with the model indicate that the model possesses statistical robustness with excellent internal and external predictive ability as well as free from chance correlations. Additionally, the Williams plot specifies that the model is statistically acceptable (see Figure 2d). Therefore, it fulfils all the OECD recommended guidelines for creating a useful QSAR model.

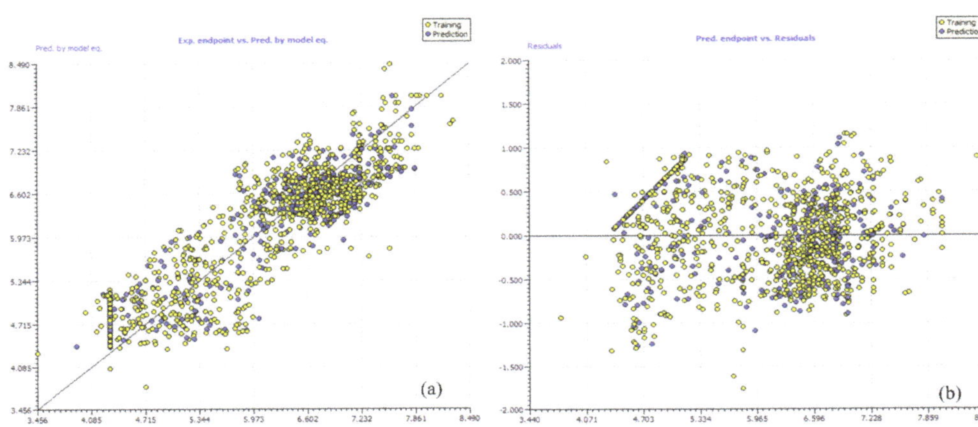

Figure 2. *Cont.*

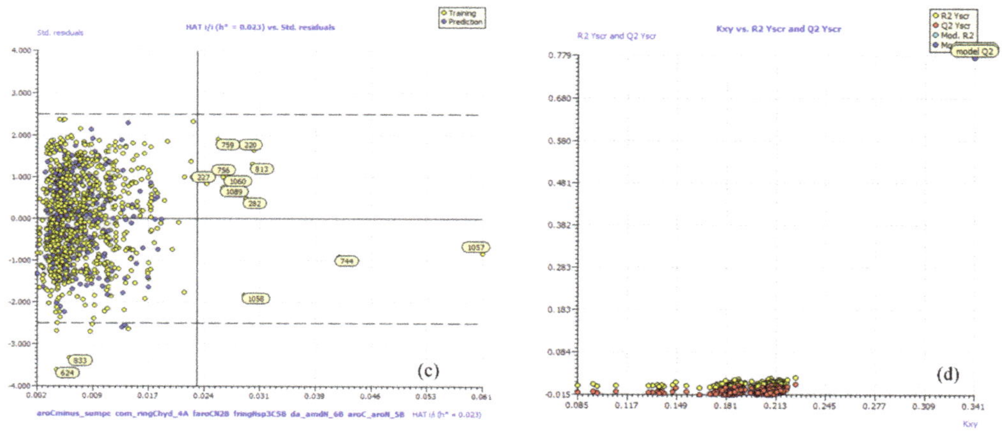

Figure 2. Different graphs associated with model-A: (**a**) experimental vs. predicted pIC_{50} (the solid line represents the regression line), (**b**) experimental vs. residuals, (**c**) Williams plot for applicability domain (the vertical solid line represents h* = 0.023 and horizontal dashed lines represent the upper and lower boundaries for applicability domain), and (**d**) Y-randomization.

3. Discussion

Mechanistic Interpretation of QSAR Model

A very crucial aspect of a useful QSAR analysis is to gain deep insight into the pharmacophore or structure-oriented linking of molecular descriptors [17,32]. This not only helps throughout the drug discovery process, but also expands the information and understanding of mechanistic aspects of different types of molecules. Though, in the present work, a specific molecular descriptor was used to equate the pIC_{50} values of different molecules, but an extending or reverse influence of unknown factors or other molecular descriptors, having a dominant effect in deciding the final pIC_{50} value of a molecule, cannot be ignored. To simplify, a single molecular descriptor (in turn structure feature) cannot decide the overall experimental pIC_{50} value of a molecule. In other words, the effective use of an appropriately validated QSAR model depends on the synchronous consideration of all constituent molecular descriptors. Interestingly, in model-A, all the molecular descriptors have positive coefficients, which indicates that increasing their value could result in a better Hsp90 inhibitory activity.

The descriptor **com_ringChyd_4A** represents the total number of hydrophobic ring carbons, having partial charge in the range ±0.2, within 4Å from the com (center of mass) of the molecule. From this, it appears that mere total number of ring carbons is very important, but replacing **com_ringChyd_4A** with **nringC** (number of ring carbon atoms) or **naroC** (number of aromatic carbon atoms) significantly reduced the statistical performance of the model (R^2 = 0.72). To add further, **com_ringChyd_4A** has a positive correlation of R = 0.488 with pIC_{50}, whereas **nringC** and **naroC** have a correlation of R = 0.461 and 0.405, respectively. **com_ringChyd_3A** and **com_ringChyd_5A** represent the total number of ring carbons, having partial charge in the range ±0.2, within 3Å and 5Å from the com (center of mass) of the molecule, respectively. Replacement of **com_ringChyd_4A** with **com_ringChyd_3A** or **com_ringChyd_5A** resulted in slightly reduced performance of the model with R^2 = 0.75 and 0.76, respectively. This indicates that the optimum distance is 4Å.

The importance of hydrophobic ring carbon atoms is supported by the X-ray-resolved structure of a good number of Hsp90 inhibitors because the active site of Hsp90 consists of lipophilic side chains of Leu48, Ile91, Val186, Leu315, Ile388, and Val391 [33,34], which favors the presence of hydrophobic moiety in the inhibitors. For example, a comparison of molecule 988 (pIC_{50} = 6.009, **com_ringChyd_4A** = 10) with 1007 (pIC_{50} = 6.481,

com_ringChyd_4A = 15) highlights the importance of **com_ringChyd_4A**. Another pair of molecules, viz. 794 and 814, also supports this observation. The molecular descriptor **com_ringChyd_4A** is depicted in Figure 3 for different molecules.

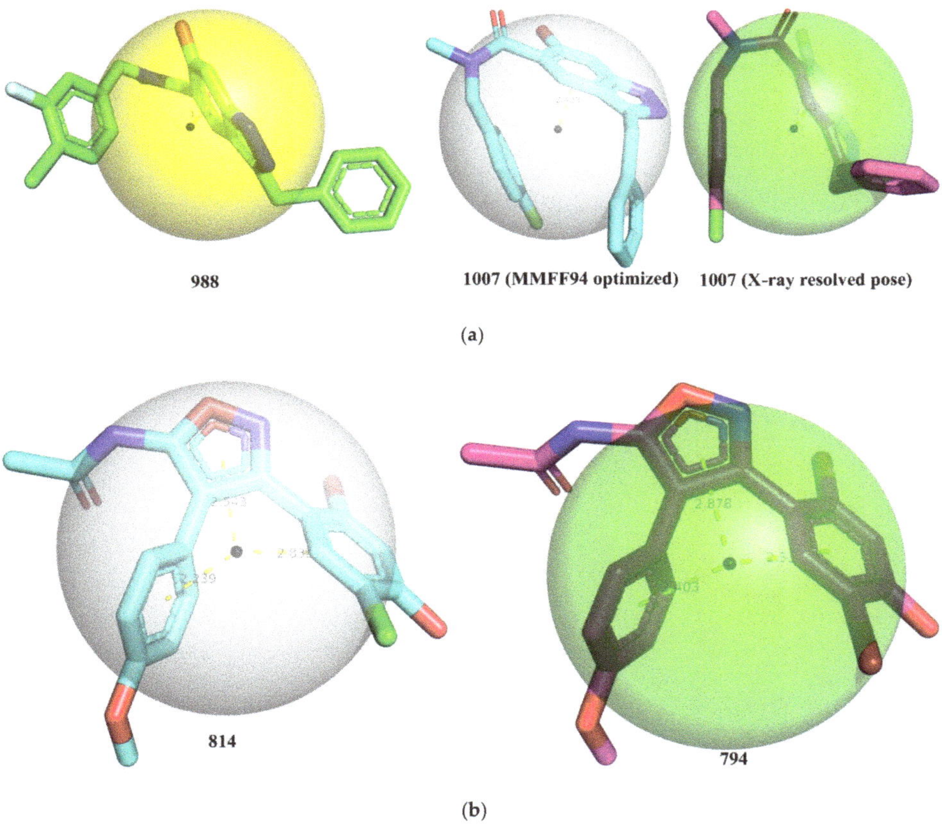

Figure 3. Depiction of **com_ringChyd_4A** using different molecules: (**a**) molecules 988, 1007 (MMFF94 optimized), and 1007 (X-ray resolved dock pose from pdb 6EY8); (**b**) molecules 794 and 814 (both X-ray-resolved poses from pdb 5XR9 and 4LWE, respectively). The small black sphere represents the com (center of mass) and the bigger transparent sphere represents the distance of 4Å from the center of mass. The dotted yellow line represents the distance (Å) of com from the centers of the different nearest rings.

From Figure 3, it is clear that the lowest energy conformer of molecule 988 has **com_ringChyd_4A** = 10 due to the closer presence of com (distance 1.206 Å) to the benzene ring of indazole ring. In case of molecule 1007 (MMFF94-optimized and X-ray-resolved pose from pdb 6EY8), the com is located slightly away from the benzene ring of Indazole ring at a distance > 2.40 due to specific conformation, thereby increasing the value of **com_ringChyd_4A** to 15. This could be a plausible reason for the difference in the bioactivity of these two compounds. Similarly, a better Hsp90 inhibitory activity of molecule 794 than 814 could be attributed to difference in their **com_ringChyd_4A** values.

Another molecular descriptor that has a positive effect on Hsp90 activity is **faroCN2B**, which signifies the presence of nitrogen exactly at two bonds from aromatic carbon atoms. If the same nitrogen atom is also present at two or less bonds from any other aromatic carbon atom, then it was excluded while calculating **faroCN2B**. This descriptor highlights the importance of nitrogen atoms separated from aromatic ring (Benzene, etc.) by two bonds. As the majority of nitrogen atoms act as either an H-bond donor or acceptor; therefore, the presence of nitrogen atoms in the vicinity of aromatic rings could be useful in enhancing interactions with the polar residues of receptor (Hsp90). Additionally, the descriptor further points out the crucial role played by the aromatic rings undoubtedly due to their lipophilic nature. Taken together, the descriptor **faroCN2B** signifies the importance of two important structural features: aromatic rings and their vicinal nitrogen atoms.

This observation is confirmed when we compare the X-ray-resolved structures of molecule 727 (pIC_{50} = 6.654, **faroCN2B** = 1, pdb = 4O09) with 725 (pIC_{50} = 7.137, **faroCN2B** = 2, pdb = 4O05) depicted in Figure 4. The nitrogen atoms responsible for **faroCN2B** are highlighted by blue dotted circles. From Figure 4, it is clear that the aromatic ring B of both the molecules is responsible for hydrophobic interactions with the residue Met98. The nitrogen atom of ring A present in both the molecules is not only a constituent of **faroCN2B,** but also responsible for H-bonding with the residue Asp93. Thus, such a combination of aromatic carbons and nitrogen is highly beneficial to enhance the interactions with the receptor. In case of molecule 733, an additional nitrogen atom is present in ring F, which is a constituent of **faroCN2B**, and responsible for the H-bond interaction with the nearby water molecule. Thus, the present QSAR analysis revealed an important structural feature, which is also visible in X-ray-resolved structures of the same inhibitors with the same target enzyme Hsp90.

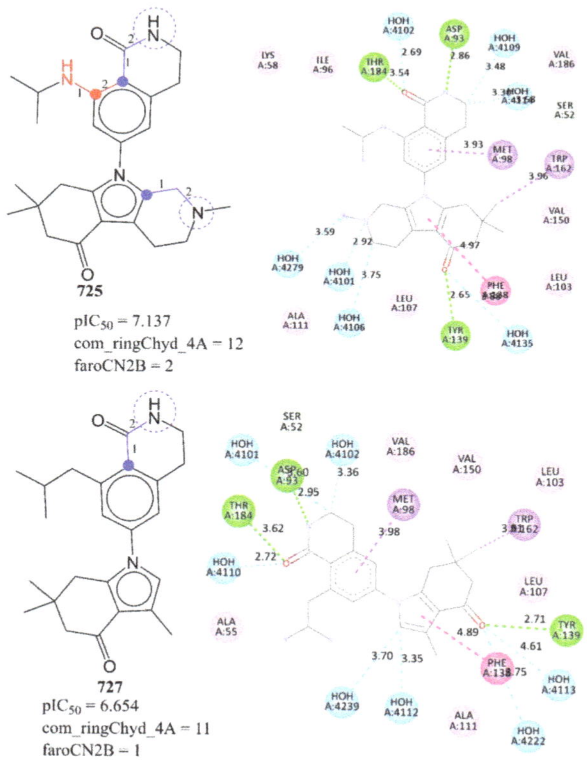

Figure 4. Depiction of **faroCN2B** using representative examples only.

A comparison of the following pairs of molecules further vindicates the importance of **faroCN2B** in determining the bioactivity: 213 (pIC_{50} = 6.523, **faroCN2B** = 2) with

212 (pIC_{50} = 6.469, **faroCN2B** = 1) and 758 (pIC_{50} = 7.444, **faroCN2B** = 2) with 759 (pIC_{50} = 7.569, **faroCN2B** = 3).

The importance of aromatic carbon atoms is further emphasized with the presence of **aroCminus_sumpc** as a constituent variable of model-A. The molecular descriptor **aroCminus_sumpc** represents the sum of partial charges on negatively charged aromatic carbon atoms. The positive coefficient for **aroCminus_sumpc** indicates that the higher the value of this descriptor, the better the activity profile. The sum of partial charges on negatively charged aromatic carbon atoms will always be negative; therefore, in reality, this descriptor actually decreases the pIC_{50} value. Further, the replacement of **aroCminus_sumpc** by **aroCplus_sumpc** (sum of partial charges on positively charged aromatic carbon atoms) led to a model with almost identical statistical performance (R^2_{tr} = 0.772, Q^2_{LMO} = 0.767, R^2_{ex} = 0.78, CCC_{ex} = 0.876). In fact, **aroCplus_sumpc** has a better correlation (R = 0.33) with pIC_{50} than **aroCminus_sumpc** (R = 0.10). From this it is clear that, if aromatic carbons are positively charged than the molecule possesses better Hsp90 inhibitory activity. Therefore, the best strategy is to attach atoms or groups that enhance lipophilic and mild polar interactions with the receptor (for example -Cl, etc.) to the aromatic carbon atoms. In short, substituted aromatic rings are preferable for better activity. This observation is supported by comparing following pairs of molecules: 2 with 3, 1054 with 1059, and 214 with 212.

aroC_aroN_5B, which represents the total number of aromatic carbon atoms within five bonds from aromatic nitrogen atoms, again points out the key role played by aromatic carbon atoms in deciding Hsp90 inhibitory activity. It also underlines the usefulness of aromatic nitrogen atoms. This descriptor has a positive correlation with pIC_{50} with R = 0.63. Therefore, an increase in number of aromatic carbon atoms within five bonds from aromatic nitrogen atoms leads to better Hsp90 inhibitory activity. The following pairs of the molecules support this observation: 888 (pIC_{50} = 7.523, **aroC_aroN_5B** = 22) with 887 (pIC_{50} = 6.046, **aroC_aroN_5B** = 20) and 107 (pIC_{50} = 5.953, **aroC_aroN_5B** = 13) with 108 (pIC_{50} = 4.874, **aroC_aroN_5B** = 10), to mention a few. Further, the 50 most active molecules possess relatively higher value of **aroC_aroN_5B** (range 8–17) than the 50 least active molecules (range 0–8).

fringNsp3C5B stands for the number of sp^3-hybridized carbon atoms exactly at five bonds from the ring nitrogen atom. If the same sp^3-hybridized carbon atom is also present at four or less bonds from any other ring nitrogen atom, then it was excluded while calculating **fringNsp3C5B**. It is interesting to note that the 50 most active molecules, except molecule 618, possess at least one or more of such a combination of carbon and ring nitrogen, whereas the 50 least active molecules either lack it or have **fringNsp3C5B** = 1. In the majority of compounds, the sp^3-hybridized carbon atoms are present either as a linker between two rings or as a substituent, which therefore enhances conformational flexibility of the molecule to adopt a bioactive conformer or lipophilic characters of the molecule. A comparison of 895 (pIC_{50} = 7.071, **fringNsp3C5B** = 2) with 896 (pIC_{50} = 6.777, **fringNsp3C5B** = 1), 859 (pIC_{50} = 7.237, **fringNsp3C5B** = 2) with 896 (pIC_{50} = 7.071, **fringNsp3C5B** = 1), 326 (pIC_{50} = 6.921, **fringNsp3C5B** = 1) with 328 (pIC_{50} = 7.046, **fringNsp3C5B** = 2), and 412 (pIC_{50} = 7.155, **fringNsp3C5B** = 1) with 411 (pIC_{50} = 6.959, **fringNsp3C5B** = 0) and 410 (pIC_{50} = 6.854, **fringNsp3C5B** = 0) confirms the importance of **fringNsp3C5B** in deciding the activity.

A molecular descriptor that identifies the relation of total number amide nitrogen atoms within six bonds from the H-bond donor and acceptor atoms is **da_amdN_6B**. In the majority of compounds in the present dataset, the amide group is present as a substituent on aromatic ring or as a linker between two rings. The descriptor **da_amdN_6B** suggests the significance of amide group and its correlation with the H-bond donor and acceptor atoms. This observation is confirmed on comparing molecule **A** with molecules **B** and **C** (see Figure 5).

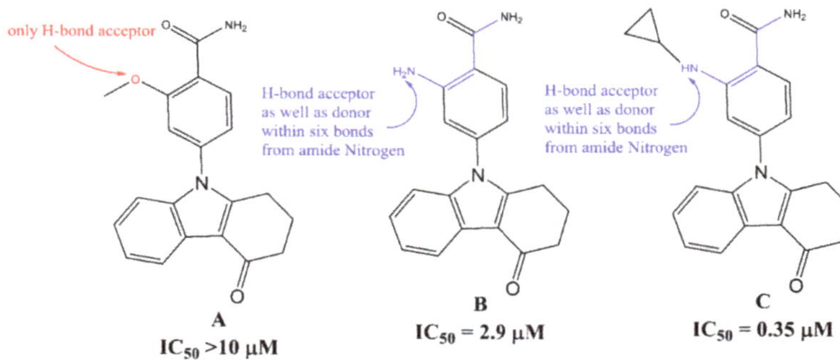

Figure 5. Pictorial representation of **da_amdN_6B** using representative examples only.

A good number of researchers have also pointed out that the amide group is crucial for Hsp90 inhibitors to establish H-bonding with residues of the active site (see pdb 4AWO). For example, Zhao et al. [4] pointed out that the distance between the nitrogen atoms on the piperidine ring and the amide are important for Hsp90 inhibition. Similarly, Baruchello and co-workers [35] studied a library of 3,4-isoxazole diamides for Hsp90 binding and found that a substantial reduction in Hsp90 binding affinity when the amide was replaced with substituted amines. In addition, a H-bond donor at the C-4 position on the isoxazole is vital for retaining the activity. Davies et al. [36] observed that S-acetamide derivatives of compounds have better bioactivity profile than the S-alkylamines. The importance of **da_amdN_6B** was further confirmed by comparing following pair of the molecules: 856 (pIC_{50} = 6.848, **da_amdN_6B** = 0) with 861 (pIC_{50} = 7.114, **da_amdN_6B** = 1). The earlier work identified the role of amide group, and in the present work, we successfully identified that a combination of amide group with H-bond donor/acceptor within six bonds is a better strategy to have better Hsp90 inhibitory activity. Therefore, such a combination of the amide nitrogen atom and H-bond donor/acceptor should be retained in future optimizations.

In short, three molecular descriptors emphasize the importance of ring carbon atoms, especially aromatic carbon atoms. This could be attributed to the lipophilic character of the active site of Hsp90. Likewise, four molecular descriptors underline the significance of different types of nitrogen atoms, which are responsible for the establishment of the polar or H-bond interactions with polar residues and water molecules present inside the active site of Hsp90. Hence, the present work is successful in identifying reported as well as novel pharmacophoric features of Hsp90 inhibitors.

4. Materials and Methods

The OECD (Organization for Economic Cooperation and Development) guidelines and a standard protocol recommended by different researchers [11–13,16,18,25,26,29,30,37] involve the sequential execution of (1) data collection and its curation, (2) structure generation and calculation of molecular descriptors, (3) objective feature selection (OFS), (4) splitting the dataset into training and external validation sets, (5) subjective feature selection involving building a regression model and validation of the developed model, which have all been followed to build a widely applicable QSAR model for Hsp-90 inhibitory activity. This also ensures thorough validation and successful application of the model.

4.1. Data Collection and Its Curation

The dataset of Hsp-90 inhibitory activity used for building, training, and validating the QSAR model in the present work was downloaded from BindingDB (https://www.bindingdb.org/bind/index.jsp, accessed on 24 December 2021), which is a free and publicly accessible database. Initially, the dataset comprised 1839 molecules. Then, as a part of data curation, entries with ambiguous IC_{50} values, duplicates, salts, metal-based inhibitors, etc.

were omitted [11–13,16,18,25,26,29,30,37]. The final dataset comprises 1141 structurally diverse molecules with remarkable variation in structural scaffolds, which were tested experimentally for potency in terms of IC_{50} (nM) (see the MS Excel file 'SupplementaryMaterial-Final' in the Supplementary Materials). The dataset includes N-terminal inhibitors of Hsp90. The experimental IC_{50} values have a sufficient variation ranging from 5 to 350,000 nM. After that, IC_{50} values were converted to their negative logarithmic value ($pIC_{50} = -\log_{10}IC_{50}$) so that a comparison of their values became easier. In Table 1 and Figure 6, some of the most and least active molecules are included as examples only.

Table 1. SMILES notation, IC_{50} (nM) and pIC_{50} (M) of the five most and least active molecules of the selected dataset.

S.N.	Ligand SMILES	IC_{50} (nM)	pIC_{50} (M)
308	COc1cccc(n1)-c1cc(F)ccc1[C@H]1Cc2nc(N)nc(C)c2C(NOC2C[C@H](O)[C@H](O)C2)=N1	5	8.301
908	CCNC(=O)c1noc(c1NC(=O)[C@H]1CC[C@H](CNS(=O)(=O)c2ccc(F)cc2)CC1)-c1cc(C(C)C)c(O)cc1O	5.4	8.268
770	CCNC(=O)c1nnn(c1-c1ccc(CNC2CCCCC2)cc1)-c1cc(C(C)C)c(O)cc1O	6.8	8.167
767	CCNC(=O)c1nnn(c1-c1ccc(CN2CCCCC2CCO)cc1)-c1cc(C(C)C)c(O)cc1O	10	8
749	CCNC(=O)c1nnn(c1-c1ccc(CNCCCN(CC)CC)cc1)-c1cc(C(C)C)c(O)cc1O	12	7.921
775	Oc1cc(O)c2C[C@@H](OC(=O)[C@H]3CC[C@H](F)CC3)[C@H](Oc2c1)c1ccc(O)c(O)c1	69,000	4.161
1073	COC(COCCOc1ccc(Br)cc1)CN1CCN(CC1)c1ccccc1C(C)(C)C	70,430	4.152
1141	CO[C@H]1C[C@H](C)Cc2c(OC)c(O)cc3NC(=O)\C(C)=C\[C@H](O)C[C@H](OC)[C@@H](OC(N)=O)\C(C)=C\[C@H](C)[C@H]1Oc23	96,000	4.018
778	Oc1cc(O)c2C[C@H](OC(=O)c3ccccc3)[C@H](Oc2c1)c1ccccc1	120,000	3.921
207	CSc1nc(C)nc(N)n1	350,000	3.456

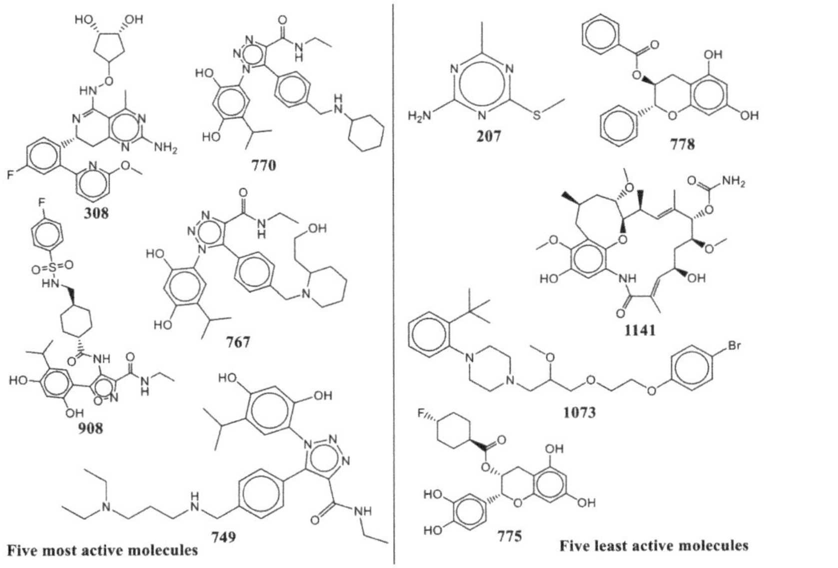

Figure 6. Representative examples from the selected dataset (the five most active and five least active molecules).

4.2. Calculation of Molecular Descriptors and Objective Feature Selection (OFS)

A crucial step before the calculation of molecular descriptors is to convert the SMILES notations to 3D-optimized structures and partial charge assignment, which was accomplished using OpenBabel 3.1 [38] using MMFF94 force field. In the present work, the X-ray-resolved structure of molecule **1007** (pdb 6YE8) was used to identify the parameter tuning in OpenBabel, required to get a better optimized structure, until there was a high similarity between the MMFF94-optimized structure and X-ray-resolved structure. This enhances the chances of getting a bioactive conformer, which in turn is highly beneficial for further optimization of Hsp90 inhibitors in the drug discovery pipeline. A comparison of the X-ray-resolved structures of molecules **1007** and **33** (pdb 2VCJ) and their respective MMFF94-optimized structures are represented in Figure 7.

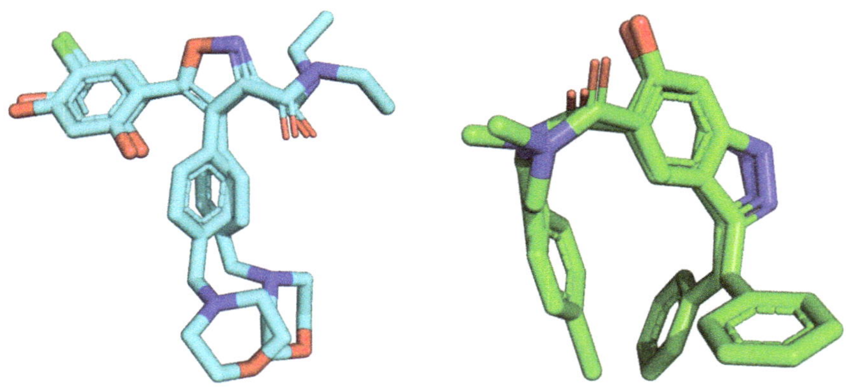

An overlap of 33 (MMFF94 optimized) and its X-ray resolved pose pdb 2VCJ (RMSD = 0.74)

An overlap of 1007 (MMFF94 optimized) and its X-ray resolved pose pdb 6EY8) (RMSD = 0.65)

Figure 7. A comparison of X-ray-resolved and MMFF94-optimized structures of molecules 1007 and 33.

From Figure 7, it is clear that there is a high similarity between the X-ray-resolved and MMFF94-optimized structure of molecules **1007** and **33**, which indicates that appropriate parameter tuning was achieved to optimize the rest of the molecules. That is, the same parameter tuning in OpenBabel was used to optimize the other molecules of the selected dataset. The parameters are as follows: geometry optimization, steepest descent, number of steps: 1500; cut off: 0.01.

In the next step, the 3D-optimized structures of all molecules in the dataset were used to calculate a good number of molecular descriptors. It is important to note that calculation of diverse molecular descriptors enhances the chances of a successful QSAR analysis and significantly helps in mechanistic interpretation. However, descriptor pruning is very useful as it further strengthens the diminished risk of overfitting from noisy redundant descriptors. To fulfil these objectives, more than 40,000 molecular descriptors were generated using *PyDescriptor* [39]. After that, OFS involved elimination of the near constant (90% molecules) and highly intercorrelated ($|R| > 0.90$) molecular descriptors. For this, QSARINS-2.2.4 was used. The final set of molecular descriptors comprises 1228 molecular descriptors, which still comprise manifold descriptors (1D- to 3D-), leading to coverage of a broad descriptor space.

4.3. Splitting the Dataset into Training and External Sets and SFS (Subjective Feature Selection)

Subjective feature selection involves selection of appropriate number and set of molecular descriptors to build a model using suitable algorithm. Prior to SFS, it is essential to divide the dataset into training and test (also known as external or prediction set) sets with a proper composition and proportions to circumvent information leakage and to verify the predictive ability of a model [11–13,16,18,25,26,29,30,37]. Hence, the dataset was randomly split into training (80% = 915 molecules) and prediction or external (20% = 226 molecules) sets. It is to be noted that the training set was used for the selection of optimum number of molecular descriptors, and the sole purpose of prediction/external set was to validate the external predictive ability of the model (Predictive QSAR). A GA-MLR-based QSAR model is free from over-fitting if it comprises an optimum number of molecular descriptors. Therefore, in the present work, a simple yet effective method of identifying the breaking point was used. Generally, the continuous inclusion of molecular descriptors in the GA-MLR model significantly increases the value of Q^2_{LOO}, but after the breaking point, the value of Q^2_{LOO} does not increase significantly [24]. The number of molecular descriptors corresponding to the breaking point was considered optimum for model building. A graph (see Figure 8) was plotted between the number of molecular descriptors involved in the model and Q^2_{LOO} values, which indicated that the breaking point agreed with the six molecular descriptors. Consequently, QSAR models comprising more than six descriptors were not considered. For SFS, the set of molecular descriptors was selected using the genetic algorithm integrated with multilinear regression (GA-MLR) method available in QSARINS-2.2.4 (generations per size: 10,000; population size: 50; mutation rate: 60; significance level: 0.05; fitness parameter: Q^2_{LOO}).

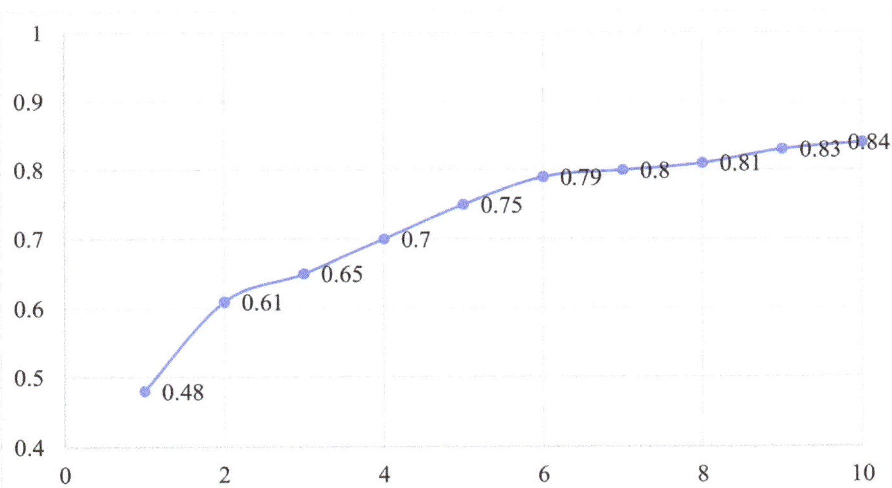

Figure 8. Plot of number of descriptors against leave-one-out coefficient of determination Q^2_{LOO} to identify the optimum number of descriptors.

4.4. Building Regression Model and Its Validation

The GA-MLR approach resulted in the generation of a good number of models having good to excellent statistical performance. Therefore, the following stringent parameters and criteria suggested by different researchers were used to select the best model [11–13,16,18,25,26,29,30,37,40]: $R^2_{tr} \geq 0.6$, $Q^2_{loo} \geq 0.5$, $Q^2_{LMO} \geq 0.6$, $R^2 > Q^2$, $R^2_{ex} \geq 0.6$, $RMSE_{tr} < RMSE_{cv}$, $\Delta K \geq 0.05$, $CCC \geq 0.80$, $Q^2\text{-}F^n \geq 0.60$, $r^2_m \geq 0.5$, $(1\text{-}r^2/r_o^2) < 0.1$, $0.9 \leq k \leq 1.1$ or $(1\text{-}r^2/r'^2_o) < 0.1$, $0.9 \leq k' \leq 1.1$, $| r_o^2 - r'^2_o | < 0.3$, $RMSE_{ex}$, MAE_{ex}, R^2_{ex}, Q^2_{F1}, Q^2_{F2}, and Q^2_{F3}, and low R^2_{Yscr}, RMSE, and MAE. The details of these statistical parameters are available in the Supplementary Materials. An important aspect of validation of a QSAR model is to identify the applicability domain. In the present work, the William's plot was plotted to assess the applicability domain of the QSAR model [11–13,16,18,25,26,29,30,37,41,42].

5. Conclusions

In the present work, a relatively large and structurally diverse dataset of 1141 Hsp90 inhibitors was used for developing a six-descriptor-based and extensively validated GA–MLR QSAR model with $R^2_{tr} = 0.78$, $Q^2_{LMO} = 0.77$, $R^2_{ex} = 0.78$, and $CCC_{ex} = 0.88$. The inclusion of easily understandable descriptors resulted in identification of important pharmacophoric features that are correlated with Hsp90 inhibitory activity. The present QSAR analysis effectively captured a mixture of reported as well as novel significant structural features. The analysis vindicates that ring and aromatic carbons are important in deciding the activity. In addition, different types of nitrogen atoms in correlation with different types of carbon atoms influence the Hsp90 inhibitory activity. A good balance of external predictive ability and mechanistic interpretations, which are further supported by the reported crystal structures of Hsp90 inhibitors, make the QSAR model useful for the future optimization of molecules in the pipeline as a better Hsp90 inhibitor.

Supplementary Materials: The following are available online at https://www.mdpi.com/article/10.3390/ph15030303/s1.

Author Contributions: Conceptualization, V.H.M., M.E.A.Z. and S.A.A.-H.; formal analysis and data curation, V.H.M. and V.M.P.; writing, M.E.A.Z., V.H.M., M.M.R., S.N.A.B. and S.D.T.; Revisions, M.E.A.Z., V.H.M., S.D.T., M.M.R. and S.N.A.B.; editing and proofreading, V.H.M., M.E.A.Z. and S.N.A.B. All authors have read and agreed to the published version of the manuscript.

Funding: The authors acknowledge the Deanship of Scientific Research at Imam Mohammad Ibn Saud Islamic University, Riyadh, Saudi Arabia, for its support of this research through research group number RG-21-09-76.

Institutional Review Board Statement: Not applicable.

Informed Consent Statement: Not applicable.

Data Availability Statement: Data is contained within the article and Supplementary Materials.

Acknowledgments: The authors acknowledge the Deanship of Scientific Research at Imam Mohammad Ibn Saud Islamic University, Riyadh, Saudi Arabia, for its support of this research through research group number RG-21-09-76. V. H. Masand is thankful to Paola Gramatica (Italy) and her team for providing the free copy of QSARINS 2.2.4.

Conflicts of Interest: The authors declare no conflict of interest.

Abbreviations

SMILES	Simplified molecular-input line-entry system
GA	Genetic algorithm
MLR	Multiple linear regression
QSAR	Quantitative structure–activity relationship
WHO	World Health Organization
ADMET	Absorption, distribution, metabolism, excretion, and toxicity
OLS	Ordinary least square
QSARINS	QSAR Insubria
OECD	Organization for Economic Cooperation and Development

References

1. Ho, N.; Li, A.; Li, S.; Zhang, H. Heat Shock Protein 90 and Role of Its Chemical Inhibitors in Treatment of Hematologic Malignancies. *Pharmaceuticals* **2012**, *5*, 779–801. [CrossRef]
2. Li, L.; Wang, L.; You, Q.-D.; Xu, X.-L. Heat Shock Protein 90 Inhibitors: An Update on Achievements, Challenges, and Future Directions. *J. Med. Chem.* **2019**, *63*, 1798–1822. [CrossRef]
3. Bhat, R.; Tummalapalli, S.R.; Rotella, D.P. Progress in the Discovery and Development of Heat Shock Protein 90 (Hsp90) Inhibitors. *J. Med. Chem.* **2014**, *57*, 8718–8728. [CrossRef] [PubMed]

4. Zhao, H.; Moroni, E.; Colombo, G.; Blagg, B.S.J. Identification of a New Scaffold for Hsp90 C-Terminal Inhibition. *ACS Med. Chem. Lett.* **2013**, *5*, 84–88. [CrossRef]
5. Li, Y.; Zhang, T.; Schwartz, S.J.; Sun, D. New developments in Hsp90 inhibitors as anti-cancer therapeutics: Mechanisms, clinical perspective and more potential. *Drug Resist. Updates* **2009**, *12*, 17–27. [CrossRef]
6. Hoter, A.; El-Sabban, M.; Naim, H. The HSP90 Family: Structure, Regulation, Function, and Implications in Health and Disease. *Int. J. Mol. Sci.* **2018**, *19*, 2560. [CrossRef]
7. Zuehlke, A.D.; Moses, M.A.; Neckers, L. Heat shock protein 90: Its inhibition and function. *Philos. Trans. R. Soc. B Biol. Sci.* **2017**, *373*, 20160527. [CrossRef]
8. Biamonte, M.A.; Van de Water, R.; Arndt, J.W.; Scannevin, R.H.; Perret, D.; Lee, W.-C. Heat Shock Protein 90: Inhibitors in Clinical Trials. *J. Med. Chem.* **2009**, *53*, 3–17. [CrossRef] [PubMed]
9. Patil, V.M.; Masand, N.; Gupta, S.P.; Blagg, B.S.J. QSAR Studies to Predict Activity of HSP90 Inhibitors. *Curr. Top. Med. Chem.* **2021**, *21*, 2272–2291. [CrossRef] [PubMed]
10. Jhaveri, K.; Taldone, T.; Modi, S.; Chiosis, G. Advances in the clinical development of heat shock protein 90 (Hsp90) inhibitors in cancers. *Biochim. Biophys. Acta BBA Mol. Cell Res.* **2012**, *1823*, 742–755. [CrossRef] [PubMed]
11. Gramatica, P. Principles of QSAR Modeling. *Int. J. Quant. Struct.-Prop. Relatsh.* **2020**, *5*, 61–97. [CrossRef]
12. Cherkasov, A.; Muratov, E.N.; Fourches, D.; Varnek, A.; Baskin, I.I.; Cronin, M.; Dearden, J.; Gramatica, P.; Martin, Y.C.; Todeschini, R.; et al. QSAR modeling: Where have you been? Where are you going to? *J. Med. Chem.* **2014**, *57*, 4977–5010. [CrossRef]
13. Gramatica, P. On the development and validation of QSAR models. *Methods Mol. Biol.* **2013**, *930*, 499–526. [CrossRef]
14. Gramatica, P.; Cassani, S.; Roy, P.P.; Kovarich, S.; Yap, C.W.; Papa, E. QSAR Modeling is not Push a Button and Find a Correlation: A Case Study of Toxicity of (Benzo-)triazoles on Algae. *Mol. Inform.* **2012**, *31*, 817–835. [CrossRef]
15. Li, J.; Gramatica, P. The importance of molecular structures, endpoints' values, and predictivity parameters in QSAR research: QSAR analysis of a series of estrogen receptor binders. *Mol. Divers.* **2010**, *14*, 687–696. [CrossRef]
16. Muratov, E.N.; Bajorath, J.; Sheridan, R.P.; Tetko, I.V.; Filimonov, D.; Poroikov, V.; Oprea, T.I.; Baskin, I.I.; Varnek, A.; Roitberg, A.; et al. QSAR without borders. *Chem. Soc. Rev.* **2020**, *49*, 3525–3564. [CrossRef]
17. Fujita, T.; Winkler, D.A. Understanding the Roles of the "Two QSARs". *J. Chem. Inf. Model.* **2016**, *56*, 269–274. [CrossRef]
18. Zaki, M.E.A.; Al-Hussain, S.A.; Masand, V.H.; Sabnani, M.K.; Samad, A. Mechanistic and Predictive QSAR Analysis of Diverse Molecules to Capture Salient and Hidden Pharmacophores for Anti-Thrombotic Activity. *Int. J. Mol. Sci.* **2021**, *22*, 8352. [CrossRef]
19. Zhao, H.; Moroni, E.; Yan, B.; Colombo, G.; Blagg, B.S.J. 3D-QSAR-Assisted Design, Synthesis, and Evaluation of Novobiocin Analogues. *ACS Med. Chem. Lett.* **2012**, *4*, 57–62. [CrossRef]
20. Barta, T.E.; Veal, J.M.; Rice, J.W.; Partridge, J.M.; Fadden, R.P.; Ma, W.; Jenks, M.; Geng, L.; Hanson, G.J.; Huang, K.H.; et al. Discovery of benzamide tetrahydro-4H-carbazol-4-ones as novel small molecule inhibitors of Hsp90. *Bioorg. Med. Chem. Lett.* **2008**, *18*, 3517–3521. [CrossRef]
21. Bussenius, J.; Blazey, C.M.; Aay, N.; Anand, N.K.; Arcalas, A.; Baik, T.; Bowles, O.J.; Buhr, C.A.; Costanzo, S.; Curtis, J.K.; et al. Discovery of XL888: A novel tropane-derived small molecule inhibitor of HSP90. *Bioorg. Med. Chem. Lett.* **2012**, *22*, 5396–5404. [CrossRef]
22. Abbasi, M.; Sadeghi-Aliabadi, H.; Amanlou, M. Prediction of new Hsp90 inhibitors based on 3,4-isoxazolediamide scaffold using QSAR study, molecular docking and molecular dynamic simulation. *DARU J. Pharm. Sci.* **2017**, *25*, 17. [CrossRef]
23. Gramatica, P. External Evaluation of QSAR Models, in Addition to Cross-Validation Verification of Predictive Capability on Totally New Chemicals. *Mol. Inform.* **2014**, *33*, 311–314. [CrossRef]
24. Gramatica, P.; Chirico, N.; Papa, E.; Cassani, S.; Kovarich, S. QSARINS: A new software for the development, analysis, and validation of QSAR MLR models. *J. Comput. Chem.* **2013**, *34*, 2121–2132. [CrossRef]
25. Chirico, N.; Gramatica, P. Real external predictivity of QSAR models. Part 2. New intercomparable thresholds for different validation criteria and the need for scatter plot inspection. *J. Chem. Inf. Model.* **2012**, *52*, 2044–2058. [CrossRef]
26. Chirico, N.; Gramatica, P. Real external predictivity of QSAR models: How to evaluate it? Comparison of different validation criteria and proposal of using the concordance correlation coefficient. *J. Chem. Inf. Model.* **2011**, *51*, 2320–2335. [CrossRef]
27. Gramatica, P.; Pilutti, P.; Papa, E. Approaches for externally validated QSAR modelling of Nitrated Polycyclic Aromatic Hydrocarbon mutagenicity. *SAR QSAR Environ. Res.* **2007**, *18*, 169–178. [CrossRef]
28. Gramatica, P. Principles of QSAR models validation internal and external. *QSAR Comb. Sci.* **2007**, *26*, 694–701. [CrossRef]
29. Martin, T.M.; Harten, P.; Young, D.M.; Muratov, E.N.; Golbraikh, A.; Zhu, H.; Tropsha, A. Does rational selection of training and test sets improve the outcome of QSAR modeling? *J. Chem. Inf. Model.* **2012**, *52*, 2570–2578. [CrossRef]
30. Tropsha, A.; Gramatica, P.; Gombar, V.K. The Importance of Being Earnest Validation is the Absolute Essential for Successful Application and Interpretation of QSPR Models. *QSAR Comb. Sci.* **2003**, *22*, 69–77. [CrossRef]
31. Golbraikh, A.; Shen, M.; Xiao, Z.; Xiao, Y.D.; Lee, K.H.; Tropsha, A. Rational selection of training and test sets for the development of validated QSAR models. *J. Comput.-Aided Mol. Des.* **2003**, *17*, 241–253. [CrossRef]
32. Polishchuk, P. Interpretation of Quantitative Structure–Activity Relationship Models: Past, Present, and Future. *J. Chem. Inf. Model.* **2017**, *57*, 2618–2639. [CrossRef]
33. Jackson, S.E. Hsp90: Structure and Function. In *Molecular Chaperones*; Springer: Berlin/Heidelberg, Germany, 2012; pp. 155–240.

34. Vallée, F.; Carrez, C.; Pilorge, F.; Dupuy, A.; Parent, A.; Bertin, L.; Thompson, F.; Ferrari, P.; Fassy, F.; Lamberton, A.; et al. Tricyclic Series of Heat Shock Protein 90 (Hsp90) Inhibitors Part I: Discovery of Tricyclic Imidazo[4,5-c]pyridines as Potent Inhibitors of the Hsp90 Molecular Chaperone. *J. Med. Chem.* **2011**, *54*, 7206–7219. [CrossRef]
35. Baruchello, R.; Simoni, D.; Grisolia, G.; Barbato, G.; Marchetti, P.; Rondanin, R.; Mangiola, S.; Giannini, G.; Brunetti, T.; Alloatti, D.; et al. Novel 3,4-Isoxazolediamides as Potent Inhibitors of Chaperone Heat Shock Protein 90. *J. Med. Chem.* **2011**, *54*, 8592–8604. [CrossRef]
36. Davies, N.G.M.; Browne, H.; Davis, B.; Drysdale, M.J.; Foloppe, N.; Geoffrey, S.; Gibbons, B.; Hart, T.; Hubbard, R.; Jensen, M.R.; et al. Targeting conserved water molecules: Design of 4-aryl-5-cyanopyrrolo[2,3-d]pyrimidine Hsp90 inhibitors using fragment-based screening and structure-based optimization. *Bioorg. Med. Chem.* **2012**, *20*, 6770–6789. [CrossRef]
37. Fourches, D.; Muratov, E.; Tropsha, A. Trust, but verify: On the importance of chemical structure curation in cheminformatics and QSAR modeling research. *J. Chem. Inf. Model.* **2010**, *50*, 1189–1204. [CrossRef]
38. O'Boyle, N.M.; Banck, M.; James, C.A.; Morley, C.; Vandermeersch, T.; Hutchison, G.R. Open Babel: An open chemical toolbox. *J. Cheminform.* **2011**, *3*, 33. [CrossRef]
39. Masand, V.H.; Rastija, V. PyDescriptor: A new PyMOL plugin for calculating thousands of easily understandable molecular descriptors. *Chemom. Intell. Lab. Syst.* **2017**, *169*, 12–18. [CrossRef]
40. Zaki, M.E.A.; Al-Hussain, S.A.; Masand, V.H.; Akasapu, S.; Bajaj, S.O.; El-Sayed, N.N.E.; Ghosh, A.; Lewaa, I. Identification of Anti-SARS-CoV-2 Compounds from Food Using QSAR-Based Virtual Screening, Molecular Docking, and Molecular Dynamics Simulation Analysis. *Pharmaceuticals* **2021**, *14*, 357. [CrossRef]
41. Kar, S.; Roy, K.; Leszczynski, J. Applicability Domain: A Step Toward Confident Predictions and Decidability for QSAR Modeling. In *Computational Toxicology*; Humana Press: New York, NY, USA, 2018; pp. 141–169.
42. Gramatica, P.; Kovarich, S.; Roy, P.P. Reply to the comment of S. Rayne on "QSAR model reproducibility and applicability: A case study of rate constants of hydroxyl radical reaction models applied to polybrominated diphenyl ethers and (benzo-)triazoles". *J. Comput. Chem.* **2013**, *34*, 1796. [CrossRef]

pharmaceuticals

MDPI

Article

Drug Discovery of New Anti-Inflammatory Compounds by Targeting Cyclooxygenases

Shady Burayk [1], Kentaro Oh-hashi [2] and Mahmoud Kandeel [1,3,*]

1 Department of Biomedical Sciences, College of Veterinary Medicine, King Faisal University, Al-Hofuf 31982, Saudi Arabia; drshady1@live.com
2 Department of Chemistry and Biomolecular Science, Faculty of Engineering, Gifu University, 1-1 Yanagido, Gifu 501-1193, Japan; oohashi@gifu-u.ac.jp
3 Department of Pharmacology, Faculty of Veterinary Medicine, KafrelShaikh University, Kafr El-Shaikh 33516, Egypt
* Correspondence: mkandeel@kfu.edu.sa

Abstract: The goal of achieving anti-inflammatory efficacy with the fewest possible adverse effects through selective COX-2 inhibition is still being investigated in order to develop drugs with safe profiles. This work shows the efficacy and safety profile of two novel benzimidazole piperidine and phenoxy pyridine derivatives in reaching this goal, which would be considered a major achievement in inflammatory therapy. The compounds were evaluated by virtual screening campaign, in vitro cyclooxygenase 1 and 2 (COX-1 and COX-2) inhibition, in vivo carrageenan-induced rat paw edema assay, cytotoxicity against Raw264.7 cells, and histopathological examination of rat paw and stomach. Two new compounds, compound **1** ([(2-{[3-(4-methyl-1H-benzimidazol-2-yl)piperidin-1-yl]carbonyl}phenyl)amino]acetic acid) and compound **2** (ethyl 1-(5-cyano-2-hydroxyphenyl)-4-oxo-5-phenoxy-1,4-dihydropyridine-3-carboxylate) showed high selectivity against COX-2, favourable drug-likeness and ADME descriptors, a lack of cytotoxicity, relived paw edema, and inflammation without noticeable side effects on the stomach. These two compounds are promising new NSAIDs.

Keywords: docking; non-steroidal anti-inflammatory drugs; drug discovery; lipoxygenase; cyclooxygenase

Citation: Burayk, S.; Oh-hashi, K.; Kandeel, M. Drug Discovery of New Anti-Inflammatory Compounds by Targeting Cyclooxygenases. *Pharmaceuticals* **2022**, *15*, 282. https://doi.org/10.3390/ph15030282

Academic Editor: Osvaldo Andrade Santos-Filho

Received: 7 January 2022
Accepted: 14 February 2022
Published: 24 February 2022

1. Introduction

Inflammation is a chain of physiological responses involving a wide range of different molecules and cellular responses [1]. The mediators that emerge from two routes are particularly interesting from the perspective of drug research. Leukotrienes (LTs) are the first class of mediators that contribute to the inflammatory process, and they play a significant part in the inflammatory process overall. LTs are produced by the enzyme Arachidonate 5-lipoxygenase (5-LOX) [2,3]. The second set is more diverse and comes in effect after the activity of COXs that convert arachidonic acid to prostaglandin. PGE2 and PGI2 increase blood flow in inflamed areas by their potent vasodilator action. Prostacyclin (PGI2) is responsible for platelet aggregation and vascular endothelium inhibition. The vasodilation effect of Prostacyclin E2 and Prostacyclin I2 contributes to the protection of the gastric mucosa by boosting mucus secretion and preventing an increase in acidity and pepsin content in the stomach. In kidneys, PGE and PGI play roles in increasing the flow of the blood and regulation of the glomerular filtration rate [4,5].

Nonsteroidal anti-inflammatory drugs (NSAIDs) are a type of prescription that, when taken in sufficient amounts, can reduce pain, inflammation, blood clotting, and fever. NSAIDs may cause several side effects in patients, however, the most dangerous side effects include gastrointestinal ulcers, kidney problems, heart attacks, and bleeding [6]. Despite a few side effects, the drug's benefits outweigh the risks, making it a viable therapeutic option. NSAIDs are the gold standard in the treatment of inflammatory episodes due to their ability to block the arachidonic acid pathways [7]. NSAIDs act by selective or non-selective inhibition of both enzymes COX-1and COX-2 [8,9]. In addition to lowering inflammation, non-selective medicines work by inhibiting the aggregation of platelets. Additionally, the medication raises the risk of stomach ulcers and bleeding. Gastrointestinal side effects are a prominent concern associated with the use of NSAIDs. These medications cause both direct and indirect irritation of the digestive tract. The acidic components of NSAIDs produce direct irritation of the stomach mucosa as well as inhibit COX-1, resulting in a decrease in prostaglandin levels. Prostaglandin secretion is suppressed throughout the gastrointestinal tract, which increases the formation of stomach acid and decreases the synthesis of mucus, bicarbonates, and the tropical effects of mucosa and epithelial cells [10]. To some extent, all NSAIDs can impair neutrophil activity, but indomethacin, piroxicam, ibuprofen, and all salicylates have the most dramatic effect [11]. There are fewer side effects with selective COX-2 inhibitors, and their gastrointestinal ulcerogenic properties are decreased as well [12]. The pursuit for a less toxic NSAID resulted in the release of two selective COX-2 inhibitors in 1999, celecoxib and rofecoxib [11]. No NSAID is a complete COX-1 or COX-2 inhibitor; rather, each enzyme is inhibited to varying degrees. Given the tremendous load posed by NSAIDs, COX-2 inhibitors appear to be a viable alternative for reducing the risk of major GI bleeding [11].

Therapeutic development will continue to rely extensively on computational tools to aid in the identification and validation of potential drug targets, which will help to accelerate the process [13–16]. The field of bioinformatics is at the forefront of our efforts to better comprehend the workings of the cell. In order to produce hypotheses for testing, it is necessary to integrate enormous volumes of knowledge from numerous subdisciplines within molecular and cell biology into a cellular model that can be tested. We used such a compilation of methods to deliver new NSAIDs. The selection of such novel compounds was based on their general high selectivity on COX-2, ability to pass drug-likeness and ADME evaluations, strong anti-inflammatory activity, no stomach side effects, and safety when tested in human cell culture.

2. Results

2.1. Molecular Docking of Compounds

The rationale behind this study was to discover new selective COX-2 inhibitors utilizing virtual screening of a library of chemical compounds that consisted of 1.2 million compounds from the Chembridge Inc core library. Following a two-step, virtual screening procedure that included standard precision docking (SP) followed by extreme precision docking (XP), the compounds with the highest docking scores were obtained from the database (Figure 1). The compound docking scores and ligand efficiency are displayed in Table 1. The compounds are accompanied by favourable hydrogen bonds and lipophilic scores as indicated by the negative values of Glide lipo and Hbond.

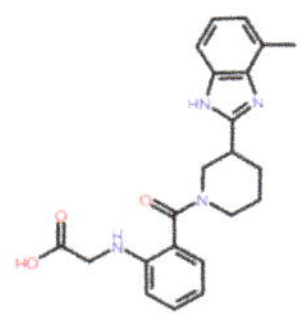

Compound 1
(90161657)

[(2-{[3-(4-methyl-1H-benzimidazol-2-yl)piperidin-1-yl]carbonyl}phenyl)amino]acetic acid

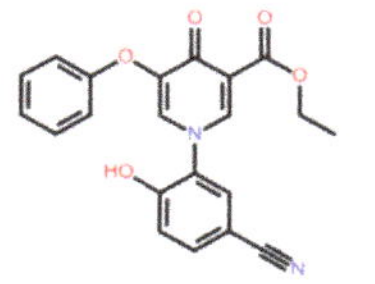

Compound 2
(35262215)

ethyl 1-(5-cyano-2-hydroxyphenyl)-4-oxo-5-phenoxy-1,4-dihydropyridine-3-carboxylate

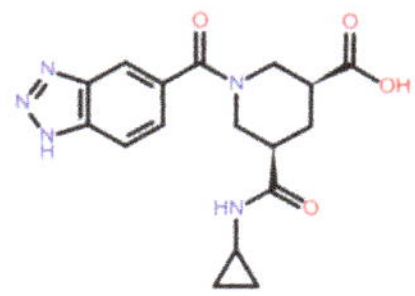

Compound 3
(14428593)

(3S,5R)-1-(1H-1,2,3-benzotriazol-5-ylcarbonyl)-5-[(cyclopropylamino)carbonyl]-3-piperidinecarboxylic acid

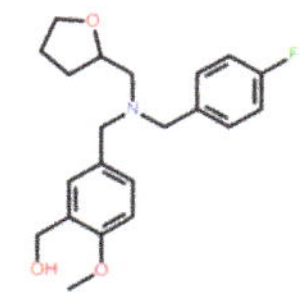

Compound 4
(43255511)

(5-{[(4-fluorobenzyl)(tetrahydrofuran-2-ylmethyl)amino]methyl}-2-methoxyphenyl)methanol

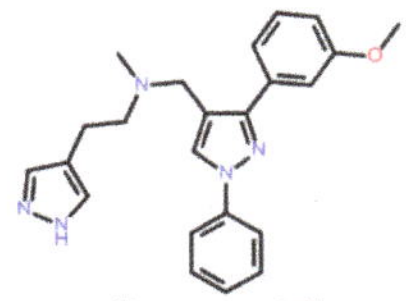

Compound 5
(20053063)

N-{[3-(3-methoxyphenyl)-1-phenyl-1H-pyrazol-4-yl]methyl}-N-methyl-2-(1H-pyrazol-4-yl)ethanamine

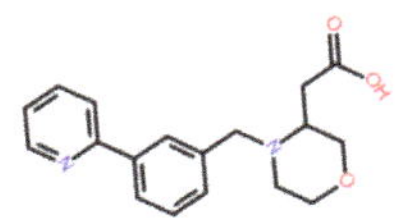

Compound 6
(21586151)

{4-[3-(2-pyridinyl)benzyl]-3-morpholinyl}acetic acid

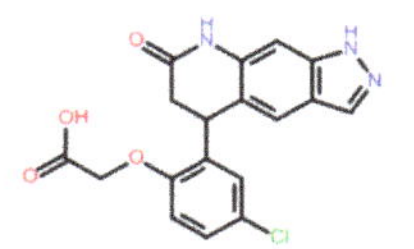

Compound 7
(86480078)

[4-chloro-2-(7-oxo-5,6,7,8-tetrahydro-1H-pyrazolo[4,3-g]quinolin-5-yl)phenoxy]acetic acid

Figure 1. Compounds' chemical names, structures, and IDs. The compounds were purchased from Chembridge (San Diego, CA, USA).

Table 1. The obtained compounds with the highest docking score after virtual screening using PDB ID 5IKQ.

Compound #	Docking Score (kcal/mol)	Glide H Bond	Glide Lipo	Glide Ligand Efficiency
1	−13.645	−0.908	−3.705	−0.471
2	−12.442	−0.172	−5.079	−0.444
3	−12.523	−0.73	−3.433	−0.482
4	−12.41	0	−5.106	−0.477
5	−13.14	−0.87	−5.373	−0.453
6	−13.408	0	−3.123	−0.583
7	−13.222	−0.813	−4.053	−0.509

By analyzing the ligand interactions of the docked compounds with COX-2 structure, several interaction forces maintained the complexes binding with COX-2, comprising salt bridges, stacking interactions, and hydrogen bonds (Figure 2). Compound **1** formed a hydrogen bond and salt bridge with ARG120. Compounds **2**, **3**, and **6** formed salt bridges with ARG120. Compound **4** formed a stacking interaction with TYR355 and a hydrogen bond with SER530. Compound **5** formed a stacking interaction with TYR385 and salt bridge with SER530. Compound **6** formed a hydrogen bond with ARG120. Compound **7** formed a hydrogen bond with SER530. Collectively, salt bridges with ARG120, hydrogen bonds with TYR335 and SER530, or stacking interactions with TRY385 were the major interaction of the compounds with COX-2. ARG120 and TYR355 are two major residues at the construction site of COX-2. The projected selectivity of compounds against COX-2 can be concluded from the interaction with the side pocket of COX-2 composed of ARG513, ALA516, ILE517, PHE518, VAL523, and LEU531.

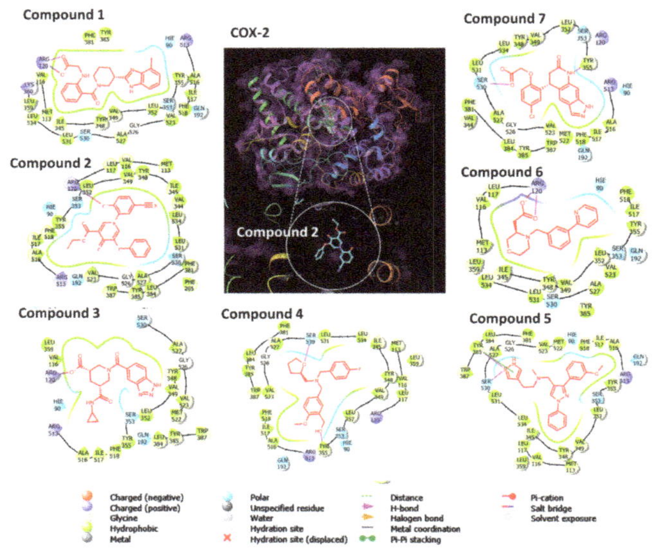

Figure 2. The docking site and ligand interactions of compounds **1**–**7**. The ligand interaction of every compound is provided. Positively charged residues are in blue, while hydrophobic residues are in green. Salt bridges are depicted as double-colored lines in blue and red. Stacking interactions are represented by green lines.

2.2. ADME Pharmacokinetic Properties and Drug-Likeness Descriptors

Table 2 shows the predicted ADME parameters for the top seven compounds. With no infractions, all compounds passed Lipinski's rule of five. All compounds showed favourable mw, donor hydrogen bonds, acceptor hydrogen bonds, human oral absorption % (>30%), predicted IC50 value for blockage of HERG K+ channels (<5), absorption from skin (QPlogKp), intestinal absorption, crossing the blood–brain barrier, water accessible surface area, as well as its hydrophilic components. A few minor violations of the prediction parameters were also observed.

Table 2. Drug-likeness and ADME properties of compounds.

	Acceptable Range	Compound 1	Compound 2	Compound 3	Compound 4	Compound 5	Compound 6	Compound 7
Mol-Mw	130–725	392.457	376.372	357.368	371.779	387.483	359.44	312.368
Donor HB	0–6	2	2	3	3	1	1	1
Accept HB	2–20	6.5	6.45	9.5	6.25	5.25	6.15	6.7
Human oral absorption %	>80 high<30 low	91.392	63.711	41.441	60.987	100	100	61.58
Rule of five	Maximum 4	0	0	0	0	0	0	0
Qplog P o/w	Maximum 3	3.886	1.274	0.168	2.367	4.446	3.65	0.623
QPlogHERG	Concern below −5	−3.629	−4.202	−1.498	−3.234	−7.581	−6.219	−4.404
QPlogKp	−8.0–−0.1	−2.236	−4.012	−5.679	−4.871	−2.982	−2.777	−4.137
QPPCaco	<25 poor>500 great	213.531	43.389	5.69	13.419	442.32	926.454	53.849
QPlogBB	−3.0–1.2	−0.742	−0.713	−2.218	−1.663	−0.232	0.089	−0.395
QPPMDCK	<25 poor>500 great	118.581	23.433	3.263	14.645	226.628	912.502	29.595
QPlogKhsa	−1.5–1.5	0.21	−0.056	−0.83	−0.067	0.77	0.211	−0.253
SASA	300–1000	640.252	624.75	609.578	586.73	712.49	655.337	584.481
FISA	7.0–330.0	112.838	122.221	265.073	239.562	78.779	44.92	112.33
Carcinogenicity in mouse	Negative	Negative	Negative	Negative	Negative	Negative	Negative	Negative
Carcinogenicity in rat	Negative	Negative	Negative	Negative	Negative	Negative	Negative	Negative

2.3. Inhibition of COXs

Within the examined seven compounds, compounds **1–3** showed the highest selectivity index. Compounds **1–3** inhibited the enzymes with compound **1** IC_{50} values of 11.68 ± 1.2 μM and 0.068 ± 0.008 for COX-1 and COX-2, respectively (Table 3). The IC_{50} for compound **2** was 12.22 ± 1.1 and 0.048 ± 0.002 μM for COX-1 and COX-2, respectively. The IC_{50} for compound **3** was 11.11 ± 1.1 and 0.06 ± 0.003 μM for COX-1 and COX-2, respectively. The selectivity index for compound **1** was 124.5 and 68.7-fold higher than indomethacin and diclofenac, respectively. In contrast, it was 1.9-fold lower than celecoxib. Compound **2** has a selectivity index of 254.5, which is higher than compound **1** and makes it the most selective COX-2 inhibitor. Compound **3** was placed second on the selectivity index, with an SI value of 194.9.

Table 3. The estimated IC50 values (μM) for Compounds **1–3** against COX-1 and COX-2. Celecoxib, rofecoxib, indomethacin, and diclofenac were used as control drugs.

	COX-1	COX-2	SI
Celecoxib	14.7 ± 1.045	0.045 ± 0.005	326.6
Rofecoxib	14.5 ± 1.125	0.025 ± 0.005	580
Indomethacin	0.1 ± 0.015	0.0725 ± 0.01	1.38
Diclofenac	0.05 ± 0.006	0.02 ± 0.001	2.5
Compound **1**	11.68 ± 1.2	0.068 ± 0.008	171.8
Compound **2**	12.22 ± 1.1	0.048 ± 0.002	254.5
Compound **3**	11.11 ± 1.1	0.06 ± 0.003	194.91
Compound **4**	7.62 ± 0.05	0.21 ± 0.01	36.3
Compound **5**	10.57 ± 0.33	0.08 ± 0.009	132.64
Compound **6**	11.52 ± 0.13	0.06 ± 0.075	190.88
Compound **7**	9.19 ± 0.046	0.097 ± 0.015	95.068

2.4. The Anti-Inflammatory Assay (Carrageenan-Induced Paw Edema in Rats)

The carrageenan-induced paw edema model was used to evaluate the compounds' anti-inflammatory activity. Only carrageenan was given to the control animals. The treatment effect was tracked by observing the improvement of rat paw edema in response to drug administration. Carrageenan injections caused rat paws to grow from 0.3 cm to 0.8 cm in size. After 1 h of dosing, diclofenac and indomethacin dramatically reduced rat paw edema (Figure 3). Compounds **1**, **2**, and **3** significantly reduced rat paw size, comparable to diclofenac and indomethacin. The size of the rat paw edema (Figure 4) decreased significantly 30 min after the compounds and drugs were administered. The growth of the rat paw progressed in a substantially comparable manner 3–4 h after injection across all chemicals and medications examined.

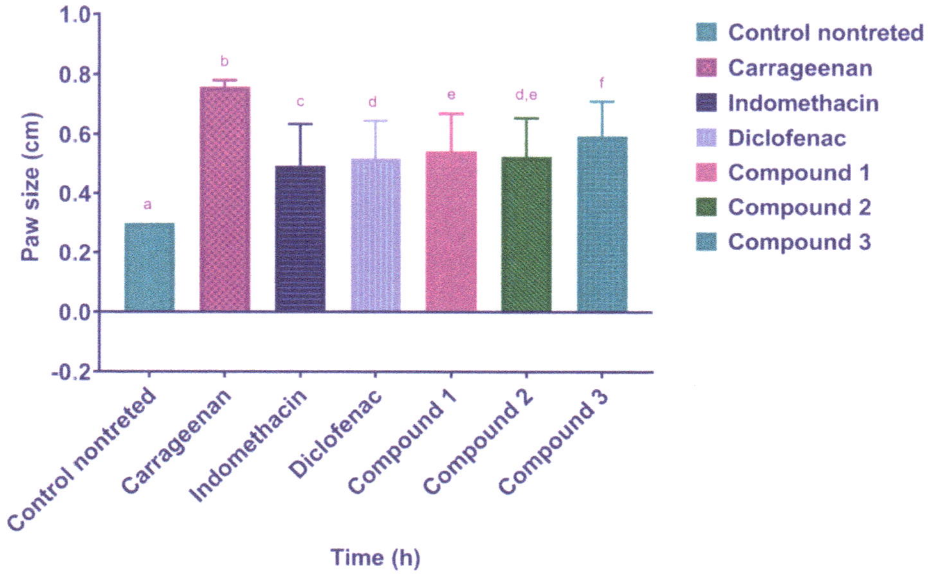

Figure 3. Average rats paw edema size (cm). The control group was treated with 0.2 mL of 1% carrageenan. Compounds **1**, **2**, and **3** were given orally at a dose rate of 10 mg/kg. The control nontreated group received NaCMC. The rat paw size was evaluated for 5 h after treatment. Each column represents the mean ± SD. Mean values in each plot followed by a different lowercase letter (a, b, c, d, e and f) are significantly different at $p \leq 0.05$.

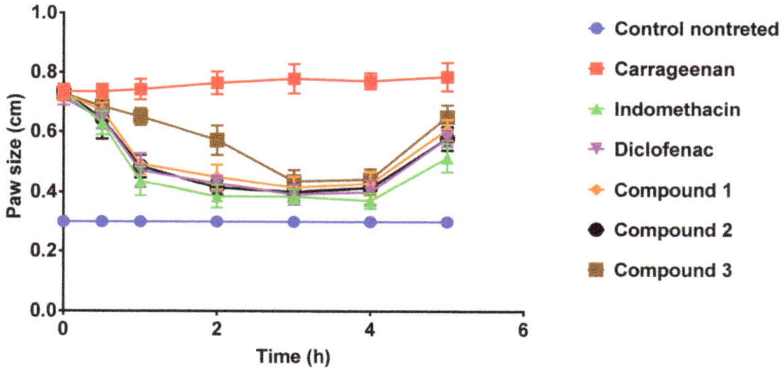

Figure 4. The progress of rat paw edema (cm) for 5 h after compounds administration. The control group was treated with 0.2 mL of 1% carrageenan. Compounds **1**, **2**, and **3** were given orally at a dose rate of 10 mg/kg. The control nontreated group received NaCMC. The measurement was performed at 0, 30 min, 1, 2, 3, 4 and 5 h after administration of the drugs.

2.5. Cytotoxicity on Mouse Macrophage-Like Cell Line (Raw264.7 Cells)

Raw264.7 cells were used to test the effects of compounds **1**, **2**, and **3** on cell viability and proliferation. Raw264.7 cells were treated for 24 h in a 96-well plate with compounds (1 µM) in the presence or absence of LPS (1 ug/mL). WST1 reagent was added to each well after treatment and incubated for an additional 2 h. Following that, the OD450/620 ratio was determined. LPS treatment had a significant impact on cell morphology and proliferation. However, all compounds had no effect on WST1 values or cell morphology in

Raw264.7 cells. Raw264.7 cells in a 96-well plate were treated with our compounds (1 uM) in the presence or absence of LPS (1 ug/mL) for 24 h. After treatment, the WST1 reagent was added into each well and incubated for an additional 2 h. After that, OD450/620 was measured.

2.6. Histopathological Examination of Rat Paw

The control group sections of rat paw displayed a healthy paw tissue structure, exhibiting a typical intact epidermal layer of stratified squamous epithelium and dermal layer with ample capillaries and connective tissue cells (Figure 5A,B). Conversely, the carrageenan-injected paw tissue section examination showed substantial histopathological changes. There was increased dermis thickness attributable to edema with a marked inflammatory cell invasion of the deep dermis compared to the control group (Figure 5C,D). However, the compound **1**-treated group exhibited marked improvement in the degree of edema and the inflammatory cell infiltration (Figure 5E,F). Interestingly, compound **2** exerted a marked anti-inflammatory effect and a pronounced decline in edema and inflammatory cell invasion (Figure 5G,H), which is almost similar to the impact of indomethacin; nevertheless, enhanced improvement in the degree of edema could be seen in the presence of compound **2**. Compound **3** showed weaker action than compounds **1** and **2** manifested by a moderate increase in cell infiltration and edema (Figure 5I,J).

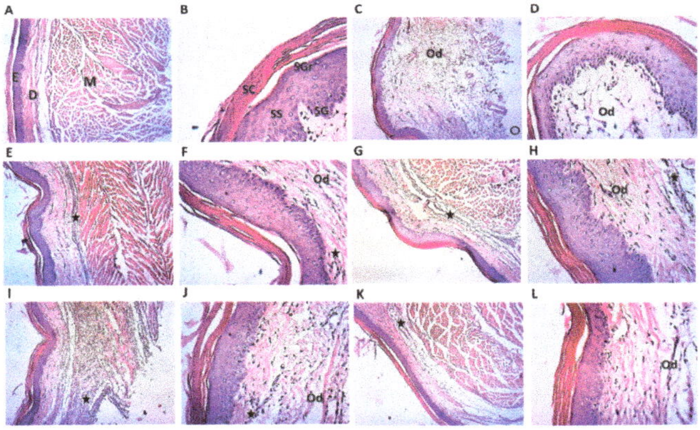

Figure 5. Histopathologic examination of rat paw stained by H&E. (**A**) Photomicrograph of control rat paw at 10× magnification showing normal epidermal layers (E), dermis (D), and muscle layer (M); notice the absence of any signs of an inflammatory reaction. (**B**) Photomicrograph of control rat paw at 40× magnification showing normal SC, stratum corneum; SGr, stratum granulosum; SS, stratum spinosum; and SG, stratum germinativum. (**C**) Photomicrograph of rat paw at 10× magnification of carrageenan-treated group showing marked thickening of the dermal layer, inflammatory reaction in the deep dermis, and wide separation between fibers due to edema (Od). (**D**) Photomicrograph of rat paw at 40× magnification of carrageenan-treated group showing edema (Od). (**E**) Photomicrograph of rat paw at 10× magnification of carrageenan-treated group followed by treatment with compound **1** showing a significant decrease in the dermal thickness, inflammatory reaction in the deep dermis (black star), and moderate improvements in edema (Od). (**F**) Photomicrograph of rat paw at 40× magnification of carrageenan-treated group followed by treatment with compound **1** showing slight inflammatory reaction (black star) and edema (Od). (**G**) Photomicrograph of rat paw at 10× magnification of carrageenan-treated group followed by treatment with compound **2** showing a substantial decrease in both the inflammatory reaction (black star) and edema (Od). (**H**) Photomicrograph of rat paw at 40× magnification of carrageenan-treated group followed by treatment with compound **2** showing slight inflammatory reaction (black star) and

edema (Od). (**I**) Photomicrograph of rat paw at 10× magnification of carrageenan-treated group followed by treatment with compound **3** showing a significant decrease in the degree of inflammatory reaction (black star) and a moderate decrease in edema (Od). (**J**) Photomicrograph of rat paw at 40× magnification of carrageenan-treated group followed by treatment with compound **3** showing moderate inflammatory reaction (black star) and edema (Od). (**K**) Photomicrograph of rat paw at 10× magnification of carrageenan-treated group followed by treatment with indomethacin showing a significant decrease in the degree of inflammatory reaction (black star) and a moderate decrease in edema (Od). (**L**) Photomicrograph of rat paw at 40× magnification of carrageenan-treated group followed by treatment with indomethacin showing slight inflammatory reaction (black star) and edema (Od).

The degree of collagen deposition was investigated by Masson's stain as a qualitative indicator. Blue-green stained collagen was used for the purpose of assessing collagen deposition progression; the cytoplasm, red blood cells, and muscle were stained red. The density of the blue-green collagen is consistent with the relative amount of deposited total collagen fiber, which represents collagen synthesis, degradation, and remodeling. As shown by Masson's stain, there were more collagen fibers in the carrageenan group compared with the normal group (Figure 6A). Besides, among the treated groups, the collagen deposition was almost similar to the control nontreated group, except for compound **3**. The quantity of collagen formation was the lowest in the compound **2**-treated group and was better than indomethacin (Figure 6B–E).

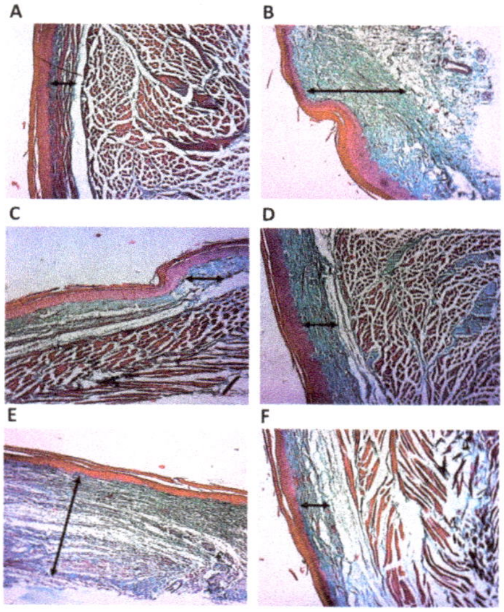

Figure 6. Histopathologic examination of rat paw stained by Masson's Trichrome stain. Collagen fibrils are stained blue-green. The double-headed arrow represents collagen fibrils thickness between epidermis and dermis. (**A**) Photomicrograph of control rat paw at 10× magnification showing normal collagen deposition. (**B**) Photomicrograph of rat paw at 10× magnification of carrageenan-treated group showing intense collagen deposition. (**C**) Photomicrograph of rat paw at 10× magnification of carrageenan-treated group followed by treatment with compound **1** showing slight collagen deposition (**D**). Photomicrograph of rat paw at 10× magnification of carrageenan-treated group followed by treatment with compound **2** showing slight collagen deposition. (**E**) Photomicrograph of rat paw at 10× magnification of carrageenan-treated group followed by treatment with compound **3** showing significant collagen deposition. (**F**) Photomicrograph of rat paw at 10× magnification of carrageenan-treated group followed by treatment with indomethacin showing slight collagen deposition.

2.7. Histopathological Examination of Rat Stomach

The control group stomach sections displayed a healthy gastric tissue structure, exhibiting typical intact villi of gastric mucosa with no signs of hemorrhages or congestion; also there is no exfoliation in the mucosal epithelium or inflammatory cell infiltration (Figure 7A,B). Interestingly, compound **1**, compound **2**, compound **3**, and indomethacin-treated groups did not show apparent histopathological changes (Figure 7C–J). The collagen deposition was almost similar to control nontreated animals in compounds **1** and **2** (Figure 8A–F). Conversely, compound **3** and indomethacin exerted a mild increase in collagen deposition (Figure 8G–J).

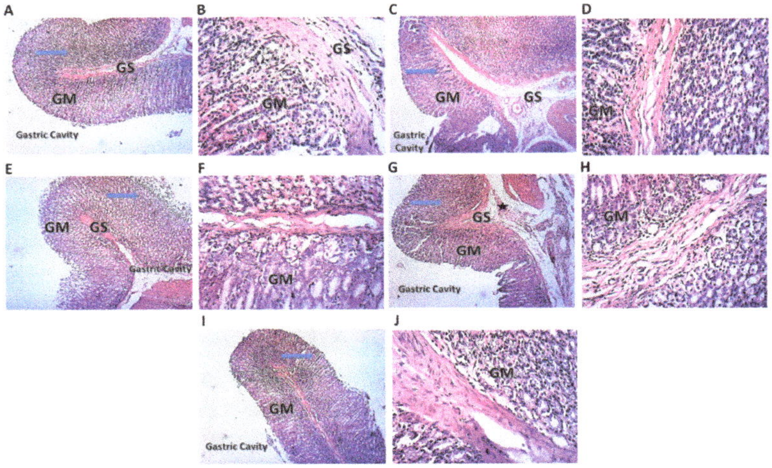

Figure 7. Histopathologic examination of rat stomach stained by H&E. (**A**) Photomicrograph of control rat stomach at 10× magnification showing normal gastric layers. Blue arrow shows intact appearance of histological structure of the epithelium and mucosa layer; GM, Gastric Mucosa; GS, Gastric Submucosa. (**B**) Photomicrograph of control rat stomach at 40× magnification showing absence of any signs of an inflammatory reaction. (**C**) Photomicrograph of rat stomach at 10× magnification of treatment with compound **1** showing normal gastric layers. Blue arrow shows intact appearance of histological structure of the epithelium and mucosa layer; GM, Gastric Mucosa; GS, Gastric Submucosa. (**D**) Photomicrograph of rat stomach at 40× magnification of treatment with compound **1** showing absence of any signs of an inflammatory reaction. (**E**) Photomicrograph of rat stomach at 10× magnification of treatment with compound **2** showing normal gastric layers. Blue arrow shows intact appearance of histological structure of the epithelium and mucosa layer; GM, Gastric Mucosa; GS, Gastric Submucosa. (**F**) Photomicrograph of rat paw at 40× magnification of treatment with compound **2** showing absence of any signs of an inflammatory reaction. (**G**) Photomicrograph of rat stomach at 10× magnification of treatment with compound **3** showing slight degeneration of gastric layers. (**H**) Photomicrograph of rat paw at 40× magnification of treatment with compound **3** showing absence of any signs of an inflammatory reaction. (**I**) Photomicrograph of rat stomach at 10× magnification of treatment with indomethacin, showing slight degeneration of gastric layers. (**J**) Photomicrograph of rat paw at 40× magnification of treatment with indomethacin showing absence of any signs of an inflammatory reaction.

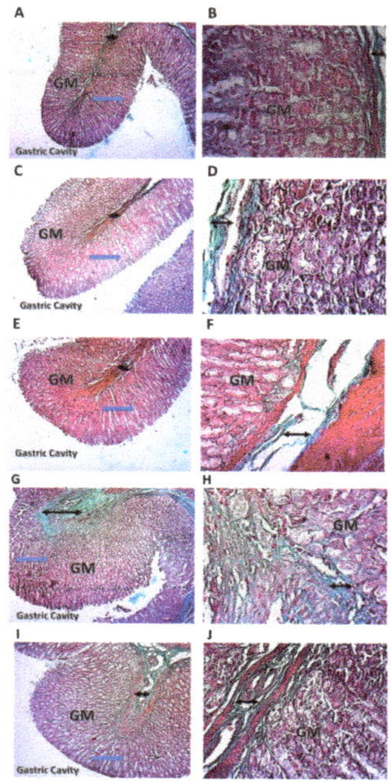

Figure 8. Histopathologic examination of rat stomach stained by Masson's Trichrome. Collagen fibrils are stained blue-green. The double-headed arrow represents collagen fibrils thickness in the submucosa. (**A**) Photomicrograph of control rat stomach at 10× magnification showing normal collagen deposition. (**B**) Photomicrograph of rat stomach at 40× magnification of control group showing normal collagen deposition. (**C**) Photomicrograph of rat stomach at 10× magnification of treatment with compound **1** showing normal collagen deposition. (**D**) Photomicrograph of rat stomach at 40× magnification of treatment with compound **1** showing normal collagen deposition. (**E**) Photomicrograph of rat stomach at 10× magnification of treatment with compound **2** showing slight collagen deposition. (**F**) Photomicrograph of rat stomach at 40× magnification of treatment with compound **2** showing slight collagen deposition. (**G**) Photomicrograph of rat stomach at 10× magnification of treatment with compound **3** showing significant collagen deposition. (**H**) Photomicrograph of rat stomach at 40× magnification of treatment with compound **3** showing significant collagen deposition. (**I**) Photomicrograph of rat stomach at 10× magnification of treatment with indomethacin showing significant collagen deposition. (**J**) Photomicrograph of rat stomach at 40× magnification of treatment with indomethacin showing collagen deposition.

3. Discussion

Despite the presence of several NSAIDs, the development of new NSAIDs is attractive, owing to the diverse inflammatory conditions and the need for optimized application in relation to disease and patient conditions. The recent development of NSAIDs comprises modified methyl sulphonyl [17]; pyrimidine-5-carbonitrile hybrids [18], pyrazole derivatives [19], indanone containing spiroisoxazoline derivatives [20], triazole, and oxadiazole compounds [21,22]. Despite the growing repository of newly synthesized NSAIDs, the development of new compounds is strictly required due to the side effects of the currently approved NSAIDs. For instance, even in short-term applications, a high dose of ibuprofen resulted in jejunal perforations [23]; naproxen affects bowel and jejunal integrity [24]. Within days of intake, diclofenac has been proven to raise the risk of heart attacks and strokes by 50% [25].

The intricate interplay between injured tissues and inflammatory cells, which results in the release of inflammatory mediators such as interleukins, necrotic factors, and enzymes such as cyclooxygenases and lipoxygenases, is a crucial aspect of inflammation [26]. The overexpression of COX-1 and COX-2 during inflammatory processes is crucial for the inflammatory signaling system [27]. Controlling inflammation can prevent excessive injury from an aggressive immune response or the development of chronic illness [28].

Drug molecules meet several membrane barriers on their kinetic voyage through the body, including the blood–brain barrier, gastrointestinal epithelial cells, and the membrane target cell. Predicting permeability behind barriers will aid in the prediction of pharmacokinetic parameters and the knowledge of chemical behavior within the body. QikProp estimates and predicts molecular characteristics and provides results for ADME (absorption, distribution, metabolism, and excretion) [29]. Lipinski's "Rule of Five" and the "Jorgensen Rule-of-Three" were used to determine drug-likeness. The "Jorgensen Rule-of-Three" is based on the qualities of over 90% of 1700 oral medications and meets the "rule of five", indicating that these molecules can be utilized as potent drugs/inhibitors [30]. The basic drug-likeness and ADME qualities of compounds **1–3** indicated generally acceptable parameters, particularly the absence of breaches of Lipinski's rule of five, good oral absorption, and lack of carcinogenic potential. This was further demonstrated experimentally by the absence of any harmful effect on Raw264.7 cells.

Compounds **1–3** were compared to selective and nonselective COX inhibitors for cyclooxygenases inhibition. Compounds **1–3** inhibited COX-1 less well than indomethacin and diclofenac but were comparable to the selective medicines celecoxib and rofecoxib. When compared to the nonselective medication indomethacin, compounds **1–3** had at least a 100-fold lower impact on COX-1. Furthermore, all compounds inhibited COX-2 at lower concentrations than indomethacin and diclofenac, particularly compound 2, which was comparable to the selective drug celecoxib. The overall selectivity index was in the following order: rofecoxib < celecoxib < compound **2** <compound **3** < compound **1** < diclofenac < indomethacin. This discovery lends credence to the usage of chemicals 1 and 2 as anti-inflammatory medicines. They have no adverse effects on the gastric mucosa and may have no negative effects on the body due to their high selectivity for COX-2 inhibition. Because of their anti-inflammatory efficacy and low gastrointestinal toxicity, COX-2 selective medications have become the most common anti-inflammatory therapy [31]. However, it was quickly discovered that long-term use of COXIBs in arthritic patients was linked to cardiac adverse effects [32]. This has resulted in the withdrawal of some COXIBs, such as rofecoxib, and a warning label for usage in patients with cardiovascular difficulties for other COXIBs, like celecoxib [33]. In this context, the strong selectivity for COX-2 could be linked to such results. In our investigation, compounds **1–3** showed medium selectivity between highly selective COXIBs and nonselective COX inhibitors. Because of their lower selectivity index than celecoxib and rofecoxib, these compounds may have an advantage because they have been proven to be kinder on the gastric mucosa and are anticipated to have a lower impact on the cardiovascular system.

In this work, the anti-inflammatory properties of the compounds were evaluated using the carrageenan-induced rat paw swelling test. Carrageenan stimulates exudate release and edema by increasing COX-2 expression, making this model excellent for testing COX-2 inhibitors [28]. The acute carrageenan-induced inflammation in the rat paw corresponds to the findings of in vitro enzymatic tests. Rat paw edema was significantly reduced after treatment with compounds **1–3**, indomethacin, and celecoxib. Edema in the paws of rats has two stages. The first stage lasts 2 h and includes histamine and serotonin release. During the second stage, inflammatory exudate and enzymes such as cyclooxygenases are released, and cells are invaded [34]. As a result, the action of compounds **1–3** after 1–4 h of inflammation is consistent with cyclooxygenase inhibitory function. Compounds **1** and **2** had a better gastrointestinal safety profile than indomethacin because they did not promote degenerative alterations and exhibited normal collagen deposition in treated rats after a single high dosage. This is consistent with the in vitro COX-1/COX-2 assay's finding of COX-2 selectivity rather than COX-1. Compounds **1** and **2** appear to be potential NSAIDs based on the entire analysis. Compound **3** was found to be less effective in alleviating inflammatory cells and rat paw edema, as well as increased collagen deposition in the rat stomach.

4. Materials and Methods

4.1. Software, Chemicals and Kits

The Schrodinger Maestro molecular modeling package (Schrodinger LLC, New York, NY, USA) was used in all virtual screening modeling steps. QikProp tools are an accurate, rapid, and simple-to-use method for predicting molecular properties. GraphPad Prism 7 software was purchased from (GraphPad Software, Inc., San Diego, CA, USA). COX-1 and COX-2 inhibitor screening assay kits were obtained from Cayman Chemical (Ann Arbor, MI, USA). Indomethacin, celecoxib, carboxymethyl cellulose (NaCMC), λ-carrageenan, tris(hydroxymethyl) aminomethane, diclofenac sodium, EDTA, hematin, phenol, and hydrochloric acid were purchased from Sigma-Aldrich (St. Louis, MO, USA). Vernier calipers were manufactured by SMIEC (Shanghai, China). All compounds tested in this work were purchased from ChemBridge Inc. (La Jolla, CA, USA).

4.2. Preparation of COX-2 Structure

The protein data bank website was searched for the COX-2 structural PDB ID 5IKQ. The structure was optimized for virtual screening and docking using the protein preparation module of the Schrodinger Maestro molecular modeling tool. The solution's crystallographic compounds and water molecules were eliminated. The protein was protonated by adding polar hydrogens, and the structures were optimized and energy was decreased by employing the OPLS2005 force field. The docking grids were created using the Maestro grid-generating module, with the defined ligand-binding cavities in the studied structures serving as a starting point. A 20-nanometer grid was built around the active site of the enzyme.

4.3. Virtual Screening

To obtain the best candidates, a two-step docking run using SP followed by XP was performed. An integer value of 0.8 was chosen for Van der Waals radius scaling. Extra precision docking is intended to reduce the possibility of a false-positive outcome. Compounds with high docking scores (-12) were chosen for interaction studies with pocket residues, and their binding characteristics and pocket-filling pattern were visually examined. The docking accuracy was confirmed by the low RMSD after redocking of the co-crystallized ligand.

4.4. Drug-Likeness and ADME Pharmacokinetic Properties and Descriptors

Pharmacokinetic parameters such as absorption, distribution, metabolism, and excretion were predicted using Qikprop v4.2 tools. The molecular weight, hydrogen bond donor and acceptor, percent oral absorption in humans, an explanation for the violation of Lipinski's rule of five, and the variety of rotable bonds were among the descriptions. Expected blood/brain partition coefficient, binding to human serum, aqueous solubility (QPlogS) and octanol/water partition constant (QPlogP o/w), apparent MDCK cell permeability and skin permeability (QPlogKp), the SASA element, expected inhibitory concentration (IC50) for blocking HERG K+ Channels, and colorectal adenocarcinoma (Ca) permeability were estimated. To estimate the carcinogenicity and toxicity risk of chemicals, the preADMET web-based application was used.

4.5. Enzyme (COXs) Inhibition Assay

Following virtual screening, in vitro experiments for COX enzyme inhibition were performed on compounds with the highest docking scores (seven compounds). The inhibitory effects of compounds on COX-1 and COX-2 were determined using COX inhibitor screening test kits. The test chemicals' capacity to inhibit the conversion of arachidonic acid to prostaglandin was determined. In test tubes, 25 mM Tris–HCl, pH 8.0, containing

5 mM EDTA, phenol, and 1 mM hematin, was added. The test compounds were dissolved in dimethyl sulfoxide and added in concentrations ranging from 0.005–200 μM. Dimethyl sulfoxide alone was applied to control test containers. COX-1 or COX-2 enzymes were added to test tubes and preincubated for 10 min at 37 °C. The arachidonic acid substrate was added, and the tubes were incubated at 37 °C for 2 min. The compound immunochemical assay was used to calculate the amount of prostaglandin produced. Three separate experiments were used to calculate the *IC*50 values. The selectivity index was calculated as follows:

$$Selectivity\ index = \frac{IC50COX-1}{IC50COX-2} \tag{1}$$

4.6. Evaluation of Anti-Inflammatory Actions by Carrageenan Induced Paw Edema in Rats

Following in vitro testing, three compounds with the highest selectivity against COX-2 were chosen for in vivo investigations utilizing the rat paw edema assay. After subcutaneous carrageenan injection into the rodent's paw, plasma extravasation, tissue proliferation, plasma protein release, and neutrophilic extravasation, all of which are caused by arachidonic acid digestion, produced inflammation. Following the carrageenan infusion, the main phase lasted 2 h. The following process is remodeling, which takes 5 h and begins at the 3rd h. The main stage is distinguished by the appearance of histamine and serotonin. The development of prostaglandins, proteases, and lysosomes causes the second stage of edema. Adult male albino rats weighing 120–150 g were divided into seven groups, each with seven rats, and kept at 25 °C with a 12-h light/dark cycle. Subplantar injection of 0.2 mL of 1% carrageenan solution in 0.9 percent saline into the right hind paw of rats was used to induce swelling and inflammation. To determine the inflammation generated by carrageenan, the Vernier Caliper was used to measure the thickness of rat paws before and after injection. Compounds **1–3**, as well as indomethacin and diclofenac sodium, were suspended in 1% NaCMC in normal saline and given orally at 10 mg/kg in a total volume of 1 mL per rat, with the negative control getting 1 mL of 1% NaCMC-saline solution. Paw edema was measured at 0, 0.5, 1, 2, 3, 4, and 5 h after the drug was administered. The edema inhibition was calculated by calculating the difference in thicknesses between the treated and control groups [35,36].

4.7. Histopathological Examination

4.7.1. Rat Paw

The rats' paws were collected and washed in a saline solution after the end of rat paw experiment. Specimens were fixed in 10% natural formalin for 2 days before being washed overnight with running water. The cleaned samples were dehydrated in ethyl alcohol at increasing percentages, starting with 70% and ending with absolute alcohol. The samples were cleaned by immersing them in xylol for 2 h. For 3 h at 37 °C, the cleared samples were placed in a sealed jar containing 50% paraffin in xylol. The samples were then soaked in melting paraffin for 2 h at 48 °C before being blocked in hard paraffin and sliced into 5-micron slices. The sections were stained with hematoxylin and eosin (H&E) and Masson's trichrome. Sections were mounted with Canada balsam and covered with a coverslip in preparation for histological examination.

4.7.2. Rat Stomach and Evaluation of the Ulcerogenic Effect of Test Compounds

Compounds **1–3** were examined for ulcerogenic effects in the rat stomach after showing anti-inflammatory advantages in a rat paw test. Rats were deprived for 24 h at 25 °C with a 12 h light/dark cycle. Indomethacin was used as a control. All compounds were given in a single dose of 20 mg/kg orally. After 24 h, the rats were slaughtered, and their stomachs were removed and washed with normal saline. Binocular magnification was used to inspect each group's stomachs for the existence of a gastric lesion on the mucosa. Following that, the stomachs were kept in 10% *w*/*v* formalin for histological investigation, as previously described.

4.8. *In Vitro Cytotoxicity Using Mouse Macrophage-Like Cell Line (Raw264.7 Cells)*

Dulbecco's modified Eagle's minimum essential medium containing 5% heat-inactivated fetal bovine serum was used to maintain Raw264.7 cells (ATCC). Raw264.7 cells (0.8104 cells/100 μL) in a 96-well plate were treated for 24 h with the indicated compounds at 1 μM or vehicle (DMSO) in the presence or absence of LPS (1 μg/mL) to detect cell viability based on mitochondrial activity. WST-1 solution (Dojindo) was then added to each well and incubated at 37 °C for an additional 2 h. According to a previous study, cell viability was determined using the difference in absorbance at 450 and 620 nm as an indicator [37].

4.9. *Statistical Analysis*

All results were presented as means standard deviations (SD). Statistical analysis was performed as previously described [38]. When appropriate, statistical analysis was carried out using two-way analysis of variance (ANOVA) followed by the Bonferroni's test, or one-way ANOVA followed by the Tukey's test. p values of less than 0.05 were regarded as statistically significant. GraphPad Prism version 5.00 for Windows (San Diego, CA, USA) was used for all statistical analyses.

5. Conclusions

A virtual screening effort of 1.2 million compounds was launched in a study to uncover novel COX-2 selective NSAIDs. A docking score filtration of the compounds offered a hint for future investigation using experimental techniques. Compound **1** ([(2-{[3-(4-methyl-1H-benzimidazol-2-yl)piperidin-1-yl]carbonyl}phenyl)amino]acetic acid) and compound **2** (ethyl 1-(5-cyano-2-hydroxyphenyl)-4-oxo-5-phenoxy-1,4-dihydropyridine-3-carboxylate) showed promising anti-inflammatory activity. Compounds **1** and **2** were highly selective for COX-2, reduced rat paw edema, were non-cytotoxic on cells, decreased inflammatory cells infiltration and edema, and did not display adverse responses on rat stomach. These two compounds are recommended as new promising NSAIDs.

6. Patents

Compounds **1** and **2** in this manuscript are subject to patent application at the US patent office. USPTO application no. 17665553 (methods of treating inflammation) and attorney docket no. 32087.20.

Author Contributions: Conceptualization, M.K. and S.B.; methodology, M.K. and K.O.-h.; software, M.K.; validation, M.K. and S.B.; formal analysis, M.K., K.O.-h. and S.B.; investigation, M.K. and S.B.; resources, M.K.; writing—original draft preparation, M.K.; funding acquisition, M.K. and S.B. All authors have read and agreed to the published version of the manuscript.

Funding: This work was supported by the Deanship of Scientific Research, Vice Presidency for Graduate Studies and Scientific Research, King Faisal University, Saudi Arabia [Project No. GRANT225].

Institutional Review Board Statement: The animal study protocol was approved by the Institutional Ethics Committee of King Faisal University (approval no. KFUREC/2020-03-03, date 24 March 2020).

Informed Consent Statement: Not applicable.

Data Availability Statement: Data is contained within the article.

Acknowledgments: The authors acknowledge the College of Veterinary Medicine at King Faisal University for providing lab animal facilities and computational resources.

Conflicts of Interest: The authors declare no conflict of interest.

References

1. Eming, S.A.; Krieg, T.; Davidson, J.M. Inflammation in wound repair: Molecular and cellular mechanisms. *J. Investig. Dermatol.* **2007**, *127*, 514–525. [CrossRef] [PubMed]
2. Serhan, C.N.; Savill, J. Resolution of inflammation: The beginning programs the end. *Nat. Immunol.* **2005**, *6*, 1191–1197. [CrossRef] [PubMed]
3. Tawfik, O.; Sagrillo, C.; Johnson, D.; Dey, S. Decidualization in the bat: Role of leukotrienes and prostaglandins. *Prostaglandins Leukot. Med.* **1987**, *29*, 221–227. [CrossRef]
4. Wolfe, M.M.; Lowe, R.C. Gastric secretions. In *Yamada's Textbook of Gastroenterology*; Wiley-Blackwell: Hoboken, NJ, USA, 2015; pp. 399–419.
5. Domschke, W.; Peskar, B.; Holtermüller, K.; Dammann, H. *Prostaglandins and Leukotrienes in Gastrointestinal Diseases*; Springer Science & Business Media: Berlin/Heidelberg, Germany, 2012.
6. Osafo, N.; Agyare, C.; Obiri, D.D.; Antwi, A.O. Mechanism of action of nonsteroidal anti-inflammatory drugs. In *Nonsteroidal Anti-Inflammatory Drugs*; IntechOpen: London, UK, 2017; pp. 1–15.
7. Amadio, P., Jr.; Cummings, D.M.; Amadio, P. Nonsteroidal anti-inflammatory drugs: Tailoring therapy to achieve results and avoid toxicity. *Postgrad. Med.* **1993**, *93*, 73–97. [CrossRef]
8. Groesch, S.; Niederberger, E.; Geisslinger, G. Investigational drugs targeting the prostaglandin E2 signaling pathway for the treatment of inflammatory pain. *Expert Opin. Investig. Drugs* **2017**, *26*, 51–61. [CrossRef]
9. Bjarnason, I.; Scarpignato, C.; Holmgren, E.; Olszewski, M.; Rainsford, K.D.; Lanas, A. Mechanisms of damage to the gastrointestinal tract from nonsteroidal anti-inflammatory drugs. *Gastroenterology* **2018**, *154*, 500–514. [CrossRef]
10. Drossman, D.A.; Corazziari, E.; Delvaux, M.; Spiller, R.; Talley, N.; Thompson, W.; Whitehead, W. *Rome III: The Functional Gastrointestinal Disorders*, 3rd ed.; Degnon Associates: McLean, VA, USA, 2006.
11. Green, G.A. Understanding NSAIDs: From aspirin to COX-2. *Clin. Cornerstone* **2001**, *3*, 50–60. [CrossRef]
12. Perazella, M.A.; Eras, J. Are selective COX-2 inhibitors nephrotoxic? *Am. J. Kidney Dis.* **2000**, *35*, 937–940. [CrossRef]
13. Al-Hizab, F.; Kandeel, M. Mycophenolate suppresses inflammation by inhibiting prostaglandin synthases: A study of molecular and experimental drug repurposing. *PeerJ* **2021**, *9*, e11360. [CrossRef]
14. Kandeel, M.; Al-Nazawi, M. Virtual screening and repurposing of FDA approved drugs against COVID-19 main protease. *Life Sci.* **2020**, *251*, 117627. [CrossRef]
15. Kandeel, M.; Yamamoto, M.; Park, B.K.; Al-Taher, A.; Watanabe, A.; Gohda, J.; Kawaguchi, Y.; Oh-Hashi, K.; Kwon, H.-J.; Inoue, J.-i. Discovery of New Potent anti-MERS CoV Fusion Inhibitors. *Front. Pharmacol.* **2021**, *12*, 1241. [CrossRef]
16. Kandeel, M.; Yamamoto, M.; Tani, H.; Kobayashi, A.; Gohda, J.; Kawaguchi, Y.; Park, B.K.; Kwon, H.-J.; Inoue, J.-i.; Alkattan, A. Discovery of New Fusion Inhibitor Peptides against SARS-CoV-2 by Targeting the Spike S2 Subunit. *Biomol. Ther.* **2021**, *29*, 282. [CrossRef]
17. Sağlık, B.N.; Osmaniye, D.; Levent, S.; Çevik, U.A.; Çavuşoğlu, B.K.; Özkay, Y.; Kaplancıklı, Z.A. Design, synthesis and biological assessment of new selective COX-2 inhibitors including methyl sulfonyl moiety. *Eur. J. Med. Chem.* **2021**, *209*, 112918. [CrossRef] [PubMed]
18. Alfayomy, A.M.; Abdel-Aziz, S.A.; Marzouk, A.A.; Shaykoon, M.S.A.; Narumi, A.; Konno, H.; Abou-Seri, S.M.; Ragab, F.A. Design and synthesis of pyrimidine-5-carbonitrile hybrids as COX-2 inhibitors: Anti-inflammatory activity, ulcerogenic liability, histopathological and docking studies. *Bioorg. Chem.* **2021**, *108*, 104555. [CrossRef]
19. Abdellatif, K.R.; Abdelall, E.K.; Elshemy, H.A.; Lamie, P.F.; Elnahaas, E.; Amin, D.M. Design, synthesis of new anti-inflammatory agents with a pyrazole core: COX-1/COX-2 inhibition assays, anti-inflammatory, ulcerogenic, histopathological, molecular Modeling, and ADME studies. *J. Mol. Struct.* **2021**, *1240*, 130554. [CrossRef]
20. Abolhasani, H.; Zarghi, A.; Movahhed, T.K.; Abolhasani, A.; Daraei, B.; Dastmalchi, S. Design, synthesis and biological evaluation of novel indanone containing spiroisoxazoline derivatives with selective COX-2 inhibition as anticancer agents. *Bioorg. Med. Chem.* **2021**, *32*, 115960. [CrossRef]
21. Bekheit, M.S.; Mohamed, H.A.; Abdel-Wahab, B.F.; Fouad, M.A. Design and synthesis of new 1, 4, 5-trisubstituted triazole-bearing benzenesulphonamide moiety as selective COX-2 inhibitors. *Med. Chem. Res.* **2021**, *30*, 1125–1138. [CrossRef]
22. Nesaragi, A.R.; Kamble, R.R.; Dixit, S.; Kodasi, B.; Hoolageri, S.R.; Bayannavar, P.K.; Dasappa, J.P.; Vootla, S.; Joshi, S.D.; Kumbar, V.M. Green synthesis of therapeutically active 1, 3, 4-oxadiazoles as antioxidants, selective COX-2 inhibitors and their in silico studies. *Bioorg. Med. Chem. Lett.* **2021**, *43*, 128112. [CrossRef] [PubMed]
23. Yehiyan, A.; Barman, S.; Varia, H.; Pettit, S. Short-course high-dose ibuprofen causing both early and delayed jejunal perforations in a non-smoking man. *BMJ Case Rep.* **2017**, *2017*. [CrossRef]
24. Risty, G.M.; Najarian, M.M.; Shapiro, S.B. Multiple indomethacin-induced jejunal ulcerations with perforation: A case report with histology. *Am. Surg.* **2007**, *73*, 344–346. [CrossRef]
25. Schmidt, M.; Sørensen, H.T.; Pedersen, L. Diclofenac use and cardiovascular risks: Series of nationwide cohort studies. *BMJ Clin. Res. Ed.* **2018**, *362*, k3426. [CrossRef] [PubMed]
26. Goldstein, I.M.; Snyderman, R.; Gallin, J.I. *Inflammation: Basic Principles and Clinical Correlates*; Raven Press: Ely, MN, USA, 1992.
27. Gunaydin, C.; Bilge, S.S. Effects of nonsteroidal anti-inflammatory drugs at the molecular level. *Eurasian J. Med.* **2018**, *50*, 116. [CrossRef] [PubMed]

28. Yonezawa, Y.; Kihara, T.; Ibi, K.; Senshu, M.; Nejishima, H.; Takeda, Y.; Imai, K.; Ogawa, H. Olive-derived hydroxytyrosol shows anti-inflammatory effect without gastric damage in rats. *Biol. Pharm. Bull.* **2019**, *42*, 1120–1127. [CrossRef] [PubMed]
29. Schrödinger, Inc. Maestro. 2017. Available online: https://www.schrodinger.com/products/maestro (accessed on 13 February 2022).
30. Jorgensen, W.L.; Duffy, E.M. Prediction of drug solubility from structure. *Adv. Drug Deliv. Rev.* **2002**, *54*, 355–366. [CrossRef]
31. Zarghi, A.; Arfaei, S. Selective COX-2 Inhibitors: A Review of Their Structure-Activity Relationships. *Iran. J. Pharm. Res. IJPR* **2011**, *10*, 655–683. [PubMed]
32. Patrono, C. Cardiovascular effects of cyclooxygenase-2 inhibitors: A mechanistic and clinical perspective. *Br. J. Clin. Pharmacol.* **2016**, *82*, 957–964. [CrossRef] [PubMed]
33. Bello, A.E.; Holt, R.J. Cardiovascular risk with non-steroidal anti-inflammatory drugs: Clinical implications. *Drug Saf.* **2014**, *37*, 897–902. [CrossRef]
34. Posadas, I.; Bucci, M.; Roviezzo, F.; Rossi, A.; Parente, L.; Sautebin, L.; Cirino, G. Carrageenan-induced mouse paw oedema is biphasic, age-weight dependent and displays differential nitric oxide cyclooxygenase-2 expression. *Br. J. Pharmacol.* **2004**, *142*, 331–338. [CrossRef]
35. Winter, C.A.; Risley, E.A.; Nuss, G.W. Carrageenin-induced edema in hind paw of the rat as an assay for antiinflammatory drugs. *Proc. Soc. Exp. Biol. Med.* **1962**, *111*, 544–547. [CrossRef]
36. Tries, S.; Neupert, W.; Laufer, S. The mechanism of action of the new antiinflammatory compound ML3000: Inhibition of 5-LOX and COX-1/2. *Inflamm. Res.* **2002**, *51*, 135–143. [CrossRef]
37. Oh-Hashi, K.; Soga, A.; Naruse, Y.; Takahashi, K.; Kiuchi, K.; Hirata, Y. Elucidating post-translational regulation of mouse CREB3 in Neuro2a cells. *Mol. Cell. Biochem.* **2018**, *448*, 287–297. [CrossRef] [PubMed]
38. Barbosa, L.M.; Amaral-Machado, L.; Félix-Silva, J.; Oliveira, W.N.; Alencar, É.N.; Rocha, K.B.; da Cunha Medeiros, A.; Rocha, H.A.; Fernandes-Pedrosa, M.F.; Egito, E.S. Bullfrog Oil Reduces the Carrageenan-induced Edema in Wistar Rats by in vitro Reduction of Inflammatory Mediators. *J. Oleo Sci.* **2020**, *69*, 133–142. [CrossRef] [PubMed]

pharmaceuticals

Article

Re-Exploring the Ability of Common Docking Programs to Correctly Reproduce the Binding Modes of Non-Covalent Inhibitors of SARS-CoV-2 Protease M^{pro}

Davide Bassani , Matteo Pavan , Giovanni Bolcato, Mattia Sturlese and Stefano Moro *

Molecular Modeling Section (MMS), Department of Pharmaceutical and Pharmacological Sciences, University of Padova, 35131 Padova, Italy; davide.bassani.1@studenti.unipd.it (D.B.); matteo.pavan.7@phd.unipd.it (M.P.); giovanni.bolcato.1@phd.unipd.it (G.B.); mattia.sturlese@unipd.it (M.S.)
* Correspondence: stefano.moro@unipd.it

Abstract: In the latest few decades, molecular docking has imposed itself as one of the most used approaches for computational drug discovery. Several docking benchmarks have been published, comparing the performance of different algorithms in respect to a molecular target of interest, usually evaluating their ability in reproducing the experimental data, which, in most cases, comes from X-ray structures. In this study, we elucidated the variation of the performance of three docking algorithms, namely GOLD, Glide, and PLANTS, in replicating the coordinates of the crystallographic ligands of SARS-CoV-2 main protease (M^{pro}). Through the comparison of the data coming from docking experiments and the values derived from the calculation of the solvent exposure of the crystallographic ligands, we highlighted the importance of this last variable for docking performance. Indeed, we underlined how an increase in the percentage of the ligand surface exposed to the solvent in a crystallographic complex makes it harder for the docking algorithms to reproduce its conformation. We further validated our hypothesis through molecular dynamics simulations, showing that the less stable protein–ligand complexes (in terms of root-mean-square deviation and root-mean-square fluctuation) tend to be derived from the cases in which the solvent exposure of the ligand in the starting system is higher.

Keywords: molecular docking; molecular dynamics; SARS-CoV-2; main protease, M^{pro}; docking benchmark

Citation: Bassani, D.; Pavan, M.; Bolcato, G.; Sturlese, M.; Moro, S. Re-Exploring the Ability of Common Docking Programs to Correctly Reproduce the Binding Modes of Non-Covalent Inhibitors of SARS-CoV-2 Protease M^{pro}. *Pharmaceuticals* **2022**, *15*, 180. https://doi.org/10.3390/ph15020180

Academic Editor: Osvaldo Andrade Santos-Filho

Received: 3 January 2022
Accepted: 28 January 2022
Published: 31 January 2022

1. Introduction

In the 1980s, with the first study provided by Kuntz et. al [1], the computational technique of molecular docking had its birth. The efficiency, speed, and robustness of this method make its presence a constant in every structure-based drug-discovery pipeline [2]. To give a brief explanation, molecular docking consists of a multistep computational process that aims to find the best conformation of a molecule to bind to another to form a stable complex [3]. In the field of medicinal chemistry, as is deductible, its main application is finding the best molecules to bind in a firm way to the desired target (a protein, a nucleic acid, etc.). The algorithm starts with the exploration of the conformations space of the ligands (exploiting the so-called "search algorithm"). The conformations (called "poses") are then classified by a "scoring function", which attributes a numeric value to the goodness of the interaction according to energetical and/or geometrical function.

After a series of iterations, the final conformations are presented from the program to the user and ranked by the internal scoring function [4].

In the last 30 years, many docking programs have been developed. Among them, GOLD [5] (a genetic docking algorithm developed by the Cambridge Crystallographic Data Center—CCDC), Glide [6] (a systematic docking program released under license by Schrödinger), AutoDock [7] (a non-commercial genetic algorithm from The Scripps

Research Institute), AutoDock VINA [8] (created by the same organization and released for non-commercial use), and PLANTS [9] (an algorithm based on an "Ant Colony Optimization" method) have gained popularity.

The performance of molecular docking programs can be measured by evaluating their ability to reproduce the experimental structural data, such as the crystallographic coordinates of a ligand into its binding site [10]. This ability has been evaluated in several benchmarks [11,12] to rank the performance of different algorithms regarding a specific target, usually using as the key parameter the root-mean-square deviation (RMSD) between the coordinates of the different poses given by the program and the crystallographic ones.

The ability to reproduce a crystallographic conformation strongly relies on different factors. First, the geometrical characteristics of the binding site, such as extension and shape, play a very important role; it is known that the performance of the algorithms has been improved to dock molecules in "cavities" or "pockets", rather than surfaces of proteins [13]. Second, the nature and the dimensions of the ligand are also crucial. Indeed, very small ligands may explore different places in a binding site, and the interactions that they can establish are usually few in number, reducing the "synergism" which could induce a molecule to keep a peculiar shape in a pocket [14]. On the other hand, even if drug-like molecules generally have higher conformational freedom, their dimensions force them to be oriented into a site in a more conserved way, so they have less roto-translational freedom.

In this study, we examined the ability of three docking programs characterized by diverse conformational sampling algorithms to efficiently reproduce the crystallographic pose of different ligands bound in different sites of a protein. To accomplish this task, a target in which several crystal structures were solved with the ligands located in different sites of the macromolecule itself was needed. To this scope, we considered a very recent and relevant target in the current pharmaceutical scenario, namely the SARS-CoV-2 main protease (M^{pro}).

In the last couple of years, with the pandemic spreading of the SARS-CoV-2 virus, the world of medical sciences had found itself fighting a new and dangerous adversary [15,16]. This biological entity, which is part of the coronavirus family, has been demonstrated to cause a pulmonary infection which eventually leads to serious complications, as witnessed by the high number of deaths that have already been linked to it (more than 5 million, at the present day [17]). The replication cycle of this virus strongly relies on the activity of its main protease (known as M^{pro} or $3CL^{pro}$, a crystallographic structure example is reported in Figure 1) [18]. Indeed, this protein is responsible for the cleavage of the propeptide transcribed by the viral genome. In this way, the formation of all the functional proteins for the building of new virions takes place, and so the viral infection can proceed. Even if many molecules have been shown to bind to M^{pro} [19] and inhibit its activity, and even if a molecule is currently in phase III clinical trial for this purpose (PF-07321332, from Pfizer [20,21]), no drug has already been approved by the European Medicinal Agency for the treatment of SARS-CoV-2 (also called "COVID-19"). Computational methods have already proven to be beneficial in the research for new potential inhibitors for M^{pro}, as the literature witnesses [22,23]. In this work, we decided to implement a molecular-docking-based approach relying on the programs GOLD, Glide, and PLANTS. These algorithms are considered "orthogonal" because they are characterized by diverse placing and scoring algorithms to obtain the best solution to the "protein–ligand posing problem". Each of these programs was used to dock each of the different non-covalent ligands of the various crystal structures of M^{pro}, and this allowed us to evaluate the factors which influence the variability in reproducing the crystallographic poses. A self-docking protocol similar to the one herein reported had already been developed by our laboratory, with the name "DockBench". This program was implemented with success in several workflows, as the literature assesses [24,25]. In this study, a slightly modified version of that tool was used, which exploits only three docking programs at the present moment but can expand the analysis of the results obtained.

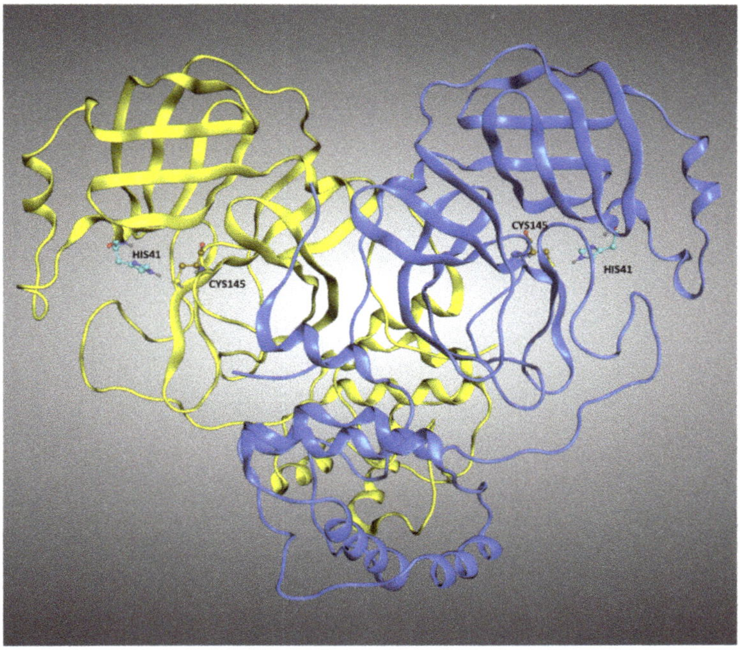

Figure 1. Representation of the crystal structure of M^{pro} (PDB:7L10). The two monomers composing the protein are colored differently, while the residues of the catalytic dyad, Cys145, and His41 are labeled in each of the monomers.

Looking at the docking benchmarking protocols on M^{pro}, we see that a remarkable study has already been conducted and published by Zev et al. [26]. In that specific work, six different docking programs were evaluated in their performance in reproducing the M^{pro} non-covalent ligands' crystallographic poses, and three of those algorithms have also been compared in their ability to correctly place M^{pro} covalent ligands into their proper binding site. In our work, we decided to expand the considerations brought by that study, evaluating specifically how docking performance changes in respect of the crystallographic data that have to be reproduced.

Indeed, we considered in our calculations parameters such as the solvent exposure of the ligand and the influence of the crystallographic water molecules in docking calculations, focusing our evaluations just on non-covalent M^{pro} ligands. We executed the experiment in two different scenarios, one which excluded the crystallographic waters from the calculation (which we will name "Scenario 1"), and one which induced the docking programs to consider them (called "Scenario 2"). After that, we compared the docking results with the percentage of solvent exposure of the crystallographic pose of the ligand, successfully confirming that a higher solvent exposure tendentially reflects a worsening in the ability to reproduce the crystallographic pose by the algorithms (that, as already mentioned, are better trained for "cavities" rather than "surfaces"). To further investigate this aspect, we expanded our computational analysis by performing a molecular dynamics (MD) experiment, in which each crystallographic ligand was left free to move for 5ns (three replicas per system). This approach (known as "MD post-docking") has already become part of our computational protocol [27,28] and is based on the fact that the conformations of the ligands, which are less prone to be displaced from their initial position during the simulation, are related to higher stability and binding strength with the target. In the case presented, this principle was applied directly to the crystallographic conformations of the ligands rather than to docking poses. This was performed because the goal was not to select the most promising molecules in binding to a specific region of the protein; instead, the objective was to elucidate which are the features of the crystallographic ligands that tend to guarantee a tighter binding with the receptor. Our evaluation demonstrated that the molecules bound to the orthosteric pocket of M^{pro} keep their position much stronger than the molecules crystallized on other sites, further validating our solvent exposure-based theory. A representation of the M^{pro} ligands crystallized in the various sites of the protein is given in Figure 2.

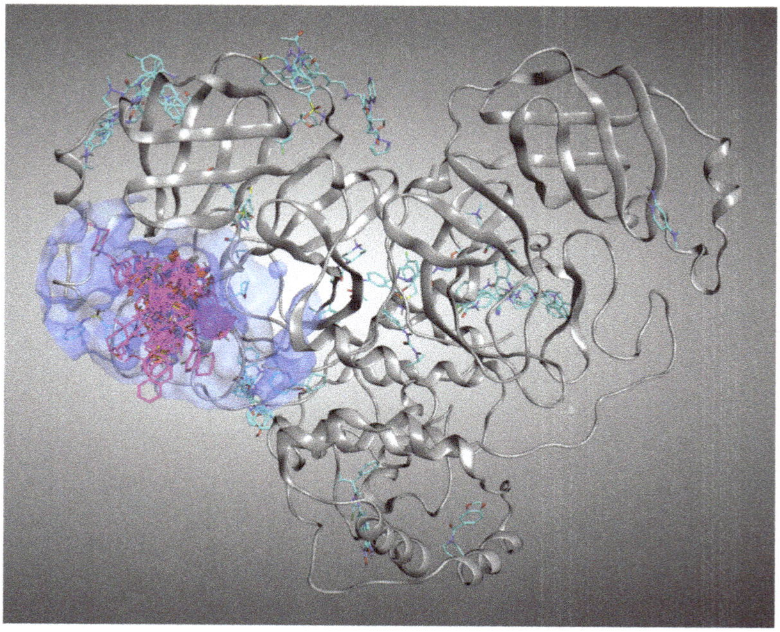

Figure 2. Representation of all the crystallographic ligands of M^{pro} superposed. To give a better view, just one protein structure is represented (the one coming from PDB:7L10). The ligands which are crystallized inside the catalytic pocket are colored in magenta, while all the small molecules crystallized outside the orthosteric binding site are colored in cyan.

2. Results and Discussion

2.1. Scenario 1—Docking Calculations without Considering the Crystallographic Water Molecules

The results of our docking protocol for this section (which are numerically reported in the Supplementary Materials File "Selfdocking_scenario1.csv") are graphically represented with colormaps. All the colormaps present in this study are based on a colorimetric scale delineating the RMSD values, starting from 0 Å, which corresponds to a molecular docking pose exactly super posable to the crystallographic one (maximum docking performance, represented by the dark blue color), and reaching values of 5 Å or higher (minimum docking performance, all represented by the dark red color), corresponding to a very low level of overlap between the coordinates of the pose produced and the ones of the crystallographic conformation. The colormaps in Figure 3 show the self-docking results obtained on the different M^{pro} crystal structures in the case in which water molecules are not considered in the calculation. As is depicted, the RMSD values were far lower for all the complexes in which the crystallographic ligand is located in the orthosteric pocket.

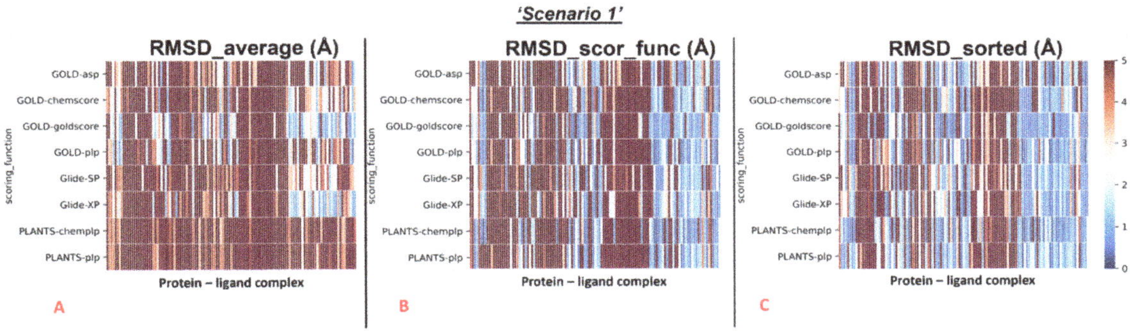

Figure 3. Colormaps represent the results of the self-docking experiments in the case in which the crystallographic water molecules are not considered during the docking runs. (**A**) Results coming from the average of the RMSDs of all the poses for each docking run. (**B**) Results derived just from the RMSD between the crystallographic ligand coordinates and the pose classified as the best from the scoring function. (**C**) Results of the self-docking experiments if just the pose showing the best RMSD value between its coordinates and the crystallographic ones are retained. The *x*-axis lists all the different protein–ligand complexes, which are plotted against the different pairs docking program-scoring function used for this study, reported in the *y*-axis.

To give a better resolution of this, we separated each map into two different colormaps, one grouping all the 78 proteins in which the ligand is located into the catalytic pocket, and one including all other cases (41 complexes).

We analyzed the data coming from the calculations, and we determined that, looking at all the complexes with all the different couples docking program-scoring functions, we see that the average values of all the RMSDs obtained was 5.76Å ("RMSD_average"). Looking at the average of the RMSDs coming from the poses which were scored as the best ones from the algorithms' scoring functions ("RMSD_scor_func"), we see that the value was 5.10Å. If the lowest RMSD values only are taken into account for each docking run ("RMSD_sorted"), the mean of the values was 3.70Å.

The average values were also calculated separately for all the complexes in which the crystallographic ligand is located in the catalytic pocket, and for all other cases. The colormaps for these different conditions are reported in Figures 4 and 5.

First, the analysis focused on the complexes having the crystallographic ligand located within the orthosteric pocket. For this set of systems, we calculated the average RMSD value of all the poses ("RMSD_average"), which was revealed to be 4.54Å. Then we computed the average of the RMSD values coming from the poses which were ranked with the best score from the scoring functions ("RMSD_scor_func"), and its value was 3.43Å. Finally, the average RMSD value of the poses with the lowest RMSD in each run was calculated ("RMSD_sorted"), and its measure was 2.45Å.

Second, the same steps were performed for the rest of the protein–ligand complexes, which are the ones in which the crystallographic ligand is located outside the orthosteric binding site. Moreover, in this case, the first passage involved the calculation of the average RMSD value of all the poses generated for these systems ("RMSD_average"), and its measure was 8.08Å. Then, the mean of the RMSD values coming from the poses which received the highest rank from the scoring functions was calculated ("RMSD_scor_func") and was revealed to be 8.29Å. In the end, the average value of the lowest RMSDs of each run was computed ("RMSD_sorted"), and its measure was shown to be 6.08Å.

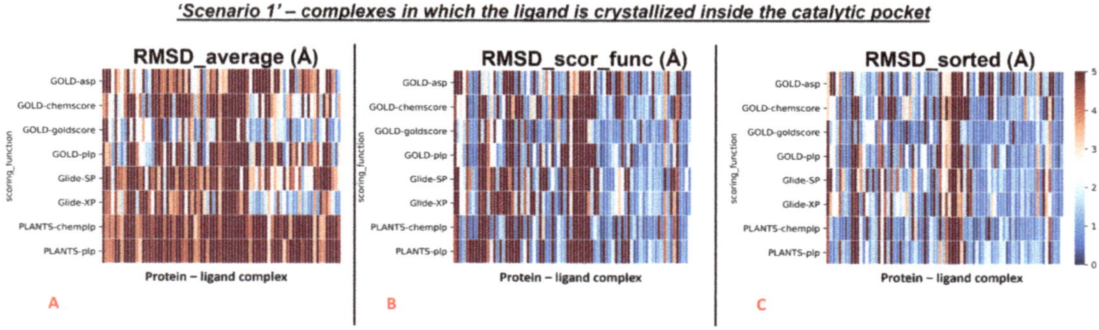

Figure 4. Colormaps represent the results of the self-docking experiments just for the ligands crystallized inside the orthosteric pocket in the situation in which the crystallographic water molecules are not considered during the docking runs. (**A**) Results coming from the average of the RMSDs of all the poses for each docking run. (**B**) Results derived just from the RMSD between the crystallographic ligand coordinates and the pose classified as the best from the scoring function. (**C**) Results of the self-docking experiments if just the pose showing the best RMSD value between its coordinates and the crystallographic ones is retained. The *x*-axis lists all the different protein–ligand complexes, which are plotted against the different pairs docking program-scoring function used for this study, reported in the *y*-axis.

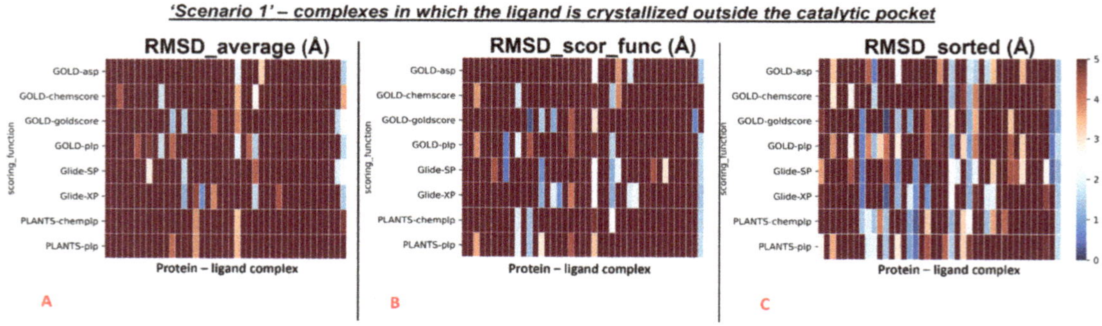

Figure 5. Colormaps represent the results of the self-docking experiments just for the ligands crystallized outside the orthosteric pocket in the case in which the crystallographic water molecules are not considered during the docking runs. (**A**) Results coming from the average of the RMSDs of all the poses for each docking run. (**B**) Results derived just from the RMSD between the crystallographic ligand coordinates and the pose classified as the best from the scoring function. (**C**) Results of the self-docking experiments if just the pose showing the best RMSD value between its coordinates and the crystallographic ones is retained. The *x*-axis lists all the different protein–ligand complexes, which are plotted against the different pairs docking program-scoring function used for this study, reported in the *y*-axis.

The results obtained for Scenario 1 are summarized in Table 1.

Table 1. Table representing the self-docking results obtained for Scenario 1.

Results for Scenario 1—Docking Calculations Executed without Considering the Water Molecules			
	RMSD_Average (Å)	**RMSD_Scor_Func (Å)**	**RMSD_Sorted (Å)**
All the 119 protein–ligand complexes	5.76	5.10	3.70
The 78 complexes with the ligand inside the catalytic pocket	4.54	3.43	2.45
The 41 complexes with the ligand outside the catalytic pocket	8.08	8.29	6.08

2.2. Scenario 2—Docking Calculations Considering the Crystallographic Water Molecules

The outcomes of our molecular docking experiment for this section (which are reported in the Supplementary Materials File "Selfdocking_scenario2.csv") are graphically represented with colormaps, which were created with the same criteria listed in the previous paragraph. The results reported in the colormaps in Figures 6–8 reveal the self-docking performance obtained on the different M^{pro} crystal structures in the case in which the crystallographic water molecules within 5 Å from the ligand were retained during the calculation. Moreover, in this case, it is easy to notice that the values result in being far better for the complexes in which the small molecule of interest is in the orthosteric binding site.

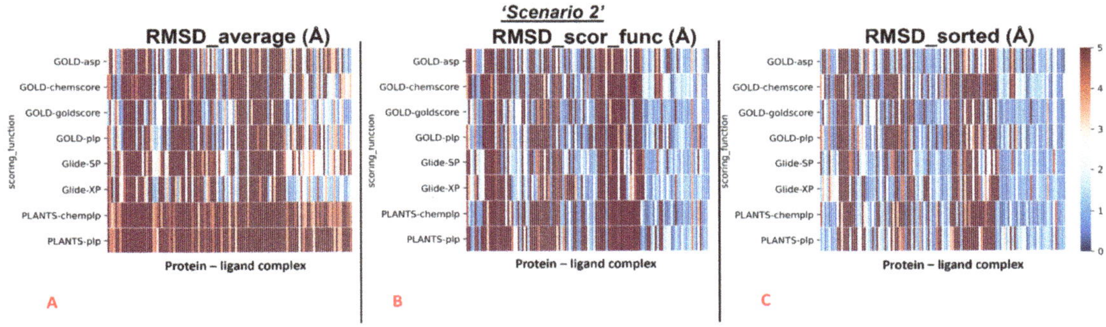

Figure 6. Colormaps represent the results of the self-docking experiments in the case in which the crystallographic water molecules at 5 Å or nearer to the ligand itself are taken into account during the docking runs. (**A**) Results coming from the average of the RMSDs of all the poses for each docking run. (**B**) Results derived just from the RMSD between the crystallographic ligand coordinates and the pose classified as the best from the scoring function.(**C**)Results of the self-docking experiments if just the pose showing the best RMSD value between its coordinates and the crystallographic ones is retained. The *x*-axis lists all the different protein–ligand complexes, which are plotted against the different pairs docking program-scoring function used for this study, reported in the *y*-axis.

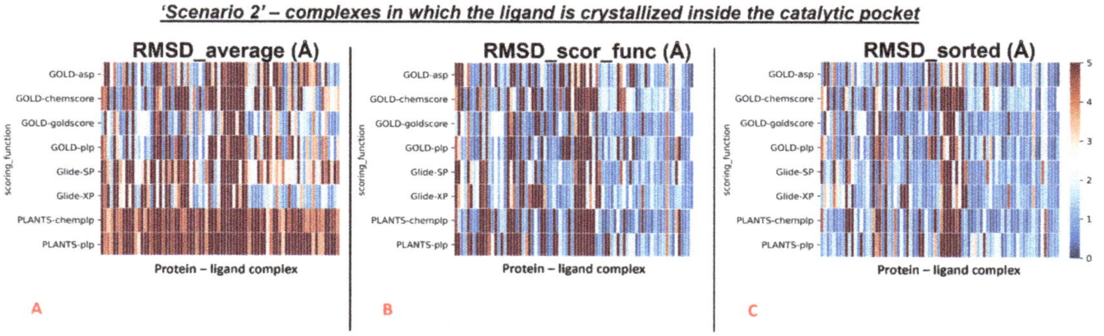

Figure 7. Colormaps represent the results of the self-docking experiments just for the ligands crystallized inside the orthosteric pocket in the situation in which the crystallographic water molecules at 5 Å or nearer to the ligand itself are taken into account during the docking runs. (**A**) Results coming from the average of the RMSDs of all the poses for each docking run. (**B**) Results derived just from the RMSD between the crystallographic ligand coordinates and the once of the pose classified as the best from the scoring function. (**C**) Results of the self-docking experiments if just the pose showing the best RMSD value between its coordinates and the crystallographic ones are retained. The *x*-axis lists all the different protein–ligand complexes, which are plotted against the different pairs docking program-scoring function used for this study, reported in the *y*-axis.

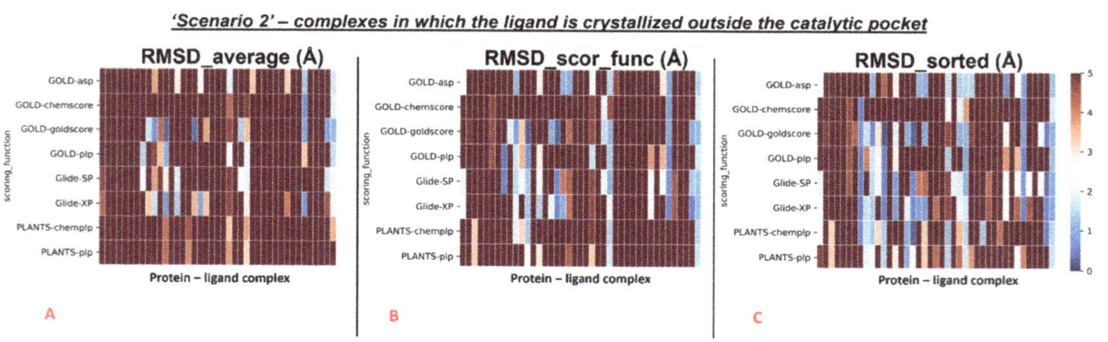

Figure 8. Colormaps represent the results of the self-docking experiments only for the ligands crystallized outside the orthosteric pocket in the situation in which the crystallographic water molecules at 5 Å or nearer to the ligand itself are taken into account during the docking runs. (**A**) Results coming from the average of the RMSDs of all the poses for each docking run. (**B**) Results derived just from the RMSD between the crystallographic ligand coordinates and the once of the pose classified as the best from the scoring function. (**C**) Results of the self-docking experiments if just the pose showing the best RMSD value between its coordinates and the crystallographic ones are retained. The *x*-axis lists all the different protein–ligand complexes, which are plotted against the different pairs docking program-scoring function used for this study, reported in the *y*-axis.

Similar to the first scenario, we divided each colormap into two sets, one with the 78 proteins having the ligand located into the catalytic pocket, and the other including all the remaining cases (41 proteins). Considering all the protein–ligand complexes with all the different pairs docking program-scoring function, the mean values of all the RMSDs obtained ("RMSD_average") was 5.64Å, but focusing only on the mean of the RMSDs derived from the poses which were given the highest rank from the algorithms ("RMSD_scor_func"), the value resulted to be 4.83Å. Looking only at the best RMSDs for each docking run ("RMSD_sorted"), we see that the average of the values was 3.68 Å.

As already performed for Scenario 1, also in Scenario 2, the analysis was divided between the complexes in having the crystallographic ligand crystallized into the catalytic pocket, and for all other situations.

We reported the colormaps which resulted from this evaluation, and those are represented in Figures 7 and 8.

We started from the complexes in which the ligand is located inside the catalytic pocket in the crystal. For those systems, the mean of the RMSD values coming from all the poses("RMSD_average") resulted in being 4.22Å. Then, the average of the RMSDs derived from the scoring function highest-ranked poses in all the docking runs ("RMSD_scor_func") was computed, and its value was 3.11Å. In the end, also the average value between the lowest of the RMSDs in each docking run was calculated ("RMSD_sorted") and was revealed to be 2.26Å.

Second, we repeated the analysis for all the complexes in which the crystallographic ligand is located outside the orthosteric pocket. For these systems, the average of the RMSD coming from all the poses collected in the docking runs ("RMSD_average") was calculated to be 8.32Å. Next, we computed the mean of the RMSD values derived from the poses which received the highest score (from the scoring functions) in each run ("RMSD_scor_func"), and this value was 8.11Å. Last, also the average value between the lowest of the RMSDs in each docking run was calculated ("RMSD_sorted"), giving 6.36 Å.

The results obtained for Scenario 1 are summarized in Table 2.

Table 2. Table representing the self-docking results obtained for Scenario 2.

Results for Scenario 2—Water Molecules 5 Å or Nearer to the Ligand Considered in Docking Calculations			
	RMSD_Average (Å)	**RMSD_Scor_Func (Å)**	**RMSD_Sorted (Å)**
All the 119 protein–ligandcomplexes	5.64	4.83	3.68
The 78 complexes with the ligand inside the catalytic pocket	4.22	3.11	2.26
The 41 complexes with the ligand outside the catalytic pocket	8.32	8.11	6.36

Just analyzing the numbers coming from the average values allows us to see how the performance of the docking programs dramatically increases when the ligand is docked inside the catalytic pocket rather than on the surface of the protein, in line with the fact that the molecules have a limitation in the conformation that they can explore into a binding site. Together with this, the ligands can exploit their accessible surface area to interact with the protein more efficiently, following the principle of "complementarity" [29,30].

2.3. Solvent Exposure Analysis

The results of the docking calculations were then analyzed in light of the data coming from the solvent exposure analysis. For each docking program-scoring function pair, the best RMSDs given by the docking calculation were evaluated against the solvent exposure of the ligand in its crystallographic pose. The results were reported in different plots, one for each couple docking program-scoring function, also in this case dividing the graphs in respect to the "scenario" from which the docking result was coming. To give an example, we reported in this article the plots for the pair GOLD-goldscore for each of these cases (Figures 9 and 10).

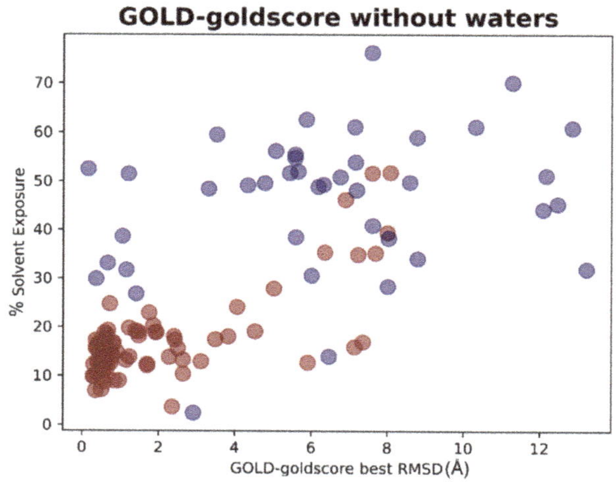

Figure 9. Scatter plots showing the different distribution of the RMSD values between the coordinates of the best pose from the GOLD-goldscore docking experiment in respect to the solvent exposure of the corresponding crystallographic ligands. The red dots represent the values having the ligand crystallized inside the catalytic pocket while the blue dots represent the ligands crystallized on the other sites of M^{pro}. As can be noticed, the molecules showing the best values of RMSD are, in most cases, located inside the orthosteric pocket and characterized by low solvent exposure. This plot depicts part of the results of Scenario 1, and so the crystallographic water molecules are not considered in the docking runs of which the outcomes are here represented.

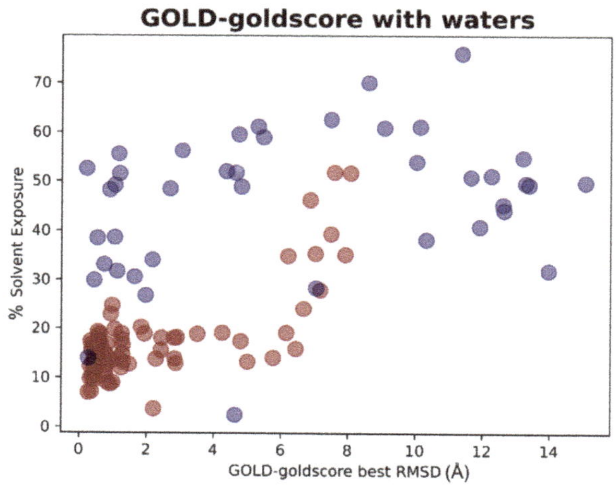

Figure 10. Scatter plots showing the different distribution of the RMSD values between the coordinates of the best pose from the GOLD-goldscore docking experiment in respect to the solvent exposure of the corresponding crystallographic ligands. The red dots represent the ligands that are originally crystallized inside the catalytic pocket, while the blue dots represent the ligands crystallized in the other parts of M^{pro}. As can be noticed, the molecules showing the best values of RMSD are in most cases located inside the orthosteric pocket and characterized by low solvent exposure. This plot depicts part of the results of Scenario 2, meaning that the crystallographic water molecules at 5 Å or nearer to the ligand are also considered in the docking runs of which the outcomes are here represented.

The plots arising from all other docking program-scoring function pairs, both in Scenario 1 and Scenario 2, are reported in Supplementary Materials Figure S1. From these graphs, we can easily see how the best RMSDs values tended to be derived from protein–ligand complexes in which the solvent exposure of the ligand is low, and, most of the time, this means that the small molecule is crystallized in the binding pocket (indicated with the red dots in the plots). There are some cases in which the mean RMSD values were suboptimal also for this kind of ligands, and this can be due to several reasons. In some situations, of which the complexes 5REH, 5RE9, 5RGK (represented in Figure 11), and 7AVD are an example, the solvent exposure was tendentially higher in respect to the other orthosteric ligands, while, in other cases, the increase in RMSD can be attributable to the small dimensions of the ligand itself, making it harder for the docking algorithms to reproduce the reference pose in a pocket of such considerable volume (the complexes 5R82 and 5RG0 are an example for this) [31].

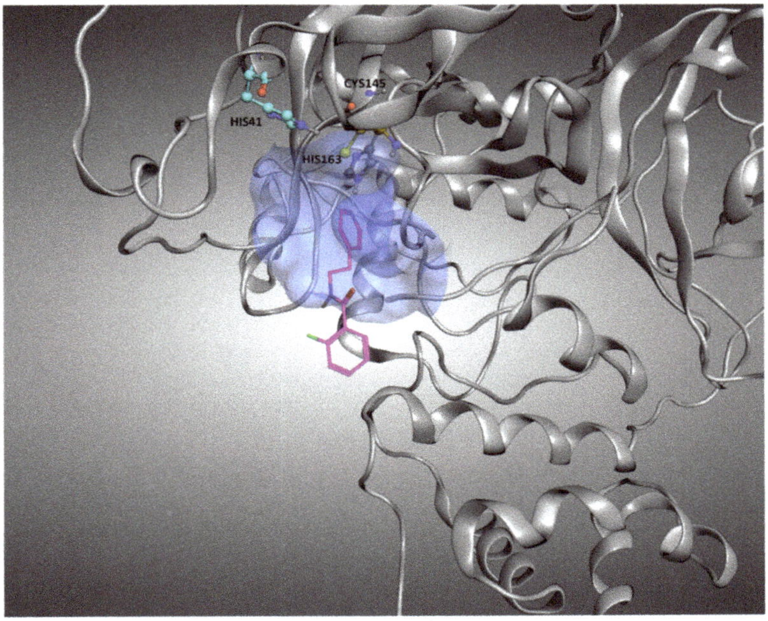

Figure 11. Representation of the crystallographic complex conformation of 5RGK, one of the protein–ligand complexes in which the crystallographic ligand is located inside the orthosteric binding site, but the docking calculation results in high RMSD values. This is mainly due to the high level of solvent exposure that characterizes this ligand, which locates just a small portion of its structure inside the pocket, leaving the rest in an outer zone. The ligand is represented with stick representation (C-atom are colored in magenta), and the catalytic dyad (Cys145 and His41) is highlighted, as well as the His163 and the binding site residue interacting with the ligand. To give a better representation, the surface of the protein in a 5 Å radius from the ligand is represented and colored in blue.

On the other hand, there are also some cases in which the best RMSD given by the protocol was pretty low, even if the crystallographic ligand was not placed inside the orthosteric pocket. This is the case, for example, of 7LFP (the crystallographic pose is reported in Figure 12); the ligand was placed at the interface between the monomers, and so its solvent exposure and RMSDs values were low, even if was marked to be "outside the catalytic pocket". A similar situation is observed on 5RF0, where the ligand, even if not located into the orthosteric pocket, is not situated in the peripheral part of the protease.

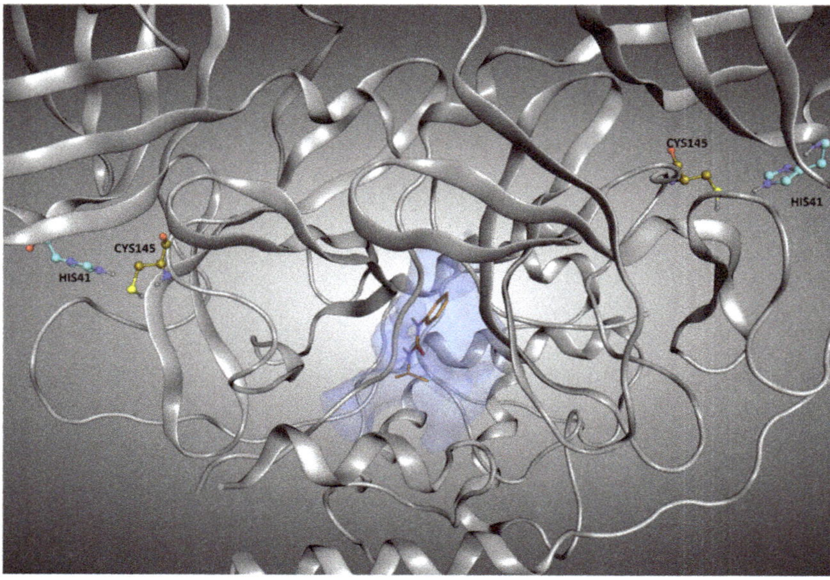

Figure 12. Representation of the crystallographic pose of 7LFP, which is one of the protein–ligand complexes in which, even if the crystallographic ligand is located outside the orthosteric binding site, the RMSD values between the original coordinates and the ones given from the docking runs are considerably low. The reason for this can be found in the very low solvent exposure of this ligand, which is located in the interface between the monomers, and so is shielded by them. The ligand is represented in orange, and the catalytic dyad (Cys145 and His41) of both monomers is highlighted. To give a better representation, the surface of the protein in a 5 Å radius from the ligand is represented and colored in blue.

2.4. Molecular Dynamics Simulations

For each of the 119 crystallographic complexes, three different molecular dynamics simulations (MD) of 5 ns each were collected to examine the behavior of the ligands in a dynamic environment. The trajectories were wrapped, aligned to the first frame and the root-mean-square fluctuation (RMSF) of the ligand, as well as the RMSD between its crystallographic and final coordinates ("RMSD_final"), and were calculated for every single experiment. For each protein, the values coming from the average of the RMSFs and "RMSD_final" derived from the replicas were considered. Considering all the simulations collected, the average of all the ligand RMSF values was calculated to be 5.28 Å, while the average of the RMSD values between the coordinates of the crystallographic conformation of the ligand and the ones coming from the last frame of the trajectory ("RMSD_final") was of 8.89 Å.

As already performed for the docking results analysis, we first focused on the complexes in which the crystallographic ligand is originally located inside the orthosteric pocket. For these systems, the average of all the RMSFs coming from the simulations was 2.19 Å. The mean value of the RMSDs of the ligands in the last frame of each trajectory ("RMSD_final") was instead calculated to be 4.43 Å.

Second, we concentrated on the systems in which the crystallographic position of the ligand (and so its initial location) is outside the catalytic pocket. For these systems, the average value of all the ligand RMSFs during the trajectories was calculated to be 11.15Å. Then the RMSD value between the final coordinates of the ligands and their crystallographic ones ("RMSD_final") were considered. The average of these values, for all the trajectories collected for these complexes, was 17.66Å. The output files of the molecular dynamics simulation geometric analysis are available in Supplementary Materials "MD_data.csv".

As already performed for the docking experiments, also for MD results, the average values of RMSF and "RMSD_final" were plotted against the percentage of solvent exposure of the crystallographic conformation of the ligand, and the plots that were obtained are reported in Figures 13 and 14.

As expected, the complexes in which the ligand is crystallized in the orthosteric site (marked with the red dots in the scatter plot) tended to fluctuate much less than the ligands which are complexed in the external parts of the protease (represented with the blue dots in the graphs). As depicted, MD analysis confirms that the best values in terms of RMSF and "RMSD_final", which are correlated to a more energetically stable situation for the protein–ligand complex, come from the systems in which the crystallographic ligand is localized inside the catalytic pocket and are characterized by a low percentage of solvent exposure. These outcomes further support the already-mentioned hypothesis about the correlation between the improvement of the docking performances in the case in which the binding site is a pocket rather than a surface.

The overall results obtained with molecular dynamics simulations are summarized in Table 3. A graphical representation of the molecular dynamics simulations is reported in Supplementary Materials "Video_S1.mp4". In this video, the ligands crystallized into the catalytic pocket are colored in magenta, while the other ligands are colored in cyan.

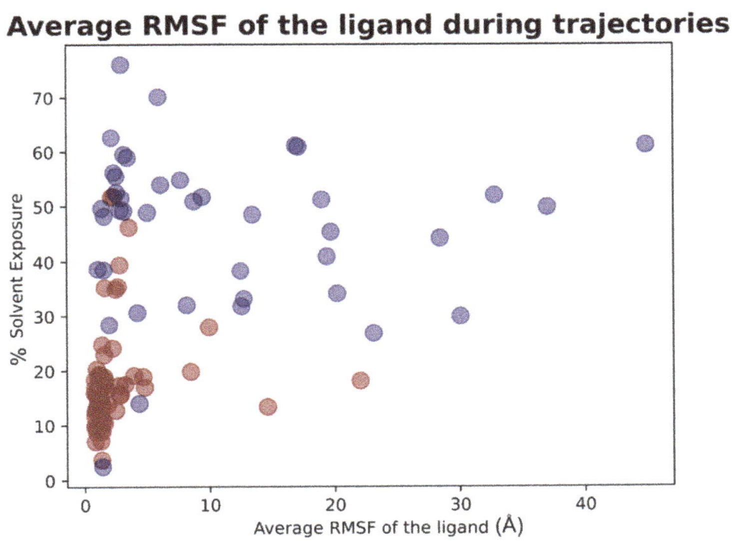

Figure 13. Scatter plots showing the different distribution of the mean RMSF values between the coordinates of the M^{pro} ligands compared to crystallographic ones after the molecular dynamics simulations in respect to the solvent exposure of the corresponding crystallographic ligands. The red dots represent the ligands thatwere originally crystallized inside the catalytic pocket, while the blue dots represent the ligands crystallized in the other parts of M^{pro}. As can be noticed, the molecules showing the best values of RMSF after the analysis of the trajectories are mainly located inside the catalytic pocket and characterized by a low solvent exposure of the original crystallographic pose.

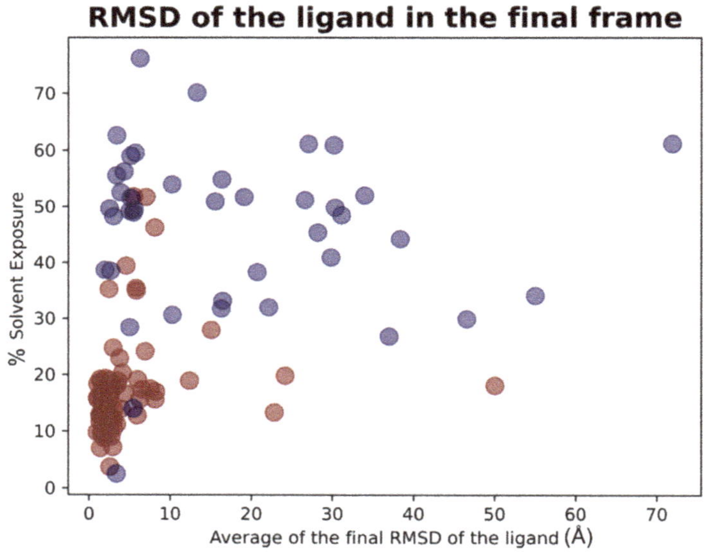

Figure 14. Scatter plots showing the different distribution of the mean RMSD values between the final coordinates of the M^{pro} ligands compared to crystallographic ones after the molecular dynamics simulations in respect to the solvent exposure of the corresponding crystallographic ligands. The red dots represent the ligands thatwere originally crystallized inside the catalytic pocket, while the blue dots represent the ligands crystallized in the other parts of M^{pro}. As can be noticed, the molecules showing the best values of RMSF after the analysis of the trajectories are mainly located inside the catalytic pocket and characterized by a low solvent exposure of the original crystallographic pose.

Table 3. Results of the molecular dynamics experiments.

Results of the Molecular Dynamics Simulations		
	RMSD_Final (Å)	**RMSF_Average (Å)**
All the 119 protein–ligandcomplexes	8.98	5.28
The 78 complexes with the ligand inside the catalytic pocket	4.43	2.19
The 41 complexes with the ligand outside the catalytic pocket	17.66	11.15

3. Materials and Methods

3.1. Software Overview

The molecular modeling operations were executed with the Molecular Operating Environment (MOE) suite (version 2019.01) [32]. The molecular docking calculations were carried out with CCDC GOLD (version 2020), Schrodinger Glide (from the Schrödinger suite 2021.3), and PLANTS. The solvent exposure calculation was performed with a series of SVL commands (exploiting "moebatch" of the MOE suite) implemented into a python script. The systems for molecular dynamics simulations were prepared by using tleap [33] and VMD [34]. The simulations were then carried out with ACEMD3 [35](version 3.3.0), a licensed program based upon OpenMM [36] (version 7.4.0). The modeling and docking calculations were performed on a 12 CPU (Intel Xeon E5-1620 3.50 GHz) Linux Workstation, while the MD simulations were carried out on a GPUs-cluster based composed of 20 NVIDIA GPUs.

3.2. Structure Preparation for Docking Calculations

The different crystal structures of M^{pro} were collected from the Protein Data Bank [37]. Among these, the proteins which did not present any ligand, or which were complexed with a covalent ligand, were excluded. This way, only the non-covalent protein–ligand complexes were retained, and the complete list of all the 119 complexes used is available in Supplementary Material Table S1. The structures were grouped into a database and were prepared with MOE "QuickPrep" tool. With this tool, each complex was properly prepared to recreate the small missing loops in the structure, assigning the proper conformation to the residues with alternate orientation (based on occupancy) and adding the hydrogens to the system (this last passage was performed with the MOE "Protonate 3D" tool). The hydrogens added this way were then minimized by using the AMBER10:EHT force field implemented in MOE [38].

After these preliminary but crucial steps, each complex was manually examined and treated to eliminate every molecule, except for the crystallographic waters and the main ligand. Each complex was then independently saved.

3.3. Docking Calculations

For each of the complexes prepared, the crystallographic ligand was separated from the protein and self-docked into its binding site. For each docking program, all the scoring functions available were used for separate runs, and in each run, 5 poses were collected for the ligand. GOLD supports 4 different scoring functions: goldscore, chemscore, asp, and plp; Glide supports two main functions for docking, which are Glide-SP and Glide-XP, while PLANTS implements plp and chemplp.

For each docking-program-scoring function couple, the docking calculation was carried out in two different scenarios: one in which the crystallographic water molecules were not considered (which we refer to as Scenario 1) and one in which also the water molecules 5 Å or nearer from the ligand atoms were taken into account into the computation (which we refer to as Scenario 2).

When all the docking calculations were executed, the ligand root-mean-square deviation (RMSD) between the coordinates of each one of the poses and the crystallographic conformations were computed. The data of major interest were the RMSD in respect to the pose which is marked with the highest score by the program (RMSD_scor_func), the lowest RMSD of the docking run (RMSD_sorted), and the average of the RMSDs of all the poses generated (RMSD_average). The output files of the self-docking experiments executed are available in the Supplementary Materials ("Selfdocking_scenario1.csv" and "Selfdocking_scenario2.csv").

3.4. Solvent Exposure Calculation

For each M^{pro} complex, the solvent exposure of the main crystallographic ligand was calculated with an SVL script based on MOE "moebatch". The output of such calculation was the percentage of the ligand surface which is exposed to the solvent in the protein–ligand crystallographic complex. All the percentages obtained are presented in Supplementary Materials Table S2.

3.5. Molecular Dynamics Simulations Setup and Execution

All the protein–ligand M^{pro} systems were independently prepared for molecular dynamics simulations. The program tleap was used for the creation of the simulation box, which was set to be cubic and characterized by a 15 Å padding. The solvation model used was the explicit TIP3P, and the neutralization of the system was performed by adding Na^+ and Cl^- ions until the salt concentration inside the box reached the value of 0.154 M.

The systems then underwent a two-passage equilibration. In the first one, both protein and ligand atoms were subjected to a harmonic position restrain of 5 kcal/mol. The length of this step was set to 0.1 ns, and the ensemble used was the canonical one (NVT). During the second equilibration step, the ensemble was set to NPT (isothermal–isobaric), the length was 0.5 ns, and the harmonic restrains (always 5 kcal/mol) were applied both on the ligand and on the alpha-carbons of the protein backbone.

After these preliminary steps, 3 replicas of 5 ns each were collected for each system; the ensemble was again the NVT one, and no restraints were applied. At the end of the simulations, the average root-mean-square fluctuation (RMSF) of the ligand during the trajectory, as well as the RMSD betweencrystallographic coordinates of the ligand and the ones coming from the last frame of the trajectory, were collected.

4. Conclusions

In this study, we evaluated the performance of three orthogonal docking algorithms in reproducing the crystallographic pose of several ligands located in different parts of the same target, which, in our case, was the SARS-CoV-2 main protease (M^{pro}). Our analysis revealed how, even if the docking programs used operate in different ways to give the final conformations to the user, all of them perform much better in the case in which the ligands are located in a binding pocket rather than crystallized outside of it. Specifically, we reported that their performance tends to decrease with the increment of the exposure of the crystallographic pose to the solvent. This was confirmed both from the experiments executed without considering the crystallographic water molecules in the docking calculations and from the ones taking into account the waters 5 Å or nearer to the ligand. Molecular dynamics simulations further give credit to our study, demonstrating how the less-fluctuating ligands (and so the most stable) through the trajectories were the ones crystallized inside the orthosteric binding site of M^{pro}.

Supplementary Materials: The following are available online at https://www.mdpi.com/article/10.3390/ph15020180/s1: "Supplementary_material.docx" (containing Table S1, Table S2, and Figure S1), the CSV files "Selfdocking_scenario1.csv", "Selfdocking_scenario2.csv" and "MD_data.csv", "Video_S1.mp4".

Author Contributions: Conceptualization, D.B. and S.M.; methodology, D.B.; formal analysis, D.B., M.S. and S.M.; writing—original draft preparation, D.B.; writing—review and editing, M.P., G.B., M.S. and S.M.; supervision, S.M. All authors have read and agreed to the published version of the manuscript.

Funding: This work was supported by Fondazione Cariparo (An Integrated Strategy for the Fast Discovery of SARS-CoV-2 Main Protease (M^{pro}) Inhibitors, No. 55812).

Institutional Review Board Statement: Not applicable.

Informed Consent Statement: Not applicable.

Data Availability Statement: Data are contained within the article and Supplementary Materials.

Acknowledgments: MMS lab is very grateful to Chemical Computing Group, OpenEye, and Acellera for the scientific and technical partnership. MMS lab gratefully acknowledges the support of NVIDIA Corporation with the donation of the Titan V GPU used for this research.

Conflicts of Interest: The authors declare no conflict of interest.

References

1. Kuntz, I.D.; Blaney, J.M.; Oatley, S.J.; Langridge, R.; Ferrin, T.E. A geometric approach to macromolecule-ligand interactions. *J. Mol. Biol.* **1982**, *161*, 269–288. [CrossRef]
2. Meng, X.-Y.; Zhang, H.-X.; Mezei, M.; Cui, M. Molecular Docking: A Powerful Approach for Structure-Based Drug Discovery. *Curr. Comput. Aided-Drug Des.* **2011**, *7*, 146–157. [CrossRef] [PubMed]
3. Lengauer, T.; Rarey, M. Computational methods for biomolecular docking. *Curr. Opin. Struct. Biol.* **1996**, *6*, 402–406. [CrossRef]
4. Kitchen, D.B.; Decornez, H.; Furr, J.R.; Bajorath, J. Docking and scoring in virtual screening for drug discovery: Methods and applications. *Nat. Rev. Drug Discov.* **2004**, *3*, 935–949. [CrossRef] [PubMed]
5. Jones, G.; Willett, P.; Glen, R.C.; Leach, A.R.; Taylor, R. Development and validation of a genetic algorithm for flexible docking. *J. Mol. Biol.* **1997**, *267*, 727–748. [CrossRef]
6. Halgren, T.A.; Murphy, R.B.; Friesner, R.A.; Beard, H.S.; Frye, L.L.; Pollard, W.T.; Banks, J.L. Glide: A New Approach for Rapid, Accurate Docking and Scoring. 2. Enrichment Factors in Database Screening. *J. Med. Chem.* **2004**, *47*, 1750–1759. [CrossRef]

7. Morris, G.M.; Huey, R.; Lindstrom, W.; Sanner, M.F.; Belew, R.K.; Goodsell, D.S.; Olson, A.J. AutoDock4 and AutoDockTools4: Automated docking with selective receptor flexibility. *J. Comput. Chem.* **2009**, *30*, 2785–2791. [CrossRef]
8. Trott, O.; Olson, A.J. AutoDock Vina: Improving the speed and accuracy of docking with a new scoring function, efficient optimization, and multithreading. *J. Comput. Chem.* **2009**, *31*, 455–461. [CrossRef]
9. Korb, O.; Stützle, T.; Exner, T.E. PLANTS: Application of Ant Colony Optimization to Structure-Based Drug Design. In Proceedings of the ANTS: International Workshop on Ant Colony Optimization and Swarm Intelligence, Brussels, Belgium, 4–7 September 2006; pp. 247–258.
10. Yusuf, D.; Davis, A.M.; Kleywegt, G.J.; Schmitt, S. An Alternative Method for the Evaluation of Docking Performance: RSR vs RMSD. *J. Chem. Inf. Model.* **2008**, *48*, 1411–1422. [CrossRef]
11. Boittier, E.D.; Tang, Y.Y.; Buckley, M.E.; Schuurs, Z.P.; Richard, D.J.; Gandhi, N.S. Assessing Molecular Docking Tools to Guide Targeted Drug Discovery of CD38 Inhibitors. *Int. J. Mol. Sci.* **2020**, *21*, 5183. [CrossRef]
12. Wang, Z.; Sun, H.; Yao, X.; Li, D.; Xu, L.; Li, Y.; Tian, S.; Hou, T. Comprehensive evaluation of ten docking programs on a diverse set of protein–ligand complexes: The prediction accuracy of sampling power and scoring power. *Phys. Chem. Chem. Phys.* **2016**, *18*, 12964–12975. [CrossRef]
13. Ramirez, U.D.; Myachina, F.; Stith, L.; Jaffe, E.K. Docking to Large Allosteric Binding Sites on Protein Surfaces. In *Advances in Experimental Medicine and Biology*; Springer: New York, NY, USA, 2010; pp. 481–488.
14. Jacquemard, C.; Drwal, M.N.; Desaphy, J.; Kellenberger, E. Binding mode information improves fragment docking. *J. Cheminform.* **2019**, *11*, 24. [CrossRef] [PubMed]
15. Fan, Y.; Zhao, K.; Shi, Z.-L.; Zhou, P. Bat Coronaviruses in China. *Viruses* **2019**, *11*, 210. [CrossRef] [PubMed]
16. Lotfi, M.; Hamblin, M.R.; Rezaei, N. COVID-19: Transmission, prevention, and potential therapeutic opportunities. *Clin. Chim. Acta* **2020**, *508*, 254–266. [CrossRef] [PubMed]
17. World Health Organization (WHO). WHO Coronavirus (COVID-19) Dashboard. Available online: https://covid19.who.int/ (accessed on 8 November 2021).
18. Jin, Z.; Du, X.; Xu, Y.; Deng, Y.; Liu, M.; Zhao, Y.; Zhang, B.; Li, X.; Zhang, L.; Peng, C.; et al. Structure of Mpro from SARS-CoV-2 and discovery of its inhibitors. *Nature* **2020**, *582*, 289–293. [CrossRef] [PubMed]
19. Zhang, C.-H.; Stone, E.A.; Deshmukh, M.; Ippolito, J.A.; Ghahremanpour, M.M.; Tirado-Rives, J.; Spasov, K.A.; Zhang, S.; Takeo, Y.; Kudalkar, S.N.; et al. Potent Noncovalent Inhibitors of the Main Protease of SARS-CoV-2 from Molecular Sculpting of the Drug Perampanel Guided by Free Energy Perturbation Calculations. *ACS Central Sci.* **2021**, *7*, 467–475. [CrossRef] [PubMed]
20. Owen, D.R.; Allerton, C.M.N.; Anderson, A.S.; Aschenbrenner, L.; Avery, M.; Berritt, S.; Boras, B.; Cardin, R.D.; Carlo, A.; Coffman, K.J.; et al. An oral SARS-CoV-2 M pro inhibitor clinical candidate for the treatment of COVID-19. *Science* **2021**, *374*, 1586–1593. [CrossRef]
21. Pavan, M.; Bolcato, G.; Bassani, D.; Sturlese, M.; Moro, S. Supervised Molecular Dynamics (SuMD) Insights into the mechanism of action of SARS-CoV-2 main protease inhibitor PF-07321332. *J. Enzym. Inhib. Med. Chem.* **2021**, *36*, 1645–1649. [CrossRef]
22. Rudrapal, M.; Celik, I.; Khan, J.; Ansari, M.A.; Alomary, M.N.; Yadav, R.; Sharma, T.; Tallei, T.E.; Pasala, P.K.; Sahoo, R.K.; et al. Identification of bioactive molecules from Triphala (Ayurvedic herbal formulation) as potential inhibitors of SARS-CoV-2 main protease (Mpro) through computational investigations. *J. King Saud Univ. Sci.* **2022**, *34*, 101826. [CrossRef]
23. Di Sarno, V.; Lauro, G.; Musella, S.; Ciaglia, T.; Vestuto, V.; Sala, M.; Scala, M.C.; Smaldone, G.; Di Matteo, F.; Novi, S.; et al. Identification of a dual acting SARS-CoV-2 proteases inhibitor through in silico design and step-by-step biological characterization. *Eur. J. Med. Chem.* **2021**, *226*, 113863. [CrossRef]
24. Cuzzolin, A.; Sturlese, M.; Malvacio, I.; Ciancetta, A.; Moro, S. DockBench: An Integrated Informatic Platform Bridging the Gap between the Robust Validation of Docking Protocols and Virtual Screening Simulations. *Molecules* **2015**, *20*, 9977–9993. [CrossRef] [PubMed]
25. Bolcato, G.; Cuzzolin, A.; Bissaro, M.; Moro, S.; Sturlese, M. Can We Still Trust Docking Results? An Extension of the Applicability of DockBench on PDBbind Database. *Int. J. Mol. Sci.* **2019**, *20*, 3558. [CrossRef] [PubMed]
26. Zev, S.; Raz, K.; Schwartz, R.; Tarabeh, R.; Gupta, P.K.; Major, D.T. Benchmarking the Ability of Common Docking Programs to Correctly Reproduce and Score Binding Modes in SARS-CoV-2 Protease Mpro. *J. Chem. Inf. Model.* **2021**, *61*, 2957–2966. [CrossRef] [PubMed]
27. Bolcato, G.; Bissaro, M.; Sturlese, M.; Moro, S. Comparing Fragment Binding Poses Prediction Using HSP90 as a Key Study: When Bound Water Makes the Difference. *Molecules* **2020**, *25*, 4651. [CrossRef]
28. Bolcato, G.; Cescon, E.; Pavan, M.; Bissaro, M.; Bassani, D.; Federico, S.; Spalluto, G.; Sturlese, M.; Moro, S. A Computational Workflow for the Identification of Novel Fragments Acting as Inhibitors of the Activity of Protein Kinase CK1δ. *Int. J. Mol. Sci.* **2021**, *22*, 9741. [CrossRef]
29. Yan, Y.; Huang, S.-Y. Pushing the accuracy limit of shape complementarity for protein-protein docking. *BMC Bioinform.* **2019**, *20*, 696. [CrossRef]
30. Gabb, H.A.; Jackson, R.M.; Sternberg, M.J.E. Modelling protein docking using shape complementarity, electrostatics and biochemical information. *J. Mol. Biol.* **1997**, *272*, 106–120. [CrossRef]
31. Verdonk, M.L.; Giangreco, I.; Hall, R.J.; Korb, O.; Mortenson, P.N.; Murray, C.W. Docking Performance of Fragments and Druglike Compounds. *J. Med. Chem.* **2011**, *54*, 5422–5431. [CrossRef]

32. Chemical Computing Group ULC. *Molecular Operating Environment (MOE)*; 2019.01; Chemical Computing Group ULC: Montreal, QC, Canada, 2021.
33. Case, D.A.; Walker, R.C.; Cheatham, T.E., III; Simmerling, C.; Roitberg, A.; Merz, K.M.; Luo, R.; Li, P.; Darden, T.; Sagui, C.; et al. *Amber 2021*; University of California: San Francisco, CA, USA, 2021.
34. Humphrey, W.; Dalke, A.; Schulten, K. VMD: Visual molecular dynamics. *J. Mol. Graph.* **1996**, *14*, 33–38. [CrossRef]
35. Harvey, M.; Giupponi, G.; De Fabritiis, G. ACEMD: Accelerating Biomolecular Dynamics in the Microsecond Time Scale. *J. Chem. Theory Comput.* **2009**, *5*, 1632–1639. [CrossRef]
36. Eastman, P.; Swails, J.; Chodera, J.D.; McGibbon, R.T.; Zhao, Y.; Beauchamp, K.A.; Wang, L.-P.; Simmonett, A.C.; Harrigan, M.P.; Stern, C.D.; et al. OpenMM 7: Rapid development of high performance algorithms for molecular dynamics. *PLoS Comput. Biol.* **2017**, *13*, e1005659. [CrossRef] [PubMed]
37. Berman, H.M.; Westbrook, J.; Feng, Z.; Gilliland, G.; Bhat, T.N.; Weissig, H.; Shindyalov, I.N.; Bourne, P.E. The Protein Data Bank. *Nucleic Acids Res.* **2000**, *28*, 235–242. [CrossRef] [PubMed]
38. Case, D.A.; Darden, T.; Cheatham, T.E., III; Simmerling, C.; Wang, J.; Duke, R.E.; Luo, R.; Crowley, M.; Walker, R.; Zhang, W.; et al. *Amber 10*; University of California: San Francisco, CA, USA, 2008.

pharmaceuticals

Article

Evaluation of Docking Machine Learning and Molecular Dynamics Methodologies for DNA-Ligand Systems

Tiago Alves de Oliveira [1,2,*], Lucas Rolim Medaglia [1], Eduardo Habib Bechelane Maia [2], Letícia Cristina Assis [1], Paulo Batista de Carvalho [3], Alisson Marques da Silva [2] and Alex Gutterres Taranto [1,4,*]

1 Department of Bioengineering, Federal University of Sao Joao del-Rei, Praça Dom Helvecio, 74, Fabricas, Sao Joao del-Rei 36301-1601, MG, Brazil; lucas.medaglia@hotmail.com (L.R.M.); leticiaassisquimica@hotmail.com (L.C.A.)
2 Federal Center for Technological Education of Minas Gerais, Department of Informatics, Management and Design, CEFET MG, Campus Divinopolis, Rua Alvares de Azevedo, 400, Bela Vista, Divinopolis 35503-822, MG, Brazil; habib@cefetmg.br (E.H.B.M.); alisson@cefetmg.br (A.M.d.S.)
3 Feik School of Pharmacy, University of the Incarnate Word, 4301 Broadway, San Antonio, TX 78209, USA; pcarvalh@uiwtx.edu
4 Faculty of Computing, University of Latvia (UL), Raina Boulevard 19 Center District, LV-1050 Riga, Latvia
* Correspondence: tiago@cefetmg.br (T.A.d.O.); professortaranto@hotmail.com (A.G.T.); Tel.: +55-(37)99969-6735 (T.A.d.O.); +55-(37)98808-6168 (A.G.T.)

Citation: de Oliveira, T.A.; Medaglia, L.R.; Maia, E.H.B.; Assis, L.C.; de Carvalho, P.B.; da Silva, A.M.; Taranto, A.G. Evaluation of Docking Machine Learning and Molecular Dynamics Methodologies for DNA-Ligand Systems. *Pharmaceuticals* **2022**, *15*, 132. https://doi.org/10.3390/ph15020132

Academic Editor: Osvaldo Andrade Santos-Filho

Received: 29 November 2021
Accepted: 17 January 2022
Published: 22 January 2022

Abstract: DNA is a molecular target for the treatment of several diseases, including cancer, but there are few docking methodologies exploring the interactions between nucleic acids with DNA intercalating agents. Different docking methodologies, such as AutoDock Vina, DOCK 6, and Consensus, implemented into Molecular Architect (MolAr), were evaluated for their ability to analyze those interactions, considering visual inspection, redocking, and ROC curve. Ligands were refined by Parametric Method 7 (PM7), and ligands and decoys were docked into the minor DNA groove (PDB code: 1VZK). As a result, the area under the ROC curve (AUC-ROC) was 0.98, 0.88, and 0.99 for AutoDock Vina, DOCK 6, and Consensus methodologies, respectively. In addition, we proposed a machine learning model to determine the experimental ΔT_m value, which found a 0.84 R^2 score. Finally, the selected ligands mono imidazole lexitropsin (**42**), netropsin (**45**), and *N,N′*-(1H-pyrrole-2,5-diyldi-4,1-phenylene)dibenzenecarboximidamide (**51**) were submitted to Molecular Dynamic Simulations (MD) through NAMD software to evaluate their equilibrium binding pose into the groove. In conclusion, the use of MolAr improves the docking results obtained with other methodologies, is a suitable methodology to use in the DNA system and was proven to be a valuable tool to estimate the ΔT_m experimental values of DNA intercalating agents.

Keywords: computer drug design; molecular docking; molecular dynamic simulation; virtual screening; MolAr; DNA intercalating agents

1. Introduction

Drugs interacting with DNA are among the most effective anticancer agents [1], but their low selectivity makes them highly toxic, a major drawback that calls for new studies and strategies to develop drugs selective towards DNA in cancerous cells [2].

One of the strategies for the development of new drugs is to identify small molecules through a systematic analysis of large groups of compounds with drug-like properties. An experimental approach commonly used is the high throughput screening (HTS), an automated process using robots for a systematic search. It is a costly technique due to the number of compounds to be acquired, the cost of purchase and operation of sophisticated robots [3], and experimental considerations such as stability and solubility of the compounds.

An alternative to HTS is the virtual high-throughput screening (vHTS or VS), an in silico method to test large groups of compounds, including databases available online containing millions of molecules. This technique also allows the design and virtual testing of theoretical compounds prior to synthesis or acquisition, reducing the cost and time required to find compounds with a high potential for further development [3,4]. VS methods use molecular docking to study the interaction between small molecules and their receptors [5], a method that has been evaluated for protein-ligand systems, and more recently have been used to model DNA-ligand complexes [6–8]. However, most docking programs use algorithms that are not suitable for modeling DNA due to its high charge density [1], prompting the need for a more adequate in silico model for nucleic acids.

Several studies have been done trying to develop a molecular docking software appropriate for DNA modeling. Ricci and Netz [9] developed a method to predict the binding mode of small molecules to DNA using AutoDock 4.0 [10], which used distinct DNA receptors in the most common conformations related to the most common binding poses to suppress the importance of the receptor's flexibility in the algorithm.

Srivastava et al. [11] described a systematic computational analysis of 57 DNA ligands through four docking protocols, with the following root-mean-square deviation (RMSD) for the best ligands: GOLD [12] (1.24 Å), Glide [13] (1.23 Å), CDOCKER [14] (1.44 Å), and AutoDock [10] (1.57 Å). GOLD and GLIDE, with similar values, were shown to have a better performance and being the most suitable for modeling nucleic acid-ligand complexes. Molecular dynamics simulations showed that the DNA duplex skeleton underwent minor deviations in the complex, supporting docking protocols even though the receptor is kept rigid. However, the area under the ROC curve (AUC) of these methodologies was not evaluated. ROC curve is an important metric to check the capacity of methodology to distinguish false positive results. Fong and Wong [15] evaluated four scoring functions (AutoDock [10], ASP@GOLD [16], ChemScore@GOLD [17], and GoldScore@GOLD [12]) for DNA-ligand complexes, and the scoring functions reproduced the experimental crystallographic structure complexes. It is noteworthy that these previous studies improved their results by combining more than one scoring function.

Good RMSD results were obtained in previous studies, but the ranking capacity of these docking methods was not evaluated. Our study used Molecular Architecture (MolAr) [18] software to predict DNA-ligand poses. MolAr is a docking workflow that allows an integrated and automated virtual screening (VS) process, from protein preparation (homology modeling and protonation state) to virtual screening with different methods. MolAr is open access and free of charge (available at http://www.drugdiscovery.com.br, accessed on 20 May 2020), allowing users to perform all the docking steps in a unique interface with a simple and intuitive operation. It uses AutoDock Vina [19], DOCK 6 [20], and Consensus Virtual Screening (CVS) docking protocols. AutoDock Vina uses a hybrid scoring function that combines knowledge-based and empiric scoring function features. DOCK 6 offers physics-based energy score functions based on force fields and score functions (GRID and AMBER scores). CVS is a ranking normalized combination of the results of AutoDock Vina and DOCK 6, reducing the chance of false positive results [18]. Our results were evaluated for DNA-ligand model systems [11] through visual inspection of the RMSD and ROC curves. In addition, docking binding energy and descriptor values of ligands were used as a predictor to calculate the ΔT_m experimental values of 11 DNA ligands previously reported. Dynamic molecular simulations were also used to clarify their intermolecular interactions with DNA.

2. Results

A visual inspection was performed on the 1VZK structure to identify the principal forces for molecular recognition. Figure 1 shows the 3D structure of the target 1VZK and a 2D diagram with its crystallographic ligand (D1B). The ligand is complexed into the minor groove of DNA (Figure 1a) through hydrogen bonds between amidinic moieties and the carbonyl oxygen of nitrogenous bases. Hydrophobic interactions can also be observed between the benzimidazole and aromatic and with nitrogenous bases (Figure 1b).

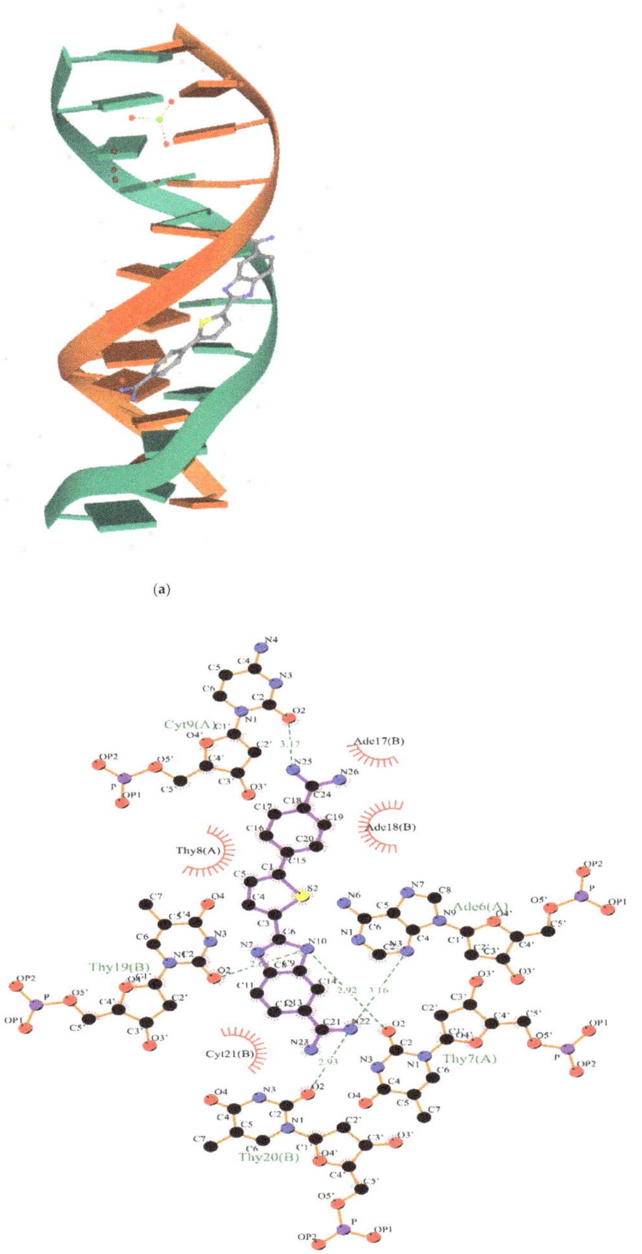

(a)

(b)

Figure 1. (**a**) The crystallographic structure of molecular target under PDB code 1VZK; (**b**) a close view of the intermolecular interactions between ligand (D1B) in the minor DNA groove of the 1VZK. The red circles and ellipses in each plot indicate protein residues. Hydrogen bonds are shown as green dotted lines, while the spoked arcs represent residues making van der Waals interactions with the ligand generated with LigPlot+.

In general, redocking is the first evaluation method to be used in the docking process. This process shows (i) the correct elaboration of grid box parameters; (ii) the capacity of the docking method of reproducing the crystallographic binding pose; (iii) the acquisition of binding energies that can be used to rank the compounds. Usually, the redocking is evaluated by the RMSD value between the crystallographic binding pose and redocking results. The RMSD value between 1VZK and D1B ligand was 0.65 Å by AutoDock Vina, while the threshold value is 2.0 Å [20]. This result was better than previous docking methodologies, GOLD, GLIDE, CDOCKER, and AUTODOCK, which had values ranging from 1.23 Å to 1.57 Å [11].

2.1. Molecular Docking

The docking performance was evaluated by calculating the AUC-ROC, EF values, and BedROC. AUC-ROC has been used to check if the docking method can distinguish false positives from true positives [21]. The AUC-ROC values for our test compounds were 0.98, 0.88, and 0.99 for AutoDock Vina, DOCK 6 (Amber Score), and CVS, respectively. Moreover, the enrichment factor (EF) value [22] reflects the ability of the docking calculations to find true positives throughout the background database compared to random selection. Thus, it indicates how good the set formed by the top x% ranked compounds is compared to a set of equal size selected randomly from the entire collection of compounds. EFs values are calculated utilizing a percentage of the data set. For example, EF5% represents the value obtained when 5% of the database was screened. The EF value is defined by:

$$\text{EF }\% = \frac{\text{actives }\%}{\text{compounds }\%} \times \frac{\text{total compounds}}{\text{total actives}} \quad (1)$$

Previous reports show CVS having the best EF values, compared to DOCK 6 and AutoDock Vina, which can be explained by the use of AutoDock Vina output as the input for DOCK 6. Consequently, AUC-ROC had values corroborated by the EF values; in other words, the EF validates AUC-ROC results, especially with the performance at EF 1%, showing the CVS method could distinguish 100% of molecules [18].

The BedROC [23] value was calculated to confirm these AUC-ROC and EF results. BedROC uses exponential weighting to give early rankings more weight than the latest rankings of active compounds. The BedROC values were 0.60, 0.52, and 0.83 for AutoDock Vina, DOCK 6 (Amber Score), and CVS, respectively. As in AUC-ROC and EF the values of CVS are better than AutoDock Vina and DOCK6 (Amber Score).

Finally, Machine Learning was used to develop a model to predict ΔTm experimental values. ΔT_m represents the change in the melting temperature of DNA upon drug binding, being directly correlated with the binding energy, and is a valuable tool to evaluate the docking results. Six algorithms of linear regression were implemented as follows: (i) Gradient Boosting Regressor [24]; (ii) Random Forest Regressor [25]; (iii) Linear Regressor [26]; (iv) Voting Regressor [27] between algorithms (i), (ii) and (iii), (v) Lasso [28] and (vi) Elastic Net [29]. The results are summarized in Table 1, with Mean Squared Error (MSE) and R^2 score information. The Gradient Boosting Regressor shows the best result, with an R^2 score of 0.84, and the worst is the Random Forest Regressor with an R^2 score of 0.33.

Table 1. Regression Linear values calculated for the Prediction of ΔT_m values.

Algorithm	MSE	R^2 Score
Gradient Boosting Regressor	3.06	0.84
Random Forest Regressor	13.05	0.33
Linear Regressor	6.18	0.68
Voting Regressor	4.48	0.77
Lasso	7.88	0.59
Elastic Net	7.18	0.63

2.2. Molecular Dynamics

The five best CVS results and the original ligand were chosen for simulation and presented in Figure 2, where the conformation changes of each of these ligands during the MD simulation were analyzed.

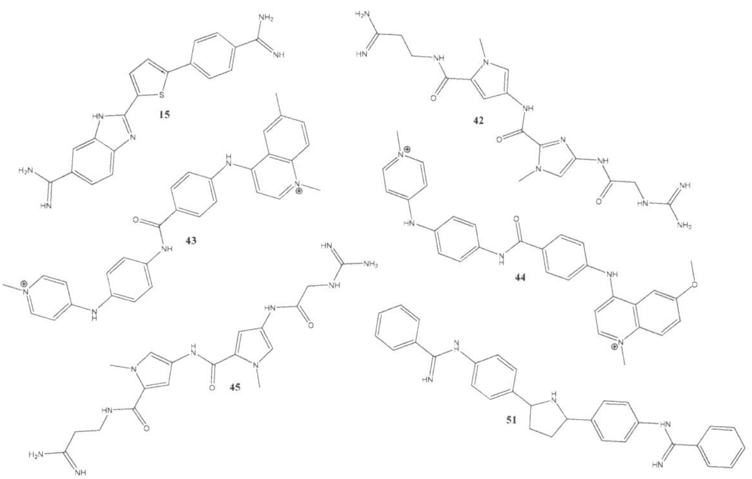

Figure 2. Ligands chosen for MD simulations after docking simulation.

The average energy for the total system, in Kcal/mol was −55,067.1, −55,473.3, −55,507.2, −55,137.1, −54,524.8, and −54,988.1 to ligands **51**, **42**, **45**, **15**, **43**, and **44**, respectively. The total energy graph shown in Figure 3 demonstrates an example of how the energy has a minimal variation. All energy graphs (available in the Supplementary Material, Figure S3) remained in equilibrium throughout the entire MD simulation.

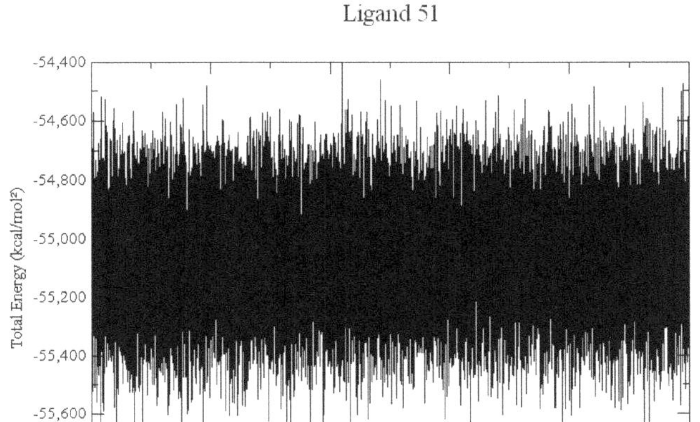

Figure 3. Example of Total Energy (Kcal/mol) calculated in Dynamic Molecular Simulation for interactions with DNA and ligand **51**.

The simulations were carried out in 50 ns to observe if there were significant conformational changes during the trajectory, with the results summarized in Figure 4. As can be observed, the ligands 42, 45, and 51 have the best results with an RMSD variation below

1Å. The original ligand and ligands **43** and **44** showed a major variation of approximately 2, 5, and 4 Å, respectively.

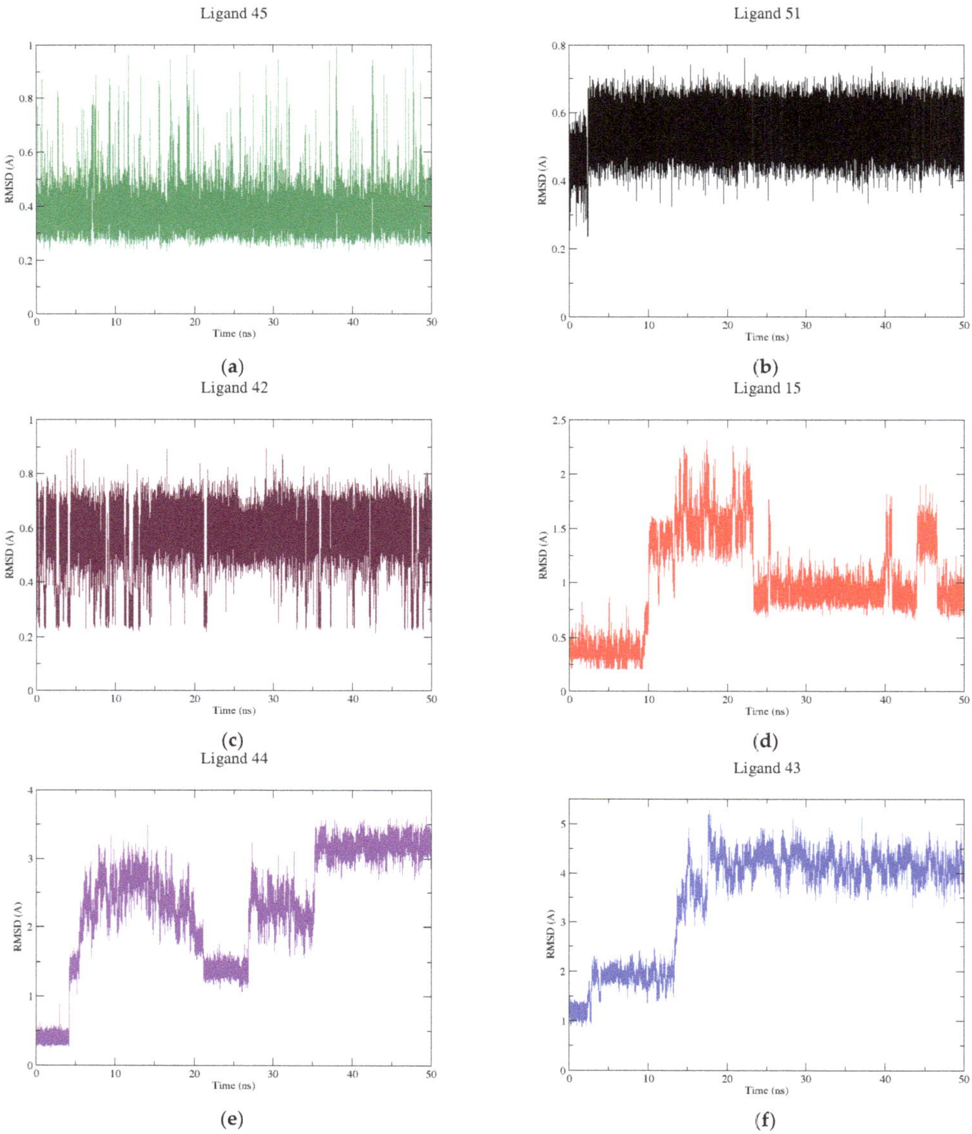

Figure 4. RMSD graphs for: (**a**) **45**; (**b**) **51**; (**c**) **42**; (**d**) **15**; (**e**) **44**; (**f**) **43** ligands complexed with DNA during 50 ns.

The intermolecular interactions of structures in equilibrium can be observed in Figure 5. As can be observed, the ligands **45** (5a), **51** (5b), **42** (5c), **15** (5d) were able to form hydrogen bonds and van der Waals interactions; whereas the ligands **44** (5e) and **43** (5f) carried out van der Waals interactions with nucleic acids.

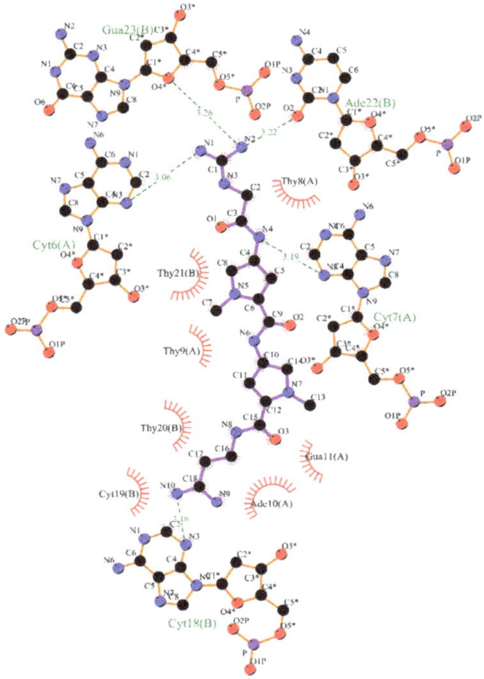

(**a**)

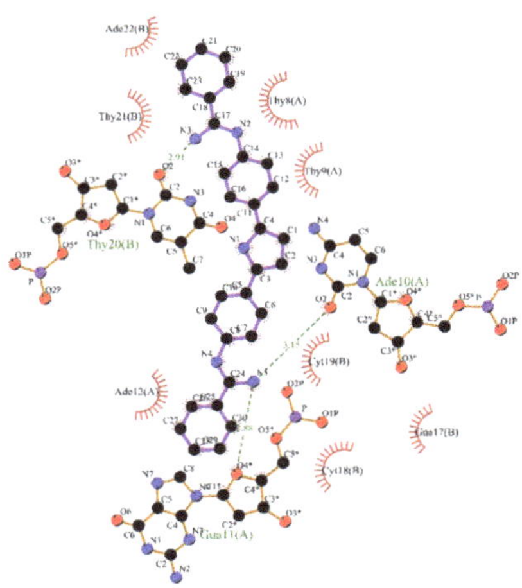

(**b**)

Figure 5. *Cont.*

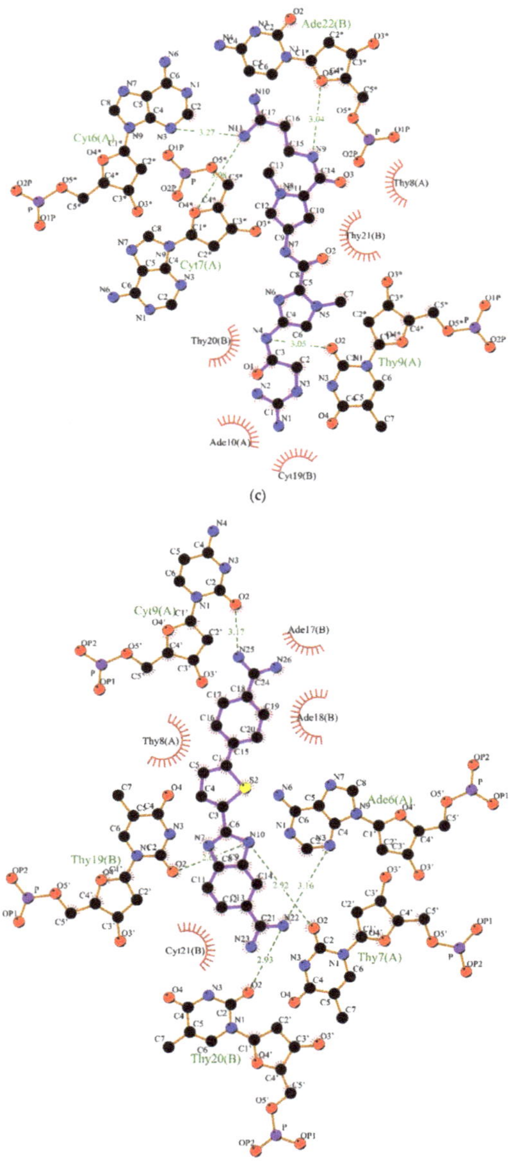

(c)

(d)

Figure 5. *Cont.*

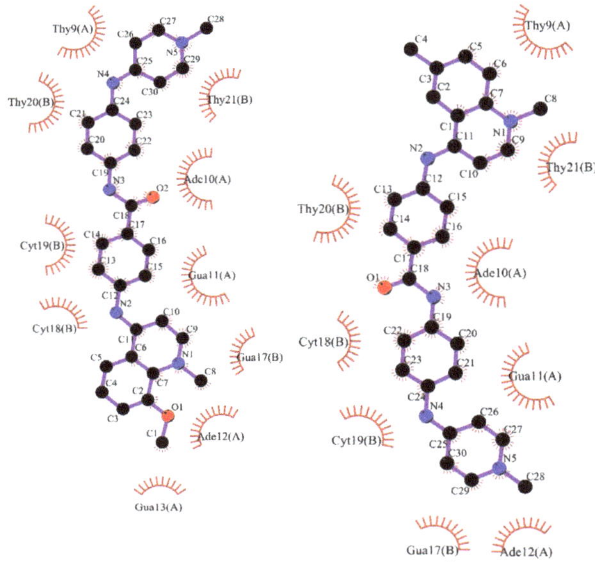

(e) (f)

Figure 5. 2D interaction diagram obtained by LigPlot+ in Dynamic Molecular Simulation for interactions with DNA and ligand: (**a**) **45**; (**b**) **51**; (**c**) **42**; (**d**) **15**; (**e**) **44**; (**f**) **43**. The red circles and ellipses in each plot indicate protein residues. Hydrogen bonds are shown as green dotted lines, while the spoked arcs represent residues making van der Waals interactions with the ligand.

Finally, to improve the analysis of RMSD values fluctuation, the heat map was plotted with the best ligands using VMD software. Figure 6 shows the heat map for ligands **45**, **51**, **45**, and **15**, Figure 6a–d, respectively. In general, the DNA structure is kept rigid during the MD trajectory with low variation. However, the highest fluctuation can be observed for all ligands reaching values ranging from 1.2 to 8.27.

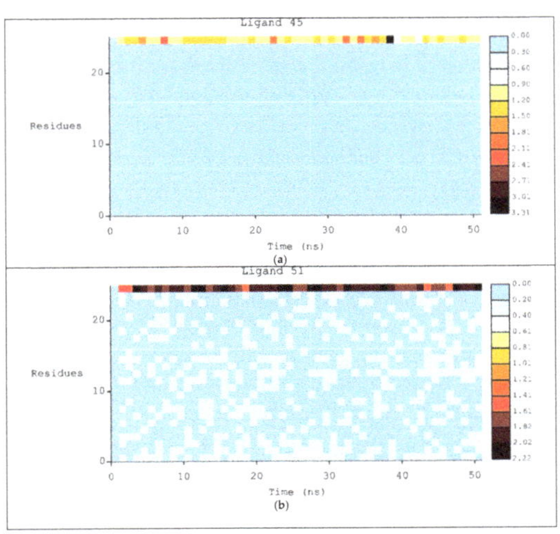

Figure 6. *Cont.*

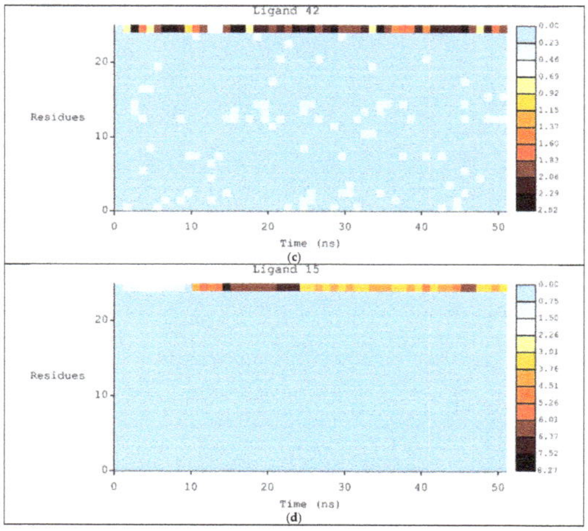

Figure 6. Heat Map for MD simulations generated with HeatMap plugin in VMD with ligand: (**a**) **45**; (**b**) **51**; (**c**) **42**; (**d**) **15**.

3. Discussion

3.1. The Best Docking Methodologies to Study the DNA System

In this study, we use AUC-ROC, EF, and BedROC to evaluate the best docking methodology for DNA intercalating agents, comparing AutoDock Vina, DOCK6, and CVS. AutoDock Vina is an important tool to find the correct pose of ligand into the binding site [19]; however, the ranking among the ligands has not been carried out properly. In addition, the score function of AutoDock Vina does not consider the charges. On the other hand, the score function of DOCK 6 [20], Amber score, includes the AM1-BCC charges of the system. Consequently, the AM1-BCC charges have been determined for a start pose obtained from AutoDock Vina output, improving the accuracy of charge calculations.

AUC-ROC was used to check if the docking method can distinguish false positives from true positives. AUC values close to 1 suggest good discrimination between false and true positives, whereas values closer to 0.5 show a random process, and values higher than 0.7 represent a good distinguishing power [21].

EF indicates how good the set formed by the top x% ranked compounds is when compared to a set of equal size selected randomly from the entire collection of compounds. EF corroborates AUC-ROC [18], yielding even better results with CVS methodology. BedROC calculated values were 0.60, 0.52, and 0.83 for AutoDock Vina, DOCK 6 (Amber Score), and CVS, respectively, confirming that CVS is the best methodology.

The model of linear regression summarized in Table 1 shows the results of the implementation of six linear regressors. The Gradient Boosting Regressor shows the best result, with an R^2 score of 0.84, and the worst is the Random Forest Regressor with an R^2 score of 0.33. Gradient Boosting Regressor (GBR) is a generalization of boosting to arbitrary differentiable loss functions. GBR is an accurate and effective off-the-shelf procedure that can be used for both regression and classification problems in a variety of areas. Our GBR's result is better than Srivastava's studies [11], which used docking information from GOLD, GLIDE, CDOCKER, AUTODOCK 4, Average Information Content level 2, and chemical hardness. Thus, our Machine Learning model was able to estimate ΔT_m value with more accuracy than previous reports.

3.2. Molecular Dynamics Simulations

MD simulations were performed to obtain information about the ligands' interaction and stability into the DNA groove. According to the results of total energy, ligand **51** obtained the lower energy; whereas ligand **44** obtained the highest energy value. Figure 3 demonstrates the lower variation of the system in simulation.

Figure 4 shows the RMSD results of MS simulations. Ligands **15, 42, 45,** and **51** showed a RMSD average variation below 1 Å. Both ligands **42** and **45** achieved the equilibrium state in the beginning of the process (Figure 4a,c). Noteworthy that ligand **51** (Figure 4b) showed a RMSD average value of 0.5 Å, indicating an absence of conformational changes for this inhibitor, suggesting a better molecular recognition between DNA and ligand in the DNA groove. In addition, **15** showed an RMSD average variation of 1 Å and stabilized in the DNA groove after 20 ns of simulation, as shown in Figure 4d. Visual inspection of the MD simulation path of **15** showed a decrease in the intermolecular interaction forces until 20 ns, followed by complete filling of the binding site during the rest of the process. **43** and **44** showed RMSD values higher than 2 Å, and it was observed that the 2-thienyl-1H-benzimidazole portion of **43** was more exposed to the solvent, resulting in a higher degree of freedom and consequent adoption of various conformations. **43** presented an RMSD value of 5.0 Å (Figure 4f), but reached equilibrium after 20 ns. **44** behaved similarly to **43**, reaching equilibrium at 35 ns (Figure 4e). **44** had the quinolinium group outside the major DNA groove, obtaining an RMSD value of 3.5 Å.

Summarizing, all ligands achieved equilibrium within 50 ns of simulation, characterizing molecular recognition. Although compounds ligand 43 and ligand 44 presented good docking results at 15 and 28 nanoseconds of dynamic simulation, respectively, the structures presented conformational changes, resulting from parts of the ligands leaving the DNA groove suggesting hydrogen bonding with the solvent.

MD results corroborate the molecular docking results, with compounds **42**, **45**, and **51** interacting and accommodating themselves better in the smaller groove of DNA, presenting themselves as promising compounds for further studies as anticancer drugs. Compounds **43** and **44** can be considered weak DNA intercalators because, despite good docking results, they had a higher variation of RMSD values during MD.

The molecular interactions are depicted on Figure 5. **45, 51, 42,** and **15** have hydrogen bonding acceptors and donors and were recognized by DNA through hydrogen bonds and van der Waals interactions (Figure 5a–d). For instance, Figure 4a shows the intermolecular interactions between compound **45** with DNA. This compound carried out hydrogen bonding with CytA:7, ThyA:9, AdeB:22 and hydrophobic interactions with ThyA:8, AdeA:10, and ThyB:20. Compound **51** (Figure 5b) was better recognized by the DNA minor groove by performing a higher number of intermolecular interactions, such as hydrogen bonding with AdeA:10, GuaA:11, and ThyB:20; and van der Waals interactions with ThyA:8, ThyA:9, AdeA:12, GuaB:17, CytB:19, and AdeB:22. Compound **42** (Figure 5c) is able to perform hydrogen bonding with CytA:6, CytA:7, ThyA:9, and AdeB:22; and hydrophobic interactions with ThyA:8, AdeA:10, CytB:19, and ThyB:20. It is noteworthy that the guanidinium groups of the **15** performed hydrogen bonds with CytA:6, CytA:7, CytB:18, AdeB:22, GuaB:23, beyond several hydrophobic interactions, such as GuaA:11, ThyB:20, and ThyB:21 (Figure 5d). These interactions with these nitrogenous bases are essential components for intercalation within the minor DNA groove, which indicates that this inhibitor remained well accommodated in the DNA during the dynamic's simulation.

In contrast, both compounds **44** and **43** were not able to perform hydrogen bonding with DNA. **44** (Figure 5e) carried out hydrophobic interactions, for instance, with ThyA:9, AdeA:10, GuaA:11, AdeA:12, GuaA:13, GuaB:17, CytB:18, CytB:19, ThyB:20 and ThyB:21. Similarly, **43** performed hydrophobic interactions with ThyA:9, AdeA:10, GuaA:11, AdeA:12, GuaB:17, CytB:18, CytB:19 and ThyB:20, as shown in Figure 4f. These missing hydrogen bonding interactions can explain the higher RMSD fluctuations value during MD simulations, once this interaction has an important hole in the molecular recognition and stabilization of the ligand within the DNA groove. These findings highlight the structure-activity relationship of guanidinium groups in the development of antineoplastic compounds.

Through the analysis of RMSD plots using heat map graphs (Figure 6) it is possible to confirm the results generated by RMSD and interactions maps. **51** presented the smallest RMSD variation (max of 2.22 Å), best RMSD graphics and total energy. **42**, **45**, and **15** demonstrated RMSD variation of 2.52 Å, 3.31 Å, and 8.27 Å, respectively.

4. Materials and Methods

4.1. Molecular Docking

The three-dimensional structures of 57 ligands were constructed using Marvin Sketch [30] and 150 decoys were generated by the DUD-E platform [31]. The DNA molecular target was obtained from the Protein Data Bank (PDB-1VZK). These ligands and targets were described in a previous report [11] and are available in the Supplementary Material, Figure S1 [31]. The ligands were refined by Run_Mopac [32] software using Parametric Method 7 (PM7) [33] and Eigenvector Following routine [34].

The target was prepared by Chimera [35] by:

- removing water molecules and magnesium ions;
- adjusting the protonation state at pH 7.4;
- assigning charges using AMBERff14SB and AM1-BBC;
- minimizing the structure using 100 steps for steepest descent and 10 steps for conjugate gradient, each step measuring 0.02 Å.

Finally, all compounds were docked against the 1VZK molecular target at the minor groove position using a grid box with 20 × 20 × 26 Å and atomic coordinates centered to 14.44 Å, 20.57 Å, and 8.64 Å, for x, y, and z, respectively. In order to evaluate the best docking methods for DNA docking, three virtual screening simulations using MolAr were performed through AutoDock Vina, DOCK 6 (Amber Score), and CSV. All methodologies were double-checked by redocking, measurement of the area under the Receiver Characteristic Operator (ROC) curve (AUC-ROC), Enrichment Factor (EF), and Boltzmann-Enhanced Discrimination (BedROC). The redocking process consisted of removing the crystallographic ligand, with subsequent docking of the ligands into the same binding site.

In addition, we developed a machine learning model with the docking binding energy results and molecular descriptors of the molecules hereby tested to calculate the ΔT_m experimental values. The data frame was elaborated using the 57 compounds described previously, from which only 11 had their ΔT_m values calculated [11]. The descriptors were obtained using the Mordred library [36], a molecular descriptor calculator. Afterward, six Linear Regression algorithms were performed with the following descriptors: Molecular Weight, cLogP, cLogS, Total Surface Area, Relative Polar Surface Area, Polar Surface Area, AutoDock Vina with major groove, AutoDock Vina with minor groove, E_{homo}, E_{homo}^{-1}, E_{lumo}, E_{homo}^{+1}, DOCK 6 with Amber Score, Consensus with Grid and Amber Score, Structural Information Content level 1, Bond Information Content level 1, and chemical hardness $[\eta = (E_{lumo} - E_{homo})/2)]$.

4.2. Molecular Dynamics

The five best-docked ligands (according to MolAr Consensus with Amber score) were chosen for MD simulations among the crystallographic reference ligands (PDB-ID 1VZK) to characterize the molecular recognition between ligands and DNA. The ligands (PDB-IDs 1VZK, 1LEY, 1ZPH, 1ZPI, 261D, and 2GYX) are shown in the Supplementary Material, Figure S2. All ligands and the energy values for all configurations are presented in the Supplementary Material, respectively, in Figure S1 and Table S1.

The ligand-DNA complexes were inserted into a 74.15 × 52.33 × 55.58 Å simulation box and solvated with TIP3P model water molecules [37]. Sodium chloride ions were added to neutralize the system charge. Each system was energetically minimized with 5000 cycles using the Conjugate Gradient algorithm [38]. The nucleic acid atoms had position restraints with an exponent of energy function of 2 and scaling of 1.0 applied to them during the first 4000 cycles and no restraints during the last 1000 cycles. After the energy minimization, the systems were heated to 310 K during a 30 ps equilibration conducted under an isothermal-isochoric ensemble (NVT), followed by a 500 ps simulation under an isothermal-isobaric ensemble (NPT) using the Langevin piston method [39] to maintain the total pressure to an average of 1 bar. The final production had a total of 50 ns. Water stretching and bending motions were constrained by the SETTLE algorithm [40]. Electrostatic interactions were treated via the Particle-Mesh Ewald method [41,42] with a 12 Å cutoff radius. All simulations were performed using the CHARMM36 [41,43,44] force field implemented into NAMD software [33], version 2.13. Analysis was performed using VMD, version 1.9.3 [45].

5. Conclusions

Even though DOCK 6 and AutoDock Vina showed different results, the overall result was improved when they were combined and subjected to the MolAr CVS approach. AUC-ROC, BedROC, and EF values showed the combination was able to generate more reliable results and a better prediction of the ligand conformation. MD is a critical methodology to confirm the interactions between ligands and nucleic acids, showing that MolAr CVS virtual screening can rank ligands in the DNA intercalating compounds. It is noteworthy that CVS has a low computational cost when compared with MD simulations.

In this study, two different approaches were carried out to predict the activity of compounds capable of binding to the minor groove of DNA. The first approach, structure-based drug design, was carried out to rank compounds for their ability to dock with the 1VZK molecular target at the minor groove position using docking and MD simulations. The second approach, ligand-based drug design through Machine Learning methods, ranked the six selected structures based on their binding energy. These methods were able to properly describe the intermolecular interactions between intercalating agents and DNA and build a machine learning model able to predict the ΔT_m experimental values. The application of docking machine learning and molecular dynamics methodologies suggests compounds **51**, **42**, and **45** as leads for the development of improved anticancer compounds.

Supplementary Materials: The following supporting information can be downloaded at: https://www.mdpi.com/article/10.3390/ph15020132/s1, Figure S1: Structure of all ligands with their PDB code and docking results values, Table S1: Docking Results with all configurations with energy values in Kcal/mol, Figure S2: Ligands chosen for MD simulations after docking. Figure S3. Total Energy (Kcal/mol) calculated in Dynamic Molecular Simulation for interactions with DNA and ligands: (a) **45**; (b) **51**; (c) **42**; (d) **15**; (e) **44**; (f) **43**.

Author Contributions: Conceptualization, A.G.T. and A.M.d.S.; methodology, A.G.T.; software, T.A.d.O. and E.H.B.M.; validation, A.G.T. and A.M.d.S.; formal analysis, T.A.d.O. and L.C.A.; investigation, T.A.d.O., L.C.A., L.R.M. and E.H.B.M.; resources, A.G.T. and A.M.d.S.; data curation, A.G.T. and A.M.d.S.; writing—original draft preparation, T.A.d.O.; writing—review and editing, A.G.T., A.M.d.S., E.H.B.M. and P.B.d.C.; visualization, T.A.d.O. and L.R.M.; supervision, A.G.T.; project administration, A.G.T.; funding acquisition, A.G.T. and A.M.d.S. All authors have read and agreed to the published version of the manuscript.

Funding: This research was funded by PPBE and PPGCF/UFSJ; Research Support Foundation of the State of Minas Gerais-FAPEMIG-Brazil, grant CDS-APQ-02742-17, grant APQ-00855-19, and grant APQ-01733-21; and National Council for Scientific and Technological Development-CNPq-Brazil, grant 305117/2017-3, grant 426261/2018-6; and by fellowship of 2021 (grant 310108/2020-9).

Institutional Review Board Statement: Not applicable.

Informed Consent Statement: Not applicable.

Data Availability Statement: Date is contained in the article and supplementary materials.

Acknowledgments: The authors would like to thank the Federal University of Sao Joao del-Rei (UFSJ) and the Federal Center for Technological Education of Minas Gerais (CEFET-MG) for providing the physical infrastructure.

Conflicts of Interest: The authors declare no conflict of interest.

References

1. Gilad, Y.; Senderowitz, H. Docking Studies on DNA Intercalators. *J. Chem. Inf. Modeling* **2014**, *54*, 96–107. [CrossRef] [PubMed]
2. Silverman, R.B. *The Organic Chemistry of Drug Design and Drug Action*, 2nd ed.; Elsevier: Evanston, IL, USA, 2004. ISBN 9780080513379.
3. Plewczynski, D.; Philips, A.; von Grotthuss, M.; Rychlewski, L.; Ginalski, K. HarmonyDOCK: The Structural Analysis of Poses in Protein-Ligand Docking. *J. Comput. Biol.* **2014**, *21*, 247–256. [CrossRef] [PubMed]
4. Bielska, E.; Lucas, X.; Czerwoniec, A.; Kasprzak, J.M.; Kaminska, K.H.; Bujnicki, J.M.; Biology, C.; Bielska, E.; Lucas, X.; Czerwoniec, A.; et al. Virtual Screening Strategies in Drug Design—Methods and Applications. *Biotechnologia* **2011**, *92*, 249–264. [CrossRef]
5. Chen, Y.-C. Beware of Docking! *Trends Pharmacol. Sci.* **2015**, *36*, 78–95. [CrossRef] [PubMed]
6. Mitra, A.; Saikh, F.; Das, J.; Ghosh, S.; Ghosh, R. Studies on the Interaction of a Synthetic Nitro-Flavone Derivative with DNA: A Multi-Spectroscopic and Molecular Docking Approach. *Spectrochim. Acta Part A Mol. Biomol. Spectrosc.* **2018**, *203*, 357–369. [CrossRef]
7. Lebedeva, A.Y.; Fedorova, O.A.; Tsvetkov, V.B.; Grinberg, V.Y.; Grinberg, N.; Burova, T.; Dubovik, A.S.; Babievsky, K.K.; Fedorov, Y. Novel 18-Crown-6-Ether Containing Mono- and Bisstyryl Dyes Derived from Pyridine Moiety as Fluorescent Dyes for Non-Covalent Interaction with DNA. *Dye. Pigment.* **2018**, *157*, 80–92. [CrossRef]
8. Althaga, I.; Elghalban, M.G.; Saad, F.; Al-fahemi, J.H.; El-metwaly, N.M.; Bondock, S.; Almazroai, L.; Saleh, K.A.; Al-hazmi, G.A. Spectral Characterization, CT-DNA Binding, DFT/B3LYP, Molecular Docking and Antitumor Studies for New Nano-Sized VO (II)-Hydrazonoyl Complexes. *J. Mol. Liq.* **2017**, *242*, 662–677. [CrossRef]
9. Ricci, C.G.; Netz, P.A. Docking Studies on DNA-Ligand Interactions: Building and Application of a Protocol to Identify the Binding Mode. *J. Chem. Inf. Modeling* **2009**, *49*, 1925–1935. [CrossRef] [PubMed]
10. Österberg, F.; Morris, G.M.; Sanner, M.F.; Olson, A.J.; Goodsell, D.S. Automated Docking to Multiple Target Structures: Incorporation of Protein Mobility and Structural Water Heterogeneity in AutoDock. *Proteins Struct. Funct. Bioinform.* **2002**, *46*, 34–40. [CrossRef]
11. Srivastava, H.K.; Chourasia, M.; Kumar, D.; Sastry, G.N. Comparison of Computational Methods to Model DNA Minor Groove Binders. *J. Chem. Inf. Modeling* **2011**, *51*, 558–571. [CrossRef]
12. Jones, G.; Willett, P.; Glen, R.C.; Leach, A.R.; Taylor, R. Development and Validation of a Genetic Algorithm for Flexible Docking. *J. Mol. Biol.* **1997**, *267*, 727–748. [CrossRef]
13. Friesner, R.A.; Banks, J.L.; Murphy, R.B.; Halgren, T.A.; Klicic, J.J.; Mainz, D.T.; Repasky, M.P.; Knoll, E.H.; Shelley, M.; Perry, J.K.; et al. Glide: A New Approach for Rapid, Accurate Docking and Scoring. 1. Method and Assessment of Docking Accuracy. *J. Med. Chem.* **2004**, *47*, 1739–1749. [CrossRef] [PubMed]
14. Wu, G.; Robertson, D.H.; Brooks, C.L.; Vieth, M. Detailed Analysis of Grid-Based Molecular Docking: A Case Study of CDOCKER—A CHARMm-Based MD Docking Algorithm. *J. Comput. Chem.* **2003**, *24*, 1549–1562. [CrossRef]
15. Fong, P.; Wong, H.-K. Evaluation of Scoring Function Performance on DNA-Ligand Complexes. *Open Med. Chem. J.* **2019**, *13*, 40–49. [CrossRef]
16. Mooij, W.T.M.; Verdonk, M.L. General and Targeted Statistical Potentials for Protein-Ligand Interactions. *Proteins Struct. Funct. Genet.* **2005**, *61*, 272–287. [CrossRef] [PubMed]
17. Eldridge, M.D.; Murray, C.W.; Auton, T.R.; Paolini, G.v.; Mee, R.P. Empirical Scoring Functions: I. The Development of a Fast Empirical Scoring Function to Estimate the Binding Affinity of Ligands in Receptor Complexes. *J. Comput. Aided Mol. Des.* **1997**, *11*, 425–445. [CrossRef] [PubMed]
18. Maia, E.H.B.; Medaglia, L.R.; da Silva, A.M.; Taranto, A.G. Molecular Architect: A User-Friendly Workflow for Virtual Screening. *ACS Omega* **2020**, *5*, 6628–6640. [CrossRef] [PubMed]
19. Trott, O.; Olson, A.J. AutoDock Vina: Improving the Speed and Accuracy of Docking with a New Scoring Function, Efficient Optimization, and Multithreading. *J. Comput. Chem.* **2010**, *31*, 455–461. [CrossRef]
20. Allen, W.J.; Balius, T.E.; Mukherjee, S.; Brozell, S.R.; Moustakas, D.T.; Lang, P.T.; Case, D.A.; Kuntz, I.D.; Rizzo, R.C. DOCK 6: Impact of New Features and Current Docking Performance. *J. Comput. Chem.* **2015**, *36*, 1132–1156. [CrossRef] [PubMed]
21. Hamza, A.; Wei, N.-N.; Zhan, C.-G. Ligand-Based Virtual Screening Approach Using a New Scoring Function. *J. Chem. Inf. Modeling* **2012**, *52*, 963–974. [CrossRef]
22. Lätti, S.; Niinivehmas, S.; Pentikäinen, O.T. Rocker: Open Source, Easy-to-Use Tool for AUC and Enrichment Calculations and ROC Visualization. *J. Cheminform.* **2016**, *8*, 45. [CrossRef] [PubMed]
23. Zhao, W.; Hevener, K.E.; White, S.W.; Lee, R.E.; Boyett, J.M. A Statistical Framework to Evaluate Virtual Screening. *BMC Bioinform.* **2009**, *10*, 225. [CrossRef]
24. Friedman, J.H. Greedy Function Approximation: A Gradient Boosting Machine. *Ann. Stat.* **2001**, *29*, 1189–1232. [CrossRef]
25. Breiman, L. Random Forests. *Mach. Learn.* **2001**, *45*, 5–32. [CrossRef]
26. Zou, K.H.; Tuncali, K.; Silverman, S.G. Correlation and Simple Linear Regression. *Radiology* **2003**, *227*, 617–622. [CrossRef] [PubMed]
27. Breiman, L. Stacked Regressions. *Mach. Learn.* **1996**, *24*, 49–64. [CrossRef]
28. Kwon, S.; Han, S.; Lee, S. A Small Review and Further Studies on the LASSO. *J. Korean Data Inf. Sci. Soc.* **2013**, *24*, 1077–1088. [CrossRef]

29. Liu, W.; Li, Q. An Efficient Elastic Net with Regression Coefficients Method for Variable Selection of Spectrum Data. *PLoS ONE* **2017**, *12*, e0171122. [CrossRef] [PubMed]
30. ChemAxon Marvin Version 21.17.0. Available online: https://chemaxon.com/products/marvin (accessed on 27 December 2021).
31. Mysinger, M.M.; Carchia, M.; Irwin, J.J.; Shoichet, B.K. Directory of Useful Decoys, Enhanced (DUD-E): Better Ligands and Decoys for Better Benchmarking. *J. Med. Chem.* **2012**, *55*, 6582–6594. [CrossRef] [PubMed]
32. Stewart, J.J.P. MOPAC2016TM. Available online: http://openmopac.net/MOPAC2016.html (accessed on 14 October 2016).
33. Stewart, J.J.P. Optimization of Parameters for Semiempirical Methods VI: More Modifications to the NDDO Approximations and Re-Optimization of Parameters. *J. Mol. Modeling* **2013**, *19*, 1–32. [CrossRef]
34. Baker, J. An Algorithm for the Location of Transition States. *J. Comput. Chem.* **1986**, *7*, 385–395. [CrossRef]
35. Pettersen, E.F.; Goddard, T.D.; Huang, C.C.; Couch, G.S.; Greenblatt, D.M.; Meng, E.C.; Ferrin, T.E. UCSF Chimera—A Visualization System for Exploratory Research and Analysis. *J. Comput. Chem.* **2004**, *25*, 1605–1612. [CrossRef] [PubMed]
36. Moriwaki, H.; Tian, Y.S.; Kawashita, N.; Takagi, T. Mordred: A Molecular Descriptor Calculator. *J. Cheminform.* **2018**, *10*, 4. [CrossRef] [PubMed]
37. Jorgensen, W.L.; Chandrasekhar, J.; Madura, J.D.; Impey, R.W.; Klein, M.L. Comparison of Simple Potential Functions for Simulating Liquid Water. *J. Chem. Phys.* **1983**, *79*, 926–935. [CrossRef]
38. Kumar, S.; Huang, C.; Zheng, G.; Bohm, E.; Bhatele, A.; Phillips, J.C.; Yu, H.; Kale, L.V. Scalable Molecular Dynamics with NAMD on the IBM Blue Gene/L System. *IBM J. Res. Dev.* **2008**, *52*, 177–188. [CrossRef]
39. Feller, S.E.; Zhang, Y.; Pastor, R.W.; Brooks, B.R. Constant Pressure Molecular Dynamics Simulation: The Langevin Piston Method. *J. Chem. Phys.* **1995**, *103*, 4613. [CrossRef]
40. Miyamoto, S.; Kollman, P.A. Settle: An Analytical Version of the SHAKE and RATTLE Algorithm for Rigid Water Models. *J. Comput. Chem.* **1992**, *13*, 952–962. [CrossRef]
41. Hart, K.; Foloppe, N.; Baker, C.M.; Denning, E.J.; Nilsson, L.; MacKerell, A.D. Optimization of the CHARMM Additive Force Field for DNA: Improved Treatment of the BI/BII Conformational Equilibrium. *J. Chem. Theory Comput.* **2012**, *8*, 348–362. [CrossRef]
42. Phillips, J.C.; Braun, R.; Wang, W.; Gumbart, J.; Tajkhorshid, E.; Villa, E.; Chipot, C.; Skeel, R.D.; Kalé, L.; Schulten, K. Scalable Molecular Dynamics with NAMD. *J. Comput. Chem.* **2005**, *26*, 1781–1802. [CrossRef]
43. MacKerell, A.D.; Banavali, N.K. All-Atom Empirical Force Field for Nucleic Acids: II. Application to Molecular Dynamics Simulations of DNA and RNA in Solution. *J. Comput. Chem.* **2000**, *21*, 105–120. [CrossRef]
44. MacKerell, A.D.; Feig, M.; Brooks, C.L. Improved Treatment of the Protein Backbone in Empirical Force Fields. *J. Am. Chem. Soc.* **2004**, *126*, 698–699. [CrossRef] [PubMed]
45. Humphrey, W.; Dalke, A.; Schulten, K. VMD: Visual Molecular Dynamics. *J. Mol. Graph.* **1996**, *14*, 33–38. [CrossRef]

pharmaceuticals

Article

In Silico Design, Synthesis and Biological Evaluation of Anticancer Arylsulfonamide Endowed with Anti-Telomerase Activity

Giulia Culletta [1,2], Mario Allegra [2], Anna Maria Almerico [2], Ignazio Restivo [2] and Marco Tutone [2,*]

1 Dipartimento di Scienze Chimiche, Biologiche, Farmaceutiche e Ambientali, Università di Messina, 98166 Messina, Italy; giulia.culletta@unime.it
2 Dipartimento di Scienze e Tecnologie Biologiche Chimiche e Farmaceutiche, Università degli Studi di Palermo, 90123 Palermo, Italy; mario.allegra@unipa.it (M.A.); annamaria.almerico@unipa.it (A.M.A.); ignazio.restivo@unipa.it (I.R.)
* Correspondence: marco.tutone@unipa.it

Abstract: Telomerase, a reverse transcriptase enzyme involved in DNA synthesis, has a tangible role in tumor progression. Several studies have evidenced telomerase as a promising target for developing cancer therapeutics. The main reason is due to the overexpression of telomerase in cancer cells (85–90%) compared with normal cells where it is almost unexpressed. In this paper, we used a structure-based approach to design potential inhibitors of the telomerase active site. The MYSHAPE (Molecular dYnamics SHared PharmacophorE) approach and docking were used to screen an *in-house* library of 126 arylsulfonamide derivatives. Promising compounds were synthesized using classical and green methods. Compound 2C revealed an interesting IC_{50} (33 ± 4 μM) against the K-562 cell line compared with the known telomerase inhibitor BIBR1532 IC_{50} (208 ± 11 μM) with an SI ~10 compared to the BALB/3-T3 cell line. A 100 ns MD simulation of 2C in the telomerase active site evidenced Phe494 as the key residue as well as in BIBR1532. Each moiety of compound 2C was involved in key interactions with some residues of the active site: Arg557, Ile550, and Gly553. Compound 2C, as an arylsulfonamide derivative, is an interesting hit compound that deserves further investigation in terms of optimization of its structure to obtain more active telomerase inhibitors

Keywords: sulfonamides; arylsulfonamide; anticancer compounds; telomerase inhibitors; structure-based drug design; pharmacophore modeling; docking; molecular dynamics

Citation: Culletta, G.; Allegra, M.; Almerico, A.M.; Restivo, I.; Tutone, M. In Silico Design, Synthesis and Biological Evaluation of Anticancer Arylsulfonamide Endowed with Anti-Telomerase Activity. *Pharmaceuticals* **2022**, *15*, 82. https://doi.org/10.3390/ph15010082

Academic Editor: Osvaldo Andrade Santos-Filho

Received: 6 December 2021
Accepted: 5 January 2022
Published: 10 January 2022

1. Introduction

The nuclear protein complex, Telomere, defends the terminal ends of chromosomes from degradation, end-to-end fusion, and recombination [1–3]. The telomere structure is subject to several changes. After each cell division cycle, the telomere gradually shortens until the chromosomal DNA is exposed, inducing a DNA damage response [4,5]. This event helps to maintain the stability of genetic information and protects the genome in a "time-bomb" manner [6]. When the length of telomeres reaches a critical point, cells reach the cycle of termination, aging, and death [5,6]. Normal cells cannot survive this progressive shortening. Sometimes, cells can extend telomeres by reactivating telomerase activity or through a telomere replacement elongation mechanism (ALT) to help cells survive the crisis [7]. The reactivation of telomerase is observed in 85–90% of human tumor cells [8]. Telomerase is a reverse transcriptase that contains an RNA template (TER) with its binding domain (TRBD) and reverse transcriptase unit (TERT). Telomerase is a challenging but appealing target, because the inhibition of its activity can be achieved by acting at different stages and using various mechanisms [9–11]. A first but now less popular used approach is based on inhibiting telomerase access to DNA by stabilizing G-quadruplexes formed by a 3′ DNA overhang, which has the task to block telomere elongation [11–15]. Another approach includes the use of inhibitors of the enzymatic active site of telomerase including antisense compounds to TER [16,17]. But the most promising approach is possibly the use of compounds that are able to block the active center of the enzyme in the catalytic subunit, directly. BIBR1532, which selectively inhibits telomerase activity, was first proposed in 2001 and has been patented as a potential anticancer drug [18,19]. As reported in a recent review, structure-based drug design strategies can be used to design potential inhibitors of the telomerase active site [20]. The first structure showing a co-crystallized inhibitor was published in 2015, revealing the *Tribolium castaneum* full-length catalytic subunit of telomerase in complex with the compound BIBR1532 (PDB 5CQG), which showed that the studied ligand interacts outside of the active center [21]. This experimental crystal structure changed the understanding of the expected mechanism of activity of this compound and possibly other active site-directed molecules. BIBR1532 binds to a highly conserved hydrophobic pocket (FVYL) motif on the outer surface of the thumb domain of telomerase.

Several other compounds designed using in silico approaches have been tested as potential inhibitors of the catalytic subunit of telomerase such as benzylidene–hydrazone analogs [22], dihydropyrazole [23–29], dibenzopyrroles [30], flavone pyridines [31], 1,3,4-oxadiazole derivatives [32–36], pyrazole-5-carboxamides and pyrazole-pyrimidines [37], spiroketals [37], celastrol derivatives [38], myricetin derivatives [39], indolyl-2′-deoxynucleotide analogs [40], flavonoid derivatives [41], and chrolactomycin derivatives [42]. Other classes of compounds developed as telomerase inhibitors are reported in two recent reviews [43,44]. Thus, considering the direct inhibition of TERT as the most promising approach for blocking the action of telomerase and the lack of an approved drug (Imetelstat is the only one to reach clinical trials [20])makes the search for new and effective inhibitors a hot topic of the pharmaceutical sciences. To the best of our knowledge, there is just one piece of evidence of arylsulfonamide derivatives (SEW05920) as an inhibitor of the TERT [45]. Exploiting our previous experience and outcomes in the use of computational approaches [46–50], we developed a structure-based computational approach to performing a virtual screening of an *in-house* arylsulfonamides library. Some arylsulfonamides have been identified as hits, also synthesized using green chemistry approaches and tested against three cancer cell lines K-562, HCT-116, and MCF-7. The results determined compound 2C as more active than the reference compound BIBR1532. The identification of this novel scaffold, which will undergo optimization, could help to identify new potent telomerase inhibitors.

2. Results

2.1. In Silico Modeling and Virtual Screening

In this study, we performed a structure-based virtual screening by using MD pharmacophore modeling and docking studies to identify potential telomerase inhibitors in our *in-house* library of arylsulfonamide compounds. Firstly, the *Tribolium castaneum* full-length catalytic subunit of telomerase in complex with the compound BIBR1532 (PDB 5CQG) was selected. The crystal structure was optimized by completing and refining the entire structure and optimizing amide groups of asparagine (Asn) and glutamine (Gln) as well as the imidazole ring in histidine (His); then, we predicted the protonation states of histidine, (His), aspartic acid (Asp), glutamic acid (Glu), and the tautomeric states of histidine. Starting from the PDB coordinates set of BIBR1532, a static pharmacophore model was created by using LigandScout containing six features (Figure 1A):

- Four hydrophobic features;
- One H-bond acceptor;
- One anionic feature.

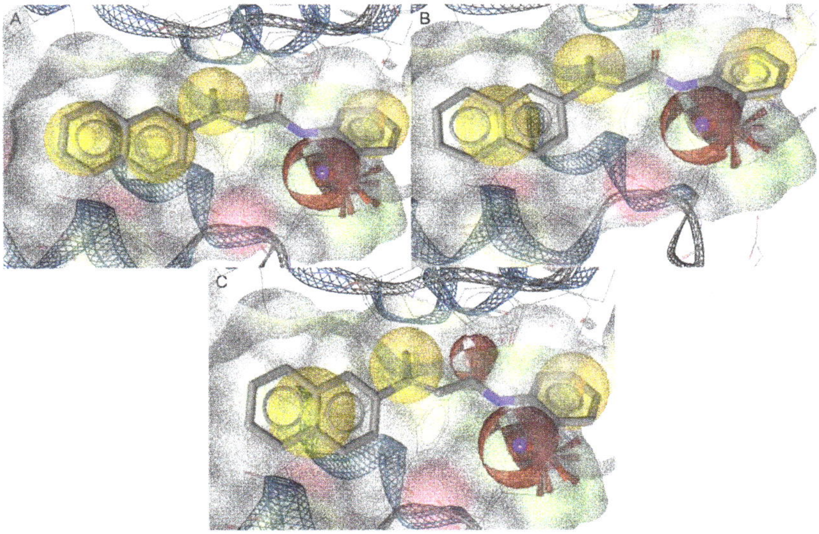

Figure 1. Pharmacophore models derived from the X-ray pose of BIBR1532 (PDB ID: 5CQG): (**A**) static pharmacophore model from the PDB with six features—4 hydrophobic features (yellow spheres), 1 H-bond acceptor (red sphere), and one anionic feature (red star); (**B**) static pharmacophore model after fusing with 5 features—3 hydrophobic features (yellow spheres), 1 H-bond acceptor (red sphere), and 1 anionic feature (red star); (**C**) MYSHAPE pharmacophore model—3 hydrophobic features (yellow spheres), 2 H-bond acceptors (red spheres), and 1 anionic feature (red star).

The pharmacophore features were decreased to five, the two hydrophobic features on the naphthyl ring of BIBR1532 were fused into one, and the tolerance radius for the new pharmacophore feature was increased by 0.15 Å to compensate for small deviations (Figure 1B). To improve the performance of the virtual screening (VS) process, the recent MYSHAPE (Molecular dYnamics SHared PharmacophorE) approach was used [51,52]. According to this approach, the exploration of the protein conformations by molecular dynamics coupled with the pharmacophore modeling improved the result of the VS concerning the corresponding model generated from the PDB coordinates set. To build the MYSHAPE model, 20 ns of molecular dynamics simulation of the BIBR1532–protein complex was run. A new interaction was retrieved such as a hydrogen bond interaction of the carbonyl group of BIBR1532 with the Met482 by a water bridge. The new MYSHAPE pharmacophore feature was added to the original pharmacophore model. In addition, in this case, the tolerance radius for the added pharmacophore feature was increased by 0.15 Å to compensate for small deviations in the 3D coordinates of the different conformations.

The MYSHAPE pharmacophore model had six features (Figure 1C):

- Three hydrophobic features;
- Two H-bond acceptors;
- One anionic feature.

This model was used to screen the *in-house* library of arylsulfonamide derivatives.

At the same time as the pharmacophore modeling, standard precision (SP) molecular docking studies were performed using Glide [53], considering the conserved hydrophobic pocket (FVYL motif) where BIBR1532 binds. The docking studies were performed centering the docking boxes on the 3D coordinates of BIBR1532. The RMSD of BIBR1532 was calculated showing a value of 0.2 Å. The residues that characterized the binding site were Phe478, Met482, Met483, Arg486, Phe494, Gly495, Ile497, Trp498, Ile550, Tyr551, Gly553, Lys552, Leu554, and Arg557. BIBR1532 established an H-bond interaction and a salt bridge between the oxygen of the amide group and Arg486 and aromatic H-bond interactions between the naphthyl ring and Phe494 and Ile550 (Figure 2).

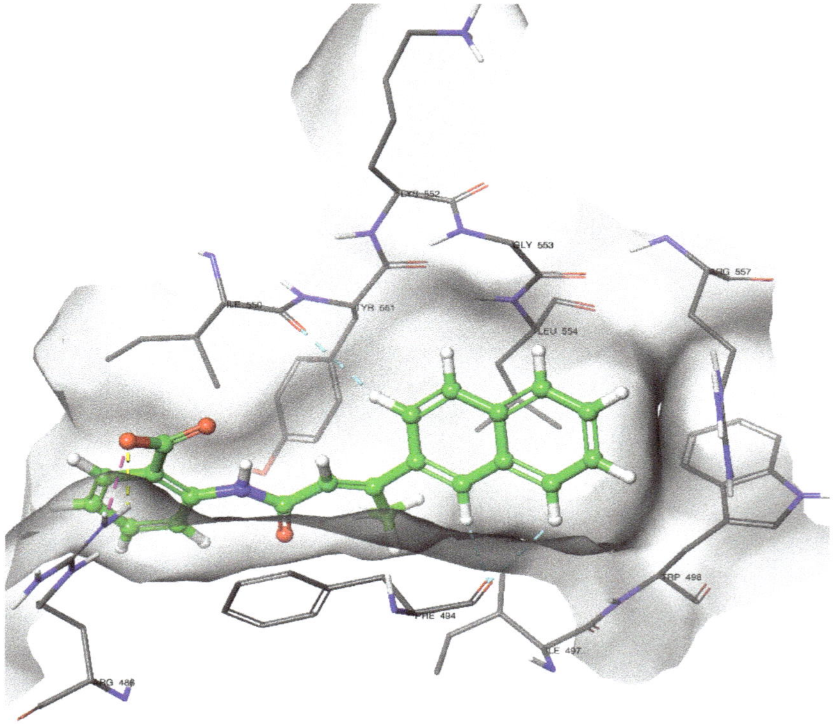

Figure 2. Binding mode after re-docking of BIBR1532: the yellow, dashed lines represent the H-bond interaction and, the purple, dashed lines represent the salt bridge between the O of the carboxyl group and Arg486, and the light blue dashed lines represent the aromatic H-bond interactions between the naphthyl ring and Phe494 and Ile550.

The *in-house* library was used to perform the VS by docking. MM–GBSA-binding free energy calculations were performed for the molecules obtained from the VS and compared with BIBR1532. Hit compounds that exhibited ΔG binding values (1A, 1B, 1C, 1E, 1G, 2B, and 2C, −70.75/−62.97 kcal/mol) lower than that obtained for BIBR1532 (−62.76 kcal/mol) were selected for synthesis and in vitro tests together with hit compounds retrieved using the MYSHAPE approach (1D, 1F, and 2A) (Figure 3).

2.2. *Synthesis*

For the preparation of sulfonamide compounds of type 1 and 2 (Figure 3), several procedures are present in the literature [54–61], and a few of them were also proposed recently in light of using more environmentally friendly green chemistry approaches [62–66].

Our approach to targeting derivatives of type 1 and 2 involved reactions of the sulfonyl chloride 3 and suitable benzylamines 4 or amine 5, according to Schemes 1 and 2. The benzylamines were commercially available, whereas the 1-(4-aminophenyl)-3,5-dimethylpyrazole (5) was prepared in two steps from acetylacetone and 4-nitrophenylhydrazine and the subsequent reduction of the nitro group with H_2 and Pd/C, using standard literature methodology (see Section 4).

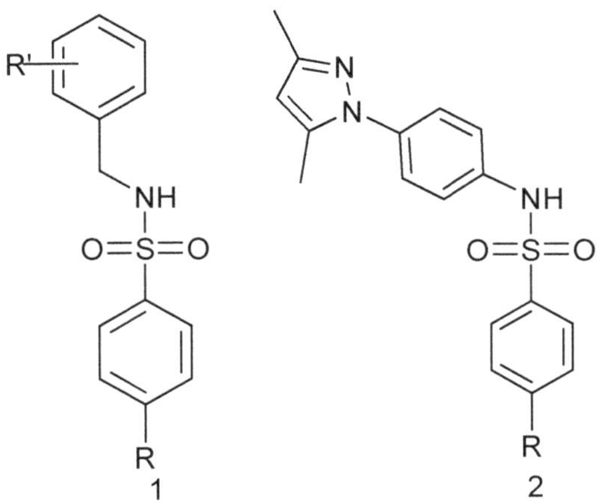

1 2

Figure 3. Structures of sulfonamides 1 and 2 prepared in this work (R = Me, NHAc; NO_2; NH_2), (R′ = 4 Cl; 4-OMe; 2,5-diOMe).

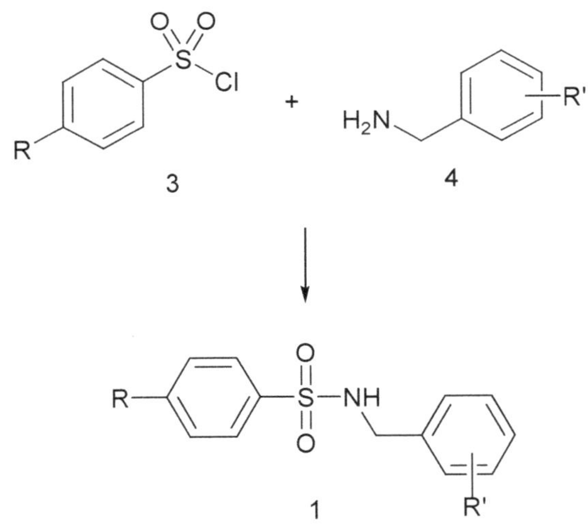

1	R	R′
A	Me	4-Cl
B	NHAc	4-Cl
C	NO_2	4-Cl
D	Me	4-OMe
E	NHAc	4-OMe
F	Me	2,5-di-OMe
G	NO_2	2,5-di-OMe

Scheme 1. The general method for the synthesis of benzyl-sulfonamides of type 1.

In all cases, initially, the reactions were carried out under classical literature conditions, according to Methods X or Y (see Section 4) affording derivatives 1 in good to high isolated yields (64–97%) and slightly lower (49%) only in the case of 1E, probably because of the solubility problem of the starting material (Scheme 1).

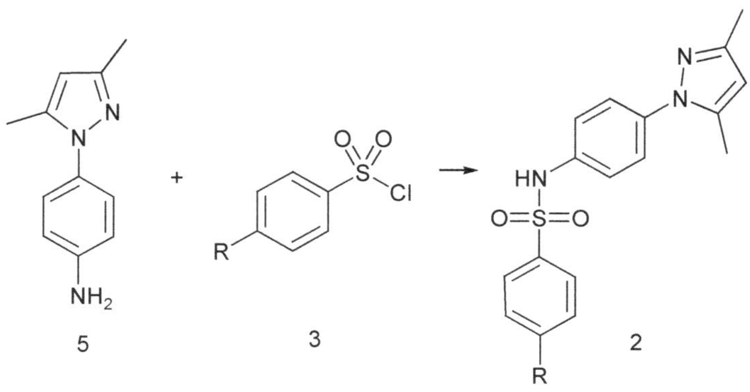

Scheme 2. General method for the synthesis of sulfonamide 2, R = Me (2A); NO2 (2B); NH2 (2C).

The aminophenyl-3,5-dimethylpyrazole 5 also reacted with sulfonylchloride 3 in anhydrous THF in the presence of an equimolar amount of triethylamine, affording sulfonamides 2A,B (Scheme 2).

The possibility of avoiding the use of dangerous/dry solvents was also considered. The pilot reaction of benzylamine and para-toluensulfonyl chloride, in Schotten–Baumann conditions under pH control with Na_2CO_3, as discussed in [67], was explored, but the result was the incomplete conversion to the desired sulfonamide. Recently, a new environmentally safe methodology was reported for the preparation of a wide range of aliphatic- and aryl-sulfonamides [68], and although the methodology was not extended to investigate the reactivity of benzylamines, we decided to explore whether this kind of amine resulted in a suitable substrate to prepare sulfonamides via this route. The green method afforded yields from good to quantitative, giving in some cases a similar efficient conversion of the reactants into products, if compared to Method X (Table 1). The major concern of this methodology is the competitive reactions leading to bis-sulfonylation which, however, in the case benzylamines were not observed, suggesting that this procedure has preferable results, especially when electron-withdrawing groups are present in both the reactants (as in the case of entry 1C).

Table 1. Comparison of the yields obtained using classical and green chemistry methods.

1	R	R′	Method X	No Solvent *
C	NO_2	4-Cl	78	100
D	Me	4-OMe	100	60
E	NHAc	4-OMe	80	70

* According to [68], the amine (2 mmol) and anhydrous $NaHCO_3$ (approximately 1 g) were ground together into a fine powder, and arylsulfonyl chloride (2 mmol) was added under vigorous stirring at room temperature. The progress of the reaction was monitored by TLC until the conversion of the amine was completed.

Compound 2C was prepared by reduction of the corresponding nitro compound with H_2/Pd in ethanol a quantitative yield.

2.3. *Cytotoxic Activity and Selectivity Index*

To select the most promising cytotoxic agents, the newly synthesized compounds were initially evaluated on human colorectal carcinoma (HCsT-116) [69,70], human breast adenocarcinoma (MCF-7) [70,71], and human chronic myeloid leukemia (K-562) [71,72] cell lines that express the active telomerase.

As shown in Table 2, except for compound 2C, the antiproliferative efficacy of the compounds was modest and only evident at the highest micro-submillimolar concentrations. Moreover, compounds 1B, 1D, 1E, 1F, 1G, and 2B exhibited solubility issues that prevented the evaluation of their cytotoxicity.

Table 2. Cytotoxicity of the synthesized compounds on human tumor cell lines HCT-116, MCF-7, and K-562. Cells were treated for 24 h in the absence or the presence of the compound tested at the indicated concentration, and cell viability was assessed by an MTT test as reported in Section 4. Values are expressed as the mean ± SD of three separate experiments conducted in triplicate. * Sol: solubility issue.

Compound	% Inhibition Cell Proliferation														
	HCT-116					MCF-7					K-562				
	Compound Concentration (μm)														
	10	75	150	300	400	10	75	150	300	400	10	75	150	300	400
1A	0	0	19 ± 2	29 ± 3	40 ± 2	0	0	0	12 ± 1	13 ± 1	0	0	0	33 ± 2	38 ± 2
1B	0	5 ± 0.2	23 ± 2	* Sol	* Sol	0	15 ± 1	21 ± 2	* Sol	* Sol	0	5 ± 0.3	21 ± 1	* Sol	* Sol
1C	0	0	2 ± 0.1	8 ± 0.2	15 ± 2	0	5 ± 0.1	15 ± 1	19 ± 1	30 ± 2	0	12 ± 1	13 ± 1	16 ± 1	25 ± 1
1D	0	0	0	* Sol	* Sol	0	0	0	* Sol	* Sol	0	0	0	* Sol	* Sol
1E	0	5 ± 0.1	* Sol	* Sol	* Sol	0	20 ± 2	* Sol	* Sol	* Sol	0	16 ± 1	* Sol	* Sol	* Sol
1F	0	0	6 ± 0.3	* Sol	* Sol	0	0	0	* Sol	* Sol	0	0	0	* Sol	* Sol
1G	0	5 ± 0.2	28 ± 2	* Sol	* Sol	0	12 ± 1	35 ± 2	* Sol	* Sol	0	2 ± 0.1	37 ± 3	* Sol	* Sol
2A	0	5 ± 0.1	30 ± 1	44 ± 2	55 ± 3	0	0	0	0	0	0	13 ± 1	42 ± 2	55 ± 3	60 ± 3
2B	0	0	37 ± 2	* Sol	* Sol	0	17 ± 1	34 ± 2	* Sol	* Sol	0	19 ± 1	23 ± 2	* Sol	* Sol
2C	15 ± 2	31 ± 2	56 ± 2	75 ± 2	91 ± 4	10 ± 1	19 ± 3	59 ± 2	76 ± 2	85 ± 2	35 ± 2	70 ± 3	76 ± 1	80 ± 3	85 ± 2
BIBR-1532	25 ± 2	47 ± 3	56 ± 3	89 ± 2	95 ± 5	12 ± 2	23 ± 2	57 ± 3	74 ± 2	91 ± 3	10 ± 2	19 ± 3	32 ± 1	62 ± 3	79 ± 2

On the other hand, compound 2C revealed an interesting activity, and it was possible to calculate its IC_{50} (Table 3). Interestingly, this value on K-562 cells appeared 3.6-fold lower than that on HCT-116 and 4.2-fold lower than that on MCF-7 cells. Moreover, in the K-562 cell line tested, compound 2C showed an IC_{50} 6.8-fold lower than the reference compound BIBR1532, and an IC_{50} comparable to BIBR1532 in the MCF-7 cell line.

Table 3. IC_{50} of 2C against HCT-116, MCF-7, K-562, and BALB/3-T3 cell lines. Values were calculated by plotting the percentage viability versus concentration on a logarithmic graph and are expressed as the mean ± SD of three separate experiments conducted in triplicate.

Compound	IC_{50} (μm)			
	HCT-116	**MCF-7**	**K-562**	**BALB/3-T3**
BIBR-1532	70 ± 4	120 ± 8	208 ± 11	N/A
2C	109 ± 8	127 ± 9	33 ± 4	324 ± 15

Selective cytotoxicity is a pivotal requirement for anticancer drugs. To determine the selectivity of compound 2C, its cytotoxicity against the cancer cell lines employed (i.e., HCT-116, MCF-7, and K-562) was compared with that against the non-cancerous, murine, embryonic, fibroblast cell line BALB/3-T3. As shown in Table 3, the IC_{50} of compound 2C on BALB/3-T3 cells was remarkably higher than those on the tumoral cell lines tested. Moreover, the calculated selectivity indexes (SIs) of compound 2C for HCT-116, MCF-7, and K-562 cells were 2.9, 2.5, and 9.8, respectively. Relevantly, these values are above the accepted threshold for antitumor drugs (SI = 2.0) [72,73].

Although selectivity for cancer cells cannot be easily derived from the comparison of toxicity parameters in different cell cultures, these data indicate that compound 2C shows preferential toxicity towards cancer cells. Along these lines, the potential use of compound 2C as a novel lead molecule for the development of more potent and selective antiproliferative agents can, therefore, be envisaged.

2.4. Docking of Compound 2C

Analysis of the best docking pose of compound 2C showed a pi–pi stacking interaction between Phe494 and the central aromatic ring as observed in BIBR1532, where the same residue is involved in two H-aromatic bonds with the naphthyl ring (Figure 2). The same residues Phe494, Asp493, and Gly495 establish positive van der Waals (vdW) contacts with the aniline group of 2C. Other positive vdW contacts are formed by the sulfonamide moiety of 2C and Ile550, Gly553, and Leu554. The major part of positive vdW contacts are established by the dimethylpyrazolyl moiety with Met482, Met483, Arg486, Phe494, and Ile550 (Figure 4).

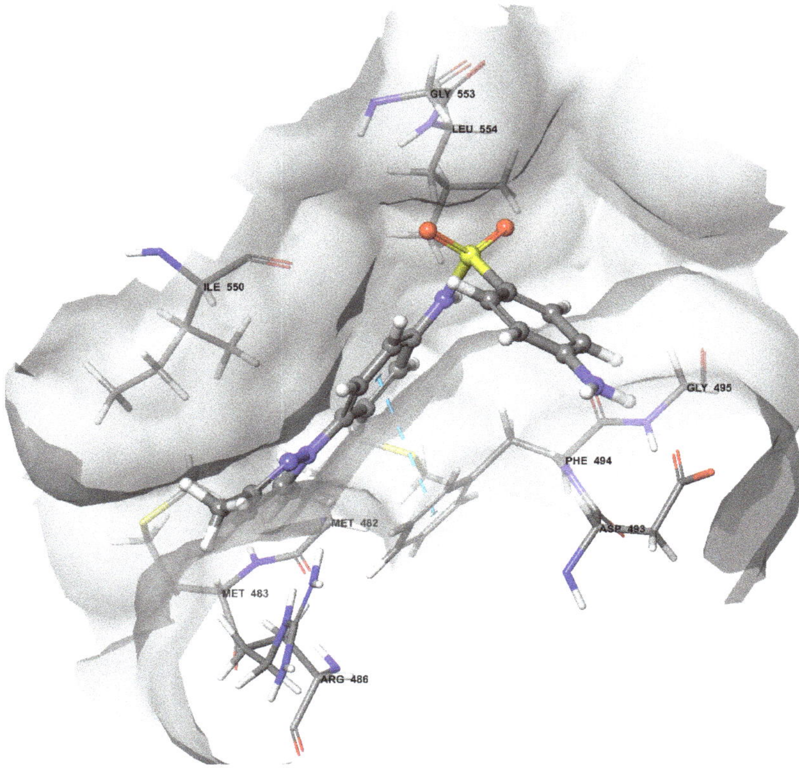

Figure 4. Binding mode of the best docking pose of 2C after the docking study. The light blue, dashed lines represent the pi–pi stacking. The displayed residues establish positive vdW contacts with the compound.

2.5. Molecular Dynamics Simulation

The running of dynamics simulations of protein–ligand complexes over time could be considered a major step toward accuracy in computer-assisted drug design. In this study, an unbiased molecular dynamics simulation was performed to investigate the conformational stability and the time-dependent binding capability of 2C in the active site of the telomerase. Additionally, we tried to understand if the protein target undergoes conformational alteration after interacting with 2C. Therefore, starting from the previous docking, 100 ns of MD simulation was carried out. Various analyses, such root mean square deviation (RMSD), root mean square fluctuation (RMSF), and determination of the number and types of protein–ligand contacts, were performed to obtain a more detailed analysis of the 2C–target complex.

2.5.1. Stability Analysis

The RMSD was selected as a criterion to evaluate the dynamic stability of the ligand-bound system [73]. The RMSD values of the protein's atoms and ligand are reported in Figure 5. The system reached equilibrium quickly and fluctuated around the average RMSD value of <3 Å. The average value of ligand vs. protein RMSD of ~6.4 Å indicated a strong stability of 2C in the binding pocket compared to the ligand vs. ligand RMSD of ~1.81 Å.

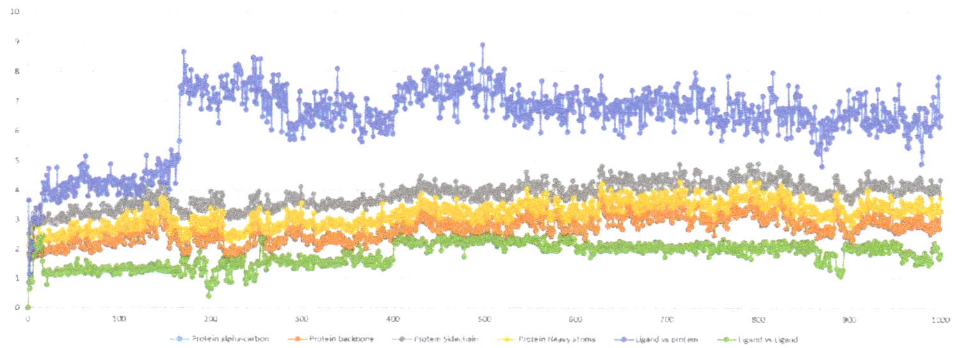

Figure 5. Compound 2C and protein RMSD during MD simulation (100 ns). The x-axis is expressed by the number of snapshots extracted, and 1 snapshot = 100 ps; the y-axis is expressed in Å.

2.5.2. Residue Mobility and Protein–Ligand Contact Analyses

To examine the structural flexibility effect of 2C upon TERT per residue, the main chain average of the root mean square fluctuation (RMSF) of the complex was calculated for the entire 100 ns of simulation. The residue-wise fluctuation of the complexes was plotted and is presented in Figure 6. As reported, the RMSF plot was low for the identified residues involved in the interactions with 2C in the docking analysis.

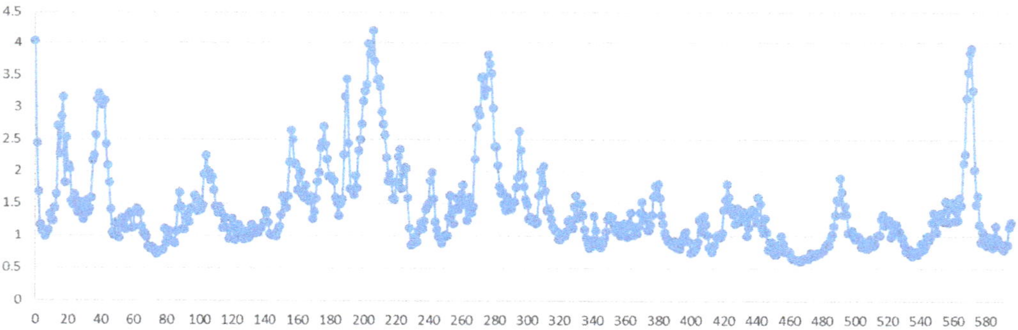

Figure 6. Protein RMSF during MD simulation (100 ns). The x-axis reports the number of the residues of TERT, and the y-axis is expressed in Å.

Evaluation of the protein interactions provides a measure of the interaction power between the ligands and the protein and can be categorized by type and summarized as represented in Figure 7. In Figure 7A, the interactions that occurred for more than 10% of the simulation time are reported. In Figure 7B, a timeline representation of the interactions and contacts (H-bonds, hydrophobic, ionic, and water bridges) summarize the total number of specific contacts the protein makes with the ligand throughout the simulation. The bottom panel of Figure 7B shows which residues interact with the ligand in each trajectory frame. Some residues make more than one specific contact with the ligand, and they are represented by a darker shade of orange, according to the scale to the right of the plot. Protein–ligand contacts are categorized into four types: hydrogen bonds, hydrophobic, ionic, and water bridges. The stacked bar charts are normalized throughout the trajectory: a value of 1.0 suggests that 100% of the simulation time, the specific interaction is maintained.

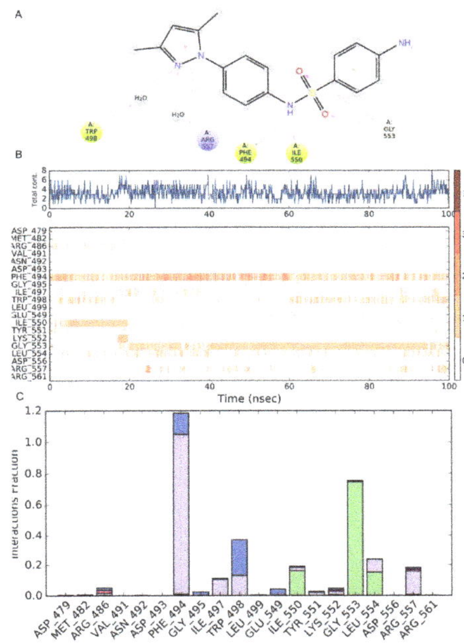

Figure 7. Protein–compound 2C contacts: (**A**) the interactions that occur for more than 10% of the simulation time are reported; (**B**) a timeline representation of the interactions and contacts (H-bonds, hydrophobic, ionic, and water bridges) during the simulation; (**C**) histogram of protein–compound 2C interactions fractions: hydrogen bonds (green), hydrophobic (purple), ionic (red), and water bridges (blue).

The analysis of the trajectory evidenced that the pi-stacking interaction between the aniline ring of 2C and Phe494 occurred at 57%. This output evidences a shifting in the pi-stacking interaction with respect to the docking where the central phenyl ring was involved, but it clearly defines Phe494 as a key residue in the inhibition pattern. As also reported in Figure 7B,C, Phe494 established at least one contact for the entire duration of the simulation and, for a major part of the time, 2–3 contacts with the phenyl ring of 2C. Gly553 showed for 57% and 17% of the time two H-bonds interactions with the oxygen of the sulfonamide group emerging after ~18 ns of simulation. Interestingly, after 22 ns of the simulation a new in pi–cation interaction appeared for 14% of the time between Arg557 and the pyrazole ring, even though it was in a spotted fashion. During the first 20 ns (16% of the total time), the protein–ligand interaction stabilized with an H-bond between Ile550 and the NH of the sulfonamide group. It is interesting evidence of the role of a water molecule as a water bridge between Trp498 and the pyrazole ring. Other residues involved in the protein–ligand interaction but with a minor role were Arg486, Ile497, Trp498, Tyr551, Lys552, and Leu554.

2.5.3. ADME Calculation for Compound 2C

ADME calculation for compound 2C was performed using the SwissADME web tool [74]. In the hexagon drug-likeness graph (Figure 8), each vertex represents a parameter that defines a bioavailable drug. The pink regions represent the optimum range of the following six properties: lipophilicity = 2.53 (XLOGP3 between −0.7 and +5.0), size = 342.42 g/mol (MW between 150 and 500 g/mol), polarity = 98.39 Å^2 (TPSA between 20 and 130 Å^2), solubility (log S not higher than 6), saturation = 0.12 (fraction of carbons in the sp3 hybridization not less than 0.25), and flexibility (no more than nine rotatable bonds). It was found that compound 2C was slightly outside the pink area on one side due to the inconformity of its insaturation. The pharmacokinetics analysis showed that compound 2C is probably not a P-glycoprotein (P-gp) substrate and not BBB permeant. It has potentially good gastrointestinal (GI) absorption and ABS, up to nearly 70%. The %ABS, a very functional physiochemical variable, defines a drug's transport properties. It was calculated according to the equation %ABS = 109 − (0.345 × TPSA) [75,76]. TPSA values below 98.39 Å^2 characterize a significant permeability in the cellular plasma membrane. It has a bioavailability score of 0.55, which means good pharmacokinetic properties according to the Rule of 5 by Lipinski [77].

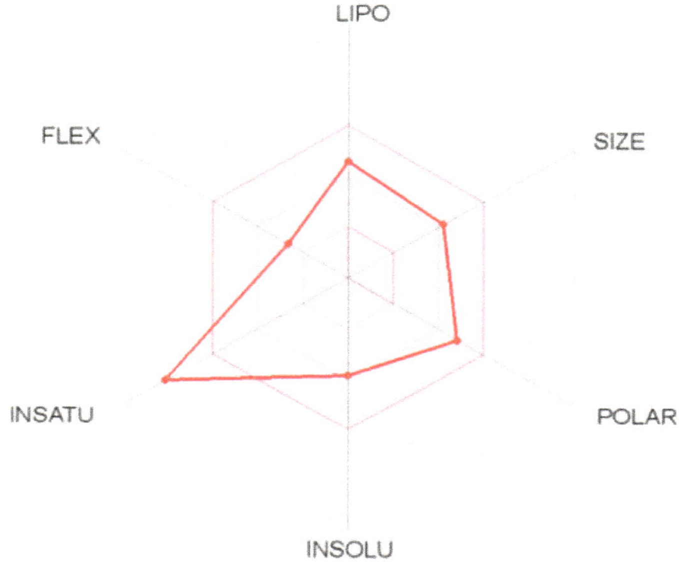

Figure 8. The bioavailability radar (the pink area exhibits the optimal range of a particular property) for compound 2C (LIPO = lipophilicity as in XLOGP3; SIZE = size as in molecular weight; POLAR = polarity as TPSA (topological polar surface area); INSOLU = insolubility in water by log S scale; INSATU = insaturation per fraction of carbons in the sp3 hybridization; FLEX = flexibility per rotatable bonds).

3. Discussion

In the past decade, there has been tangible progress in the definition of the role of telomerase in tumor progression. Several studies evidenced telomerase as a promising target for developing cancer therapeutics. The main reason is due to the overexpression of telomerase in cancer cells (85–90%) compared with normal cells where it is almost unexpressed. Despite the fact that efforts have allowed for the identification of several small molecules, oligonucleotides, natural products, and immunotherapeutics, no telomerase-based cancer drugs have yet been approved by the FDA due to the long lag time between administration of the drug and clinical response. For these reasons, the identification and then the optimization of new small molecules, such as telomerase inhibitors, remain a crucial point that deserves to be further explored. A structure-based drug design approach could be used to design potential inhibitors of the telomerase active site. Exploiting the experimental structure of TERT showing a known inhibitor co-crystallized, we developed a combined structure-based strategy to screen an *in-house* library of 126 arylsulfonamide derivatives. The combined computational strategy was performed using the MYSHAPE approach, first, to identify hit compounds. Successively, docking and calculation of the binding free energy using the MM-GBSA method identified other hits. These approaches guided the selection of the most promising compounds for synthesis and in vitro tests.

As described in Section 2.2., the compounds were initially prepared using classical methodologies. To explore the possibility of avoiding using dangerous and/or dry solvents, a reported green procedure was successfully utilized in the case of derivatives listed in Table 1, affording yields from good to quantitative for a major part of the compounds.

With the aim of identifying the most promising cytotoxic agents, the selected hits, newly synthesized, were evaluated on three cancer lines: human colorectal carcinoma (HCT-116), human breast adenocarcinoma (MCF-7), and human chronic myeloid leukemia (K-562) cell lines, considering the known telomerase inhibitor BIBR1532 as the reference compound. One of the major problems faced during the in vitro test was the poor solubility for some of the tested compounds, which prevented the evaluation of the cytotoxicity and gave results in micro-submillimolar concentrations. In general, the pyrazole derivatives (2A, 2B, and 2C) seems to show a higher activity on the tested cell lines, probably even due to the major solubility

One of the selected hits (2C) revealed an interesting IC_{50} in all three cell lines. In particular, the IC_{50} results were comparable with BIBR1532 for the HCT-116 cell line and the MCF7 cell line, but several times lower in the K-562 cell lines. These findings were confirmed by the evidence of the selective cytotoxicity against the non-cancerous, murine, embryonic, fibroblast cell line BALB/3-T3. The IC_{50} of compound 2C on BALB/3-T3 cells was remarkably higher than those on the tumoral cell lines tested. Another interesting concern regarding the data was the absence of the solubility issue encountered during the in vitro test for the compound 2C in addition to the calculated ADME values that seemed to exclude a binding with the P-gp, an important parameter for the insurgence of resistance issues. In the end, compound 2C showed a good calculated pharmacokinetic profile. Further, the MD simulation of compound 2C at the telomerase active site showed good stability and evidenced Phe494 as the key residue also in BIBR1532. But the more interesting evidence of the simulation regarded that each moiety of compound 2C was involved in key interactions with some residues of the active site: the pyrazole moiety in a cation–pi-stacking interaction with Arg557, the two phenyl rings in the pi-stacking interaction with Phe494, and the sulfonamide moiety in the H-bond interaction with Ile550 and Gly553. Compound 2C as arylsulfonamide derivative is an interesting hit compound that deserves, for the reasons stated above, further investigation in terms of the optimization of its structure to obtain more active telomerase inhibitors.

4. Materials and Methods

4.1. Library and Protein Preparation

The library used for this experimental work comprised a series of 126 sulfonamide derivates. The sulfonamide and BIBR1532 structures were built using the builder panel in Maestro, and ligand preparation was carried out by LigPrep (Schrödinger, LLC, New York, NY, USA, 2021). The force field adopted was OPLS4 [78] and Epik 5.5 (Schrödinger, 2021-1) was selected as an ionization tool at pH 7.2 ± 0.2. Tautomer generation was unflagged, and the maximum number of conformers generated was set at 32. For the purpose of this study, the 2.30 Å resolution crystal structure of *Tribolium castaneum* telomerase in complex with the highly specific inhibitor BIBR1532 (PDB ID: 5CQG) [21] was used. The structure was optimized using the Protein Preparation Wizard in Maestro (Schrödinger, 2021-1) adding bond orders and hydrogen atoms to the crystal structure using the OPLS4 force field. The remaining settings are reported in [79].

4.2. Docking Studies

The library was submitted to a docking study using Glide v9.0 [80] in standard precision (SP) with the OPLS4 force field. The grid box was built considering the BIBR1532 as the centroid of the grid. The study was performed using no constraints. Van der Waals radii were set at 0.8, and the partial cutoff was 0.15 with flexible ligand sampling. Bias sampling torsion penalization for amides with non-planar conformation and Epik state penalties were added to the docking score.

4.3. MYSHAPE Approach

MYSHAPE [51] is an approach in which the pharmacophore model is built using only the common pharmacophore feature patterns that the ligands exhibit during MD simulations. The evaluation of the ligand–protein interaction patterns during the MD simulation was investigated using the data recorded employing the MD simulation (exactly 1001 frames for each simulation). The MYSHAPE model was used to distinguish this type of model from the "default" pharmacophore models that were generated using the crystal structure of the ligand–protein complex. For the newly added pharmacophore features, the tolerance radius was increased by 0.15 Å to compensate for small deviations in the 3D coordinates. The computational details are reported in previously published papers [51,52]

4.4. MM-GBSA Free Energy Calculations

The output of docking was used to calculate the ΔG values of the BIBR1532 and molecules using MM-GBSA (molecular mechanics generalized-born surface area) (Prime, Schrödinger, LLC, New York, NY, USA, 2021). Protein–ligand binding free energy using MM-GBSA was calculated as the difference between the energy of the bound complex and the energy of the unbound protein and ligand. The entropy term $-T\Delta S$ was not calculated to reduce computational time as previously reported [79,81–83]. The VSGB solvation model was chosen using OPLS4 force field with the minimized sampling method.

4.5. Molecular Dynamic Simulations

A 100 ns MD simulation was carried out using a Desmond 6.5 (Desmond Molecular Dynamics System, D. E. Shaw Research, New York, NY, USA, 2021) using the OPLS4 force field for the complex TERT/2C. The complex was solvated in a cubic box using the TIP3P. Ions were added to neutralize charges. The systems were minimized and equilibrated at a temperature of 303.15 K and a pressure of 1.013 bar. The system was simulated as an NPT ensemble; a Nose–Hover thermostat and Martyna–Tobia–Klein barostat were used. The integration time step was chosen to be 2 fs. To keep the hydrogen-heavy atom bonds rigid, the SHAKE algorithm was used. A 9 Å cutoff radius was set for the short-range Coulomb interactions, and smooth particle mesh Ewald was used for the long-range interactions. The detection ranges for energy were 1.2 ps, and 5.0 ps for the trajectory.

4.6. ADME Prediction

Drug-likeness, physicochemical properties, lipophilicity, solubility, and pharmacokinetics properties were analyzed by the SwissADME web tool (http://www.swissadme.ch/index.php (accessed on 30 November 2021)). SwissADME is a new comprehensive tool run by the Swiss Institute of Bioinformatics (SIB) enabling estimation of ADME (absorption, distribution, metabolism, and excretion) parameters of drug candidates. 2D structural models of the compound were drawn in the molecular sketcher into the ChemAxon's Marvin JS window and transferred to the SMILES (simplified molecular-input line-entry system) format to predict suitable properties [74].

4.7. Chemistry

All melting points were taken on a Büchi melting point M-560 apparatus and were uncorrected. IR spectra were recorded in Bromoform with a JASCO FT-IR spectrophotometer. 1H and 13C NMR spectra were measured at 200 and 50.0 MHz, respectively, in DMSO-d_6 solution and TMS as an internal standard, using a Bruker Avance II Series 200 MHz spectrometer or at 300 and 75 MHz (APT) with a Bruker AC-E spectrometer. Column chromatography was performed with Merck silica gel (230–400 mesh ASTM). Elemental analyses (C, H, and N) were within ±0.4% of theoretical values. The substituted benzylamine derivatives were commercially available and were used without further purification. For all the compounds already cited in the literature, the IR and NMR spectra results were identical to those reported (1A–E). The 1H and 13C NMR spectra of new synthesized compounds (1F,G and 2A–C) are reported in the Supplementary Materials.

4.7.1. General Methods for the Preparation of *N*-(R′-Benzyl)-4-R-benzenesulfonamides of Type 1

Method X: To a stirred solution of amino derivative (1.5 mmol) in anhydrous THF (20 mL), an equimolar amount of triethylamine (0.21 mL) and the suitable sulfonylchloride were added. The reaction mixture was stirred for the appropriate time-lapse until the disappearance of the starting amine (TLC monitoring). The ammonium salt was collected and taken up with 20 mL H_2O. The aqueous solution was extracted using DCM. The organic layers were combined with the organic mother liquor, dried over Na_2SO_4, and concentrated under reduced pressure to yield the desired sulfonamide of type 1.

Method Y: The amino derivative (5 mmol) was dissolved in dry pyridine, and the suitable sulfonylchloride (5 mmol) was added. The reaction mixture was stirred for the appropriate time-lapse until the disappearance of starting amine (TLC monitoring). The mixture was poured onto ice/water and the solid precipitate was collected by filtration, air-dried, and recrystallized from ethanol.

N-(4-Chlorobenzyl)-4-methylbenzenesulfonamide (1A)

This compound was prepared according to Method X. The reaction mixture was stirred for 24 h at room temperature. Yield 70%. Mp 98 °C ([84] 107–108 °C; [85] 106.1 °C). 1H NMR ppm: 2.43 (s, 3H, Me), 4.06 (d, J = 6.4 Hz, 2H, CH_2), 5.18 (t, J = 6.0 Hz, 1H, NH), 7.11 (d, J = 8.4 Hz, 2H, Ar-H), 7.20 (d, J = 8.4 Hz, 2H, Ar-H), 7.27 (d, J = 8.0 Hz, 2H, Ar-H), 7.70 (d, J = 8.4 Hz, 2H, Ar-H). 13C NMR ppm: 21.6, 46.6, 127.2, 128.8, 129.3, 129.9, 133.7, 135.1, 136.9, and 143.8.

N-(4-Chlorobenzyl)-4-acetylaminobenzenesulfonamide (1B)

This compound was prepared according to Method X. The reaction mixture was stirred for 24 h at room temperature and under reflux for an additional 4 h. Yield 64%. Mp 152°C [56] 172–174 °C). 1H NMR ppm: 2.10 (s, 3H, Me), 3.08 (bs, 1H, NH), 3.96 (s, 2H, CH_2), 7.30–8.11 (m, 8H, Ar-H), 10.42 (bs, 1H, NH). 13C NMR ppm: 24.1, 45.5, 118.6, 127.6, 128.5, 129.4, 131.6, 134.1, 136.9, 142.5, and 169.0.

N-(4-Chlorobenzyl)-4-nitrobenzenesulfonamide (1C)

This compound was prepared according to Method X. The reaction mixture was stirred under reflux for 4.5 h. Yield 78%. Mp 174–176 °C ([86] 168–170 °C). 1H NMR ppm: 3.80 (d, J = 6.0 Hz, 2H, CH2), 6.61 (d, J = 8.0 Hz, 2H, Ar-H), 6.85 (d, J = 8.0 Hz, 2H, Ar-H), 7.15 (d, J = 8.0 Hz, 2H, Ar-H), 7.45 (d, J = 8.0 Hz, 2H, Ar-H), 7.56 (t, J = 6.0 Hz, 1H, NH). 13C NMR ppm: 45.5, 112.6, 113.5, 125.5, 128.4, 128.9, 129.8, 152.4, and 158.3.

N-(4-Methoxybenzyl)-4-methylbenzenesulfonamide (1D)

This compound was prepared according to Method X. The reaction mixture was stirred for 3 h at room temperature. Yield 71%. Mp 122–123 °C ([87] 114–117 °C; [88] 122–123 °C from EtOAc). 1H NMR (300 MHz, DMSO) ppm: 2.38 (s, 3H, Me), 3.72 (s, 3H, Me), 3.89 (s, 2H, CH_2), 6.85 (d, J = 8.4 Hz, 2H, Ar-H), 7.17 (d, J = 8.4 Hz, 2H, Ar-H), 7.38 (d, J = 8.0 Hz, 2H, Ar-H), 7.71 (d, J = 8.4 Hz, 2H, Ar-H), 8.03 (bs, 1H, NH). 13C NMR ppm: 20.9, 45.8, 55.0, 113.6, 126.5, 128.9, 129.4, 129.5, 137.8, 142.5, and 158.4.

N-(4-Methoxybenzyl)-4-acetylaminobenzenesulfonamide (1E)

This compound was prepared according to Method Y. The reaction mixture was stirred for 1 h at room temperature and under reflux for an additional 2 h. Yield 49%. Mp 192–193 °C ([87] 164–167 °C). 1H NMR ppm: 1.84 (s, 2H, CH_2), 2.12 (s, 3H, Me), 4.46 (sa, 1H, NH), 7.74 (d, J = 8.5 Hz, 2H), 7.79 (d, J = 8.5 Hz, 2H), 9.41 (sa, 1H, NH). 13C NMR ppm: 24.2, 45.6, 55.2, 113.6, 118.6, 127.6, 129.1, 129.5, 134.0, 142.9, 158.5, and 169.4

N-(2,5-Dimethoxybenzyl)-4-methylbenzenesulfonamide (1F)

This compound was prepared according to Method Y. The reaction mixture was stirred for 10 h at room temperature. Yield 80%. Mp 110–111 °C. IR ν: 3268 (NH) cm^{-1}. 1H-NMR ppm: 2.37 (3H, s, Me), 3.65 (6H, s, Me), 3.91 (2H, t, J = 3.9 Hz, CH_2), 6.77–6.83 (3H, m, ArH), 7.10 (2H, d, J = 8.5 Hz), 7.36 (2H, d, J = 7.6 Hz), 7.68 (2H, d, J = 7.6 Hz), 7.89 (1H, t, J = 3.9 Hz, NH). 13C NMR ppm: 21.4, 41.3, 55.8, 56.1, 111.8, 113.0, 115.0, 126.7, 127.0, 130.0, 138.2, 143.0, 150.9, and 153.4.

N-(2,5-Dimethoxybenzyl)-4-nitrobenzenesulfonamide (1G)

This compound was prepared according to Method X. The reaction mixture was stirred for 24 h at room temperature. Yield 97%. Mp 129–132°C. ir ν: 3268 (NH), 1523 and 1348 (NO_2) cm^{-1}. 1H NMR ppm: 3.35 (s, 3H, Me), 3.63 (s, 3H, Me), 4.03 (s, 2H, CH_2), 6.65–6.86 (m, 3H, Ar), 7.96 (2H, d, J = 8.8 Hz), 8.34 (2H, d, J = 8.8 Hz). 13C NMR ppm: 46.0, 55.7, 56.1, 111.8, 113.2, 115.5, 124.7, 125.9, 128.4, 147.0, 149.8, 151.0, and 153.2.

4.7.2. Preparation of 1-(4-Aminophenyl)-3,5-dimethylpyrazole

A solution of acetylacetone (10 mmol) and 4-nitrophenylhydrazine (10 mmol) in acetic acid was heated under reflux for 9 h. The reaction mixture was cooled to room temperature and poured onto ice/water to give a solid precipitate. Purification by column chromatography (eluant DCM/EtOAc 4:1) gave the nitro compound. Yield 80%, mp 100 °C ([89] 102 °C from EtOH). 1-(4-Nitrophenyl)-3,5-dimethylpyrazole (0.56 mg) dissolved in EtOH (20 mL) Pd/C was added, and the mixture was reduced overnight at room temperature in an H2 atmosphere (50 psi) in a Parr apparatus. The catalyst was filtered off, and the solution was evaporated under reduced pressure. The amino derivatives were isolated as white crystals. Yield 100%. Mp 84 °C ([90] 82–84 °C from benzene).

4.7.3. General Method for the Preparation of *N*-[4-(3,5-Dimethyl-1H-pyrazol-1-yl)phenyl]-4- R-benzenesulfonamide of Type 2

To a stirred solution of 1-(4-aminophenyl)-3,5-dimethylpyrazole (1.5 mmol) in anhydrous THF (20 mL), an equimolar amount of triethylamine (0.21 mL) and the suitable sulfonylchloride were added. The reaction mixture was stirred for the appropriate timelapse until the disappearance of the starting amine (TLC monitoring). The ammonium salt was collected and taken up with 20 mL H_2O. The aqueous solution was extracted using DCM. The organic layers were combined with the organic mother liquor, dried over Na_2SO_4, and concentrated under reduced pressure to yield the desired sulfonamide.

N-[4-(3,5-Dimethylpyrazol-1-yl)phenyl]-4-methylbenzenesulfonamide (2A)

The reaction mixture was stirred for 30 h at room temperature. Yield 96%. Mp 167 °C ir ν: 3392 (NH) cm^{-1}. 1H NMR ppm: 2.09 (s, 3H, Me), 2.13 (s, 3H, Me), 2.28 (s, 3H, Me), 6.00 (s, 1H, pyrazole-CH), 7.20 (dd, 4H, ArH), 7.27 (d, 2H, ArH), 7.64 (d, 2H, ArH), 10.41 (s, 1H, NH). 13C NMR ppm: 12.3, 13.4, 21.3, 107.5, 120.7, 125.5, 125.8, 127.2, 128.8, 130.3, 136.7, 134.0, 144.2, and 148.6.

N-[4-(3,5-Dimethylpyrazol-1-yl)phenyl]-4-nitrobenzenesulfonamide (2B)

The reaction mixture was stirred for 3 h at room temperature. The solid residue was recrystallized from ethanol. Yield 57%. Mp 219 °C. ir ν: 3392 (NH), 1532, and 1348 (NO_2) cm^{-1} 1H NMR ppm: 2.12 (s, 3H, Me), 2.21 (s, 3H, Me), 6.02 (s, 1H, pyrazole-CH), 7.27 (dd, 4H, ArH) 8.19 (dd, 4H, ArH), 10.81 (s, 1H, NH). 13C NMR ppm: 12.0, 13.2, 107.0, 120.9, 124.7, 125.0, 128.3 132.2, 135.5, 136.2, 139.0, 147.7, and 149.9.

Preparation of *N*-[4-(3,5-Dimethylpyrazol-1-yl)phenyl]-4-aminobenzenesulfonamide (2C)

To the nitro derivative, 2B dissolved was in EtOH (20 mL), Pd/C was added, and the mixture was reduced overnight at room temperature in an H_2 atmosphere (50 psi) in a Parr apparatus. The catalyst was filtered off, and the solution was evaporated under reduced pressure. The amino derivative was isolated as white crystals. Yield 100%. Mp 106–110 °C. ir ν: 3482 and 3380 (NH_2), 3234 (NH) cm^{-1}. 1H NMR ppm: 1.92 (s, 3H, Me), 2.33 (s, 3H, Me), 6.00 (s, 1H, pyrazole-CH), 7.30–7.35 (m, 4H, Ar-H), 7.42–7.46 (m, 4H, Ar-H), 13C NMR ppm: 12.0, 13.2, 112.6, 119.5, 122.6, 124.8, 125.0, 128.3, 130.3, and 152.9.

4.8. Cell Proliferation Assay

Cell Culturing and MTT Assay

Unless stated otherwise, all reagents were from Merck (Milan, Italy) and of the highest purity grade commercially available. All synthesized compounds were dissolved in dimethyl sulfoxide (DMSO) and then diluted in a culture medium so that the effective DMSO concentration did not exceed 0.1% (*v*/*v*). HCT-116, MCF-7, K-562, and BALB/3-T3 cell lines were purchased from the American Type Culture Collection, Rockville, MD, USA. Except for BALB/3-T3 cells, which were grown in DMEM, all other cells were cultured in the RPMI-1640 medium. Both DMEM and RPMI-1640 were supplemented with L-glutamine (2 mM), 10% fetal bovine serum (FBS), penicillin (100 U/mL), streptomycin (100 μg/mL), and gentamicin (5 μg/mL). Cells were maintained in the log phase by seeding them twice a week at a density of 3×10^5 cells/mL, in humidified 5% CO_2 atmosphere at 37 °C.

The cytotoxic activity of the synthesized compounds against all the cell lines employed was determined by the MTT colorimetric assay as previously reported [91]. The assay is based on the reduction of 3-(4,5-dimethyl-2-thiazolyl)bromide-2,5-diphenyl-2-*H*-tetrazolium to purple formazan by the mitochondrial dehydrogenases of living cells. Briefly, cells at the passage that did not exceed the number 20, were seeded into 96-well plates (Corning, New York, NY, USA) at a density of 2.0×10^4 cells/cm^2, incubated overnight, and then treated with either the compounds or the vehicle (control) for 24 h. Afterward, the medium was carefully removed, and 200 μL of 5 mg/mL MTT was added. The supernatant was discarded after a 2 h of incubation at 37 °C, and the formazan blue formed dissolved in DMSO. The absorbance at 565 nm of the formazan product was measured using a microplate reader (LTek, INNO, Seongnam, South Korea), and the value of control cells was taken as 100% of viability. Each experiment was repeated three times in triplicate to obtain the mean values. No differences were found between cells treated with DMSO 0.1% and untreated cells in terms of cell number and viability.

The growth inhibition activity of the tested compounds was defined as the IC_{50} value that represents the concentration of the compound that inhibits 50% of cell viability. IC_{50} values were calculated using the dose–response inhibition model in Prism 8 (GraphPad Software, San Diego, CA, USA). The SI, a measure of the therapeutic potential of the tested compound, was calculated by dividing the IC_{50} for normal BALB/3-T3 cells by the IC_{50} for HCT-116, MCF-7, and K-562 cancer cells.

Two hundred milliliters (6.0×104 cells/cm^2) of a K-562 cell suspension were plated in each well of a 96-well plate and treated with different concentrations of compounds. An equal volume of DMSO was added to the control well, and the cells were cultured for an additional 24 h; then, 20 μL MTT (5 mg/mL) in the growth medium was added per well, and the plates were incubated at 37 °C for 4 h as reported in [91] with some modifications. Plates were then centrifuged at 400× *g* for 10 min. Supernatants were removed from the wells, and the reduced MTT dye in each well was solubilized in 200 μL DMSO. Absorbance was measured in a microplate reader (LTek, INNO, Seongnam, Korea), and the value of the control cells was taken as 100% of viability.

Supplementary Materials: The following supporting information can be downloaded at: https://www.mdpi.com/article/10.3390/ph15010082/s1, 1H and 13C NMR spectra of new derivatives synthetized and tested in this work.

Author Contributions: Conceptualization, M.T.; methodology, M.T., G.C. and M.A.; software, G.C. and M.T.; synthesis G.C. and A.M.A.; biological evaluation M.A. and I.R.; data curation, M.T. and

M.A.; writing—original draft preparation, M.T.; writing—review and editing, M.T., M.A. and A.M.A. All authors have read and agreed to the published version of the manuscript.

Funding: This research received no external funding.

Institutional Review Board Statement: Not applicable.

Informed Consent Statement: Not applicable.

Data Availability Statement: The data presented in this study are available in article and Supplementary Material.

Conflicts of Interest: The authors declare no conflict of interest.

References

1. Cong, Y.-S.; Wright, W.E.; Shay, J.W. Human Telomerase and Its Regulation. *Microbiol. Mol. Biol. Rev.* **2002**, *66*, 407–425. [CrossRef]
2. Wojtyla, A.; Gladych, M.; Rubis, B. Human telomerase activity regulation. *Mol. Biol. Rep.* **2011**, *38*, 3339–3349. [CrossRef]
3. Wang, F.; Podell, E.R.; Zaug, A.J.; Yang, Y.; Baciu, P.; Cech, T.R.; Lei, M. The POT1-TPP1 telomere complex is a telomerase processivity factor. *Nature* **2007**, *445*, 506–510. [CrossRef]
4. Masutomi, K.; Yu, E.Y.; Khurts, S.; Ben-Porath, I.; Currier, J.L.; Metz, G.B.; Brooks, M.W.; Kaneko, S.; Murakami, S.; DeCaprio, J.A.; et al. Telomerase maintains telomere structure in normal human cells. *Cell* **2003**, *114*, 241–253. [CrossRef]
5. Shay, J.W.; Wright, W.E. Role of telomeres and telomerase in cancer. *Semin. Cancer Biol.* **2011**, *21*, 349–353. [CrossRef] [PubMed]
6. Blackburn, E.H. Telomere states and cell fates. *Nature* **2000**, *408*, 53–56. [CrossRef] [PubMed]
7. Ramlee, M.K.; Wang, J.; Toh, W.X.; Li, S. Transcription regulation of the human telomerase reverse transcriptase (hTERT) gene. *Genes* **2016**, *7*, 50. [CrossRef] [PubMed]
8. Hanahan, D.; Weinberg, R.A. Hallmarks of cancer: The next generation. *Cell* **2011**, *144*, 646–674. [CrossRef] [PubMed]
9. Ruden, M.; Puri, N. Novel anticancer therapeutics targeting telomerase. *Cancer Treat. Rev.* **2013**, *39*, 444–456. [CrossRef]
10. Arndt, G.M.; MacKenzie, K. New prospects for targeting telomerase beyond the telomere. *Nat. Rev. Cancer* **2016**, *16*, 508–524. [CrossRef]
11. Jäger, K.; Walter, M. Therapeutic Targeting of Telomerase. *Genes* **2016**, *7*, 39. [CrossRef]
12. Neidle, S. Human telomeric G-quadruplex: The current status of telomeric G-quadruplexes as therapeutic targets in human cancer. *FEBS J.* **2009**, *277*, 1118–1125. [CrossRef]
13. Islam, M.K.; Jackson, P.J.; Rahman, K.M.; Thurston, D.E. Recent advances in targeting the telomeric G-quadruplex DNA sequence with small molecules as a strategy for anticancer therapies. *Futur. Med. Chem.* **2016**, *8*, 1259–1290. [CrossRef] [PubMed]
14. Rahman, K.M.; Tizkova, K.; Reszka, A.P.; Neidle, S.; Thurston, D.E. Identification of novel telomeric G-quadruplex-targeting chemical scaffolds through screening of three NCI libraries. *Bioorg. Med. Chem. Lett.* **2012**, *22*, 3006–3010. [CrossRef] [PubMed]
15. Lauria, A.; Terenzi, A.; Bartolotta, R.; Bonsignore, R.; Perricone, U.; Tutone, M.; Martorana, A.; Barone, G.; Almerico, A.M. Does ligand symmetry play a role in the stabilization of DNA g-quadruplex host-guest complexes? *Curr. Med. Chem.* **2014**, *21*, 2665–2690. [CrossRef] [PubMed]
16. Barata, P.; Sood, A.K.; Hong, D.S. RNA-targeted therapeutics in cancer clinical trials: Current status and future directions. *Cancer Treat. Rev.* **2016**, *50*, 35–47. [CrossRef]
17. Asai, A.; Oshima, Y.; Yamamoto, Y.; Uochi, T.; Kusaka, H.; Akinaga, S.; Yamashita, Y.; Pongracz, K.; Pruzan, R.; Wunder, E.; et al. A novel telomerase template antagonist (GRN163) as a potential anticancer agent. *Cancer Res.* **2003**, *63*, 3931–3939.
18. Damm, K.; Hemmann, U.; Garin-Chesa, P.; Hauel, N.; Kauffmann, I.; Priepke, H.; Niestroj, C.; Daiber, C.; Enenkel, B.; Guilliard, B.; et al. A highly selective telomerase inhibitor limiting human cancer cell proliferation. *EMBO J.* **2001**, *20*, 6958–6968. [CrossRef] [PubMed]
19. Man, R.-J.; Chen, L.-W.; Zhu, H.-L. Telomerase inhibitors: A patent review (2010–2015). *Expert Opin. Ther. Patents* **2016**, *26*, 679–688. [CrossRef] [PubMed]
20. Baginski, M.; Serbakowska, K. In silico design of telomerase inhibitors. *Drug Discov. Today* **2020**, *25*, 1213–1222. [CrossRef]
21. Bryan, C.; Rice, C.; Hoffman, H.; Harkisheimer, M.; Sweeney, M.; Skordalakes, E. Structural Basis of Telomerase Inhibition by the Highly Specific BIBR1532. *Structure* **2015**, *23*, 1934–1942. [CrossRef]
22. Alam, M.S.; Lee, D.-U. Synthesis, biological evaluation, drug-likeness, and in silico screening of novel benzylidene-hydrazone analogues as small molecule anticancer agents. *Arch. Pharmacal Res.* **2015**, *39*, 191–201. [CrossRef] [PubMed]
23. Cai, Z.-Y.; Yang, Y.; Liu, X.-H.; Qi, X.-B. Novel 3-(1-acetyl-5-(substituted-phenyl)-4,5-dihydro-1H-pyrazol-3-yl)-7-fluoro-2H-chromen-2-one Derivatives: Synthesis and Anticancer Activity. *Lett. Drug Des. Discov.* **2010**, *7*, 640–643. [CrossRef]
24. Liu, X.-H.; Li, J.; Shi, J.B.; Song, B.-A.; Qi, X.-B. Design and synthesis of novel 5-phenyl-N-piperidine ethanone containing 4,5-dihydropyrazole derivatives as potential antitumor agents. *Eur. J. Med. Chem.* **2012**, *51*, 294–299. [CrossRef] [PubMed]
25. Liu, X.-H.; Liu, H.-F.; Chen, J.; Yang, Y.; Song, B.-A.; Bai, L.-S.; Liu, J.-X.; Zhu, H.-L.; Qi, X.-B. Synthesis and molecular docking study of novel coumarin derivatives containing 4,5-dihydropyrazole moiety as potential antitumor agents. *Bioorg. Med. Chem. Lett.* **2010**, *20*, 5705–5708. [CrossRef] [PubMed]

26. Luo, Y.; Zhang, S.; Qiu, K.-M.; Liu, Z.-J.; Yang, Y.-S.; Fu, J.; Zhong, W.-Q.; Zhu, H.-L. Synthesis, biological evaluation, 3D-QSAR studies of novel aryl-2H-pyrazole derivatives as telomerase inhibitors. *Bioorg. Med. Chem. Lett.* **2013**, *23*, 1091–1095. [CrossRef] [PubMed]
27. Luo, Y.; Zhou, Y.; Fu, J.; Zhu, H.-L. 4,5-Dihydropyrazole derivatives containing oxygen-bearing heterocycles as potential telomerase inhibitors with anticancer activity. *RSC Adv.* **2014**, *4*, 23904–23913. [CrossRef]
28. Chen, Y.Y.; Wu, X.Q.; Tang, W.J.; Shi, J.B.; Li, J.; Liu, X.H. Novel dihydropyrazole-chromen: Design and modulates hTERT inhibition proliferation of MGC-803. *Eur. J. Med. Chem.* **2016**, *110*, 65–75. [CrossRef]
29. Xiao, X.; Ni, Y.; Jia, Y.-M.; Zheng, M.; Xu, H.-F.; Xu, J.; Liao, C. Identification of human telomerase inhibitors having the core of N -acyl-4,5-dihydropyrazole with anticancer effects. *Bioorg. Med. Chem. Lett.* **2016**, *26*, 1508–1511. [CrossRef] [PubMed]
30. Kalathiya, U.; Padariya, M.; Baginski, M. Molecular Modeling and Evaluation of Novel Dibenzopyrrole Derivatives as Telomerase Inhibitors and Potential Drug for Cancer Therapy. *IEEE/ACM Trans. Comput. Biol. Bioinform.* **2014**, *11*, 1196–1207. [CrossRef] [PubMed]
31. Liu, X.-H.; Liu, H.-F.; Shen, X.; Song, B.-A.; Bhadury, P.S.; Zhu, H.-L.; Liu, J.-X.; Qi, X.-B. Synthesis and molecular docking studies of novel 2-chloro-pyridine derivatives containing flavone moieties as potential antitumor agents. *Bioorg. Med. Chem. Lett.* **2010**, *20*, 4163–4167. [CrossRef] [PubMed]
32. Zheng, Q.-Z.; Zhang, X.-M.; Xu, Y.; Cheng, K.; Jiao, Q.-C.; Zhu, H.-L. Synthesis, biological evaluation, and molecular docking studies of 2-chloropyridine derivatives possessing 1,3,4-oxadiazole moiety as potential antitumor agents. *Bioorg. Med. Chem.* **2010**, *18*, 7836–7841. [CrossRef] [PubMed]
33. Zhang, X.M.; Qiu, M.; Sun, J.; Zhang, Y.B.; Yang, Y.S.; Wang, X.L.; Tang, J.F.; Zhu, H.L. Synthesis, biological evaluation, and molecular docking studies of 1,3,4-oxadiazole derivatives possessing 1,4-benzodioxan moiety as potential anticancer agents. *Bioorg. Med. Chem.* **2011**, *19*, 6518–6524. [CrossRef]
34. Zhang, F.; Wang, X.-L.; Shi, J.; Wang, S.-F.; Yin, Y.; Yang, Y.-S.; Zhang, W.-M.; Zhu, H.-L. Synthesis, molecular modeling, and biological evaluation of N-benzylidene-2-((5-(pyridin-4-yl)-1,3,4-oxadiazol-2-yl)thio)acetohydrazide derivatives as potential anticancer agents. *Bioorg. Med. Chem.* **2014**, *22*, 468–477. [CrossRef] [PubMed]
35. Sun, J.; Zhu, H.; Yang, Z.M.; Zhu, H.L. Synthesis, molecular modeling and biological evaluation of 2-aminomethyl-5-(quinolin-2-yl)-1,3,4-oxadiazole-2(3H)-thione quinolone derivatives as novel anticancer agent. *Eur. J. Med. Chem.* **2013**, *60*, 23–28. [CrossRef] [PubMed]
36. Tutone, M.; Pecoraro, B.; Almerico, A.M. Investigation on Quantitative Structure-Activity Relationships of 1,3,4-Oxadiazole Derivatives as Potential Telomerase Inhibitors. *Curr. Drug Discov. Technol.* **2020**, *17*, 79–86. [CrossRef]
37. Shi, J.B.; Tang, W.J.; Qi, X.B.; Li, R.; Liu, X.H. Novel pyrazole-5-carboxamide and pyrazole-pyrimidine derivatives: Synthesis and anticancer activity. *Eur. J. Med. Chem.* **2015**, *90*, 889–896. [CrossRef] [PubMed]
38. Tang, W.J.; Wang, J.; Tong, X.; Shi, J.B.; Liu, X.H.; Li, J. Design and synthesis of celastrol derivatives as anticancer agents. *Eur. J. Med. Chem.* **2015**, *95*, 166–173. [CrossRef] [PubMed]
39. Xue, W.; Song, B.A.; Zhao, H.J.; Qi, X.B.; Huang, Y.J.; Liu, X.H. Novel myricetin derivatives: Design, synthesis and anticancer activity. *Eur. J. Med. Chem.* **2015**, *97*, 155–163. [CrossRef]
40. Hernandez-Sanchez, W.; Huang, W.; Plucinsky, B.; Garcia-Vazquez, N.; Robinson, N.J.; Schiemann, W.P.; Berdis, A.J.; Skordalakes, E.; Taylor, D.J. A non-natural nucleotide uses a specific pocket to selectively inhibit telomerase activity. *PLoS Biol.* **2019**, *17*, e3000204. [CrossRef]
41. Fan, Z.F.; Ho, S.T.; Wen, R.; Fu, Y.; Zhang, L.; Wang, J.; Hu, C.; Shaw, P.C.; Liu, Y.; Cheng, M.S. Design, synthesis and molecular docking analysis of flavonoid derivatives as potential telomerase inhibitors. *Molecules* **2019**, *24*, 3180. [CrossRef]
42. Betori, R.C.; Liu, Y.; Mishra, R.K.; Cohen, S.B.; Kron, S.J.; Scheidt, K.A. Targeted Covalent Inhibition of Telomerase. *ACS Chem. Biol.* **2020**, *15*, 706–717. [CrossRef]
43. Saraswati, A.P.; Relitti, N.; Brindisi, M.; Gemma, S.; Zisterer, D.; Butini, S.; Campiani, G. Raising the bar in anticancer therapy: Recent advances in, and perspectives on, telomerase inhibitors. *Drug Discov. Today* **2019**, *24*, 1370–1388. [CrossRef]
44. Chen, X.; Tang, W.-J.; Shi, J.B.; Liu, M.M.; Liu, X.-H. Therapeutic strategies for targeting telomerase in cancer. *Med. Res. Rev.* **2020**, *40*, 532–585. [CrossRef]
45. Wong, L.H.; Unciti-Broceta, A.; Spitzer, M.; White, R.; Tyers, M.; Harrington, L. A Yeast Chemical Genetic Screen Identifies Inhibitors of Human Telomerase. *Chem. Biol.* **2013**, *20*, 333–340. [CrossRef] [PubMed]
46. Pibiri, I.; Lentini, L.; Melfi, R.; Tutone, M.; Baldassano, S.; Ricco Galluzzo, P.; Di Leonardo, A.; Pace, A. Rescuing the CFTR protein function: Introducing 1,3,4-oxadiazoles as translational readthrough inducing drugs. *Eur. J. Med. Chem.* **2018**, *159*, 126–142. [CrossRef] [PubMed]
47. Almerico, A.M.; Tutone, M.; Lauria, A. Docking and multivariate methods to explore HIV-1 drug-resistance: A comparative analysis. *J. Comput.-Aided Mol. Des.* **2008**, *22*, 287–297. [CrossRef]
48. Tutone, M.; Pibiri, I.; Lentini, L.; Pace, A.; Almerico, A.M. Deciphering the Nonsense Readthrough Mechanism of Action of Ataluren: An *in Silico* Compared Study. *ACS Med. Chem. Lett.* **2019**, *10*, 522–527. [CrossRef] [PubMed]
49. Tutone, M.; Virzì, A.; Almerico, A.M. Reverse screening on indicaxanthin from Opuntia ficus-indica as natural chemoactive and chemopreventive agent. *J. Theor. Biol.* **2018**, *455*, 147–160. [CrossRef]

50. Tutone, M.; Pibiri, I.; Perriera, R.; Campofelice, A.; Culletta, G.; Melfi, R.; Pace, A.; Almerico, A.M.; Lentini, L. Pharmacophore-Based Design of New Chemical Scaffolds as Translational Readthrough-Inducing Drugs (TRIDs). *ACS Med. Chem. Lett.* **2020**, *11*, 747–753. [CrossRef] [PubMed]
51. Perricone, U.; Wieder, M.; Seidel, T.; Langer, T.; Padova, A.; Almerico, A.M.; Tutone, M. A Molecular Dynamics–Shared Pharmacophore Approach to Boost Early-Enrichment Virtual Screening: A Case Study on Peroxisome Proliferator-Activated Receptor α. *ChemMedChem* **2017**, *12*, 1399–1407. [CrossRef] [PubMed]
52. Culletta, G.; Almerico, A.M.; Tutone, M. Comparing molecular dynamics-derived pharmacophore models with docking: A study on CDK-2 inhibitors. *Chem. Data Collect.* **2020**, *28*, 100485. [CrossRef]
53. Halgren, T.A.; Murphy, R.B.; Friesner, R.A.; Beard, H.S.; Frye, L.L.; Pollard, W.T.; Banks, J.L. Glide: A New Approach for Rapid, Accurate Docking and Scoring. 2. Enrichment Factors in Database Screening. *J. Med. Chem.* **2004**, *47*, 1750–1759. [CrossRef]
54. Doobary, S.; Sedikides, A.T.; Caldora, H.P.; Poole, D.L.; Lennox, A.J.J. Electrochemical Vicinal Difluorination of Alkenes: Scalable and Amenable to Electron-Rich Substrates. *Angew. Chem. Int. Ed.* **2019**, *59*, 1155–1160. [CrossRef]
55. Yang, Y.; Meng, X.; Zhu, B.; Jia, Y.; Cao, X.; Huang, S. A Micellar Catalysis Strategy for Amidation of Alkynyl Bromides: Synthesis of Ynamides in Water. *Eur. J. Org. Chem.* **2019**, *2019*, 1166–1169. [CrossRef]
56. Ge, S.; Zhong, H.; Ma, X.; Zheng, Y.; Zou, Y.; Wang, F.; Wang, Y.; Hu, Y.; Li, Y.; Liu, W.; et al. Discovery of secondary sulphonamides as IDO1 inhibitors with potent antitumour effects in vivo. *J. Enzyme Inhib. Med. Chem.* **2020**, *35*, 1240–1257. [CrossRef]
57. Peng, H.; Ma, J.; Luo, W.; Zhang, G.; Yin, B. Methyl-triflate-mediated dearylmethylation of N -(arylmethyl)carboxamides via the retro-Mannich reaction induced by electrophilic dearomatization/rearomatization in an aqueous medium at room temperature. *Green Chem.* **2019**, *21*, 2252–2256. [CrossRef]
58. Li, M.B.; Tang, X.L.; Tian, S.K. Cross-coupling of Grignard reagents with sulfonyl-activated sp3 carbon-nitrogen bonds. *Adv. Synth. Catal.* **2011**, *353*, 1980–1984. [CrossRef]
59. Kiruthika, S.E.; Nandakumar, A.; Perumal, P.T. Synthesis of pyrrolo-/indolo[1,2-a]quinolines and naphtho[2,1- b]thiophenes from gem -dibromovinyls and sulphonamides. *Org. Lett.* **2014**, *16*, 4424–4427. [CrossRef] [PubMed]
60. Baraldi, P.G.; Moorman, A.R.; Borea, P.A. Novel Adenosine A3 Receptor Agonists. U.S. Patent 20090233878A1, 17 September 2009.
61. Nardi, M.; Cano, N.H.; Costanzo, P.; Oliverio, M.; Sindona, G.; Procopio, A. Aqueous MW eco-friendly protocol for amino group protection. *RSC Adv.* **2015**, *5*, 18751–18760. [CrossRef]
62. Huang, M.; Li, Y.; Liu, J.; Lan, X.B.; Liu, Y.; Zhao, C.; Ke, Z. A bifunctional strategy for N-heterocyclic carbene-stabilized iridium complex-catalyzed: N -alkylation of amines with alcohols in aqueous media. *Green Chem.* **2019**, *21*, 219–224. [CrossRef]
63. Li, Q.Q.; Xiao, Z.F.; Yao, C.Z.; Zheng, H.X.; Kang, Y.B. Direct Alkylation of Amines with Alcohols Catalyzed by Base. *Org. Lett.* **2015**, *17*, 5328–5331. [CrossRef] [PubMed]
64. Zhang, C.; Chen, Y.; Yuan, G. Electrosynthesis of Arylsulfonamides from Amines and Sodium Sulfinates Using H2O-NaI as the Electrolyte Solution at Room Temperature. *Chin. J. Chem.* **2016**, *34*, 1277–1282. [CrossRef]
65. Wang, H.; Wei, W.; Zhu, H.; Cui, H.; Wang, L. A Kind of Ethod of Sulfamide Compound. China Patent CN107033106A, 11 August 2017.
66. Vicente, D.A.; Galdino, D.; Navarro, M.; Menezes, P.H. Electrochemical synthesis of sulfonamides in a graphite powder macroelectrode. *Green Chem.* **2020**, *22*, 5262–5266. [CrossRef]
67. Deng, X.; Mani, N.S. A facile, environmentally benign sulfonamide synthesis in water. *Green Chem.* **2006**, *8*, 835–838. [CrossRef]
68. Massah, A.; Kazemi, F.; Azadi, D.; Farzaneh, S.; Aliyan, H.; Naghash, H.; Momeni, A. A Mild and Chemoselective Solvent-Free Method for the Synthesis of N-Aryl and N-Alkylsulfonamides. *Lett. Org. Chem.* **2006**, *3*, 235–241. [CrossRef]
69. Myung, K.; Ghosh, G.; Fattah, F.J.; Li, G.; Kim, H.; Dutia, A.; Pak, E.; Smith, S.; Hendrickson, E.A. Regulation of Telomere Length and Suppression of Genomic Instability in Human Somatic Cells by Ku86. *Mol. Cell. Biol.* **2004**, *24*, 5050–5059. [CrossRef]
70. Raymond, E.; Sun, D.; Izbicka, E.; Mangold, G.; Silvas, E.; Windle, B.; Sharma, S.; Soda, H.; Laurence, R.; Davidson, K.; et al. A human breast cancer model for the study of telomerase inhibitors based on a new biotinylated-primer extension assay. *Br. J. Cancer* **1999**, *80*, 1332–1341. [CrossRef]
71. Akiyama, M.; Yamada, O.; Kanda, N.; Akita, S.; Kawano, T.; Ohno, T.; Mizoguchi, H.; Eto, Y.; Anderson, K.C.; Yamada, H Telomerase overexpression in K562 leukemia cells protects against apoptosis by serum deprivation and double-stranded DNA break inducing agents, but not against DNA synthesis inhibitors. *Cancer Lett.* **2002**, *178*, 187–197. [CrossRef]
72. Badisa, R.B.; Darling-Reed, S.F.; Joseph, P.; Cooperwood, J.S.; Latinwo, L.M.; Goodman, C.B. Selective cytotoxic activities of two novel synthetic drugs on human breast carcinoma MCF-7 cells. *Anticancer Res.* **2009**, *29*, 2993–2996.
73. Le, M.-T.; Mai, T.T.; Huynh, P.N.H.; Tran, T.-D.; Thai, K.-M.; Nguyen, Q.-T. Structure-based discovery of interleukin-33 inhibitors: A pharmacophore modelling, molecular docking, and molecular dynamics simulation approach. *SAR QSAR Environ. Res.* **2020**, *31*, 883–904. [CrossRef]
74. Daina, A.; Michielin, O.; Zoete, V. SwissADME: A free web tool to evaluate pharmacokinetics, drug-likeness and medicinal chemistry friendliness of small molecules. *Sci. Rep.* **2017**, *7*, 42717. [CrossRef]
75. Azam, F.; Madi, A.M.; Ali, H.I. Molecular Docking and Prediction of Pharmacokinetic Properties of Dual Mechanism Drugs that Block MAO-B and Adenosine A2A Receptors for the Treatment of Parkinson's Disease. *J. Young Pharm.* **2012**, *4*, 184–192 [CrossRef] [PubMed]
76. Zhao, Y.H.; Abraham, M.H.; Le, J.; Hersey, A.; Luscombe, C.N.; Beck, G.; Sherborne, B.; Cooper, I. Rate-limited steps of human oral absorption and QSAR studies. *Pharm. Res.* **2002**, *19*, 1446–1457. [CrossRef]

77. Lipinski, C.A.; Lombardo, F.; Dominy, B.W.; Feeney, P.J. Experimental and computational approaches to estimate solubility and permeability in drug discovery and development settings. *Adv. Drug Deliv. Rev.* **1997**, *23*, 3–25. [CrossRef]
78. Lu, C.; Wu, C.; Ghoreishi, D.; Chen, W.; Wang, L.; Damm, W.; Ross, G.A.; Dahlgren, M.K.; Russell, E.; Von Bargen, C.D.; et al. OPLS4: Improving force field accuracy on challenging regimes of chemical space. *J. Chem. Theory Comput.* **2021**, *17*, 4291–4300. [CrossRef]
79. Allegra, M.; Tutone, M.; Tesoriere, L.; Attanzio, A.; Culletta, G.; Almerico, A.M. Evaluation of the IKKβ Binding of Indicaxanthin by Induced-Fit Docking, Binding Pose Metadynamics, and Molecular Dynamics. *Front. Pharmacol.* **2021**, *12*. [CrossRef] [PubMed]
80. Friesner, R.A.; Murphy, R.B.; Repasky, M.P.; Frye, L.L.; Greenwood, J.R.; Halgren, T.A.; Sanschagrin, P.C.; Mainz, D.T. Extra precision glide: Docking and scoring incorporating a model of hydrophobic enclosure for protein-ligand complexes. *J. Med. Chem.* **2006**, *49*, 6177–6196. [CrossRef] [PubMed]
81. Hou, T.; Yu, R. Molecular dynamics and free energy studies on the wild-type and double mutant HIV-1 protease complexed with amprenavir and two amprenavir-related inhibitors: Mechanism for binding and drug resistance. *J. Med. Chem.* **2007**, *50*, 1177–1188. [CrossRef] [PubMed]
82. Massova, I.; Kollman, P.A. Combined molecular mechanical and continuum solvent approach (MM-PBSA/GBSA) to predict ligand binding. *Perspect. Drug Discov. Des.* **2000**, *18*, 113–135. [CrossRef]
83. Culletta, G.; Gulotta, M.R.; Perricone, U.; Zappalà, M.; Almerico, A.M.; Tutone, M. Exploring the SARS-CoV-2 Proteome in the Search of Potential Inhibitors via Structure-Based Pharmacophore Modeling/Docking Approach. *Computation* **2020**, *8*, 77. [CrossRef]
84. Jiang, Y.; Wang, Q.Q.; Liang, S.; Hu, L.-M.; Little, R.D.; Zeng, C.-C. Electrochemical Oxidative Amination of Sodium Sulfinates: Synthesis of Sulfonamides Mediated by NH4I as a Redox Catalyst. *J. Org. Chem.* **2016**, *81*, 4713–4719. [CrossRef] [PubMed]
85. Shi, F.; Kin Tse, M.; Zhou, S.; Pohl, M.-M.; Radnik, J.; Hübner, S.; Jähnisch, K.; Brückner, A.; Beller, M. Green and Efficient Synthesis of Sulfonamides Catalyzed by Nano-Ru/Fe3O4. *J. Am. Chem. Soc.* **2009**, *131*, 1775–1779. [CrossRef] [PubMed]
86. Lai, Y.; Ge, S.; Zheng, Y.; Zou, Y.; Wang, F.; Xu, Q.; Guo, W.; Wang, Y.; Hu, Y. Benzene sulfonamide IDO1 inhibitor, its preparation method and application. China Patent CN106928101A, 7 July 2017.
87. Molander, G.A.; Fleury-Brégeot, N.; Hiebel, M.-A. Synthesis and Cross-Coupling of Sulfonamidomethyltrifluoroborates. *Org. Lett.* **2011**, *13*, 1694–1697. [CrossRef] [PubMed]
88. Martínez-Asencio, A.; Ramón, D.J.; Yus, M. N-Alkylation of poor nucleophilic amines and derivatives with alcohols by a hydrogen autotransfer process catalyzed by copper(II) acetate: Scope and mechanistic considerations. *Tetrahedron* **2011**, *67*, 3140–3149. [CrossRef]
89. Burness, D.M. β-Keto Acetals. I. Synthesis of Pyrazoles and Pyrimidines and the Steric Inhibition of Resonance in 5-Alkyl-1-p-nitrophenylpyrazoles. *J. Org. Chem.* **1956**, *21*, 97–101. [CrossRef]
90. Bouchet, P. *Bulletin de la Societe Chimique de France*; Société chimique de France: Paris, France, 1976; Volume 5–6, pp. 839–844.
91. Allegra, M.; De Cicco, P.; Ercolano, G.; Attanzio, A.; Busà, R.; Cirino, G.; Tesoriere, L.; Livrea, M.A.; Ianaro, A. Indicaxanthin from Opuntia Ficus Indica (L. Mill) impairs melanoma cell proliferation, invasiveness, and tumor progression. *Phytomedicine* **2018**, *50*, 19–24. [CrossRef]

pharmaceuticals

Article

A Review on Parallel Virtual Screening Softwares for High-Performance Computers

Natarajan Arul Murugan [1,*,†], Artur Podobas [1], Davide Gadioli [2], Emanuele Vitali [2], Gianluca Palermo [2] and Stefano Markidis [1,*]

1 Department of Computer Science, School of Electrical Engineering and Computer Science, KTH Royal Institute of Technology, SE-10044 Stockholm, Sweden; podobas@kth.se
2 Dipartimento di Elettronica, Infomazione e Bioingegneria, Politecnico di Milano, 20133 Milano, Italy; davide.gadioli@polimi.it (D.G.); emanuele.vitali@polimi.it (E.V.); gianluca.palermo@polimi.it (G.P.)
* Correspondence: arul.murugan@iiitd.ac.in or murugan@kth.se (N.A.M.); markidis@kth.se (S.M.)
† Present address: Department of Computational Biology, Indraprastha Institute of Information Technology (IIIT-Delhi), New Delhi 110020, India.

Abstract: Drug discovery is the most expensive, time-demanding, and challenging project in biopharmaceutical companies which aims at the identification and optimization of lead compounds from large-sized chemical libraries. The lead compounds should have high-affinity binding and specificity for a target associated with a disease, and, in addition, they should have favorable pharmacodynamic and pharmacokinetic properties (grouped as ADMET properties). Overall, drug discovery is a multivariable optimization and can be carried out in supercomputers using a reliable scoring function which is a measure of binding affinity or inhibition potential of the drug-like compound. The major problem is that the number of compounds in the chemical spaces is huge, making the computational drug discovery very demanding. However, it is cheaper and less time-consuming when compared to experimental high-throughput screening. As the problem is to find the most stable (global) minima for numerous protein–ligand complexes (on the order of 10^6 to 10^{12}), the parallel implementation of in silico virtual screening can be exploited to ensure drug discovery in affordable time. In this review, we discuss such implementations of parallelization algorithms in virtual screening programs. The nature of different scoring functions and search algorithms are discussed, together with a performance analysis of several docking softwares ported on high-performance computing architectures.

Keywords: computational drug discovery; virtual screening; molecular docking; chemical space; parallelization; high-performance computers and accelerators

Citation: Murugan, N.A.; Podobas, A.; Vitali, E.; Gadioli, D.; Palermo, G.; Markidis, S. A Review on Parallel Virtual Screening Softwares for High-Performance Computers. *Pharmaceuticals* **2022**, *15*, 63. https://doi.org/10.3390/ph15010063

Academic Editor: Osvaldo Andrade Santos-Filho

Received: 21 November 2021
Accepted: 28 December 2021
Published: 4 January 2022

1. Introduction

Drug discovery is one of the most highly challenging, time-consuming and expensive projects in the healthcare sector. The usual time involved in bringing a drug from basic research to market is 12–16 years, and the cost associated is about 2.5 billion dollars [1–4]. To meet one of the EU Sustainable Development Goals [5] aimed at the good health and wellbeing for everyone, drugs should be made available to common people at an affordable price, and the current protocols in drug development need to be redesigned to make the discovery process economically sustainable. One of the most promising techniques to accelerate the drug discovery process, and to make it more cost-effective, is to perform in silico virtual screening, and to exploit the computational power of large high-performance computing (HPC) systems.

One of the major contributing factors to the cost and time associated with the discovery is that it has been reported [6,7] that only one in 10,000 compounds subjected to research and development (R&D) turns out to be successful. The drug discovery involves various steps such as target discovery, lead identification, lead optimization, ADMET (absorption, distribution, metabolism, excretion, toxicity) properties optimization, and clinical trials [8].

Once a valid target is known for a disease, compounds from different chemical libraries are subjected to high-throughput screening against this target. If the number of compounds used for screening can be narrowed down to a few hundred, the cost and time associated with a drug discovery process can be drastically reduced. Using computational approaches, many of the steps involved in the drug discovery projects can be made to be cost-effective and less time-consuming. For example, in the case of protein tyrosine phosphatase-1B [9], the experimental high-throughput screening of a chemical library with 400,000 compounds yielded a success rate of 0.021% in identifying the ligands that can inhibit the enzyme with IC_{50} values less than 100 µM. However, with the use of a preliminary screening phase using a computational approach, the success rate turned out to be 34.8% starting from a chemical library of 235,000 compounds.

To summarize, the experimental high-throughput screening is not suitable to deal with modern chemical spaces as they are composed of up to billions of molecules. To solve this problem, it is common to use computational approaches on HPC systems. In this review, we highlight various currently available implementations of virtual screening softwares suitable for high-performance computers. Below, we provide general introduction to virtual screening (VS) problems and discuss the possibilities for the parallelization so that it can be effectively implemented for computing facilities offered by HPCs.

The paper is organized as follows. Section 2 introduces the computational VS with details on scoring functions and search algorithms. Section 2.2 presents details on the major breakthroughs obtained in VS and Section 3 presents the main parallelization techniques used in VS and why they target HP systems. In Section 4, we provide an overview about the implementations of different VS softwares. Finally, we discuss the opportunities offered by reconfigurable architectures such as FPGAs.

2. The In Silico Virtual Screening Problem

In general, the computational approaches for molecular docking have two main components: sampling and scoring. Sampling refers to generation of various conformations and orientations for the ligand within a target binding site (defined usually by a grid box). Scoring refers to evaluating the binding/docking energies for various configurations of the ligand within the binding site. The most stable configuration of the ligand is referred to as binding pose. The VS protocol where molecular dockings are carried out for all the ligands from a chemical library includes a third component referred to as ranking, where different ligands are ranked with respect to their binding potential. Overall, the VS identifies the ligand with the topmost binding affinity (which is based on the docking energies of different ligands) for a given biomolecular target. In addition, the most stable binding mode/pose for each of the ligands within the binding site is found (which is based on the relative docking energies of different configurations of the same ligand). Figure 1 shows the general workflow of computer-aided drug discovery where the VS approach is used to identify lead compounds. It shows the steps involved in the binding pose identification of ligands within the binding site, and the ranking of different ligands is subsequently carried out to identify the lead compounds. Most of the VS schemes do not include the flexibility for the target protein, and only the sampling over translational, rotational, and torsional degrees of freedom of ligand is accounted for.

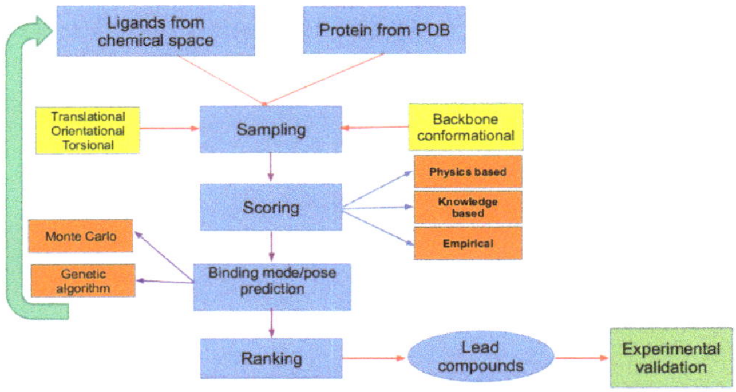

Figure 1. Workflow for computer-aided drug discovery where the lead compounds are identified using VS. It shows that the various configurations of the ligands within binding sites are generated using sampling, which is scored using a scoring function to identify the most stable binding mode/pose. The docking energies of the most stable configurations of all the ligands are used in ranking them to identify a list of lead compounds which are taken for further experimental validation. As the sampling and scoring need to be performed for all the ligands in the chemical library, these steps are shown within a loop.

2.1. Scoring Functions

The reliability and accuracy of the scoring functions used for screening compounds are the most important parameters that dictate the success rate of the computational screening approaches. The scoring functions are mostly defined to be proportional to the binding affinity of the ligand towards a target. The scoring functions are often classified as *physics-based*, *knowledge-based*, and *empirical*.

(i) *Physics-based* (also referred to as force-field based) scoring functions are based on the binding free energies which are the sum of various interactions between protein–ligand subsystems such as van der Waals, electrostatic, hydrogen bonding, solvation energy, and entropic contributions.
(ii) The *knowledge-based* scoring functions are based on the available protein–ligand complex structural data from which the distributions of different atom–atom pairwise contacts are estimated. The frequency of appearance of different pairwise contacts are used to compute potential mean force which is used for ranking protein–ligand complexes.
(iii) Finally, the *empirical scoring* functions, as the name implies, are based on empirical fitting of binding affinity data to potential functions whose weights are computed using a reference test system. Modern scoring functions mainly fall into this class, including the machine learning-based approaches built based on the available information on the protein–ligand 3D structures and inhibition/dissociation constants [10].

As discussed above, there are different scoring functions developed, and this section mainly focuses on implementations available in open-source softwares such as Dock [11], Autodock4.0 [12,13], Autodock Vina [14,15], and Gnina [16]. The docking energy defined to rank protein–ligand complexes (sf) in Autodock4.0 is classified as physics-based and is defined as the sum of van der Waals, electrostatic, hydrogen bonding, and desolvation energy, as shown in Equation (1).

$$sf = W_{vdw}\sum_{i,j}(\frac{A_{ij}}{r_{ij}^{12}} - \frac{B_{ij}}{r_{ij}^{6}}) + W_{HB}\sum_{i,j}(\frac{C_{ij}}{r_{ij}^{12}} - \frac{D_{ij}}{r_{ij}^{10}}) + W_{elec}\sum_{i,j}(\frac{q_i q_j}{\epsilon(rij)r_{ij}}) + W_{ds}\sum_{i,j}(S_iV_j + S_jV_i)(exp\frac{-r_{ij}^2}{2\sigma^2}) \quad (1)$$

In addition, the entropic contribution which is proportional to number of rotatable bonds is also added to the docking energy. In the equation, r_{ij} refers to the distance between the two atoms, i and j, centered on protein and ligand subsystems. Similarly, q_i and q_j refer to charges on these atoms. A_{ij} and B_{ij} are the coefficients of the potential energy functions describing van der Waals interaction. C_{ij} and D_{ij} are the coefficients of the potential energy functions describing hydrogen bonding interaction. The terms S_i and V_i refer to the solvation parameter and fragmental volume of atom i, respectively.

Because the protein–ligand complexes are considered to be in an aqueous environment, the binding free energies need to account for this, and solvation energy adds the binding free energy differences due to vacuum to aqueous-like environments. In particular, the last term in the equation accounts for this solvation effect (refer to Equation (1)).

In general, the entropic contributions can be due to translational, rotational, and torsional degrees of freedom. However, the docking energies implemented in the aforementioned molecular docking softwares only account for the contributions due to torsional degrees of freedom. The contributions due to other degrees of freedom are assumed to be negligible in ranking different ligands. It is worth noting that certain free energy calculation tools such as MMPBSA.py estimate the entropic contributions due to all degrees of freedom based on normal mode analysis [17]. The entropic contributions due to torsional degrees of freedoms in molecular docking softwares are oversimplified and they are estimated from the number of rotatable bonds (each bond contributes with 0.2–0.5 kcal/mol) [18]. In the case of Autodock Vina, the scoring function can be majorly classified as empirical in nature and it is a sum of various distance-dependent pairwise interactions [14]. It includes terms for describing steric, hydrophobic, and hydrogen bond interactions. The values for different parameters and weights for different terms of potential functions were obtained from nonlinear regression of the PDBbind 2007 dataset. In other words, the empirical scoring functions can have the same mathematical expression as in Equation (1), but the weights/coefficients for different types of interactions are obtained from fitting to experimental binding potentials. The knowledge-based scoring functions [19] (sf_{kb}) have the following form:

$$sf_{kb} = \sum_{i}^{L}\sum_{j}^{R} -k_B T ln[g(r_{ij})] \tag{2}$$

Here, the summation runs over the ligand and receptor atoms, and $g(r_{ij})$ refers to the relative probability distribution of distances of a specific types of protein–ligand atom pairs in the docked complex structure when compared to reference experimental complex structure.

Recently, deep learning networks have been proposed to provide scoring functions. For instance, Gnina uses convolutional neural network (CNN)-based scoring function to rank the protein–ligand complexes [16]. The neural networks were trained using three-dimensional protein–ligand complex structures from the PDBbind database. In particular, the dataset contained two sets of poses for the ligands within the binding site. The group of positive poses had root mean square deviation (RMSD) value below 2 Å, when compared to the crystallographic poses, while the rest were considered as a group of negative poses. Here, RMSD is the root mean square deviation in atomic positions in the predicted pose when compared to reference pose, as in the crystal structure. The positive and negative poses were generated using the experimental protein–ligand three-dimensional structures by adopting a random conformation generation algorithm. The CNN model was trained using the 4D grid (which was constructed using the protein–ligand coordinates within the grid box and atom types) to classify the poses.

2.2. Search Algorithms

The search algorithms aim at finding the protein–ligand structure corresponding to the global minimum in a potential energy surface. However, this is a very challenging problem and many search algorithms end up in a local minima. Therefore, molecular docking software uses several techniques, such as deterministic search [20], genetic algorithm, Monte Carlo with simulated annealing [21], particle swarm optimization [22], or Broyden–Fletcher–Goldfarb–Shanno (BFGS) [14]. Deterministic approaches apply techniques such as gradient descent, and they focus on a reproducible sequence of pose evaluations. Monte Carlo algorithms generate numerous poses by using random values for translational, rotational, and torsional degrees of freedom of the ligand. In Monte Carlo-simulated annealing, the heating step allows the system to escape from the local minimum (during which it can sample high-energy regions of the potential energy surface). In genetic algorithms, each pose is defined by a vector of genes that correspond to translational, rotational, and torsional degrees of freedom. By varying these values in the genes, new poses can be generated. The fitness function aims at finding the minimum energy of the pose.

2.3. Validation of Molecular Docking Approaches

As discussed above, molecular docking approaches employ different types of scoring functions, and before implementation they were validated rigorously against available experimental data. In particular, two properties obtained from molecular docking can be considered in general for benchmarking:

(i) RMSD computed for the predicted binding pose against the crystallographic pose obtained experimentally.
(ii) Binding free energies/docking energies which are proportional to experimental inhibition/dissociation constants.

The RMSD in the above list is computed from the experimental and predicted protein–ligand complex structures and provides an estimate of how well the molecular docking software is capable of producing the most stable binding mode and binding pose of the ligand within the target biomolecule. An RMSD value of <2 Å is considered as a threshold value for the correct prediction of complex structures [23].

A benchmark study using Autodock4.0 and Autodock Vina on the complex structures (190 in number) from PDBbind showed that the latter could predict structures within the threshold value (i.e., <2 Å) for about 78% complexes while the former one achieved 42% [14]. A recent study compared the performance of Autodock4.0 and Autodock Vina in discriminating the active compounds and decoys using a dataset of 102 protein targets, 22,432 active compounds, and 1,380,513 decoy molecules [24], The study showed that Autodock4.0 was better in discriminating actives and decoys in the targets having hydrophobic binding sites, while the Autodock Vina's performance was better for those targets having binding sites with polar and charged residues [24]. There are other studies reported in the literature which compared the performance of various molecular docking softwares such as AutoDock, DOCK, FlexX, GOLD, and ICM, and the ICM turned out to be the superior performer, with structures predicted for 93% complexes within the acceptable accuracy [23].

The other set of quantities used for benchmarking the molecular docking approaches are the inhibition constants, dissociation constants, IC_{50} and pIC_{50}, which are available from experimental binding assay studies. All these quantities refer to the binding potential or inhibiting potential of ligands to a specific biomolecular target. The dissociation constants and binding free energies are related to each other through the following equation:

$$\Delta G = RTlnK_d \tag{3}$$

where R is the gas constant (equal to 1.987 cal K^{-1} mol^{-1}) and T refers to temperature (set to 298.15 K). Thanks to this equation, the computed docking energies can be directly validated using the experimental binding assay results.

2.4. Computational Cost Associated with Virtual Screening

In a computational drug discovery project, high-affinity lead compounds against a target biomolecule (can be an enzyme, membrane protein, DNA, RNA, Quadruplex, membrane, or fibril aggregates) are identified using a reliable scoring function. One can identify lead compounds for a target from various chemical spaces. The popular chemical spaces are ZINC, Cambridge, Chemspider, ChEMBL, Pubchem, Pubmed, DrugBank, TCM, IMPPAT, and GDB13-17. Refer to Table 1 for a list of different chemical libraries with their properties [25]. The estimate for the size of chemical space for carbon-based compounds with molecular mass <500 daltons is 10^{60}, which clearly indicates that there are limitless possibilities for designing a therapeutic compound. As can be seen, even the use of the top supercomputers with exascale computing speed (which can perform 10^{18} floating point operations per second running the high-performance Linpack benchmark) for screening these compounds will take a universal lifetime. Therefore, it is reasonable to use certain filters to reduce the number of compounds before subjecting to screening. Recently, a filtering procedure based on Bayesian optimization algorithm, referred to as MolPAL, was used to identify the top 50% compounds by developing a model with data of explicit screening of less than 5% compounds of the chemical space [26].

Otherwise, it is reasonable to use other chemical libraries having compounds that are easy to synthesize and having favourable pharmacokinetic (ADMET) properties. The chemical library with the largest number of compounds is GDB17, which contains 166 billion organic molecules made of just 17 atoms of C, O, N, S and halogens [27]. Most of the drug discovery applications use the DrugBank database, Enamine database, ZINC15, [28], and Cambridge, and the number of compounds in these chemical libraries are listed in Table 1. As can be seen, the compounds range from tens of thousands to billions, and the computational cost associated with screening is enormous, which requires use of the HPCs and accelerators.

To demonstrate the computational demand associated with virtual screening, we describe an application below. In the case of the AmpC target, Lyu et al. docked 99 million molecules. For each compound, 4000 orientations on average were generated. Further, for each orientation, about 280 conformations were generated [29]. Therefore, for each ligand, 1.1 M docking energy calculations were carried out, and given that the number of compounds considered were 99 M, a total of 10^{13} of such calculations were carried out. This will be further increased in the flexible receptor docking where the sampling over side-chain conformations of residues needs to be accounted for [29]. As can be seen, the computational demand is really huge with such virtual screening applications, and so it is inevitable to develop parallel algorithms and to use HPCs to accomplish such screenings within affordable time.

Table 1. Top chemical spaces available for VS.

Chemical Library	NO of Compounds	Features
Virtual compounds	10^{60}	Molecular mass $\leq$ 500 daltons
GDB17 [25]	166 B	17 heavy atoms of type C, O, N, S and halogens
REAL DB (Enamine) [30]	1.95 B	Synthesizeable compounds M $\leq$ 500, Slogd $\leq$ 5, HB $\leq$ 10, HB $\leq$ 5 rotatable bond $\leq$ 10, and TPS $\leq$ 140
ZINC15 [28]	980 M	Synthesizable, available in ready-to-dock format
Pubchem [31]	90 M	Literature-derived bioactive compounds
Chemspider [32]	63 M	Curated database with chemical structure and physicochemical properties
ChEMBL [33]	2 M	Manually-curated drug-like bioactive molecules

3. Milestones in Virtual Screening

The first virtual screening using 3D structures of chemical compounds was carried out in 1990 against the target, dopamine D2 agonists based on which agonist with pKi 6.8 was successfully found [34]. A similar search against other targets, such as alpha-amylase, thermolysin, and HIV-I protease, yielded inhibitors with significant inhibition potential [34,35]. The top compounds obtained from screening were found to be potential inhibitors, and with further optimization of the lead compounds, the inhibition potential increased considerably. With the use of more accurate scoring functions and large-sized chemical libraries and powerful computers, the computer-aided drug discovery can become a potential route to narrow down the search space before subjecting to experimental high-throughput screening. Thanks to the currently available Petaflop/s computing facilities, one can screen a billion compounds in a day. The latest record on the high-speed virtual screening is reported by Jens Claser et al. [36], where the authors screened a billion compounds within 21 h.

The number of compounds screened against various targets keeps increasing with time. As the chance for a compound with better binding affinity increases with size of the chemical library, such screening procedures result in identifying highly potent compounds. We here list a few example cases (refer to Table 2): The screening study by J. Lyu et al. [29] yielded an active compound (339204163), which had 20 times more potency than the known inhibitors for AmpC target. The most potent inhibitor for the same target was designed by the same research group by optimizing the lead compound (the end compound was referred to as 549719643). Similarly, 10-fold more potent agonists (465129598, 270269326, and 464771011) were identified for the D4 receptor [29]. The most potent compound with 180 pM binding affinity, 621433144, for the same target has been identified by the same group. Using the multistage docking workflow, referred to as Virtual Flow for Virtual Screening (VFVS) (where different docking softwares such as Quickvina2, Smina vinardo, and Autodock Vina were used in sequence), the inhibitors for KEAP1 target were recently identified from the chemical space of 1.4 billion compounds (made of Enamine Real database and ZINC15) [37]. The first round of scoring was carried out using Quickvina2, while the rescoring was carried out for the top 3 million compounds using Smina vinardo and Autodock Vina. An inhibitor, iKEAP1 with dissociation constant 114 nM, was identified which is shown to interrupt the interaction between the KEAP1 and transcription factor NRF2 [37].

Thanks to parallel implementations of molecular docking software, not only has the number of compounds used for screening increased drastically, but the time required to accomplish the high-throughput screening has also reduced considerably. The inhibitors for the targets Purine Nucleoside Phosphorylase and Heat Shock Protein 90 were identified from the REAL enamine database (1.4 B compounds) using CPU-enabled Orion software [38]. The recent screening of compounds from Enamine database against the enzyme targets from SARS-CoV-2 was carried out in 21 h instead of 43 days with the use of parallel implementation of Autodock4.0 (referred to as Autodock-GPU) on the Summit supercomputer [39,40]. Currently, the largest experiment ever run was achieved using the EXSCALATE platform based on LIGEN software. It virtual-screened a library of 71.6 B compounds against 15 docking sites of 12 viral proteins of SARS-CoV-2. The experiment was carried out on the CINECA-Marconi100 and ENI-HPC5 supercomputers, and it lasted 60 h [41], performing more than 1 trillion docking evaluations overall. A list of megadocking and gigadocking screening calculations on large-sized chemical libraries is presented in Table 2.

Table 2. Topmost mega or gigadocking applications reported in the literature.

NO	Year	Target	No of Compounds	Docking Tool
1	2019	enzyme AmpC	99 M	Dock3.7
2	2019	D4 dopamine receptor	138 M	Dock3.7
3	2019	Purine Nucleoside Phosphorylase	1.43 B	Orion
4	2019	Heat Shock Protein 90	1.43 B	Orion
5	2020	KEAP1	1.4 B	Quickvina2
6	2021	Mpro	1.37 B	Autodock-GPU
7	2021	12 SARS-CoV-2 Proteins	71.6 B	LiGen

4. High-Performance Computing

Molecular docking for a single chemical compound involves sampling and scoring. This refers to sampling over the configurational phase space for the compound in the target binding site and computing the scoring functions for each of these configurations generated. In the case of virtual screening, compounds from a chemical library are ranked against a single target with respect to their binding affinities, and this additional component is referred to as ranking (refer to Figure 1). As discussed in the previous section, this is computationally very demanding and can highly benefit from the use of the parallel algorithms which can run on high-performance computers with different (shared memory and/or distributed) architectures [42,43]. Nowadays, the massively parallel computing units, referred as graphical processing units (GPUs) and field programmable gate arrays (FPGAs), are accessible to research groups or even individuals, and with the development of parallel virtual screening software, drug discovery projects can be offloaded to such groups, making the drug discovery economically sustainable. Below, we highlight the opportunities for the parallelization of VS protocol.

4.1. Parallelization Strategies of Virtual Screening for High-Performance Computers

As we discussed above, the virtual screening involves three key steps:

(i) Sampling over configurational phase space of ligands within the binding site.
(ii) Estimating the scoring function for each of the configurations of the chemical compound within the target binding site to identify the most stable binding mode/pose.
(iii) Ranking of compounds with respect to their relative binding potentials.

Each of these key steps can be parallelized, as the computations can be carried out independently.

The estimate of scoring function for each binding mode/pose within the protein binding site involves the computation of docking energies or binding free energies or any other empirical potentials. We need to find the most stable binding mode for each of the ligands in the target binding site (which corresponds to a global minimum in the protein–ligand potential energy surface). Therefore, for each ligand, millions of configurations (each configuration is a point in the ligand configurational phase space) are generated and the scoring functions are estimated for these structures. As discussed above, the configurations can be generated by changing the translational, rotational, or torsional degrees of freedom. These changes can be performed with a deterministic methodology or by using random-driven approaches such as Monte Carlo simulations or genetic algorithms. The estimate of energies for each of these configurations can be carried out independently; these can be distributed to different computing units.

In the virtual screening, the aforementioned procedure is repeated for all the ligands in the chemical library, and even this can be carried out independently, and so can be distributed to different computing units. Finally, even the calculation of the energy of a single conformation can be parallelized, as it needs to estimate the interactions of all the ligand–protein atoms couples. Overall, the parallelization of the virtual screening approach can be implemented in the following three steps, as we also show in Figure 2.

(i) **Low-level parallelization (LLP)**: Parallelizing the energy calculation.
(ii) **Mid-level parallelization (MLP)**: Parallelizing the conformer evaluations and scoring.

(iii) **High-level parallelization (HLP)**: Parallelizing the ligands evaluations on different computing units.

These three different levels have different efficiencies, as the amount of data transfer between the computing units is very different and may become a strong overhead. Moreover, it is also possible to combine more of these strategies in a single application to address different level of parallelism available (such as, for example, HLP for multi-node and MLP for multi-core architectures). The low-level parallelism approach is, however, usually not appealing, since the computed docking energies for different docking poses need to be compared, and this involves frequent data transfer between different computing units. The docking energy calculation involves summation over the pairwise interactions of the atoms centered on protein and ligand subsystems. In case of flexible targets, the intramolecular energies also need to be computed, which is obtained from a double summation over the number of atoms in the target. The non-bonded interaction calculation (sum of electrostatic and van der Waals) is the most time-consuming part of the energy calculation (by 80%) [42]. Stone et al. showed a 100-times speed-up for the non-bonded energy calculation using GPUs, while Harvey et al. showed 200-times increased performance [44,45]. A more sophisticated algorithm which effectively distributed the tasks to CPUs and GPUs for computing non-bonded interactions was developed by Gine's D. Guerrero et al. [46]. In this case, each atom of the receptor was assigned to a single thread in GPUs, which handle computing its interaction with all the ligand atoms [46]. Each thread was provided with necessary ligand and receptor atom coordinates and charges. The speed-up due to this algorithm was up to 280 times.

The parallelization of scoring function calculation is the most problematic approach, as it requires to sum all the atom contributions that are evaluated by different compute units (see Figure 2). This introduces frequent small data transfers that may be limiting the scaling behavior For this reason, the other two techniques are the most used in parallelizing VS software. Indeed, computing the energy for different configurations of the ligand can be carried out independently. Similarly, finding the global minimum structure for each of the ligands as well can be carried out independently. Each molecular docking step involves generation of millions of configurations, and the scoring functions for all the conformers can be calculated independently by assigning the tasks to different computing units. The energies for conformers can be gathered and checked for the least energy configuration corresponding to global minimum in the protein–ligand free energy surface.

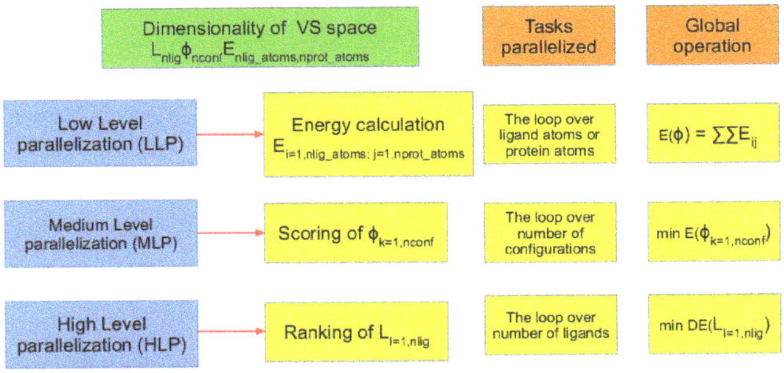

Figure 2. Various parallelization opportunities in virtual screening. The terms nlig, nconf, nlig_atoms, and nprot_atoms refer to number of ligands in a chemical library, number of configurations (specific to each ligand and dictated by number of rotatable bonds), number of ligand atoms, and number of protein atoms, respectively.

4.2. HPCs and Accelerator Technology as Problem Solvers

Parallel computing architectures can be classified based on the memory availability to computing units:

(i) In the shared memory architectures, a set of processors use the same memory segment.

(ii) In the case of distributed memory architectures, each computing unit has its own memory.

In general, a high-performance computing environment is usually made of both architectures where the shared-memory multi-core CPUs are connected through high-performance network connections. The memory in different nodes are local and are available to those cores within the specific node. The parallel execution of tasks in a shared memory architecture can be achieved by compiler directives such as OpenMP pragmas or libraries such as pthreads.

On the other hand, the parallel implementation of tasks in distributed memory architectures requires to handle the communication manually, using libraries such as Message Passing Interface (MPI) between different nodes of the machine.

As most of the supercomputers have both shared memory behavior (on a single node) and distributed memory behavior, as they are multi-node machines, it is easy to see the usage of both programming libraries for parallelizing the VS. In addition to multiple CPUs, recent HPCs also are integrated with accelerators such as graphical processing units, which have their own memory unit. The programming languages for CPU+GPU supercomputers are CUDA, OpenACC, and OpenCL. To use the accelerators, it is mandatory to move the data between the host and the device memory, which means that the developer needs to copy the data on the device before performing the computation and the result from the device after the computation is done. In addition, the tasks distribution to GPU cores and synchronization of the task execution in CPU and GPUs are achieved.

In virtual screening, the docking of different ligands can be carried out independently from each other. The procedure can be effectively parallelized on supercomputers with thousands of multiprocessor nodes, as well as in multi-CPU+GPU computers. As discussed above, there are different possibilities for running the virtual screening in HPCs. The molecular docking procedure for each ligand can be parallelized by distributing the docking energy calculations for different conformers of the ligand in a target binding site. In this case, the receptor coordinates and ligand coordinates and their charges need to be provided to all computing units (i.e., server nodes or GPU cards). In the second scenario, the molecular docking workload for different ligands is distributed to different computing units. In this case, the receptor coordinates and charges should be made available to all the computing units, while the ligand coordinates can be made available to the specific computing unit handling this specific ligand. The main disadvantage in this way of distributing tasks is that the ligands can have different sizes and so a rank assigned with the smaller sized ligand completes the task and waits until the molecular docking procedure is completed for all the ligands in different ranks to accept the tasks of second-round screening. This way, the computing time in this specific node is wasted. Thus, it is usually recommended to sort the ligands in terms of their size, and then the distribution of ligands can be carried out from the list. In this way, all the ranks will have more-or-less equivalent-sized tasks, and the wall time in different ranks is efficiently used. The next section provides an overview of the different software targeting HPC systems, also highlighting the type of parallelization employed.

5. Current Implementation of VS Available for Workstations, Accelerators, and HPCs

Currently, there are many parallel implementations for performing virtual screening in multicore machines, clusters, and accelerators. As discussed above, different strategies were adopted for parallel virtual screening. Only a few virtual screening softwares, such as Flexscreen, use the parallel implementation of docking energy calculation. The remaining perform the parallelization by distributing the conformational sampling/scoring or the ligands ranking segments over different computing units.

Table 3 shows a comparison of the analyzed software under some key features. As we can notice, most of the available softwares have the possibility to scale on multiple nodes, thus are able to exploit the whole HPC machine. All of them are able to fully utilize a node, while only a few have the support for the GPU acceleration. Moreover, as we already anticipated, all of them use an MLP (parallel conformational search) or HLP (parallel ligand evaluations) or both strategies to parallelize the computation, while none of them uses a low-level parallelism (parallel energy evaluations).

We now analyze, one by one, more in detail, these softwares: we focus on their performance in massively parallel architectures and accelerators when compared to CPU implementation. Wherever possible, the accuracy of the docking results (in terms of reproducing the experimental protein–ligand complex structure and experimental inhibition constants) will be discussed.

Table 3. Different parallel virtual screening softwares and important features.

Software	Parallelization Segment	Programming Language	Scoring Function	Minimization	Multi Thread	Multi Node	GPU
Dock 5,6	Conformational search	C++, C, Fortran77, MPI	Physics-based and hybrid	Monte Carlo	Yes	Yes	No
DOVIS2.0	Ligand screening	C++, Perl, Python	Physics-based	Monte Carlo&GA	Yes	Yes	No
Autodock Vina	Conformational search	C++, OpenMP	Hybrid	Monte Carlo	Yes	No	No
VSDocker	Ligand screening	C++, Perl, Python	Physics-based	Monte Carlo&GA	Yes	Yes	No
MPAD4	Ligand screening, Conformational search	C++, MPI, OpenMP	Physics-based	Lamarckian GA	Yes	Yes	No
VinaLC	Ligand screening, Conformational search	C++, MPI, OpenMP	Hybrid	Monte Carlo	Yes	Yes	No
VinaMPI	Ligand screening, Conformational search	C++, MPI, OpenMP	Hybrid	Monte Carlo	Yes	Yes	No
Ligen Docker-HT	Ligand screening, Conformational search	C++, MPI, CUDA	Empirical	Deterministic	Yes	Yes	Yes
GeauxDock	Ligand screening, Conformational search	C++, OpenMP, CUDA	Physics- and knowledge-based	Monte Carlo	Yes	Yes	Yes
POAP	Ligand screening	bash	Same as parent docking software	Same as parent Docking software	Yes	Yes	No
GNINA	Conformational search	C++	Empirical and CNN ML	Monte Carlo	Yes	Yes	Yes
Autodock-GPU	Ligand screening	C++ and OpenCL	Physics-based	MC/ LGA	Yes	No	Yes

5.1. Dock5,6

Dock5 and 6 [47,48] are the parallel implementations of virtual screening program written in C++ with MPI libraries. They are based on the original version referred to as Dock1, which was developed by Kuntz and coworkers [11]. The Dock1 used a geometric shape-matching approach for identifying the lead compounds for a given protein target. The subsequent versions adopted physics-based scoring functions for ranking and had improvement over the thoroughness of sampling and accounted for the ligand flexibility. The recent version allowed using multiple scoring functions where the solvation energies are computed using different implicit models, such as Zou GB/SA [49], Hawkins GB/SA [50], PB/SA [51], and generalized solvent models as implemented in Amber16. The benchmarking study to evaluate the performance of recent Dock6 (V6.7) used SB2012 dataset [52] which is a collection of crystallographic structures for about 1043 receptor–ligand complexes. It was able to reproduce the crystallographic poses in this dataset to an extent of 73.3% (i.e., RMSD between the experimental and predicted binding poses was <2 Å), which is due to reduction in the sampling failure of previous Dock versions. There is also a report in the literature on the offloading of Dock6 to CPU+GPU architectures using CUDA [53]. Only the ranking using amber scoring was offloaded to GPU architectures. In this offloading, the coordinates, gradients, and velocities are copied to host (CPU) memory to device (GPU) memory and the results are copied back from GPU to CPU memory. As the GPU could only handle single-precision numbers, the original data in double-precision were converted to single-precision numbers before transfer. Overall, the study reported about a 6.5-speedup for the amber scoring in Dock6 in GPU (NVIDIA GeForce 9800 GT) when compared to AMD dual-core CPU [53].

5.2. DOVIS2.0 VSDocker2.0

Both these parallel VS softwares use Autodock4.0 as docking engine. The former one has been developed for the multi-CPU systems with Linux operating system (OS), while the latter one is for parallel computer system running with MS Windows OS. DOVIS2.0 [54] uses multithreading, SSH, and batch system for parallelization, while C++ library, Perl, and Python are used for ligand format conversion, virtual screening workflow, and receptor grid files preparation, respectively. Instead of preparing the receptor grid files for each ligand, the program reuses them, and so the I/O file operation is reduced drastically. As the program employs dynamic job controlling, the load balancing due to different size of the ligands is effectively handled. Once the docking of block of ligands assigned to a CPU is completed, the results are written to project directory. Subsequently, the CPU requests for newer assignment for screening. This way, the CPUs are continuously in action until all the ligands are ranked and the results are written to shared directory. During a virtual screening for 2.3 M ligands from ZINC database on 256 CPUs, the DOVIS2.0 achieved a ranking speed of 670 ligands/CPU/day. The VSDocker program is developed to carry parallel virtual screening in both multiprocessor computing clusters and work stations running MS windows OS. The program is written in C++ and parallel library mpi.h [55]. In this VS implementation, the receptor map file generation and analysis of docking results for different ligands are carried out sequentially while the docking of different ligands are carried out in parallel. The performance of VSDocker has been tested using a chemical library of 86,775 ligands from ZINC database against a target made of 145 amino acids. The speed-up was comparable to that of DOVIS2.0, which is similar to VSDocker in implementation, but is suited for Linux running computer clusters.

5.3. Autodock Vina

Autodock4.0 is the most widely used molecular docking software based on physics-based scored function, but the original version is sequential in nature. However, the Autodock Vina, which is also from the same developers at Scripps Institute, can use multiple cores simultaneously for carrying out the docking. The calculations can be executed with single-threaded or multithreading options. The implementation uses C++ with Boost thread libraries. In the multithreading version, mutiple Monte Carlo simulations are initiated with different random number seed to explore different areas of conformational space of the ligand within the binding site. In a benchmarking study, for the same protein–ligand complex, the Autodock Vina [14] with single thread ran 62 times faster than the Autodock4.0. Further, running Autodock Vina with multithreading option in eight CPU machines yielded a 7.3-times-faster (when compared to single-threaded option) completion of molecular docking. The performance of single-threaded Autodock Vina compared to Autodock should be attributed to the difference in the computational cost of scoring functions. The more than 7-times speed-up with multithreading option in an eight-core machine shows that the molecular docking calculation scales well with the number of cores. Autodock Vina relies on OpenMP for distributing tasks to different threads and so is suitable for workstations with multiple cores. However, for the supercomputers with distributed memory, this version of Autodock Vina is not suitable, and rather more robust programs that allow the data transfer and communication between different nodes need to be used. It is also worth mentioning that there are updated versions of Autodock Vina, namely, Qvina 1 and Qvina 2, which showed some speedup due to the improvement in local search algorithm. SMINA [56] is a fork of Autodock Vina with a number of additional features such as user-specified scoring function, creating grid box for docking based on the coordinates of ligand bound to target, improved minimization, feasibility to include residues for flexible docking, and possibility to print more than 20 poses. In terms of speed-up in HPCs, this did not contribute to any improvement.

5.4. MPAD4

MPAD4 [57] is a parallel implementation of Autodock4.0, and the important features when compared to parent code are listed as follows: (i) It uses MPI to distribute docking jobs across the cluster; (ii) The grid maps generated for receptor are reused for all the docking calculations while in the default version, and these files are generated for each ligand docking with the target receptor and loaded into memory and released at the completion of docking. In MPAD4, The maps are loaded into memory of the node at the beginning of tasks and are used for all remaining docking calculations. This greatly reduces I/O usage, contributing to speed-up in the performance; (iii) The OpenMP is used for the node-level parallelization in executing the LGA for finding the global minimum. Overall, it allows system-level and node-level parallelization. The performance analysis of MPI version and MPI+OpenMP version can be studied by setting OMP to 1 and 4, respectively. The computers used for the initial performance analysis were IBM Blue gene/P and shared-memory 32-core POWER7 p755 server. The dataset used for performance analysis was

HIV protease target and 9000 compounds from a druglike subset of ZINC8 database (which has 34,481 ligands in total). The performance analysis in Blue gene/P with 2048 (8192) node (core) showed that grid map reuse has reduced single-threaded execution time by 17.5%. Multithreaded execution of the code yielded 25% improvement in the overall performance. The execution of the code on nodes ranging from 512–4096 showed near-linear scaling behavior for symmetric multiprocessing (SMP) mode (OMP = 4). In particular, for 16,384 core system, the speed gained was 92% compared to that of the ideal case. The virtual node (VN) mode (OMP = 1) with the grid map "reuse" option showed, however, 72% speed-up when compared to the ideal case. The gain in the performance of SMP mode should be attributed to multithreading. The node utilization can be further improved with the use of preordering ligands with decreasing number of torsional angles.

5.5. *VinaLC*

VinaLC [58] is an Autodock Vina extension to use MPI library for parallelization in large supercomputers. This implementation is very similar to VinaMPI (which is described below) and uses MPI and multithreading hybrid scheme for parallelization across nodes and within node, respectively. The computational cost of each docking calculation depends on the size of the ligand, receptors, and the grid box. If the calculations are distributed on all MPI processes due to this uneven size of the input systems, there can be MPI load imbalance where the processes are waiting for other processes to complete the task. This load imbalance is tackled effectively by the master–slave MPI scheme where the master process handles the inputs, and outputs job allocation to the slave processes. The tasks in the master slaves are handled by three loops: (i) the first loop is over each combination of receptor–target ligand which assigns docking task to a free slave; (ii) The second loop collects the docking results from slave processes and the new tasks are assigned in case of unfinished calculations; (iii) The third loop frees the slave processes. In the slave processes, an infinite whole loop is initiated which ends when the "job finished" signal is received from the master. The ideal slave processes are identified from the MPI_ANY_source tag and docking tasks are assigned upon the completion of previous task. In this way, the computing resources available in different processes are utilized efficiently. To make the communication effective, all the inputs needed for a single docking calculation are sent by single MPI_Send call. Therefore, coordinates of the receptor and ligand and grids (which are computed on the fly in the master process) are sent to the slave process. The outputs from the slave processes are collected by the master process into a few files instead of generating file for each ligands (which will generate a million or billion files depending upon the size of the chemical library). The benchmarking study was carried out using the two datasets, namely ZINC and DUD (directory of useful decoys). The target was chosen as Thermus thermophilus gyrase B ATP-binding domain. The benchmarking calculations were carried out on HPC machines at Lawrence Livermore National Laboratory, and the number of cores used were in the range 600–15,408. The study showed that the average CPU time per docking was closer to ideal average CPU time. The VinaLC was shown to scale well up to 15 K cores. The percentage of I/O activity was reported to be negligible when compared to the total computing time. For aforementioned target using 15 K cores, VinaLC could screen about one million compounds from Zinc15 database in 1.4 h. This can be extrapolated to 17 million compounds per day which suggests the suitability of VinaLC for the most time-taking mega- or gigadocking screening applications.

5.6. *VINAMPI*

VinaMPI is another implementation of Autodock Vina for distributed computing architectures [59]. It is written in C and for communication between the nodes, it uses MPI libraries. In order to avoid poor scaling behavior of the parent-child (or master-slave) distribution scheme in massively parallel supercomputers, this implementation uses all-worker scheme. It is worth recalling that rather VinaLC used Master-slave scheme for distributing tasks. In this code, each worker (or each MPI rank) deals with its own protein-ligand complex and within each rank the computation (related to search of global minimum) is carried out using multithreading. Due to this reason it is also suitable for the virtual screening for more than one targets. Further the computations are sorted out in terms of complexity so that the work loads at a given round of screening can be distributed equivalently. The computational complexity is measured based on the number of rotatable bonds and size of the ligands which is used to sort the tasks in the beginning of the screening. As a benchmark, the dockings were carried out for targets namely ACE (angiotensin-converting enzyme), ER AGONIST (estrogen receptor agonist), VEGFR2 (vascular endothelial growth factor receptor kinase), and PARP (poly(ADP-ribose) polymerase) with a chemical library of 98,164 compounds (comprised of ligands and decoys). Running this screening in a 516 cores supercomputer costed about 103 s [59]. It is expected that the same implementation in a supercomputer with 0.3 M cores can be used to screen 250 M compounds in 24 h.

5.7. LiGen Docker-HT

LiGen [60] is a VS software that leverages CPU and GPU to perform the required computation. Several versions of the tool have been developed, starting from a CPU-only application [20,60,61], then the main kernels have been ported to the GPU by [62] using OpenACC. Finally, it has been optimized using CUDA for the GPU kernels and this last version has been used to perform a large VS experiment in the search of a therapeutic cure for COVID-19 screening 71.6 B compounds against 15 binding sites from 12 Sars-Cov2 viral proteins on two supercomputers, accounting for 81PFlops [41]. LiGen uses deterministic algorithms to generate the different conformers of a ligand, and an empirical scoring function to select the best molecule. The Docker-HT application is the version of LiGen that is designed targeting a large VS campaign, and it is able to leverage multi-node, multi-core, and heterogeneous systems. In particular, it uses MPI to perform the multi-node communication, which is limited as much as possible by the algorithm to avoid large communication overheads [63]. Indeed, the amount of data that needs to be processed by every node is divided beforehand, and it may create load-balancing issues as there is no mechanism to rebalance it during the execution of the application. On the single node, it leverages the C++ thread library. Finally, it uses CUDA to support GPU acceleration. Within each node, the program uses pipeline parallelism and work-stealing to process the ligands.

5.8. Geauxdock

This is a parallel implementation of virtual screening available for multicore CPU, GPU, and Xeon Phi-computers. The software uses a common code for front-end computations in all these computers [64]. However, the back-end codes have one version for CPU and Xeon Phi architectures, and another for GPU. The code for CPU and Xeon Phi architectures written in C++, OpenMP and IntelSIMD pragmas. The GPU version is written in C++ and CUDA. The program uses the Monte Carlo approach for conformational search and for identifying the global minimum of the protein–ligand complex. The scoring function is based on physics-based energy terms combined with statistical and knowledge-based potentials. The performance of the code has been tested in multi-core CPUs and massively parallel architectures, namely Xeon Phi and NVIDIA GPUs. The testing using CCDC/Astex dataset showed a 1.9-times increase in performance for Xeon Phi when compared to 10-core Xeon CPU. Further, on the GeForce GTX 980 GPU accelerator, the performance was 3.5 times higher when compared to the CPU version.

5.9. POAP

Poap is a GNU parallel-based multithreaded pipeline for preprocessing ligands, for virtual screening, and for postprocessing the docking results [65]. It also allows the minimal use of memory through optimized dynamic file-handling protocol. It has also been optimized in a way that erroneous ligand input does not affect the workflow. It can be integrated with any of other sequential or multithreaded molecular docking softwares, such as Autodock4.0, Autodock Vina, or AutodockZn. In the case of Autodock-based virtual screening, the map files are generated for each ligand in the datasets. In the case of POAP, the map files are directed to a common hub directory and so occupancy of space due to redundant atom types in ligands is overcome. The number of threads to be used should be mentioned when the Autodock Vina is used as a docking software. In the case of Autodock and AutodockZn, the number of parallel jobs to be executed (which can be equal to the number of CPU threads) should be defined by the user. The performance of POAP has been tested using the virtual screening for the targets namely Human ROCK I, HTH-type transcriptional regulator, Polyketide synthase, and PqsA (Anthranilate-coenzyme A ligase) using the ligands from the chemical library, DrugBank. Since POAP does not have any serial code, the speed-up (theoretical estimate) is directly proportional to the number of processors used. The performance analysis of Autodock in a T5510 DELL workstation with Intel Xeon(R) CPU E5-2620V2, 2.10 GHz clock speed (12 Cores, 24 threads) with 62.9 GB RAM showed a 12.4-times speed-up when compared to serial mode (the number of parallel jobs specified is 24). Similarly, the Autodock Vina showed 2.4-times speed when compared to default mode (which is already multithreaded) and here, the number of jobs was set to three.

5.10. GNINA

GNINA is a fork of SMINA [56] and Autodock Vina [16]. When compared to the hybrid scoring function employed in Autdock Vina, it provides options to use various built-in scoring functions (such as Vina, Vinardo) along with user-customized scoring functions. More importantly, it provides a machine learning-based scoring function to rank the complexes. The default scoring function (called "none" option) is the same as used in Vina or Smina, while the rescoring (called "rescoring" option) allows the topmost ligand poses to be ranked using machine learning-based scoring functions.

In particular, this scoring function is based on convolutional neural networks trained using 3D protein–ligand complex structures (as reported in PDBBind or BindingDB) and corresponding experimental inhibition constants. They were trained to reproduce binding pose and the binding affinity. There are multiple machine learning functions (namely, crossdock_default2018, dense, general_default2018, redock_default2018, and default2017) provided by GNINA, and these have been developed using different datasets. The CNN-based scoring function outperforms the scoring function implemented in Vina in reproducing the binding poses. The RMSDs for the predicted poses in the unseen examples are below 2 Å in as many cases as 56%. Further, the binding prediction of poses within this cutoff improves to 79% if the redocking is performed.

When compared to Autodock Vina, the grid box center can be provided with the help of a ligand file. For the conformational search, GNINA uses Monte Carlo sampling scheme. The sampling is carried out over the ligand translational, rotational, and torsional degrees of freedom. In the case of flexible docking, the sampling is also carried out over the residue side-chain conformations. Unlike Smina, GNINA performs computing in single-precision (32 bit) which allows the possibility of offloading the CNN scoring tasks to GPUs. Even though GNINA can be used in massively parallel supercomputers and HPCs with accelerators, there is no performance analysis or profiling when compared to other docking softwares reported in the literature.

5.11. AUTODOCK-GPU

Autodock4.0 is one of the most widely used molecular docking softwares, but it is a serial code which runs on a single thread so cannot be effectively used in high-performance computing environments with multiple CPUs and GPUs. Autodock-GPU [66] is the version of Autodock developed for multiple node parallel computers with GPU accelerators. It is worth recalling that the above discussed MPAD4 was developed for multi-CPU architectures. This program has been developed using the application programming interface, OpenCL, as it allows portability to hybrid platforms with CPUs and GPUs. When compared to Autodock4.0, the local search algorithm uses derivatives of energies with respect to translations, rotations, and torsions (this implementation of gradient-based local search is referred to as ADADELTA). In the case of CPU+GPU architectures, the workflow consists of a sequence of host and device functions. In analogy to biological gene, the state of the protein–ligand complex is represented by a sequence of variables. In the case of a rigid docking (where the protein framework is treated as a rigid body), the variables represent positions, orientations, and conformation of the ligand. The number of variables are 6+Nrot, where Nrot is the number of rotatable bonds. The docking is aimed at finding the genotype which corresponds to the global minimum in the protein–ligand potential energy surface and the ranking is dictated by the scoring function.

The performance of Autodock-GPU has been tested using the diverse data set of 140 protein–ligand complexes from Astex Diversity Set [67], CASF-2013 [68], and protein databank. The reference docking calculations were performed using the single-threaded Autodock4.2.6. The speedup performance was dependent on the minimization algorithm used for the local search (whether Solis–Wets or ADADELTA), GPU type, and the type of protein used in the docking. With the use of Solis–Wets local search algorithm, the speed-up was 30 to 350 times in GPUs, with the M2000 showing the least performance and with TITAN V showing the best. However, with the use of ADADELTA local search, the speed-up was only 2 to 80 times improved, which has to be attributed to the computationally expensive calculation of gradients and difficulties associated with the parallelization of this local minimization step. In general, TITAN V cards showed 10 times higher speed-up when compared to M2000 versions. The performance analysis in multiple-core CPUs showed a similar trend where for the Solis–Wets search, the speed-up was in the range 5 to 33 times (the number of cores employed 8–36), while for the ADADELTA local search the speed-up was 2–20 times better.

5.12. Other VS Tools

The focus of this review was mostly about the open-source parallel VS softwares which are summarized in Table 3 along with some important features. The details about the year they were introduced and source URL pages are listed in Table 4. Many of these softwares such as GeauxDock, Autodock-GPU, and GNINA, were introduced in recent years and so their capacity in the lead compounds identification from huge chemical libraries needs to be validated extensively. Meanwhile, many already existing virtual screening softwares have contributed to successful lead compound identification and lead optimization over the years. In particular, the softwares such as FlexX, DOCK (the sequential version of above discussed Dock6), SLIDE, Fred (OpenEye), GOLD, LigandFit, PRO_LEADS, ICM, GLIDE, LUDI, and QXP are worth mentioning [69]. Among these, LigandFit and QXP employ Monte Carlo for sampling, while SLIDE and Fred employ conformational ensembles approach. GOLD, ICM, and GLIDE, respectively, adopt genetic algorithm, pseudo-Brownian sampling/local minimization, and exhaustive search for sampling. Finally, Dock and FlexX use incremental build approach for identifying the most stable binding mode/pose for the ligand. There are other VS softwares, such as RosettaDock [70], Surflex [71], and LIDAEUS [72], which are not discussed here as the review focuses on those with parallellism capability. It is also worth mentioning Spark-VS [73] software, which uses Google's MapReduce to run parallel virtual screening in distributed cloud resources. The parallel efficiency of Spark-VS against a chemical library of 2.2 M compounds is reported to be 87% when compared to a public cloud environment [73]. This opens up another possibility of using cloud computing resources for parallel virtual screening without a need to buy our own HPCs and accelerators.

Table 4. Timeline for different parallel virtual screening software and source URLs (with accessed dates in bracket).

No	Year	Parallel VS	Source
1	2006	Dock5&6	http://dock.docking.org/ (1 August 2021)
2	2008	DOVIS2.0	http://www.bioanalysis.org/downloads/DOVIS-2.0.1-installer.tar.gz (15 December 2021)
3	2009	Autodock Vina	http://vina.scripps.edu/ (1 August 2021)
4	2010	VSDocker	http://www.bio.nnov.ru/projects/vsdocker2/ (15 December 2021)
5	2011	MPAD4	http//autodock.scripps.edu/downloads/multilevel-parallel-autodock4.2 (15 August 2021)
6	2013	vinaMPI	https://github.com/mokarrom/mpi-vina (1 June 2021)
7	2013	vinaLC	https://github.com/XiaohuaZhangLLNL/VinaLC (10 June 2021)
8	2016	GeauxDock	http://www.brylinski.org/geauxdock (20 June 2021)
9	2018	POAP	https://github.com/inpacdb/POAP (21 June 2021)
10	2021	Autodock-GPU	https://github.com/ccsb-scripps/AutoDock-GPU (10 September 2021)
11	2021	GNINA	https://github.com/gnina/gnina (1 November 2021)

6. Emerging Reconfigurable Architectures for Molecular Docking

In prior sections, we have focused exclusively on reviewing methods of virtual screening and molecular docking that target modern central processing unit (CPU) and graphics processing unit (GPU) solutions (refer to Figure 3). At the same time, we know that Moore's law (transistor scaling) is terminating, which could motivate (or even necessitate) the search for alternative computing platforms that can continue the performance trend that molecular docking has come to rely upon. Among the many (so-called) post-Moore technologies [74], reconfigurable architectures are perhaps the most noticeable, partially because they are readily available today. A reconfigurable architecture, such as a field-programmable gate array (FPGA) or coarse-grained reconfigurable array (CGRAs) [75] is a system which aspires to retain some of the silicon plasticity that is lost when manufacturing an application-specific integrated circuit (ASIC). In turn, users can leverage reconfigurable systems to perfectly match the hardware to the application, which in turn can lead to improvement in performance and reduction in energy costs. For example, the expensive von Neumann bottleneck associated with the decoding of instructions in CPUs can be virtually eliminated. Traditionally, reconfigurable architectures such as FPGAs have been programmed using complex, low-level hardware description languages (HDLs) such as VHDL or Verilog. This, in turn, has limited exposure of using these devices to specialized hardware and is thus out of reach for typical HPC users. However, with the increase in maturity of high-level synthesis (HLS) [76] tools in the past decade, today, programmers can describe their hardware in abstract languages such as C/C++ and directive-driven models (e.g., OpenCL [77] or OpenMP [78]) and automatically translate the code down to specialized hardware. Modern HLS has, in turn, facilitated the accelerated use and research of FPGAs in other HPC applications such as computational fluid dynamics, neuroscience, and molecular docking.

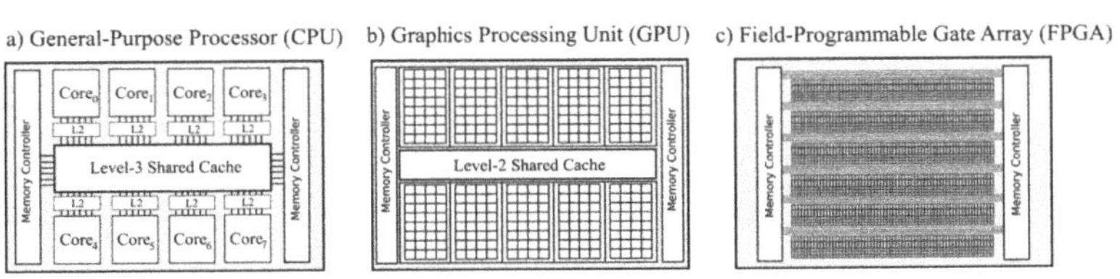

Figure 3. A conceptual picture of different processors and accelerators, showing (**a**) CPUs, which are latency-focused architectures with few processing units and large (and deep) memory hierarchies, (**b**) a GPU, which is a throughput-focused architecture with more processing units (contra CPUs) and a shallower memory hierarchy, and (**c**) FPGAs, which offer much more parallelism compared to both CPUs and GPUs, with finer control over individual unit types (here shown in different controls), but is harder to use.

Pechan et al. [79] evaluated and compared the use of FPGAs against both GPU and CPU solutions of the popular Autodock software. They created a custom RTL-based three-stage FPGA accelerator that computes the performance-critical sections of the Autodock algorithm. More specifically, the custom accelerator has four modules capable of exploiting MLP (see Section 4.1), while LLP is exploited inside each module (through pipelining); the accelerator relies on other methods to exploit HLP. They compared their solution against a custom (CUDA-based) GPU solution (GT220 and GTX260) and a CPU (Intel Xeon 3.2 GHz) version on the `1hvr` and `2cpp` protein pairs (from the Protein Data Bank). The overall results showed that FPGAs outperformed the CPUs for both use-cases independent of the number of dockings that were used. The GPU, however, had a clear advantage when a large number of dockings were executed, and the FPGA was only preferable when a few number of docking runs were executed. Recent work by Solis-Vasquez et al. [80,81] focused particularly on using OpenCL HLS tools to create custom accelerators that target FPGAs. Aside from disseminating their design process, they also vary several different architectural properties in their accelerator. For example, they consider both floating-point and fixed-point representation for various phases of the computation, which demonstrates an advantage that FPGAs can provide over more general-purpose approaches. The accelerator runs at a fairly high frequency (between 172 MHz and 215 MHz) on a Intel Arria 10, and consumes a varying amount of resources (subject to their design-space exploration). They compare their accelerator against the single-threaded Autodock software on five protein targets, and show that they reach between 1.73× and 2.77× speed up.

Today, there is a remarkably small number of published work that leverages FPGAs in the Autodock software (for surveys using FPGAs on other molecular algorithms, see [82,83]). Even more surprising is that (to the authors' knowledge) CGRAs have been largely unexplored in this domain. With both FPGAs and CGRAs emerging as performance (and, more importantly, *greener*) alternatives to traditional CPUs and GPUs, we believe that these systems will come to play a much larger role in molecular docking and virtual screening in the future than they have so far.

7. The Advent of Quantum Computing for Molecular Docking

With the advent of publicly available quantum computers via cloud computing, such as the IBM, Righetti, Google, and D-Wave quantum systems [84], quantum computing is becoming a promising approach to support and accelerate molecular docking computations.

A study of a molecular docking implementation on a photonic quantum computer was presented in [85]. The authors used a Gaussian boson sampler (GBS) which is a special model of photonic quantum computer where the computation is realized via the interference of identical photons that are passing through a circuit or a network of beam splitters and phase shifters. In this work, the binding interaction graph between ligands and receptor is used to generate the ligand orientations within the protein pocket. A simplified pharmacophore representation is used, limiting the graph size from all-molecular model of the ligand and receptor to a set of points having large influence on the interactions, i.e., negative/positive-charged atoms, hydrogen bond donor/acceptor atoms, hydrophobic characteristics, and aromatic ring positions. The docking problem has been formalized by mapping it to the identification of large clusters in a weighted graph. The GBS device was used to search for the largest cliques while considering the graph weights. The method shows very good results compared to solving the same problem in a classical way; however, it cannot be used alone in a virtual screening process unless to pair it with classical data postprocessing techniques (scoring) thus generating a hybrid-quantum approach.

The usage of quantum annealers to understand the capabilities of these devices to improve the quality and the throughput of molecular docking methods is presented in [86]. In particular, the paper focused on a specific phase of the molecular docking, consisting of ligand manipulation in terms of its rotatable bonds. The authors propose a quantum annealing approach to molecular docking by formulating it as a high-order unconstrained binary optimization (HUBO), which was possible to solve on the latest D-Wave annealing hardware (2000Q and Advantage). The work demonstrated how a lot of simplifications have to be taken into consideration during the problem formulation and embedding phase, even with small molecules. The results show that despite that the current hardware is not yet mature to solve the molecular docking problem on real-life scales, there is a clear positive trend in that direction.

8. Conclusions

The parallel implementation virtual screening algorithms in massively parallel computers with multiple CPUs and/or GPUs have the high potential to speed up the exploration of gigantic chemical spaces (having compounds in the range 10^9 to 10^{12}) in real time. In a serial version of virtual screening software, it may take many years of CPU hours for such tasks. The current regard for gigantic docking is the screening of billions of compounds from ZINC15 and Enamine databases with the use of Autodock GPU in Summit HPC computers in less than a day. The parallel implementations and reliable scoring functions will increase the success rates in the lead compounds identification for drug discovery. This makes the drug discovery less time-consuming and economically sustainable. Further, as the chemical spaces are really huge, the drugs with entirely different scaffold geometry can be identified. The speed-up of the virtual screening software is found to be dependent on the number of factors: energy minimization algorithm, scoring function, biomolecular target, and computer architecture. More elaborate studies will allow us to develop highly optimized virtual screening software in the future. The implementation of VS for FPGAs and quantum computing is still in its infancy, and a dedicated research is needed for adopting such architectures for drug discovery projects.

Author Contributions: Conceptualization, N.A.M. and S.M.; writing—original draft preparation, N.A.M., A.P. and S.M.; writing—review and editing, N.A.M., A.P., D.G., E.V., G.P. and S.M.; funding acquisition, S.M. All authors have read and agreed to the published version of the manuscript.

Funding: Funding for the work is received from the European Commission H2020 program, Grant Agreement No. 801039 (EPiGRAM-HS). We also acknowledge funding from EuroHPC-JU under grant agreement No 956137 (LIGATE) and European Commission H2020 program.

Institutional Review Board Statement: Not applicable.

Informed Consent Statement: Not applicable.

Data Availability Statement: The data has been presented in main text.

Conflicts of Interest: The authors declare no conflict of interest.

Abbreviations

The following abbreviations are used in this manuscript:

ADMET	Absorption, Distribution, Metabolism, Excretion, Toxicity
CUDA	Compute Unified Device Architecture
CGRA	Coarse-Grained Reconfigurable Arrays
GPU	Graphical processing unit
FPGA	Field programmable gate array
HPC	High-Performance Computing
OS	Operating system
PDB	Protein data bank
RMSD	Root Mean Square Deviation
VS	Virtual screening

References

1. Clark, D.E. What has virtual screening ever done for drug discovery? *Expert Opin. Drug Discov.* **2008**, *3*, 841–851. [CrossRef] [PubMed]
2. Morgan, S.; Grootendorst, P.; Lexchin, J.; Cunningham, C.; Greyson, D. The cost of drug development: A systematic review. *Health Policy* **2011**, *100*, 4–17. [CrossRef] [PubMed]
3. Dickson, M.; Gagnon, J.P. The cost of new drug discovery and development. *Discov. Med.* **2009**, *4*, 172–179.
4. Mullin, R. Drug development costs about $1.7 billion. *Chem. Eng. News* **2003**, *81*, 8. [CrossRef]

5. Rickels, W.; Dovern, J.; Hoffmann, J.; Quaas, M.F.; Schmidt, J.O.; Visbeck, M. Indicators for monitoring sustainable development goals: An application to oceanic development in the European Union. *Earths Future* **2016**, *4*, 252–267. [CrossRef]
6. Petrova, E. Innovation in the pharmaceutical industry: The process of drug discovery and development. In *Innovation and Marketing in the Pharmaceutical Industry*; Springer: Berlin/Heidelberg, Germany, 2014; pp. 19–81.
7. Kiriiri, G.K.; Njogu, P.M.; Mwangi, A.N. Exploring different approaches to improve the success of drug discovery and development projects: A review. *Future J. Pharm. Sci.* **2020**, *6*, 27. [CrossRef]
8. Frazier, K. *Biopharmaceutical Research & Development: The Process Behind New Medicines*; PhRMA: Washington, DC, USA, 2015.
9. Doman, T.N.; McGovern, S.L.; Witherbee, B.J.; Kasten, T.P.; Kurumbail, R.; Stallings, W.C.; Connolly, D.T.; Shoichet, B.K. Molecular docking and high-throughput screening for novel inhibitors of protein tyrosine phosphatase-1B. *J. Med. Chem.* **2002**, *45*, 2213–2221. [CrossRef]
10. Li, H.; Sze, K.H.; Lu, G.; Ballester, P.J. Machine-learning scoring functions for structure-based drug lead optimization. *Wiley Interdiscip. Rev. Comput. Mol. Sci.* **2020**, *10*, e1465. [CrossRef]
11. DesJarlais, R.L.; Sheridan, R.P.; Seibel, G.L.; Dixon, J.S.; Kuntz, I.D.; Venkataraghavan, R. Using shape complementarity as an initial screen in designing ligands for a receptor binding site of known three-dimensional structure. *J. Med. Chem.* **1988**, *31*, 722–729. [CrossRef]
12. Morris, G.M.; Goodsell, D.S.; Halliday, R.S.; Huey, R.; Hart, W.E.; Belew, R.K.; Olson, A.J. Automated docking using a Lamarckian genetic algorithm and an empirical binding free energy function. *J. Comput. Chem.* **1998**, *19*, 1639–1662. [CrossRef]
13. Cosconati, S.; Forli, S.; Perryman, A.L.; Harris, R.; Goodsell, D.S.; Olson, A.J. Virtual screening with AutoDock: Theory and practice. *Expert Opin. Drug Discov.* **2010**, *5*, 597–607. [CrossRef]
14. Trott, O.; Olson, A.J. AutoDock Vina: Improving the speed and accuracy of docking with a new scoring function, efficient optimization, and multithreading. *J. Comput. Chem.* **2010**, *31*, 455–461. [CrossRef]
15. Jaghoori, M.M.; Bleijlevens, B.; Olabarriaga, S.D. 1001 Ways to run AutoDock Vina for virtual screening. *J. Comput.-Aided Mol. Des.* **2016**, *30*, 237–249. [CrossRef]
16. McNutt, A.T.; Francoeur, P.; Aggarwal, R.; Masuda, T.; Meli, R.; Ragoza, M.; Sunseri, J.; Koes, D.R. GNINA 1.0: Molecular docking with deep learning. *J. Cheminform.* **2021**, *13*, 1–20. [CrossRef] [PubMed]
17. Miller, B.R., III; McGee, T.D., Jr.; Swails, J.M.; Homeyer, N.; Gohlke, H.; Roitberg, A.E. MMPBSA. py: An efficient program for end-state free energy calculations. *J. Chem. Theory Comput.* **2012**, *8*, 3314–3321. [CrossRef] [PubMed]
18. Poongavanam, V.; Namasivayam, V.; Vanangamudi, M.; Al Shamaileh, H.; Veedu, R.N.; Kihlberg, J.; Murugan, N.A. Integrative approaches in HIV-1 non-nucleoside reverse transcriptase inhibitor design. *Wiley Interdiscip. Rev. Comput. Mol. Sci.* **2018**, *8*, e1328. [CrossRef]
19. Dittrich, J.; Schmidt, D.; Pfleger, C.; Gohlke, H. Converging a knowledge-based scoring function: DrugScore2018. *J. Chem. Inf. Model.* **2018**, *59*, 509–521. [CrossRef] [PubMed]
20. Beccari, A.R.; Cavazzoni, C.; Beato, C.; Costantino, G. *LiGen: A High Performance Workflow for Chemistry Driven De Novo Design*; ACS Publications: Washington, DC, USA, 2013.
21. Nayeem, A.; Vila, J.; Scheraga, H.A. A comparative study of the simulated-annealing and Monte Carlo-with-minimization approaches to the minimum-energy structures of polypeptides: [Met]-enkephalin. *J. Comput. Chem.* **1991**, *12*, 594–605. [CrossRef]
22. Kennedy, J.; Eberhart, R. Particle swarm optimization. In Proceedings of the ICNN'95-International Conference on Neural Networks, Perth, Australia, 27 November–1 December 1995; Volume 4, pp. 1942–1948.
23. Bursulaya, B.D.; Totrov, M.; Abagyan, R.; Brooks, C.L. Comparative study of several algorithms for flexible ligand docking. *J. Comput.-Aided Mol. Des.* **2003**, *17*, 755–763. [CrossRef]
24. Vieira, T.F.; Sousa, S.F. Comparing AutoDock and Vina in ligand/decoy discrimination for virtual screening. *Appl. Sci.* **2019**, *9*, 4538. [CrossRef]
25. Walters, W.P. Virtual chemical libraries: Miniperspective. *J. Med. Chem.* **2018**, *62*, 1116–1124. [CrossRef]
26. Graff, D.E.; Shakhnovich, E.I.; Coley, C.W. Accelerating high-throughput virtual screening through molecular pool-based active learning. *Chem. Sci.* **2021**, *12*, 7866–7881. [CrossRef] [PubMed]
27. Ruddigkeit, L.; Van Deursen, R.; Blum, L.C.; Reymond, J.L. Enumeration of 166 billion organic small molecules in the chemical universe database GDB-17. *J. Chem. Inf. Model.* **2012**, *52*, 2864–2875. [CrossRef] [PubMed]
28. Sterling, T.; Irwin, J.J. ZINC 15—Ligand discovery for everyone. *J. Chem. Inf. Model.* **2015**, *55*, 2324–2337. [CrossRef] [PubMed]
29. Lyu, J.; Wang, S.; Balius, T.E.; Singh, I.; Levit, A.; Moroz, Y.S.; O'Meara, M.J.; Che, T.; Algaa, E.; Tolmachova, K.; et al. Ultra-large library docking for discovering new chemotypes. *Nature* **2019**, *566*, 224–229. [CrossRef]
30. Shivanyuk, A.; Ryabukhin, S.; Tolmachev, A.; Bogolyubsky, A.; Mykytenko, D.; Chupryna, A.; Heilman, W.; Kostyuk, A. Enamine real database: Making chemical diversity real. *Chem. Today* **2007**, *25*, 58–59.
31. Kim, S.; Thiessen, P.A.; Bolton, E.E.; Chen, J.; Fu, G.; Gindulyte, A.; Han, L.; He, J.; He, S.; Shoemaker, B.A.; et al. PubChem substance and compound databases. *Nucleic Acids Res.* **2016**, *44*, D1202–D1213. [CrossRef]
32. Williams, A.J.; Tkachenko, V.; Golotvin, S.; Kidd, R.; McCann, G. ChemSpider-building a foundation for the semantic web by hosting a crowd sourced databasing platform for chemistry. *J. Cheminform.* **2010**, *2*, O16. [CrossRef]
33. Gaulton, A.; Bellis, L.J.; Bento, A.P.; Chambers, J.; Davies, M.; Hersey, A.; Light, Y.; McGlinchey, S.; Michalovich, D.; Al-Lazikani, B.; et al. ChEMBL: A large-scale bioactivity database for drug discovery. *Nucleic Acids Res.* **2012**, *40*, D1100–D1107. [CrossRef]
34. Martin, Y.C. Accomplishments and challenges in integrating software for computer-aided ligand design in drug discovery. *Perspect. Drug Discov. Des.* **1995**, *3*, 139–150. [CrossRef]

35. Martin, Y.C. 3D database searching in drug design. *J. Med. Chem.* **1992**, *35*, 2145–2154. [CrossRef]
36. Glaser, J.; Vermaas, J.V.; Rogers, D.M.; Larkin, J.; LeGrand, S.; Boehm, S.; Baker, M.B.; Scheinberg, A.; Tillack, A.F.; Thavappiragasam, M.; et al. High-throughput virtual laboratory for drug discovery using massive datasets. *Int. J. High Perform. Comput. Appl.* **2021**, *35*, 452–468. [CrossRef]
37. Gorgulla, C.; Boeszoermenyi, A.; Wang, Z.F.; Fischer, P.D.; Coote, P.W.; Das, K.M.P.; Malets, Y.S.; Radchenko, D.S.; Moroz, Y.S.; Scott, D.A.; et al. An open-source drug discovery platform enables ultra-large virtual screens. *Nature* **2020**, *580*, 663–668. [CrossRef] [PubMed]
38. LeGrand, S.; Scheinberg, A.; Tillack, A.F.; Thavappiragasam, M.; Vermaas, J.V.; Agarwal, R.; Larkin, J.; Poole, D.; Santos-Martins, D.; Solis-Vasquez, L.; et al. GPU-accelerated drug discovery with docking on the summit supercomputer: Porting, optimization, and application to COVID-19 research. In Proceedings of the 11th ACM International Conference on Bioinformatics, Computational Biology and Health Informatics, Virtual, 21–24 September 2020; pp. 1–10.
39. OpenEye Scientific, GigaDocking™—Structure Based Virtual Screening of over 1 Billion Molecules Webinar. Available online: https://www.eyesopen.com/ (accessed on 1 August 2020).
40. Acharya, A.; Agarwal, R.; Baker, M.B.; Baudry, J.; Bhowmik, D.; Boehm, S.; Byler, K.G.; Chen, S.; Coates, L.; Cooper, C.J.; et al. Supercomputer-based ensemble docking drug discovery pipeline with application to COVID-19. *J. Chem. Inf. Model.* **2020**, *60*, 5832–5852. [CrossRef] [PubMed]
41. Gadioli, D.; Vitali, E.; Ficarelli, F.; Latini, C.; Manelfi, C.; Talarico, C.; Silvano, C.; Cavazzoni, C.; Palermo, G.; Beccari, A.R. EXSCALATE: An extreme-scale in-silico virtual screening platform to evaluate 1 trillion compounds in 60 h on 81 PFLOPS supercomputers. *arXiv* **2021**, arXiv:2110.11644.
42. Dong, D.; Xu, Z.; Zhong, W.; Peng, S. Parallelization of molecular docking: A review. *Curr. Top. Med. Chem.* **2018**, *18*, 1015–1028. [CrossRef] [PubMed]
43. Perez-Sanchez, H.; Wenzel, W. Optimization methods for virtual screening on novel computational architectures. *Curr. Comput.-Aided Drug Des.* **2011**, *7*, 44–52. [CrossRef]
44. Stone, J.E.; Phillips, J.C.; Freddolino, P.L.; Hardy, D.J.; Trabuco, L.G.; Schulten, K. Accelerating molecular modeling applications with graphics processors. *J. Comput. Chem.* **2007**, *28*, 2618–2640. [CrossRef]
45. Harvey, M.; De Fabritiis, G. An implementation of the smooth particle mesh Ewald method on GPU hardware. *J. Chem. Theory Comput.* **2009**, *5*, 2371–2377. [CrossRef]
46. Guerrero, G.D.; Pérez-Sánchez, H.; Wenzel, W.; Cecilia, J.M.; García, J.M. Effective parallelization of non-bonded interactions kernel for virtual screening on gpus. In Proceedings of the 5th International Conference on Practical Applications of Computational Biology & Bioinformatics (PACBB 2011), Salamanca, Spain, 6–8 April 2011; Springer: Berlin/Heidelberg, Germany, 2011; pp. 63–69.
47. Moustakas, D.T.; Lang, P.T.; Pegg, S.; Pettersen, E.; Kuntz, I.D.; Brooijmans, N.; Rizzo, R.C. Development and validation of a modular, extensible docking program: DOCK 5. *J. Comput.-Aided Mol. Des.* **2006**, *20*, 601–619. [CrossRef]
48. Allen, W.J.; Balius, T.E.; Mukherjee, S.; Brozell, S.R.; Moustakas, D.T.; Lang, P.T.; Case, D.A.; Kuntz, I.D.; Rizzo, R.C. DOCK 6: Impact of new features and current docking performance. *J. Comput. Chem.* **2015**, *36*, 1132–1156. [CrossRef] [PubMed]
49. Liu, H.Y.; Kuntz, I.D.; Zou, X. Pairwise GB/SA scoring function for structure-based drug design. *J. Phys. Chem. B* **2004**, *108*, 5453–5462. [CrossRef]
50. Hawkins, G.D.; Cramer, C.J.; Truhlar, D.G. Parametrized models of aqueous free energies of solvation based on pairwise descreening of solute atomic charges from a dielectric medium. *J. Phys. Chem.* **1996**, *100*, 19824–19839. [CrossRef]
51. Grant, J.A.; Pickup, B.T.; Nicholls, A. A smooth permittivity function for Poisson–Boltzmann solvation methods. *J. Comput. Chem.* **2001**, *22*, 608–640. [CrossRef]
52. Mukherjee, S.; Balius, T.E.; Rizzo, R.C. Docking validation resources: Protein family and ligand flexibility experiments. *J. Chem. Inf. Model.* **2010**, *50*, 1986–2000. [CrossRef] [PubMed]
53. Yang, H.; Zhou, Q.; Li, B.; Wang, Y.; Luan, Z.; Qian, D.; Li, H. GPU acceleration of Dock6's Amber scoring computation. In *Advances in Computational Biology*; Springer: Berlin/Heidelberg, Germany, 2010; pp. 497–511.
54. Jiang, X.; Kumar, K.; Hu, X.; Wallqvist, A.; Reifman, J. DOVIS 2.0: An efficient and easy to use parallel virtual screening tool based on AutoDock 4.0. *Chem. Cent. J.* **2008**, *2*, 18. [CrossRef]
55. Prakhov, N.D.; Chernorudskiy, A.L.; Gainullin, M.R. VSDocker: A tool for parallel high-throughput virtual screening using AutoDock on Windows-based computer clusters. *Bioinformatics* **2010**, *26*, 1374–1375. [CrossRef]
56. Koes, D.R.; Baumgartner, M.P.; Camacho, C.J. Lessons learned in empirical scoring with smina from the CSAR 2011 benchmarking exercise. *J. Chem. Inf. Model.* **2013**, *53*, 1893–1904. [CrossRef]
57. Norgan, A.P.; Coffman, P.K.; Kocher, J.P.A.; Katzmann, D.J.; Sosa, C.P. Multilevel parallelization of AutoDock 4.2. *J. Cheminform.* **2011**, *3*, 1–9. [CrossRef]
58. Zhang, X.; Wong, S.E.; Lightstone, F.C. Message passing interface and multithreading hybrid for parallel molecular docking of large databases on petascale high performance computing machines. *J. Comput. Chem.* **2013**, *34*, 915–927. [CrossRef]
59. Ellingson, S.R.; Smith, J.C.; Baudry, J. VinaMPI: Facilitating multiple receptor high-throughput virtual docking on high-performance computers. *J. Comput. Chem.* **2013**, *34*, 2212–2221. [CrossRef] [PubMed]
60. Beato, C.; Beccari, A.R.; Cavazzoni, C.; Lorenzi, S.; Costantino, G. Use of experimental design to optimize docking performance: The case of ligendock, the docking module of ligen, a new de novo design program. *J. Chem. Inf. Model.* **2013**, *53*, 1503–1517. [CrossRef] [PubMed]

61. Gadioli, D.; Palermo, G.; Cherubin, S.; Vitali, E.; Agosta, G.; Manelfi, C.; Beccari, A.R.; Cavazzoni, C.; Sanna, N.; Silvano, C Tunable approximations to control time-to-solution in an HPC molecular docking Mini-App. *J. Supercomput.* **2021**, *77*, 841–869 [CrossRef]
62. Vitali, E.; Gadioli, D.; Palermo, G.; Beccari, A.; Silvano, C. Accelerating a geometric approach to molecular docking with OpenACC. In Proceedings of the 6th International Workshop on Parallelism in Bioinformatics, Barcelona, Spain, 23 September 2018, pp. 45–51.
63. Markidis, S.; Gadioli, D.; Vitali, E.; Palermo, G. Understanding the I/O Impact on the Performance of High-Throughput Molecular Docking. In Proceedings of the IEEE/ACM Sixth International Parallel Data Systems Workshop (PDSW), St. Louis, MO, USA 15 November 2021.
64. Fang, Y.; Ding, Y.; Feinstein, W.P.; Koppelman, D.M.; Moreno, J.; Jarrell, M.; Ramanujam, J.; Brylinski, M. GeauxDock: Accelerating structure-based virtual screening with heterogeneous computing. *PLoS ONE* **2016**, *11*, e0158898. [CrossRef]
65. Samdani, A.; Vetrivel, U. POAP: A GNU parallel based multithreaded pipeline of open babel and AutoDock suite for boosted high throughput virtual screening. *Comput. Biol. Chem.* **2018**, *74*, 39–48. [CrossRef]
66. Santos-Martins, D.; Solis-Vasquez, L.; Tillack, A.F.; Sanner, M.F.; Koch, A.; Forli, S. Accelerating AutoDock4 with GPUs and gradient-based local search. *J. Chem. Theory Comput.* **2021**, *17*, 1060–1073. [CrossRef] [PubMed]
67. Hartshorn, M.J.; Verdonk, M.L.; Chessari, G.; Brewerton, S.C.; Mooij, W.T.; Mortenson, P.N.; Murray, C.W. Diverse, high-quality test set for the validation of protein-ligand docking performance. *J. Med. Chem.* **2007**, *50*, 726–741. [CrossRef] [PubMed]
68. Li, Y.; Han, L.; Liu, Z.; Wang, R. Comparative assessment of scoring functions on an updated benchmark: 2. Evaluation methods and general results. *J. Chem. Inf. Model.* **2014**, *54*, 1717–1736. [CrossRef]
69. Lyne, P.D. Structure-based virtual screening: An overview. *Drug Discov. Today* **2002**, *7*, 1047–1055. [CrossRef]
70. Marze, N.A.; Roy Burman, S.S.; Sheffler, W.; Gray, J.J. Efficient flexible backbone protein–protein docking for challenging targets *Bioinformatics* **2018**, *34*, 3461–3469. [CrossRef]
71. Jain, A.N. Surflex: Fully automatic flexible molecular docking using a molecular similarity-based search engine. *J. Med. Chem* **2003**, *46*, 499–511. [CrossRef] [PubMed]
72. Taylor, P.; Blackburn, E.; Sheng, Y.; Harding, S.; Hsin, K.Y.; Kan, D.; Shave, S.; Walkinshaw, M. Ligand discovery and virtual screening using the program LIDAEUS. *Br. J. Pharmacol.* **2008**, *153*, S55–S67. [CrossRef]
73. Capuccini, M.; Ahmed, L.; Schaal, W.; Laure, E.; Spjuth, O. Large-scale virtual screening on public cloud resources with Apache Spark. *J. Cheminform.* **2017**, *9*, 15. [CrossRef] [PubMed]
74. Vetter, J.S.; DeBenedictis, E.P.; Conte, T.M. Architectures for the post-Moore era. *IEEE Micro* **2017**, *37*, 6–8. [CrossRef]
75. Podobas, A.; Sano, K.; Matsuoka, S. A survey on coarse-grained reconfigurable architectures from a performance perspective *IEEE Access* **2020**, *8*, 146719–146743. [CrossRef]
76. Nane, R.; Sima, V.M.; Pilato, C.; Choi, J.; Fort, B.; Canis, A.; Chen, Y.T.; Hsiao, H.; Brown, S.; Ferrandi, F.; et al. A survey and evaluation of FPGA high-level synthesis tools. *IEEE Trans. Comput.-Aided Des. Integr. Circuits Syst.* **2015**, *35*, 1591–1604. [CrossRef]
77. Czajkowski, T.S.; Aydonat, U.; Denisenko, D.; Freeman, J.; Kinsner, M.; Neto, D.; Wong, J.; Yiannacouras, P.; Singh, D.P. From OpenCL to high-performance hardware on FPGAs. In Proceedings of the 22nd international conference on field programmable logic and applications (FPL), Oslo, Norway, 29–31 August 2012; pp. 531–534.
78. Podobas, A. Accelerating parallel computations with openmp-driven system-on-chip generation for fpgas. In Proceedings of the IEEE 8th International Symposium on Embedded Multicore/Manycore SoCs, Aizu-Wakamatsu, Japan, 23–25 September 2014 pp. 149–156.
79. Pechan, I.; Fehér, B.; Bérces, A. FPGA-based acceleration of the AutoDock molecular docking software. In Proceedings of the 6th Conference on Ph.D. Research in Microelectronics & Electronics, Berlin, Germany, 18–21 July 2010; pp. 1–4.
80. Solis-Vasquez, L.; Koch, A. A case study in using opencl on fpgas: Creating an open-source accelerator of the autodock molecular docking software. In Proceedings of the FSP Workshop 2018; Fifth International Workshop on FPGAs for Software Programmers Dublin, Ireland, 31 August 2018; pp. 1–10.
81. Solis Vasquez, L. Accelerating Molecular Docking by Parallelized Heterogeneous Computing—A Case Study of Performance Quality of Results, and Energy-Efficiency Using CPUs, GPUs, and FPGAs. Ph.D. Thesis, Technische Universität, Darmstadt Germany, 2019. [CrossRef]
82. Majumder, T.; Pande, P.P.; Kalyanaraman, A. Hardware accelerators in computational biology: Application, potential, and challenges. *IEEE Des. Test* **2013**, *31*, 8–18. [CrossRef]
83. Pechan, I.; Fehér, B. Hardware Accelerated Molecular Docking: A Survey. Bioinformatics, Horacio Pérez-Sánchez, IntechOpen 2012, Volume 133. Available online: https://www.intechopen.com/chapters/41236 (accessed on 1 August 2020). [CrossRef]
84. Castelvecchi, D. Quantum computers ready to leap out of the lab in 2017. *Nat. News* **2017**, *541*, 9. [CrossRef]
85. Banchi, L.; Fingerhuth, M.; Babej, T.; Ing, C.; Arrazola, J.M. Molecular docking with Gaussian boson sampling. *Sci. Adv.* **2020** *6*, eaax1950. [CrossRef]
86. Mato, K.; Mengoni, R.; Ottaviani, D.; Palermo, G. Quantum Molecular Unfolding. *arXiv* **2021**, arXiv:2107.13607.

pharmaceuticals

MDPI

Article

Discovery of Small Molecules as Membrane-Bound Catechol-*O*-methyltransferase Inhibitors with Interest in Parkinson's Disease: Pharmacophore Modeling, Molecular Docking and In Vitro Experimental Validation Studies

Pedro Cruz-Vicente [1,2,†], Ana M. Gonçalves [1,2,3,†], Octávio Ferreira [1], João A. Queiroz [1], Samuel Silvestre [1,4,5,*], Luís A. Passarinha [1,2,3,5,*] and Eugenia Gallardo [1,5,*]

1 CICS-UBI, Health Sciences Research Centre, Universidade da Beira Interior, 6201-001 Covilha, Portugal; pedromvcruz@hotmail.com (P.C.-V.); ggmargarida@gmail.com (A.M.G.); octavioferreira.2@gmail.com (O.F.); jqueiroz@ubi.pt (J.A.Q.)
2 UCIBIO—Applied Molecular Biosciences Unit, Departamento de Química, Faculdade de Ciências e Tecnologia, Universidade NOVA de Lisboa, 2829-516 Caparica, Portugal
3 Associate Laboratory i4HB—Institute for Health and Bioeconomy, NOVA School of Science and Technology, Universidade NOVA de Lisboa, 2819-516 Caparica, Portugal
4 CNC—Center for Neuroscience and Cell Biology, University of Coimbra, 3004-504 Coimbra, Portugal
5 Laboratório de Fármaco-Toxicologia—UBIMedical, Universidade da Beira Interior, 6200-001 Covilha, Portugal
* Correspondence: sms@ubi.pt (S.S.); lpassarinha@fcsaude.ubi.pt (L.A.P.); egallardo@fcsaude.ubi.pt (E.G.); Tel.: +351-275-329-002 (S.S. & L.A.P. & E.G.)
† These authors contributed equally to this paper.

Citation: Cruz-Vicente, P.; Gonçalves, A.M.; Ferreira, O.; Queiroz, J.A.; Silvestre, S.; Passarinha, L.A.; Gallardo, E. Discovery of Small Molecules as Membrane-Bound Catechol-*O*-methyltransferase Inhibitors with Interest in Parkinson's Disease: Pharmacophore Modeling, Molecular Docking and In Vitro Experimental Validation Studies. *Pharmaceuticals* **2022**, *15*, 51. https://doi.org/10.3390/ph15010051

Academic Editor: Osvaldo Andrade Santos-Filho

Received: 30 November 2021
Accepted: 28 December 2021
Published: 31 December 2021

Publisher's Note: MDPI stays neutral with regard to jurisdictional claims in published maps and institutional affiliations.

Abstract: A pharmacophore-based virtual screening methodology was used to discover new catechol-*O*-methyltransferase (COMT) inhibitors with interest in Parkinson's disease therapy. To do so, pharmacophore models were constructed using the structure of known inhibitors and then they were used in a screening in the ZINCPharmer database to discover hit molecules with the desired structural moieties and drug-likeness properties. Following this, the 50 best ranked molecules were submitted to molecular docking to better understand their atomic interactions and binding poses with the COMT (PDB#6I3C) active site. Additionally, the hits' ADMET properties were also studied to improve the obtained results and to select the most promising compounds to advance for in-vitro studies. Then, the 10 compounds selected were purchased and studied regarding their in-vitro inhibitory potency on human recombinant membrane-bound COMT (MBCOMT), as well as their cytotoxicity in rat dopaminergic cells (N27) and human dermal fibroblasts (NHDF). Of these, the compound ZIN27985035 displayed the best results: For MBCOMT inhibition an IC_{50} of 17.6 nM was determined, and low cytotoxicity was observed in both cell lines (61.26 and 40.32 μM, respectively). Therefore, the promising results obtained, combined with the structure similarity with commercial COMT inhibitors, can allow for the future development of a potential new Parkinson's disease drug candidate with improved properties.

Keywords: Parkinson's disease; catechol-*O*-methyltransferase; inhibitors; bioinformatics; pharmacophore modeling; molecular docking; cytotoxicity

1. Introduction

With the increasing life expectancy of the population, neurodegenerative disorders (ND) such as Alzheimer's and Parkinson's disease (PD), are becoming more common and recognized as a social problem to modern societies [1]. PD is characterized by a progressive neurodegeneration in the central nervous system (CNS) that involves a loss of dopaminergic neurons in the brain and nowadays is considered one of the main causes of disability and mortality [2]. The current drug therapy mostly targets symptomatic relief, mainly aiming to restore dopaminergic function [2]. However, this strategy is not capable of stopping the progression of the disease and the advance of neurodegeneration and symptom aggravation [2]. To date, the most effective drug combination used in PD treatment is levodopa (*L*-DOPA) combined with aromatic *L*-amino acid decarboxylase and catechol-*O*-methyltransferase (COMT) inhibitors to restore dopaminergic brain levels [2]. However, their long-term administration is generally associated with harmful side effects that affect the patient's quality of life, and a loss in pharmacological effect is usually observed over time [3]. Therefore, there is an increasing demand to develop novel PD drug candidates. Considering the active role that COMT holds in *L*-DOPA metabolism, both in the periphery and in CNS, converting more than 90% of administered *L*-DOPA before reaching the brain, the discovery of a novel COMT inhibitor with low toxicity, high inhibitory potency, and selectivity towards the CNS is of high interest. Specifically, COMT is a magnesium-dependent enzyme that mediates the removal of a methyl group from *S*-adenosyl-L-methionine (SAM) to a catecholic substrate, affording *O*-methylated products and *S*-adenosylhomocysteine (AdoHcy) [4]. Physiologically, this enzyme appears as two distinct isoforms, a soluble isoform (SCOMT) mainly expressed in the peripheric systems, such as the liver, kidney, and intestines, and a membrane-bound (MBCOMT) isoform with a major prevalence in the central nervous system (CNS) [5–7]. Despite the high similarity shared by both isoforms, SCOMT has a higher enzymatic activity capacity, whereas MBCOMT has a higher substrate affinity (Km), especially towards catecholamines like dopamine and epinephrine [2,5]. Since the discovery of the pharmacological benefit of COMT inhibition, several families of molecules have been reported in the literature. The first generation was composed of molecules with a high structure similarity with known COMT substrates, bearing a catechol moiety [8,9]. However, despite some promising in-vitro results, in in-vivo testing, the compounds displayed a high toxicity and low inhibitory potency [8]. So, a new group of inhibitors was proposed, mainly formed by di-substituted catechols, where entacapone and tolcapone, commercial COMT inhibitors used in a clinical setting at the moment, were included [9]. These compounds showed enhanced potency, generally in the nanomolar range, especially caused by the presence of electron-withdrawing groups at the *ortho* position to a hydroxyl group of the catechol moiety [8]. Despite its clinical use and pharmacological properties, including the capacity to cross the blood–brain barrier (BBB) and thus inhibit central COMT, tolcapone is also associated with high hepatoxicity, limiting its use in more advanced cases of PD progression. In contrast, entacapone, a strictly peripheric inhibitor, is less potent, but has less toxicity and was considered as the first line of treatment for many years [10]. Recently, another peripheric COMT inhibitor, opicapone, was approved for clinical use. This drug displays a higher bioavailability than other commercial inhibitors and leads to stable and sustained *L*-DOPA plasma levels for over 24 h periods, which allows for a big improvement in the life quality of PD patients [11]. Regardless of the intense research to improve levodopa bioavailability, only a couple of novel adjunct compounds acting through COMT inhibition have been approved in the last few decades [3]. So, it is imperative to find new COMT inhibitors with the ability to cross the BBB and promote a synergic effect (peripheral/central) with a high safety profile. Considering the need to combine new technologies to support the design of novel drugs, bioinformatics is gaining outstanding relevance in almost all therapeutical areas. It is no different for COMT inhibition, and since the 1990s many researchers have employed some of these tools to discover and/or aid in the design of new molecules. In this context, Vidgren et al. were one of the first research groups to employ the use of computational tools to study the molecular interactions of potential inhibitors with the COMT catalytic site [12]. The acidity of both catechol hydroxyl groups and the lipophilicity of the inhibitors side chains were demonstrated to play an important role in the molecules' binding affinity, later confirmed by the determination of the first COMT crystal structure [13]. Lautala et al. [14], by comparing unsubstituted catechol and pyrogallol, first-generation inhibitors, and their substituted derivatives, demonstrated that the turnover rate modification of the molecules was inversely proportional to their binding affinity to the protein active site. Moreover, several research groups studied the inhibitory potential of flavonoids through molecular docking [15], dynamic simulations [16], and QSAR (quantitative structure–activity relationship) studies [17]. Similar strategies were employed for the "second generation" inhibitors, as reported by Palma et al., who applied molecular docking to understand the molecular interactions of nebicapone [18], a nitrocatechol inhibitor, and the *O*-regioselectivity of the enzyme for BIA 3-228 and BIA 8-176, two other nitrocatecholic-type inhibitors [19]. Another class of inhibitors that was studied was the bisubstrate inhibitors, molecules that target simultaneously both the SAM and the substrate binding sites [20]. In fact, both Lerner et al. [21] and Paulini et al. [22] used molecular docking to evaluate the effect of several substituents on the binding affinity with COMT. Moreover, Lee et al., through homology modeling of the 3D structure of rat COMT, developed several bisubstrate inhibitors performed molecular docking to analyze putative binding affinities [23]. Furthermore, Ellerman et al. used structure-based drug design (SBDD) methodologies to evaluate the binding affinity of multiple compounds with the COMT 3D structure [24,25]. Recently, garcinol, a natural product with an in-vitro effect identical to the one observed with tolcapone, was also studied in silico and it was shown that it can form identical atomic interactions with COMT when compared to tolcapone [26]. A slightly different approach was used by Jatana et al. by employing pharmacophore modeling and ligand screening analysis to obtain molecules with a high potential to interact with COMT [27]. All studies were performed with the soluble isoform of mouse or human COMT. So, due to the difficulty of obtaining the 3D structure of membrane proteins, bioinformatics approaches have been extensively used to explore the conformational space of a ligand in the binding pocket of the selected target protein. At present, more than 100 3D SCOMT crystal structures can be found in the Protein Data Bank (https://www.rcsb.org/, accessed on 27 November 2021), and they provided essential information about the atomic interactions formed between the protein active site and substrates/inhibitors. Nevertheless, the MBCOMT structure has not been solved to date and no structures between SCOMT and MBCOMT coupled to new molecules have been reported in the literature. So, in this work, the resolution of the crystal structure of the SCOMT variant [28] was the base for structure-based virtual screening and pharmacophore modeling studies to find potential COMT inhibitors with increased selectivity towards MBCOMT. This study, using a combination of structure- and ligand-based drug design approaches to select new promising candidates to be studied in-vitro for both MBCOMT inhibition and cell line cytotoxicity, aims to discover novel PD drug candidates with interest for further studies.

2. Results

2.1. Pharmacophore Modeling

Employing a ligand-based molecular modeling strategy, a pharmacophore containing the main structural moieties of the training set (Figure 1) was generated to find new potential COMT inhibitor drug candidates. By merging the essential features of the selected molecules (Figure 1), the model explored the number of hydrogen bond donors/acceptors as well as the aromatic and hydrophobic groups involved in the interaction with the COMT active site, generating a model very similar to the interactions performed by the commercial COMT inhibitor tolcapone, as shown in Figure 2 [29].

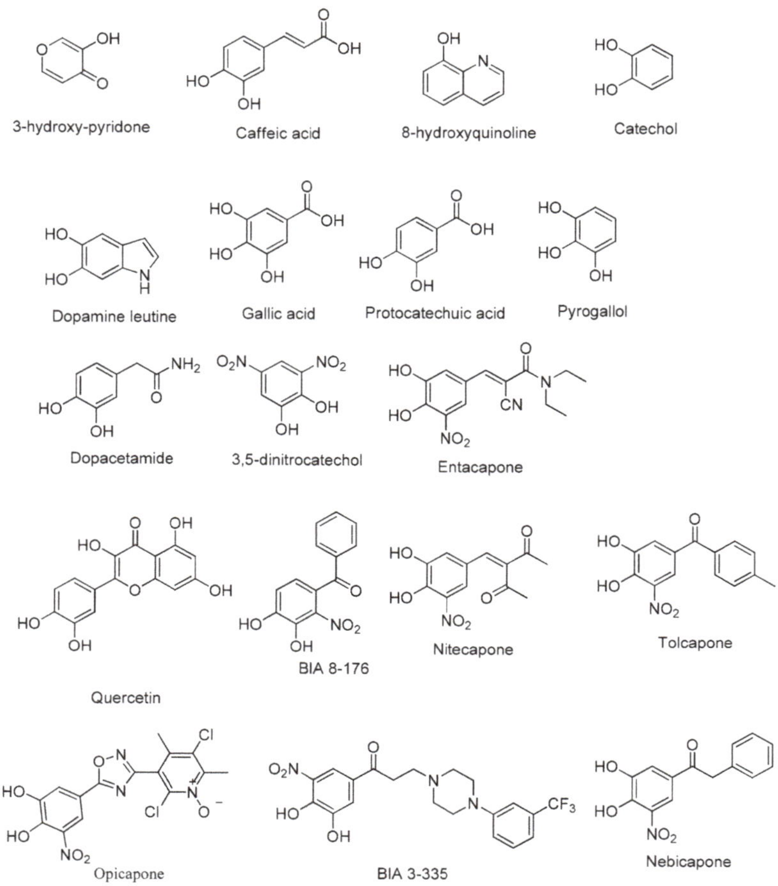

Figure 1. 2D structures of the selected COMT inhibitor training set.

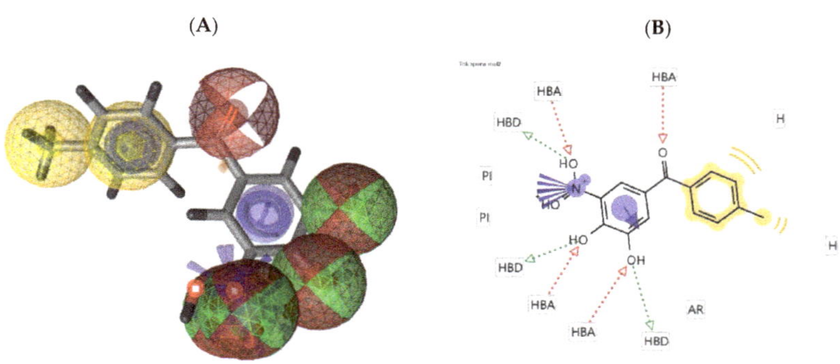

Figure 2. (**A**) Pharmacophore model of tolcapone generated by LigandScout (hydrogen bond donor: green sphere, hydrogen bond acceptor: red sphere, ionizable area: blue asterisk, and aromatic rings: yellow); (**B**) 2D representation of the pharmacophore features of tolcapone.

2.2. Database Searching

From the 10 best scored hypotheses, only the best scored model was selected to advance for further studies. The selected pharmacophore was loaded into the ZINCPharmer software and a virtual screening of the ZINC purchasable database was performed, selecting the 100 best scored hit molecules. These 100 compounds were selected considering literature data, with a focus on the knowledge of the main molecules with COMT inhibitory effects (e.g., compounds presented in Figure 1). From an initial set of 21,777,093 compounds, the compounds with RMSD (root-mean-square deviation) ranging from 0.5 to 1.5 Å were the best ranked compounds, and commercial COMT inhibitors like tolcapone and opicapone were also considered hit molecules, improving the reliability of the obtained data. In Supplementary Material Table S1 the RMSDs, molecular weight, and routable bonds of some of the hit molecules selected are displayed.

2.3. Molecular Docking Studies

Molecular docking was used to better comprehend and validate the provisional results obtained in Section 2.2, filtering potential false negatives and studying in detail the atomic interactions formed with the COMT active site. To do so, the 3D structure of COMT (PDB#6I3C) co-crystallized with the cofactors SAM and Mg^{2+} ions and the inhibitor 3,5-DNC, identified as the reference compound, was used [28]. To date, this structure has the best resolution of all the structures of COMT deposited in PDB (data checked on 27 November 2021). Structurally, the COMT catalytic site is surrounded by the "gatekeeper" residues Trp143 and Pro174, which ensure the correct orientation of the substrate, the Mg^{2+} ions, and the SAM cofactors, as well as residues Lys144 and Glu199, which are involved in substrate binding [30]. The methodology used was validated through a re-docking of the co-crystallized reference COMT inhibitor 3,5-DNC into the protein active site through AutoDock Tools software, obtaining an RMSD value of 1.6 Å and a binding energy of −4.85 kcal/mol. These results indicate that the procedure used was able to reproduce the crystallographic complexes in a very precise approach. The hit molecules were also subjected to the same procedure and were ranked based on their molecular interactions formed with the COMT active site by both hydrophobic and electrostatic interactions, as summarized in Supplementary Material Table S2. In Table 1 the atomic interactions of some of the most promising scoring molecules are displayed in more detail, as well as in Figures 3–12. A special focus was brought to the molecules that could form interactions with the most important amino acids of the protein active site, mainly with Lys144 and Glu199 by hydrogen bonding and with Trp38, Trp143, and Trp174 by hydrophobic interactions. Additionally, the binding energy values were also evaluated, namely, in comparison with the reference compound 3,5-DNC.

2.4. ADMET Property Prediction

The ADMET properties were predicted for the 50 best scored compounds in the virtual screening. Table 2 summarizes the results for the 10 most relevant selected molecules in several categories, such as absorption, distribution, metabolism, excretion, and predicted toxicity, obtained in the webserver pkCSM. These included the BBB (blood–brain barrier) and CNS (central nervous system) permeability, which are considered important attributes of a PD drug, where most of the tested compounds were in the lower limit of being considered a permeable drug. The human intestinal potential absorption is indicative of higher intestinal absorption, which is a factor to take into account in cases of oral drug administration (the results were in most cases percentages above 80%, a very positive result). Regarding the PgP (P-glycoprotein) interaction, a protein involved in cells' internal efflux mechanisms for xenobiotic substances, the compound properties both as a substrate and/or inhibitor were assessed, yielding positive data due to low indications of an interaction with these proteins. The inhibition of several cytochrome P450 enzymes was also predicted, specifically for the CYP2C9, CYP2D6, CYP3A4, CYP1A2, and CYP2C19 variants, where most compounds did not inhibit any of these enzymes, with the exception of CYP2C19, where almost half of the studied compounds inhibited this isoenzyme. For AMES toxicity, which states the mutagenicity of a compound evaluated, we concluded that only a few compounds were predicted as being potentially mutagenic. The compounds LD_{50} (median lethal dose) and LOAEL (lowest observed adverse effect level) were predicted as being similar to other clinically used drugs, such as some of the commercial COMT inhibitors. Finally, hepatotoxicity was also studied, with only one negative result observed, for the compound ZINC825166420. These results, despite being in-silico data, are very interesting, with some very positive results that can potentially indicate some of the in-vitro and in-vivo results. However, they can only be validated with further testing.

Table 1. Hit molecule predicted values of the binding affinities and main interactions with the target.

Compound	Binding Energy	Main Interactions
ZINC825166420	−7.48	Met40, Pro174, Glu199
ZINC1547205762	−7.39	Trp38, Met40, Pro174, Mg^{2+}
ZINC98288	−6.98	Trp38, Met40, Lys144, Pro174, Glu199
ZINC95473053	−6.79	Trp38, Met40, Asp141, Trp143, Lys144, Asn170, Pro174, Glu199, Mg^{2+}
ZINC302226	−6.63	Met40, Pro174, Glu199, Mg^{2+}
ZINC27985035	−6.26	Met40, Asp141, Lys144, Asn170, Pro174,
ZINC78496496	−6.12	Trp38, Met40, Pro174, Leu198, Glu199, Mg^{2+}
ZINC38175059	−6.04	Trp38, Met40, Asp141, Lys144, Asn170, Pro174, Leu198, Glu199
ZINC605706834	−6.24	Trp38, Trp143, Pro174
ZINC68675288	−5.90	Met40, Asn170, Pro174, Glu199

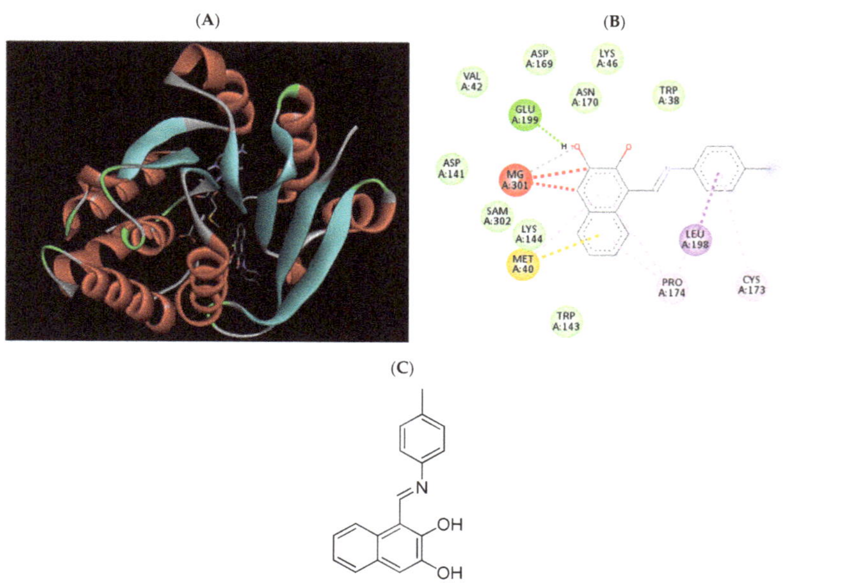

ZINC825166420

Figure 3. (**A**) Binding modes of ZINC825166420 with the crystal structure of human COMT complexed with SAM and Mg^{2+}, (**B**) receptor–ligand interactions, (**C**) 2D representation of ZINC825166420.

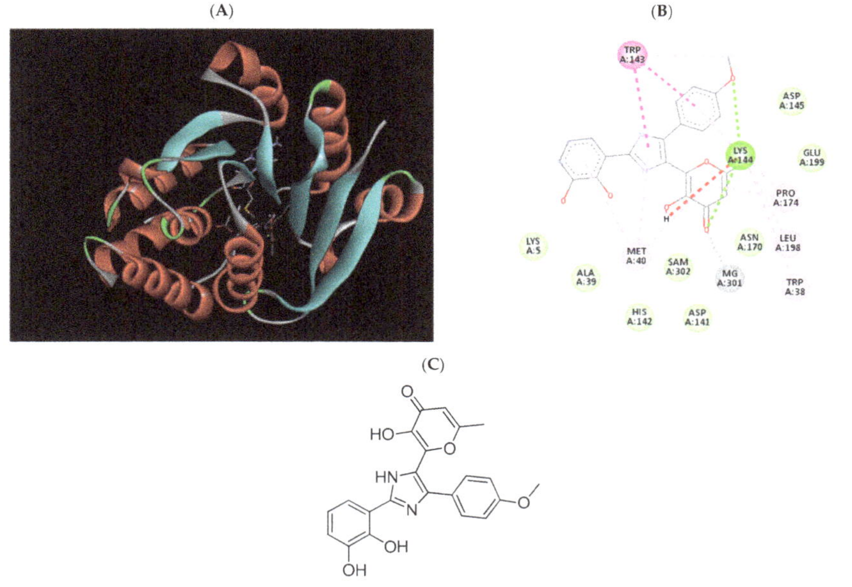

ZINC1547205762

Figure 4. (**A**) Binding modes of ZINC1547205762 with the crystal structure of human COMT complexed with SAM and Mg^{2+}, (**B**) receptor–ligand interactions, (**C**) 2D representation of ZINC1547205762.

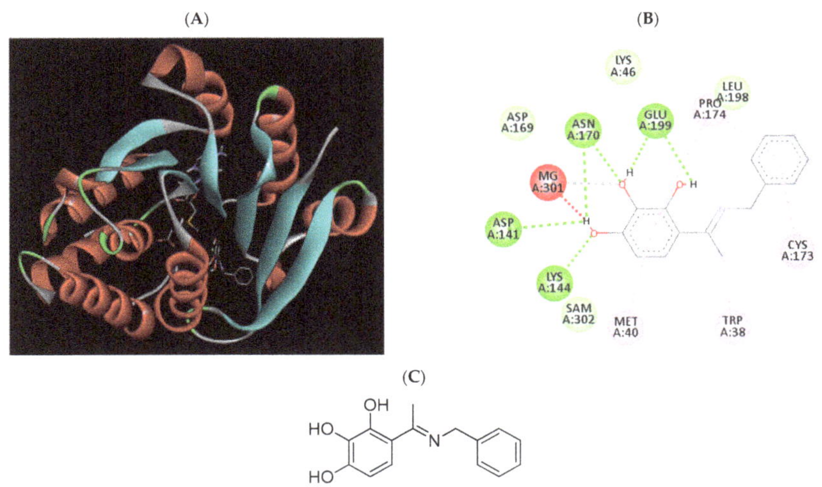

ZINC98288

Figure 5. (**A**) Binding modes of ZINC98288 with the crystal structure of human COMT complexed with SAM and Mg^{2+}, (**B**) receptor–ligand interactions, (**C**) 2D representation of ZINC98288.

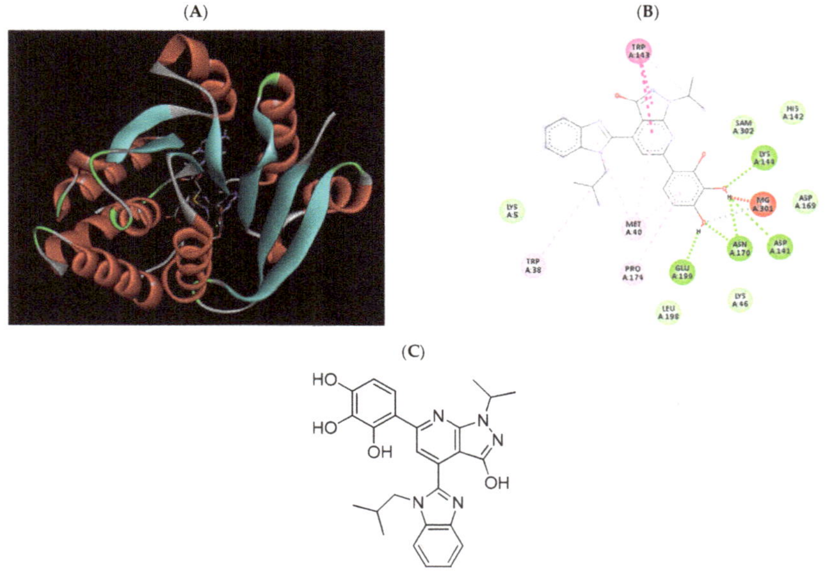

ZINC95473053

Figure 6. (**A**) Binding modes of ZINC95473053 with the crystal structure of human COMT complexed with SAM and Mg^{2+}, (**B**) receptor–ligand interactions, (**C**) 2D representation of ZINC95473053.

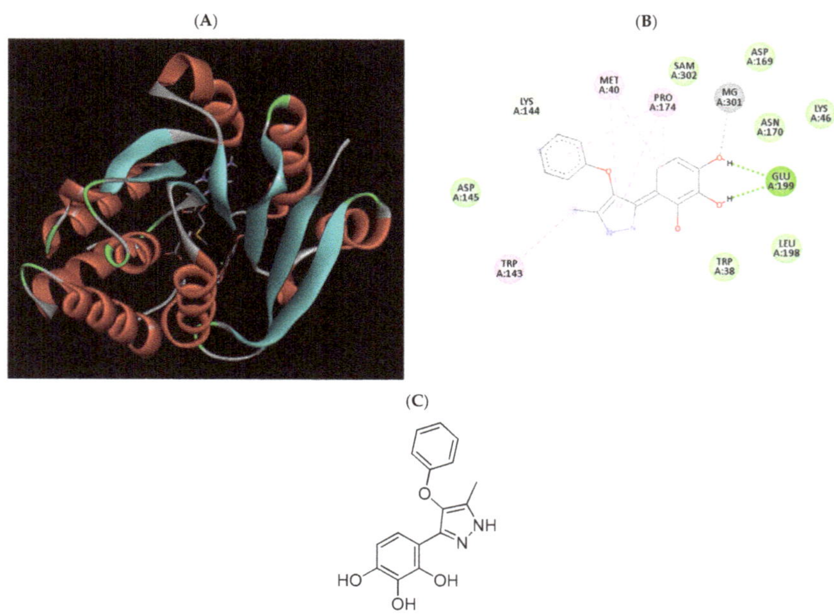

ZINC302226

Figure 7. (**A**) Binding modes of ZINC302226 with the crystal structure of human COMT complexed with SAM and Mg^{2+}, (**B**) receptor–ligand interactions, (**C**) 2D representation of ZINC302226.

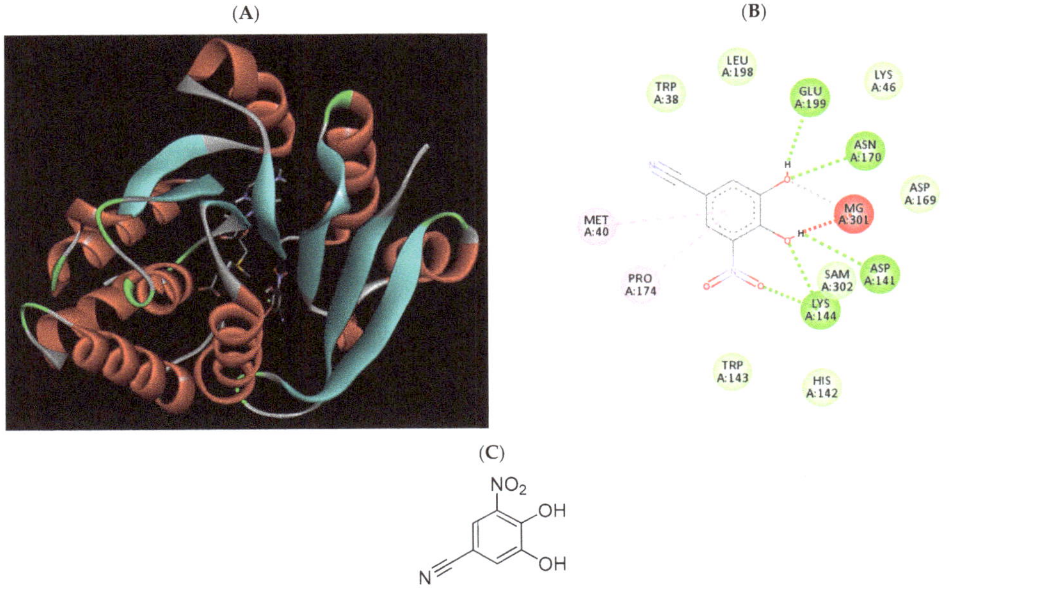

ZINC27985035

Figure 8. (**A**) Binding modes of ZINC27985035 with the crystal structure of human COMT complexed with SAM and Mg^{2+}, (**B**) receptor–ligand interactions, (**C**) 2D representation of ZINC27985035.

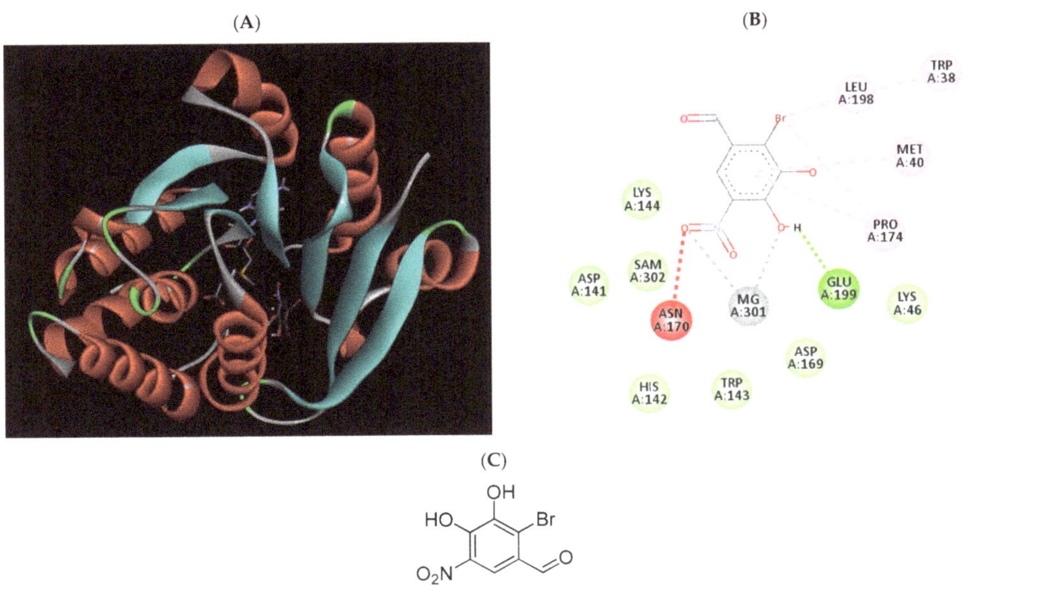

ZINC78496496

Figure 9. (**A**) Binding modes of ZINC78496496 with the crystal structure of human COMT complexed with SAM and Mg^{2+}, (**B**) receptor–ligand interactions, (**C**) 2D representation of ZINC78496496.

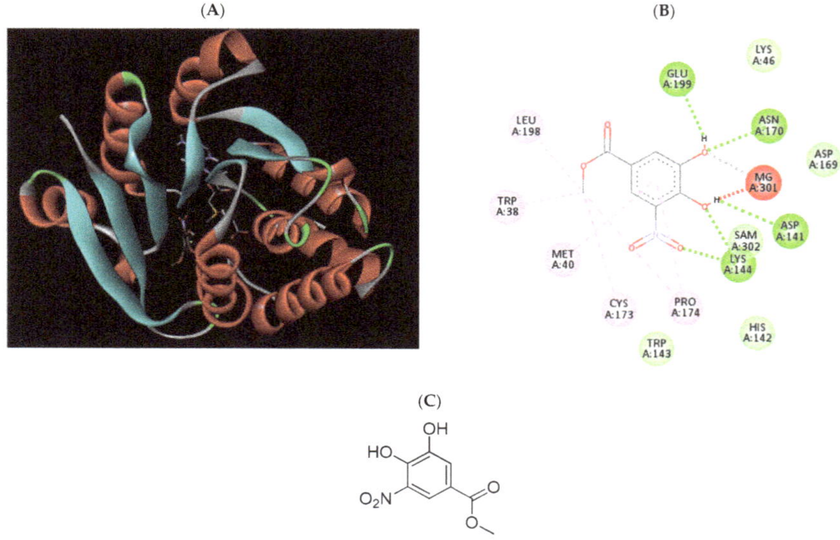

ZINC38175059

Figure 10. (**A**) Binding modes of ZINC38175059 with the crystal structure of human COMT complexed with SAM and Mg^{2+}, (**B**) receptor–ligand interactions, (**C**) 2D representation of ZINC38175059.

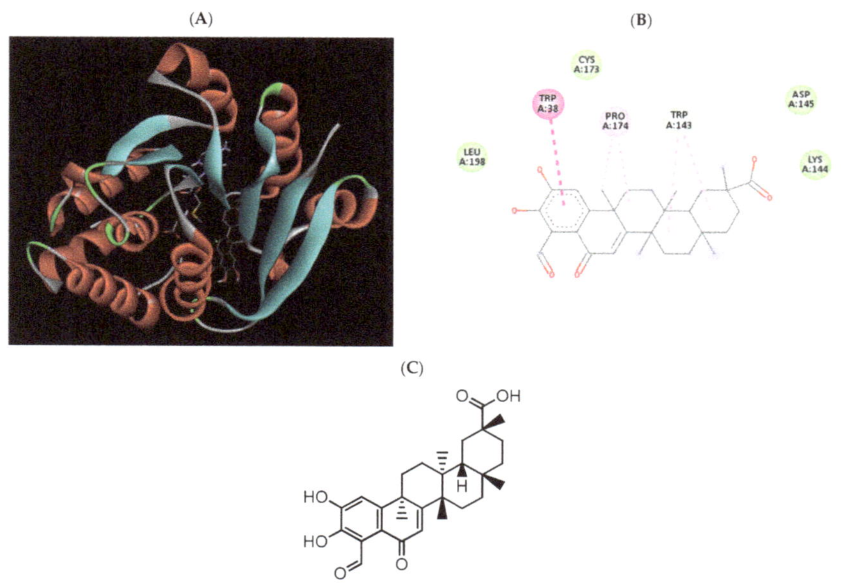

ZINC605706834

Figure 11. (**A**) Binding modes of ZINC605706834 with the crystal structure of human COMT complexed with SAM and Mg^{2+}, (**B**) receptor–ligand interactions, (**C**) 2D representation of ZINC605706834.

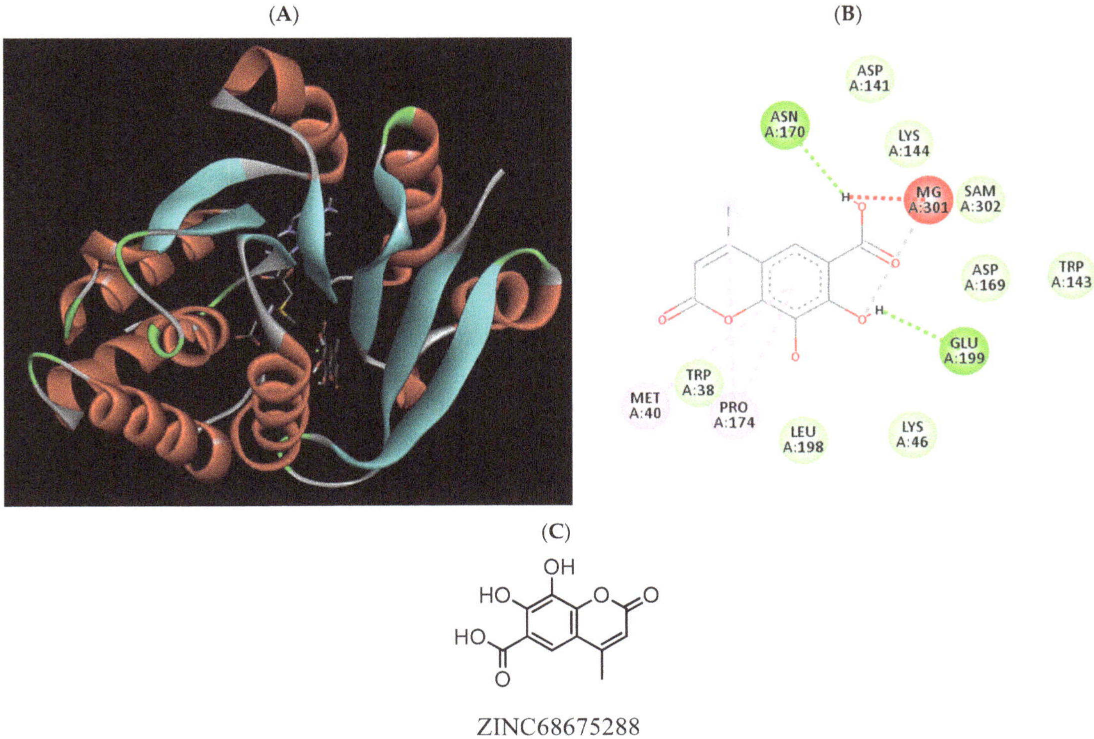

Figure 12. (**A**) Binding modes of ZINC68675288 with the crystal structure of human COMT complexed with SAM and Mg^{2+}, (**B**) receptor–ligand interactions, (**C**) 2D representation of ZINC68675288.

After this analysis, based on binding energies and atomic interactions formed with the COMT active site (Section 2.3), commercial availability, and the structure similarity with commercial or previously reported COMT inhibitors, 10 compounds were selected to be tested further.

2.5. In-Vitro MBCOMT Assays

Despite structural-based drug design tools being able to predict the binding modes and affinity of new molecules to the targets with significant accuracy and efficiency [31], an in-vitro validation of the best modeling results must be performed. Therefore, according to the best hits given by the computational models, 10 compounds were chosen to perform the enzymatic inhibition assay (Supplementary Material Table S3). As previously mentioned, our group purchased the most promising compounds with purity above 99.5% according to the manufacturer. The compounds used in this study are presented in Figure 13, with the respective identification.

From these previous studies, a first screening of MBCOMT inhibitory effects allowed us to select the compounds with the five best inhibitory profiles for concentration-response studies to calculate IC_{50} values, which are presented in Table 3. From the analysis of the results, the lowest IC_{50} was determined for the compound ZINC27985035, followed by ZINC78496496.

Table 2. ADMET prediction for the most promising compounds.

Compound	Intestinal Absorption (%)	PgP Sub-strate	PgP I/II Inhibitor	BBB Permeability (logBB)	CNS Permeability (log PS)	CYP2D6 Substrate	CYP3A4 Substrate	CYP1A2 Inhibitor	CYP2C19 Inhibitor	CYP2C9 Inhibitor	CYP2D6 Inhibitor	AMES Toxicity	LD50 (mol/kg)	LOAEL	Hepatoxicity
ZINC825166420	91.048	Yes	No/No	−0.013	−1.625	No	Yes	Yes	Yes	Yes	No	Yes	2.563	2.278	Yes
ZINC1547205762	84.913	Yes	No/No	−1.601	−3.777	No	No	Yes	Yes	Yes	Yes	No	2.346	2.323	No
ZINC98288	88.908	Yes	No/No	−0.722	−2.205	No	No	Yes	Yes	No	No	No	2.017	2.085	No
ZINC95473053	97.282	Yes	Yes/Yes	−1.467	−3.022	No	Yes	Yes	Yes	Yes	Yes	Yes	2.444	2.511	No
ZINC302226	69.066	Yes	No/No	−1.669	−2.427	No	No	Yes	No	Yes	No	No	2.67	3.036	No
ZINC27985035	76.88	Yes	No/No	−0.356	−2.587	No	No	No	No	No	No	Yes	2.044	2.407	No
ZINC78496496	77.717	Yes	No/No	−0.603	−2.601	No	No	No	Yes	No	No	Yes	2.154	2.329	No
ZINC38175059	71.419	Yes	No/No	−0.569	−2.78	No	No	No	No	No	No	Yes	1.804	2.158	No
ZINC605706834	63.604	Yes	No/No	−0.813	−2.724	No	No	No	No	No	No	No	2.655	2.538	No
ZINC68675288	53.332	Yes	No/No	−1.278	−4.074	No	No	No	No	No	No	No	2.474	2.537	No

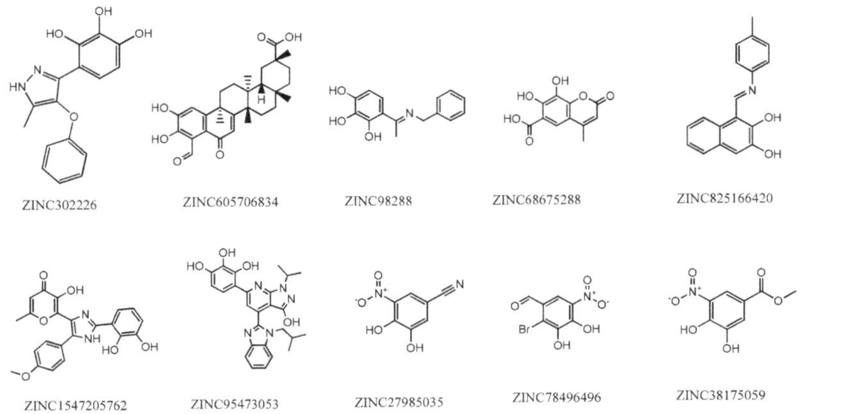

Figure 13. Structure and identification of the studied compounds.

Table 3. Estimated IC_{50} values (nM) for selected compounds with MBCOMT performed in this work in comparison with previous ones reported in the literature. Values are means with 95% confidence (n = 2 to 3).

Sample	Compound	IC50 (nM)	Reference
Recombinant SCOMT	3,5-DNC	13.26 (10.7 to 16.44)	[32]
	Entacapone	4.224 (2.949 to 6.050)	
Brain MBCOMT	Tolcapone	2 (1 to 2)	[33]
Liver MBCOMT	Tolcapone	123 (52 to 292)	
Liver SCOMT	Pyrazoline derivate	48	[34]
	Entacapone	230	
Recombinant MBCOMT	ZINC302226	1083 (879.9 to 1333)	This work
	ZINC98288	943.8 (816 to 1092)	
	ZINC825166420	1538 (1254 to 1888)	
	ZINC27985035	17.6 (13.53 to 22.96)	
	ZINC78496496	470 (401.4 to 550.4)	

2.6. Cytotoxicity Studies

The neuronal cytotoxicity is an important parameter to evaluate considering the target organ of action of anti-Parkinsonian agents, namely, for potential COMT inhibitors. Therefore, the effect of the selected compounds was evaluated against dopaminergic neuronal cells (N27) by the 3-(4,5-dimethylthiazol-2-yl)-2,5-diphenyltetrazolium bromide (MTT) colorimetric assay, as previously described [35]. To do so, the cells were exposed to different concentrations of the compounds during 48 h, and after the MTT assay (Supplementary Material Figures S1 and S2), their half maximal inhibitory concentrations (IC_{50}) were calculated by considering the data from concentration-response curves (Table 4). In addition, the cytotoxicity of these compounds to normal human dermal fibroblasts (NHDF) was also assessed by the same methodology to obtain further data on the in-vitro safety to non-tumoral cells existing outside of the CNS. The clinical drug 5-fluorouracil (5-FU) was included in the study for comparative purposes.

Table 4. Estimated IC_{50} values (μM) for selected compounds in dopaminergic neuronal (N27) and normal fibroblast (NHDF) cells [a].

Compound	N27	NHDF
ZINC302226	52.50	>100
ZINC98288	69.78	>100
ZINC825166420	16.98	12.14
ZINC27985035	61.26	40.31
ZINC78496496	>100	92.90
5-FU	4.28	5.16

[a] Cells were treated with different concentrations (0.1, 1, 10, 30, 50, and 100 μM) during 48 h. The cell proliferation effects were determined by the MTT assay. The data shown are representative of at least two independent experiments. 5-FU: 5-fluorouracil.

3. Discussion

Aiming to discover new compounds with potential interest in PD therapy, we employed a previously described crystal structure of SCOMT [28] to develop a pharmacophore to find potential new COMT inhibitors with higher selectivity to MBCOMT. Then, we used the pharmacophore developed to computationally find molecules of interest at the ZINC purchasable database. Next, the 100 best scored compounds achieved in this database search were evaluated for their drug-likeness properties and by molecular docking followed by an analysis of relevant ADMET parameters. Considering the results of these studies as well as commercial availability, 10 compounds were selected and acquired for further in-vitro studies, taking into account the obtained binding energy and the main interaction promoted with the target amino acids (Supplementary Material Table S2). Therefore, by a combination of in-silico structure- and ligand-based drug design strategies, new hit molecules were selected. In this context, it is important to mention that structural-based drug design tools are being widely used to predict the position and affinity of new molecules to the target protein with considerable accuracy and efficiency, among other studies [31]. Nevertheless, despite extensive in-silico studies, the in-vitro validation of the best predicted modeling results must be performed. To do so, we carried out experiments to evaluate the inhibition of MBCOMT activity (Table 3) as well as the cytotoxicity (Table 4) of the compounds with higher relevancy in dopaminergic and fibroblast cells, and we observed interesting results that are discussed below.

COMT inhibitors can be divided into the "first generation," associated with toxic properties and weak or nonselective activity, and the "second generation," with nitrocatecholic structure, which includes the inhibitors 3,5-dinitrocatechol (3,5-DNC), opicapone, nitecapone, nebicapone, entacapone, and tolcapone [36,37]. The last two proved to be potent COMT inhibitors with similar IC_{50}s of approximately 250 nM [36]. Although entacapone has been considered relatively safe, it only acts peripherally [10]. In contrast, tolcapone, the only commercial COMT inhibitor able to cross the BBB, is used with caution due to safety concerns regarding liver toxicity [38]. In this work, the MBCOMT inhibition potencies of the five selected compounds were determined based on the sigmoidal curve of dose vs. response drawn and expressed as IC_{50} values. As shown in Table 3, the majority of the tested compounds in this work presented an IC_{50} value below 1000 nM, with the compound ZINC825166420 presenting the highest IC_{50} (1538 nM), followed by ZINC302226. Although the compound ZINC302226 was computationally predicted to be the strongest inhibitor to be tested, it presented a relatively high IC_{50} value (1083 nM) compared to the reported values for entacapone or tolcapone [2,5,6]. On the other hand, the compounds ZINC98288, ZINC27985035, and ZINC78496496 had the lowest IC_{50} values (below 1 μM). In fact, the derivative ZINC27985035 presented the lowest IC_{50} value achieved (17.6 nM), similar to that determined for 3,5-DNC when the recombinant SCOMT was used. However, if we consider liver S- and MBCOMT as the protein source, the obtained value is much lower than those reported for both entacapone and tolcapone, which share structural similarities with ZINC27985035. A detailed analysis of the scientific literature also allowed for the identification of compounds with a structure similar to ZINC302226 [37] and ZINC78496496 [39] as COMT inhibitors. For the last one, the only difference was the presence a chlorine group instead of bromine. In addition, via a deep bibliographic search and analysis, we found that the compound ZINC27985035, the structure with the highest MBCOMT inhibition in our studies, has already been described as a COMT inhibitor [39,40]. Despite this, it is important to mention that the structural similarity of ZINC302226 and ZINC78496496 to previously described COMT inhibitors and that ZINC27985035 was already published as an inhibitor of this enzyme can be considered a support to our in-silico strategy applied to discovering new compounds targeting this enzyme. In addition, and more importantly, the inhibition studies performed for these three compounds were performed against the enzyme isolated from animal tissues and not for cell extracts of recombinant human MBCOMT. However, we did not find any information in the literature concerning the compounds ZINC98288 and ZINC825166420 as COMT inhibitors. Therefore, taking into account the results described in the present work and despite the inhibition levels observed in our assays and the need for more studies, especially at the in-vitro and in-vivo levels, we consider that these compounds may have potential interest in the context of PD and can be new skeletons for further exploration in the medicinal chemistry of COMT inhibitors.

Concerning the cytotoxicity (Table 4), overall, with the exception of ZINC825166420, it can be considered that the majority of the tested compounds did not exhibit relevant cytotoxicity in both cell lines. The lowest IC_{50} values were observed for 5-FU, as expected.

Therefore, these results can be of high interest, revealing a marked selectivity when considering the effects of the studied compounds on MBCOMT inhibition in comparison with their cytotoxicity.

Overall, considering the pros and cons of the existing commercial COMT inhibitors, with further structural optimization, pharmacokinetics, and bioavailability studies, these molecules could have potential to improve the day-to-day life of PD patients. However, more studies are needed to address this possibility.

4. Materials and Methods

4.1. Ligand Selection

From an initial set of 100 molecules with known COMT inhibitory properties, the 18 most promising compounds were selected to integrate into the study training set (Figure 1) [9]. This selection was carried out based on the compounds' structure and existing in-silico data regarding their interaction with COMT, including molecular docking and molecular dynamics interactions with the protein active site [29] and the ADMET (absorption, distribution, metabolism, excretion, and toxicity) property prevision, as well as their in-vitro and in-vivo COMT inhibitory potency and bioavailability [9]. The 18 selected most promising compounds, used as the training set, were drawn in ChemDraw (v. 12.0), and their conformational energies were minimized using the MM2 force field in Chem3D (v. 12.0) to improve the reliability of the obtained results. Moreover, the 3D protein structure determined by X-ray diffraction of human SCOMT (PDB#6I3C) was retrieved from the Protein Data Bank (PDB) [28]. This COMT structure was determined with an atomic resolution of 1.34 Å, contained 232 amino acids in a single chain, and was co-crystallized with the cofactors Mg^{2+}, SAM, and the inhibitor 3,5-DNC [28]. For this study, the computational 3D protein structure was prepared using Chimera (v. 1.13), removing the crystallographic water molecules, adding the hydrogen atoms, and minimizing the conformational energy using the Amber ff99SB force field of Chimera [41]. At this point, the structure was considered ready for protein–ligand docking.

4.2. Pharmacophore Generation

Furthermore, the ligands were aligned using the alignment perspective tool in LigandScout (v. 4.4), their key structural features were merged, and various pharmacophore models were generated based on their multi-conformer [42]. To do so, the FAST settings and the Pharmacophore RDF-Code Similarity algorithms were applied to obtain all the hypotheses [42]. Additionally, the pharmacophore fit, the number of omitted structures, and the atom overlaps were set to 4, limiting only the best scoring models for further studies and rejecting the remaining worst scored models [43].

4.3. Virtual Screening and ADMET Virtual Filtration

Next, the obtained models were submitted for screening as a 3D query in the ZINCPharmer search database (http://zincpharmer.csb.pitt.edu/, accessed on 14 September 2021), specifically the ZINC purchasable subsection from a training set with over 21,777,093 compounds [44]. This software provided the results based on the predicted binding affinity of the database ligands against the protein (PDB#6I3C) using docking algorithms. To filter the selection, only the ligands with all the desired structural moieties shared with the training set were considered hit molecules. Moreover, to enhance the possibilities of discovering potential new drug-like leads, the results were also subjected to a Lipinski's Rule of Five properties filter to improve the results obtained [45,46], analyzing the compounds' molecular weight, their logP, and the number of rotatable bonds and hydrogen bond acceptor/donor groups. From there, 100 hit molecules were selected to be further analyzed by molecular docking and to study their predicted ADMET properties to screen for potential false positive.

4.4. Molecular Docking

To further improve the reliability of the model, a redocking of the top 100 hit molecules was performed using the AutoDock Tools 4 software (v. 4.2.6) [47]. This study allowed for the screening of potential false positive hits, as well as to better understand the ligands' interactions with the COMT active site. The 3D grid box (x = 40; y = 40; z = 40) was optimized to fit all the study hits using a grid spacing of 0.375 Å and was centered in the protein active site, identified by the binding site of the inhibitor 3,5-DNC. The binding poses were generated using the Lamarckian genetic computational algorithm. The hits were ranked based on their binding energies and their binding free energy (ΔG), expressed in kcal/mol by the software, and their atomic interactions were further studied using the PMV (v. 1.5.6) tool and the Discovery Studios (v. 4.5) program to better visualize and identify the most important atomic interactions [29].

4.5. ADMET Property Analysis

The ADMET properties were predicted using the webserver pkCSM (http://biosig unimelb.edu.au/pkcsm/prediction, accessed on 3 October 2021) [48]. This server compares the data from approved FDA drugs and experimental compounds to predict the compounds' main pharmacokinetic features. These include the BBB and CNS permeability, the drug's potential human intestinal absorption, whether it is a P-glycoprotein substrate/inhibitor, and its hepatoxicity, among other properties used to filter potentially toxic drugs.

4.6. Materials, Reagents, and Solutions for In-Vitro Studies

Ultrapure reagent-grade water was obtained with a Milli-Q system (Milipore/Waters) Yeast nitrogen base (YNB), glucose, agar, yeast extract, peptone, glycerol, dithiotreitol (DTT), protease inhibitor cocktail, *S*-adenosyl-L-methionine (SAM), epinephrine (bitartrate salt), *DL*-methanephrine hydrochloride, citric acid monohydrate, and glass beads (500 µm) were purchased from Sigma Chemical Co. (St. Louis, MO, USA). The tested compounds ZINC302226, ZINC98288, ZINC825166420, ZINC27985035, and ZINC78496496 were purchased from MolPort (Riga, Latvia). All chemicals used were of analytical grade, commercially available, and used without further purification.

The five selected tested compounds (Table 5) to be studied were dissolved in DMSO in a final concentration of 10 mM and stored at 4 °C with protection from light. From this solution, several dilutions were prepared in order to obtain the final desired concentrations to be tested. The final DMSO concentrations used were 1% (cytotoxic assays) and 5% (enzymatic assays), concentrations with no significant effect on cytotoxicity studies and enzyme bioactivity, as previously tested (data not shown).

Table 5. Compounds and concentrations to be used in the in-vitro studies of enzymatic activity and cytotoxicity.

Compound	Concentrations for Cytotoxicity Assays (μM)	Concentrations for Bioactivity Assays (μM)
ZINC302226	0.1 to 100	0.125 to 10
ZINC98288		0.0315 to 10
ZINC 825166420		0.125 to 20
ZINC27985035		0.0078 to 0.5
ZINC78496496		0.125 to 10

4.7. *In-Vitro MBCOMT Inhibition Assays*

4.7.1. Biosynthesis and Recuperation of MBCOMT

The production of the human recombinant MBCOMT was performed according to the procedure described by Pedro et al. [49]. Briefly, transformed *Komagataella pastoris* X33 with the expression vector was grown for 72 h at 30 °C in yeast extract peptone dextrose (YPD) medium plates with 200 μg/mL of Zeocin. A single colony was inoculated in 100 mL of buffered minimal glycerol medium (BMGH) in 500 mL shake flasks. Cells were grown at 30 °C and 250 rpm to a cell density of 600 nm (OD_{600}) of 6.0 units. Afterwards, an aliquot was introduced into 100 mL of buffered minimal methanol medium (BMMH) in 500 mL shake flasks, with an initial OD_{600} fixed to 1.0 unit. After 24 h of growth at 30 °C and 250 rpm, cells were collected by centrifugation (1500× *g*, 10 min, 4 °C). The cells were resuspended in lysis buffer (150 mmol L^{-1} NaCl, 10 mmol L^{-1} DTT, 50 mmol L^{-1} Tris, 1 mmol L^{-1} $MgCl_2$, pH 8.0) supplemented with protease inhibitor cocktail. Then, a mechanical treatment with glass beads (7 cycles of vortexing for 1 min with 1 min of interval on ice) was applied to disrupt the cells. Cell suspensions were centrifuged (500× *g*, 5 min, 4 °C). The supernatant was removed, and the pellet obtained was resuspended in the same lysis buffer, without DTT. The samples were stored at 4 °C until use for further assays.

4.7.2. MBCOMT Enzymatic Assay

The methylation efficiency of MBCOMT, alone or in the presence of the tested compounds, was evaluated by the amount of metanephrine converted from the substrate epinephrine, as described by Vieira-Coelho and Soares-da-Silva, with minor alterations [33]. Briefly, MBCOMT lysates with a fixed concentration of 1 mg/mL were preincubated at 37 °C for 20 min with increasing concentrations of the selected tested compounds (Table 5) before the addition of the substrate epinephrine (after 15 min) in the presence of SAM, EGTA, and sodium phosphate buffer (pH 7.8). The reaction was then stopped with 2 M of perchloric acid. After 1 h at 4 °C, samples were centrifuged (6000 rpm, 10 min, 4 °C) and the supernatant was filtered through a 0.22 μm cellulose acetate pore filter. The metanephrine levels in the sample were determined by HPLC with coulometric detection, as previously described [50]. All data analysis was performed using Prism 6 (GraphPad Software Inc. San Diego, CA, USA).

4.8. Cytotoxicity Studies

4.8.1. Cell Cultures

The cell lines used were normal human dermal fibroblasts (NHDF) and an N27 rat dopaminergic neural cell line (N27), both obtained from American Type Culture Collection (ATCC). The cultures were performed in 75 cm^3 culture flasks in an incubator at 37 °C under a humidified atmosphere with 5% carbon dioxide. The NHDF cell line was cultured in Roswell Park Memorial Institute (RPMI) 1640 culture medium (Sigma Aldrich, St. Louis, MO, USA) supplemented with 10% fetal bovine serum (FBS), 2 mM of *L*-glutamine, 10 mM of HEPES, 1 mM of sodium pyruvate, and 1% antibiotic Ab (Sigma Aldrich; 10,000 U/mL of penicillin G, 100 mg/mL of streptomycin, and 25 µg/mL of amphotericin B). The N27 cell line was cultured in RPMI 1640 culture medium with 10% FBS, 2 mM of *L*-glutamine, and 1% antibiotic Sp (Sigma Aldrich; 10,000 U/mL of penicillin G, 100 mg/mL of streptomycin). The medium was renewed every 2–3 days for NHDF and every day for N27 until cell confluence was 90–95%. Then, cells were incubated for 2–3 min with a solution of trypsin (0.5 g/L trypsin with 0.02 g/L of ethylene diamine tetra-acetic acid (EDTA)) to detach cells from the bottom of the culture flask. Afterwards, the suspension of cells in trypsin solution was diluted with an appropriate medium and centrifuged for 5 min at 125 G. Then, cells were counted by Trypan-blue exclusion method using a Neubauer chamber, resuspended, and seeded at 2×10^4 cells/mL density in 96-well culture plates (VWR) with a volume of 100 µL per well. The cells were kept in culture for a period of 48 h for cell adherence and growth before cytotoxicity studies.

4.8.2. MTT Assay

The cytotoxicity was assessed by the 3-(4,5-dimethylthiazol-2-yl)-2,5-diphenyltetrazolium bromide (MTT) colorimetric assay, performed as previously described [51]. For this, after adherence and growth, cells were exposed during 48 h to the compounds under study as well as 5-fluorouracil (5-FU; positive control) at different concentrations (0.1, 1, 10, 30, 50, and 100 µM) for dose-response studies. These solutions were prepared from stock solutions at 10 mM in DMSO by dilution in the appropriate cell culture medium. Then, the experimental medium was replaced with 100 µL per well of an MTT solution (1 mg/mL of MTT concentration, 20% phosphate buffer saline (PBS), and 80% culture medium without FBS and antibiotics). After 4 h of incubation, the MTT solution was replaced by DMSO to solubilize formazan crystals. The absorbance of each well was measured at 570 nm using a microplate spectrophotometer Bio-Rad xMark. The results are expressed as relative cell viability (%) normalized to negative control and considering standard deviation. At least two independent assays in quadruplicate were performed for each stimulus. Differences between treatments were analyzed with Student's *t*-test and the results were considered statistically significant when the p-value < 0.05. Half maximal inhibitory concentrations (IC_{50}) were determined through sigmoidal dose-response curve fit considering a 95% confidence interval.

5. Conclusions

PD is the second most common neurodegenerative disorder, and in most situations its cause is unknown. Its prevalence is between 100 and 300/100,000 inhabitants, and the number of PD patients is expected to double by 2030 [52]. The search for new drugs that improve the patient's quality of life and prevent the progression of the disease is ceaseless on the part of the pharmaceutical industry. The advantage of the use of computational chemistry in comparison with experimental laboratory methods is that it reduces expenses derived from the purchase of materials as well as the production of polluting compounds, and allows the research process to be accelerated, for example, in the preclinical stages of drug development. In the present work, a set of molecules with potential interest in PD acting as COMT inhibitors was discovered through a computational-based approach. The five selected molecules for in-vitro studies revealed relevant and selective MBCOMT inhibitory effects. In addition, cytotoxicity evaluation in dopaminergic (N27) and fibroblast

(NHDF) cells evidenced that selected hits have relatively low toxicity. Within this group, the best results were observed for the compound ZINC27985035, with an IC_{50} of 17.6 nM determined for MBCOMT inhibition and low cytotoxicity observed in both cell lines (61.26 and 40.31 μM, respectively). Despite this compound having been previously described as a COMT inhibitor, no studies have been performed on membrane COMT isoform. In addition, the other four selected compounds have not been previously studied against this target to our knowledge, which can open new medicinal chemistry possibilities in the design of new COMT inhibitors. The relevant results obtained, combined with the similarity in structure to the commercial COMT inhibitor entacapone, may allow the future development of potential new drug candidates for PD with improved properties.

Supplementary Materials: The following supporting information can be downloaded at: https://www.mdpi.com/article/10.3390/ph15010051/s1. Table S1. Characteristics of the studied compounds; Table S2. Virtual screening results of the hit molecules obtained in ZINCPharmer; Table S3. Results of in vitro MBCOMT inhibition evaluation of the 10 best scored selected compounds by in silico studies; Figure S1. Graphics of concentration-response studies in dopaminergic N27 cell line; Figure S2. Graphics of concentration-response studies in normal human dermal fibroblasts (NHDF).

Author Contributions: Conceptualization, S.S., L.A.P. and E.G. sample preparation, P.C.-V., A.M.G. and O.F.; methodology, P.C.-V., A.M.G. and O.F.; pharmacophore modeling and molecular docking analysis, P.C.-V.; chromatographic analysis, in-vitro assays, and data, A.M.G. and O.F.; formal analysis, P.C.-V., A.M.G., O.F.; J.A.Q., S.S., L.A.P. and E.G.; investigation, P.C.-V., A.M.G., O.F., J.A.Q., S.S., L.A.P. and E.G.; writing—original draft preparation, P.C.-V., A.M.G. and O.F.; writing—review and editing, P.C.-V., A.M.G., O.F.; S.S., L.A.P. and E.G.; supervision, S.S., L.A.P. and E.G.; funding acquisition, S.S., L.A.P. and E.G. All authors have read and agreed to the published version of the manuscript.

Funding: This work is part of the project "Design of new Catechol-O-methyltransferase inhibitors with therapeutic potential for diseases of the central nervous system—Project Centro-01-0145-FEDER-000019—C4—Centro de Competências em Cloud Computing" supported by the European Regional Development Fund through the "Programa Operacional Regional do Centro (Centro 2020)—Sistema de Apoio à Investigação Científica e Tecnológica—Programas Integrados de IC&DT (Covilhã)." This work was developed within the scope of the CICS-UBI projects UIDB/00709/2020 and UIDP/00709/2020, and financed by national funds through the Portuguese Foundation for Science and Technology (FCT)/MCTES. It was also supported by the Applied Molecular Biosciences Unit UCIBIO (UIDB/04378/2020 and UIDP/04378/2020) and the Associate Laboratory Institute for Health and Bioeconomy—i4HB (project LA/P/0140/2020), which are financed by national funds from FCT/MCTES. Ana Margarida Gonçalves and Octávio Ferreira acknowledge the PhD fellowships from FCT (SFRH/BD/147519/2019 and SFRH/BD/141900/2018, respectively).

Institutional Review Board Statement: Not applicable.

Informed Consent Statement: Not applicable.

Data Availability Statement: Data is contained within the article.

Conflicts of Interest: The authors declare no conflict of interest.

References

1. Dong, J.; Cui, Y.; Li, S.; Le, W. Current Pharmaceutical Treatments and Alternative Therapies of Parkinson's Disease. *Curr. Neuropharmacol.* **2016**, *14*, 339–355. [CrossRef]
2. Jankovic, J.; Tan, E.K. Parkinson's disease: Etiopathogenesis and treatment. *J. Neurol. Neurosurg. Psychiatry* **2020**, *91*, 795–808. [CrossRef]
3. McFarthing, K.; Buff, S.; Rafaloff, G.; Dominey, T.; Wyse, R.K.; Stott, S.R.W. Parkinson's Disease Drug Therapies in the Clinical Trial Pipeline: 2020. *J. Parkinsons Dis.* **2020**, *10*, 757–774. [CrossRef] [PubMed]
4. Axelrod, J.; Tomchick, R. Enzymatic O-methylation of epinephrine and other catechols. *J. Biol. Chem.* **1958**, *233*, 702–705. [CrossRef]
5. Guldberg, H.C.; Marsden, C.A. Catechol-O-Methyl Transferase: Pharmacological Aspects and Physiological Role. *Pharmacol. Rev.* **1975**, *27*, 135–206.

6. Chen, J.; Lipska, B.K.; Halim, N.; Ma, Q.D.; Matsumoto, M.; Melhem, S.; Kolachana, B.S.; Hyde, T.M.; Herman, M.M.; Apud, J.; et al. Functional analysis of genetic variation in catechol-O-methyltransferase (COMT): Effects on mRNA, protein, and enzyme activity in postmortem human brain. *Am. J. Hum. Genet.* **2004**, *75*, 807–821. [CrossRef]
7. Schott, B.; Frischknecht, R.; Debska-Vielhaber, G.; John, N.; Behnisch, G.; Düzel, E.; Gundelfinger, E.; Seidenbecher, C. Membrane-Bound Catechol-O-Methyl Transferase in Cortical Neurons and Glial Cells is Intracellularly Oriented. *Front. Psychiatry* **2010**, *1*, 142. [CrossRef]
8. Bonifácio, M.J.; Palma, P.N.; Almeida, L.; Soares-da-Silva, P. Catechol-O-methyltransferase and its inhibitors in Parkinson's disease. *CNS Drug Rev.* **2007**, *13*, 352–379. [CrossRef]
9. Kiss, L.E.; Soares-da-Silva, P. Medicinal chemistry of catechol O-methyltransferase (COMT) inhibitors and their therapeutic utility. *J. Med. Chem.* **2014**, *57*, 8692–8717. [CrossRef]
10. Najib, J. Entacapone: A catechol-O-methyltransferase inhibitor for the adjunctive treatment of Parkinson's disease. *Clin. Ther.* **2001**, *23*, 802–832. [CrossRef]
11. Vokurka, P.; Barron, A.; Sumaria, S.; Stockford, L.; Jarman, P.; Bhatia, K.; Farmer, S.; Saifee, T.; Warner, T.; Weil, R.; et al. Opicapone Efficacy and Tolerability in Parkinson's Disease Patients Reporting Insufficient Benefit/Failure of Entacapone. *Mov. Disord. Clin. Pract.* **2020**, *7*, 955–960. [CrossRef]
12. Vidgren, J. X-ray crystallography of catechol O-methyltransferase: Perspectives for target-based drug development. *Adv. Pharmaco.* **1998**, *42*, 328–331.
13. Vidgren, J.; Svensson, L.A.; Liljas, A. Crystal structure of catechol O-methyltransferase. *Nature* **1994**, *368*, 354–358. [CrossRef]
14. Lautala, P.; Ulmanen, I.; Taskinen, J. Molecular mechanisms controlling the rate and specificity of catechol O-methylation by human soluble catechol O-methyltransferase. *Mol. Pharmacol.* **2001**, *59*, 393–402. [CrossRef]
15. Chen, D.; Wang, C.Y.; Lambert, J.D.; Ai, N.; Welsh, W.J.; Yang, C.S. Inhibition of human liver catechol-O-methyltransferase by tea catechins and their metabolites: Structure-activity relationship and molecular-modeling studies. *Biochem. Pharmacol.* **2005**, *69*, 1523–1531. [CrossRef] [PubMed]
16. Cao, Y.; Chen, Z.J.; Jiang, H.D.; Chen, J.Z. Computational studies of the regioselectivities of COMT-catalyzed meta-/para-O methylations of luteolin and quercetin. *J. Phys. Chem. B* **2014**, *118*, 470–481. [CrossRef]
17. Monteiro, A.F.M.; Viana, J.O.; Nayarisseri, A.; Zondegoumba, E.N.; Mendonça Junior, F.J.B.; Scotti, M.T.; Scotti, L. Computational Studies Applied to Flavonoids against Alzheimer's and Parkinson's Diseases. *Oxidative Med. Cell. Longev.* **2018**, *2018*, 7912765. [CrossRef]
18. Palma, P.N.; Bonifácio, M.J.; Loureiro, A.I.; Wright, L.C.; Learmonth, D.A.; Soares-da-Silva, P. Molecular modeling and metabolic studies of the interaction of catechol-O-methyltransferase and a new nitrocatechol inhibitor. *Drug Metab. Dispos.* **2003**, *31*, 250–258. [CrossRef]
19. Palma, P.N.; Rodrigues, M.L.; Archer, M.; Bonifácio, M.J.; Loureiro, A.I.; Learmonth, D.A.; Carrondo, M.A.; Soares-da-Silva, P. Comparative study of ortho- and meta-nitrated inhibitors of catechol-O-methyltransferase: Interactions with the active site and regioselectivity of O-methylation. *Mol. Pharmacol.* **2006**, *70*, 143–153. [CrossRef] [PubMed]
20. Moschovou, K.; Melagraki, G.; Mavromoustakos, T.; Zacharia, L.C.; Afantitis, A. Cheminformatics and virtual screening studies of COMT inhibitors as potential Parkinson's disease therapeutics. *Expert Opin.Drug Discov.* **2020**, *15*, 53–62. [CrossRef]
21. Lerner, C.; Ruf, A.; Gramlich, V.; Masjost, B.; Zürcher, G.; Jakob-Roetne, R.; Borroni, E.; Diederich, F. X-ray Crystal Structure of a Bisubstrate Inhibitor Bound to the Enzyme Catechol-O-methyltransferase: A Dramatic Effect of Inhibitor Preorganization on Binding Affinity We thank F. Hoffmann-La Roche for generous support of this work. We are grateful to P. Malherbe for the cloning of COMT, P. Caspers for the expression of COMT, A. Cesura for enzyme purification, B. Wipf for fermentation, and H. W. Lahm for sequencing. *Angew. Chem. Int. Ed. Engl.* **2001**, *40*, 4040–4042.
22. Paulini, R.; Lerner, C.; Jakob-Roetne, R.; Zürcher, G.; Borroni, E.; Diederich, F. Bisubstrate inhibitors of the enzyme catechol O-methyltransferase (COMT): Efficient inhibition despite the lack of a nitro group. *Chembiochem* **2004**, *5*, 1270–1274. [CrossRef]
23. Lee, J.Y.; Kim, Y.M. Comparative Homology Modeling and Ligand Docking Study of Human Catechol-O-Methyltransferase for Antiparkinson Drug Design. *Bull. Korean Chem. Soc.* **2005**, *26*, 1695–1700. [CrossRef]
24. Ellermann, M.; Jakob-Roetne, R.; Lerner, C.; Borroni, E.; Schlatter, D.; Roth, D.; Ehler, A.; Rudolph, M.G.; Diederich, F. Molecular recognition at the active site of catechol-o-methyltransferase: Energetically favorable replacement of a water molecule imported by a bisubstrate inhibitor. Angew. *Chem. Int. Ed. Engl.* **2009**, *48*, 9092–9096. [CrossRef] [PubMed]
25. Ellermann, M.; Paulini, R.; Jakob-Roetne, R.; Lerner, C.; Borroni, E.; Roth, D.; Ehler, A.; Schweizer, W.B.; Schlatter, D.; Rudolph, M.G.; et al. Molecular recognition at the active site of catechol-O-methyltransferase (COMT): Adenine replacements in bisubstrate inhibitors. *Chemistry* **2011**, *17*, 6369–6381. [CrossRef] [PubMed]
26. Deb, S.; Phukan, B.C.; Mazumder, M.K.; Dutta, A.; Paul, R.; Bhattacharya, P.; Sandhir, R.; Borah, A. Garcinol, a multifaceted sword for the treatment of Parkinson's disease. *Neurochem. Int.* **2019**, *128*, 50–57. [CrossRef]
27. Jatana, N.; Sharma, A.; Latha, N. Pharmacophore modeling and virtual screening studies to design potential COMT inhibitors as new leads. *J. Mol. Graph. Model.* **2013**, *39*, 145–164. [CrossRef] [PubMed]
28. Czarnota, S.; Johannissen, L.O.; Baxter, N.J.; Rummel, F.; Wilson, A.L.; Cliff, M.J.; Levy, C.W.; Scrutton, N.S.; Waltho, J.P.; Hay, S. Equatorial Active Site Compaction and Electrostatic Reorganization in Catechol-O-methyltransferase. *ACS Catal.* **2019**, *9*, 4394–4401. [CrossRef]

29. Cruz-Vicente, P.; Passarinha, L.A.; Silvestre, S.; Gallardo, E. Recent Developments in New Therapeutic Agents against Alzheimer and Parkinson Diseases: In-Silico Approaches. *Molecules* **2021**, *26*, 2193. [CrossRef]
30. Ma, Z.; Liu, H.; Wu, B. Structure-based drug design of catechol-O-methyltransferase inhibitors for CNS disorders. *Br. J. Clin. Pharmacol.* **2014**, *77*, 410–420. [CrossRef]
31. Wang, X.; Song, K.; Li, L.; Chen, L. Structure-Based Drug Design Strategies and Challenges. *Curr. Top. Med.Chem.* **2018**, *18*, 998–1006. [CrossRef] [PubMed]
32. Pedro, A.Q.; Correia, F.F.; Santos, F.M.; Espírito-Santo, G.; Gonçalves, A.M.; Bonifácio, M.J.; Queiroz, J.A.; Passarinha, L.A. Biosynthesis and purification of histidine-tagged human soluble catechol-O-methyltransferase. *J. Chem. Technol. Biotechnol.* **2016**, *91*, 3035–3044. [CrossRef]
33. Vieira-Coelho, M.A.; Soares-da-Silva, P. Effects of tolcapone upon soluble and membrane-bound brain and liver catechol-O-methyltransferase. *Brain Res.* **1999**, *821*, 69–78. [CrossRef]
34. Hitge, R.; Smit, S.; Petzer, A.; Petzer, J.P. Evaluation of nitrocatechol chalcone and pyrazoline derivatives as inhibitors of catechol-O-methyltransferase and monoamine oxidase. *Bioorg. Med. Chem. Lett.* **2020**, *30*, 127188. [CrossRef]
35. Matias, M.; Campos, G.; Silvestre, S.; Falcão, A.; Alves, G. Early preclinical evaluation of dihydropyrimidin(thi)ones as potential anticonvulsant drug candidates. *Eur. J. Pharm. Sci.* **2017**, *102*, 264–274. [CrossRef]
36. Haasio, K. Toxicology and safety of COMT inhibitors. *Int. Rev. Neurobiol.* **2010**, *95*, 163–189.
37. Kiss, L.E.; Ferreira, H.S.; Torrão, L.; Bonifácio, M.J.; Palma, P.N.; Soares-da-Silva, P.; Learmonth, D.A. Discovery of a long-acting, peripherally selective inhibitor of catechol-O-methyltransferase. *J. Med. Chem.* **2010**, *53*, 3396–3411. [CrossRef]
38. Antonini, A.; Abbruzzese, G.; Barone, P.; Bonuccelli, U.; Lopiano, L.; Onofrj, M.; Zappia, M.; Quattrone, A. COMT inhibition with tolcapone in the treatment algorithm of patients with Parkinson's disease (PD): Relevance for motor and non-motor features. *Neuropsychiatr. Dis. Treat.* **2008**, *4*, 1–9. [CrossRef]
39. Borgulya, J.; Bruderer, H.; Bernauer, K.; Zürcher, G.; Prada, M.D. Catechol-O-methyltransferase-inhibiting pyrocatechol derivatives: Synthesis and structure-activity studies. *Helv. Chim. Acta* **1989**, *72*, 952–968. [CrossRef]
40. Backstrom, R.; Honkanen, E.; Pippuri, A.; Kairisalo, P.; Pystynen, J.; Heinola, K.; Nissinen, E.; Linden, I.B.; Mannisto, P.T. Synthesis of some novel potent and selective catechol O-methyltransferase inhibitors. *J. Med. Chem.* **1989**, *32*, 841–846. [CrossRef]
41. Pettersen, E.F.; Goddard, T.D.; Huang, C.C.; Couch, G.S.; Greenblatt, D.M.; Meng, E.C.; Ferrin, T.E. UCSF Chimera–a visualization system for exploratory research and analysis. *J. Comput. Chem.* **2004**, *25*, 1605–1612. [CrossRef]
42. Wolber, G.; Langer, T. LigandScout: 3-D pharmacophores derived from protein-bound ligands and their use as virtual screening filters. *J. Chem. Inf. Modeling* **2005**, *45*, 160–169. [CrossRef]
43. Chen, Z.; Li, H.L.; Zhang, Q.J.; Bao, X.G.; Yu, K.Q.; Luo, X.M.; Zhu, W.L.; Jiang, H.L. Pharmacophore-based virtual screening versus docking-based virtual screening: A benchmark comparison against eight targets. *Acta Pharmacol. Sin.* **2009**, *30*, 1694–1708. [CrossRef]
44. Irwin, J.J.; Sterling, T.; Mysinger, M.M.; Bolstad, E.S.; Coleman, R.G. ZINC: A free tool to discover chemistry for biology. *J. Chem. Inf. Modeling* **2012**, *52*, 1757–1768. [CrossRef] [PubMed]
45. Lipinski, C.A. Lead- and drug-like compounds: The rule-of-five revolution. *Drug Discov. Today Technol.* **2004**, *1*, 337–341. [CrossRef] [PubMed]
46. Lipinski, C.A. Rule of five in 2015 and beyond: Target and ligand structural limitations, ligand chemistry structure and drug discovery project decisions. *Adv. Drug Deliv. Rev.* **2016**, *101*, 34–41. [CrossRef]
47. Morris, G.M.; Huey, R.; Lindstrom, W.; Sanner, M.F.; Belew, R.K.; Goodsell, D.S.; Olson, A.J. AutoDock4 and AutoDockTools4: Automated docking with selective receptor flexibility. *J. Comput. Chem.* **2009**, *30*, 2785–2791. [CrossRef] [PubMed]
48. Pires, D.E.; Blundell, T.L.; Ascher, D.B. pkCSM: Predicting Small-Molecule Pharmacokinetic and Toxicity Properties Using Graph-Based Signatures. *J. Med. Chem.* **2015**, *58*, 4066–4072. [CrossRef] [PubMed]
49. Pedro, A.Q.; Oppolzer, D.J.; Bonifácio, M.J.; Maia, C.J.; Queiroz, J.A.; Passarinha, L.A. Evaluation of MutS and Mut+Pichia pastoris Strains for Membrane-Bound Catechol-O-Methyltransferase Biosynthesis. *Appl. Biochem. Biotechnol.* **2015**, *175*, 3840–3855. [CrossRef]
50. Pedro, A.Q.; Rf, S.; Oppolzer, D.J.; Santos, F.M.; La, R.; Gonçalves, A.M.; Bonifácio, M.J.; Queiroz, J.A.; Gallardo, E.; Passarinha, L.A. An Improved HPLC Method for Quantification of Metanephrine with Coulometric Detection. *J. Chromatogr. Sep. Tech.* **2014**, *5*, 17–24.
51. Canário, C.; Matias, M.; Brito, V.; Santos, A.O.; Falcão, A.; Silvestre, S.; Alves, G. New Estrone Oxime Derivatives: Synthesis, Cytotoxic Evaluation and Docking Studies. *Molecules* **2021**, *26*, 2687. [CrossRef] [PubMed]
52. Elbaz, A.; Carcaillon, L.; Kab, S.; Moisan, F. Epidemiology of Parkinson's disease. *Rev. Neurol.* **2016**, *172*, 14–26. [CrossRef] [PubMed]

pharmaceuticals

MDPI

Article

Unravelling the Interaction of Piperlongumine with the Nucleotide-Binding Domain of HSP70: A Spectroscopic and In Silico Study

Ana Paula Ribeiro Povinelli [1], Gabriel Zazeri [1], Alan M. Jones [2,*] and Marinônio Lopes Cornélio [1,*]

[1] Departamento de Física, Instituto de Biociências, Letras e Ciências Exatas (IBILCE), Universidade Estadual Paulista (UNESP), Rua Cristovão Colombo 2265, São José do Rio Preto 15054-000, Brazil; ana.povinelli@unesp.br (A.P.R.P.); gabriel.zazeri@unesp.br (G.Z.)

[2] School of Pharmacy, University of Birmingham, Edgbaston, Birmingham B15 2TT, UK

* Correspondence: a.m.jones.2@bham.ac.uk (A.M.J.); m.cornelio@unesp.br (M.L.C.)

Abstract: Piperlongumine (PPL) is an alkaloid extracted from several pepper species that exhibits anti-inflammatory and anti-carcinogenic properties. Nevertheless, the molecular mode of action of PPL that confers such powerful pharmacological properties remains unknown. From this perspective, spectroscopic methods aided by computational modeling were employed to characterize the interaction between PPL and nucleotide-binding domain of heat shock protein 70 (NBD/HSP70), which is involved in the pathogenesis of several diseases. Steady-state fluorescence spectroscopy along with time-resolved fluorescence revealed the complex formation based on a static quenching mechanism. Van't Hoff analyses showed that the binding of PPL toward NBD is driven by equivalent contributions of entropic and enthalpic factors. Furthermore, IDF and Scatchard methods applied to fluorescence intensities determined two cooperative binding sites with K_b of $(6.3 \pm 0.2) \times 10^4\ M^{-1}$. Circular dichroism determined the thermal stability of the NBD domain and showed that PPL caused minor changes in the protein secondary structure. Computational simulations elucidated the microenvironment of these interactions, showing that the binding sites are composed mainly of polar amino acids and the predominant interaction of PPL with NBD is Van der Waals in nature.

Keywords: heat shock protein; HSP70; nucleotide-binding domain; piperlongumine; fluorescence spectroscopy; circular dichroism; molecular docking; molecular dynamics; molecular mechanics Poisson–Boltzmann surface area

Citation: Povinelli, A.P.R.; Zazeri, G.; Jones, A.M.; Cornélio, M.L. Unravelling the Interaction of Piperlongumine with the Nucleotide-Binding Domain of HSP70: A Spectroscopic and In Silico Study. *Pharmaceuticals* **2021**, *14*, 1298. https://doi.org/10.3390/ph14121298

Academic Editor: Osvaldo Andrade Santos-Filho

Received: 17 November 2021
Accepted: 7 December 2021
Published: 13 December 2021

1. Introduction

Living organisms, regardless of their kingdom, are constantly subjected to stressful situations and respond to these stimuli through changes in cellular metabolism, activating their defence mechanisms [1]. The stress response includes heat shock proteins (HSPs), which is one of the primary cellular protection responses [2,3].

HSPs are part of the large family of proteins known as molecular chaperones, so called because they have the ability to interact reversibly with other proteins, helping in formation, folding and trans-membrane transport [4]. HSP70 is the 70 kDa heat shock protein, composed of a conserved N-terminal nucleotide binding domain (NBD) with ATPase activity, a substrate binding domain (SBD) and a C-terminal domain. Among the domains, NBD is a 40 kDa ATP binding domain [5] with a highly flexible chain.

The HSP70 was found to be over expressed in various cancers in response to the stressful environment of tumors, leading to tumor protection and consequently to therapeutic resistance. Recently, the set of functions of heat shock proteins (HSP) has been extended based on studies that have shown that HSP70 is also found in the extracellular environment and exhibits potent cytokine activity, with the ability to activate the nuclear factor-kappaB (NF-κB) and consequently regulate the expression of pro-inflammatory cytokines [6–8]. Due to the involvement of HSP70 in the pathogenesis of several diseases, this macromolecule has become a potential molecular target for the development of pharmacotherapies [9]. Much effort has been dedicated to the search for small ligands that are able to inhibit the chaperone function of HSP70, mostly through the interaction with ADP binding site [5,10]. However, to the best of our knowledge the decrease of HSP70 inflammatory activity due to the binding of small ligands has not been investigated.

Piperlongumine (PPL) is a small molecule that has been reported to have a multitude of biological activities such as anti-inflammatory, anti-carcinogenic, anti-atherosclerotic, amongst others [11–14]. PPL is an alkaloid isolated from long pepper that is widely used in Indian traditional medicine [15,16]. This molecule is characterized by the presence of electrophilic motifs [12] including an α,β-unsaturated amide acting as a Michael acceptor (inset of Figure 1) [17]. As a potential drug scaffold, PPL has no Lipinski or lead-like rule violations [18]. Biological studies have shown that the anti-inflammatory and anti-carcinogenic activities of PPL are a consequence of the inhibition of NF-κB pathway [17,19–21]. However, to the best of our knowledge there are no studies to date regarding the molecular interaction of PPL and NBD/HSP70.

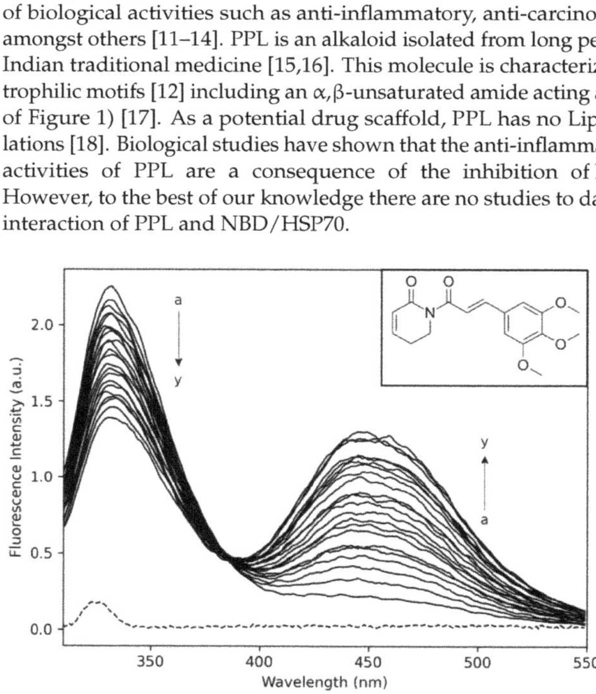

Figure 1. NBD fluorescence emission spectra obtained from titration experiments with increments in the concentration of PPL (pH 7.4, T = 283 K, $\lambda_{excitation}$ = 295 nm). [*NBD*] = 4.0 μM; PPL titrations with increments of −1.0 μM (a → y = 0 μM → 24 μM). Inset: Chemical structure of PPL.

In the present work we bring a detailed biophysical characterization of the interaction of PPL with NBD to support further drug discovery efforts. The experimental characterization is based on multi-pronged spectroscopic approaches. Fluorescence and circular dichroism spectroscopy were employed to disclose the number of binding sites, the mode of binding, the binding affinity, the thermodynamic parameters of interaction and the protein conformational changes due to these interactions. To have a complete description of the complex, molecular docking and dynamics parameterized by experimental results were employed to predict the binding sites and to disclose the molecular interactions in the microenvironments.

2. Results and Discussion

2.1. Fluorescence Spectroscopy

Figure 1 shows the fluorescence emission spectra of Trp90 NBD domain at 330 nm in the absence (a) and the presence of PPL (→y). Furthermore, Figure 1 shows PPL fluorescence emission band at 450 nm while the molecule was added to the solution (→y) The full-width half maximum (FWHM) of ±30 nm for the band of Trp90 and ±45 nm for the band of PPL showed that PPL fluorescence emission intensity did not influence NBD fluorescence emission spectra intensity, which allows for further analyses of the quenching mechanism. The interaction of NBD with PPL was monitored following the intensity of Trp90 emission spectra at 330 nm. Analysis of the spectra revealed the NBD fluorescence was quenched with the addition of PPL in the sample, demonstrating the existence of the quenching effect upon the Trp90 emission.

The quenching mechanism may be classified as dynamic (diffusive encounters) or static (complex formation) processes. It is possible to differentiate them by analysing the dependence of Stern–Volmer constant (K_{SV}) with temperature (Equation (1)) [22]. In general terms, static quenching reflects a decrease in K_{SV} with the increase in temperature, while dynamic quenching may provoke an increase in K_{SV} with the increase in temperature. Another method to determine the quenching mechanism involves comparing the ratio of fluorescence signals (F_0/F) with the ratio of the lifetime values (τ_0/τ). For dynamic quenching, the relation $F_0/F = \tau_0/\tau$ has to be observed for the system, otherwise collisions are not observed and the quenching is static [23]. The analysis of the bimolecular quenching rate constant (k_q) is another method that can also be used to confirm the quenching mechanism. To have the system ruled by collisions (dynamic quenching), the bimolecular constant cannot exceed the limit of 10^{10} $M^{-1}{\cdot}s^{-1}$ [23].

$$\frac{F_0}{F} = 1 + K_{SV}{\cdot}[PPL] = 1 + k_q{\cdot}\tau_0{\cdot}[PPL] \quad (1)$$

The Stern–Volmer plots (Figure 2) presented a linear response to the increment of PPL concentration. At temperatures 283 K, 293 K and 303 K, the K_{SV} constant showed a noticeable decrease by the drop in slope of the linear regression, which is strong evidence of the static quenching process [24]. The quenching mechanism obtained by steady-state fluorescence results was confirmed by time-resolved experiments as a second experimental method. In this experiment, the NBD tryptophan lifetime of excited states were measured in the absence (τ_0) and presence (τ) of different concentrations of PPL (Figure S1 and Table S1). The ratio (τ_0/τ) of fluorescence lifetime, plotted at the right ordinate of Figure 2, remained close to unity and did not present equivalence with F_0/F, which indicated that PPL poorly affects the NBD tryptophan fluorescence lifetime and confirms that the quenching mechanism is static [22]. To further confirm this result, the values of bimolecular constants k_q were calculated, all k_q are in the order of magnitude of 10^{12} $M^{-1}{\cdot}s^{-1}$ which exceeded the limit of 10^{10} $M^{-1}{\cdot}s^{-1}$ observed for dynamic quenching. In conclusion, these results characterize the quenching mechanism as static, which means that a complex has been formed by the PPL and NBD.

Table 1 shows the data for the Stern–Volmer constants and the bimolecular constant at different temperatures.

Table 1. Stern–Volmer constant (K_{SV}), bimolecular constants (k_q) and binding constant (K_a) for the complex NBD and PPL at 283, 293 and 303 K.

T (K)	K_{SV} ($\times 10^4$ M^{-1})	K_q ($\times 10^{12}$ $M^{-1}{\cdot}s^{-1}$)	K_a ($\times 10^4$ M^{-1})
283	1.9 ± 0.1	8.9 ± 0.1	2.5 ± 0.8
293	1.5 ± 0.1	6.9 ± 0.1	2.2 ± 0.5
303	1.0 ± 0.1	4.3 ± 0.1	1.8 ± 0.2

Once it was determined that a complex formation occurred, the association constant also known as binding constant (K_a) was calculated. The variables K_a were obtained by linearizing the function of the plot of Figure 3 using the double-logarithm equation (Equation (2)) that relates the quenching fluorescence intensities to the total concentration of PPL.

$$log\left(\frac{F_0 - F}{F}\right) = n{\cdot}log\ K_a - n{\cdot}log\left(\frac{1}{[PPL] - \left(\frac{F_0 - F}{F_0}\right){\cdot}[NBD]}\right) \quad (2)$$

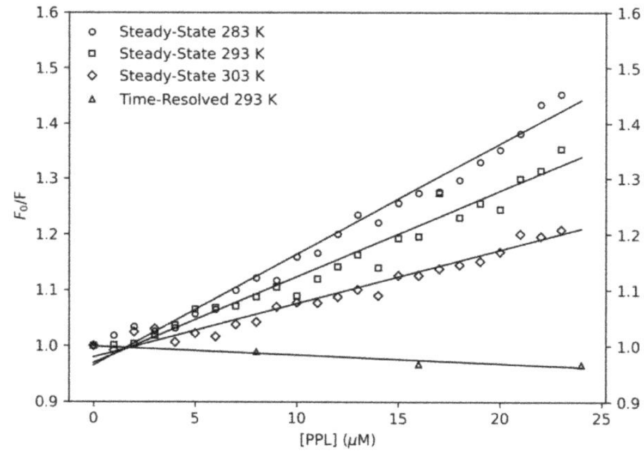

Figure 2. Left ordinate: Stern–Volmer plots at three temperatures, 283 K, 293 K, and 303 K. Right ordinate: Time-resolved fluorescence lifetime plot at 293 K; $[NBD] = 4.0$ μM, $[PPL] = 0$–24.0 μM. PPL was added to the sample in increments of 1.0 μM.

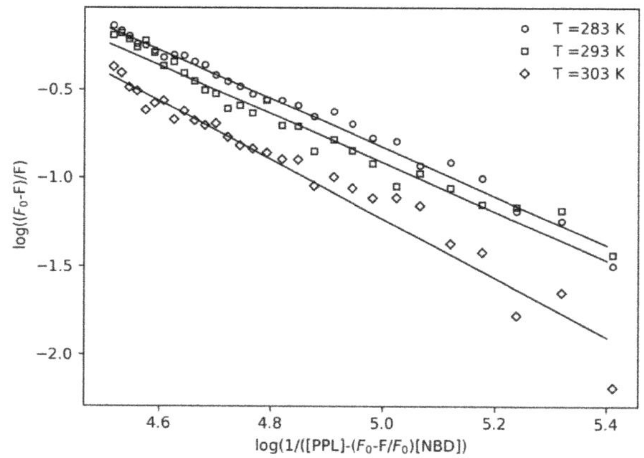

Figure 3. Double-log plots for the fluorescence quenching of NBD (4.0 μM) by the presence of PPL at 283 K, 293 K, and 303 K.

The results of K_a at different temperatures obtained for the first order model (n~1) are shown in Table 1. The binding constants found for different temperatures are in the order of magnitude of 10^4 M^{-1}. As shown in Table 1, the affinity of the complex is influenced by temperature, since the results of the binding equilibrium experiments showed that K_a decreased while the temperature increased.

2.1.1. Thermodynamic Parameters

To obtain a description of the thermodynamic of complex formation, the thermodynamic parameters ΔS (entropy variation) and ΔH (enthalpy variation) were determined by linear regression of the data shown in Figure 4, using the Van't Hoff equation (Equation (3)). ΔG (Gibbs free variation) was obtained according to Equation (4).

$$ln\ K_a = -\frac{\Delta H}{R \cdot T} + \frac{\Delta S}{R} \quad (3)$$

$$\Delta G = \Delta H - T\Delta S \quad (4)$$

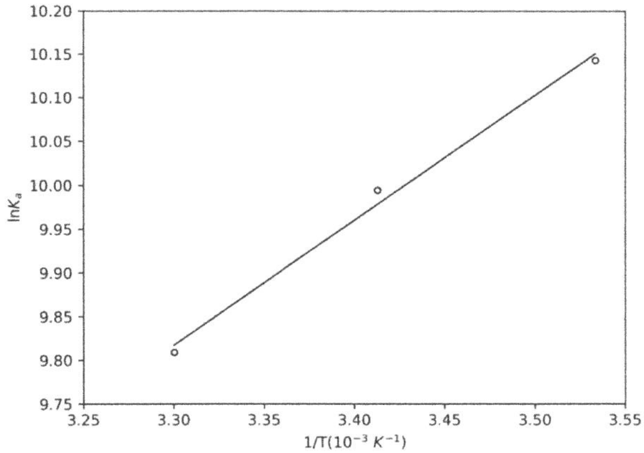

Figure 4. Van't Hoff plot for the complex NBD-PPL at 283 K, 293 K, and 303 K.

According to the results of the thermodynamic parameters gathered in Table 2, the values of ΔG exhibited negative values at the three temperatures, which showed the spontaneity of the complex formation process. Besides that, $\Delta H < 0$ characterized the complexation as an exothermic process. Furthermore, the positive values of ΔS may be an effect of water molecules displacement due to PPL entrance into the protein [25]. The thermodynamic balance of ΔH and $T{\cdot}\Delta S$ indicated the Van der Waals interactions as the major contribution to the complexation [26].

Table 2. Thermodynamic parameters of the complex NBD-PPL at the temperatures of 283, 293 and 303 K.

T (K)	ΔG (kJ·mol^{-1})	ΔH (kJ·mol^{-1})	ΔS (J·mol^{-1}·K^{-1})	$T{\cdot}\Delta S$ (kJ·mol^{-1})
283	-23.7 ± 1.3			11.9 ± 0.9
293	-24.2 ± 1.3	-11.9 ± 0.9	42.4 ± 3.4	12.4 ± 0.9
303	-24.6 ± 1.3			12.8 ± 1.0

2.1.2. Interaction Density Function (IDF)

As a second method, IDF was also applied in fluorescence data in order to obtain a complete description of the system. Differently from the binding equilibrium model, IDF does not make use of any model a priori [27] and the advantage of applying IDF is the possibility of not only determining the number of binding sites but also identifying cooperativity occurrence among them. IDF considers that, if the free ligand concentration ($[PPL]_{free}$) is the same for two at different concentrations of total protein ([NBD]), the average interaction density (Σv_i) will also be the same, and consequently the system will have the same variation on the percentage of quenching (ΔF). The percentage of fluorescence quenching is given by Equation (5). Where F is the observed fluorescence signal in the presence of PPL and F_0 is the observed fluorescence signal for free protein. Figure 5 shows the plot of ΔF per log $[PPL]$ for two known concentrations of NBD adjusted by a sigmoidal function.

$$\Delta F = \frac{|F - F_0|}{F_0} \tag{5}$$

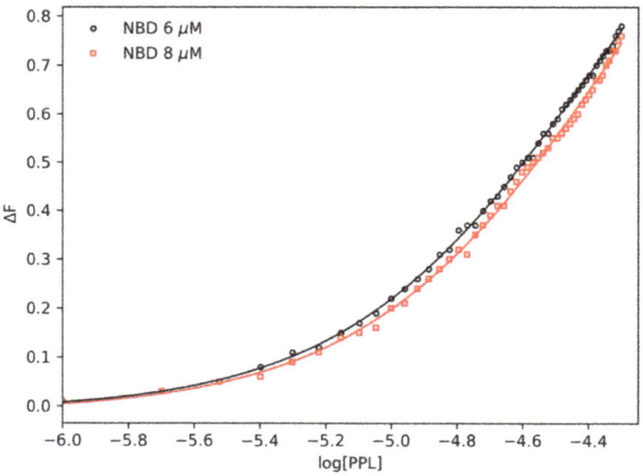

Figure 5. Plot of ΔF versus Log $[PPL]$ obtained from PPL titration experiments with NBD concentrations of 6.0 μM and 8.0 μM at 293 K.

Free ligand concentration and the average of interaction density are related to each other through the expression of mass conservation (Equation (6)).

$$[PPL] = [PPL]_{free} + (\sum \nu_i).[NBD] \quad (6)$$

By means of the plot shown on Figure 5, the values of $[NBD]$ and $[PPL]$ for each ΔF were obtained. According to the IDF results, a Scatchard plot was built (Figure 6a) This plot presented a concave function, revealing positive cooperativity between the NBD binding sites [28]. Interestingly, we reported recently that the interaction of piperine with NBD led to a cooperative mode of binding [29]. These results showed that different ligands can induce similar modes of binding in NBD structure.

The number of sites (n) and the binding constant (K_b) were obtained using Hill's model, based on Equation (7). Another parameter obtained through this model was the cooperativity, indicated by Hill's coefficient (h) [30].

$$\sum \nu_i = \frac{n \cdot (K_b[PPL]_{free})^h}{1 + (K_b[PPL]_{free})^h} \quad (7)$$

The Hill's plot (Figure 6b) shows the variation of the average interaction density ($\sum \nu_i$) with the free ligand concentration ($[PPL]_{free}$). With the mathematical fitting of these results, the number of sites (n) and the binding constant (K_b) were found to be 2.2 ± 0.1 and (6.3 ± 0.2) × 10^4 M^{-1}, respectively. Besides that, the fitting also revealed the Hill's coefficient (h) as 1.4 ± 0.1, confirming the cooperative binding of PPL toward NBD, previously detected in Scatchard plot.

These results showed that both methods applied in the analysis of fluorescence quenching (binding equilibrium model and IDF) are in agreement with respect to the order of magnitude of K_b, since binding equilibrium model revealed the binding constant as (2.2 ± 0.5) × 10^4 M^{-1}.

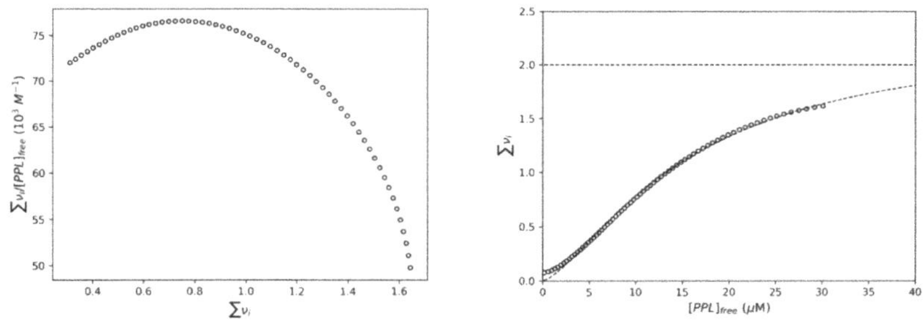

(a) (b)

Figure 6. (**a**) Scatchard plot for the interaction of NBD and PPL obtained at 293 K based on IDF data. (**b**) Hill's plot for the interaction of NBD and PPL.

2.2. Circular Dichroism

Circular Dichroism (CD) is a suitable method to analyse secondary structure of proteins in different conditions. In this way, CD experiments were performed to obtain both the thermal structural stability of the domain NBD (Figure 7) and possible secondary conformational changes due to the PPL interaction (Figure 8). Considering that NBD structure is predominantly composed by alpha-helices in solution with two CD characteristic bands centred at 208 nm (π-π*) and at 222 nm (n-π*) [31], the wavelength of 222 nm was followed to monitor the thermal transition (Figure 7b) of NBD. According to the results obtained (Figure 7b), NBD experienced a transition from folded to unfolded state at ~314 K. Similar results were obtained from calorimetric and spectroscopic methods applied to bacterial HSP (DnaK) [32,33].

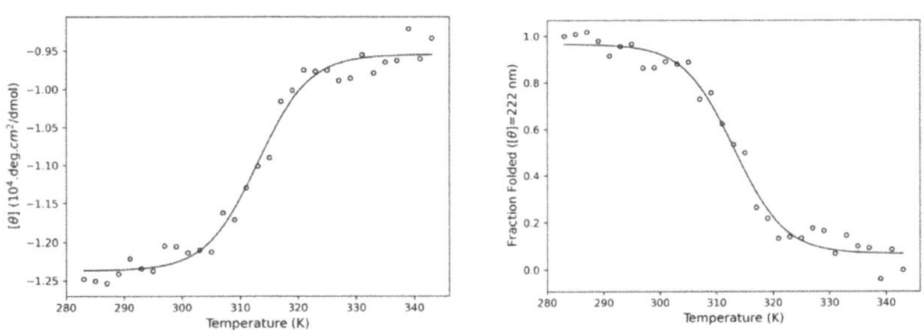

(a) (b)

Figure 7. Denaturation curve of NBD monitored at 222 nm with a melting temperature of 314 K. (**a**) The plot shows the ellipticity $[\theta]$ versus temperature and (**b**) The plot shows the fraction folded calculated with Equation (12).

Figure 8 shows the CD spectrum of pure NBD and in the presence of PPL at stoichiometry of 1:12, the same stoichiometry reached in the IDF experiment. According to the results, the deconvolution of pure NBD spectrum presented 38% of alpha-helices, 14% of β-sheet, 20% of turn and 28% of coil, which is in a good agreement with the results obtained by Zazeri et al. [29] at a similar temperature. After PPL addition, NBD underwent some secondary conformational changes, being 33% of α-helices, 17% of β-sheet, 19% of turn and 31% of coil. Interestingly, while the percentage of α-helices decreased by 5%, the percentage of β-sheet increased by 3%. Despite the smaller secondary structural changes found in this work compared to those reported by Zazeri et al. [29] for the interaction of NBD and piperine, the same behavior for α-helices and β-sheet changes were observed. Furthermore, although the results showed a maximum secondary structure change of 4%

(related to α-helices), it is not statistically significant in terms of conformational changes, such changes may modulate the biochemical activity [34].

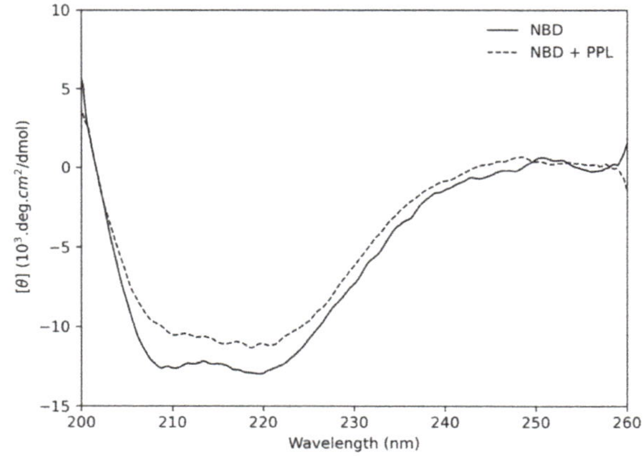

Figure 8. Circular Dichroism of free NBD (solid lines) and NBD + PPL at the stoichiometry 1:12 (dotted lines) at 293 K.

2.3. Molecular Docking

The structure of NBD obtained from PDB 1S3X was directly subjected to molecular docking that disclosed several possible pockets where PPL can interact with NBD (Figure S2), with energy ranked from (7.2 to 5.0 kcal). The analysis of the poses from cluster "a" to "g" (Figure S3) revealed that they are in the environment of the binding site accessed by the ADP molecule, represented in black. The next cluster analyzed was "h", which is not in the proximity of the ADP binding site, as shown in Figure S3. The next clusters were not considered once they were less populated than the previous ones. For the next analyses, we will consider the coordinates from cluster "a" and "h" as being Site 1 and 2, respectively (Figure 9).

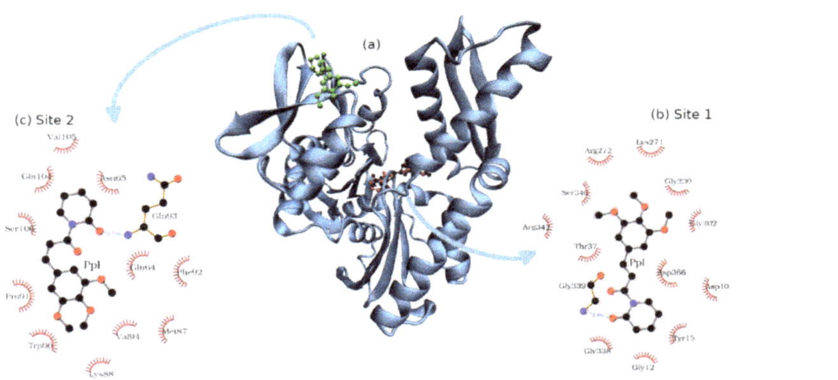

Figure 9. Bind sites of NBD accessed by PPL: (**a**) NBD structure with PPL in Site 1 (red) and in Site 2 (green), in this picture ADP molecule is represented in black. (**b**) The amino acids composition of Site 1 and the interactions between PPL and NBD, where one hydrogen bond was found between Gly339 and PPL (blue dashed line). (**c**) The amino acids composition of Site 2 and the interactions between PPL and NBD, where one hydrogen bond was found between Gln93 and PPL (blue dashed line).

The composition of the bind sites was organized in Table 3, which shows that Site 1 is rich in glycine and presents a generous number of polar amino acids (whether charged or not). Ligplot software detected a hydrogen bond between PPL and the nitrogen atom of Gly339 which is part of the backbone of NBD. It is worth noting that such analysis was made based on a fixed pose calculated by molecular docking; a more holistic analysis of hydrogen bonds will be presented based on molecular dynamics results.

Table 3. The characteristics of amino acids that compose the microenvironment of Sites 1 and 2 obtained by molecular docking.

Binding Sites	Amino Acids			
	Non-Polar	Positively Charged	Negatively Charged	Polar
1	Gly12, 202, 230, 338, 339	Lys271; Arg272, 342	Asp10, 366	Tyr15; Thr37; Ser340
2	Val94, 105; Met87; Pro91; Trp90; Phe92	Lys88	-	Asn65; Gln64; 93, 104; Ser106

Site 2 presents an equilibrated balance of polar and non-polar amino acids. No negatively charged residues were found in the environment, which favors the interaction with PPL with protein since its structure presents charge delocalization that concentrates negative charges in the extremities of the molecule [35]. Besides that, the interaction of PPL with Site 2 includes one hydrogen bond with Gln93.

2.4. Molecular Dynamics

The equilibration and stability of the complexes formed by NBD and PPL in Sites 1 and 2 was verified through the parameters obtained from molecular dynamics (Figure 10). The root mean square deviation (RMSD) of NBD with PPL in Site 1 and 2 remained stable during the simulation, fluctuating around 0.25 nm. Similar behavior was found to the RMSD calculated for PPL atoms when bound in Site 1 and 2, which remained stable, fluctuating around 0.1 nm, i.e., PPL remained in the Sites 1 and 2 throughout the simulation.

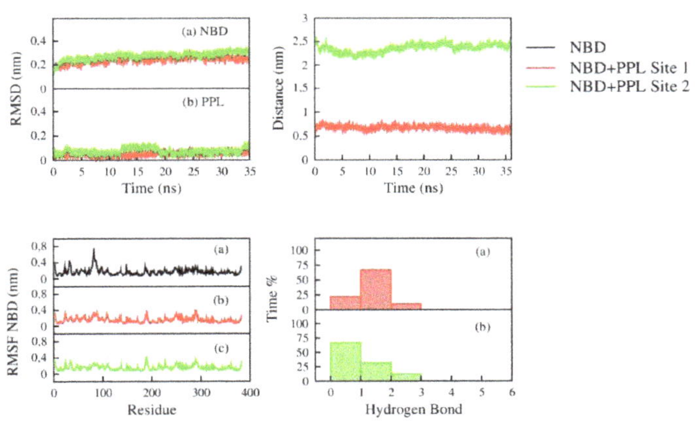

Figure 10. Parameters obtained from the molecular dynamics simulation of the NBD (black), NBD with PPL in Site 1 (red) and Site 2 (green). **Top Left**: The RMSD of (a) protein NBD and (b) molecule PPL. **Top Right**: Distance between COG of NBD and COG of PPL in Sites 1 and 2. **Bottom Left**: The RMSF of the residues of (a) NBD, (b) NBD when interacting with PPL in Site 1 and (c) NBD when interacting with PPL in Site 2. **Bottom Right**: The hydrogen bonds performed between NBD and PPL in (a) Site 1 and (b) Site 2.

Another helpful parameter used to verify the stability of the protein-ligand complex is the distance from the centre of geometry (COG) of protein to the COG of ligand.

The distance calculated for the complex formed by NBD and PPL in Site 1 remained around 0.7 nm, as expected, since the molecule is located close to the centre of geometry of NBD (Figure 9). For Site 2, the distance fluctuated around 2.5 nm, confirming that PPL remained in the binding site located in the periphery of NBD (Figure 9).

The root mean square fluctuation (RMSF) of the residues of NBD free, bound to PPL in site 1 and 2 was calculated to verify possible changes in the dynamics of the protein caused by the interaction with ligand. No drastic change was observed in the RMSF of NBD with PPL in Sites 1 and 2 when compared to RMSF of free NBD. A slight change was observed for residues 78–87 that compose an α-helix close to Site 1. However, the change in the dynamics is not necessarily due to the interaction of PPL in Site 1 since the dynamics of such residues also presented low fluctuation in the analysis of NBD with PPL in Site 2.

The analyses of hydrogen bonds showed that in Site 1 PPL performs between 1 and 2 H-bond with residues of NBD 72% of the simulation time. Hydrogen bonds are less observed in the interaction of PPL with Site 2. Molecular dynamics revealed that the number of the H-bond was between 0 and 1 in 73% of the simulation time. Hydrogen bonds give an enthalpic contribution to the thermodynamic balance. Application of the Van't Hoff model to the experimental data (Table 2) gave insight into an equilibrated balance between entropic and enthalpic interactions. Molecular dynamics corroborated this result since a moderate formation of H-bonds in both sites was detected.

Figure 11 shows the results of MMPBSA calculations applied to the trajectory from molecular dynamics simulations. According to the results, the binding sites have similar binding energy (-58 ± 3 kJ·mol^{-1} and -49 ± 3 kJ·mol^{-1} for Site 1 and 2, respectively) Moreover, the results revealed the Van der Waals as the predominant interaction of the complex, which reinforced the result obtained from Van't Hoff analyses.

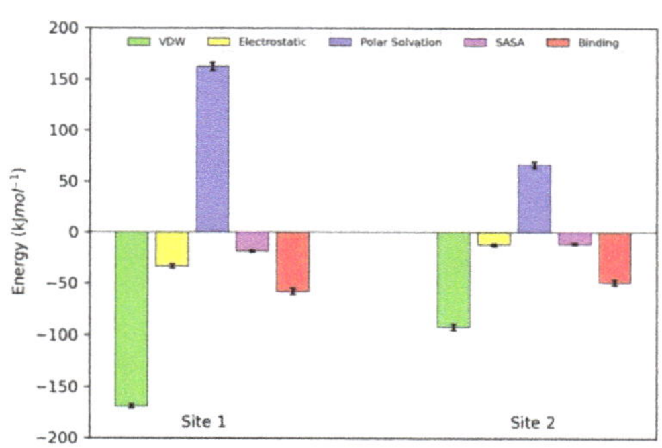

Figure 11. Energy decomposition obtained by MMPBSA for the interactions of NBD with PPL for Site 1 and 2. Contributions of Van der Waals (VDW), electrostatic, polar solvation (P.Solvation), and solvent accessible area (SASA) to the final binding energy (Binding).

3. Materials and Methods

3.1. Reagents

Piperlongumine (>97%) was purchased from Sigma-Aldrich Chemical Co. (Schnelldorf, Germany), as dibasic sodium phosphate (>99%) reagents, anhydrous citric acid (>99%), and sodium chloride (>99%). Lyophilised Nucleotide Binding Domain of Heat Shock Protein 70 kDa (>97%) was purchased from GenScript. Methanol was purchased from Dynamics Química Contemporânea LTDA (Indaiatuba, SP, Brazil). All the materials purchased were used as supplied. Ultrapure water was prepared by a Millipore water purification system–Direct-Q UV-3 (Merck KGaA, Darmstadt, Germany). Lyophilized NBD was reconstituted in a 50 mM phosphate buffer containing 150 mM sodium chloride, and the pH was adjusted to 7.4 with anhydrous citric acid. Stock solutions of PPL were prepared in methanol. The concentrations of PPL and NBD solutions were determined by UV-Vis experiments performed on Biospectro spectrophotometer (Biospectro, Curitiba, PR, Brazil) using the extinction coefficient of 18,700 $M^{-1} \cdot cm^{-1}$ at 326 nm for PPL and 20,525 $M^{-1} \cdot cm^{-1}$ at 280 nm for NBD.

3.2. Experimental Methods

3.2.1. Steady-State Fluorescence Spectroscopy

Fluorescence experiments were performed on the Lumina (Thermo Fisher Scientific, Waltham, MA, USA) stationary state spectrofluorimeter equipped with thermal bath and Xenon lamp. A 100 μL quartz cuvette with 2 mm × 10 mm optical path was used in the experiments. The widths of the excitation and the emission slits were adjusted to 10 nm. The wavelength of 295 nm was used to excite the single tryptophan residue of NBD (Trp90). The emission spectra were obtained in the range from 305 to 500 nm with a resolution of 1.0 nm ± 5.0 nm. Each emission point collected was the average of 15 accumulations. The software ScanWave was used to collect the measured data.

In the binding equilibrium experiments, aliquots of PPL (increment of 1.0 μM) were added in NBD solution at 4.0 μM. Measurements were performed at 283 K, 293 K, and 303 K. In the interaction density function analysis, aliquots of PPL (increments of 1.0 μM) were added in NBD solutions at 6.0 μM and 8.0 μM at a fixed temperature (293 K). In all experiments, the final volume of methanol in the buffer was <1.0%.

The correction of the inner filter effects was done with Equation (8), where F_{corr} and F_{obs} are corrected and observed fluorescence intensities, and A_{ex} and A_{em} are the absorbance of the sample in a 10 mm optical path cuvettes at the excitation and the emission wavelengths, respectively [22].

$$F_{corr} = F_{obs} \cdot 10^{\frac{(5 \cdot A_{ex} + A_{em})}{10}} \quad (8)$$

3.2.2. Time-Resolved Fluorescence

Fluorescence lifetime measurements were performed using a Mini-tau filter-based fluorescence lifetime spectrometer coupled to a Time-Correlated Single Photon Counting (TCSPC) system (Edinburgh Instruments, Livingston, UK). Aliquots of PPL were added in the NBD solution from 0 to 24 μM. Experiments were carried out at 293 K.

The sample was excited at 295 nm using a picosecond pulsed light emitting diode (LED), and fluorescence decay was collected using a 340 nm filter. The fluorescence decay profile (Figure S1) was fitted using multiexponential decay (Equation (9)), where τ_i is the lifetime of each component, and α_i is the contribution of each component to total fluorescence decay. The average lifetime $<\tau_{avg}>$ was calculated using Equation (10) (Table S1).

$$I_T = \sum_{i=1}^{n} \alpha_i . e^{\frac{-T}{\tau_i}} \quad (9)$$

$$\tau_{avg} = \frac{\alpha_1 \tau_1{}^2 + \alpha_2 \tau_2{}^2}{\alpha_1 \tau_1 + \alpha_2 \tau_2} \quad (10)$$

3.2.3. Circular Dichroism

Circular dichroism spectra were recorded on a Jasco J-815 spectropolarimeter model DRC-H (Jasco, Easton, MD, USA) equipped with a demountable quartz cell with a 0.01 cm optical path length. The CD spectra were recorded from the 200 to 260 nm range with a scan rate of 20 nm/min and a spectral resolution of 0.1 nm. For each spectrum, 15 accumulations were performed. For the denaturation experiments, the spectra were recorded in the temperature range of 280 and 340 K. The ellipticity θ collected in millidegrees was converted to mean residue ellipticity $[\theta]$ (deg·cm^2·$dmol^{-1}$) using Equation (11) and the protein denatured fractions were determined with Equation (12) where $[\theta]^{nat}$ is the $[\theta]$ at 280 K and $[\theta]^{den}$ is $[\theta]$ at the 340 K. For the interaction experiments, the molar ratio NBD:PPL was 1:12, the buffer spectrum was subtracted, and the temperature was kept at 293 K. The secondary structures percentages were calculated with CDPro applying the CONTIN method with the SP43 protein library [36].

$$[\theta] = \frac{\theta(mdeg)}{10 \cdot [P] \cdot l \cdot n} \tag{11}$$

$$f = \frac{([\theta]^{obs} - [\theta]^{den})}{([\theta]^{nat} - [\theta]^{den})} \tag{12}$$

3.3. *Computational Methods*

3.3.1. Molecular Docking

PPL structure used in molecular docking was obtained from ab initio calculations from our previous work [31]. The AutoDockTools [37] software of the MGL program Tools 1.5.4 was used to prepare the NBD (PDB 1S3X) by adding polar hydrogen atoms and Gasteiger charges. The maps were generated by the AutoGrid 4.2 program [38] with a spacing of 0.541 Å, a dimension of 126 × 126 × 126 points, and grid center coordinates of 51.315, 42.946, and 49.437 for x, y, and z coordinates, respectively. The AutoDock 4.2 program [37] was used to investigate the NBD binding sites using the Lamarckian Genetic Algorithm (LGA) with a population size of 150, a maximum number of generations of 27,000, and energy evaluations equal to 2.5×10^6. All other parameters were selected as software defaults. To generate different conformations, the total number of runs was set to 100. (Figure S2). The final conformations were visualized on VMD [39]. The binding microenvironment was generated by LigPlot [40].

3.3.2. Molecular Dynamics

The simulations of the complex NBD/PPL were performed with GROMOS53a6 force field [41] by Gromacs v.5.1.4 [42]. The complex was placed in a rectangular box, solvated with the simple point charge water (SPC) [43] and neutralized with NaCl in a concentration of 150 mM. The energy minimization was performed with the steepest descent algorithm with 5000 steps and a tolerance of 10 $kJ \cdot mol^{-1}$. The cut-off for small-range interactions was set to 10 Å and the long-range electrostatic interactions were treated with particle mesh Ewald (PME) [44]. Then, the heavy atoms were restrained with a force constant of 1000 kJ mol^{-1} nm^{-2} and the system was submitted to the first stage of equilibration for 100 ps in the NVT ensemble coupled to V-rescale thermostat at 293 K [45]. All bonds were constrained with the LINCS algorithm [46]. Random velocities were generated by the Maxwell–Boltzman distribution. The second stage of equilibration was performed in the NPT ensemble for 100 ps of simulation coupled to Parrinello–Rahman barostat [47] at 1 atm. Finally, the restrictions were turned off and the molecular dynamics simulations were performed with steps of 2 fs using the leap-frog algorithm to integrate the equations of motion. The hydrogen bonds were calculated by *gmx hbond*. The results presented are an average of three independent simulations.

The free energy of the binding process of PPL toward NBD was calculated by G_mmpbsa tool [48], using the molecular mechanics Poisson–Boltzmann surface area (MM/PBSA) method applied to the snapshots obtained from molecular dynamics simulations. The snapshots were extracted in intervals of 500 ps from the trajectory after the system reached the equilibrium, which was verified by the root mean square deviation (RMSD) and the distance from the center of geometry of NBD to PPL, obtained by the programs *gmx rms* and *gmx distance*, respectively (Figure 10). The coarse grid-box (cfac) was set as 2 and the finer grid-box (fadd) was set as 20. The concentration of positive and negative ions was set as 0.150, being the positive and negative radii set as 0.95 and 1.81 Å, which correspond to sodium and chloride atoms, respectively. The values for the vacuum (vdie) and solvent (sdie) dielectric constants were set and 1 and 80, respectively. The solute dielectric constant (pdie) was set as 4.

4. Conclusions

Multi-pronged spectroscopic analyses aided by computational modeling elucidated in detail the main features of the NBD/PPL interaction for the first time. Steady state fluorescence spectroscopy and time-resolved fluorescence results revealed the complex formation via static quenching mechanism. The use of binding equilibrium and IDF methods to treat the fluorescence quenching resulted in a binding affinity with an order of magnitude of 10^4 M^{-1}. Besides that, IDF method revealed two cooperative binding sites for PPL in NBD. Van't Hoff analyses showed through the thermodynamic balance that the complexation between NBD and PPL is an exothermic and spontaneous process, with Van der Waals as the key interaction to stabilize the complex. Molecular docking and molecular dynamics disclosed the main features of the microenvironments of interaction. In this context, the microenvironments are rich in polar (charged or non-charged) amino acids. Moreover, MMPBSA data reinforced the experimental results, confirming the equivalence of the binding sites and that Van der Waals interactions were predominant in the complex interaction. Although the environments disclosed by the analyses are highly polar, an elevated number of H-bonds was not observed. Further chemical modifications on the PPL structure aimed at increasing the affinity for the NBD binding sites would benefit from the insertion of hydrogen bond donors to reach the acceptors present in these sites. In conclusion, this work brings the key aspects involved in NBD and PPL interaction, which will further the drug development of PPL.

Supplementary Materials: The following are available online at https://www.mdpi.com/article/10.3390/ph14121298/s1, Figure S1: Time-dependent fluorescence decay of NBD with PPL concentration range from 0 to 24 μM. [NBD] = 10 μM, T = 298 K and λexc = 295 nm, Figure S2: Molecular docking clusters with their respective binding energy scores, Figure S3: Representation of the clusters a-h calculated by molecular docking. ADP molecule is represented in black, cluster a, b, c, d, e, f, g and h are represented in red, yellow, silver, tan, blue, orange and green, respectively, Table S1: Tryptophan lifetime in different stoichiometries HSP70:PPL obtained through biexponential decay.

Author Contributions: Conceptualization, A.P.R.P., G.Z., A.M.J. and M.L.C.; experimental methodology, A.P.R.P. and G.Z.; computational methodology, A.P.R.P. and G.Z.; formal analysis, A.P.R.P. and G.Z.; investigation, A.P.R.P., G.Z. and M.L.C.; resources, A.M.J. and M.L.C.; writing—original draft preparation, A.P.R.P., G.Z., A.M.J. and M.L.C.; writing—review and editing, A.P.R.P., G.Z., A.M.J. and M.L.C.; supervision, A.M.J. and M.L.C.; project administration, M.L.C.; funding acquisition, A.M.J. and M.L.C. All authors have read and agreed to the published version of the manuscript.

Funding: The authors A.P.R.P. and G.Z. were recipients of scholarships from Coordenação de Aperfeiçoamento de Pessoal de Nível Superior—(CAPES), Brazil-Finance Code 001, and Conselho Nacional de Desenvolvimento Científico e Tecnológico (CNPq), Brazil—(Grant 141953/2017-9), respectively. The author M.L.C. acknowledges the financial support from Fundação de Amparo à Pesquisa do Estado de São Paulo-FAPESP (Grant 2017/08834-9), Brazil.

Institutional Review Board Statement: Not applicable.

Informed Consent Statement: Not applicable.

Data Availability Statement: Data is contained within the article and Supplementary Materials.

Acknowledgments: Molecular Dynamics simulations were performed at the Center for Scientific Computing (NCC/GridUNESP) of São Paulo State University (UNESP), Brazil. The authors thank João Ruggiero Neto for availability of spectropolarimeter, Valdecir Ximenes for availability of fluorescence lifetime spectrometer and Marcelo de Freitas Lima for availability of stationary state spectrofluorimeter.

Conflicts of Interest: The authors declare no conflict of interest.

References

1. Meyer, T.N.; Da Silva, A.L. Resposta celular ao estresse. *Rev. Assoc. Med. Bras.* **1999**, *45*, 181–188. (In Portuguese) [CrossRef] [PubMed]
2. Lindquist, S.; Craig, E.A. The heat-shock proteins. *Annu. Rev. Genet.* **1988**, *22*, 631–677. [CrossRef]

3. Ritossa, F. A new puffing pattern induced by temperature shock and DNP in Drosophila. *Cell. Mol. Life Sci.* **1962**, *18*, 571–573 [CrossRef]
4. Karp, G. *Biologia Celular e Molecular: Conceitos e Experimentos*, 1st ed.; Manole: Barueri, Brazil, 2005; pp. 53–54. (In Portuguese)
5. Jones, A.M.; Westwood, I.M.; Osborne, J.D.; Matthews, T.P.; Cheeseman, M.D.; Rowlands, M.G.; Jeganathan, F.; Burke, R.; Lee, D. Kadi, N.; et al. A fragment-based approach applied to a highly flexible target: Insights and challenges towards the inhibition of HSP70 isoforms. *Sci. Rep.* **2016**, *6*, 34701. [CrossRef]
6. Somensi, N.; Brum, P.O.; de Miranda Ramos, V.; Gasparotto, J.; Zanotto-Filho, A.; Rostirolla, D.C.; da Silva Morrone, M.; Moreira J.C.F.; Gelain, D.P. Extracellular HSP70 activates ERK1/2, NF-kB and pro-inflammatory gene transcription through binding with RAGE in A549 human lung cancer cells. *Cell. Physiol. Biochem.* **2017**, *42*, 2507–2522. [CrossRef] [PubMed]
7. Hulina, A.; Rajković, M.G.; Despot, D.J.; Jelić, D.; Dojder, A.; Čepelak, I.; Rumora, L. Extracellular Hsp70 induces inflammation and modulates LPS/LTA-stimulated inflammatory response in THP-1 cells. *Cell Stress Chaperones* **2018**, *23*, 373–384. [CrossRef] [PubMed]
8. Tukaj, S. Heat shock protein 70 as a double agent acting inside and outside the cell: Insights into autoimmunity. *Int. J. Mol. Sci* **2020**, *21*, 5298. [CrossRef] [PubMed]
9. Yang, S.; Xiao, H.; Cao, L. Recent advances in heat shock proteins in cancer diagnosis, prognosis, metabolism and treatment *Biomed. Pharmacother.* **2021**, *142*, 112074. [CrossRef]
10. Cheeseman, M.D.; Westwood, I.M.; Barbeau, O.; Rowlands, M.; Dobson, S.; Jones, A.M.; Jeganathan, F.; Burke, R.; Kadi, N. Workman, P.; et al. Exploiting protein conformational change to optimize adenosine-derived inhibitors of HSP70. *J. Med. Chem* **2016**, *59*, 4625–4636. [CrossRef] [PubMed]
11. Bezerra, D.P.; Pessoa, C.; de Moraes, M.O.; Saker-Neto, N.; Silveira, E.R.; Costa-Lotufo, L.V. Overview of the therapeutic potential of piplartine (piperlongumine). *Eur. J. Pharm. Sci.* **2013**, *48*, 453–463. [CrossRef]
12. Adams, D.J.; Dai, M.; Pellegrino, G.; Wagner, B.K.; Stern, A.M.; Shamji, A.F.; Schreiber, S.L. Synthesis, cellular evaluation, and mechanism of action of piperlongumine analogs. *Proc. Natl. Acad. Sci. USA* **2012**, *109*, 15115–15120. [CrossRef]
13. Piska, K.; Gunia-Krzyżak, A.; Koczurkiewicz, P.; Wójcik-Pszczoła, K.; Pękala, E. Piperlongumine (piplartine) as a lead compound for anticancer agents—Synthesis and properties of analogues: A mini-review. *Eur. J. Med. Chem.* **2018**, *156*, 13–20. [CrossRef]
14. Wu, Y.; Min, X.; Zhuang, C.; Li, J.; Yu, Z.; Dong, G.; Yao, J.; Wang, S.; Liu, Y.; Wu, S.; et al. Design, synthesis and biological activity of piperlongumine derivatives as selective anticancer agents. *Eur. J. Med. Chem.* **2014**, *82*, 545–551. [CrossRef] [PubMed]
15. Prasad, S.; Tyagi, A.K. Historical spice as a future drug: Therapeutic potential of piperlongumine. *Curr. Pharm. Des.* **2016**, *22*, 4151–4159. [CrossRef] [PubMed]
16. Zazeri, G.; Povinelli, A.P.R.; Le Duff, C.S.; Tang, B.; Cornelio, M.L.; Jones, A.M. Synthesis and spectroscopic analysis of piperine and piperlongumine-inspired natural product scaffolds and their molecular docking with IL-1β and NF-κB proteins. *Molecules* **2020**, *25*, 2841. [CrossRef]
17. Sun, L.-D.; Wang, F.; Dai, F.; Wang, Y.-H.; Lin, D.; Zhou, B. Development and mechanism investigation of a new piperlongumine derivative as a potent anti-inflammatory agent. *Biochem. Pharmacol.* **2015**, *95*, 156–169. [CrossRef]
18. Zheng, J.; Son, D.J.; Gu, S.M.; Woo, J.R.; Ham, Y.W.; Lee, H.P.; Kim, W.J.; Jung, J.K.; Hong, J.T. Piperlongumine inhibits lung tumor growth via inhibition of nuclear factor kappa B signaling pathway. *Sci. Rep.* **2016**, *6*, 26357. [CrossRef]
19. Ginzburg, S.; Golovine, K.V.; Makhov, P.B.; Uzzo, R.G.; Kutikov, A.; Kolenko, V.M. Piperlongumine inhibits NF-κB activity and attenuates aggressive growth characteristics of prostate cancer cells. *Prostate* **2014**, *74*, 177–186. [CrossRef]
20. Si, D.; Wang, Y.; Zhou, Y.-H.; Guo, Y.; Wang, J.; Zhou, H.; Li, Z.-S.; Fawcett, J.P. Mechanism of CYP2C9 inhibition by flavones and flavonols. *Drug Metab. Dispos.* **2009**, *37*, 629–634. [CrossRef] [PubMed]
21. Gu, S.M.; Lee, H.P.; Ham, Y.W.; Son, D.J.; Kim, H.Y.; Oh, K.W.; Han, S.-B.; Yun, J.; Hong, J.T. Piperlongumine improves lipopolysaccharide-induced amyloidogenesis by suppressing NF-KappaB pathway. *Neuromol. Med.* **2018**, *20*, 312–327. [CrossRef]
22. Lakowicz, J.R. *Principles of Fluorescence Spectroscopy*; Springer: Berlin/Heidelberg, Germany, 2004. Available online: https //www.academia.edu/34533342/Principles_of_Fluorescence_Spectroscopy_Third_Edition (accessed on 6 December 2021).
23. Lakowicz, J.R.; Weber, G. Quenching of fluorescence by oxygen. Probe for structural fluctuations in macromolecules. *Biochemistry* **1973**, *12*, 4161–4170. [CrossRef] [PubMed]
24. Povinelli, A.P.R.; Zazeri, G.; Cornélio, M.L. Molecular Mechanism of Flavonoids Using Fluorescence Spectroscopy and Computational Tools. In *Flavonoids a Coloring Model for Cheering Up Life*; IntechOpen: London, UK, 2019.
25. Caruso, Í.P.; Vilegas, W.; de Oliveira, L.C.; Cornélio, M.L. Fluorescence spectroscopic and dynamics simulation studies on isoorientin binding with human serum albumin. *Spectrochim. Acta Part A Mol. Biomol. Spectrosc.* **2020**, *228*, 117738. [CrossRef]
26. Ross, P.D.; Subramanian, S. Thermodynamics of protein association reactions: Forces contributing to stability. *Biochemistry* **1981** *20*, 3096–3102. [CrossRef] [PubMed]
27. Lohman, T.M.; Bujalowski, W. Thermodynamic methods for model-independent determination of equilibrium binding isotherms for protein-DNA interactions: Spectroscopic approaches to monitor binding. *Methods Enzymol.* **1991**, *208*, 258–290.
28. Scatchard, G. The attractions of proteins for small molecules and ions. *Ann. N. Y. Acad. Sci.* **1949**, *51*, 660–672. [CrossRef]
29. Zazeri, G.; Povinelli, A.P.R.; de Freitas Lima, M.; Cornélio, M.L. Detailed Characterization of the Cooperative Binding of Piperine with Heat Shock Protein 70 by Molecular Biophysical Approaches. *Biomedicines* **2020**, *8*, 629. [CrossRef]
30. Bordbar, A.K.; Saboury, A.A.; Moosavi-Movahedi, A.A. The shapes of Scatchard plots for systems with two sets of binding sites *Biochem. Educ.* **1996**, *24*, 172–175. [CrossRef]

31. Zazeri, G.; Povinelli, P.A.; de Freitas Lima, M.; Cornélio, L.M. Experimental Approaches and Computational Modeling of Rat Serum Albumin and Its Interaction with Piperine. *Int. J. Mol. Sci.* **2019**, *20*, 2856. [CrossRef]
32. Montgomery, D.; Jordan, R.; McMacken, R.; Freire, E. Thermodynamic and structural analysis of the folding/unfolding transitions of the Escherichia coli molecular chaperone DnaK. *J. Mol. Biol.* **1993**, *232*, 680–692. [CrossRef] [PubMed]
33. Palleros, D.R.; Reid, K.L.; McCarty, J.S.; Walker, G.C.; Fink, A.L. DnaK, hsp73, and their molten globules. Two different ways heat shock proteins respond to heat. *J. Biol. Chem.* **1992**, *267*, 5279–5285. [CrossRef]
34. Zazeri, G.; Povinelli, A.P.R.; de Freitas Lima, M.; Cornélio, M.L. The Cytokine IL-1β and Piperine Complex Surveyed by Experimental and Computational Molecular Biophysics. *Biomolecules* **2020**, *10*, 1337. [CrossRef] [PubMed]
35. Povinelli, A.P.R.; Zazeri, G.; de Freitas Lima, M.; Cornélio, M.L. Details of the cooperative binding of piperlongumine with rat serum albumin obtained by spectroscopic and computational analyses. *Sci. Rep.* **2019**, *9*, 15667. [CrossRef] [PubMed]
36. Sreerama, N.; Woody, R.W. Estimation of protein secondary structure from circular dichroism spectra: Comparison of CONTIN, SELCON, and CDSSTR methods with an expanded reference set. *Anal. Biochem.* **2000**, *287*, 252–260. [CrossRef] [PubMed]
37. Morris, G.M.; Huey, R.; Lindstrom, W.; Sanner, M.F.; Belew, R.K.; Goodsell, D.S.; Olson, A.J. AutoDock4 and AutoDockTools4: Automated docking with selective receptor flexibility. *J. Comput. Chem.* **2009**, *30*, 2785–2791. [CrossRef]
38. Morris, G.M.; Goodsell, D.S.; Pique, M.E.; Lindstrom, W.; Huey, R.; Forli, S.; Hart, W.E.; Halliday, S.; Belew, R.; Olson, A.J. User Guide AutoDock Version 4.2. Automated Docking of Flexible Ligands to Flexible Receptors. 2010. Available online: https://autodock.scripps.edu/wp-content/uploads/sites/56/2021/10/AutoDock4.2.6_UserGuide.pdf (accessed on 6 December 2021).
39. Humphrey, W.; Dalke, A.; Schulten, K. VMD: Visual molecular dynamics. *J. Mol. Graph.* **1996**, *14*, 33–38. [CrossRef]
40. Wallace, A.C.; Laskowski, R.A.; Thornton, J.M. LIGPLOT: A program to generate schematic diagrams of protein-ligand interactions. *Protein Eng. Des. Sel.* **1995**, *8*, 127–134. [CrossRef]
41. Oostenbrink, C.; Villa, A.; Mark, A.E.; Van Gunsteren, W.F. A biomolecular force field based on the free enthalpy of hydration and solvation: The GROMOS force-field parameter sets 53A5 and 53A6. *J. Comput. Chem.* **2004**, *25*, 1656–1676. [CrossRef]
42. Van Der Spoel, D.; Lindahl, E.; Hess, B.; Groenhof, G.; Mark, A.E.; Berendsen, H.J.C. GROMACS: Fast, flexible, and free. *J. Comput. Chem.* **2005**, *26*, 1701–1718. [CrossRef]
43. Wu, Y.; Tepper, H.L.; Voth, G.A. Flexible simple point-charge water model with improved liquid-state properties. *J. Chem. Phys.* **2006**, *124*, 24503. [CrossRef]
44. Batcho, P.F.; Case, D.A.; Schlick, T. Optimized particle-mesh Ewald/multiple-time step integration for molecular dynamics simulations. *J. Chem. Phys.* **2001**, *115*, 4003–4018. [CrossRef]
45. Bussi, G.; Donadio, D.; Parrinello, M. Canonical sampling through velocity rescaling. *J. Chem. Phys.* **2007**, *126*, 14101. [CrossRef]
46. Hess, B.; Bekker, H.; Berendsen, H.J.C.; Fraaije, J.G.E.M. LINCS: A linear constraint solver for molecular simulations. *J. Comput. Chem.* **1997**, *18*, 1463–1472. [CrossRef]
47. Parrinello, M.; Rahman, A. Polymorphic transitions in single crystals: A new molecular dynamics method. *J. Appl. Phys.* **1981**, *52*, 7182–7190. [CrossRef]
48. Kumari, R.; Kumar, R.; Consortium, O.S.D.D.; Lynn, A. g_mmpbsa—A GROMACS tool for high-throughput MM-PBSA calculations. *J. Chem. Inf. Model.* **2014**, *54*, 1951–1962. [CrossRef] [PubMed]

pharmaceuticals

Article

Fragment-Based Ligand Discovery Applied to the Mycolic Acid Methyltransferase Hma (MmaA4) from *Mycobacterium tuberculosis*: A Crystallographic and Molecular Modelling Study

Romain Galy [1], Stéphanie Ballereau [2], Yves Génisson [2], Lionel Mourey [1], Jean-Christophe Plaquevent [2] and Laurent Maveyraud [1,*]

1 Institut de Pharmacologie et de Biologie Structurale, Université Toulouse III—Paul Sabatier, Centre National de la Recherche Scientifique, 31077 Toulouse, France; lionel.mourey@ipbs.fr
2 Laboratoire de Synthèse et Physico-Chimie de Molécules d'Intérêt Biologique, Université Toulouse III—Paul Sabatier, Centre National de la Recherche Scientifique, 31062 Toulouse, France; ballereau@chimie.ups-tlse.fr (S.B.); genisson@chimie.ups-tlse.fr (Y.G.)
* Correspondence: laurent.maveyraud@ipbs.fr; Tel.: +33-561-17-54-35

Abstract: The mycolic acid biosynthetic pathway represents a promising source of pharmacological targets in the fight against tuberculosis. In *Mycobacterium tuberculosis*, mycolic acids are subject to specific chemical modifications introduced by a set of eight S-adenosylmethionine dependent methyltransferases. Among these, Hma (MmaA4) is responsible for the introduction of oxygenated modifications. Crystallographic screening of a library of fragments allowed the identification of seven ligands of Hma. Two mutually exclusive binding modes were identified, depending on the conformation of residues 147–154. These residues are disordered in *apo*-Hma but fold upon binding of the S-adenosylmethionine (SAM) cofactor as well as of analogues, resulting in the formation of the short η1-helix. One of the observed conformations would be incompatible with the presence of the cofactor, suggesting that allosteric inhibitors could be designed against Hma. Chimeric compounds were designed by fusing some of the bound fragments, and the relative binding affinities of initial fragments and evolved compounds were investigated using molecular dynamics simulation and generalised Born and Poisson–Boltzmann calculations coupled to the surface area continuum solvation method. Molecular dynamics simulations were also performed on *apo*-Hma to assess the structural plasticity of the unliganded protein. Our results indicate a significant improvement in the binding properties of the designed compounds, suggesting that they could be further optimised to inhibit Hma activity.

Keywords: *Mycobacterium tuberculosis*; mycolic acid methyltransferases; fragment-based ligand discovery; binding energies; molecular modelling

Citation: Galy, R.; Ballereau, S.; Génisson, Y.; Mourey, L.; Plaquevent, J.-C.; Maveyraud, L. Fragment-Based Ligand Discovery Applied to the Mycolic Acid Methyltransferase Hma (MmaA4) from *Mycobacterium tuberculosis*: A Crystallographic and Molecular Modelling Study. *Pharmaceuticals* **2021**, *14*, 1282. https://doi.org/10.3390/ph14121282

Academic Editor: Osvaldo Andrade Santos-Filho

Received: 9 November 2021
Accepted: 5 December 2021
Published: 8 December 2021

1. Introduction

Mycobacterium tuberculosis (Mtb), the causative agent of tuberculosis (TB), remains one of the deadliest infectious agents worldwide: it claimed 1.5 million deaths in 2020, and an estimated 10 million new cases were reported [1]. This remarkable efficacy as a human pathogen relies in part on the structure of its thick, atypical, highly hydrophobic cell wall [2], which limits antibiotic penetration [3], protects Mtb from the host immune system [4,5], and provides important virulence factors [6,7]. This cell wall is formed by the mycomembrane, or mycobacterial outer membrane, which surrounds arabinogalactan and peptidoglycan [2]. The inner leaflet of the mycomembrane comprises mycolic acids (MAs) covalently bound to arabinogalactan, whereas trehalose-bound mycolic acids are found in the outer leaflet [8].

Mycolic acids, long-chain 2-alkyl, 3-hydroxy fatty acids, are an idiosyncrasy of the genus *Mycobacterium* [6], and, as such, their metabolism is a relevant target in the fight against Mtb [9,10]. Indeed, isoniazid, one of the most widely used antitubercular drugs, targets this biosynthetic pathway [11–13]. The biosynthesis of MAs starts with the synthesis of C_{16}–C_{18} fatty acids (FAs), by the multifunctional fatty acid synthase (FAS) I enzyme, which are further elongated up to C_{48}–C_{62} by the FAS-II multienzyme system, while being decorated at two distinct positions by a set of eight MA S-adenosylmethionine (SAM) dependent methyltransferases (MAMTs). The enzyme Pks13 condensates these long modified FAs, called a meromycolic chain, with a C_{24}–C_{26} long FA, also generated by FAS-I [14]. The resulting decorated MAs are translocated to the periplasm by the membrane transporter MmpL3 [15].

The introduction of decorations at the distal and proximal positions on the meromycolic chain necessitates the presence of *cis* double bonds. The exact mechanism that leads to the presence of these double bonds is subject to debate [6]. These *cis* double bonds can be converted at the distal and proximal positions into cyclopropane by MmaA2 [16] and PcaA [17], respectively, into a *trans* double bond with a vicinal methyl by UmaA1 [18], or hydrated into a hydroxylated compound by MmaA4/Hma [19,20]. The resulting hydroxymycolates can be further modified to keto- and methoxy-MAs by MmaA3 [19,21,22]. The catalytic mechanisms of CmaA2, MmaA4, and MmaA1 have been studied by QM/MM steered molecular dynamics [23]. It would begin with the formation of a carbocation at the olefin site that would spontaneously convert into a methyl alcohol in the case of Hma/MmaA4 [23]. Deletion of individual genes encoding SAM-dependent MAMTs is not lethal and affects the mycomembrane structure and/or virulence of Mtb to varying extent [16–18,24]. On the other hand, simultaneous inactivation of all eight genes encoding MAMTs resulted in a viable but highly attenuated and hyperinflammatory Mtb [25]. Furthermore, chemical inhibition of MAMTs was found to be bactericidal [24,26]. All these results suggest that MAMTs are attractive targets in the fight against TB.

Among these, MmaA4/Hma is particularly interesting, as it has been shown that it is necessary and sufficient for the introduction of oxygenated modifications on MAs [19,20,27] and that oxygenated MAs participate in the virulence of Mtb in mice [19], modulate IL12 production in macrophages [28], and trigger the differentiation of macrophages into foamy macrophages in granulomas in vitro [29]. In continuation of our previous work on the 3D structure of Hma in the presence of SAM and of cofactor analogues [26,30], we screened a small library of fragments against Hma using X-ray crystallography. Molecular dynamics simulations were performed for the experimentally observed bound fragments to estimate their binding energies. Based on the observed structures, evolved fragments were designed and their binding energies were also estimated.

2. Results

2.1. Crystallographic Structures of Fragment-Bound Hma

Soaking experiments at 20 mM were performed with 126 fragments (average molecular weight 153 ± 29 Da, 0–3 hydrogen bond donors, 0–5 hydrogen bond acceptors, 1–3 cycles and 0–4 rotatable bonds), providing as many crystals that were flash cooled in a stream of nitrogen gas at 100 K. Diffraction data could be collected for 109 crystals, resulting in 66 datasets with resolution better than 2.5 Å. After a preliminary refinement with dimple the PanDDA procedure [31,32] identified seven datasets corresponding to possible bound fragments (Figure 1), which were further refined (Table 1). In the case of compound ZT260 as low ligand occupation was observed, a second soaking experiment was performed with 100 mM of compound. Four distinct binding sites were observed (Figure 2): two binding sites are buried in a profound crevice, which has been shown to accommodate the cofactor [30] and the substrate [26], and the other two are on the surface of the protein involving in one case residues of a neighbouring protein in the crystal.

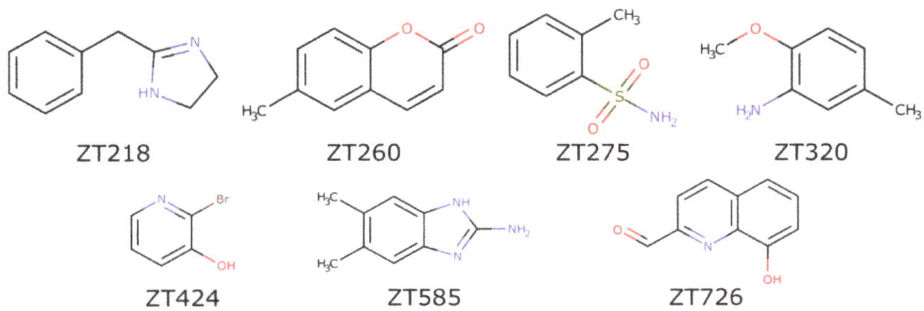

Figure 1. Structures of the fragments bound to Hma.

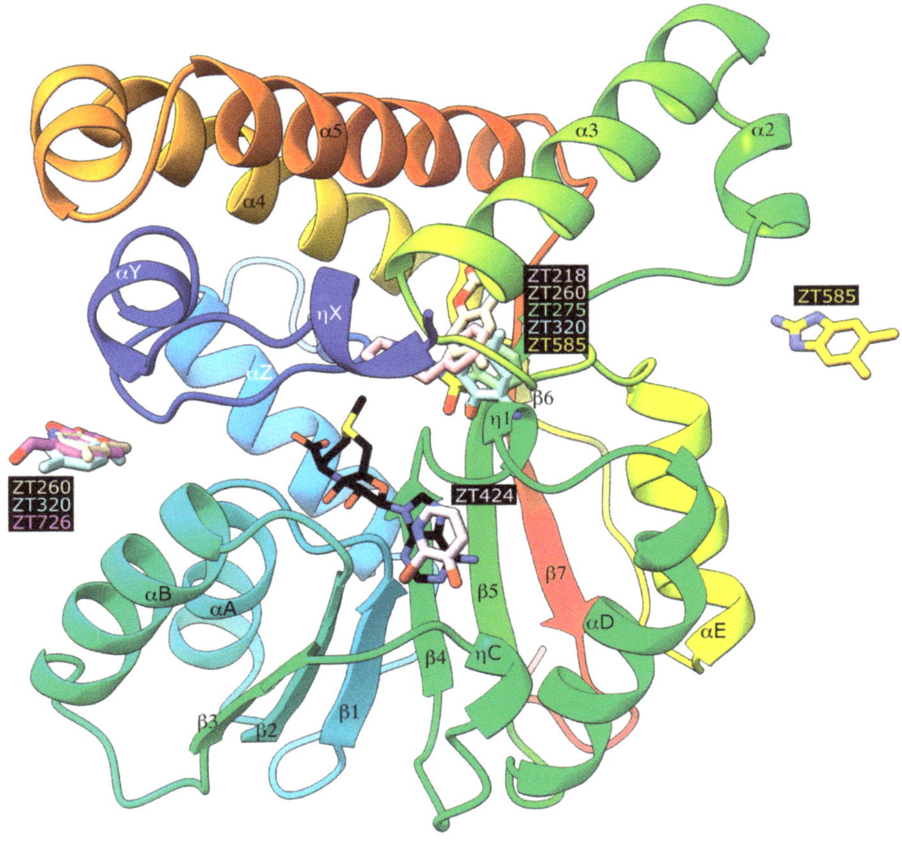

Figure 2. Ribbon representation of the Hma protein (PDB ID 2FK8) in the presence of the S-adenosylmethionine cofactor, represented as sticks with black carbon atoms, with all observed bound fragments represented as sticks with coloured carbon atoms. The protein is represented as a ribbon coloured from blue at the N-terminus to red at the C-terminus and secondary structure elements are labelled according to [30].

Table 1. Data collection and refinement statistics.

	ZT218	ZT260	ZT275	ZT320	ZT424	ZT585	ZT726
PDB code	7Q2B	7Q2C	7Q2H	7Q2D	7Q2E	7Q2F	7Q2G
Data Collection							
Beamline	ESRF, ID14-4	ESRF, ID14-4	ESRF, ID23-1	ESRF, ID29	ESRF, ID29	SOLEIL, PX1	ESRF, ID14-4
Spacegroup	$P3_121$	$P3_121$	$P3_121$	$P3_121$	$P3_121$	$P3_121$	$P3_121$
Unit cell a, c (Å)	57.29, 206.00	57.11, 205.90	56.62, 207.67	57.02, 207.35	55.77, 207.02	57.11, 204.46	57.06, 205.93
Resolution range (Å) [1]	40.21–1.85 (1.96–1.85)	35.66–1.85 (1.96–1.85)	49.03–1.75 (1.86–1.75)	49.38–1.90 (2.02–1.90)	49.17–2.00 (2.12–2.00)	49.46–1.85 (1.88–1.85)	40.10–2.00 (2.12–2.00)
No. unique reflections	34,449 (5438)	33,875 (5254)	40,075 (6368)	31,853 (5032)	27,163 (4292)	33,526 (1649)	27,352 (4359)
Completeness (%)	99.8 (99.7)	98.4 (96.7)	99.5 (99.7)	100.0 (100.0)	99.6 (99.7)	98.3 (99.9)	99.9 (99.9)
Redundancy	6.0 (6.0)	5.1 (3.7)	8.9 (8.8)	11.4 (11.8)	6.7 (6.5)	5.9 (5.2)	7.5 (7.6)
$<I/\sigma(I)>$	11.5 (1.8)	15.1 (1.0)	13.7 (2.6)	16.2 (2.6)	17.3 (2.4)	7.2 (1.4)	11.4 (1.3)
R_{merge} (%)	8.2 (95.5)	5.1 (109.3)	8.9 (75.8)	8.1 (90.9)	5.2 (70.8)	15.8 (116.7)	9.1 (133.9)
CC(1/2)	99.6 (75.2)	99.9 (59.1)	99.6 (89.0)	99.8 (89.2)	99.9 (84.2)	98.3 (53.1)	99.6 (81.4)
Refinement							
Resolution range (Å)	40.25–1.85	35.66–1.85	49.03–1.75	49.38–1.90	49.17–2.00	49.46–1.85	40.10–2.00
No. reflections (work/test)	29,899/1703	28,298/1619	35,907/2034	28,849/1645	26,984/1545	30,090/1718	20,616/1191
R_{work}/R_{free}	0.1668/0.2059	0.1792/0.2256	0.1782/0.2105	0.1856/0.2281	0.1847/0.2375	0.1894/0.2293	0.1926/0.2538
No. of non-hydrogen atoms	2484	2472	2525	2440	2385	2480	2339
Protein	2298	2310	2305	2305	2281	2291	2264
Fragment	12	24	11	20	8	24	13
Solvent	174	138	209	115	96	165	62
Rms deviations							
Bond length (Å)	0.007	0.004	0.003	0.005	0.005	0.004	0.008
Bond angles (°)	1.338	1.233	1.164	1.225	1.296	1.199	1.226
Ramachandran plot							
Most favoured (%)	98	98	98	96	98	98	97
Allowed/Outliers (%)	2/0	2/0	2/0	4/0	2/0	2/0	3/0

[1] Values in parentheses are for the highest resolution shell.

2.1.1. Fragments ZT218, ZT260, ZT275, ZT320, and ZT585 Bind at the Substrate Binding Site

Five fragments were found to bind Hma at the substrate binding site (Figure 2), where the lipophilic moiety of S-adenosyl-N-decyl-aminoethyl (SADAE) has been observed in Hma [26], as well as didecyldimethylammonium bromide (DDDMAB) and cetyltrimethylammonium bromide (CTAB) in the structures of homologous CmaA1 and CmaA2, respectively [33].

The binding modes of ZT218, ZT260, and ZT585 (Figure 1) share common features: these fragments are buried between residues Ile204, Phe209, Tyr274, and Cys278 on one side and residues Glu149, Ser178, and Leu214 on the other side (Figures 3 and 4). Water-mediated hydrogen bonds are observed in all three structures, albeit at longer distance in the case of ZT260: a water molecule, occupying an almost identical position in all three structures, connects the fragments to Glu146OE2 (2.5–2.7 Å), Glu149OE2 (2.5–2.7 Å), and Ser178OG (2.6–2.7 Å). In the case of ZT218, an additional water-mediated hydrogen bond to the imidazole group of His150 is found (Figures 3 and 4). Protein residues interacting with these fragments display a conformation almost identical to that observed in the structures of Hma in the presence of the SAM cofactor or analogues. In the *apo*-Hma structure, residues 151–153 were found to be disordered, resulting in a dramatically different conformation for residues 147–150: the phenyl group of Phe148 in *apo*-Hma is approximately 12.5 Å from the position it occupies in the structures of these complexes. The conformation of residues 147–150 observed in the *apo*-Hma structure would not be compatible with the binding of these fragments. It is likely that the binding of ZT218, ZT260, and ZT585 fragments leads to structuration of residues 147–153, resulting in folding of the helix η1, as already observed upon binding of the SAM cofactor or analogues [26,30].

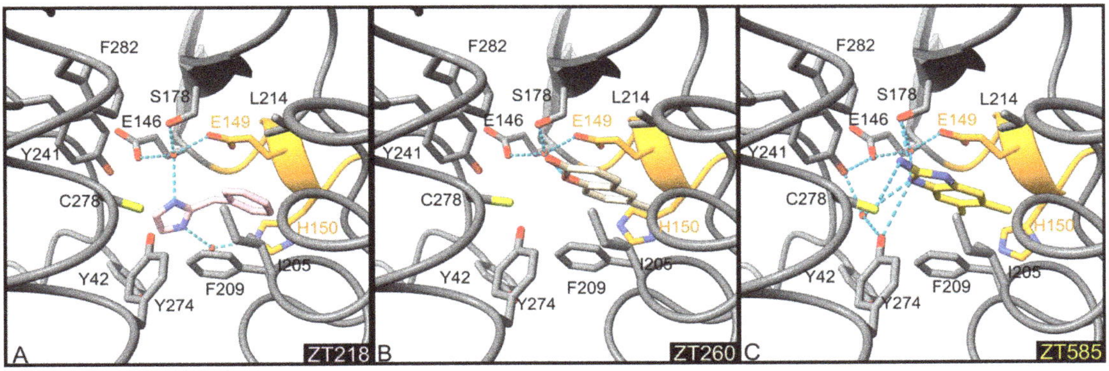

Figure 3. Detailed representation of binding of ZT218 (**A**, pink), ZT260 (**B**, beige), and ZT585 (**C**, yellow) at the substrate binding site. The protein backbone is represented as a tube, the side chains of residues involved in ligand binding are shown as sticks and labelled, water molecules as red spheres, and hydrogen bonds as blue dotted lines. Residues 148–151 forming helix η1 are coloured orange.

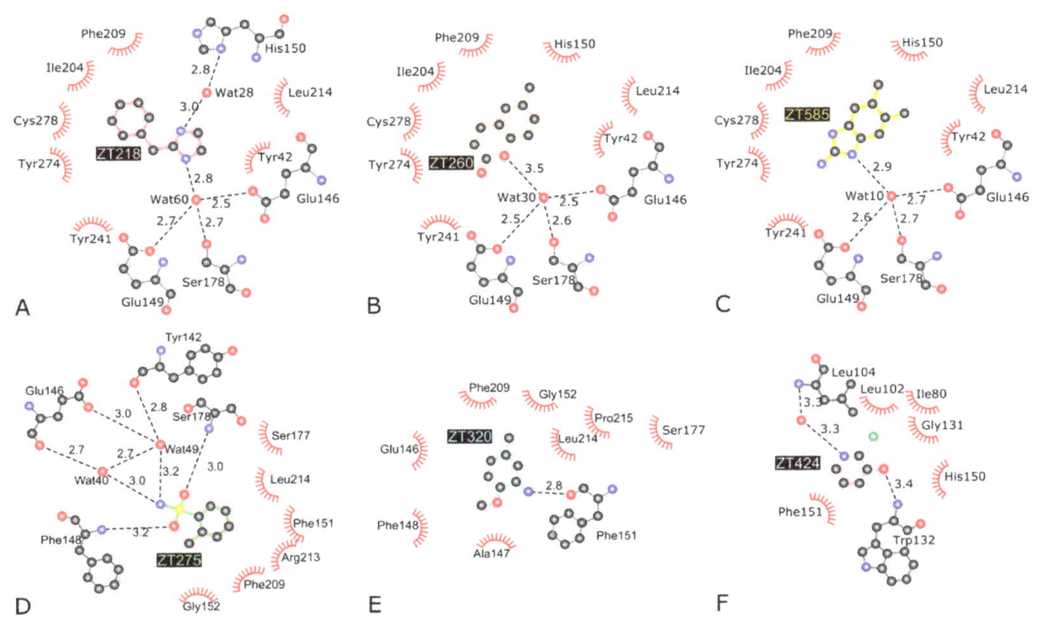

Figure 4. 2D interaction maps of fragments ZT218 (**A**), ZT260 (**B**), ZT585 (**C**), ZT275 (**D**), ZT320 (**E**), and ZT424 (**F**) bound to the Hma protein. Hydrogen bonds are represented with dashed black lines and their lengths are indicated. Residues/atoms involved in van der Waals contacts are represented by notched semicircles (figure adapted from LigPlot+ [34]).

Although ZT275 and ZT320 (Figure 1) also bind to Hma at the substrate binding site (Figure 2), they induce a previously unobserved conformation for residues 147–154 These two fragments establish van der Waals contacts with Phe148, Gly152, Phe209, and Leu214 (Figures 4 and 5). The oxygen atoms of the sulphonamide group of ZT275 form a hydrogen bond with the main-chain nitrogen atom of Phe148 (3.2 Å) and Ser178 (3.0 Å). In the case of ZT320, the nitrogen atom of the amine moiety forms a hydrogen bond with the oxygen atom of the main chain of Phe151 (2.8 Å, Figures 4 and 5). In both cases, binding results in a modified conformation for residues 147–154. The three-residue long helix η1 (Phe148–His150), observed in the presence of the SAM cofactor or the ZT218, ZT260, or ZT585 fragments, is pushed away from the fragment binding site, reorganises, and includes Phe151. In this new position, Phe148 is about 10 Å away from the position it occupies in the structure of the other complexes: the main-chain atoms are in a position similar to that observed in the *apo*-Hma structure, but the position of the side chain is different, as a result of a 110° rotation of the χ1 dihedral angle. In addition, Glu149 and His150 are found at the position where the adenine moiety of the cofactor resides when bound to Hma [26,30]. Therefore, binding of ZT275 or ZT320 induces a new conformation that would not be compatible with the presence of the cofactor.

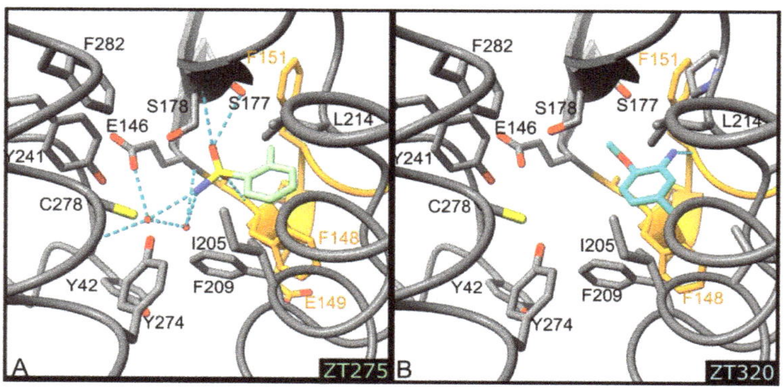

Figure 5. Detailed representation of binding of ZT275 ((**A**), pale green) and ZT320 ((**B**), turquoise) at the substrate binding site. The protein is represented as a ribbon, the side chains of residues involved in ligand biding are shown as sticks and labelled, water molecules as red spheres, and hydrogen bonds as blue dotted lines. Residues 148–151 forming helix η1 are coloured orange.

2.1.2. Fragment ZT424 Binds at the Cofactor Adenine Site

Binding of ZT424 (Figure 1) is observed at the position where the adenine moiety of the SAM cofactor and its analogues were located [26,30] (Figure 2). ZT424 establishes van der Waals contacts with the side chains of Leu104, Trp132, His150, and Phe151 (Figures 4 and 6). The bromine atom of ZT424 makes a weak halogen bond [35] with the main-chain oxygen atom of Leu102 (4.0 Å), while the ring nitrogen atom of the fragment interact with a water molecule (3.3 Å), which is also hydrogen bonded to the main-chain nitrogen atom of Leu104 (3.3 Å). The hydroxyl group of ZT424 makes a weak hydrogen bond with the main-chain nitrogen atom of Trp132 (3.4 Å) and with the carboxylate group of Glu133 (3.4 Å). In this structure, residues 147–154 display the same conformation as that found in the structures of Hma in the presence of the SAM cofactor or analogues, as well as those obtained in the presence of ZT218, ZT260, and ZT585.

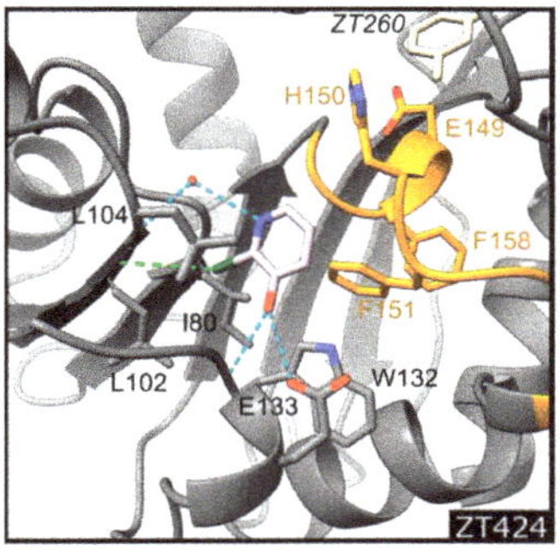

Figure 6. Detailed representation of binding of ZT424 (light pink) at the cofactor binding site. The protein is represented as a ribbon, the side chains of residues involved in ligand biding are shown as sticks and labelled, water molecules as red spheres, and hydrogen and halogen bonds as blue and green dotted lines, respectively. Residues 148–151 forming helix η1 are coloured orange. The position of ZT260, coloured beige, in the substrate binding site is also indicated for easier comparison with Figures 4 and 5.

2.1.3. Fragments ZT260, ZT320, ZT585, and ZT726 Bind at the Protein Surface

Two fragment binding sites are observed on the surface of Hma (Figure 2). The first is delineated by Arg40, Arg111, and Trp84. A second molecule of the ZT260 and ZT320 fragments is located at this position, as well as ZT726 (Figure 1). The planar aromatic ring of ZT260, ZT320, and ZT726 is intercalated between the guanidinium groups of the two arginine residues and forms a perpendicular aromatic–aromatic interaction with the indole moiety of Trp84 (Figure 7). Broad, planar, and ill-defined electron density peaks were observed at this position in several of the structures obtained in this study, but they did not allow the unambiguous positioning of the corresponding fragments.

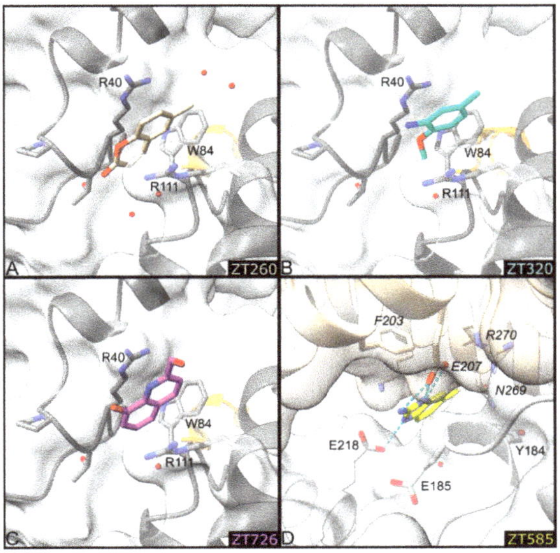

Figure 7. Detailed representation of binding of ZT260 (**A**), ZT320 (**B**), ZT726 (**C**), and ZT585 (**D**) at the protein surface. The protein is represented as a ribbon, the side chains of residues involved in ligand biding are shown as sticks and labelled, water molecules as red spheres, and hydrogen bonds as blue dotted lines. Residues 148–151 forming helix η1 are coloured orange. In D, the symmetry-related molecule is represented in beige and labelled in italics.

A second surface binding site is also observed in the case of ZT585, located between two protein molecules in the crystal, near helix α2 (Figure 7). ZT585 makes van der Waals contacts with the side chain of Tyr184 and hydrogen bonding with the side chain of Glu218. ZT585 is also hydrogen-bonded to the side chain of Glu207 and within van der Waals distance of the main-chain atoms of Asn269 and Arg270, all belonging to a symmetry-related molecule in the crystal. The binding of ZT585 induces significant conformational changes. Indeed, in all Hma structures determined so far, the α2 helix comprises residues 183–188 and a two-residue long loop (residues 189–190) connects the α2 and α3 (residues 191–208) helices. In the presence of ZT585, the α2 helix is shortened at residues 183–185 and the α3 helix is extended with an additional turn at its N-terminus (188–208).

2.2. Chimeric Compounds

As several fragments bind to the substrate binding site, chimeric compounds were designed to mimic the simultaneous binding of two fragments and thus improve binding affinities. Superimposition of fragments suggested that chimeric compounds could be derived from the fusion of ZT218 with ZT260 or ZT585. Indeed, replacement of the phenyl ring of ZT218 with the aromatic core of ZT260 or ZT585 results in the series 218260x and 218585x (Figure 8). On the other hand, ZT275 could be merged with ZT320 to give the compounds 275320x (Figure 8). Additionally, compound 320sadae was designed by the addition of a lipophilic C_7 chain to the aromatic nucleus of ZT320, in order to mimic the binding of SADAE [26]. The chimeric compounds were manually positioned in the appropriate structure of Hma using Coot.

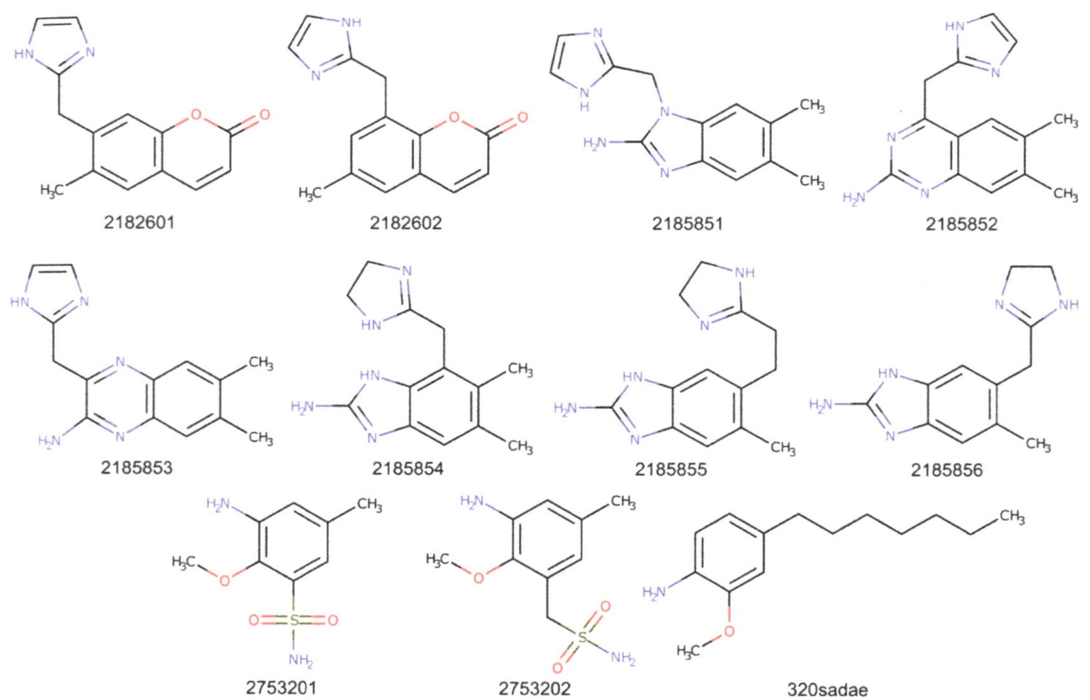

Figure 8. Chimeric compounds derived from merged fragments.

2.3. Molecular Dynamics Simulations

2.3.1. *Apo*-Hma

In the crystallographic structure of *apo*-Hma, residues 151–153 were found to be disordered [30] suggesting that the 146–155 loop, connecting strand β4 to helix αD, was mobile, at least partially. In the presence of the SAM cofactor [30] and analogues [26], this loop displays decreased mobility, and residues 148–150 form the short η1 helix. A similar conformation of the η1 helix was also observed in the structures of complexes of Hma with ZT218, ZT260, and ZT585 bound in the substrate binding site and with ZT424 bound in the cofactor binding site. On the other hand, a very different conformation was observed in the presence of ZT275 and ZT320 in the substrate binding site. This new conformation would not be compatible with cofactor binding, as Glu149 and His150 are displaced to the position occupied by the adenine moiety. Molecular dynamics simulations were performed for *apo*-Hma, using the two observed conformations of the loop, for a simulation time of 1.2 μs. The calculations were performed in triplicate. The all-atoms root-mean-square fluctuation (RMSF) per residue monitored throughout the simulation indicates that some parts of the protein are indeed more flexible (Figure S1). In both cases, four regions of higher mobility can be identified. Indeed, the N- and C-terminal extremities (residues 19–28 and 298–301, respectively) and residues 152–155 and 182–195 display an average RMSF greater than 1.5 Å for more than three consecutive residues. Residues 152–155 are part of the disordered loop observed in the *apo*-Hma structure that folds upon cofactor binding and residues 182–195 are part of helices α2 and α3. These residues are displaced upon binding of ZT585 at the protein surface (see above). Although the RMSF profiles are comparable for the two starting conformations, residues 129–136 display greater mobility in the conformation compatible with the presence of the cofactor (average RMSF of 1.5 Å compared to 0.9 Å).

The root-mean-square deviation (RMSD) from the starting conformation was also analysed, after removing the global rotational and translational displacement and ignoring the parts of the protein with the highest RMSF, i.e., residues 19–28, 152–155, 182–195, and 298–301. The variations of the RMSD in function of the simulation time (Figure S2) display a homogeneous behaviour independent of the starting conformation. The RMSD converges to about 1.2–1.7 Å after 0.2 μs in each case.

The possibility of a transition between the two conformations observed for residues 147–154 was also investigated. To this end, some distances were monitored during the simulation. This was the case for the distance between the centre of mass of the aromatic side chains of Phe148 and Phe160, which was measured to be 5.7 and 16.2 Å in the crystallographic structures of the cofactor-compatible and cofactor-incompatible conformation, respectively. Similarly, the distances from the centre of mass of the imidazole group of His150 to the Cα atom of Gly131 or to the centre of mass of the aromatic ring of Tyr42 was also monitored. Initial values were 11.5 Å and 9.3 Å, respectively, in the cofactor-compatible conformation, and 4.7 Å and 14.4 Å, respectively, in the cofactor-incompatible conformation. Representative profiles of the variation of these distances over the course of the simulation are shown in Figure S3.

2.3.2. Hma in the Presence of Fragments or of Chimeric Compounds

Molecular dynamics simulations were also performed with Hma in the presence of fragments, starting from observed crystallographic structures, or chimeric compounds, starting from manually generated structures. In the case of the fragments ZT218, ZT260, and ZT585, for which water molecules mediate hydrogen bonds to the protein, two simulations were performed, with or without these water molecules. Simulations were also performed in the presence of the cofactor or analogues of the cofactor, starting from the coordinates of the complexes found at the PDB [26,30].

2.4. Estimation of Binding Energies for Fragments and Chimeric Compounds

For the estimation of binding energies, 2000 consecutive frames were selected from the trajectories of the molecular dynamics simulation, after an equilibrium was reached, visualised by the stabilisation of the main-chain RMSD. One frame out of two was used for the calculation of the binding energies, according to the generalised Born method and the Poisson–Boltzmann method coupled to the surface area continuum solvation method (hereafter GBSA and PBSA, respectively). Both approaches approximate the enthalpic term of the binding Gibbs energy and neglect the entropic term, which would be complicated and time consuming to evaluate. Nevertheless, this simplification allows compounds to be ranked in a drug design perspective and the impact of chemical modifications of the ligand on binding to be assessed [36,37]. The PBSA approach is generally considered more accurate in calculating absolute free energies, but it is more time consuming and appears to be more dependent on the system under study, whereas the GBSA approach is better at ranking binding affinities [37]. PBSA and GBSA terms were evaluated for all ligands investigated, including the SAM cofactor and its analogues SAH, SADAE, and sinefungin which have been shown to bind Hma [26,30]. The binding energies evaluated using the PBSA method are consistently lower than those obtained with the GBSA method (Table 2 and Figure S4). However, as a good correlation was found between the two methods (R^2 = 0.983, Figure S4), the values obtained with the GBSA method will be considered.

Table 2. Estimated binding energies and standard deviations (kcal/mol) for all ligands mentioned in this study.

Ligand	GBSA	PBSA
ZT218	−22.8 ± 2.2	−11.9 ± 2.6
ZT218 *	−22.2 ± 1.8	−10.2 ± 2.2
ZT260	−18.0 ± 1.8	−12.0 ± 2.1
ZT260 *	−22.2 ± 1.8	−10.2 ± 2.2
ZT275	−17.9 ± 2.1	−7.0 ± 2.1
ZT320	−23.0 ± 2.1	−12.8 ± 2.2
ZT424	−18.9 ± 1.7	−9.7 ± 1.9
ZT585	−26.8 ± 1.7	−14.8 ± 2.0
ZT585 *	−26.2 ± 1.7	−14.0 ± 2.0
ZT726	−19.2 ± 1.8	−11.4 ± 2.1
2182601	−29.9 ± 2.5	−10.7 ± 3.0
2182601 *	−33.9 ± 2.2	−19.6 ± 2.2
2182602	−30.5 ± 1.8	−14.2 ± 2.1
2182602 *	−31.5 ± 2.1	−15.6 ± 2.7
2753201	−24.9 ± 2.9	−12.5 ± 2.2
2753202	−18.9 ± 3.8	−5.3 ± 2.6
2185851	−32.4 ± 2.1	−12.2 ± 2.3
2185852	−32.3 ± 2.6	−13.2 ± 2.8
2185853	−34.4 ± 2.0	−14.5 ± 2.4
2185854	−34.3 ± 2.2	−18.2 ± 2.4
2185855	−35.1 ± 2.2	−18.6 ± 2.6
2185856	−35.0 ± 2.3	−19.7 ± 2.5
320sadae	−35.7 ± 2.2	−20.3 ± 2.5
SAM	−45.7 ± 4.9	−25.0 ± 4.1
SAH	−40.2 ± 3.4	−21.8 ± 3.2
Sinefungin	−39.6 ± 3.8	−24.8 ± 3.6
SADAE	−67.7 ± 3.5	−35.8 ± 3.1

*An asterisk following the name of the fragment indicates that experimentally observed bridging water molecules were conserved in the molecular dynamics simulations.

As expected, the estimated binding energies for the fragments are significantly higher (−17.9 to −26.8 kcal/mol) than the values obtained for the SAM cofactor and its analogues (−39.6 to −67.7 kcal/mol). SAM, SAH (the reaction product), and sinefungin display comparable values (−45.7, −40.2, and −39.6 kcal/mol, respectively) while SADAE shows an extremely favourable binding energy (−67.7 kcal/mol). The chimeric compounds resulting from the fusion of the fragments exhibit binding energies ranging from −18.9 to −35.7 kcal/mol, intermediate between values found with the original fragments or the cofactor and its analogues. The most favourable chimeric compounds are 320sadae (−35.7 kcal/mol), which combines ZT320 with a C_7 alkyl chain reminiscent of the C_{10} alkyl chain of SADAE, and 218585x (−32.3 to −35.1 kcal/mol) resulting from the fusion of ZT218 and ZT585. The chimeric compounds 218260x and 218585x show more favourable binding energies (between −29.9 and –35.1 kcal/mol) than the individual original fragments (−22.8 kcal/mol for ZT218, −18.0 kcal/mol for ZT260, and −26.8 kcal/mol for ZT585), which is not the case for the chimeric compounds 275320x, which exhibit comparable binding energies (between −18.9 and −24.9 kcal/mol) to those found for ZT275 (−17.9 kcal/mol) and ZT320 (−23.0 kcal/mol).

3. Discussion

3.1. Crystallographic Screening

X-ray crystallography is a powerful technique for fragment screening, as high concentrations of fragments can be achieved in co-crystallisation or soaking experiments, as long as the crystals are resistant to the treatment [38–40]. High concentrations are required to provide clear electron density for bound fragments, despite the expected low affinity resulting from their low molecular weights [41,42]. Nevertheless, weak binding is often observed, and specific ligand detection procedures have to be used in order to detect those fragments. In this regard, the use of the PanDDA procedure [31,43] was instrumental in this study to visualise the binding of the ZT275, ZT320, ZT424, and ZT726 fragments that were barely visible in conventional electron density maps.

Crystallographic screening of 126 fragments identified 7 bound fragments, corresponding to a hit rate of 5.5%, in the lower range of what is usually observed in a fragment screening [43–46]. Among the seven positive hits, five were found to bind in the substrate binding site and one in the cofactor binding site at the adenine position.

3.2. Molecular Plasticity of Hma

Comparison of the structure of *apo*-Hma [30] with those of Hma in the presence of the SAM cofactor or analogues [26,30] showed that the 146–155 loop was highly mobile in the absence of ligands and stabilised upon binding of the cofactor or analogues. This is also confirmed by our structures in the presence of the ZT218, ZT260, ZT424, and ZT585 fragments, since the 146–155 loop adopts a similar conformation to that observed in the presence of the cofactor. Surprisingly, while the ZT275 and ZT320 fragments also bind at the substrate binding site, albeit deeper in the crevice, they induce a different conformation of the 146–155 loop. Notably, in this new conformation, Glu149 and His150 occupy the position of the adenine portion of the cofactor. Hence, this new conformation is likely to be incompatible with the presence of the cofactor.

Molecular dynamics simulation of *apo*-Hma, starting with either of the two conformations observed for the 146–155 loop, was run in triplicate for simulation time of 1.2 µs to assess the structural plasticity of each conformation and the possible exchange between them. RMSD analysis along the simulation indicates that both conformations reach an equilibrium state with RMSD values of approximately 1.5 Å relative to the starting conformation (Figure S2). The RMSFs along the protein backbone also display a homogeneous behaviour: in addition to the N- and C-terminal ends, two regions display higher mobility, namely, residues 147–156 and 188–200, as previously observed in the case of the other mycolic acid methyltransferases CmaA2 and CmaA3, which are responsible for the cyclopropanation of MAs [47]. A notable exception occurs for residues 129–137 for which a greater mobility is observed in the case of the cofactor-compatible conformation (average RMSF of 1.5 Å compared to 0.9 Å) (Figure S1). These residues border the cofactor binding site and interact with its adenine moiety [30]. In the cofactor-compatible conformation of *apo*-Hma, this site is filled with water molecules, and residues 129–136 are not restrained. In the cofactor-incompatible conformation, this site is occupied by His150, which makes a water-mediated hydrogen bond with the carboxylate group of Glu133. An additional hydrogen bond is observed between the main-chain oxygen atom of His153 and the side-chain nitrogen atom of Trp132 (2.9 Å). These interactions likely decrease the mobility of residues 129–136. In the presence of the SAM cofactor or analogues, it is the adenine moiety that similarly limits the mobility of residues 129–136 (Figure S1).

The crystallographic structures presented here indicate that the substrate binding site of Hma is capable of adopting at least two distinct conformations, depending on the ligand bound. Interestingly, one of these conformations is not compatible with the presence of the SAM cofactor in its binding site, which, from the perspective of inhibiting the enzyme activity, appears particularly interesting. It seems that there is no transition between the two conformations, at least during the 1.2 μs of the simulation. However, the evolution of inter-residue distances throughout the simulation of *apo*-Hma (Figure S3) suggests that the cofactor-incompatible conformation displays less structural variability than the cofactor-compatible conformation.

3.3. Computed Binding Energies of Fragments and Chimeric Compounds

As expected for low molecular weight fragments, the calculated binding energies are rather high (−19.1 kcal/mol on average), suggesting that the interactions are indeed tenuous. The explicit inclusion of experimentally observed water molecules involved in the interactions with the fragment and the protein does not significantly alter the binding energies. Indeed, although the presence of these water molecules might have an effect on the position of the fragment during the dynamics, and thus indirectly affect the estimation of binding energies, they do not directly contribute to the binding energy estimation, as the calculation relies on an implicit solvent model.

Although five of the identified fragments bind to the substrate binding site, they can be divided into two binding modes. Binding of the ZT218, ZT260, or ZT585 fragments induces a conformation for residues 146–155 similar to that observed in the Hma structures obtained in the presence of the SAM cofactor and analogues. Furthermore, from a steric point of view, the binding of these fragments would not prevent cofactor binding. Thus, the inhibitors derived from these fragments would compete with the enzyme substrate. On the other hand, binding of ZT275 and ZT320 fragments induces a different conformation for residues 146–155, resulting in residues 149 and 150 occupying the position where the adenine part of the cofactor is located. Thus, inhibitors derived from these fragments would simultaneously prevent binding of the substrate and cofactor, in a manner similar to that observed for SADAE [26,48]. However, unlike SADAE, which competes for binding with both substrate and cofactor, the inhibitors derived from the ZT275 and ZT320 fragments would act as competitive inhibitors for the substrate but as allosteric inhibitors for the cofactor.

Based on the observed structures, several chimeric compounds were designed by fusion of the identified bound fragments. The 218260x and 218585x series were derived from merging fragments ZT218 with ZT260, and ZT218 with ZT585, respectively, and compounds 275320x resulted from merging ZT275 and ZT320. Binding energies of chimeric compounds were evaluated in the same way as for those of original fragments. Among those chimeric compounds, compounds 2753201 and 2753202 display binding energies of the same order of magnitude as those of the original fragments (−18.9 and −24.9 kcal/mol). This could be related to the low molecular complexity of these compounds, comparable to that of the original fragments. The chimeric compounds 218260x and 218585x display much more favourable binding energies (−31.5 and −33.9 kcal/mol, on average, respectively).

SADAE is a SAM analogue that was shown to inhibit *Escherichia coli* cyclopropane fatty acid synthase (CFAS) both in vivo and in vitro [48], as well as Hma in vitro [26].

Furthermore, SADAE also inhibited the growth of Mtb and *M. smegmatis*, indicating that it is able to cross the cell wall of mycobacteria [26]. The efficacy of SADAE has been attributed partly to the lipophilic C_{10} chain, which is thought to mimic the lipophilic chain of CFAS and Hma substrates [26,48]. The calculated binding energy for SADAE is extremely favourable, due to the numerous van der Waals interactions resulting from the presence of the lipophilic chain. It should be noted, however, that for a compound with such a degree of freedom, neglecting the entropic term is likely to lead to significant approximations. The chimeric compound 320sadae was designed by adding a C_7-chain to ZT320 to occupy the substrate binding site. It exhibits the lowest binding energy (−35.7 kcal/mol), compared to other chimeric compounds, marginally better than the values obtained for compounds of the 218585x series. Compared to the binding energy of the original ZT320 fragment (−23.0 kcal/mol), the observed gain is, however, important, even considering the uncertainty resulting from neglecting the entropic term.

These results suggest that at least two strategies are conceivable to inhibit Hma, and potentially other mycolic acid methyltransferases, which share high structural similarities [33,49]. First, elaborating from the ZT275 and ZT320 fragments would yield compounds that simultaneously interfere with substrate binding, as they occupy the substrate binding site, and prevent cofactor binding, as they induce structural modifications of the protein that are not compatible with the presence of SAM. Secondly, the addition of a lipophilic moiety would optimise the occupation of the substrate binding site, and would contribute to improve the specificity of the compounds towards methyltransferases acting on long aliphatic compound, such as lipids. In this regard, the functionalisation of the aliphatic chain that would mimic reaction intermediates would further improve the inhibitors' affinity and specificity.

4. Materials and Methods

4.1. Expression, Purification, and Crystallisation of Hma

The Hma protein was expressed and purified as previously described [26,48]. In summary, a pET15b plasmid (Novagen) containing the *hma* cDNA was used for transformation of *Escherichia coli* BL21(DE3)pLysS bacteria. This construct exchanges the first three residues of Hma with a 20-residue cleavable His-tag. Expression of the recombinant protein was induced by the addition of 1 mM Isopropyl β-D-1-thiogalactopyranoside (IPTG) at 310 K for 3 h. After sonication and centrifugation, the soluble fraction was loaded onto a nickel affinity column (Amersham Biosciences, Amersham, UK) and the His-tagged protein was eluted with a 5–500 mM imidazole gradient in a buffer consisting of 50 mM MES, pH 6.5, and 300 mM NaCl. A final size exclusion chromatography step, using a Sephadex 75 HiLoad column (Amersham Biosciences), yielded a pure protein for structural studies.

The purified Hma protein was crystallised at 285 K by vapor diffusion using the hanging drop technique. The crystallisation conditions were optimised from those published previously [26,30] to reproducibly provide sufficient quantities of good quality crystals. A 3 µL droplet was prepared by mixing 2 µL of a 3–4 mg/mL of Hma solution (MES 50 mM, NaCl 50 mM, pH 6.5) with 1 µL of reservoir solution (BisTris 50 mM, PEG 3350 4% (*w*/*v*), pH 6.5). Under these conditions, seeding of crushed crystal fragments was necessary because the protein concentration in the drop was not sufficient to allow spontaneous nucleation. This procedure yielded reproducibly 5 to 10 single crystals per drop, bipyramidal in shape, and about 200 µm long in their largest dimension, suitable for soaking experiments.

4.2. Fragments

A 352-fragment library was acquired from Zenobia Therapeutics. The molecular fragments (average molecular weight 154 ± 29 Da, 0–3 hydrogen bond donors, 0–6 hydrogen bond acceptors, 0–3 cycles, and 0–5 rotatable bonds) were formulated at 200 mM in pure DMSO. Fragments were used without prior purification or characterisation.

4.3. Crystallographic Screening

Crystallographic screening was performed by soaking Hma crystals overnight in 20 mM fragment solutions in 50 mM BisTris, PEG 3350 4% (*w*/*v*), pH 6.5, at 285 K. Soaked crystals were cryoprotected by immersion for 2 min in the crystallisation solution supplemented with 20% (*v*/*v*) glycerol before cooling in a stream of nitrogen gas at 100 K.

Diffraction data were collected at ALBA (Barcelona, Spain, beamline XALOC), SOLEIL (Saclay, France, beamline PX1), and European Synchrotron Radiation Facility (ESRF, Grenoble, France, beamlines ID14-1, ID14-2, ID23-1, ID23-2, and ID29), and processed with XDS [50] and AutoProc [51]. Preliminary refinement was performed using the dimple pipeline of the CCP4 Program Suite [52] starting with *apo*-Hma coordinates [30] before identifying structures with potentially bound fragments with the PanDDA procedure [31]. These structures were further refined with REFMAC5 [53], Buster [54], and Coot [55]. The fragment dictionaries were generated using MarvinSketch [56] and the Grade Server [57].

4.4. Molecular Dynamics Simulation

Available crystallographic structures of the apo protein and of complexes [26,30] including those described here, as well as models of complexes generated in the presence of the chimeric compounds, were used as starting point for molecular dynamics simulations. The chimeric compounds were drawn and converted in 3D with MarvinSketch [56].

The tleap module for AMBER-20 [58] was used to generate a periodic cubic box extending 10 Å around the protein, containing the structure of the protein, the ligand if present, water molecules represented with the TIP3P model, and sodium cations to neutralise the system. The GPU version of the PMEMD module available in AMBER-20 was used for energy minimisation and molecular dynamics calculations. An initial energy minimisation was performed, with progressively reduced constraints on protein atom positions, followed by a 150 ps equilibration MD and a 100 ns production run. In the case of *apo*-Hma and of the SAM-Hma complex, the production simulations were extended to 1 µs. Analysis of trajectories, as well as monitoring of interactions and of inter-residue distances along the trajectories were performed using CCPTRAJ [59].

4.5. Relative Binding Affinity Evaluation

Molecular dynamics (MD) simulation was coupled with the MM-GB/PBSA post processing method [60] to estimate the interaction energies of fragments, cofactor and cofactor analogues, and chimeric compounds derived from the identified bound fragments. This procedure relies on frames extracted from an all-atom molecular dynamics simulation of a protein–ligand complex, after removal of solvent molecules, since these methods rely on an implicit solvent model. The enthalpic term of the Gibbs free energy of binding is approximated from the force-field energy, and the entropic term is usually neglected as it is extremely time consuming to calculate [61]. Therefore, this procedure does not provide true binding energies, but it can still estimate relative binding energies between ligands as the entropy term should be dominated by the protein contribution, which should be comparable for the different ligands. The MMPBSA.py.MPI program [60] was used for the calculations.

5. Conclusions

The crystallographic screening of a fragment library allowed for the identification of 7 fragments bound to Hma. The presence of bound fragments in the substrate binding site of Hma induced two distinct conformations of residues 147–154. One of these conformations would be incompatible with the presence of the SAM cofactor in its binding site. Second generation chemical compounds were designed based on the observed positions of the fragments. Binding energies of initial fragments, of second generations molecules and of the SAM cofactor and analogues were estimated using MM-GBSA/PBSA methods. Whereas bonding energies of fragments were high, as would be expected for low molecular weight compounds, some of the second generations compounds displayed binding ener gies close to that found for cofactor analogues. These results suggest that our compounds could be further improved to inhibit Hma, and possibly other MAMTs. Additionally, our findings allow to envision the possibility of allosteric inhibition of cofactor binding.

Supplementary Materials: The following are available online at https://www.mdpi.com/article/10.3390/ph14121282/s1, Figure S1: Root-mean-square fluctuation along the MD simulation of *apo*-Hma. The per residue main-chain atom fluctuations are average of three independent 1.2 μs simulations of *apo*-Hma starting either from the cofactor-compatible conformation (orange) or from the conformation observed in the presence of ZT275 or ZT320 that would be incompatible with the binding of the cofactor (blue). For comparison, the per residue main-chain atom fluctuations of the structure of Hma in complex with SAM (averaged from 2 independent 1.2 μs simulations) is shown in grey. Secondary structures elements are indicated, labelled and coloured as in Figure 2. Figure S2: Evolution of the root-mean-square deviation along the MD simulation of *apo*-Hma. RMS deviations (Å) were computed using main-chain atoms of residues 29–151, 156–181, and 196–297 on the whole trajectory and plotted as a function of time for the 1.2 μs simulation of *apo*-Hma starting either from the cofactor-compatible conformation (blue) or from the cofactor-incompatible, ZT320-bound conformation (orange). For clarity, only one in 10 values is plotted. A single representative curve is displayed for each simulation performed in triplicate. Figure S3: Variations of selected inter-residues distances along the simulation trajectory of *apo*-Hma. Distances were measured between the centre of mass of the aromatic side chain of Phe160 and of Phe148 (blue) and between the centre of mass of the imidazole group of His150 and either the Cα atom of Gly131 (orange) or the centre of mass of the aromatic ring of Tyr42 (grey). Distances are plotted as a function of time for the simulation starting from the cofactor-compatible conformation (top) and from the cofactor-incompatible, ZT320-bound conformation (bottom). Simulations were performed in triplicate, curves from a single simulation are shown. Figure S4: Comparison of binding affinities as evaluated using the GBSA or the PBSA approach. The linear fit is indicated. Initial fragments are represented with red dots, chimeric compounds with blue dots and SAM and analogues with green dots. An asterisk following the name of the fragment indicates that experimentally observed bridging water molecules were conserved in the molecular dynamics simulations. Abbreviation: SIN, sinefungin. A straight line is fitted to all the points, passing at the origin. The square of the Pearson correlation coefficient is indicated.

Author Contributions: Conceptualisation, L.M. (Lionel Mourey) and L.M. (Laurent Maveyraud); validation, R.G., L.M. (Lionel Mourey), and L.M. (Laurent Maveyraud); formal analysis, R.G. and L.M. (Laurent Maveyraud); investigation, R.G., Y.G., S.B., J.-C.P., L.M. (Lionel Mourey), and L.M. (Laurent Maveyraud); resources, J.-C.P. and L.M. (Lionel Mourey); writing—original draft preparation, R.G. and L.M. (Laurent Maveyraud); writing—review and editing, L.M. (Lionel Mourey), Y.G., S.B., and L.M. (Laurent Maveyraud); supervision, J.-C.P. and L.M. (Laurent Maveyraud); project administration, L.M. (Lionel Mourey); funding acquisition, L.M. (Lionel Mourey). All authors have read and agreed to the published version of the manuscript.

Funding: This project was supported by the Centre National de la Recherche Scientifique (CNRS). RG was supported by a fellowship from the Scientific Council of the Université Paul Sabatier, Université de Toulouse.

Institutional Review Board Statement: Not applicable.

Informed Consent Statement: Not applicable.

Data Availability Statement: The atomic coordinates and crystallographic structure factors of complexes described in this work have been deposited in the Protein Data Bank (www.rcsb.org) with accession codes as follows: Hma-ZT218 7Q2B; Hma-ZT260 7Q2C; Hma-ZT275 7Q2H; Hma-ZT320 7Q2D; Hma-ZT424 7Q2E; Hma-ZT585 7Q2F; and Hma-ZT726 7Q2G.

Acknowledgments: We thank the scientific staff at the European Synchrotron Radiation Facility (Grenoble, France) SOLEIL (Saclay, France) and ALBA (Barcelona, Spain) for the use of their excellent data collection facilities. We particularly thank the staff of beamlines ID14-4, ID23-1, and ID29 at the European Synchrotron Radiation Facility and beamline PX1 at SOLEIL where the crystallographic data presented here were collected. The macromolecular crystallography equipment used in this study are part of the Integrated Screening Platform of Toulouse (PICT, IBiSA).

Conflicts of Interest: The authors declare no conflict of interest. The funders had no role in the design of the study; in the collection, analyses, or interpretation of data; in the writing of the manuscript, or in the decision to publish the results.

References

1. World Health Organization. *Global Tuberculosis Report 2021*; World Health Organization: Geneva, Switzerland, 2021; ISBN 978-92-4-003702-1.
2. Daffé, M.; Marrakchi, H. Unraveling the Structure of the Mycobacterial Envelope. *Microbiol. Spectr.* **2019**, *7*, GPP3-0027-2018. [CrossRef] [PubMed]
3. Jarlier, V.; Nikaido, H. Mycobacterial Cell Wall: Structure and Role in Natural Resistance to Antibiotics. *FEMS Microbiol. Lett.* **1994**, *123*, 11–18. [CrossRef] [PubMed]
4. Cambier, C.J.; Takaki, K.K.; Larson, R.P.; Hernandez, R.E.; Tobin, D.M.; Urdahl, K.B.; Cosma, C.L.; Ramakrishnan, L. Mycobacteria Manipulate Macrophage Recruitment through Coordinated Use of Membrane Lipids. *Nature* **2014**, *505*, 218–222. [CrossRef]
5. Batt, S.M.; Minnikin, D.E.; Besra, G.S. The Thick Waxy Coat of Mycobacteria, a Protective Layer against Antibiotics and the Host's Immune System. *Biochem. J.* **2020**, *477*, 1983–2006. [CrossRef]
6. Marrakchi, H.; Lanéelle, M.-A.; Daffé, M. Mycolic Acids: Structures, Biosynthesis, and Beyond. *Chem. Biol.* **2014**, *21*, 67–85. [CrossRef]
7. Jackson, M. The Mycobacterial Cell Envelope—Lipids. *Cold Spring Harb. Perspect. Med.* **2014**, *4*, a021105. [CrossRef]
8. McNeil, M.; Daffé, M.; Brennan, P.J. Location of the Mycolyl Ester Substituents in the Cell Walls of Mycobacteria. *J. Biol. Chem.* **1991**, *266*, 13217–13223. [CrossRef]
9. Abrahams, K.A.; Besra, G.S. Mycobacterial Cell Wall Biosynthesis: A Multifaceted Antibiotic Target. *Parasitology* **2018**, *145*, 116–133. [CrossRef] [PubMed]
10. North, E.J.; Jackson, M.; Lee, R.E. New Approaches to Target the Mycolic Acid Biosynthesis Pathway for the Development of Tuberculosis Therapeutics. *Curr. Pharm. Des.* **2014**, *20*, 4357–4378. [CrossRef]
11. Banerjee, A.; Dubnau, E.; Quémard, A.; Balasubramanian, V.; Um, K.S.; Wilson, T.; Collins, D.; de Lisle, G.; Jacobs, W.R. InhA, a Gene Encoding a Target for Isoniazid and Ethionamide in *Mycobacterium tuberculosis*. *Science* **1994**, *263*, 227–230. [CrossRef]
12. Quémard, A.; Lanéelle, G.; Lacave, C. Mycolic Acid Synthesis: A Target for Ethionamide in Mycobacteria? *Antimicrob. Agents Chemother.* **1992**, *36*, 1316–1321. [CrossRef]
13. Takayama, K.; Wang, L.; David, H.L. Effect of Isoniazid on the In Vivo Mycolic Acid Synthesis, Cell Growth, and Viability of *Mycobacterium tuberculosis*. *Antimicrob. Agents Chemother.* **1972**, *2*, 29–35. [CrossRef]
14. Portevin, D.; de Sousa-D'Auria, C.; Houssin, C.; Grimaldi, C.; Chami, M.; Daffé, M.; Guilhot, C. A Polyketide Synthase Catalyzes the Last Condensation Step of Mycolic Acid Biosynthesis in Mycobacteria and Related Organisms. *Proc. Natl. Acad. Sci. USA* **2004**, *101*, 314–319. [CrossRef]
15. Varela, C.; Rittmann, D.; Singh, A.; Krumbach, K.; Bhatt, K.; Eggeling, L.; Besra, G.S.; Bhatt, A. MmpL Genes Are Associated with Mycolic Acid Metabolism in Mycobacteria and Corynebacteria. *Chem. Biol.* **2012**, *19*, 498–506. [CrossRef] [PubMed]
16. Glickman, M.S. The *MmaA2* Gene of *Mycobacterium tuberculosis* Encodes the Distal Cyclopropane Synthase of the α-Mycolic Acid. *J. Biol. Chem.* **2003**, *278*, 7844–7849. [CrossRef]
17. Glickman, M.S.; Cox, J.S.; Jacobs, W.R. A Novel Mycolic Acid Cyclopropane Synthetase Is Required for Cording, Persistence, and Virulence of *Mycobacterium tuberculosis*. *Mol. Cell* **2000**, *5*, 717–727. [CrossRef]
18. Laval, F.; Haites, R.; Movahedzadeh, F.; Lemassu, A.; Wong, C.Y.; Stoker, N.; Billman-Jacobe, H.; Daffé, M. Investigating the Function of the Putative Mycolic Acid Methyltransferase UmaA: Divergence between the *Mycobacterium smegmatis* and *Mycobacterium tuberculosis* Proteins. *J. Biol. Chem.* **2008**, *283*, 1419–1427. [CrossRef]
19. Dubnau, E.; Chan, J.; Raynaud, C.; Mohan, V.P.; Lanéelle, M.-A.; Yu, K.; Quémard, A.; Smith, I.; Daffé, M. Oxygenated Mycolic Acids Are Necessary for Virulence of *Mycobacterium tuberculosis* in Mice. *Mol. Microbiol.* **2000**, *36*, 630–637. [CrossRef]
20. Dinadayala, P.; Laval, F.; Raynaud, C.; Lemassu, A.; Lanéelle, M.-A.; Lanéelle, G.; Daffé, M. Tracking the Putative Biosynthetic Precursors of Oxygenated Mycolates of *Mycobacterium tuberculosis*. Structural Analysis of Fatty Acids of a Mutant Strain Devoid of Methoxy- and Ketomycolates. *J. Biol. Chem.* **2003**, *278*, 7310–7319. [CrossRef] [PubMed]
21. Dubnau, E.; Marrakchi, H.; Smith, I.; Daffé, M.; Quémard, A. Mutations in the CmaB Gene are Responsible for the Absence of Methoxymycolic Acid in *Mycobacterium bovis* BCG Pasteur. *Mol. Microbiol.* **1998**, *29*, 1526–1528. [PubMed]
22. Yuan, Y.; Crane, D.C.; Musser, J.M.; Sreevatsan, S.; Barry, C.E. MMAS-1, the Branch Point Between Cis- and Trans-Cyclopropane-Containing Oxygenated Mycolates in *Mycobacterium tuberculosis*. *J. Biol. Chem.* **1997**, *272*, 10041–10049. [CrossRef]
23. Felipe, L.A.; Osman, F.; Marti, M.A.; Turjanski, A.G. Structural and mechanistic comparison of the Cylopropane Mycolic Acid Synthases (CMAS) protein of *Mycobacterium tuberculosis*. *Biochem. Biophys. Res. Commun.* **2018**, *598*, 288–295. [CrossRef]
24. Barkan, D.; Liu, Z.; Sacchettini, J.C.; Glickman, M.S. Mycolic Acid Cyclopropanation Is Essential for Viability, Drug Resistance, and Cell Wall Integrity of *Mycobacterium tuberculosis*. *Chem. Biol.* **2009**, *16*, 499–509. [CrossRef] [PubMed]
25. Barkan, D.; Hedhli, D.; Yan, H.-G.; Huygen, K.; Glickman, M.S. *Mycobacterium tuberculosis* Lacking all Mycolic Acid Cyclopropanation is Viable but Highly Attenuated and Hyperinflammatory in Mice. *Infect. Immun.* **2012**, *80*, 1958–1968. [CrossRef] [PubMed]

26. Vaubourgeix, J.; Bardou, F.; Boissier, F.; Julien, S.; Constant, P.; Ploux, O.; Daffé, M.; Quémard, A.; Mourey, L. S-Adenosyl-N-Decyl-Aminoethyl, a Potent Bisubstrate Inhibitor of *Mycobacterium tuberculosis* Mycolic Acid Methyltransferases. *J. Biol. Chem.* **2009**, *284*, 19321–19330. [CrossRef] [PubMed]
27. Laval, F.; Lanéelle, M.A.; Déon, C.; Monsarrat, B.; Daffé, M. Accurate Molecular Mass Determination of Mycolic Acids by MALDI-TOF Mass Spectrometry. *Anal. Chem.* **2001**, *73*, 4537–4544. [CrossRef]
28. Dao, D.N.; Sweeney, K.; Hsu, T.; Gurcha, S.S.; Nascimento, I.P.; Roshevsky, D.; Besra, G.S.; Chan, J.; Porcelli, S.A.; Jacobs, W.R., Jr. Mycolic Acid Modification by the MmaA4 Gene of *M. tuberculosis* Modulates IL-12 Production. *PLoS Pathog.* **2008**, *4*, e1000081. [CrossRef]
29. Peyron, P.; Vaubourgeix, J.; Poquet, Y.; Levillain, F.; Botanch, C.; Bardou, F.; Daffé, M.; Emile, J.; Marchou, B.; Cardona, P.; et al. Foamy Macrophages from Tuberculous Patients' Granulomas Constitute a Nutrient-Rich Reservoir for *M. tuberculosis* Persistence. *PLoS Pathog.* **2008**, *4*, e1000204. [CrossRef]
30. Boissier, F.; Bardou, F.; Guillet, V.; Uttenweiler-Joseph, S.; Daffé, M.; Quémard, A.; Mourey, L. Further Insight into S-Adenosylmethionine-Dependent Methyltransferases: Structural Characterization of Hma, an Enzyme Essential for the Biosynthesis of Oxygenated Mycolic Acids in *Mycobacterium tuberculosis*. *J. Biol. Chem.* **2006**, *281*, 4434–4445. [CrossRef]
31. Pearce, N.M.; Krojer, T.; Bradley, A.R.; Collins, P.; Nowak, R.P.; Talon, R.; Marsden, B.D.; Kelm, S.; Shi, J.; Deane, C.M.; et al. A Multi-Crystal Method for Extracting Obscured Crystallographic States from Conventionally Uninterpretable Electron Density. *Nat. Commun.* **2017**, *8*, 15123. [CrossRef]
32. Pearce, N.M.; Krojer, T.; von Delft, F. Proper Modelling of Ligand Binding Requires an Ensemble of Bound and Unbound States. *Acta Crystallogr. Sect. D Biol. Crystallogr.* **2017**, *73*, 256–266. [CrossRef] [PubMed]
33. Huang, C.; Smith, C.V.; Glickman, M.S.; Jacobs, W.R.; Sacchettini, J.C. Crystal Structures of Mycolic Acid Cyclopropane Synthases from *Mycobacterium tuberculosis*. *J. Biol. Chem.* **2002**, *277*, 11559–11569. [CrossRef] [PubMed]
34. Laskowski, R.A.; Swindells, M.B. LigPlot+: Multiple Ligand–Protein Interaction Diagrams for Drug Discovery. *J. Chem. Inf. Model.* **2011**, *51*, 2778–2786. [CrossRef]
35. Sirimulla, S.; Bailey, J.B.; Vegesna, R.; Narayan, M. Halogen Interactions in Protein–Ligand Complexes: Implications of Halogen Bonding for Rational Drug Design. *J. Chem. Inf. Model.* **2013**, *53*, 2781–2791. [CrossRef]
36. Genheden, S.; Ryde, U. The MM/PBSA and MM/GBSA Methods to Estimate Ligand-Binding Affinities. *Expert Opin. Drug Discov.* **2015**, *10*, 449–461. [CrossRef]
37. Wang, E.; Sun, H.; Wang, J.; Wang, Z.; Liu, H.; Zhang, J.Z.H.; Hou, T. End-Point Binding Free Energy Calculation with MM/PBSA and MM/GBSA: Strategies and Applications in Drug Design. *Chem. Rev.* **2019**, *119*, 9478–9508. [CrossRef]
38. Maveyraud, L.; Mourey, L. Protein X-ray Crystallography and Drug Discovery. *Molecules* **2020**, *25*, 1030. [CrossRef] [PubMed]
39. Price, A.J.; Howard, S.; Cons, B.D. Fragment-Based Drug Discovery and its Application to Challenging Drug Targets. *Essays Biochem.* **2017**, *61*, 475–484. [CrossRef]
40. Caliandro, R.; Belviso, D.B.; Aresta, B.M.; de Candia, M.; Altomare, C.D. Protein Crystallography and Fragment-Based Drug Design. *Future Med. Chem.* **2013**, *5*, 1121–1140. [CrossRef]
41. Hajduk, P.J.; Greer, J. A Decade of Fragment-Based Drug Design: Strategic Advances and Lessons Learned. *Nat. Rev. Drug Discov.* **2007**, *6*, 211–219. [CrossRef]
42. Hartshorn, M.J.; Murray, C.W.; Cleasby, A.; Frederickson, M.; Tickle, I.J.; Jhoti, H. Fragment-Based Lead Discovery Using X-ray Crystallography. *J. Med. Chem.* **2005**, *48*, 403–413. [CrossRef]
43. Pearce, N.M.; Bradley, A.R.; Krojer, T.; Marsden, B.D.; Deane, C.M.; von Delft, F. Partial-Occupancy Binders Identified by the Pan-Dataset Density Analysis Method Offer New Chemical Opportunities and Reveal Cryptic Binding Sites. *Struct. Dyn.* **2017**, *4*, 032104. [CrossRef] [PubMed]
44. McIntyre, P.J.; Collins, P.M.; Vrzal, L.; Birchall, K.; Arnold, L.H.; Mpamhanga, C.; Coombs, P.J.; Burgess, S.G.; Richards, M.W.; Winter, A.; et al. Characterization of Three Druggable Hot-Spots in the Aurora-A/TPX2 Interaction Using Biochemical, Biophysical, and Fragment-Based Approaches. *ACS Chem. Biol.* **2017**, *12*, 2906–2914. [CrossRef] [PubMed]
45. Huschmann, F.U.; Linnik, J.; Sparta, K.; Ühlein, M.; Wang, X.; Metz, A.; Schiebel, J.; Heine, A.; Klebe, G.; Weiss, M.S.; et al. Structures of Endothiapepsin–Fragment Complexes from Crystallographic Fragment Screening Using a Novel, Diverse and Affordable 96-Compound Fragment Library. *Acta Crystallogr. Sect. F Struct. Biol. Cryst. Commun.* **2016**, *72*, 346–355. [CrossRef]
46. Xue, Y.; Guo, H.; Hillertz, P. Fragment Screening of RORγt Using Cocktail Crystallography: Identification of Simultaneous Binding of Multiple Fragments. *ChemMedChem* **2016**, *11*, 1881–1885. [CrossRef]
47. Annaraj, P.D.; Kadirvel, P.; Subramanian, A.; Anishetty, S. Free Enzyme Dynamics of CmaA3 and CmaA2 Cyclopropane Mycolic Acid Synthases from *Mycobacterium tuberculosis*: Insights into Residues with Potential Significance in Cyclopropanation. *J. Mol. Graph. Model.* **2019**, *91*, 61–71. [CrossRef]
48. Guianvarc'h, D.; Guangqi, E.; Drujon, T.; Rey, C.; Wang, Q.; Ploux, O. Identification of Inhibitors of the *E. coli* Cyclopropane Fatty Acid Synthase from the Screening of a Chemical Library: In Vitro and in Vivo Studies. *Biochim. Biophys. Acta Proteins Proteom.* **2008**, *1784*, 1652–1658. [CrossRef] [PubMed]
49. Goulding, C.W.; Apostol, M.; Anderson, D.H.; Gill, H.S.; Smith, C.V.; Kuo, M.R.; Yang, J.K.; Waldo, G.S.; Suh, S.W.; Chauhan, R.; et al. The TB Structural Genomics Consortium: Providing a Structural Foundation for Drug Discovery. *Curr. Drug Targets Infect. Disord.* **2002**, *2*, 121–141. [CrossRef]
50. Kabsch, W. XDS. *Acta Crystallogr. Sect. D Biol. Crystallogr.* **2010**, *66*, 125–132. [CrossRef] [PubMed]

51. Vonrhein, C.; Flensburg, C.; Keller, P.; Sharff, A.; Smart, O.; Paciorek, W.; Womack, T.; Bricogne, G. Data Processing and Analysis with the AutoPROC Toolbox. *Acta Crystallogr. Sect. D Biol. Crystallogr.* **2011**, *67*, 293–302. [CrossRef]
52. Winn, M.D.; Ballard, C.C.; Cowtan, K.D.; Dodson, E.J.; Emsley, P.; Evans, P.R.; Keegan, R.M.; Krissinel, E.B.; Leslie, A.G.; Airlie, M.; et al. Overview of the CCP4 Suite and Current Developments. *Acta Crystallogr. Sect. D Biol. Crystallogr.* **2011**, *67*, 235–242 [CrossRef]
53. Murshudov, G.N.; Skubák, P.; Lebedev, A.A.; Pannu, N.S.; Steiner, R.A.; Nicholls, R.A.; Winn, M.D.; Long, F.; Vagin, A.A REFMAC5 for the Refinement of Macromolecular Crystal Structures. *Acta Crystallogr. Sect. D Biol. Crystallogr.* **2011**, *67*, 355–367 [CrossRef]
54. Bricogne, G.; Blanc, E.; Brandl, M.M.; Flensburg, C.C.; Keller, P.; Paciorek, W.; Roversi, P.; Sharff, A.; Smart, O.S.; Vonrhein, C., et al. *BUSTER Version 2.10.3*; Global Phasing: Cambridge, UK, 2017.
55. Emsley, P.; Cowtan, K. Coot: Model-Building Tools for Molecular Graphics. *Acta Crystallogr. Sect. D Biol. Crystallogr.* **2004**, *60*, 2126–2132. [CrossRef] [PubMed]
56. MarvinSketch Version 20.8.0, ChemAxon, 2020. Available online: https://www.chemaxon.com (accessed on 18 August 2021).
57. Smart, O.S.; Womack, T.O.; Sharff, A.; Flensburg, C.; Keller, P.; Paciorek, W.; Vonrhein, C.; Bricogne, G. *Grade, Version 1.2*; Global Phasing Ltd.: Cambridge, UK, 2020; Available online: https://www.globalphasing.com (accessed on 18 August 2021).
58. Case, D.A.; Betz, R.M.; Cerutti, D.S.; Cheatham, T.E., III; Darden, T.A.; Duke, R.E.; Giese, T.J.; Gohlke, H.; Goetz, A.W.; Homeyer N.; et al. *AMBER 2016*; University of California: San Francisco, CA, USA, 2016.
59. Roe, D.R.; Cheatham, T.E. PTRAJ and CPPTRAJ: Software for Processing and Analysis of Molecular Dynamics Trajectory Data. *J Chem. Theory Comput.* **2013**, *9*, 3084–3095. [CrossRef] [PubMed]
60. Miller, B.R.; McGee, T.D.; Swails, J.M.; Homeyer, N.; Gohlke, H.; Roitberg, A.E. MMPBSA.Py: An Efficient Program for End-State Free Energy Calculations. *J. Chem. Theory Comput.* **2012**, *8*, 3314–3321. [CrossRef] [PubMed]
61. Menchon, G.; Maveyraud, L.; Czaplicki, G. Molecular Dynamics as a Tool for Virtual Ligand Screening. In *Computational Drug Discovery and Design*; Methods in Molecular Biology; Gore, M., Jagtap, U.B., Eds.; Springer: New York, NY, USA, 2018; pp. 145–178, ISBN 978-1-4939-7756-7.

pharmaceuticals

Article

A Deep-Learning Proteomic-Scale Approach for Drug Design

Brennan Overhoff, Zackary Falls, William Mangione and Ram Samudrala *

Department of Biomedical Informatics, Jacobs School of Medicine and Biomedical Sciences, University at Buffalo, Buffalo, NY 14203, USA; brennano@buffalo.edu (B.O.); zmfalls@buffalo.edu (Z.F.); wmangion@buffalo.edu (W.M.)
* Correspondence: ram@compbio.org

Abstract: Computational approaches have accelerated novel therapeutic discovery in recent decades. The Computational Analysis of Novel Drug Opportunities (CANDO) platform for shotgun multi-target therapeutic discovery, repurposing, and design aims to improve their efficacy and safety by employing a holistic approach that computes interaction signatures between every drug/compound and a large library of non-redundant protein structures corresponding to the human proteome fold space. These signatures are compared and analyzed to determine if a given drug/compound is efficacious and safe for a given indication/disease. In this study, we used a deep learning-based autoencoder to first reduce the dimensionality of CANDO-computed drug–proteome interaction signatures. We then employed a reduced conditional variational autoencoder to generate novel drug-like compounds when given a target encoded "objective" signature. Using this approach, we designed compounds to recreate the interaction signatures for twenty approved and experimental drugs and showed that 16/20 designed compounds were predicted to be significantly (p-value ≤ 0.05) more behaviorally similar relative to all corresponding controls, and 20/20 were predicted to be more behaviorally similar relative to a random control. We further observed that redesigns of objectives developed via rational drug design performed significantly better than those derived from natural sources (p-value ≤ 0.05), suggesting that the model learned an abstraction of rational drug design. We also show that the designed compounds are structurally diverse and synthetically feasible when compared to their respective objective drugs despite consistently high predicted behavioral similarity. Finally, we generated new designs that enhanced thirteen drugs/compounds associated with non-small cell lung cancer and anti-aging properties using their predicted proteomic interaction signatures. his study represents a significant step forward in automating holistic therapeutic design with machine learning, enabling the rapid generation of novel, effective, and safe drug leads for any indication.

Keywords: computational drug design; deep learning; multiscale; polypharmacology; autoencoder; docking; recurrent neural network

Citation: Overhoff, B.; Falls, Z.; Mangione, W.; Samudrala, R. A Deep-Learning Proteomic-Scale Approach for Drug Design. *Pharmaceuticals* **2021**, *14*, 1277. https://doi.org/10.3390/ph14121277

Academic Editor: Osvaldo Andrade Santos-Filho

Received: 24 September 2021
Accepted: 29 November 2021
Published: 7 December 2021

1. Introduction

Drug discovery—identifying chemicals with therapeutic effects against a particular indication/disease that is safe for human use—is a long, laborious, and expensive process. On average, $3 billion and about 15 years are required to bring a novel chemical entity to the market using traditional approaches [1]. Computational methods are a popular means of identifying potential leads through paradigms such as high-throughput virtual screening [2–5], where simulations are run to assess the binding affinity of a library of compounds against a therapeutic target of interest. The combinatorial explosion of binding poses [6,7] and ligand conformations [6,8,9] and the chaotic nature of such dynamical systems [10] prevent popular virtual screening methods from producing safe and effective therapeutic leads a priori. These issues are exacerbated by the fact that virtual screening studies usually consider a single protein target, whereas drugs ingested by humans go through absorption, dispersion, metabolism, and excretion (ADME) and exert their effects (and side effects or toxicity (T)) via interactions with multiple targets and systems [3,11–15]. Furthermore, the chemical space explored by virtual screening is limited to a relatively small selection of compounds when compared to the vastness of the small molecule space [4,16], thus missing more effective and safer leads.

Computational methods are efficient, accurate, holistic (i.e., take into account the entire interaction space of chemical entities), and have breadth in terms of chemical space exploration necessary to overcome the limitations of traditional approaches [2,6,12,13,17–34]. To expand compound libraries utilized in screening, combinatorial chemistry and machine-learning design pipelines have been developed to generate libraries of compounds likely to bind to a given target [35–37]. Some notable examples in machine learning include Insilico Medicine's Chemistry42 platform, which designs compounds to a binding pocket [38], or a recent transformer-based network that utilized machine translation methods to generate binding ligands for the amino acid sequence of a target protein [39]. However, to take full advantage of these leads, additional screening and in vivo work must be performed to identify off-target binding as these approaches do not address the multitarget nature of drug interactions [11,13].

Various encoder–decoder models [40–42] for conditional [43] molecular generation on multiple properties have been proposed [17,44–46], but in most cases, these properties are limited to physiochemical ones. These models, however, do show great promise in their ability to rapidly generate compounds with desired properties. The most sophisticated conditional molecular generation performed thus far to our knowledge is inducing a differential expression profile of several hundred genes [17]. In all these models, proteins, the functional molecules that are primarily bound by human-ingested drugs to ensure efficacy and ADMET, remain to be considered explicitly on a large scale. Determining interactions between drug candidates and target proteins on a proteomic scale will offer the most comprehensive predictions for bioactivity and safety as many on- and off-targets will be considered simultaneously.

We developed the Computational Analysis of Novel Drug Repurposing Opportunities (CANDO) platform for shotgun multitarget drug discovery, repurposing, and design to overcome the aforementioned limitations of traditional single-target approaches [18–29]. The platform screens and ranks drugs/compounds for every disease/indication (and adverse event) through the large-scale modeling and analytics of the interactions between comprehensive libraries of drugs/compounds and protein structures. CANDO is agonistic to the interaction scoring method used; two primary pipelines within the platform allow for rapid screening and assessment of billions of drug/compound to protein interactions with fast bioanalytic docking and machine learning affinity regression protocols. Machine learning is also used to improve performance in conjunction with preclinical data in an iterative manner. Finally, CANDO implements a variety of benchmarking protocols for shotgun repurposing, i.e., to determine how every known drug is related to every other in the context of the indications/diseases for which they are approved, which enables the evaluation of various pipelines and protocols within and external to the platform for their utility in drug discovery. The multiple fast and accurate interaction scoring/docking protocols, the proteomic scale, and rigorous all-against-all benchmarking used within the platform make it unique and ideal for the design of chemical entities that target a desired proteomic space or objective.

Here, we describe the development and rigorous benchmarking of a multi-step deep learning pipeline for drug design. These pipelines perform conditional drug design given a desired proteomic interaction signature using a generative approach to explore the vastness of the entire small molecule space, while evaluating the functional behavior of candidate designs across the proteomic space. The CANDO platform's benchmarking strategy is used in a modified fashion to determine the performance of the designed compounds relative to an objective drug. We show that the best generated designs were evaluated as being equivalent or better than a variety of controls for twenty objective drugs. Our pipeline represents a significant leap in automating holistic drug design with machine learning, with the ability to rapidly generate effective and safe drug candidates that accurately target multiple proteins within a proteome as desired.

2. Results and Discussion

2.1. Behavioral Similarity of Designed Compounds to Their Objectives

We observed excellent performance of our Reduced Conditional Variational Autoencoder (RCVAE) proteome-scale design pipeline in all our benchmarking experiments following training (see the methods Section 3.2). If this performance continues to hold following synthesis and validation, it indicates that this pipeline will greatly enhance the pharmaceutical discovery pipeline for novel treatments against a variety of simple and complex indications. A critical aspect of verifying the utility of the designs generated was to compare their predicted behavior (i.e., proteomic interaction signatures) to their intended behavior, which was input to conditional generation. If the predicted behaviors of designed compounds were highly similar to the conditional objective across objectives relative to the corresponding controls, we concluded that the RCVAE design pipeline may be used to accurately design compounds that possess any desirable bioactivity and subsequent function, given the extensive benchmarking and validation the CANDO paradigm has undergone [18,21,26,29,47–50]. This is the primary motivation and goal for using the CVAE architecture in terms of accelerating drug discovery: design with respect to arbitrary numbers of on-, off-, and anti-targets (Figure 1).

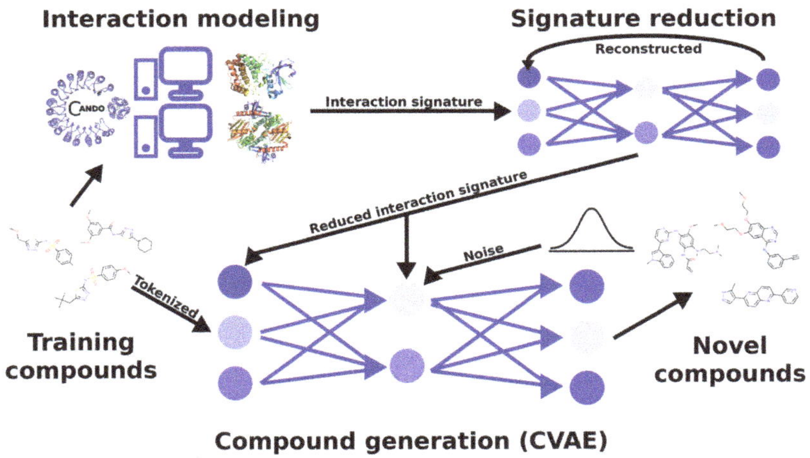

Figure 1. Deep -learning architecture and pipeline for generative drug design. We used the CANDO platform to predict interaction signatures for each compound in a training set against a library of nonredundant protein structures representing the human proteome. The interaction signatures have their dimensionality reduced in an autoencoder, which models the underlying correspondence between protein structures as they behave in the proteome. The reduced signatures are then used as labels for each training compound, which the generative conditional variational autoencoder model learns to reconstruct given a target interaction signature. This pipeline allows us to redesign behaviorally similar compounds to existing drugs based on their interaction signatures, as well as to modulate interactions on a proteomic scale as desired to generate behaviorally novel therapeutics.

We evaluated the performance primarily by the median of each distribution, indicated by the horizontal bars in the box plots in Figure 2. Lower root-mean-squared deviation (RMSD) values indicate a greater reproduction of proteomic interaction signatures for the intended and/or predicted behavior of any given compound, i.e., greater behavioral similarity. Every set of redesigns performed significantly better (p-value of ≤ 0.05) than a selection of random compounds according to this criterion. Additionally, despite being comparatively close in predicted proteomic behavior, our redesigns maintained high levels of structural diversity, as evidenced by their Tanimoto coefficients to our drug library (average ≤ 0.39). For sixteen of the objectives (excluding sirolimus, cucurbitacin Q1, digoxin, and myriocin), the redesigns significantly outperformed the corresponding top 100 and same indication controls. The top 100 control, which included several "me too" compounds (or structural analogs) for each objective [24,51], is the most rigorous one we could devise and illustrates that just generating 100 designs in many instances produces more behaviorally similar compounds to a desired interaction signature than selecting the most similar 100 compounds from a total of 13,194 (the size of the CANDO drug library). The existence of structural analogs in the top100 control indicates bias in favor of already effective compounds in an effort to break into a new market or retain market dominance by generating new intellectual property. New drugs are often derivatives of existing ones with small changes, which our design pipeline is able to overcome, particularly with a bit of extra effort (see Section 2.4 below). Overall, these results indicate that the RCVAE design pipeline produces compounds that accurately match the behavior of desired proteomic interactions relevant to drug discovery. In other words, interactions related to therapeutic efficacy, ADME, and toxicity are modulated precisely in the designed compounds, particularly for objectives from the rational sources subset.

2.2. Relative Performance Gains of Designs Relative to Controls

The bottom panel of Figure 2 compares the relative performance gains for proteomic objectives from the rational design and natural sources subsets relative to the controls. Compounds in the natural sources subset were derived from massively parallel evolutionary processes over eons of time. As a result, they exhibit evolutionary drift, resulting in complex behaviors that are suboptimal from a therapeutic discovery perspective, i.e. unnecessary off-target interactions and/or individual interactions drifting away from functional free energy minima [52]. In addition to verifying that our designs behave as intended, our benchmarking also shows that the RCVAE design pipeline accomplishes this replication of behavioral similarity through an abstraction of rational drug design. That is, the similarities of redesigns to objectives from the rational design subset were greater relative to those from the natural sources subset (Figure 2). Adopting an abstraction of rational drug design is optimal for the impact of this platform on drug discovery because if the model was merely replicating the molecular structure of design objectives and not proteomic behavior specifically, the limitations of natural products (low synthetic accessibility, poor ADMET [53]) would present themselves in the designs in addition to indicating that the model may be over-trained. This discrepancy in the similarity of redesigned natural products and rationally designed drugs, therefore, further supports the notion that the RCVAE pipeline is able to intelligently design compounds with desirable bioactivities across multiple targets.

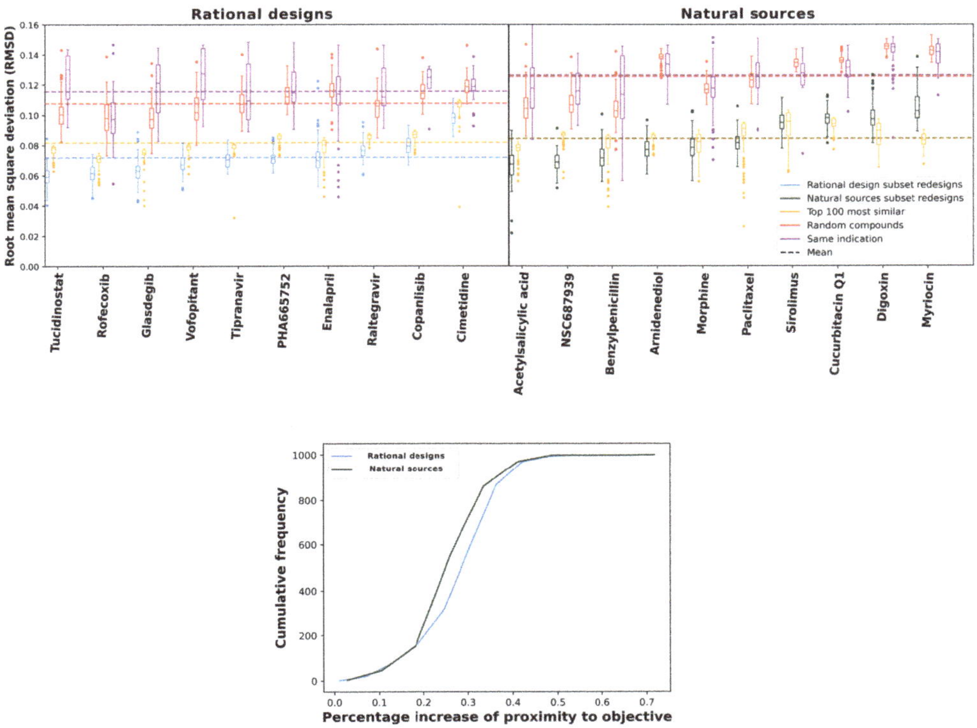

Figure 2. Performance of our deep learning drug design pipeline. To evaluate the performance of the RCVAE pipeline for drug design, we compared redesigned compounds to three controls. The root-mean-squared deviations (RMSDs) between redesigned and control interaction signatures for the rational design and natural sources subsets and the corresponding objective signatures were used to evaluate the performance, as a proxy for behavioral similarity. In the top panels, the blue and green box plots denote the distributions of RMSDs between predicted proteomic interaction signatures for 100 redesigns and the ten corresponding objectives from the rational design (left) and the natural sources (right) subsets along the horizontal axis, respectively. For each RMSD distribution box plot, the boxes indicate the first and third quartile ranges, the horizontal bar indicates the median, and the whiskers indicate non-outlier ranges, with outliers plotted as dots. As a naive control, the red box plots in both panels denote the distributions of the RMSDs between predicted proteomic interaction signatures for a set of 100 randomly selected drug-like compounds taken from the ZINC database [54] and the corresponding objectives. Yellow box plots denote the distributions of the CANDO-predicted top 100 most similar compounds by interaction signature and their corresponding RMSDs; this is a more rigorous control, which checks to see if there exists any compound in the CANDO library that could match or exceed the performance of the design pipeline. Purple box plots denote the RMSD distributions of compounds approved for the same indication as the objective; this is a third control based on phenotype. Dots represent RMSD values for outlier points for each distribution. Dashed lines show the average RMSDs of all compounds corresponding to a given color. All redesign–control distribution pairs were significantly different as indicated by Kolmogorov–Smirnov (K-S) tests and outperformed random controls. For 16/20 of the objective compounds, our redesigns were able to perform better than the top 100 and same indication controls (medians and distributions). The exceptions were four compounds from the natural sources subsets (sirolimus, cucurbitacin Q1, digoxin, and myriocin), discussed further in Sections 2.2 and 2.4. The bottom panel displays cumulative frequency graphs of percentage increases of similarities ("proximity") to the objective for rational design and natural sources subsets redesigns (see the Materials and Methods Section 3.3). Redesigns from the former subset were significantly more accurate to the objective compound than the natural sources subset when compared to the naive control, with mean percentage similarity increases of 33.4% and 32.9%, respectively (p-value $\leq 7.0 \times 10^{-6}$). This indicates that not only does the design pipeline generate compounds with the desired proteomic-scale behavior, but that it likely implements a learned abstraction of rational drug design.

2.3. Visualizing and Filtering Using t-SNE Plots

For all objectives, the redesigns greatly outperformed existing drugs approved for the desired indication when compared to the objective signature. Despite this, some Kolmogorov–Smirnov (K-S) tests indicated weaker statistical significance when differentiating between the RCVAE design and the same indication distributions. To understand the distributions of redesigned and control compounds and to provide an additional filtering mechanism to evaluate the performance of our designs as illustrated in Figure 2, we visualized the interaction signatures of all compounds (objectives, redesigns, and all controls) evaluated in our benchmarking with t-SNE plots [55] (Figure 3).

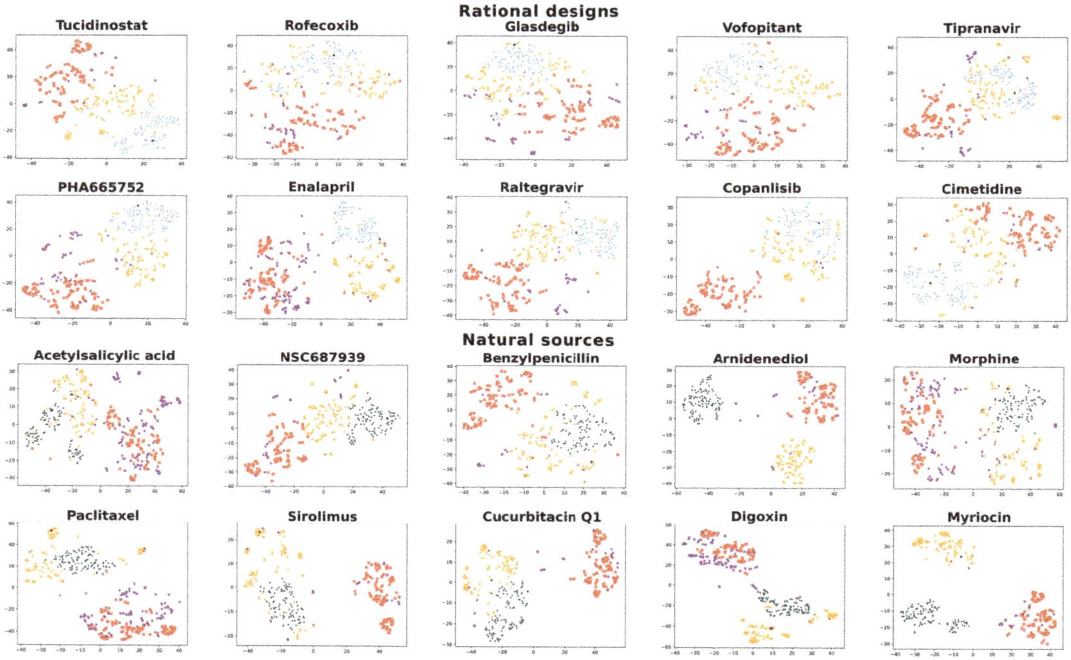

Figure 3. t-SNE visualizations for the interaction signatures of objective compounds, redesigns, and various controls with structural comparisons. t-SNE plots were generated for each of the twenty design objectives. The t-SNE algorithm was run on the interaction signatures of the objectives (black stars) and 100 redesigns (blue and green circles), as well as the 100 random (red squares), top 100 (orange triangles), and same indication (purple hexagons) control compounds. (Color coding is the same as in Figure 2.) Euclidean distances shown in t-SNE visualizations generally corroborate our findings from Figure 2 when considering the RMSD due to the maintenance of proximal points and distributions. The exceptions to this were for benzylpenicillin and paclitaxel, as Figure 2 shows greater proximity for designs than the top 100 control, whereas t-SNE plots show better clustering for the top 100 set around the objective. The generally (14/20) greater proximity of designed compound clusters to the objective point when compared to top 100, same indication, and random control compounds corroborate the behavioral similarity of designed compounds to their objective in the predicted interaction space, i.e., designed compounds are predicted to behave in the manner in which they were designed.

t-SNE plots generally corroborate the relative behavioral similarities between redesigns and controls relative to their objectives. RCVAE pipeline designs tend to cluster densely around the objective compound, as they are designed to do. The top 100 compounds cluster around these designs, with a few structural analogs very close to their objectives. Finally, the same indication and random compounds clustered the farthest from the objective. As the same indication compounds represent a group of diverse drugs approved for an indication that includes the objective, there is a general lack of clustering and they are at greater distances from their objectives. Comparing the performance of the designs relative to their objectives and controls using both Figures 2 and 3 indicates that the t-SNE plots illustrated in the latter may be used to assess the confidence in and room for improvement of the design pipeline performance for specific objectives.

2.4. Improving Cases with Sub-Optimal Performance

For eleven objectives, a handful of outliers in the top 100 or same indication controls outperformed the design distributions (Figures 2 and 3). As noted above, structural analogs create a bias when evaluating performance due to them having very similar behavioral interaction signatures. We observed that the top 10 compounds (out of the top 100 controls, covering almost all outliers) yielded an average Tanimoto coefficient of 0.51, in contrast to an average of 0.39 for all designs, relative to their objectives. We further observed that 23/200 top 10 compounds, across all 20 objectives, had a Tanimoto coefficient $\geq$0.90 with an average of 0.96, demonstrating the "me too" bias with the top 100 control. Unlike the few top 100 outliers, the designs offer a larger and more diverse selection pool for prospective validation.

Regardless, we further investigated the behavior of the RCVAE pipeline for one of the objectives (cucurbitacin Q1) where an outlier was clearly better than the best designed compound by expanding the number of designs generated by the RCVAE pipeline from 100 to 1000 compounds. We found that the RMSDs of the top 100 out of 1000 designs, far less than the 13,194 compounds that were the source for the top 100 most similar compounds control, ranged from 0.073 to 0.09. This placed the RMSD of the best designs well below the lowest RMSD outlier of the top 100 control. Altogether, this indicates that the performance of the RCVAE pipeline may be enhanced by increasing the number of designs generated and selecting for behavioral similarity. Our design pipeline offers structurally diverse lead compounds with the potential to match or exceed the behavioral similarity of the top CANDO predictions from its known drug library for noisy objectives, such as compounds from the natural sources subset.

2.5. Synthetic Feasibility of Designed Compounds

To viably demonstrate that our 2000 redesigns were synthetically feasible, we utilized a high-throughput machine-learning-based approach to predict synthetic complexity scores, called SCScore. SCScore utilizes a database of known synthetic reaction pathways for training to make predictions of how easy or difficult it is to synthesize a novel compound.

As shown in Figure 4, predicted synthetic complexities for the RCVAE pipeline redesigns are often comparable to their design objective, i.e., the objective compound's scores exist within the distribution of the scores for the redesigns. Low Tanimoto coefficients (average 0.39) between designs and objective compounds indicate that the comparable synthetic complexities of our redesigns are not due to a corresponding high structural similarity. In other words, despite the high structural diversity of the generated designs, the synthetic complexity for objective and designed compounds remains stable. This may be explained by the maintenance of functionally relevant substructures of comparable synthetic complexity that are present in any given objective and redesign that are combined differently to produce similar behaviors and low structural similarity. We are studying this phenomenon more thoroughly with larger datasets by investigating the redundancy of the substructures of all approved drugs and redesigns for publication in a future study.

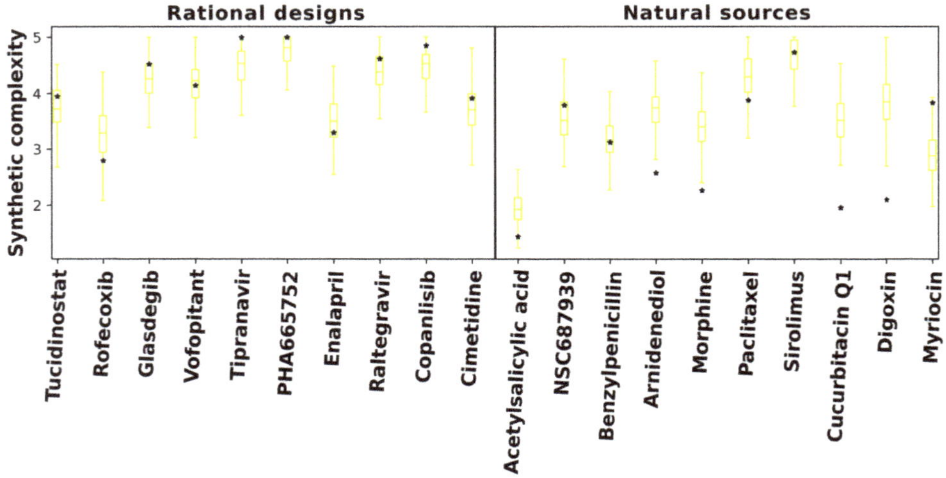

Figure 4. Predicted synthetic complexity of designs compared to objective compounds. Synthetic complexity scores for objective and RCVAE pipeline designed compounds as predicted by SCScore [56] serve as the basis for this comparison. Box plots denote the distributions of predicted synthetic complexity scores for RCVAE redesigns of objective compounds (stars). The scores of the objectives enable us to evaluate the synthetic feasibility of the redesigns relative to their corresponding objective compounds. There is a greater occurrence of low-scoring natural sources objectives in predicted synthetic complexity. This indicates that the SCScore software is biased by what is already well known or it may also highlight a potential reason why RCVAE performs better for objectives from the rational design subset: it is somewhat plausible that evolution optimizes for synthetic accessibility over binding free energies, hence the discrepancies in behavioral similarities between the designs and their objectives for the two benchmarking (rational design and natural sources) subsets (Figure 2). RCVAE designs are of similar synthetic complexity to their corresponding objective compounds as most objective complexities lie within the box plot whiskers (not outliers), with some designs being more accessible than their objectives.

Additionally, predicted synthetic complexities are typically lower for objectives and redesigns in the natural sources subset relative to the rational design one, indicating that the SCScore software may be biased by what is already well known. As objectives in the natural sources subset score similarly to their redesigns, it is somewhat plausible that evolutionary optimization towards synthetic accessibility, at the expense of macromolecular interaction free energies [52], may account for the diminished behavioral similarity of RCVAE designs between objectives in the rational design and natural sources subsets correspondingly (see Figure 2). A comprehensive analysis of this hypothesis with larger subsets is necessary to validate or falsify this hypothesis.

It is useful to note that many RCVAE designs are more synthetically accessible than the compound whose behaviors they replicate. As Figure 2 already indicates high behavioral similarity between redesigns and their objectives, the RCVAE design pipeline may serve the additional purpose of designing analogs to existing drugs that are more synthetically feasible and therefore easier and less costly to produce. This is accomplished without adding a synthetic complexity parameter to the condition vector for compound generation (Figure 4).

Finally, we routinely used several other methods to evaluate RCVAE designs such as the Quantitative Estimation of Drug-likeness (QED) [57], Synthetic Accessibility Score (SAScore) [58], and AiZynthFinder [59] to assess their chemical viability and drug-likeness. We also compared our designs to benchmarks from GuacaMol [60]. These results corroborated the outputs of our benchmarking and/or SCScore; future work will include a rigorous evaluation of drug design technologies, much as we have done for repurposing [29].

2.6. Applications to Aging and Non-Small Cell Lung Cancer

A fundamental tenet of CANDO is that evaluating all the possible interactions between a human-ingested drug/compound and the macromolecules and systems it encounters on a proteomic/interactomic scale is necessary to determine its safety and efficacy for a given indication [18–29]. The RCVAE design pipeline represents a significant step forward in early drug discovery as it allows for the virtually unlimited generation of novel putative drug candidates to treat any indication/disease by combating it on a proteomic scale. As a precursor to upcoming work, we generated designs for several objective compounds/drugs associated with human or cell longevity ("aging") [61–70] and approved for Non-Small Cell Lung Cancer (NSCLC) [71–78]. We expect our pipeline to produce redesigns that retain the proteome-scale behaviors of these objectives used to treat these complex indications/diseases, while being structurally diverse.

Figure 5 illustrates the top redesigns for the thirteen objectives covering the two indications ranked using two metrics based on the greatest similarity criterion: lowest RMSD between corresponding interaction signatures and highest Tanimoto coefficient between corresponding molecular fingerprints. Two classes of redesigns, all with the greatest behavioral similarity to their objectives, emerged when performing the comparisons illustrated in Figure 5: designs that chemically/structurally resemble their objective compound/indication (metformin, NAD+, resveratrol, curcumin, and RepSox for aging and gefitinib, erlotinib, afatinib, and dacomitinib for NSCLC, all with a Tanimoto coefficient $\geq$0.39) and those that do not. The former class is intriguing as it implies the existence of highly optimized structures for a given phenotype (indication), as shown by the convergence of redesigns to known drugs. It also demonstrates that the RCVAE design pipeline produces highly similar designs to known drugs to perform specific tasks, only from their proteomic interaction behavior and without being exposed to any similar structures in training. In other words, the proteomic-scale interaction information for a compound is enough information for our design pipeline to reliably reconstruct a chemically/structurally similar compound in some cases. The latter class demonstrates the expanse and diversity of a chemical space not yet charted by medicinal chemists, capable of replicating the interactions of known drugs. We are in the process of synthesizing the top designs from these pipelines for these indications and validating them in corresponding preclinical models via industry partners and collaborators.

2.7. Limitations and Future Work

To treat an indication in a comprehensive fashion, especially complex ones such as aging or NSCLC, entirely novel drugs will likely need to be developed that go beyond replicating the systemic effects of existing ones. This would require a thorough and accurate description of the interaction networks responsible for disease etiology, as well as compound behavior to ensure optimal efficacy and safety. The creation of these interaction networks may be accomplished by multiscale modeling, literature/database analyses, and/or high-throughput experimental studies, all of which may be incorporated within CANDO. We are currently in the process of conditioning the RCVAE design pipelines and comparing them to ones based on graph neural networks [79] using these more complex interaction networks that go beyond the information present in the linear signatures.

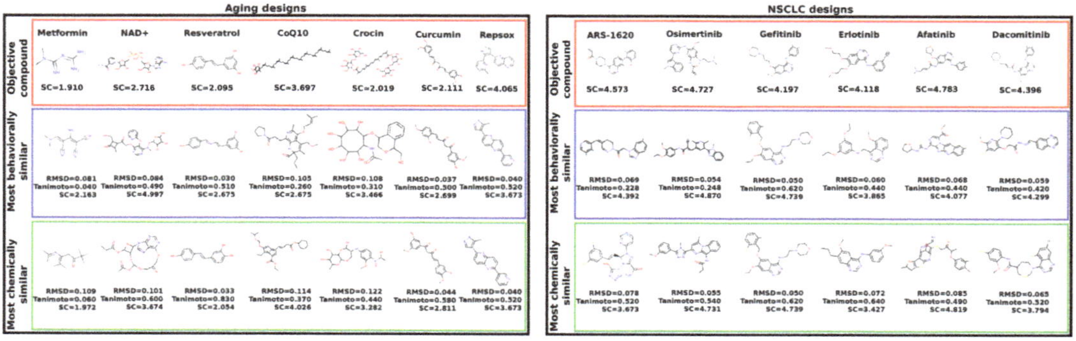

Figure 5. Analysis of the top designs generated for aging and Non-Small Cell Lung Cancer (NSCLC). The names, chemical structures, and predicted Synthetic Complexity (SC) scores of the objective compounds for aging (left) and NSCLC (right) are displayed in the top row of each panel (red border). The chemical structures of the most similar redesigns to each objective based on their interaction signatures alongside three metrics for these redesigned compounds relative to their objectives (RMSD of interaction signatures, Tanimoto coefficient, and predicted synthetic complexity) are displayed in the row below (blue border). The chemical structures of the most similar redesigns using molecular fingerprints alongside the same three metrics (RMSD, Tanimoto, and synthetic complexity) for these redesigns relative to their objectives are displayed in the bottom row (green border). The designs generated using the RCVAE pipeline retain a fair amount of structural diversity, as indicated by the fingerprint comparison scores (low Tanimoto coefficients) whilst maintaining high predicted behavioral similarity in terms of interaction signatures (low RMSDs). Other methods for evaluating our designs such as QED corroborated the above results [57]. These designs demonstrate the utility of our pipeline for designing novel compounds to combat complex indications on a proteomic scale and may be pursued further via preclinical validation studies.

We are currently exploring other scoring protocols within the CANDO platform for conditional generation to overcome the limitations of any specific interaction calculation method. For example, the interaction scoring protocol used in this work has been shown to have great utility in the context of evaluating proteomic behavioral similarity based on benchmarking performance [18–29]. However, information on agonism/antagonism, and downstream functional activity upon binding may be obtained via design pipelines that utilize gene and protein expression data, which we are incorporating into CANDO. Public gene expression data, available through the L1000 and Connectivity Map projects [80,81], highlight important genes/proteins that are upregulated and downregulated following exposure to a drug/compound. For example, if gene expression data suggest that certain downstream genes are significantly upregulated in a given pathway following interaction with a compound and that same compound is predicted to have strong interactions with multiple proteins in that pathway, it can be inferred that those are likely to cause activating/agonist behavior. The same can be inferred for downregulated genes and inhibition/antagonism. In addition, we are exploring the use of high-throughput robotic systems such as DESI-MS to generate large-scale interaction and activity data [82–90]. CANDO thus enables and illustrates the benefit of combining heterogeneous sources (gene, as well as protein expression, protein pathway databases, high-throughput binding, and activity data) to create novel types of interaction signatures/networks to produce design objectives that tackle complex indications.

The CANDO platform enables the benchmarking of any arbitrary proteome/protein library for its utility in drug discovery using a similar all-against-all process as described in Section 3.3. The generation of highly accurate modeled protein structures such as those predicted by Deepmind's AlphaFold offer an attractive representation of the full human proteome to perform such benchmarking, which we have completed and will publish separately. This allows for conditional drug design using AlphaFold interaction signatures especially giving us greater coverage and control over particular proteins and pathways to modulate with expert input for specific indications.

The benchmarking and performance evaluation of our RCVAE drug design pipeline were based on using known data as the ground truth or gold standard. While computational experiments are an important first step and indicate promising, prospective preclinical validation of the pipeline, its designs will require medicinal chemistry synthesis, binding studies, and disease models assays at multiple scales, which we are currently undertaking. Regardless, our combined work to date [18–29], including this study, indicates that novel high-throughput methods for rapidly identifying relationships between compounds, proteins, pathways, and cells are highly desirable for holistic drug discovery. As CANDO is agnostic to the specific methods used for any of its protocols, should such data become available, the RCVAE design pipeline described here would be well poised to take advantage of them for maximum drug discovery efficiency.

3. Materials and Methods

Figure 1 illustrates our overall methodology to create a new drug design pipeline. We employed the Computational Analysis of Novel Drug Opportunities (CANDO) platform to generate proteomic interaction signatures for the compounds in the training set of our learning-based model. The CANDO interaction signatures had their dimensionality reduced in an autoencoder, which models the underlying correspondence between protein structures as they function in the proteome. The reduced signatures were then used as labels for each training molecule, which the generative Conditional Variational Autoencoder (CVAE) model learns to reconstruct given a target interaction signature. We then used CANDO to benchmark the performance of the designed compounds in the context of their objectives and make predictions of novel designs for two indications for future prospective validation.

3.1. Compound–Proteome Interaction Signature Generation Using the CANDO Platform

Multiple pipelines for multiscale therapeutic discovery, repurposing, and design have been implemented in the CANDO platform [18–29]. Here, we utilized CANDO to simulate the interactions between a given drug/compound and a library of protein structures to generate the corresponding proteomic interaction signature.

The protein structure library used in this study is a set of 14,606 nonredundant structures derived from the Protein Data Bank (PDB) [91] corresponding to the human proteome fold space ("nrPDB")[92–97]. The compound–protein interaction scores in these signatures are computed using the bioanalytic docking protocol BANDOCK, which compares query compound structures to all ligands that are known or predicted to interact with a protein binding site [22,27,29].

Potential binding sites on a protein are elucidated using the COACH algorithm, which uses three different complementary algorithms and a consensus approach to consider the sequence or substructure similarity to known PDB binding sites [98]. COACH has been utilized extensively within the CANDO platform to accurately predict the binding behavior of numerous compounds against numerous targets, as demonstrated by its benchmarking performance in multiple studies (Section 3.3 and [18–29]). For each potential binding site, the COACH output includes a set of co-crystallized ligands, which are compared to a compound of interest using binary chemical fingerprinting methods that describe the presence or absence of particular molecular substructures [99]. The maximum Tanimoto coefficient between the binary fingerprints of the query compound and the set of all predicted protein binding site ligands becomes the interaction score. The better the score, the higher the likelihood of the interaction being correct due to the inferred homology. Thus, if there are proteins with multiple binding sites and corresponding ligands, the strongest interaction is used. If there are no matches, then the score returned is zero (i.e., no interaction). The final output is a vector of 14,606 scores comprising the interaction signature between a given compound and the nrPDB library. Further detail on the pipelines used to generate and benchmark the interaction signatures is given elsewhere in numerous publications [18–29].

3.2. Model Architecture and Data Generation

We selected a CVAE [45] architecture for generating novel molecular structures. Training data consisted of SMILES [100] strings labeled with predicted proteomic interaction signatures based on the nrPDB library. The training set consisted of 300,000 compounds selected at random from the ZINC database [54]. The 14,606 protein binding scores were predicted for each compound. The dimensionality of the protein interaction signatures was reduced to a 200-dimensional vector via a conventional autoencoder [101]. Following an input layer with 14,606 neurons, the encoder consisted of 10 sequential, densely connected layers with 10,000, 7750, 5500, 2250, 2000, 1250, 1000, 500, 250, and 200 neurons in each layer, respectively. This was reversed in the decoder, and a final layer with 14,606 neurons was used as the output to the network. The root-mean-squared deviation (RMSD) between the input and reconstructed signatures was used as a loss metric. This model was trained on 250,000 compounds until over-fitting was observed, which occurred after 15 epochs/iterations. Each epoch was validated on another 50,000 randomly selected compounds. The model was then used to reduce the non-redundant signatures of the training compounds. These became the labels for each SMILES string present in the CVAE training data.

Before being input into the CVAE, SMILES strings were one-hot encoded [102,103] resulting in a rank-2 tensor of size (sequence length $\times$ vocab length), where sequence length is the maximum number of characters allowed per SMILES string and vocab length is the unique number of characters represented in the input data. The reduced protein signature, c, was appended to the end of the one-hot encoding repeated at each sequence position (commonly referred to as time steps in the context of Long Short-Term Memory (LSTM) cells [102,104,105]). Similar to [45], the tensor was fed sequentially through three LSTM cells [104,105] to encode the original input. The encoder outputs to two parallel layers, one representing the mean and one for the standard deviation of the latent vector. The latent vector, z, consists of 200 dimensions and is sampled from the encoder output. The latent vector is then repeated for the total number of time steps, and the protein signature, c, is re-appended onto the resulting tensor in the prior fashion. This is input into the decoder, which also consists of three LSTM cells. Finally, this is output to a matrix of probabilities for each character in a SMILES string. Taking the maximum probability token for each character slot, one-hot encoded SMILES strings denoting reconstructions of input compounds are generated.

The loss metric used to train the CVAE is as follows:

$$E[log(P(X|z,c))] - D_{KL}[Q(z|X,c)||P(X|z,c)] \quad (1)$$

where E denotes the reconstruction error and D_{KL} denotes the relative entropy or the Kullback–Leibler divergence [106]. $P(X|z,c)$ denotes the probability density function approximated by the decoder for each character in a SMILES string given the latent and conditional vectors. $Q(z|X,c)$ denotes the probability density function approximated by the encoder given the input SMILES strings and condition vector. The CVAE was trained on 300,000 compounds until convergence. The Reduced CVAE (RCVAE) model pipeline is depicted visually in Figure 1.

3.3. Benchmarking and Analysis of the RCVAE Design Pipeline Performance

The fundamental supposition and result of benchmarking the CANDO platform is that compounds with similar interaction signatures will behave similarly. On a proteomic scale, these behaviors take the form of efficacy and ADMET for a given indication. The CANDO platform was benchmarked using known drug-indication associations [18–29] derived from the Comparative Toxicogenomics Database [107] and, more recently, drug adverse events obtained from OFFSIDES [108,109] and SIDER [109]. We recently published the best metrics to use for benchmarking drug repurposing platforms [29]. The results of benchmarking and prospectively validating CANDO indicate that the proteomic-scale interaction modeling of drugs elucidates their behaviors, and these behaviors correspond to treatments for indications for which these drugs are approved [18,21,26,29,47–50]. The benchmarking of the platform using known associations in this comprehensive all-against-all manner enables us to assess the correctness and utility of other parameters, such as the protein library composition, solved vs. modeled structures, different molecular docking and machine-learning algorithms, etc.

We performed several benchmarks of the RCVAE to verify its utility and robustness beyond that of its performance based on metrics used in training. Our benchmark set consisted of twenty approved or experimental objective drugs, comprised of subsets of ten derived from rational design and natural sources, respectively (Figure 2). These compounds and all related ones with a Tanimoto [110] coefficient $\geq$0.9 were omitted from training. Proteomic interaction signatures were computed by CANDO, and output SMILES strings were generated by the RCVAE design pipeline as described above. This resulted in SMILES strings corresponding to 100 novel redesigns for each objective drug. One-hundred compounds were selected at random from the curated ZINC database to serve as a naive control. As a second, more rigorous control, the CANDO platform was used to generate the 100 most similar compounds ("top 100") from its 13,194-sized library to each objective drug according to their proteomic interaction signatures. As a third control, the CANDO platform's indication prediction pipeline was used to predict a set of compounds for the indication associated with each objective, i.e., the indication that the objective is approved for ("same indication") [27,107]. Proteomic interaction signatures were generated for all compounds (designs and controls), which were then compared to that of the objective using the RMSDs between them. The RMSD distributions are illustrated using box plots with boxes depicting the first and third quartile ranges, horizontal bars depicting the median, whiskers representing non-outlier ranges, and outliers explicitly plotted (Figure 2, Results Section 2.1).

Kolmogorov–Smirnov (K-S) tests [111,112] were used to demonstrate statistical significance [113] between samples for each redesign–control RMSD distribution pair for each objective. We also compared the performance of the RCVAE design pipeline between objectives from the rational design and natural sources subsets, respectively. To do this, we computed the average RMSD between each naive control and the corresponding objective and compared this to the RMSD of each redesign for an objective. This yielded a percent increase of similarities to the objective for each redesign given by:

$$P = \frac{< RMSD_{control} > -RMSD_{redesign}}{< RMSD_{control} >} \quad (2)$$

where P denotes the percent increase ("proximity"), $< RMSD_{control} >$ denotes the average RMSD between the naive control and corresponding objective, and $RMSD_{redesign}$ denotes the RMSD of the redesign when compared to the objective proteomic interaction signature. This yielded 1000 total values of percent proximity increases for both the rational design and natural sources subsets. The values for both subsets were then averaged and compared using K-S tests (Figure 2, Results Section 2.1).

To better visualize the distributions of our redesigns and controls, t-distributed Stochastic Network Embedding (t-SNE) plots [55] that show the clustering of similar interaction signatures in two dimensions were generated with the interaction signatures of all objective, redesign, top 100, and same indication compounds (Figure 3, results Section 2.3).

We also computed Tanimoto coefficients for all redesigns relative to their respective objective compounds to determine structural diversity. Finally, we utilized SCScore [56], a machine-learning platform to predict the synthetic complexity of our redesigns in relation to the corresponding objectives (Figure 4, Results Section 2.5).

3.4. Generating Novel Designs for Prospective Validation

Design objectives for benchmarking were selected from a diverse set of indications and approved/experimental statuses to ensure broad coverage of the proteomic interaction signature space and to mitigate potential bias in the results. Regardless, the benchmark set was repeatedly used to parameterize the pipeline described here, which has the potential to lead to overtraining. To address this and also to apply our design pipelines to relevant real-world problems of sufficient complexity where the proteomic approach would be relevant, we selected 13 (7 + 6) objective compounds that have shown promise for aging/developmental intervention [114–118] and NSCLC [118–120] to redesign for prospective validation (Figure 5, Results Section 2.6).

4. Conclusions

We utilized the RCVAE pipeline within the CANDO platform to take advantage of multiscale compound–proteome interaction modeling and develop an attractive approach to holistic drug design. We compared the predicted behaviors of the designed compounds to those of known drugs/compounds and demonstrated that the RCVAE pipeline is capable of generating novel compounds with the desired specificity of binding on a proteomic scale. We additionally demonstrated that compounds designed by our pipeline maintained reasonable predicted synthetic complexities and were structurally diverse. We expect the compounds designed using our pipeline for aging/developmental intervention and NSCLC will serve as novel leads for safe and effective therapeutics following prospective validation. The RCVAE design pipeline generates novel compounds that are synthetically feasible and behaviorally desirable, simultaneously taking efficacy and ADMET into account by examining interactions on a proteomic scale, which is necessary to understand the science of small molecule behavior and apply it to holistic therapeutic discovery.

Author Contributions: B.O. conceived of the RCVAE pipeline, research design, approach, and methods, conducted all experiments and analyses, and drafted the manuscript. Z.F. helped with the research design, approach, and methods and editing and proofing of the manuscript. W.M. helped with the research design, approach, and methods and editing and proofing of the manuscript. R.S. conceived of the research design, approach, and methods, supervised the overall project, and edited the manuscript. All authors have read and agreed to the published version of the manuscript.

Funding: This work was supported in part by National Institutes of Health Director's Pioneer Award (DP1OD006779), National Institutes of Health Clinical and Translational Sciences Award (UL1TR001412), NIH T15 Award (T15LM012495), NCATS ASPIRE Design Challenge Award, NCATS ASPIRE Reduction-to- Practice Award, and startup funds from the Department of Biomedical Informatics at the University at Buffalo.

Institutional Review Board Statement: Not applicable.

Informed Consent Statement: Not applicable.

Data Availability Statement: All relevant data are presented/illustrated in this manuscript.

Acknowledgments: The authors would like to acknowledge the support provided by the Center for Computational Research at the University at Buffalo. In addition to all members of the Samudrala Computational Biology Group, we give special thanks to Liana Bruggemann for providing us with the list of NSCLC objectives and Mira Moukheiber for assistance with proofreading.

Conflicts of Interest: The funders had no role in the design of the study; in the collection, analyses, or interpretation of the data; in the writing of the manuscript; nor in the decision to publish the results. The authors have formed multiple startups that seek to commercialize the outputs of the CANDO platform.

References

1. Schuhmacher, A.; Gassmann, O.; Hinder, M. Changing R&D models in research-based pharmaceutical companies. *J. Transl. Med* **2016**, *14*, 105.
2. Bajorath, J. Integration of virtual and high-throughput screening. *Nat. Rev. Drug Discov.* **2002**, *1*, 882–894. [CrossRef] [PubMed]
3. Dhasmana, A.; Raza, S.; Jahan, R.; Lohani, M.; Arif, J.M. *Chapter 19-High-Throughput Virtual Screening (HTVS) of Natural Compounds and Exploration of Their Biomolecular Mechanisms: An In Silico Approach*; Academic Press: Cambridge, MA, USA 2019; pp. 523–548.
4. Graff, D.E.; Shakhnovich, E.I.; Coley, C.W. Accelerating high-throughput virtual screening through molecular pool-based active learning. *Chem. Sci.* **2021**, *12*, 7866–7881. [CrossRef]

5. Lim, J.; Ryu, S.; Park, K.; Choe, Y.J.; Ham, J.; Kim, W.Y. Predicting drug–target interaction using a novel graph neural network with 3D structure-embedded graph representation. *J. Chem. Inf. Model.* **2019**, *59*, 3981–3988. [CrossRef] [PubMed]
6. Zoete, V.; Grosdidier, A.; Michielin, O. Docking, virtual high throughput screening and in silico fragment-based drug design. *J. Cell. Mol. Med.* **2009**, *13*, 238–248. [CrossRef]
7. Ha, E.; Lwin, C.; Durrant, J. LigGrep: A tool for filtering docked poses to improve virtual-screening hit rates. *J. Cheminform.* **2020**, *12*, 69. [CrossRef]
8. Lee, H.S.; Choi, J.; Kufareva, I.; Abagyan, R.; Filikov, A.; Yang, Y.; Yoon, S. Optimization of high throughput virtual screening by combining shape-matching and docking methods. *J. Chem. Inf. Model.* **2008**, *48*, 489–497. [CrossRef]
9. Corbeil, C.R.; Moitessier, N. Docking ligands into flexible and solvated macromolecules. 3. Impact of input ligand conformation, protein flexibility, and water molecules on the accuracy of docking programs. *J. Chem. Inf. Model.* **2009**, *49*, 997–1009. [CrossRef]
10. Feher, M.; Williams, C. Numerical errors and chaotic behavior in docking simulations. *J. Chem. Inf. Model.* **2012**, *52*, 724–738. [CrossRef] [PubMed]
11. Boran, A.; Iyengar, R. Systems approaches to polypharmacology and drug discovery. *Curr. Opin. Drug Discov. Dev.* **2010**, *13*, 297–309.
12. Peyvandipour, A.; Saberian, N.; Shafi, A.; Donato, M.; Draghici, S. A novel computational approach for drug repurposing using systems biology. *Bioinformatics* **2018**, *34*, 2817–2825. [CrossRef]
13. Shafi, A.; Nguyen, T.; Peyvandipour, A.; Nguyen, H.; Draghici, S. A multi-cohort and multi-omics meta-analysis framework to identify network-based Gene signatures. *Front. Genet.* **2019**, *10*, 159. [CrossRef] [PubMed]
14. Tatonetti, N.P.; Liu, T.; Altman, R.B. Predicting drug side-effects by chemical systems biology. *Genome Biol.* **2009**, *10*, 238. [CrossRef]
15. Liu, T.; Altman, R.B. Relating essential proteins to drug side-effects using canonical component analysis: A structure-based approach. *J. Chem. Inf. Model.* **2015**, *55*, 1483–1494. [CrossRef]
16. Kirkpatrick, P.; Ellis, C. Chemical space. *Nature* **2004**, *432*, 832. [CrossRef]
17. Shayakhmetov, R.; Kuznetsov, M.; Zhebrak, A.; Kadurin, A.; Nikolenko, S.; Aliper, A.; Polykovskiy, D. Molecular generation for desired transcriptome changes with adversarial autoencoders. *Front. Pharmacol.* **2020**, *11*, 269. [CrossRef]
18. Minie, M.; Sethi, G.; Chopra, G.; Horst, J.; Roy, A.; White, G.; Samudrala, R. CANDO and the infinite drug discovery frontier. *Drug Discov. Today* **2014**, *19*, 1353–1363. [CrossRef]
19. Sethi, G.; Chopra, G.; Samudrala, R. Multiscale modelling of relationships between protein classes and drug behavior across all diseases using the CANDO platform. *Mini Rev. Med. Chem.* **2015**, *15*, 705–717. [CrossRef] [PubMed]
20. Chopra, G.; Samudrala, R. Exploring polypharmacology in drug discovery and repurposing using the CANDO platform. *Curr. Pharm. Des.* **2016**, *22*, 3109–3123. [CrossRef]
21. Chopra, G.; Kaushik, S.; Elkin, P.; Samudrala, R. Combating Ebola with repurposed therapeutics using the CANDO platform. *Molecules* **2016**, *21*, 1537. [CrossRef] [PubMed]
22. Mangione, W.; Samudrala, R. Identifying protein features responsible for improved drug repurposing accuracies using the CANDO platform: Implications for drug design. *Molecules* **2019**, *24*, 167. [CrossRef] [PubMed]
23. Falls, Z.; Mangione, W.; Schuler, J.; Samudrala, R. Exploration of interaction scoring criteria in the CANDO platform. *BMC Bioinform.* **2019**, *12*, 318. [CrossRef] [PubMed]
24. Schuler, J.; Samudrala, R. Fingerprinting CANDO: Increased accuracy with structure and ligand based shotgun drug repurposing. *ACS Omega* **2019**, *4*, 17393–17403. [CrossRef] [PubMed]
25. Fine, J.; Lacker, R.; Samudrala, R.; Chopra, G. Computational chemoproteomics to understand the role of selected psychoactives in treating mental health disorders. *Sci. Rep.* **2019**, *9*, 13155. [CrossRef] [PubMed]
26. Mangione, W.; Falls, Z.; Melendy, T.; Chopra, G.; Samudrala, R. Shotgun drug repurposing biotechnology to tackle epidemics and pandemics. *Drug Discov. Today* **2020**, *25*, 1126–1129. [CrossRef]
27. Mangione, W.; Falls, Z.; Chopra, G.; Samudrala, R. cando.py: Open source software for analyzing large scale drug-protein-disease data. *J. Chem. Inf. Model.* **2020**, *60*, 4131–4136. [CrossRef]
28. Hudson, M.; Samudrala, R. Multiscale virtual screening optimization for shotgun drug repurposing using the CANDO platform. *Molecules* **2021**, *26*, 2581–2597. [CrossRef] [PubMed]
29. Schuler, J.; Falls, Z.; Mangione, W.; Hudson, M.; Bruggemann, L.; Samdurala, R. Evaluating performance of drug repurposing technologies. *Drug Discov. Today* **2021**, in press. . [CrossRef]
30. Yang, L.; Wang, K.J.; Wang, L.S.; Jegga, A.G.; Qin, S.Y.; He, G.; Chen, J.; Xiao, Y.; He, L. Chemical-protein interactome and its application in off-target identification. *Interdiscip. Sci. Comput. Life Sci.* **2011**, *3*, 22–30. [CrossRef]
31. Liu, T.; Tang, G.; Capriotti, E. Comparative modeling: The state of the art and protein drug target structure prediction. *Comb. Chem. High Throughput Screen.* **2011**, *14*, 532–547. [CrossRef]
32. Wu, C.; Gudivada, R.C.; Aronow, B.J.; Jegga, A.G. Computational drug repositioning through heterogeneous network clustering. *BMC Syst. Biol.* **2013**, *7*, S6. [CrossRef] [PubMed]
33. Yella, J.; Yaddanapudi, S.; Wang, Y.; Jegga, A. Changing trends in computational drug repositioning. *Pharmaceuticals* **2018**, *11*, 57. [CrossRef]
34. Wang, Y.; Yella, J.; Jegga, A.G. Transcriptomic data mining and repurposing for computational drug discovery. In *Methods in Molecular Biology*; Springer: New York, NY, USA, 2018; pp. 73–95.

35. Patel, L.; Shukla, T.; Huang, X.; Ussery, D.W.; Wang, S. Machine learning methods in drug discovery. *Molecules* **2020**, *25*, 5277 [CrossRef] [PubMed]
36. Yuan, Y.; Pei, J.; Lai, L. LigBuilder V3: A multi-target de novo drug design approach. *Front. Chem.* **2020**, *8*, 142. [CrossRef]
37. Bai, Q.; Tan, S.; Xu, T.; Liu, H.; Huang, J.; Yao, X. MolAICal: A soft tool for 3D drug design of protein targets by artificial intelligence and classical algorithm. *Brief. Bioinform.* **2020**, *22*, bbaa161. [CrossRef]
38. Chemistry 42. Available online: https://insilico.com/chemistry42 (accessed on 30 July 2021).
39. Grechishnikova, D. Transformer neural network for protein-specific de novo drug generation as a machine translation problem *Sci. Rep.* **2021**, *11*, 321. [CrossRef]
40. Schmidhuber, J. Deep learning in neural networks: An overview. *Neural Netw.* **2015**, *61*, 85–117. [CrossRef]
41. Kingma, D.P.; Welling, M. Auto-Encoding Variational Bayes. *arXiv* **2014**, arXiv:1312.6114.
42. Polykovskiy, D.; Vetrov, D. Deterministic Decoding for Discrete Data in Variational Autoencoders. In Proceedings of the Machine Learning Research, Proceedings of the Twenty Third International Conference on Artificial Intelligence and Statistics, Palermo Italy, 3–5 June 2020; Chiappa, S., Calandra, R., Eds.; 2020; Volume 108, pp. 3046–3056.
43. Sohn, K.; Lee, H.; Yan, X. Learning Structured Output Representation using Deep Conditional Generative Models. In *Advances in Neural Information Processing Systems 28 (NIPS 2015)*; Curran Associates, Inc.: Red Hook, NY, USA, 2015; Volume 28.
44. Gómez-Bombarelli, R.; Wei, J.N.; Duvenaud, D.; Hernández-Lobato, J.M.; Sánchez-Lengeling, B.; Sheberla, D.; Aguilera-Iparraguirre, J.; Hirzel, T.D.; Adams, R.P.; Aspuru-Guzik, A. Automatic chemical design using a data-driven continuous representation of molecules. *ACS Cent. Sci.* **2018**, *4*, 268–276. [CrossRef] [PubMed]
45. Lim, J.; Ryu, S.; Kim, J.; Kim, W. Molecular generative model based on conditional variational autoencoder for de novo molecular design. *J. Cheminform.* **2018**, *10*, 31. [CrossRef]
46. Polykovskiy, D.; Zhebrak, A.; Sanchez-Lengeling, B.; Golovanov, S.; Tatanov, O.; Belyaev, S.; Kurbanov, R.; Artamonov, A. Aladinskiy, V.; Veselov, M.; et al. Molecular Sets (MOSES): A benchmarking platform for molecular generation models. *Front Pharmacol.* **2020**, *11*, 1931. [CrossRef]
47. Jenwitheesuk, E.; Samudrala, R. Identification of potential multitarget antimalarial drugs. *J. Am. Med. Assoc.* **2005**, *294*, 1490–1491
48. Jenwitheesuk, E.; Samudrala, R. New paradigms for drug discovery: Computational multitarget screening. *Trends Pharmacol. Sci* **2008**, *29*, 62–71. [CrossRef]
49. Costin, J.; Jenwitheesuk, E.; Lok, S.; Hunsperger, E.; Conrads, K.; Fontaine, K.; Rees, C.; Rossmann, M.; Isern, S.; Samudrala, R. et al. Structural optimization and de novo design of dengue virus entry inhibitory peptides. *PLoS Negl. Trop. Dis.* **2010**, *4*, e721 [CrossRef]
50. Palanikumar, L.; Karpauskaite, L.; Al-Sayegh, M.; Chehade, I.; Alam, M.; Hassan, S.; Maity, D.; Ali, L.; Kalmouni, M.; Hunashal Y.; et al. Protein mimetic amyloid inhibitor potently abrogates cancer-associated mutant p53 aggregation and restores tumor suppressor function. *Nat. Commun.* **2021**, *12*, 3962. [CrossRef] [PubMed]
51. MedicineNet. Available online: https://www.medicinenet.com/me-too_drug/definition.htm (accessed on 30 July 2021).
52. Cheng, G.; Qian, B.; Samudrala, R.; Baker, D. Improvement in protein functional site prediction by distinguishing structural and functional constraints on protein family evolution using computational design. *Nucleic Acids Res.* **2005**, *33*, 5861–5867. [CrossRef]
53. Xiao, Z.; Morris-Natschke, S.L.; Lee, K.H. Strategies for the optimization of natural leads to anticancer drugs or drug candidates *Med. Res. Rev.* **2016**, *36*, 32–91. [CrossRef] [PubMed]
54. Sterling, T.; Irwin, J. ZINC 15—Ligand discovery for everyone. *J. Chem. Inf. Model.* **2015**, *55*, 2324–2337. [CrossRef]
55. van der Maaten, L.; Hinton, G. Visualizing data using t-SNE. *J. Mach. Learn. Res.* **2008**, *9*, 2579–2605.
56. Coley, C.; Rogers, L.; Green, W.; Jensen, K. SCScore: Synthetic complexity Learned from a reaction corpus. *J. Chem. Inf. Model* **2018**, *58*, 251–261. [CrossRef] [PubMed]
57. Bickerton, G.R.; Paolini, G.V.; Besnard, J.; Muresan, S.; Hopkins, A.L. Quantifying the chemical beauty of drugs. *Nat. Chem.* **2012** *4*, 90–98. [CrossRef] [PubMed]
58. Ertl, P.; Schuffenhauer, A. Estimation of synthetic accessibility score of drug-like molecules based on molecular complexity and fragment contributions. *J. Cheminform.* **2009**, *1*, 8. [CrossRef]
59. Genheden, S.; Thakkar, A.; Chadimová, V.; Reymond, J.L.; Engkvist, O.; Bjerrum, E. AiZynthFinder: A fast, robust and flexible open-source software for retrosynthetic planning. *J. Cheminform.* **2020**, *12*, 70. [CrossRef] [PubMed]
60. Brown, N.; Fiscato, M.; Segler, M.H.; Vaucher, A.C. GuacaMol: Benchmarking Models for de Novo Molecular Design. *J. Chem Inf. Model.* **2019**, *59*, 1096–1108. [CrossRef]
61. Li, J.; Zhang, C.X.; Liu, Y.M.; Chen, K.L.; Chen, G. A comparative study of anti-aging properties and mechanism: Resveratrol and caloric restriction. *Oncotarget* **2017**, *8*, 65717–65729. [CrossRef] [PubMed]
62. Soukas, A.; Hao, H.; Wu, L. Metformin as anti-Aging therapy: Is it for everyone? *Trends Endocrinol. Metab.* **2019**, *30*, 745–755 [CrossRef]
63. Aman, Y.; Qiu, Y.; Tao, J.; Fang, E. Therapeutic potential of boosting NAD+ in aging and age-related diseases. *Transl. Med. Aging* **2018**, *2*, 30–37. [CrossRef]
64. Hernández-Camacho, J.; Bernier, M.; López-Lluch, G.; Navas, P. Coenzyme Q10 supplementation in aging and disease. *Front Physiol.* **2018**, *9*, 44. [CrossRef]
65. Fagot, D.; Pham, D.; Laboureau, J.; Planel, E.; Guerin, L.; Nègre, C.; Donovan, M.; Bernard, B. Crocin, a natural molecule with potentially beneficial effects against skin ageing. *Int. J. Cosmet. Sci.* **2018**, *40*, 388–400. [CrossRef] [PubMed]

66. Bielak-Zmijewska, A.; Grabowska, W.; Ciolko, A.; Bojko, A.; Mosieniak, G.; Bijoch, L.; Sikora, E. The role of curcumin in the modulation of ageing. *Int. J. Mol. Sci.* **2019**, *20*, 1239. [CrossRef]
67. Ichida, J.K.; Blanchard, J.; Lam, K.; Son, E.Y.; Chung, J.E.; Egli, D.; Loh, K.; Carter, A.C.; Di Giorgio, F.P.; Koszka, K.; et al. A small-molecule inhibitor of TGF-β signaling replaces sox2 in reprogramming by inducing nanog. *Cell Stem Cell* **2009**, *5*, 491–503. [CrossRef] [PubMed]
68. Yamoah, E.N.; Li, M.; Shah, A.; Elliott, K.L.; Cheah, K.; Xu, P.X.; Phillips, S.; Young, S.M., Jr.; Eberl, D.F.; Fritzsch, B. Using sox2 to alleviate the hallmarks of age-related hearing loss. *Ageing Res. Rev.* **2020**, *59*, 101042. [CrossRef]
69. Tominaga, K.; Suzuki, H. TGF-β signaling in cellular senescence and aging-related pathology. *Int. J. Mol. Sci.* **2019**, *20*, 5002. [CrossRef] [PubMed]
70. Kennedy, B.K.; Pennypacker, J.K. Drugs that modulate aging: The promising yet difficult path ahead. *Transl. Res.* **2014**, *163*, 456–465. [CrossRef]
71. Jiao, D.; Yang, S. Overcoming resistance to drugs targeting KRASG12C mutation. *Innovation* **2020**, *1*, 100035.
72. Shah, R.; Lester, J. Tyrosine Kinase inhibitors for the treatment of EGFR mutation-positive non-small-cell lung cancer: A clash of the generations. *Clin. Lung Cancer* **2020**, *21*, 216–228. [CrossRef] [PubMed]
73. Wu, Y.L.; Tsuboi, M.; He, J.; John, T.; Grohe, C.; Majem, M.; Goldman, J.W.; Laktionov, K.; Kim, S.W.; Kato, T.; et al. Osimertinib in resected EGFR-mutated Non–Small-Cell Lung Cancer. *N. Engl. J. Med.* **2020**, *383*, 1711–1723. [CrossRef]
74. Molina-Arcas, M.; Moore, C.; Rana, S.; van Maldegem, F.; Mugarza, E.; Romero-Clavijo, P.; Herbert, E.; Horswell, S.; Li, L.S.; Janes, M.R.; et al. Development of combination therapies to maximize the impact of KRAS-G12C inhibitors in lung cancer. *Sci. Transl. Med.* **2019**, *11*, eaaw7999. [CrossRef]
75. Moore, A.; Rosenberg, S.; McCormick, F.; Malek, S. RAS-targeted therapies: Is the undruggable drugged? *Nat. Rev. Drug Discov.* **2020**, *19*, 533–552. [CrossRef]
76. Lau, S.C.M.; Batra, U.; Mok, T.S.K.; Loong, H.H. Dacomitinib in the management of advanced Non-Small-Cell Lung Cancer. *Drugs* **2019**, *79*, 823–831. [CrossRef]
77. Keating, G.M. Afatinib: A review in advanced Non-Small Cell Lung Cancer. *Target. Oncol.* **2016**, *11*, 825–835. [CrossRef] [PubMed]
78. Piperdi, B.; Perez-Soler, R. Role of Erlotinib in the treatment of Non-Small Cell Lung Cancer. *Drugs* **2012**, *72*, 11–19. [CrossRef]
79. Zhou, J.; Cui, G.; Hu, S.; Zhang, Z.; Yang, C.; Liu, Z.; Wang, L.; Li, C.; Sun, M. Graph Neural Networks: A review of methods and applications. *arXiv* **2021**, arXiv:1812.08434.
80. Lamb, J.; Crawford, E.; Peck, D.; Modell, J.; Blat, I.; Wrobel, M.; Lerner, J.; Brunet, J.; Subramanian, A.; Ross, K.; et al. The Connectivity Map: Using gene-expression signatures to connect small molecules, genes, and disease. *Science* **2006**, *313*, 1929–1935. [CrossRef]
81. Subramanian, A.; Narayan, R.; Corsello, S.; Peck, D.; Natoli, T.; Lu, X.; Gould, J.; Davis, J.; Tubelli, A.; Asiedu, J.; et al. A next generation Connectivity Map: L1000 platform and the first 1,000,000 profiles. *Cell* **2017**, *171*, 1437–1452. [CrossRef] [PubMed]
82. Wleklinski, M.; Loren, B.; Ferreira, C.; Jaman, Z.; Avramova, L.; Sobreira, T.; Thompson, D.; Cooks, R. High throughput reaction screening using desorption electrospray ionization mass spectrometry. *Sci. Rep.* **2018**, *9*, 1647–1653. [CrossRef] [PubMed]
83. Morato, N.; Holden, D.; Cooks, R. High-throughput label-free enzymatic assays using desorption electrospray-ionization mass spectrometry. *Angew. Chem. Int. Ed. Engl.* **2020**, *59*, 20459–20464. [CrossRef]
84. Logsdon, D.; Li, Y.; Sobreira, T.; Ferreira, C.; Thompson, D.; Cooks, R. High-throughput screening of reductive amination reactions using desorption electrospray ionization mass spectrometry. *Org. Process Res. Dev.* **2020**, *24*, 1647–1657. [CrossRef]
85. Sobreira, T.; Avramova, L.; Szilagyi, B.; Logsdon, D.; Loren, B.; Jaman, Z.; Hilger, R.; Hosler, R.; Ferreira, C.; Koswara, A.; et al. High-throughput screening of organic reactions in microdroplets using desorption electrospray ionization mass spectrometry (DESI-MS): Hardware and software implementation. *Methods* **2020**, *12*, 3654–3669. [CrossRef]
86. Le, M.; Morato, N.; Kaerner, A.; Welch, C.; Cooks, R. Fragmentation of polyfunctional compounds recorded using automated high-throughput desorption electrospray ionization. *J. Am. Soc. Mass Spectrom.* **2021**, *32*, 2261–2273. [CrossRef] [PubMed]
87. Morato, N.; Le, M.; Holden, D.; Cooks, R. Automated high-throughput system combining small-scale synthesis with bioassays and reaction screening. *SLAS Technol.* **2021**, *26*, 555–571. [CrossRef]
88. Biyani, S.; Qi, Q.; Wu, J.; Moriuchi, Y.; Larocque, E.A.; Sintim, H.; Thompson, D. Use of high-throughput tools for telescoped continuous flow synthesis of an alkynylnaphthyridine anticancer agent, HSN608. *Org. Process Res. Dev.* **2020**, *24*, 2240–2251. [CrossRef]
89. Jaman, Z.; Mufti, A.; Sah, S.; Avramova, L.; Thompson, D. High Throughput Experimentation and Continuous Flow Validation of Suzuki-Miyaura Cross-Coupling Reactions. *Chem. Eur. J.* **2018**, *24*, 9546–9554. [CrossRef] [PubMed]
90. Wei, Z.; Xie, Z.; Kuvelkar, R.; Shah, V.; Bateman, K.; McLaren, D.; Cooks, R. high-throughput bioassays using "dip-and-go" multiplexed electrospray mass spectrometry. *Angew. Chem. Int. Ed. Engl.* **2019**, *58*, 17594–17598. doi:10.1002/anie.201909047. [CrossRef]
91. Berman, H.; Westbrook, J.; Feng, Z.; Gilliland, G.; Bhat, T.; Weissig, H.; Shindyalov, I.; Bourne, P. The Protein Data Bank. *Nucleic Acids Res.* **2000**, *28*, 235–242. [CrossRef] [PubMed]
92. Yang, J.; Zhang, Y. I-TASSER server: New development for protein structure and function predictions. *Nucleic Acids Res.* **2015**, *43*, W174–W181. [CrossRef]

93. Yang, J.; Yan, R.; Roy, A.; Xu, D.; Poisson, J.; Zhang, Y. The I-TASSER Suite: Protein structure and function prediction. *Nat. Methods* **2015**, *12*, 7–8. [CrossRef] [PubMed]
94. Zhang, C.; Mortuza, S.; He, B.; Wang, Y.; Zhang, Y. Template-based and free modeling of I-TASSER and QUARK pipelines using predicted contact maps in CASP12. *Proteins Struct. Funct. Genet.* **2018**, *86* (Suppl. S1), 136–151. [CrossRef]
95. Zhang, W.; Yang, J.; He, B.; Walker, S.; Zhang, H.; Govindarajoo, B.; Virtanen, J.; Xue, Z.; Shen, H.; Zhang, Y. Integration of QUARK and I-TASSER for ab initio protein structure prediction in CASP11. *Proteins Struct. Funct. Genet.* **2016**, *84* (Suppl. S1), 76–86. [CrossRef]
96. Yang, J.; Zhang, W.; He, B.; Walker, S.; Zhang, H.; Govindarajoo, B.; Virtanen, J.; Xue, Z.; Shen, H.; Zhang, Y. Template-based protein structure prediction in CASP11 and retrospect of I-TASSER in the last decade. *Proteins Struct. Funct. Genet.* **2016**, *84* (Suppl. S1), 233–246. [CrossRef]
97. Xu, D.; Zhang, J.; Roy, A.; Zhang, Y. Automated protein structure modeling in CASP9 by I-TASSER pipeline combined with QUARK-based ab initio folding and FG-MD-based structure refinement. *Proteins Struct. Funct. Genet.* **2011**, *79* (Suppl. S10), 147–160. [CrossRef] [PubMed]
98. Wu, Q.; Peng, Z.; Zhang, Y.; Yang, J. COACH-D: Improved protein-ligand binding sites prediction with refined ligand-binding poses through molecular docking. *Nucleic Acids Res.* **2018**, *46*, W438–W430. [CrossRef] [PubMed]
99. Willett, P. Similarity-based virtual screening using 2D fingerprints. *Drug Discov. Today* **2006**, *11*, 1046–1053. [CrossRef] [PubMed]
100. Weininger, D. SMILES, a chemical language and information system. 1. Introduction to methodology and encoding rules. *J. Chem. Inform. Comput. Sci.* **1988**, *28*, 31–36. [CrossRef]
101. Kramer, M. Nonlinear principal component analysis using autoassociative neural networks. *AIChE J.* **1991**, *37*, 233–243. [CrossRef]
102. Santhanam, S. Context based text-generation using LSTM networks. *arXiv* **2020**, arXiv:2005.00048.
103. Hancock, J.T.; Khoshgoftaar, T.M. Survey on categorical data for neural networks. *J. Big Data* **2020**, *7*, 28. [CrossRef]
104. Hochreiter, S.; Schmidhuber, J. Long Short-Term Memory. *Neural Comput.* **1997**, *9*, 1735–1780. [CrossRef]
105. Yu, Y.; Si, X.; Hu, C.; Zhang, J. A Review of recurrent neural networks: LSTM cells and network architectures. *Neural Comput.* **2019**, *31*, 1235–1270. [CrossRef] [PubMed]
106. Kullback, S.; Leibler, R. On information and sufficiency. *Ann. Math. Statist.* **1951**, *22*, 79–86. [CrossRef]
107. Davis, A.; Grondin, C.; Johnson, R.; Sciaky, D.; Wiegers, J.; Wiegers, T.; Mattingly, C. Comparative Toxicogenomics Database (CTD): Update 2021. *Nucleic Acids Res.* **2021**, *49*, D1138. [CrossRef]
108. Tatonetti, N.; Ye, P.; Daneshjou, R.; Altman, R. Data-driven prediction of drug effects and interactions. *Sci. Transl. Med.* **2012**, *4*, 125–129. [CrossRef]
109. Kuhn, M.; Letunic, I.; Jensen, L.; Bork, P. The SIDER database of drugs and side effects. *Nucleic Acids Res.* **2016**, *44*, D1075–D1079. [CrossRef]
110. Bajusz, D.; Rácz, A.; Héberger, K. Why is Tanimoto index an appropriate choice for fingerprint-based similarity calculations? *J. Cheminform.* **2015**, *7*, 20. [CrossRef] [PubMed]
111. Feller, W. On the Kolmogorov-Smirnov Limit Theorems for Empirical Distributions. *Ann. Math. Stat.* **1948**, *19*, 177–189. [CrossRef]
112. Karson, M. Handbook of Methods of Applied Statistics. Volume I: Techniques of Computation Descriptive Methods, and Statistical Inference. Volume II: Planning of Surveys and Experiments. I. M. Chakravarti, R. G. Laha, and J. Roy, New York, John Wiley; 1967, $9.00. *J. Am. Stat. Assoc.* **1968**, *63*, 1047–1049. [CrossRef]
113. Cox, D.R. Statistical significance tests. *Br. J. Clin. Pharmacol.* **1982**, *14*, 325–331. [CrossRef]
114. Johnson, A.A.; Shokhirev, M.N.; Wyss-Coray, T.; Lehallier, B. Systematic review and analysis of human proteomics aging studies unveils a novel proteomic aging clock and identifies key processes that change with age. *Ageing Res. Rev.* **2020**, *60*, 101070. [CrossRef]
115. Lorusso, J.S.; Sviderskiy, O.A.; Labunskyy, V.M. Emerging omics approaches in aging research. *Antioxid. Redox Signal.* **2018**, *29*, 985–1002. [CrossRef] [PubMed]
116. Gill, D.; Parry, A.; Santos, F.; Hernando-Herraez, I.; Stubbs, T.M.; Milagre, I.; Reik, W. Multi-omic rejuvenation of human cells by maturation phase transient reprogramming. *bioRxiv* **2021**. . [CrossRef]
117. Natarajan, K.N.; Teichmann, S.A.; Kolodziejczyk, A.A. Single cell transcriptomics of pluripotent stem cells: reprogramming and differentiation. *Curr. Opin. Genet. Dev.* **2017**, *46*, 66–76. [CrossRef] [PubMed]
118. Ramsay, R.R.; Popovic-Nikolic, M.R.; Nikolic, K.; Uliassi, E.; Bolognesi, M.L. A perspective on multi-target drug discovery and design for complex diseases. *Clin. Transl. Med.* **2018**, *7*, 3. [CrossRef]
119. Koomen, J.M.; Haura, E.B.; Bepler, G.; Sutphen, R.; Remily-Wood, E.R.; Benson, K.; Hussein, M.; Hazlehurst, L.A.; Yeatman, T.J.; Hildreth, L.T.; et al. Proteomic contributions to personalized cancer care. *Mol. Cell. Proteom.* **2008**, *7*, 1780–1794. [CrossRef] [PubMed]
120. Yumura, M.; Nagano, T.; Nishimura, Y. Novel multitarget therapies for lung cancer and respiratory disease. *Molecules* **2020**, *25*, 3987. [CrossRef] [PubMed]

pharmaceuticals

Article

De Novo Molecular Design of Caspase-6 Inhibitors by a GRU-Based Recurrent Neural Network Combined with a Transfer Learning Approach

Shuheng Huang [1], Hu Mei [1,*], Laichun Lu [1,*], Minyao Qiu [1], Xiaoqi Liang [1], Lei Xu [1], Zuyin Kuang [1], Yu Heng [1] and Xianchao Pan [2,*]

1 Key Laboratory of Biorheological Science and Technology (Ministry of Education), College of Bioengineering, Chongqing University, Chongqing 400044, China; shhuang@cqu.edu.cn (S.H.); 202019021051@cqu.edu.cn (M.Q.); 202019021086@cqu.edu.cn (X.L.); 201919021051@cqu.edu.cn (L.X.); 201819021101@cqu.edu.cn (Z.K.); 201819021102@cqu.edu.cn (Y.H.)

2 Department of Medicinal Chemistry, School of Pharmacy, Southwest Medical University, Luzhou 646000, China

* Correspondence: meihu@cqu.edu.cn (H.M.); lulaicq@cqu.edu.cn (L.L.); panxc@swmu.edu.cn (X.P.)

Abstract: Due to their potential in the treatment of neurodegenerative diseases, caspase-6 inhibitors have attracted widespread attention. However, the existing caspase-6 inhibitors showed more or less inevitable deficiencies that restrict their clinical development and applications. Therefore, there is an urgent need to develop novel caspase-6 candidate inhibitors. Herein, a gated recurrent unit (GRU)-based recurrent neural network (RNN) combined with transfer learning was used to build a molecular generative model of caspase-6 inhibitors. The results showed that the GRU-based RNN model can accurately learn the SMILES grammars of about 2.4 million chemical molecules including ionic and isomeric compounds and can generate potential caspase-6 inhibitors after transfer learning of the known 433 caspase-6 inhibitors. Based on the novel molecules derived from the molecular generative model, an optimal logistic regression model and Surflex-dock were employed for predicting and ranking the inhibitory activities. According to the prediction results, three potential caspase-6 inhibitors with different scaffolds were selected as the promising candidates for further research. In general, this paper provides an efficient combinational strategy for de novo molecular design of caspase-6 inhibitors.

Keywords: gated recurrent unit; recurrent neural network; machine learning; transfer learning; caspase-6; inhibitor; molecular design

Citation: Huang, S.; Mei, H.; Lu, L.; Qiu, M.; Liang, X.; Xu, L.; Kuang, Z.; Heng, Y.; Pan, X. De Novo Molecular Design of Caspase-6 Inhibitors by a GRU-Based Recurrent Neural Network Combined with a Transfer Learning Approach. *Pharmaceuticals* 2021, *14*, 1249. https://doi.org/10.3390/ph14121249

Academic Editor: Osvaldo Andrade Santos-Filho

Received: 4 November 2021
Accepted: 24 November 2021
Published: 30 November 2021

1. Introduction

Caspase is a family of cysteinyl aspartate-specific proteases, which plays a critical role in the cell regulatory networks controlling inflammation and programmed cell death [1]. Up to now, 11 functional caspase subtypes (i.e., caspase 1–10, 14) have been found in human encode proteins, of which caspase-1, -4 and -5 are related to inflammatory response, caspase-14 to keratinocyte differentiation and others to apoptosis. The apoptotic caspases are further divided into two subcategories, namely apoptotic initiator and executioner caspases according to their functions in apoptosis processes. The initiator caspases (caspases-2, -8, -9, and -10) can be recruited and activated by either death receptors or apoptosomes, while the downstream executioner caspases (caspases-3, -6, and -7) are responsible for the actual cell destruction [2–4].

Accumulated evidence has suggested that the activation of caspase-6 is responsible for neuronal apoptosis and amyloid β peptide (Aβ) deposition, which is highly involved in age-dependent axon degeneration and neurodegenerative diseases, such as Huntington's disease and Alzheimer's disease [5–7]. Due to the potencies in the treatment of neurodegenerative diseases, caspase-6 inhibitors have attracted intensive attention. Recently, a series of aza-peptides [8], acyl dipeptides [9,10], and non-peptide benzenesulfonyl chloride isatin sulfonamide [11–15], tetrafluorophenoxy methyl ketone [16], phenothiazin-5-ium derivatives [17], heteroaryl propanamido hexanoic acid [18], vinyl sulfone [19], furoyl phenylalanine derivatives [20] have been identified as caspase-6 inhibitors with nanomolar to micromolar potencies (Figure 1). However, the existing caspase-6 inhibitors showed more or less inevitable deficiencies that restrict their clinical development and applications. Therefore, there is an urgent need to develop novel caspase-6 candidate inhibitors [21].

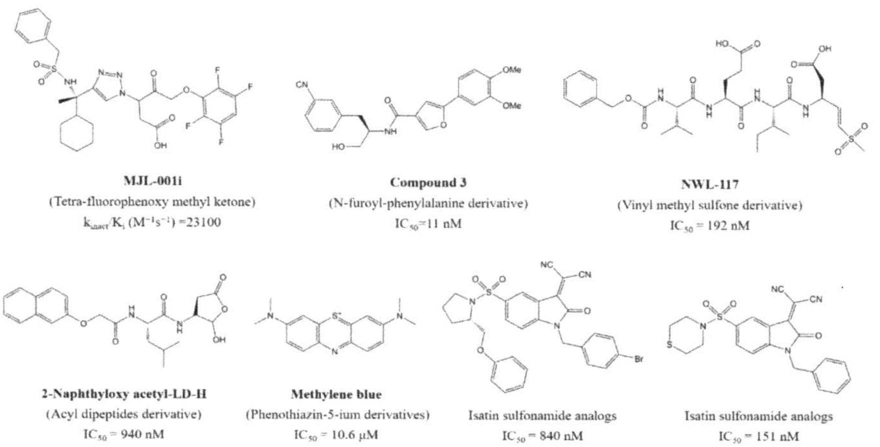

Figure 1. Representative structures of caspase-6 inhibitors.

Over the last decade, deep learning (DL) technologies, such as convolutional networks (CNN), restricted Boltzmann machines (RBM), recurrent neural networks (RNN), and generative adversarial networks (GAN) have been gradually applied in drug design and proven to be promising approaches for artificial intelligence-based drug design [22–24]. Recently, RNN-based molecular generative network has attracted particular attentions duo to its unique features in de novo molecular design [25–27]. By using variational auto-encoder (VAE), Gómez-Bombarelli et al. [28] proposed an RNN-based molecular generator which was further applied in a set of drug-like molecules and exhibited excellent predictive power when training jointly with a property prediction task. Winter et al. [29] designed neural network-based translation model and used it to translate chemical structures (e.g. SMILES) into continuous and fixed-sized low-level encodings. Additionally, the models can be used to predict several basic molecular properties for query structures without the need for re-training or including labels.

Olivecrona et al. [30] applied an RNN-based deep learning method combined with policy-based reinforcement learning to generate new molecules with potential activities against dopamine receptor type 2. The results showed that more than 95% of the generated compounds were predicted to be active. Jaques et al. [31] applied RNN and off-policy reinforcement learning methods to generate new molecular structures with desirable properties, such as cLogP and drug-likeness. Although a variety of generative models have been developed for de novo molecular generation, the structural diversity or search space computational efficiency, and synthetic accessibility, conditional molecule generation, etc need to be further investigated [32,33].

In this paper, a gated recurrent unit (GRU)-based RNN network combined with transfer learning and traditional machine learning were employed for de novo molecular design of caspase-6 inhibitors. The results showed that the established generative RNN model can generate efficiently potent caspase-6 inhibitors with the similar chemical space distribution to the known caspase-6 inhibitors, which can be easily incorporated with the traditional molecular design methods. In addition, the Surflex-dock method was employed for molecular activities prediction and ranking generated potential inhibitors. Collectively, this paper provides an efficient combinational strategy for de novo molecular design of caspase-6 inhibitors.

2. Methods

2.1. Datasets

Figure 2 shows the framework of the de novo design strategy of caspase-6 inhibitors, which mainly consists of 3 parts: (1) the generative RNN network; (2) the ML-based prediction model; (3) molecular docking-based ligand screening.

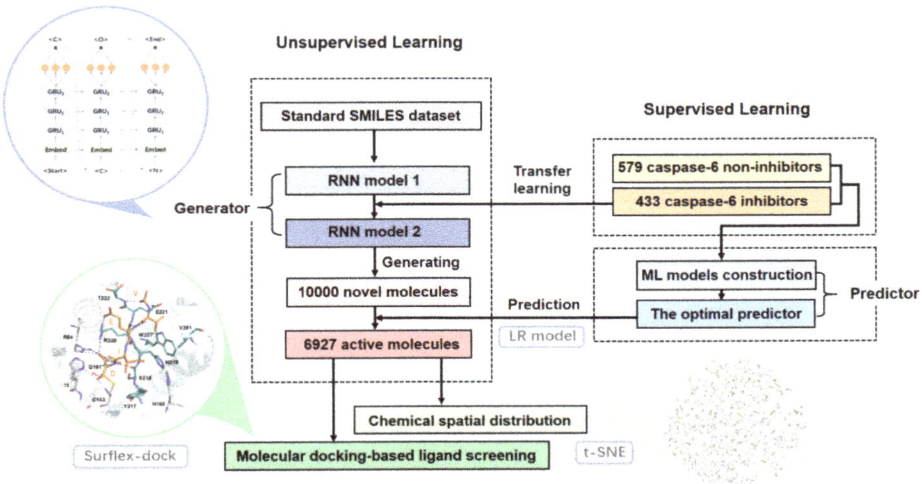

Figure 2. The flowchart of de novo molecular design of the caspase-6 inhibitors.

In this paper, about 2.4 million chemical molecules including ionic and isomeric compounds were first retrieved from PubChem database [34]. Then, all of the known caspase-6 inhibitors were removed from the dataset. In order to decrease the degree of data heterogeneity, only the molecules with a number of heavy atoms between 10 and 100 and the length of canonical SMILES string less than 140 were selected. As a result, a total of 2,393,029 molecules (SMILES strings) were retained for training the generative RNN network.

To construct a prediction model of caspase-6 inhibitors, 1656 samples consisting of 577 caspase-6 inhibitors and 1079 non-inhibitors were derived from the recent literature (Tables S1 and S2, Supplementary Materials) [9–15,35–45]. The activities of the collected caspase-6 inhibitors were mainly detected by enzyme inhibition assays and fluorescent plate reader assay.

2.2. Machine Learning Based Classification Models of Caspase-6 Inhibitors

Firstly, the 577 caspase-6 inhibitors and 1079 non-inhibitors were divided into a training/validation set (433 positives/579 negatives) and an independent test set (144 positives/500 negatives) according to Table S1. Then, the positive and negative samples in the training/validation set were further randomly divided into the training and validation sets at a ratio of 6:4, respectively. The statistic information of the datasets refers to Table S2. Lastly, a total of 200 fragmental and topological descriptors (Table S3, Supplementary Materials) generated by RDKit toolkit [46] were used for the structural description of the 1656 samples. Herein, five machine learning methods, i.e., support vector machine

(SVM), k-nearest neighbor (KNN), Gaussian Naïve Bayesian (GNB), random forest (RF) and logistic regression (LR), were used to construct binary classification models by the Scikit-Learn toolkit [47]. The ROC (receiver operating characteristic), AUC (area under the curve), Matthews correlation coefficient (MCC), accuracy (Acc), specificity (Spe), sensitivity (Sen) and random accuracy (Random Acc) were used for model evaluations [48–50].

2.3. Generative RNN Modeling and Transfer Learning

The architecture of the generative RNN model is composed of one input layer, one auto-embedding layer with 128 dimensions, three GRU layers with 512 neurons in each layer, and one output layer with softmax activation function (Figure 3). The input layer is responsible for receiving the sequential tokens of the SMILES string of a given sample and the output layer for calculating the occurrence probability of the token at the next position. In this paper, the RNN network was trained by an Adam optimizer [51], of which the initial learning rate is set to 0.001 with a decay rate of 0.05 every 300 steps. The batch size was set to 128 and the loss function was defined as negative log likelihood function. After pretrained by the 2,393,029 SMILES strings from PubChem database, the RNN network was further fine-tuned by using the 433 caspase-6 inhibitors in the training and validation datasets.

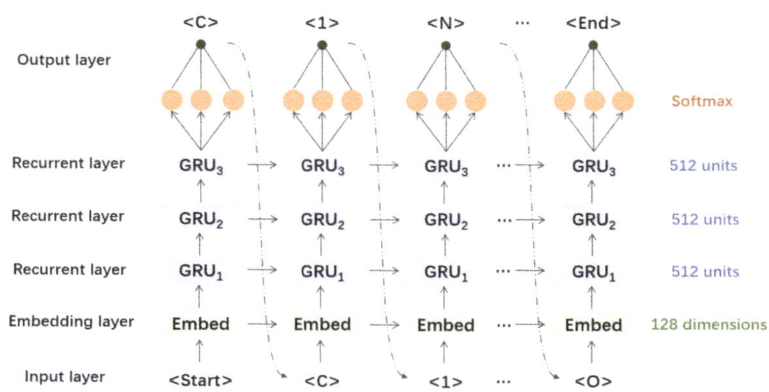

Figure 3. The architecture of the GRU-based recurrent neural network.

2.4. Molecular Docking

Surflex-dock (Sybyl 8.1, Tripos Inc., MO, USA) [52] has been proved be an efficient receptor-based drug design and virtual screening strategy, which employs a protomol to guide the generation process of putative ligand binding poses. Herein, a crystal structure of caspase-6 (PDB ID: 3OD5) was used for generating the protomol based on the residues within the 8 Å distance to the co-crystallized ligand Ac-VEID-CHO, a peptidomimetic inhibitor of caspase-6. Before docking, the structures of the ligands were charged by MMFF94 method [53] and then optimized by a Tripos force field [54] with a conjugate gradient minimizer. The maximum iteration steps and energy gradient were set to 10,000 times and 0.05 kcal/mol·Å. To promote the precision of the docking procedure, 3 additional starting conformations per ligand, self-scoring, ring flexibility, soft grid, pre- and post-dock minimizations were also considered in this paper.

3. Results and Discussion

3.1. Performances of ML Predictors

Herein, ML modeling was performed and repeated 10 times based on the randomly divided training (60%) and validation (40%) sets (Figure 4). It can be observed that most of the ML models showed satisfactory prediction performances on the training and validation datasets. In consideration of the accuracy and balanced performances on the validation set, the LR model was chosen as the optimal predictor, of which the means of AUC, MCC, Acc, Spe and Sen are 0.90 ± 0.008, 0.80 ± 0.015, 0.90 ± 0.008, 0.92 ± 0.007, 0.88 ± 0.014 for the training set, and 0.75 ± 0.012, 0.50 ± 0.025, 0.75 ± 0.013, 0.77 ± 0.023, 0.73 ± 0.025 for the validation set, respectively (Tables S4 and S5, Supplementary Materials). It should be noted that the differences in the prediction performances between the training and validation set may be caused by over-fitting in some degree due to the small training dataset.

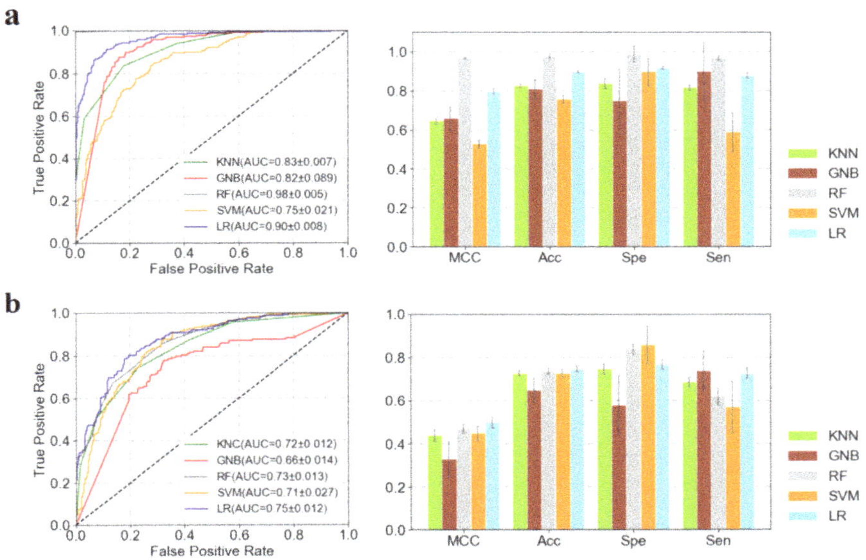

Figure 4. The performances of the 5 ML models on the training (**a**) and validation dataset (**b**). (SVM model: a radial basis function (RBF) kernel was used, of which the C and γ were set as 1 and 'auto', respectively; LR model: the inverse of regularization strength, tolerance for stopping criteria, maximum number of iterations, and penalty were set as 0.5, 0.001, 200, and "L1", respectively. Herein, default parameters were used for the ML models if not specified.)

Then, five-fold cross-validation and an independent external test by using 644 samples were also performed. The results showed that the optimal LR model achieved excellent prediction performances, of which the Acc for the five-fold cross-validation and the independent test are 0.78 ± 0.047 and 0.86, respectively (Table S6 and Table 1). Therefore, it can be concluded that the resulting LR model is a good predictor of the caspase-6 inhibitors.

Table 1. The performance of the optimal LR model on the 644 test samples.

		Confusion Matrix		Performance				
		CP	CN	Acc	Spe	Sen	MCC	Random Acc
Independent test set	PCP	102	49	0.86	0.90	0.71	0.60	0.647
	PCN	42	451					

CP: condition positive; CN: condition negative; PCP: predicted condition positive; PCN: predicted condition negative. For more details, please refer to Table S7 (Supplementary Materials).

3.2. The Generative RNN Modeling

Herein, 2,393,029 SMILES strings derived from Pubchem database were used for pre-training of the RNN models. Firstly, the effect of the number of GRU layers on the performance of the generative RNN model was investigated based on the network architecture shown in Figure 3. It can be seen that, after 14,000 steps of iterations, the loss values of the RNN models with one, two and three GRU layers reach the state of convergence (Figure 5a). At the mean time, the valid percentages of 128 SMILES strings sampled by the 3 RNN models reached 0.85, 0.90 and 0.95, respectively. Moreover, no significant improvement in the valid percentage was observed for the RNN models with more than three GRU layers. Thus, the RNN model with three GRU layers was chosen for the following transfer learning.

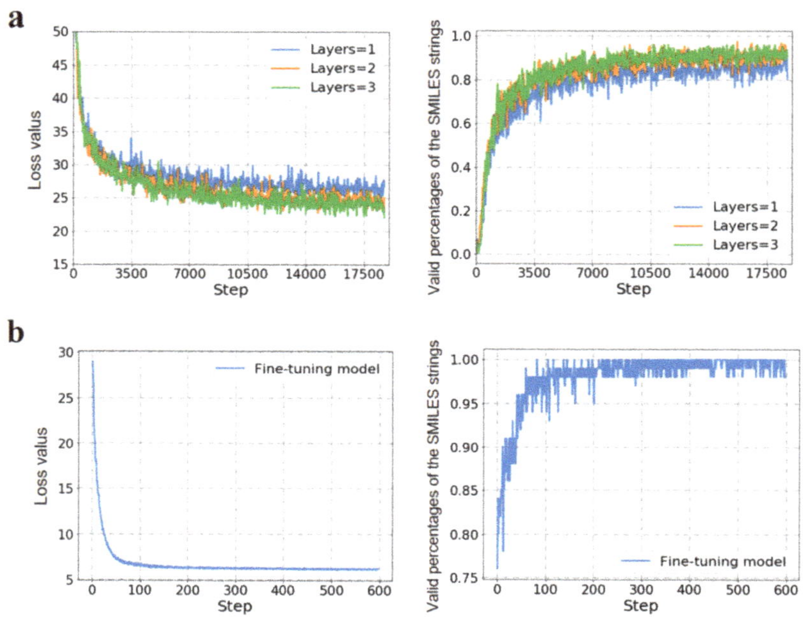

Figure 5. Performances of the pre-trained RNN models with different GRU layers (**a**) and the fine-tuned RNN model by transferred learning of 433 caspase-6 inhibitors (**b**).

In this paper, the 433 caspase-6 inhibitors in the training and validation sets (Table S2) were used for the transfer learning of the pre-trained RNN model. From Figure 5b, it can be observed that, after 200 steps of fine-tuning, the loss value tends to converge and the valid percentage of the sampled SMILES strings reached 99%. In order to evaluate the performance of the refined RNN model in generating potential caspase-6 inhibitors, a retrospective study was performed by using the 144 caspase-6 inhibitors in the test dataset (Table S2), which the RNN model had never seen before. At first, a total of 50,000 valid SMILES strings were randomly sampled by the fine-tuned RNN model. After structural description using the RDKit toolkit, the 50,000 molecules were then predicted by the LR predictor. Based on the predicted positive samples, the recall value of the 144 caspase-6 inhibitors was finally calculated. As shown in Table 2, it can be seen that the percentage of the predicted positive samples remains at a relatively high level during the whole sampling process. Additionally, it can be noticed that the recall value of the 144 caspase-6 inhibitors increases gradually from the lowest value of 2.08% to the highest value of 13.19% (Table 2). Accordingly, it can be concluded that the RNN model can generate efficiently the potential caspase-6 inhibitors after transfer learning. It should be noted that the relatively low recall value is mainly caused by the small sample size of the test caspase-6 inhibitors.

Table 2. The recall value of the 144 caspase-6 inhibitors.

Sampling Process	I	II	III	IV	V	VI	VII	VIII	IX	X
No. of SMILES strings	1000	2000	3000	4000	5000	10,000	20,000	30,000	40,000	50,000
The predicted positive samples (%)	76.0	72.7	71.4	70.7	70.6	69.3	67.1	66.2	65.5	65.0
Recall (%)	2.08	2.08	3.47	5.55	6.94	8.33	10.41	11.80	13.19	13.19

3.3. The Distribution in Chemical Space of the Potential Caspase-6 Inhibitors

According to Table 2, a total of 6927 strings (69.3%) were predicted as positive samples from the 10,000 SMILES strings generated. Herein, based on the properties of the H-Bond acceptor/donor, rotatable bonds, aromatic/aliphatic cycles, heterocycle atoms and molecular weight, the distribution of the potential 6927 caspase-6 inhibitors was explored by using the t-distributed stochastic neighbor embedding (t-SNE) method.

As shown in Figure 6, it can be seen that the distribution of the generated potential 6927 caspase-6 inhibitors in the chemical space is highly overlapped with that of the known 577 caspase-6 inhibitors. Herein, three small clusters of the samples were selected randomly to explore the structural features in detail. For each cluster, it can be observed that the generated molecules have similar molecular scaffolds with the known caspase-6 inhibitors (Figure 6). Thus, it can be inferred that the generated 6927 potential inhibitors have the similar chemical space as the known 577 caspase-6 inhibitors. The structural modification mainly involves substituent modification, scaffold hopping, and chiral transformation, etc., which are also the major means in traditional drug design.

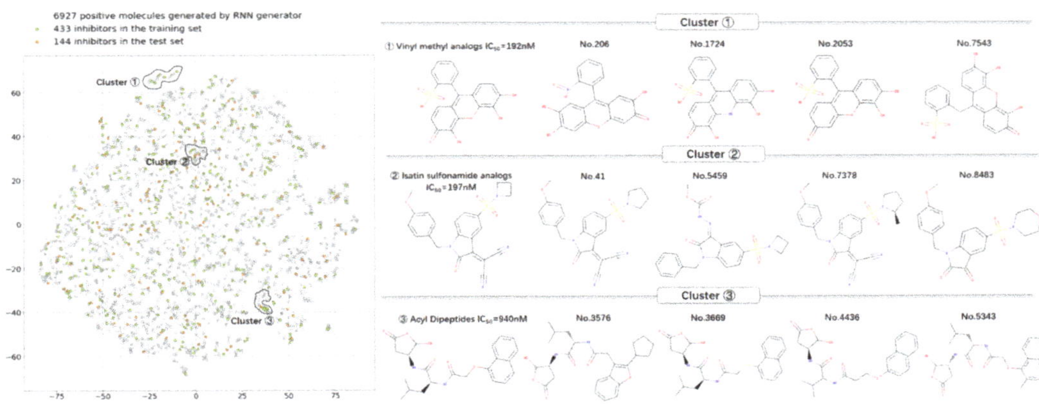

Figure 6. The distribution in the chemical space of the 6927 generated molecules (grey) and 577 known caspase-6 inhibitors (green: training samples; yellow: test samples).

3.4. Molecular Docking-Based Ligand Screening

Before docking-based screening of the caspase-6 inhibitors, the protocol of Surflex-dock was first validated by re-docking a co-crystallized ligand Ac-VEID-CHO into the binding pocket of caspase-6 (PDB: 3OD5). The results showed that the Surflex-dock can reproduce the native ligand binding conformation with a docking score of 7.67 (Figure S1, Supplementary Materials).

Based on the docking results of the 577 known caspase-6 inhibitors and the potential 6927 positive samples, the occurrence frequencies of the residues involved in the inter-molecular interactions with the 577 caspase-6 inhibitors and 6927 potential inhibitors were investigated, respectively. From Figure 7a, it can be clearly seen that the distributions in the occurrence frequencies of the binding residues are quite similar between the two cases, especially for the binding residues with occurrence frequencies larger than 50%. Therefore, it can be deduced that the potential 6927 inhibitors have similar binding modes with the known 577 caspase-6 inhibitors.

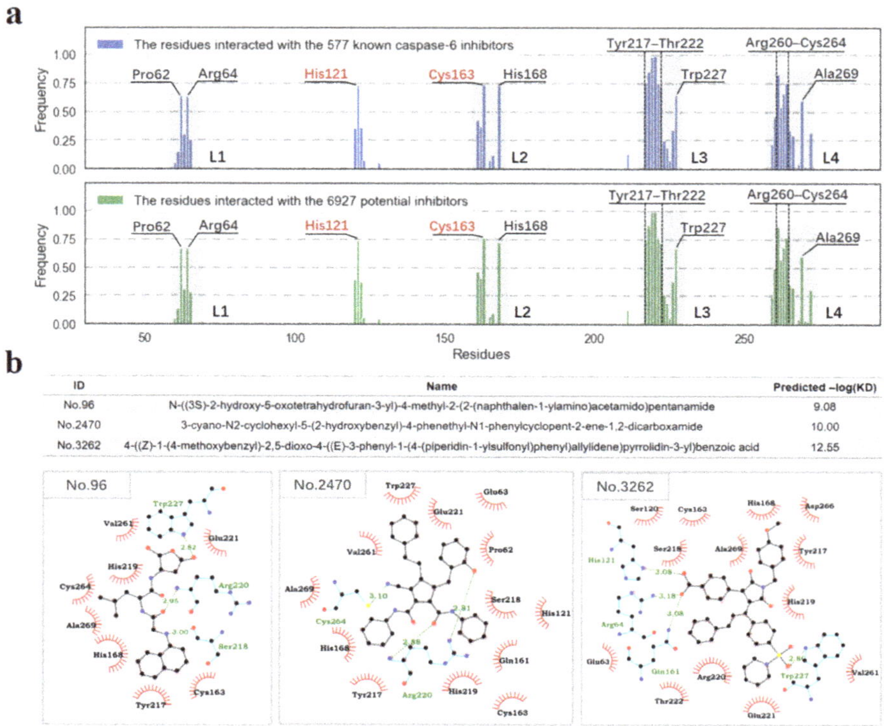

Figure 7. The binding modes of the 577 known caspase-6 inhibitors and 6927 potential inhibitors. (**a**) The occurrence frequencies of the binding residues involved in the intermolecular interactions with the binding ligands (the distance cutoff was set to 5 Å). The residues with the occurrence frequencies larger than 50% are marked, and the catalytic dyad residues His121 and Cys163 are colored in red. (**b**) Schematic diagrams of protein–ligand interactions of three representative samples. H-bonds are represented as green dashed lines. The carbon, nitrogen, oxygen, sulfur atoms are colored in black, blue, red and yellow, respectively.

Furthermore, the Surflex-dock method was employed for predicting and ranking the generated potential inhibitors. Herein, take example for three representative positive samples (ID: 96, 2470 and 3262) with different scaffolds to explore the feasibility of molecular docking-based ligand screening. The docking scores of the 3 positive samples are higher than 9.0 (-logKD), which indicate potential inhibitory activities at nanomolar level. As shown in Figure 7b, both of the sample 96 and 2470 can form strong H-bond interactions with Arg220, while sample 3262 form 3 H-bonds with Arg64, His121 and Gln161. For sample 2470 and 3262, strong π–cation interactions with Arg220 can be also observed Recent research has proved that Arg64, Gln161, and Arg220 are closely related with the substrate-specificity of caspase-6, and that His121 is a key catalytic residue for substrate hydrolysis [1]. Furthermore, all the three samples can form strong hydrophobic interactions with the hotspot residues Tyr217, Val261, Cys264 and Ala269. Collectively, the three potential caspase-6 inhibitors with nanomolar-level activities are promising candidates for further research.

4. Conclusions

In this paper, a GRU-based RNN network combined with transfer learning, ligand-based and receptor-based molecular screening strategies was employed for de novo molecular design of caspase-6 inhibitors. The results showed that the established GRU-based RNN model can accurately learn the SMILES grammars of 2.4 million chemical molecules including ionic and isomeric compounds and is capable of generating novel potential caspase-6 inhibitors with similar chemical space after transfer learning of the known 433 caspase-6 inhibitors. Based on the molecules generated by the RNN models, five ligand-based ML together with the receptor-based docking methods were employed for screening the potential caspase-6 inhibitors. The results showed that the obtained potential caspase-6 inhibitors are mainly generated by substituent modification, scaffold hopping, and chiral transformation, etc. operations from the known inhibitors on the level of SMILES stings. Three potential caspase-6 inhibitors with different scaffolds were finally selected as the most promising candidates for the further research. In general, the framework presented in this paper provides an efficient combinational strategy for de novo molecular design of caspase-6 inhibitors. However, the efficiency and application domain of the proposed molecular design pipeline still need to be tested by in vitro experiments.

Supplementary Materials: The following are available online at: https://www.mdpi.com/article/10.3390/ph14121249/s1. Table S1: The statistic information of the known caspase-6 inhibitors dataset, Table S2: The information of 1656 samples, Table S3: Definitions of 200 RDKit descriptors, Table S4: The representative confusion matrices of five machine learning models on the training set, Table S5: The representative confusion matrices of five machine learning models on the validation set, Table S6: The 5-fold cross-validation results of the ML models, Table S7: The representative confusion matrices of five machine learning models on test set, Figure S1: The result of molecular docking.

Author Contributions: Conceptualization, S.H., H.M. and X.P.; data curation, S.H. and Z.K.; funding acquisition, X.P.; investigation, L.L.; methodology, M.Q. and L.X.; project administration, X.P.; resources, Y.H.; validation, X.L.; writing—original draft, S.H. All authors have read and agreed to the published version of the manuscript.

Funding: The authors acknowledge the support of Key Projects of Technological Innovation and Application Development of Chongqing (Project No. csts2019jscx-gksbX0099), Collaborative Fund of Science and Technology Agency of Luzhou Government and Southwest Medical University (Project No. 2019LZXNYDZ05), Graduate Scientific Research and Innovation Foundation of Chongqing (Project No. CYB19042). Shuheng Huang acknowledges the financial support from the China Scholarship Council.

Institutional Review Board Statement: Not applicable.

Informed Consent Statement: Not applicable.

Data Availability Statement: Code, data, and pre-trained models are available from our GitHub: https://github.com/ShuhengH/De-Novo-Caspase-6-Inhibitors-Design-by-GRU-Based-RNN-Combined-with-Transfer-Learning-Approach (accessed date: 30 November 2020). Data is contained within the article or Supplementary Material.

Conflicts of Interest: The authors declare no conflict of interest.

References

1. Clark, A.C. Caspase Allostery and Conformational Selection. *Chem. Rev.* **2016**, *116*, 6666–6706. [CrossRef] [PubMed]
2. Slee, E.A.; Adrain, C.; Martin, S.J. Executioner caspase-3,-6, and-7 perform distinct, non-redundant roles during the demolition phase of apoptosis. *J. Biol. Chem.* **2001**, *276*, 7320–7326. [CrossRef]
3. McIlwain, D.R.; Berger, T.; Mak, T.W. Caspase functions in cell death and disease. *Cold Spring Harb. Perspect. Biol.* **2013**, *5*, a008656. [CrossRef]
4. Denecker, G.; Ovaere, P.; Vandenabeele, P.; Declercq, W. Caspase-14 reveals its secrets. *J. Cell Biol.* **2008**, *180*, 451–458. [CrossRef] [PubMed]
5. Wang, X.J.; Cao, Q.; Zhang, Y.; Su, X.D. Activation and Regulation of Caspase-6 and Its Role in Neurodegenerative Diseases. *Annu. Rev. Pharmacol. Toxicol.* **2015**, *55*, 553–572. [CrossRef]

6. LeBlanc, A.; Liu, H.; Goodyer, C.; Bergeron, C.; Hammond, J. Caspase-6 role in apoptosis of human neurons, amyloidogenesis, and Alzheimer's disease. *J. Biol. Chem.* **1999**, *274*, 23426–23436. [CrossRef]
7. Klaiman, G.; Petzke, T.L.; Hammond, J.; LeBlanc, A.C. Targets of Caspase-6 activity in human neurons and Alzheimer disease. *Mol. Cell. Proteom.* **2008**, *7*, 1541–1555. [CrossRef]
8. Sexton, K.B.; Kato, D.; Berger, A.B.; Fonovic, M.; Verhelst, S.H.L.; Bogyo, M. Specificity of aza-peptide electrophile activity-based probes of caspases. *Cell Death Differ.* **2007**, *14*, 727–732. [CrossRef]
9. Linton, S.D.; Karanewsky, D.S.; Ternansky, R.J.; Wu, J.C.; Pham, B.; Kodandapani, L.; Smidt, R.; Diaz, J.-L.; Fritz, L.C.; Tomaselli, K.J. Acyl Dipeptides as reversible caspase inhibitors. Part 1: Initial lead optimization. *Bioorg. Med. Chem. Lett.* **2002**, *12*, 2969–2971. [CrossRef]
10. Linton, S.D.; Karanewsky, D.S.; Ternansky, R.J.; Chen, N.; Guo, M.; Jahangiri, K.G.; Kalish, V.J.; Meduna, S.P.; Robinson, E.D.; Ullman, B.R.; et al. Acyl Dipeptides as reversible caspase inhibitors. Part 2: Further optimization. *Bioorg. Med. Chem. Lett.* **2002**, *12*, 2973–2975. [CrossRef]
11. Chu, W.H.; Rothfuss, J.; d'Avignon, A.; Zeng, C.B.; Zhou, D.; Hotchkiss, R.S.; Mach, R.H. Isatin sulfonamide analogs containing a michael addition acceptor: A new class of caspase 3/7 inhibitors. *J. Med. Chem.* **2007**, *50*, 3751–3755. [CrossRef]
12. Chu, W.H.; Rothfuss, J.; Chu, Y.X.; Zhou, D.; Mach, R.H. Synthesis and in Vitro Evaluation of Sulfonamide Isatin Michael Acceptors as Small Molecule Inhibitors of Caspase-6. *J. Med. Chem.* **2009**, *52*, 2188–2191. [CrossRef]
13. Chu, W.H.; Rothfuss, J.; Zhou, D.; Mach, R.H. Synthesis and evaluation of isatin analogs as caspase-3 inhibitors: Introduction of a hydrophilic group increases potency in a whole cell assay. *Bioorg. Med. Chem. Lett.* **2011**, *21*, 2192–2197. [CrossRef]
14. Limpachayaporn, P.; Schafers, M.; Schober, O.; Kopka, K.; Haufe, G. Synthesis of new fluorinated, 2-substituted 5-pyrrolidinylsulfonyl isatin derivatives as caspase-3 and caspase-7 inhibitors: Nonradioactive counterparts of putative PET-compatible apoptosis imaging agents. *Bioorg. Med. Chem.* **2013**, *21*, 2025–2036. [CrossRef]
15. Limpachayaporn, P.; Wagner, S.; Kopka, K.; Schober, O.; Schafers, M.; Haufe, G. Synthesis of 7-Halogenated Isatin Sulfonamides: Nonradioactive Counterparts of Caspase-3/-7 Inhibitor-Based Potential Radiopharmaceuticals for Molecular Imaging of Apoptosis. *J. Med. Chem.* **2014**, *57*, 9383–9395. [CrossRef] [PubMed]
16. Leyva, M.J.; Degiacomo, F.; Kaltenbach, L.S.; Holcomb, J.; Zhang, N.; Gafni, J.; Park, H.; Lo, D.C.; Salvesen, G.S.; Ellerby, L.M.; et al. Identification and evaluation of small molecule pan-caspase inhibitors in Huntington's disease models. *Chem. Biol.* **2010**, *17*, 1189–1200. [CrossRef] [PubMed]
17. Pakavathkumar, P.; Sharma, G.; Kaushal, V.; Foveau, B.; LeBlanc, A.C. Methylene Blue Inhibits Caspases by Oxidation of the Catalytic Cysteine. *Sci. Rep.* **2015**, *5*, 13730. [CrossRef] [PubMed]
18. Lee, H.; Shin, E.A.; Lee, J.H.; Ahn, D.; Kim, C.G.; Kim, J.H.; Kim, S.H. Caspase inhibitors: A review of recently patented compounds (2013–2015). *Expert Opin. Ther. Pat.* **2018**, *28*, 47–59. [CrossRef] [PubMed]
19. Pakavathkumar, P.; Noel, A.; Lecrux, C.; Tubeleviciute-Aydin, A.; Hamel, E.; Ahlfors, J.E.; LeBlanc, A.C. Caspase vinyl sulfone small molecule inhibitors prevent axonal degeneration in human neurons and reverse cognitive impairment in Caspase-6-overexpressing mice. *Mol. Neurodegener.* **2017**, *12*, 22. [CrossRef] [PubMed]
20. Heise, C.E.; Murray, J.; Augustyn, K.E.; Bravo, B.; Chugha, P.; Cohen, F.; Giannetti, A.M.; Gibbons, P.; Hannoush, R.N.; Hearn, B.R.; et al. Mechanistic and Structural Understanding of Uncompetitive Inhibitors of Caspase-6. *PLoS ONE* **2012**, *7*, e50864. [CrossRef]
21. MacKenzie, S.H.; Schipper, J.L.; Clark, A.C. The potential for caspases in drug discovery. *Curr. Opin. Drug Discov. Dev.* **2010**, *13*, 568–576.
22. Jing, Y.; Bian, Y.; Hu, Z.; Wang, L.; Xie, X.Q. Deep Learning for Drug Design: An Artificial Intelligence Paradigm for Drug Discovery in the Big Data Era. *AAPS J.* **2018**, *20*, 58. [CrossRef] [PubMed]
23. Gawehn, E.; Hiss, J.A.; Schneider, G. Deep Learning in Drug Discovery. *Mol. Inform.* **2016**, *35*, 3–14. [CrossRef] [PubMed]
24. Sellwood, M.A.; Ahmed, M.; Segler, M.H.S.; Brown, N. Artificial intelligence in drug discovery. *Future Med. Chem.* **2018**, *10*, 2025–2028. [CrossRef]
25. Xue, D.Y.; Gong, Y.K.; Yang, Z.Y.; Chuai, G.H.; Qu, S.; Shen, A.Z.; Yu, J.; Liu, Q. Advances and challenges in deep generative models for de novo molecule generation. *Wiley Interdiscip. Res. Comput. Mol. Sci.* **2019**, *9*, e1395. [CrossRef]
26. Grisoni, F.; Moret, M.; Lingwood, R.; Schneider, G. Bidirectional Molecule Generation with Recurrent Neural Networks. *J. Chem. Inf. Model.* **2020**, *60*, 1175–1183. [CrossRef]
27. Amabilino, S.; Pogany, P.; Pickett, S.D.; Green, D.V.S. Guidelines for Recurrent Neural Network Transfer Learning-Based Molecular Generation of Focused Libraries. *J. Chem. Inf. Model.* **2020**, *60*, 5699–5713. [CrossRef]
28. Gomez-Bombarelli, R.; Wei, J.N.; Duvenaud, D.; Hernandez-Lobato, J.M.; Sanchez-Lengeling, B.; Sheberla, D.; Aguilera-Iparraguirre, J.; Hirzel, T.D.; Adams, R.P.; Aspuru-Guzik, A. Automatic Chemical Design Using a Data-Driven Continuous Representation of Molecules. *ACS Cent. Sci.* **2018**, *4*, 268–276. [CrossRef]
29. Winter, R.; Montanari, F.; Noe, F.; Clevert, D.A. Learning continuous and data-driven molecular descriptors by translating equivalent chemical representations. *Chem. Sci.* **2019**, *10*, 1692–1701. [CrossRef]
30. Olivecrona, M.; Blaschke, T.; Engkvist, O.; Chen, H.M. Molecular de-novo design through deep reinforcement learning. *J. Cheminform.* **2017**, *9*, 48. [CrossRef]
31. Jaques, N.; Gu, S.; Bahdanau, D.; Hernández-Lobato, J.M.; Turner, R.E.; Eck, D. Sequence Tutor: Conservative Fine-Tuning of Sequence Generation Models with KL-control. *arXiv* **2017**, arXiv:1611.02796.

32. Benhenda, M. ChemGAN challenge for drug discovery: Can AI reproduce natural chemical diversity? *arXiv* **2017**, arXiv:1708.08227.
33. Sousa, T.; Correia, J.; Pereira, V.; Rocha, M. Generative Deep Learning for Targeted Compound Design. *J. Chem. Inf. Model.* **2021**, *61*, 5343–5361. [CrossRef]
34. Kim, S.; Thiessen, P.A.; Bolton, E.E.; Chen, J.; Fu, G.; Gindulyte, A.; Han, L.; He, J.; He, S.; Shoemaker, B.A.; et al. PubChem Substance and Compound databases. *Nucleic Acids Res.* **2016**, *44*, D1202–D1213. [CrossRef] [PubMed]
35. Wang, Y.; Huang, J.C.; Zhou, Z.L.; Yang, W.; Guastella, J.; Drewe, J.; Cai, S.X. Dipeptidyl aspartyl fluoromethylketones as potent caspase-3 inhibitors: SAR of the P-2 amino acid. *Bioorg. Med. Chem. Lett.* **2004**, *14*, 1269–1272. [CrossRef] [PubMed]
36. Choong, I.C.; Lew, W.; Lee, D.; Pham, P.; Burdett, M.T.; Lam, J.W.; Wiesmann, C.; Luong, T.N.; Fahr, B.; DeLano, W.L.; et al. Identification of potent and selective small-molecule inhibitors of caspase-3 through the use of extended tethering and structure-based drug design. *J. Med. Chem.* **2002**, *45*, 5005–5022. [CrossRef] [PubMed]
37. Asgian, J.L.; James, K.E.; Li, Z.Z.; Carter, W.; Barrett, A.J.; Mikolajczyk, J.; Salvesen, G.S.; Powers, J.C. Aza-peptide epoxides: A new class of inhibitors selective for clan CD cysteine proteases. *J. Med. Chem.* **2002**, *45*, 4958–4960. [CrossRef]
38. Lee, D.; Long, S.A.; Murray, J.H.; Adams, J.L.; Nuttall, M.E.; Nadeau, D.P.; Kikly, K.; Winkler, J.D.; Sung, C.-M.; Ryan, M.D.; et al. Potent and selective nonpeptide inhibitors of caspases 3 and 7. *J. Med. Chem.* **2001**, *44*, 2015–2026. [CrossRef] [PubMed]
39. Wang, Y.; Guan, L.F.; Jia, S.J.; Tseng, B.; Drewe, J.; Cai, S.X. Dipeptidyl aspartyl fluoromethylketones as potent caspase inhibitors: Peptidomimetic replacement of the P-2 alpha-amino acid by a alpha-hydroxy acid. *Bioorg. Med. Chem. Lett.* **2005**, *15*, 1379–1383. [CrossRef]
40. Han, Y.X.; Giroux, A.; Colucci, J.; Bayly, C.I.; Mckay, D.J.; Roy, S.; Xanthoudakis, S.; Vaillancourt, J.; Rasper, D.M.; Tam, J.; et al. Novel pyrazinone mono-amides as potent and reversible caspase-3 inhibitors. *Bioorg. Med. Chem. Lett.* **2005**, *15*, 1173–1180. [CrossRef] [PubMed]
41. Wang, Y.; Jia, S.J.; Tseng, B.; Drewe, J.; Cai, S.X. Dipeptidyl aspartyl fluoromethylketones as potent caspase inhibitors: Peptidomimetic replacement of the P-2 amino acid by 2-aminoaryl acids and other non-natural amino acids. *Bioorg. Med. Chem. Lett.* **2007**, *17*, 6178–6182. [CrossRef]
42. Thompson, C.M.; Quinn, C.A.; Hergenrother, P.J. Total Synthesis and Cytoprotective Properties of Dykellic Acid. *J. Med. Chem.* **2009**, *52*, 117–125. [CrossRef]
43. Mott, B.T.; Ferreira, R.S.; Simeonov, A.; Jadhav, A.; Ang, K.K.H.; Leister, W.; Shen, M.; Silveira, J.T.; Doyle, P.S.; Arkin, M.R.; et al. Identification and Optimization of Inhibitors of Trypanosomal Cysteine Proteases: Cruzain, Rhodesain, and TbCatB. *J. Med. Chem.* **2010**, *53*, 52–60. [CrossRef]
44. Rosse, G. Irreversible Inhibitors of Cysteine Proteases. *ACS Med. Chem. Lett.* **2013**, *4*, 163–164. [CrossRef] [PubMed]
45. Krause-Heuer, A.M.; Howell, N.R.; Matesic, L.; Dhand, G.; Young, E.L.; Burgess, L.; Jiang, C.D.; Lengkeek, N.A.; Fookes, C.J.R.; Pham, T.Q.; et al. A new class of fluorinated 5-pyrrolidinylsulfonyl isatin caspase inhibitors for PET imaging of apoptosis. *MedChemComm* **2013**, *4*, 347–352. [CrossRef]
46. Landrum, G. RDKit: Open-Source Cheminformatics. 2006. Available online: https://www.rdkit.org/ (accessed on 30 November 2020).
47. Pedregosa, F.; Varoquaux, G.; Gramfort, A.; Michel, V.; Thirion, B.; Grisel, O.; Blondel, M.; Prettenhofer, P.; Weiss, R.; Dubourg, V.; et al. Scikit-learn: Machine Learning in Python. *J. Mach. Learn. Res.* **2011**, *12*, 2825–2830.
48. Powers, D.M. Evaluation: From precision, recall and F-measure to ROC, informedness, markedness and correlation. *arXiv* **2020**, arXiv:2010.16061.
49. Lučić, B.; Batista, J.; Bojović, V.; Lovrić, M.; Kržić, A.S.; Bešlo, D.; Nadramija, D.; Vikić-Topić, D. Estimation of Random Accuracy and its Use in Validation of Predictive Quality of Classification Models within Predictive Challenges. *Croat. Chem. Acta* **2019**, *92*, 379–391. [CrossRef]
50. Batista, J.; Vikić-Topić, D.; Lučić, B. The Difference Between the Accuracy of Real and the Corresponding Random Model is a Useful Parameter for Validation of Two-State Classification Model Quality. *Croat. Chem. Acta* **2016**, *89*, 527–534. [CrossRef]
51. Kingma, D.; Ba, J. Adam: A method for stochastic optimization. *arXiv* **2014**, arXiv:1412.6980.
52. Jain, A.N. Surflex: Fully automatic flexible molecular docking using a molecular similarity-based search engine. *J. Med. Chem.* **2003**, *46*, 499–511. [CrossRef] [PubMed]
53. Halgren, T.A. Merck molecular force field. II. MMFF94 van der Waals and electrostatic parameters for intermolecular interactions. *J. Comput. Chem.* **1996**, *17*, 520–552. [CrossRef]
54. Clark, M.; Cramer, R.D.; Vanopdenbosch, N. Validation of the General-Purpose Tripos 5.2 Force-Field. *J. Comput. Chem.* **1989**, *10*, 982–1012. [CrossRef]

pharmaceuticals

Article

A Rational Design of α-Helix-Shaped Peptides Employing the Hydrogen-Bond Surrogate Approach: A Modulation Strategy for Ras-RasGRF1 Interaction in Neuropsychiatric Disorders

Maria Rita Gulotta [1,*], Riccardo Brambilla [2], Ugo Perricone [1,†] and Andrea Brancale [3,†]

1 Molecular Informatics Unit, Fondazione Ri.MED, via Filippo Marini 14, 90128 Palermo, Italy; uperricone@fondazionerimed.com
2 Neuroscience and Mental Health Research Institute (NMHRI) and Neuroscience Division, School of Biosciences, Cardiff University, Haydn Ellis Building, Maindy Road, Cardiff CF24 4HQ, UK; brambillar@cardiff.ac.uk
3 School of Pharmacy and Pharmaceutical Sciences, Cardiff University, King Edward VII Avenue, Cardiff CF10 3NB, UK; brancalea@cardiff.ac.uk
* Correspondence: mrgulotta@fondazionerimed.com
† Both authors contributed equally to this manuscript.

Citation: Gulotta, M.R.; Brambilla, R.; Perricone, U.; Brancale, A. A Rational Design of α-Helix-Shaped Peptides Employing the Hydrogen-Bond Surrogate Approach: A Modulation Strategy for Ras-RasGRF1 Interaction in Neuropsychiatric Disorders. *Pharmaceuticals* **2021**, *14*, 1099. https://doi.org/10.3390/ph14111099

Academic Editor: Osvaldo Andrade Santos-Filho

Received: 30 September 2021
Accepted: 26 October 2021
Published: 28 October 2021

Publisher's Note: MDPI stays neutral with regard to jurisdictional claims in published maps and institutional affiliations.

Abstract: In the last two decades, abnormal Ras (rat sarcoma protein)–ERK (extracellular signal-regulated kinase) signalling in the brain has been involved in a variety of neuropsychiatric disorders, including drug addiction, certain forms of intellectual disability, and autism spectrum disorder. Modulation of membrane-receptor-mediated Ras activation has been proposed as a potential target mechanism to attenuate ERK signalling in the brain. Previously, we showed that a cell penetrating peptide, RB3, was able to inhibit downstream signalling by preventing RasGRF1 (Ras guanine nucleotide-releasing factor 1), a neuronal specific GDP/GTP exchange factor, to bind Ras proteins, both in brain slices and in vivo, with an IC_{50} value in the micromolar range. The aim of this work was to mutate and improve this peptide through computer-aided techniques to increase its inhibitory activity against RasGRF1. The designed peptides were built based on the RB3 peptide structure corresponding to the α-helix of RasGRF1 responsible for Ras binding. For this purpose, the hydrogen-bond surrogate (HBS) approach was exploited to maintain the helical conformation of the designed peptides. Finally, residue scanning, MD simulations, and MM-GBSA calculations were used to identify 18 most promising α-helix-shaped peptides that will be assayed to check their potential activity against Ras-RasGRF1 and prevent downstream molecular events implicated in brain disorders.

Keywords: Ras; RasGRF1; hydrogen-bond surrogate; computational residue scanning; molecular dynamics; MM-GBSA; protein–protein interaction; ERK signalling; cocaine addiction; intellectual disability (ID); autism spectrum disorder (ASD)

1. Introduction

Maladaptive signalling mechanisms in the brain have been demonstrated in several psychiatric and neurological conditions. Amongst the most severe and poorly treated brain disorders, cocaine and psychostimulant addiction is a poorly managed chronic disease characterised by high relapse rates and compulsive drug use [1,2]. Most notably, addictive drugs exploit cellular mechanisms and signalling pathways involved in normal learning and memory processes [3–6]. Modulation of such learned associations between drug-paired cues and the rewarding effects of these drugs significantly contribute to persistently elicited drug-seeking behaviours and high rates of relapse [7–22]. The Ras (rat sarcoma protein)–ERK (extracellular signal-regulated kinase) pathway is crucially involved in both the acute and long-term effects of cocaine in experimental animal models, and previous work has shown that brain-penetrating Ras–ERK inhibitors may ameliorate the associated symptoms. Particularly relevant was the observation that Ras-RasGRF1 (Ras guanine nucleotide-releasing factor 1) interaction is responsible for the activation of the ERK cascade downstream of neurotransmitter receptor systems. Indeed, we previously showed that a cell-penetrating peptide, RB3, able to attenuate Ras-RasGRF1 binding could reduce downstream ERK signalling in response to cocaine in a mouse model. Similarly RB3 was shown to ameliorate cellular effects and behavioural symptoms in two distinct mouse models of intellectual disability (ID) and autism spectrum disorder (ASD) [23,24].

ERK signalling in most tissues responds to extracellular signals and regulates cell proliferation, differentiation, and survival [25–27]. In this context, Ras proteins act as binary switches in signalling pathways by cycling between inactive GDP- and active GTP bound states [28]. Kinetic studies highlighted that the activation of Ras protein, proceeding from the conversion of Ras-GDP to Ras-GTP, initiates through the recruitment of the guanine nucleotide exchange factors (GEFs), such as RasGRF1 and Sos (Son of sevenless protein) [29–34], that catalyse GDP release and allow its replacement by GTP [35–40]. Then the GTP molecule binds to this complex, promoting the release of the GEF protein [41]. The RasGRF1 and Sos region responsible for Ras-specific nucleotide exchange activity exhibits a Ras exchanger motif (Rem) domain of about 450 amino acids and a Cdc25 homology domain [42–46]. In addition, Sos requires allosteric activation through a second Ras-binding site that bridges the Rem and Cdc25 domains [47,48]. When Sos is activated a helical hairpin belonging to the Cdc25 domain inserts between two flexible regions of Ras, switch I (amino acids 25–40) and switch II (amino acids 57–75) [49–58], causing Ras conversion to the transient state by opening the nucleotide-binding site of Ras for GDP release [43] (Figure 1). After this event, Ras can promptly accommodate and bind GTP into the nucleotide-binding site, thus exhibiting its active state. Therefore, a potential strategy to inhibit Ras-GEF interaction should target the open—or transient—state of Ras protein by designing modulators able to bind the nucleotide-exchange region.

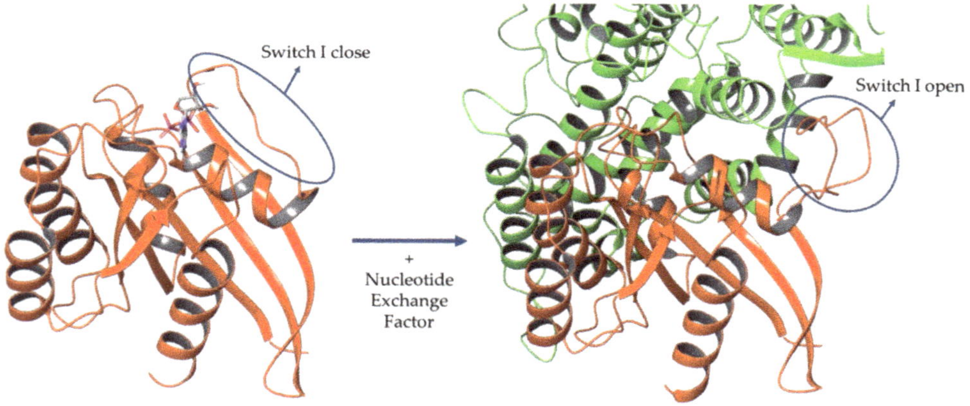

Figure 1. Inactive and transient states of the Ras protein. On the left, a Ras protein (orange chain; PDB ID: 1XD2 [48]) bound to GDP (grey ligand in stick format) exhibits its inactive state, where the Switch I region (highlighted by a blue circle) is closed; on the right, after binding to a guanine nucleotide-exchange factor (Sos protein, green chain), Ras (orange chain; PDB ID: 1XD2) exhibits a transient state, where the Switch I region is open to accommodate the GEF α-helix.

In contrast to Sos, which requires Ras binding to the allosteric site for activity, the Cdc25 domain of RasGRF1 is active on its own [33,41,47,48]. The structure of the Cdc25 domain of RasGRF1 is very similar to that of Sos, registering 30% of sequence identity between the two Cdc25 domains. The orientation and conformation of the RasGRF1 helical hairpin resemble that of Sos in its active form, with an RMSD value of 2.3 Å for the helical hairpins after superposition on the Cdc25 domain core. Moreover, distance difference matrices demonstrated that the main differences between RasGRF1 and Sos in its inactive form have been identified in the helical hairpin, even in this case confirming that the RasGRF1 Cdc25 domain is more similar to active Sos [59]. Therefore, the analysis of the Ras-Sos complex might provide crucial insights, even for RasGRF1 interaction.

1.1. Mutational Studies on Sos and Design of a Peptide-Based Ras Inhibitor

To date, no complex structure of Ras-RasGRF1 is available in the Protein Data Bank [60]; thus, provided that Sos and RasGRF1 proteins share the Ras-specific nucleotide exchange domain [59], Ras-Sos X-ray crystallographic complexes were exploited for a comparative analysis.

Over the last decades, several mutational studies were conducted on Ras and Sos proteins to determine the key amino acids. In 1998, Boriack-Sjodin et al. [43] demonstrated that the contacts between Ras and Sos are mainly mediated by the Switch I and Switch II regions of Ras [43,49–58] and are essentially hydrophobic, polar, and charge–charge contacts. Hall et al. [61] performed site-directed mutagenesis to deeply investigate these contacts. The results shed light on the hydrophobic pocket of Sos protein, consisting of residues Ile825, Leu872, and Phe929, which embed the side chain of Tyr64 of Ras through hydrophobic contacts. In addition, the contribution of Tyr64 of Ras was explored by applying a mutation to alanine (Y64A). The result was a 50-fold reduction in the apparent binding affinities of Ras to Sos, but did not provide significant nucleotide dissociation. Then, the authors performed another binding assay by using wild-type (WT) Ras and mutated Phe929 of Sos to alanine (F929A). The Sos mutant reported a decrease of more than 50-fold in binding affinity for Ras. This data indicated that Tyr64 and Phe929 mediated crucial contacts for the formation of a stable Ras-Sos complex.

On the other hand, polar and charged interactions showed to be not essential for the binding affinity of Ras to Sos. Indeed, alanine mutations on Sos residues Arg826, Thr935, and Glu1002 weakly impacted on Ras binding and activation. In addition, the mutation of Ala59 of Ras to glycine (A59G) did not significantly affect the GDP-dissociation rate, displaying more than 50% of the inhibitory effect on Sos-catalysed GTP dissociation. Finally, the contribution of two Ras amino acids involved in the Switch I region were investigated: Tyr32 of Ras that established hydrophobic contacts with Lys939 of Sos, and Tyr40 of Ras that mediated stacking interaction with His911 of Sos. Tyr32 and Tyr40 of Ras were mutated to Ser (Y32S) and Ala (Y40A), respectively. Both mutations decreased the binding of Sos to Ras and accelerated the rate of intrinsic GDP/GTP exchange, suggesting that these residues are important for Ras-Sos recognition and the nucleotide stabilization. Consistent with these results, mutations of Sos Lys939 and His911 to alanine (K939A and H911A, respectively) also caused a reduction in Ras-Sos binding. Furthermore, the Y40A mutation had no significant effect on Sos-catalysed guanine nucleotide exchange, whereas the disruption of the contact between Tyr32 of Ras and Lys939 of Sos reduced the sensitivity of Ras to the exchange activity of Sos [43].

Several efforts have been reported in the literature to design and identify Ras inhibitors to block the nucleotide exchange. However, to date, the current scientific insights on ERK signalling in drug addiction has not been transferred into clinical treatments due to the lack of drugs with relatively low IC_{50} values, toxicity, and ability to efficiently cross the blood–brain barrier (BBB) [62].

In 2016, Papale and colleagues [63] designed and generated an active cell-penetrating peptide, named RB3 [64], based on the interaction between Ras and a GEF protein; i.e., RasGRF1, able to attenuate cocaine-mediated activation of the Ras–ERK signalling cascade in vivo. Subsequently, the same peptide was successfully used, in combination with the KIM sequence containing RB1 peptide, to treat two genetic animal models of intellectual disability and autism spectrum disorder, both characterised by an abnormally high ERK signalling activity [23,24].

The cell-penetrating peptides have been shown to be promising for the treatment of neuropsychiatric disorders, especially due to their low reported toxicity and tolerability [65,66].

Although their biological activity spans a micromolar range, they usually show a potential advantage, as they are able to partially disrupt protein–protein interactions without preventing the enzymatic activity.

The RB3 peptide was designed by using molecular graphics tools, on the basis of the ternary complex consisting of Ras in its transient state bound to the Sos Cdc25 domain and Ras in its inactive state complexed with a GDP molecule (PDB ID: 1XD2) [48]. The Cdc25 domain of Sos involved in this ternary complex was compared to the crystal structure of the RasGRF1 Cdc25 domain (PDB ID: 2IJE [59]). The peptide sequence (amino acids 1173–1203 of the Cdc25 domain) includes an α-helix—from Met1181 to Glu1191—crucial for the GDP exchange activity on Ras proteins, linked to two loops—from Pro1173 to Gly1180 and from Gly1192 to Asn1203 (Figure 2).

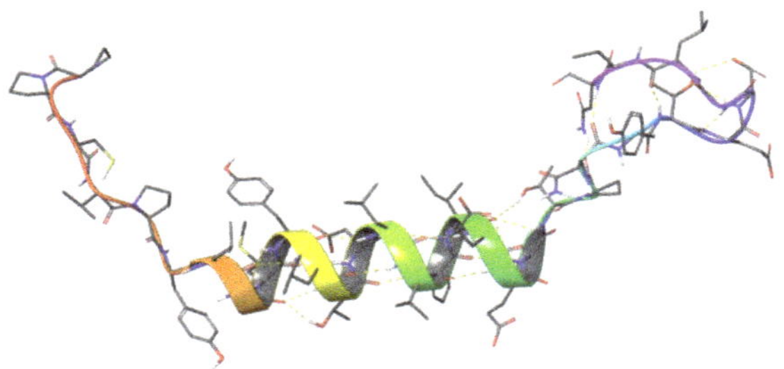

Figure 2. RB3 peptide structure including a loop from Pro1173 to Gly1180, an α-helix from Met1181 to Glu1191, and another loop from Gly1192 to Asn1203.

Moreover, Papale and colleagues [67] added to the RB3 peptide sequence a portion retrieved from the HIV TAT protein known to exhibit a translocating behaviour [68]. In this way, the final structure of the cell-penetrating peptide was created able to cross the cell membranes and the BBB [67]. Thus, the peptide sequence is below reported:

GRKKRRQRRR—PPCVPYLGMYLTDLVFIEEGTPNYTEDGLVN
TAT sequence RasGRF1 interacting region

Then, the RB3 peptide was tested in an ex vivo model of acute striatal brain slices to investigate its inhibitory potential on ERK phosphorylation after stimulation with 100 μM of glutamate. The result was a significant reduction of ERK activity, with an IC_{50} of 6 μM To deeply explore the effect of the RB3 peptide on Ras–ERK signalling pathway, Papale and colleagues investigated whether RB3 may also affect the phosphorylation of two well-characterised ERK substrates, (Ser10)-acetylated (Lys14) histone H3 (pAc-H3) and S6 ribosomal protein (pS6, Ser235/236 specific site) [69–71]. Even in this case, the peptide was effective in decreasing the phosphorylation of Ac-H3, with an IC_{50} of 5.2 μM; and pS6 levels, with an IC_{50} of 3.69 μM [63].

1.2. RB3 Peptide Modifications by Using Hydrogen-Bond Surrogates

In light of the above, the RB3 peptide was selected to enter a compound optimisation process to increase the biological activity. This work aimed to provide insights on Ras-RasGRF1 interaction and suggest novel potential modulators of this interaction based on the RB3 peptide structure, which will be further investigated through biological assays. For this purpose, multiple computational techniques were exploited to investigate modifications of the RB3 peptide in order to potentially increase its inhibitory activity of Ras-RasGRF1 interaction. Scheme 1 lists the steps of the workflow that are described in detail in the following sections.

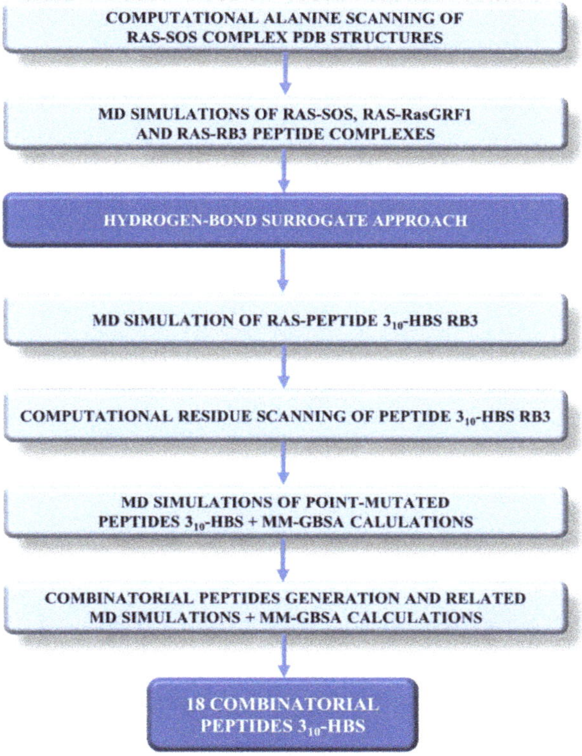

Scheme 1. Overview of the computational workflow performed to identify potential peptide-based modulators to inhibit Ras-RasGRF1 interaction.

First, a computational alanine scanning of the Ras-Sos complex available from the Protein Data Bank [60] was performed and, in parallel, molecular dynamics (MD) simulations on the three complexes (Ras-Sos, Ras-RasGRF1, and the Ras-RB3 peptide), were run to identify the most stable and frequent interactions between protein partners. Surprisingly, the RB3 peptide exhibited helicity loss, where the helical hairpin corresponding to RasGRF1 interacting region lost helicity propensity, generating instability within the complex. In order to optimise the structure of this peptide and increase the inhibitory capacity of the peptide, from the analysis of the literature, a potential strategy arose to solve this issue. Indeed, in the literature, similar cases of helicity loss have been reported and faced by exploiting the hydrogen-bond surrogate (HBS) approach [72]. This methodology was developed especially for modulating biomolecular interactions, such as protein–protein contacts, through small-molecular-weight protein secondary structure mimetics, when designing small molecules could be a very challenging strategy [73–79]. The HBS approach is based on the helix-coil transition theory for peptides, whereas α-helices composed of a few amino acids are expected to be essentially unstable due to a low nucleation probability [80,81]. This approach is expected to overwhelm the intrinsic nucleation propensities of the amino acids by providing a preorganization of the residues upstream, which triggers the helix formation initialization [82,83]. An example of a successful case of HBS use was the HBS3 peptide [62,84], a synthetic α-helix that reduced the Ras nucleotide exchange in vitro and modestly activated ERK in cells [62,84]. This peptide was basically built on the Sos sequence able to bind the Ras protein, and incorporates the HBS strategy reported in the literature [62,72,84]. On the other hand, in the literature, there is no evidence that the HBS methodology has been applied to the RB3 peptide. Thus, it appeared interesting to investigate the employment of this strategy aiming at avoiding the helicity loss of RB3 peptide.

In general, in an α-helix, the carbonyl group of the *i*th amino acid residue mediates a hydrogen bond with the amine group of the (*i* + 4)th amino acid residue by generating nucleation and stabilisation of the helical structure. Based on this evidence, the HBS strategy for generation of artificial α-helices involves the replacement of one of the main chain hydrogen bonds with a covalent linkage [73,85]. Indeed, to mimic the C=O · · · H-N hydrogen bond as closely as possible, a covalent bond of the type C=X–Y–N is included where X and Y are usually carbon atoms that would be part of the *i*th and the (*i* + 4)th residues. However, the analysis of the RB3 α-helix highlighted that the first amino acid implicated in the helix H-bond ensemble does not establish a traditional hydrogen bond with the (*i* + 4)th amino acid, while it forms a contact with the (*i* + 3)th amino acid by creating the so-called 3_{10}-helix [86]. Therefore, in this work, the RB3 peptide was modified by creating a C-C bond between the first (Tyr1178) and the fourth amino acid (Met1181) hereafter called the 3_{10}-HBS RB3 peptide. An MD simulation of the complex Ras-3_{10}-HBS RB3 peptide was run, highlighting a stable peptide helical conformation during the entire trajectory.

Then, a computational residue scanning was run on the peptide to analyse and identify the most promising mutations to be considered in terms of $\Delta\Delta G_{affinity}$ and $\Delta\Delta G_{stability}$. The point-mutated peptides, in complex with the Ras protein, were exploited to run MD simulations and MM-GBSA calculations to guide the selection of the most interesting mutations. The resulting ones were further combined with each other in the 3_{10}-HBS RB3 peptide structure to obtain 48 combinatorial peptides. Thus, these latter were investigated through MD and MM-GBSA to retrieve the calculated $\Delta G_{binding}$ average values for each couple Ras-combinatorial peptide. Finally, 18 combinatorial peptides were selected, and they will enter an experimental follow-up to further explore their potential activity against the Ras-RasGRF1 interaction. In the next sections of this manuscript, efforts to modify the peptide structure to increase the biological activity will be described.

2. Results and Discussion

2.1. Sos and RasGRF1 Binding Interfaces Analysis

To date, no PDB structures of the Ras-RasGRF1 complex are available in the literature thus the Ras-Sos complex structure was exploited to collect key information useful to guide and address the computational studies described herein. In order to deeply explore and predict the hot-spot residues of the Sos Cdc25 domain (i.e., amino acids 924 to 957), all of the six available PDB structures of the Ras-Sos complex (PDB IDs: 1XD2 [48], 1BKD [43], 1NVW, 1NVV, 1NVU, and 1NVX [47]) were examined by using the Robetta Computational Interface Alanine Scanning Server [87,88]. In Table 1, the highest ΔΔG values from the alanine mutations on the Sos binding interface are reported.

Table 1. Predicted ΔΔG values from the alanine mutations on Sos binding interface amino acids retrieved by the Robetta Computational Interface Alanine Scanning Server [87,88].

	ΔΔG (kcal/mol)					
Sos aa	1XD2	1BKD	1NVW	1NVV	1NVU	1NVX
Phe929	1.54	1.48	1.64	3.00	1.53	1.47
Thr935	2.97	1.59	1.11	n.a.	3.13	3.11
Lys939	n.a.	n.a.	n.a.	4.21	n.a.	n.a.
Glu942	n.a.	n.a.	1.10	n.a.	n.a.	n.a.
Asn944	2.51	2.63	2.35	2.66	2.63	2.70

n.a. = not available.

These predicted data were in accordance with mutational studies performed by Hall et al. [61], whereas Phe929, Thr935, and Lys939 were highlighted as Sos interact ing hot spots. In detail, from the computational alanine scanning, Phe929 and Thr935 were shared by most of the six PDB complexes as hot spots, while Lys939 resulted from the PDB 1NVV analysis. As can be seen, this computational tool pointed out another Sos hot spot not previously identified by Hall et al., Asn944, which was shared from all the six PDB complexes. Another hot spot on Glu942 was retrieved from PDB 1NVW.

These identified hot spots, both from biological assays [61] and computational alanine scanning, were considered equally important for the next steps, and were used for comparison to RasGRF1 amino acids in order to investigate similarities between the two GEF sequences (RasGRF1 and Sos). For this purpose, PDB 1XD2 [48], including Sos in complex with the Ras protein, was chosen for the low resolution, while the only available PDB structure of the RasGRF1 Cdc25 domain (PDB ID: 2IJE [59]) was used. However, the latter PDB was from *Mus musculus* as organism. Hence, before proceeding with the protein structure alignment between the Sos and RasGRF1 Cdc25 domains, a FASTA alignment was performed while considering human and murine RasGRF1 sequences through the Protein BLAST sequence alignment tool [89,90]. The resulted overall identity was 83.22%, whereas within the RasGRF1 region involved in Ras binding (i.e., from residue 1173 to 1203 of mouse sequence), the only detected difference was between Ala1198 for human and Val1187 for mouse, as illustrated in Figure S1 in the Supplementary Materials. These two amino acids exhibited side chains with very similar chemical properties, thus the PDB 2IJE was considered suitable for proceeding with this study.

Therefore, both PDB protein structures (2IJE [59] and 1XD2 [48]) were aligned through the "Protein Structure Alignment" tool of the Schrödinger suite, and the result is depicted in Figure 3. As can be seen, the two α-helices of Sos and RasGRF1 are perfectly aligned.

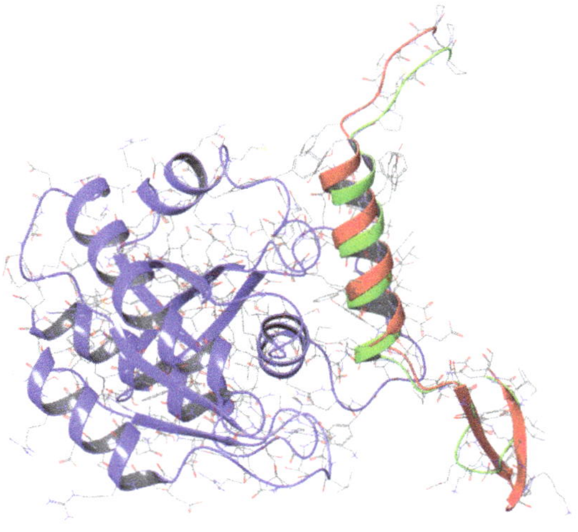

Figure 3. Superposition of the RasGRF1 binding region (green chain, retrieved from PDB 2IJE [59]), and the Sos binding region (pink chain, retrieved from PDB 1XD2 [48]) in complex with the Ras protein (blue chain from PDB 1XD2).

Furthermore, Sos and RasGRF1 binding regions share several amino acids, as shown in the sequence alignment of the Sos and RasGRF1 Cdc25 domains illustrated in Figure 4.

```
                    929          935     939    942 944
                     |            |       |      |   |
Sos       924-PPCVPFFGIYLTNILKTEEGNPEVLKRHGKELIN-957
RasGRF1  1173-PPCVPYLGMYLTDLVFIEEGTPNYTE---DGLVN-1203
                     |            |       |      |   |
                    1178         1184    1188 1191 1193
```

Figure 4. FASTA sequence alignment between the Sos and RasGRF1 regions able to bind the Ras protein.

RasGRF1 amino acids corresponding to Sos hot spots are reported in Table 2. As can be seen, the pairs Thr935-Thr1184 and Glu942-Glu1191 shared the same amino acid, while Phe929 (Sos) and Tyr1178 (RasGRF1) both presented hydrophobic side chains, and Asn944 (Sos) and Thr1193 (RasGRF1) shared polar uncharged side chains. Only Lys939 and Phe1188 were very different amino acids, whereas lysine showed an electrically charged side chain, while phenylalanine exhibited a hydrophobic side chain. The amino acids of RasGRF1 highlighted in the above-described comparison were considered for the next steps of the analysis.

Table 2. Correspondences of Sos hot-spot residues (from biological assays [61] and computational alanine scanning) to RasGRF1 amino acids identified by performing protein structures alignment.

Sos aa	Corresponding RasGRF1 aa
Phe929	Tyr1178
Thr935	Thr1184
Lys939	Phe1188
Glu942	Glu1191
Asn944	Thr1193

2.2. MD Simulations of Ras in Complex with Sos and RasGRF1 Binding Fragments

In order to investigate the importance of the computationally predicted hot spots not reported in the literature; i.e., Glu942 and Asn944, and to explore the interactions between the Ras-Sos complex, a MD simulation was run. For this purpose, PDB 1XD2 [48] was chosen, and the simulation was run for a short time of 50 ns to observe and identify the most stable and frequent contacts. The stability of the system was monitored during the entire trajectory, thus registering the RMSD plot depicted in Figure S2 in the Supplementary Materials. Then, the MD frames were clustered using the "Desmond trajectory clustering tool of the Schrödinger suite (Schrödinger Inc., New York, NY, USA, software release v2018-4) by setting five clusters to be generated, and the frame centroids representative for the clusters were analysed; i.e., frame 120, frame 540, frame 660, frame 780, and frame 820. These five frames were investigated to identify the interactions between the Ras and Sos proteins, where among the above-mentioned five Sos hot spots (please refer to Table 2), four residues established stable interactions with Ras during the trajectory; i.e., Phe929, Thr935, Glu942, and Asn944. The related interactions are listed in Table 3, and the H-bonds are plotted against the simulation time in Table S1 in the Supplementary Materials.

Table 3. Stable interactions established during MD trajectories of Ras-Sos and Ras-RasGRF1 complexes.

	MD on Ras-Sos Complex		**MD on Ras-RasGRF1 Complex**	
Ras aa	Sos aa 924–957	Interaction type	RasGRF1 aa 1173–1203	Interaction type
Tyr64	Phe929	Hydrophobic	Tyr1178	Pi–Pi stacking
	Phe930	Hydrophobic	Leu1179	Hydrophobic
			Leu1183	Hydrophobic
Tyr40	-	-	Phe1188	Hydrophobic
Gln61	Ile932	Hydrophobic	Tyr1178	1 H-bond
	Thr935	1 H-bond	Thr1184	1 H-bond
Ala59	Thr935	1 H-bond	Thr1184	1 H-bond
			Leu1183	Hydrophobic
			Val1187	Hydrophobic
			Phe1188	Hydrophobic
Ser17	Glu942	1 H-bond	Glu1191	1 H-bond
			Val1187	Hydrophobic
Ala18	Glu942	1 H-bond	Glu1191	1 H-bond
Tyr32	Asn944	2 H-bonds	Gly1192	1 H-bond
			Phe1188	Hydrophobic
Pro34	Thr940	Hydrophobic	-	-
Asp57	Lys939	1 H-bond + 1 salt bridge	-	-
Gly60	Leu934	Hydrophobic	Leu1183	Hydrophobic
Lys147	-	-	Glu1191	1 H-bond + 1 salt bridge

Based on the previously described comparison between the Sos interacting region and the RasGRF1 Cdc25 domain, an MD simulation of the Ras-RasGRF1 complex was performed through the Schrödinger suite [91] to investigate whether the five putative RasGRF1 key residues (Tyr1178, Thr1184, Phe1188, Glu1191, and Thr1193) were responsible for contacting the Ras protein and stabilising the complex.

Therefore, the protein–protein complex was generated by using the previous aligned structures involving PDBs 1XD2 [48] and 2IJE [59], where the RasGRF1 interacting region (residues 1173 to 1203) was located within the binding pocket of the Ras protein through performing a superimposition on the Sos chain, which was subsequently deleted. The complex was minimised, and the MD was run by setting 50 ns as the simulation time. The output was analysed, and the stability of the system was checked through the RMSD plot (Figure S3 in the Supplementary Materials). The trajectory was clustered by setting five clusters to be generated. Then, the MD frame centroids were analysed; that is, frame 40, frame 65, frame 110, frame 280, and frame 362. The most stable interactions between Ras and RasGRF1 were observed, and they are reported in Table 3. In Table S2 in the Supplementary Materials, the H-bonds are plotted against the simulation time. As can be observed, most of these interactions were similarly established between Ras and the corresponding Sos amino acids (please refer to Table 2) during the MD simulation. This provided interesting information to take forward in this work.

2.3. *MD Simulations of the Ras-RB3 Peptide Complex*

After collecting information about interactions between Ras and its GEFs (Sos and RasGRF1), other MD simulations were performed to explore the binding mode and the established contacts between Ras and the parental (WT) RB3 peptide.

The core sequence of this peptide (without TAT portion) corresponds to RasGRF1 sequence 1173-PPCVPYLGMYLTDLVFIEEGTPNYTEDGLVN-1203. Therefore, the complex Ras-RasGRF1 was used, and all those residues not included in the RB3 peptide sequence were deleted. Thus, this new complex, the Ras-RB3 peptide, was processed by running MD simulations of 500 ns each. The RMSD plot was generated, and it is depicted in Figure S4a in the Supplementary Materials. This plot revealed a certain instability of the systems, ranging from about 3.5 to 6.4 Å. Therefore, a second MD simulation was computed, and even in this case the RMSD plot (Figure S4b in the Supplementary Materials) showed the same trend. On the other hand, the interactions between Ras and the peptide were investigated for both trajectories. The MD frames of both simulations were grouped into five clusters each, and the frame centroids were analysed to retrieve the most stable and frequent interactions: (a) first MD → centroid frame 390, centroid frame 2340, centroid frame 1400, centroid frame 3590, and centroid frame 4270; (b) second MD → centroid frame 3610, centroid frame 4800, centroid frame 2660, centroid frame 620, and centroid frame 1280. The observed contacts between the Ras protein and the RB3 peptide from the above-listed frames are reported in Table 4.

Table 4. The most stable interactions between Ras and the RB3 peptide highlighted from the MD trajectory analyses.

First MD			Second MD		
Ras aa	**RB3 aa**	**Interaction type**	**Ras aa**	**RB3 aa**	**Interaction type**
Tyr40	Asp1185	1 H-bond	Tyr40	Asp1185	1 H-bond
Tyr40	Phe1188	Pi–Pi stacking	Tyr40	Phe1188	Pi–Pi stacking
Tyr32	Gly1192	1 H-bond	Glu31	Gly1192	1 H-bond
Gln61	Tyr1182	1 H-bond	Arg149	Glu1198	1 H-bond + 1 salt bridge
			Gln25	Gly1192	1 H-bond

The two MD simulations shared only two interactions; i.e., one hydrogen bond between Tyr40 of Ras and Asp1185 of the RB3 peptide, and a pi–pi stacking between the aromatic ring of the Tyr40 side chain of Ras and the other aromatic ring of the Phe1188 side chain of the RB3 peptide. Furthermore, all the other interactions retrieved from the MD simulations registered low stability during the entire trajectories.

Thus, a visual check of both simulations shed light on an important behaviour of the RB3 peptide α-helix; i.e., a portion of the α-helix (from Met1181 to Thr1184) began to lose helicity propensity after about 50/60 ns of simulation time, resulting in a misfolding behaviour. Indeed, not surprisingly, the two above-mentioned interactions shared by both simulations from the MD analyses were involved into the folded region of the peptide over the entire trajectories; i.e., the residues from Asp1185 to Glu1191 not exhibiting the misfolding. Figure 5 illustrates the misfolding of the RB3 α-helix after 50 ns of the first MD simulation.

Therefore, a strategy to overcome this issue was implemented by applying the hydrogen-bond surrogate approach, which had already provided successful experimental evidence [62,73–79,84]. Thus, the RB3 peptide was processed by modifying the structure. First, two portions of the peptide were deleted; i.e., the residues belonging to the two loops of the peptide (residues 1171 to 1177 and 1194 to 1203), because they showed a lack of crucial interactions according to mutational studies reported in the literature [43,61] and the MD simulations of Ras-RasGRF1 (please refer to Table 3). Thus, residues 1171 to 1177 and 1194 to 1203 were considered not important for the purpose of this work, and were deleted from the structure. Then, the analysis of the α-helix highlighted that Tyr1178, the first amino acid implicated in the helix H-bonds ensemble, did not establish a traditional hydrogen bond with the (*i* + 4)th amino acid, while it formed a contact with the (*i* + 3)th amino acid, by creating the so-called 3_{10}-helix [86].

Hence, a MD simulation of 500 ns was performed on the Ras protein in complex with the RB3 peptide modified by deleting the two loops at the N- and C-termini and creating a covalent C-C bond between the carbonyl oxygen of the Tyr1178 backbone and the amine hydrogen of the Met1181 backbone. The resulting peptide was termed 3_{10}-HBS-RB3 (Figure 6).

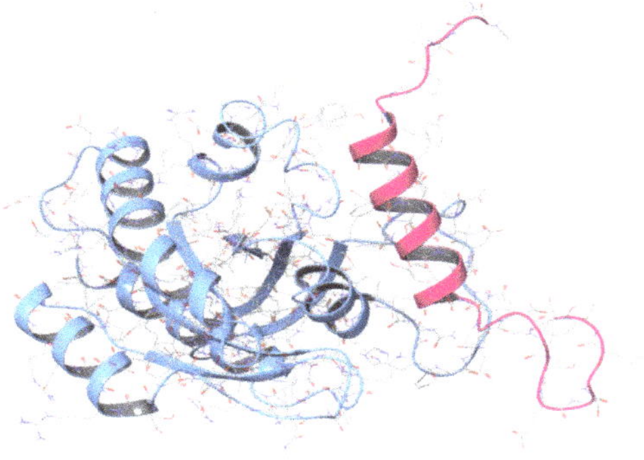

(a)

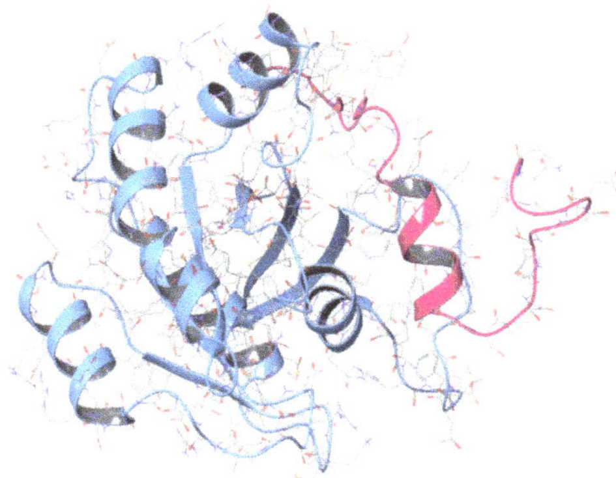

(b)

Figure 5. (**a**) Frame 0 of the first MD simulation on Ras (blue chain) in complex with a RasGRF1 fragment (pink chain, aa 1173 to 1203); (**b**) frame from the first MD simulation on Ras in complex with a RasGRF1 fragment after about 50 ns, depicting the RB3 peptide losing helicity propensity in the portion from Met1181 to Thr1184.

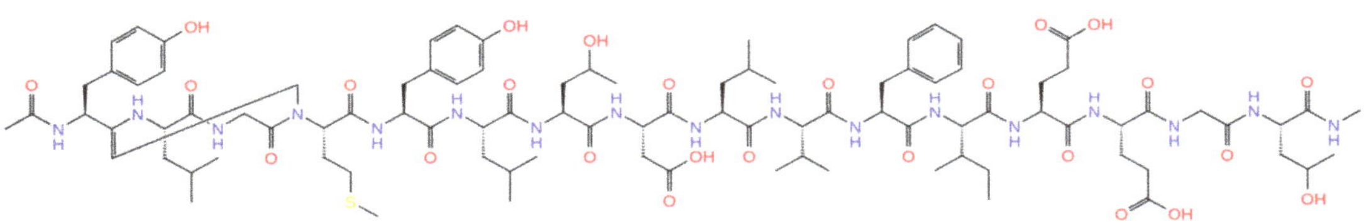

(a)

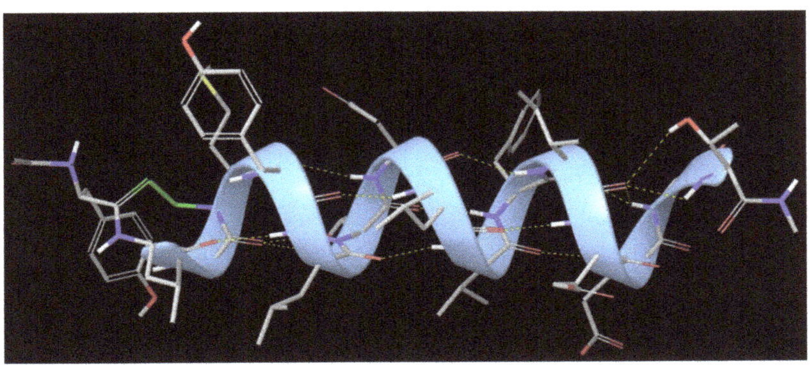

(b)

Figure 6. (**a**) Structure of the 3_{10}-HBS RB3 peptide; (**b**) the 3_{10}-HBS RB3 peptide including a covalent C-C bond (green bond) between the carbonyl oxygen of Tyr1178 backbone and the amine hydrogen of Met1181 backbone.

The analysis of the output revealed a stable trend for the α-helicity of the peptide, which held its folded conformation. Even the RMSD plot (Figure S5 in the Supplementary Materials) showed a certain stability of the system, thus the frames were analysed to retrieve information about the most stable interactions, and the results were plotted as depicted in Figure 7.

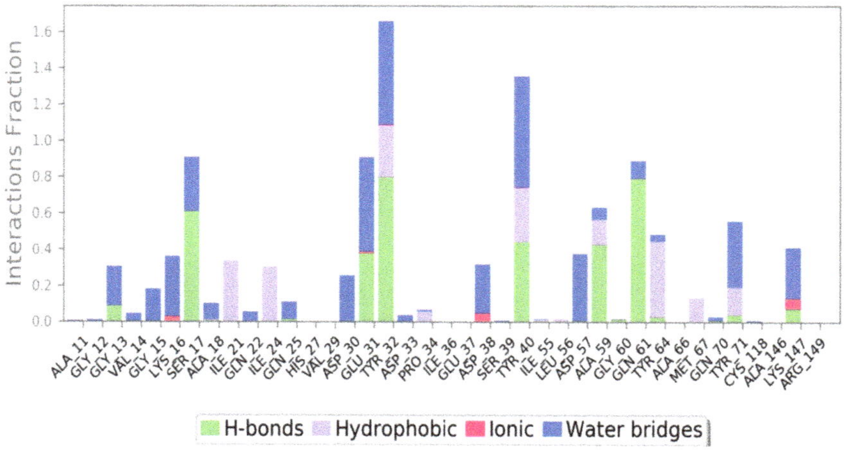

(**a**)

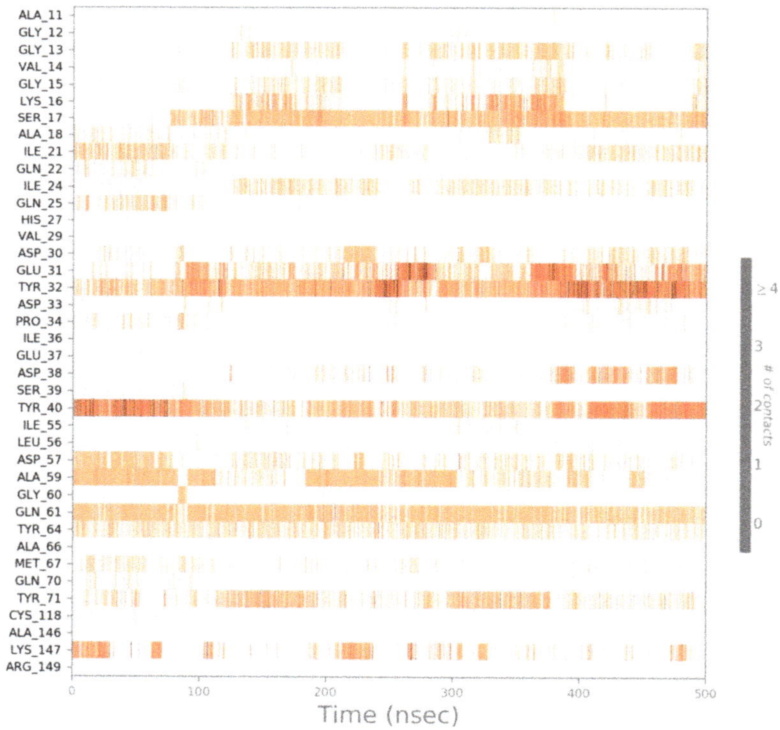

(**b**)

Figure 7. (**a**) Histogram of the interactions established between the Ras protein binding region and the 3_{10}-HBS RB3 peptide; (**b**) Plot illustrating the frequency of interaction occurrences between the Ras protein binding region and the 3_{10}-HBS RB3 peptide.

This newly designed 3_{10}-HBS RB3 peptide showed that it could establish some of the key interactions identified in the previous MD simulation between the Ras and RasGRF1 proteins (please refer to Table 3) and other contacts with Ras amino acids (Tyr32 and Tyr40) highlighted as key residues from mutational studies [61]. Finally, an MM-GBSA calculation of the MD frame was computed to obtain the $\Delta G_{binding}$ of the complex Ras-3_{10}-HBS RB3 peptide, which was −79.70 kcal/mol. This value was exploited as a reference for the peptide optimisation process described in the following sections.

2.4. Computational Residue Scanning of the 3_{10}-HBS RB3 Peptide and MD Simulations of Point-Mutated Peptides

In order to optimise the structure of the 3_{10}-HBS RB3 peptide, a computational residue scanning was performed on the amino acids of the peptide by using the "Residue scanning" tool of Bioluminate (Schrödinger Inc., software release v2018-4) [92]. The peptide was point-mutated where each residue was substituted with all the standard amino acids, and $\Delta\Delta G_{affinity}$ and $\Delta\Delta G_{stability}$ values of the new complexes were computed. The aim was to identify the most promising mutations in terms of $\Delta\Delta G_{affinity}$ and $\Delta\Delta G_{stability}$. For this purpose, only mutations reporting both $\Delta\Delta G_{affinity}$ and $\Delta\Delta G_{stability}$ values below −3 kcal/mol were considered, according to the work of Beard et al. [92], which reported a correlation between experimental results and the computationally predicted ones through the Schrödinger suite. Indeed, the authors demonstrated that a difference of 3 kcal/mol between the mutated and WT forms of a complex might be considered reliable in hot-spot prediction. Finally, 16 mutations reported $\Delta\Delta G_{affinity}$ and $\Delta\Delta G_{stability}$ values lower than −3 kcal/mol, thus they were considered for the next steps of this work (Table 5).

Table 5. Computational residue scanning results for the peptide 3_{10}-HBS RB3, highlighting 16 promising mutations.

3_{10}-HBS RB3 Peptide aa	**Mutation**	**$\Delta\Delta G_{affinity}$ (kcal/mol)**	**$\Delta\Delta G_{stability}$ (kcal/mol)**
Thr1184	Arg	−19.17	−3.67
	Met	−8.17	−3.18
Asp1185	Trp	−12.56	−7.64
	Tyr	−9.19	−3.49
	Phe	−8.26	−4.26
	Leu	−7.77	−12.61
Phe1188	Arg	−9.55	−4.12
Phe1188	His	−8.25	−8.75
Ile1189	Met	−3.59	−4.08
Glu1190	His	−3.29	−4.13
Glu1191	Ile	−6.97	−4.68
	Leu	−5.16	−3.79
	Val	−4.71	−4.08
	Thr	−4.32	−4.27
Thr1193	Arg	−3.85	−5.84
	Gln	−3.56	−5.86

These 16 mutations were used to create as many complexes involving the Ras protein and the 3_{10}-HBS RB3 point-mutated peptides that underwent MD simulations. The trajectory time was set at 100 ns for each system, since this timeframe was considered suitable to detect potential misfolding of the peptides. Indeed, the previously described MD simulations on the WT RB3 peptide exhibited misfolded conformation by losing α-helicity after about 50/60 ns of simulation. From the analysis of the MD trajectories, all the point-mutated peptides were able to keep the helical conformation, thus MM-GBSA calculations were computed, and the related $\Delta G_{binding}$ values are reported below in Table 6. Table S3 in the Supplementary Materials lists the $\Delta G_{binding}$ average values of the interaction energies and the generalized Born solvation energy for the MD trajectories of the complexes' Ras-point-mutated 3_{10}-HBS RB3 peptides. The stability of the systems was investigated by analysing the RMSD plots per each complex, resulting in suitable stationary shape for each system (Table S4 in the Supplementary Materials).

Table 6. MM-GBSA calculation results based on MD simulations of the 16 point-mutated 3_{10}-HBS RB3 peptides in complex with the Ras protein.

	First Peptide	Second Peptide	Third Peptide
Point mutation	T1184R	T1184M	D1185W
$\Delta G_{binding}$ average	−89.51 kcal/mol	−92.77 kcal/mol	−103.50 kcal/mol
$\Delta G_{binding}$ Std. Dev.	12.50	15.53	8.90
$\Delta G_{binding}$ range	−128.52 to −55.50 kcal/mol	−134.237 to −39.51 kcal/mol	−126.30 to −73.35 kcal/mol
	Fourth Peptide	**Fifth Peptide**	**Sixth Peptide**
Point mutation	D1185Y	D1185F	D1185L
$\Delta G_{binding}$ average	−102.50 kcal/mol	−94.84 kcal/mol	−82.07 kcal/mol
$\Delta G_{binding}$ Std. Dev.	22.23	8.34	9.26
$\Delta G_{binding}$ range	−145.44 to −40.67 kcal/mol	−120.13 to −52.39 kcal/mol	−109.19 to −32.63 kcal/mol
	Seventh Peptide	**Eighth Peptide**	**Ninth Peptide**
Point mutation	F1188R	F1188H	I1189M
$\Delta G_{binding}$ average	−87.49 kcal/mol	−69.58 kcal/mol	−83.12 kcal/mol
$\Delta G_{binding}$ Std. Dev.	11.60	15.23	10.89
$\Delta G_{binding}$ range	−120.32 to −57.76 kcal/mol	−111.45 to −24.94 kcal/mol	−122.63 to −44.93 kcal/mol
	Tenth Peptide	**Eleventh Peptide**	**Twelfth Peptide**
Point mutation	E1190H	E1191I	E1191L
$\Delta G_{binding}$ average	−73.36 kcal/mol	−78.65 kcal/mol	−95.11 kcal/mol
$\Delta G_{binding}$ Std. Dev.	12.64	11.67	12.89
$\Delta G_{binding}$ range	−110.79 to −39.82 kcal/mol	−115.33 to −43.76 kcal/mol	−140.50 to −49.67 kcal/mol
	Thirteenth Peptide	**Fourteenth Peptide**	**Fifteenth Peptide**
Point mutation	E1191V	E1191T	T1193R
$\Delta G_{binding}$ average	−94.42 kcal/mol	−84.50 kcal /mol	−90.18 kcal/mol
$\Delta G_{binding}$ Std. Dev.	10.69	12.71	10.85
$\Delta G_{binding}$ range	−121.24 to −58.75 kcal/mol	−116.52 to −47.48 kcal/mol	−119.87 to −59.72 kcal/mol
	Sixteenth Peptide		
Point mutation	T1193N		
$\Delta G_{binding}$ average	−97.15 kcal/mol		
$\Delta G_{binding}$ Std. Dev.	11.88		
$\Delta G_{binding}$ range	−127.15 to −53.43 kcal/mol		

As previously mentioned, the $\Delta G_{binding}$ of the complex between Ras and the WT 3_{10}-HBS RB3 peptide (−79.70 kcal/mol) was used as a reference to select the most promising mutations associated with $\Delta G_{binding}$ values lower than the reference one. In light of the above, from the MM-GBSA results, only three mutated peptides showed higher $\Delta G_{binding}$ values. Hence, the related mutations, F1188H, E1190H, and E1191I, were neglected. On the contrary, the other 13 mutations were considered for creating combinatorial peptides, as described in the next section.

2.5. Combinatorial Peptides Using 3_{10}-HBS RB3: Creation and MD Simulations

The most promising mutations on the 3_{10}-HBS RB3 peptide were combined with each other to obtain 48 mutated peptides overall, as listed below in Table 7.

Table 7. Combinatorial peptides designed based on computational residue scanning performed on the 3_{10}-HBS RB3 peptide and MM-GBSA calculations on MD simulations.

Combinatorial Peptides			
1.	YLGMYLRWLVRMELGR	25.	YLGMYLRWLVRMELGN
2.	YLGMYLMWLVRMELGR	26.	YLGMYLMWLVRMELGN
3.	YLGMYLRYLVRMELGR	27.	YLGMYLRYLVRMELGN
4.	YLGMYLMYLVRMELGR	28.	YLGMYLMYLVRMELGN
5.	YLGMYLRFLVRMELGR	29.	YLGMYLRFLVRMELGN
6.	YLGMYLMFLVRMELGR	30.	YLGMYLMFLVRMELGN
7.	YLGMYLRLLVRMELGR	31.	YLGMYLRLLVRMELGN
8.	YLGMYLMLLVRMELGR	32.	YLGMYLMLLVRMELGN
9.	YLGMYLRWLVRMEVGR	33.	YLGMYLRWLVRMEVGN
10.	YLGMYLRYLVRMEVGR	34.	YLGMYLRYLVRMEVGN
11.	YLGMYLRFLVRMEVGR	35.	YLGMYLRFLVRMEVGN
12.	YLGMYLRLLVRMEVGR	36.	YLGMYLRLLVRMEVGN
13.	YLGMYLMWLVRMEVGR	37.	YLGMYLMWLVRMEVGN
14.	YLGMYLMYLVRMEVGR	38.	YLGMYLMYLVRMEVGN
15.	YLGMYLMFLVRMEVGR	39.	YLGMYLMFLVRMEVGN
16.	YLGMYLMLLVRMEVGR	40.	YLGMYLMLLVRMEVGN
17.	YLGMYLRWLVRMETGR	41.	YLGMYLRWLVRMETGN
18.	YLGMYLRYLVRMETGR	42.	YLGMYLRYLVRMETGN
19.	YLGMYLRFLVRMETGR	43.	YLGMYLRFLVRMETGN
20.	YLGMYLRLLVRMETGR	44.	YLGMYLRLLVRMETGN
21.	YLGMYLMWLVRMETGR	45.	YLGMYLMWLVRMETGN
22.	YLGMYLMYLVRMETGR	46.	YLGMYLMYLVRMETGN
23.	YLGMYLMFLVRMETGR	47.	YLGMYLMFLVRMETGN
24.	YLGMYLMLLVRMETGR	48.	YLGMYLMLLVRMETGN

The 48 combinatorial peptides in complex with the Ras protein were processed by running MD simulations of 100 ns each to investigate helix conformational stability and the contacts formed with the Ras protein. All the trajectories were observed by generating RMSD plots to ensure the reliability of the outputs, and the interaction frequency and stability were analysed. Finally, MM-GBSA calculations of the MD simulations were computed. Thus, all those combinatorial peptides not responding to the following criteria were neglected:

1. $\Delta G_{binding}$ value higher than the reference one (−79.70 kcal/mol);
2. Loss of helical conformation.

Finally, 18 combinatorial peptides overall fulfilled the above criteria by resulting in promising $\Delta G_{binding}$ values and exhibiting a helical trend during the whole MD trajectory. Thus, Table 8 reports the MM-GBSA results of these 18 most promising combinatorial peptides, which will be considered for the follow-up of this study by carrying out biological assays. Table S5 in the Supplementary Materials lists the $\Delta G_{binding}$ average values of the interaction energies and the generalized Born solvation energy for the MD trajectories of the complexes' Ras-combinatorial peptides. The related RMSD plots and interaction diagrams of these 18 selected peptides are reported in Tables S6 and S7, respectively, in the Supplementary Materials. Based on the above-mentioned plots, these selected combinatorial peptides were able to mainly reproduce the key interactions of the 3_{10}-HBS RB3 peptide reported above in Figure 7 by establishing contacts with Ras key residues, especially Tyr32, Tyr40, and Tyr64, which were highlighted as crucial by previous experimental assays [43,61].

Table 8. MM-GBSA calculation results based on MD simulations of 3_{10}-HBS combinatorial peptides not misfolded during the simulations in complex with Ras protein, and with $\Delta G_{binding}$ values lower than the reference one (−79.70 kcal/mol).

	First Peptide	**Third Peptide**	**Eleventh Peptide**
Peptide sequence	YLGMYLRWLVRMELGR	YLGMYLRYLVRMELGR	YLGMYLRFLVRMEVGR
$\Delta G_{binding}$ average	−83.46 kcal/mol	−96.80 kcal/mol	−91.39 kcal/mol
$\Delta G_{binding}$ Std. Dev.	9.00	9.84	11.55
$\Delta G_{binding}$ range	−117.54 to −55.07 kcal/mol	−123.01 to −52.38 kcal/mol	−119.67 to −61.34 kcal/mol
	Twelfth Peptide	**Fifteenth Peptide**	**Sixteenth Peptide**
Peptide sequence	YLGMYLRLLVRMEVGR	YLGMYLMFLVRMEVGR	YLGMYLMLLVRMEVGR
$\Delta G_{binding}$ average	−92.49 kcal/mol	−79.79 kcal/mol	−92.54 kcal/mol
$\Delta G_{binding}$ Std. Dev.	10.15	14.46	7.93
$\Delta G_{binding}$ range	−129.87 to −56.49 kcal/mol	−112.94 to −41.42 kcal/mol	−116.28 to −65.18 kcal/mol
	Eighteenth Peptide	**Nineteenth Peptide**	**Twentieth Peptide**
Peptide sequence	YLGMYLRYLVRMETGR	YLGMYLRFLVRMETGR	YLGMYLRLLVRMETGR
$\Delta G_{binding}$ average	−100.34 kcal/mol	−102.63 kcal/mol	−88.71 kcal/mol
$\Delta G_{binding}$ Std. Dev.	14.21	11.01	13.50
$\Delta G_{binding}$ range	−137.53 to −65.42 kcal/mol	−130.87 to −62.69 kcal/mol	−125.02 to −50.94 kcal/mol
	Twenty-third Peptide	**Twenty-fourth Peptide**	**Twenty-fifth Peptide**
Peptide sequence	YLGMYLMFLVRMETGR	YLGMYLMLLVRMETGR	YLGMYLRWLVRMELGN
$\Delta G_{binding}$ average	−85.53 kcal/mol	−82.31 kcal/mol	−97.24 kcal /mol
$\Delta G_{binding}$ Std. Dev.	11.35	10.37	14.17
$\Delta G_{binding}$ range	−117.73 to −42.84 kcal/mol	−116.03 to −40.57 kcal/mol	−133.33 to −60.15 kcal/mol
	Twenty-ninth Peptide	**Forty-second Peptide**	**Forty-third Peptide**
Peptide sequence	YLGMYLRFLVRMELGN	YLGMYLRYLVRMETGN	YLGMYLRFLVRMETGN
$\Delta G_{binding}$ average	−86.56 kcal/mol	−89.59 kcal/mol	−123.50 kcal/mol
$\Delta G_{binding}$ Std. Dev.	11.67	10.32	20.97
$\Delta G_{binding}$ range	−124.70 to −56.47 kcal/mol	−128.75 to −60.00 kcal/mol	−161.49 to −75.91 kcal/mol
	Forty-fourth Peptide	**Forty-fifth Peptide**	**Forty-eighth Peptide**
Peptide sequence	YLGMYLRLLVRMETGN	YLGMYLMWLVRMETGN	YLGMYLMLLVRMETGN
$\Delta G_{binding}$ average	−96.31 kcal/mol	−86.04 kcal/mol	−91.80 kcal/mol
$\Delta G_{binding}$ Std. Dev.	17.98	13.60	9.51
$\Delta G_{binding}$ range	−137.97 to −57.81 kcal/mol	−124.08 to −53.76 kcal mol	−122.78 to −60.84 kcal/mol

Furthermore, other contacts appeared, especially with Asp57, Gly60, and Gln61 of Ras. Indeed, these amino acids were involved in interactions with Sos and RasGRF1 according to previous MD simulations, thus confirming that these designed peptides might bind and inhibit the interaction between the Ras protein and the guanine nucleotide exchange factors, Sos and RasGRF1. Figure 8 depicts the binding mode of the 3_{10}-HBS combinatorial peptide forty-three, which reported the lowest $\Delta G_{binding}$ average.

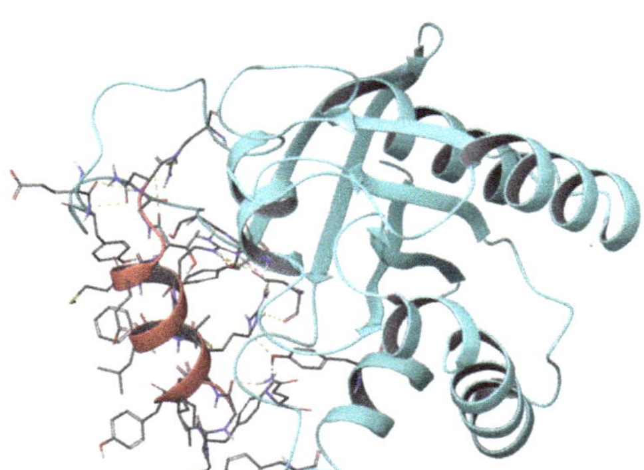

Figure 8. Frame of the MD simulation performed on the combinatorial peptide forty-three in complex with the Ras protein, depicting the binding mode of the peptide.

3. Methods

3.1. Protein Preparation

The 3D structures of the Ras-Sos complex (PDB IDs: 1XD2 [48], 1BKD [43], 1NVW, 1NVV, 1NVU, and 1NVX [47]) and RasGRF1 protein (PDB ID: 2IJE [59]) were retrieved from the Protein Data Bank [60] and optimised using the "Protein preparation" tool of the Schrödinger suite (Schrödinger Inc., New York, NY, USA) software release v2018-4) [93]. The bond orders for untemplated residues were assigned by using known HET groups based on their SMILES strings in the Chemical Component Dictionary. Hydrogens were added to the structure, zero-order bonds between metals and nearby atoms were added, and formal charges to metals and neighbouring atoms were corrected. Disulfide bonds were created according to possible geometries, and water molecules beyond 5.0 Å from any of the HET groups, including ions, were deleted. Then, protonation and metal charge states for the ligands, cofactors, and metals were generated [94,95]. Finally, PROPKA [95] was run under pH 7.0 to optimise hydroxyl groups and Asn, Gln, and His states.

3.2. MD Simulations of Ras Protein in Complex with Sos, RasGRF1, RB3 Peptide, and the Designed 3_{10}-HBS Peptides

In this work, 69 MD simulations were performed using Desmond [91,96–99], as follows: 1 MD simulation of 50 ns for the Ras-Sos complex, 1 MD simulation of 50 ns for the Ras-RasGRF1 complex, 2 MD simulations of 500 ns for Ras in complex with the WT RB3 peptide, 1 MD simulation of 500 ns for Ras in complex with the 3_{10}-HBS RB3 peptide, 16 MD simulations of 100 ns for Ras complexed with the point-mutated 3_{10}-HBS peptides, and 48 MD simulations of 100 ns for Ras in complex with the combinatorial 3_{10}-HBS peptides. All the trajectories were computed by applying the same MD settings below described. The systems were created using TIP3P [100] as a solvent model, and the orthorhombic shape box was chosen. The box side distances were set at 10 Å. The force field OPLS3e [101] was applied, and the systems were neutralized by adding Na^+ ions. The outputs were further processed by performing MD simulations with the above-reported simulation times.

The ensemble class NPT was chosen to maintain the number of atoms, the pressure, and the temperature constant for the entire trajectories. The thermostat method employed was the Nosé–Hoover chain with a relaxation time of 1.0 ps and a temperature of 300 K. The barostat method applied was Martyna–Tobias–Klein, with a relaxation time of 2.0 ps and an isotropic coupling style. The timestep for numerical integration was 2.0 fs for bonded interactions, 2.0 fs for nonbonded-near (van der Waals and short-range electrostatic interactions), and 6.0 fs for nonbonded-far (long-range electrostatic interactions). For Coulombic interactions, a cut-off radius of 9.0 Å was tuned as a short-range method. Pressure and temperature were set at 1.01325 bar and 300 K, respectively. Finally, the systems were relaxed before beginning the simulations according to the following steps:

1. Minimization with the solute restrained;
2. Minimization without restraints;
3. 12 ps in the NVT ensemble with a Berendsen thermostat, temperature of 10 K, a fast temperature relaxation constant, velocity resampling every 1 ps, and nonhydrogen solute atoms restrained;
4. 12 ps in the NPT ensemble in a Berendsen thermostat and barostat, temperature equal to 10 K and a pressure of 1 atm, a fast temperature relaxation constant, a slow pressure relaxation constant, velocity resampling every 1ps, and nonhydrogen solute atoms restrained;
5. 24 ps in the NPT ensemble with a Berendsen thermostat and barostat, temperature of 300 K and a pressure of 1 atm, a fast temperature relaxation constant, a slow pressure relaxation constant, velocity resampling every 1 ps, and nonhydrogen solute atoms restrained;

6. Final step of 24 ps of relaxation in NPT ensemble using a Berendsen thermostat and barostat, a temperature of 300 K and a pressure of 1 atm, a fast temperature relaxation constant, and a normal pressure relaxation constant.

3.3. MD Frame Clustering

In order to retrieve the key contacts between the protein partners during the entire simulations, for the MD simulations performed for Ras-Sos, Ras-RasGRF1, and Ras-RB3 peptide complexes, the frames were clustered to identify the most representative centroids to be analysed. The RMSD matrix calculation was set using the protein backbone as reference, the frequency of frames analysis was set 10, and the hierarchical cluster linkage method as average. Finally, for each MD trajectory, five clusters were generated; the analysis was reported in the Results and Discussion section.

3.4. Computational Residue Scanning of Peptide 3_{10}-HBS RB3 in Complex with Ras

The 3_{10}-HBS RB3 peptide in complex with Ras (from PDB 1XD2 [48]) was used to perform a computational residue scanning (Schrödinger Inc., software release v2018-4) to perform point mutations on the peptide residues. The predicted changes in binding affinity and stability were calculated according to Equation (1) [92]:

$$\Delta\Delta G_{Affinity} = \left(E_{A\cdot B}^{MUT} - E_{A}^{MUT} - E_{B}^{MUT}\right) - \left(E_{A\cdot B}^{WT} - E_{A}^{WT} - E_{B}^{WT}\right) \quad (1)$$

where E is the calculated energy of each protein (A and B) or complex (A·B) after refinement while considering the mutant form (MUT) and the wild-type (WT) of the protein. The resulting structures were refined by selecting side-chain prediction with backbone minimization.

For the purpose of the model, $\Delta\Delta G_{stability}$ was computed while representing the unfolded ligand as a tripeptide, A-X-B, where X is the residue that is mutated, and A and B are its neighbours, capped with ACE and NMA. The assumption was that the remaining interactions in the unfolded state were negligible. Thus, $\Delta\Delta G_{stability}$ values were calculated according to Equation (2):

$$\Delta\Delta G_{Stability} = \left(E_{L(u)}^{MUT} - E_{L(f)}^{MUT}\right) - \left(E_{L(u)}^{WT} - E_{L(f)}^{WT}\right) \quad (2)$$

where E, in this case, is the calculated energy for the unfolded parent ligand (L(u)) and the folded parent ligand (L(f)) while considering the mutant form (MUT) and the wild-type (WT) of the protein [92]. The calculations were done with Prime MM-GBSA [102,103], which employs an implicit (continuum) solvation model.

3.5. MM-GBSA Calculations of All the Complexes Used to Perform MD

The MD outputs of Ras protein in complex with 3_{10}-HBS RB3 peptide, the point-mutated peptides, and the combinatorial peptides were used to compute MM-GBSA calculations through the command line. For this purpose, the Python script "thermal_mmgbsa.py" was used. Overall, 65 MM-GBSA calculations were carried out using VSGB as a solvation model, and OLPS3 FF was set for each MD trajectory. The $\Delta G_{binding}$ values were computed for each trajectory frame according to Equation (3):

$$\Delta G_{binding} = E_{A\cdot B\ (minimized)} - E_{A\ (minimized)} - E_{B\ (minimized)} \quad (3)$$

where E is the calculated energy of complex (A·B) or each protein (A and B) after minimization [68]. Finally, the average of $\Delta G_{binding}$ values of the entire trajectories was calculated; the results were reported above in Tables 7 and 8 in the "Results and Discussion" section.

4. Conclusions

The above-described work was intended to investigate potential modifications of a patented peptide, RB3 [64], to increase its inhibitory capacity of the Ras–ERK signalling pathway involved in cocaine abuse. This peptide has been reported to work as an inhibitor targeting the interaction between Ras protein and the guanine nucleotide exchange factors [63]. In detail, assays carried out on an ex vivo model of acute striatal brain slices reported an inhibitory activity of RB3 peptide against ERK phosphorylation by significantly reducing the ERK activity, with an IC_{50} of 6 μM. The inhibitory potential of this peptide was further explored by Papale and colleagues, who highlighted that this peptide was effective in decreasing the phosphorylation of two ERK substrates, (Ser10)-acetylated (Lys14) histone H3 (pAc-H3) and S6 ribosomal protein (pS6, Ser235/236 specific site) [69–71], with an IC_{50} of 5.2 μM for pAc-H3 and 3.69 μM for pS6 [63]. Due to the increasing interest in the RB3 peptide, it was chosen for to improve and modify the structure, aiming at increasing its inhibitory activity to reduce cocaine relapses in drug-addicted patients. The below-described strategy allowed us to identify 18 peptides exploiting the peptide RB3 structure, including amino acid mutations, and employing an artificial construct, the hydrogen bond surrogate, to stabilise the helical conformation of the peptides. The MD simulations performed on these molecules in complex with the Ras protein registered stable and frequent contacts with key residues of the Ras protein, as known from the literature [43,61]. Furthermore, MM-GBSA calculation of the MD trajectories reported promising $\Delta G_{binding}$ average values, where, for example, the combinatorial peptide forty-three showed a $\Delta G_{binding}$ value of −123.50 kcal/mol. Interestingly, the selected combinatorial peptides showed an important interaction energy increase compared to the point-mutated ones, whereas the GB solvation term reported positive values (see Tables S3 and S5 in the Supplementary Materials). Thus, it seems that the presented combinatorial peptides' interaction patterns were crucial for the complex stabilisation, as also observed in the MD RMSD plots (see Table S6 in the Supplementary Materials).

Therefore, the 16 selected combinatorial peptides were chosen, and the next step of this work will be the biological screening of the ERK signalling pathway by measuring the phosphorylation rate of the two ERK substrates, pAc-H3 and pS6 [69–71]. The results of these assays will provide crucial information about the potential of these designed peptides in inhibiting Ras activation, thus preventing molecular effects' maladaptive behavioural manifestations associated with brain conditions in which this signalling pathway is abnormally enhanced, such as cocaine abuse and certain forms of ID and ASD.

Supplementary Materials: The following are available online at https://www.mdpi.com/article/10.3390/ph14111099/s1, Figure S1. FASTA sequence alignment between RasGRF1 interacting region from two different organisms (*Homo sapiens* and *Mus musculus*); Figure S2. RMSD plot of the MD simulation performed on the Ras-Sos complex (PDB 1XD2); Table S1. Plots of the H-bonds established between Ras and Sos during the MD simulation; Figure S3. RMSD plot of the MD simulation performed on the Ras-RasGRF1 complex; Table S2. Plots of the H-bonds established between Ras and RasGRF1 during the MD simulation; Figure S4. RMSD plots of first (a) and second (b) MD simulations performed on the Ras-RB3 peptide complex; Figure S5. RMSD plot of the MD simulation performed on the Ras protein in complex with the 3_{10}-HBS RB3 peptide; Table S3. ΔGbinding average values of the interaction energies and the generalized Born solvation energy for the MD trajectories of the complexes' Ras-point-mutated 3_{10}-HBS RB3 peptides; Table S4. RMSD plots of 100 ns MD simulations performed on the Ras protein in complex with the 16 point-mutated 3_{10}-HBS RB3 peptides; Table S5. ΔGbinding average values of the interaction energies and the generalized Born solvation energy for the MD trajectories of the complexes' Ras-combinatorial peptides; Table S6. RMSD plots of 100 ns MD simulations performed on the Ras protein in complex with the selected 18 3_{10}-HBS RB3 combinatorial peptides; Table S7. The bar charts of protein-ligand interactions for the 18 3_{10}-HBS RB3 combinatorial peptides (left column), and the plots illustrating the frequency of interaction occurrences between the combinatorial peptides and Ras protein (right column).

Author Contributions: Conceptualization, R.B. and A.B.; methodology, M.R.G. and A.B.; software, A.B.; formal analysis, U.P. and A.B.; investigation, M.R.G.; resources, A.B.; data curation, M.R.G.; writing—original draft preparation, M.R.G.; writing—review and editing, R.B, U.P. and A.B.; visualization, U.P. and A.B.; supervision, U.P. and A.B.; project administration, A.B.; funding acquisition, U.P. and A.B. All authors have read and agreed to the published version of the manuscript.

Funding: The research activity of M.R.G. was funded by the Regione Siciliana, Assessorship of Productive Activities—Department of Productive Activities, funds: FSC 2014/2020, project name: Computational Molecular Design e Screening—CheMISt—CUPG77B17000110001, Scientific Research within the "Patto per il sud" of the Sicily Region. The APC were funded by Regione Siciliana, Assessorship of Productive Activities—Department of Productive Activities, Action 1.1.5 of PO FESR Sicilia 2014/2020, Project n. 086202000366—"OBIND", CUP G29J18000700007 to U.P.

Institutional Review Board Statement: Not applicable.

Informed Consent Statement: Not applicable.

Data Availability Statement: Data sharing not applicable.

Conflicts of Interest: The authors declare no conflict of interest.

References

1. Everitt, B.J. Neural and psychological mechanisms underlying compulsive drug seeking habits and drug memories—Indications for novel treatments of addiction. *Eur. J. Neurosci.* **2014**, *40*, 2163–2182. [CrossRef]
2. Berhow, M.T.; Hiroi, N.; Nestler, E.J. Regulation of ERK (Extracellular Signal Regulated Kinase), Part of the Neurotrophin Signal Transduction Cascade, in the Rat Mesolimbic Dopamine System by Chronic Exposure to Morphine or Cocaine. *J. Neurosci.* **1996**, *16*, 4707–4715. [CrossRef] [PubMed]
3. Nestler, E.J. Molecular mechanisms of drug addiction. *Neuropharmacology* **2004**, *47*, 24–32. [CrossRef]
4. Miller, C.A.; Marshall, J.F. Molecular Substrates for Retrieval and Reconsolidation of Cocaine-Associated Contextual Memory. *Neuron* **2005**, *47*, 873–884. [CrossRef] [PubMed]
5. Torregrossa, M.M.; Corlett, P.R.; Taylor, J.R. Aberrant learning and memory in addiction. *Neurobiol. Learn. Mem.* **2011**, *96*, 609–623. [CrossRef] [PubMed]
6. Itzhak, Y.; Perez-Lanza, D.; Liddie, S. The strength of aversive and appetitive associations and maladaptive behaviors. *IUBMB Life* **2014**, *66*, 559–571. [CrossRef] [PubMed]
7. Belin, D.; Belin-Rauscent, A.; Murray, J.E.; Everitt, B.J. Addiction: Failure of control over maladaptive incentive habits. *Curr. Opin. Neurobiol.* **2013**, *23*, 564–572. [CrossRef] [PubMed]
8. Sanchis-Segura, C.; Spanagel, R. Behavioural assessment of drug reinforcement and addictive features in rodents: An overview. *Addict. Biol.* **2006**, *11*, 2–38. [CrossRef] [PubMed]
9. Fasano, S.; Brambilla, R. Ras-ERK Signaling in Behavior: Old Questions and New Perspectives. *Front. Behav. Neurosci.* **2011**, *5*, 79. [CrossRef]
10. Pascoli, V.; Besnard, A.; Hervé, D.; Pagès, C.; Heck, N.; Girault, J.-A.; Caboche, J.; Vanhoutte, P. Cyclic Adenosine Monophosphate–Independent Tyrosine Phosphorylation of NR2B Mediates Cocaine-Induced Extracellular Signal-Regulated Kinase Activation. *Biol. Psychiatry* **2011**, *69*, 218–227. [CrossRef]
11. Pascoli, V.; Turiault, M.; Lüscher, C. Reversal of cocaine-evoked synaptic potentiation resets drug-induced adaptive behaviour. *Nature* **2012**, *481*, 71–75. [CrossRef] [PubMed]
12. Pascoli, V.; Cahill, E.; Bellivier, F.; Caboche, J.; Vanhoutte, P. Extracellular Signal-Regulated Protein Kinases 1 and 2 Activation by Addictive Drugs: A Signal Toward Pathological Adaptation. *Biol. Psychiatry* **2014**, *76*, 917–926. [CrossRef]
13. Cahill, E.; Salery, M.; Vanhoutte, P.; Caboche, J. Convergence of dopamine and glutamate signaling onto striatal ERK activation in response to drugs of abuse. *Front. Pharmacol.* **2014**, *4*, 172. [CrossRef] [PubMed]
14. García-Pardo, M.P.; Roger-Sanchez, C.; Rodríguez-Arias, M.; Miñarro, J.; Aguilar, M.A. Pharmacological modulation of protein kinases as a new approach to treat addiction to cocaine and opiates. *Eur. J. Pharmacol.* **2016**, *781*, 10–24. [CrossRef] [PubMed]
15. Valjent, E.; Corvol, J.-C.; Pagès, C.; Besson, M.-J.; Maldonado, R.; Caboche, J. Involvement of the Extracellular Signal-Regulated Kinase Cascade for Cocaine-Rewarding Properties. *J. Neurosci.* **2000**, *20*, 8701–8709. [CrossRef] [PubMed]
16. Lu, L.; Hope, B.T.; Dempsey, J.; Liu, S.Y.; Bossert, J.M.; Shaham, Y. Central amygdala ERK signaling pathway is critical to incubation of cocaine craving. *Nat. Neurosci.* **2005**, *8*, 212–219. [CrossRef] [PubMed]
17. Valjent, E.; Corbille, A.-G.; Bertran-Gonzalez, J.; Herve, D.; Girault, J.-A. Inhibition of ERK pathway or protein synthesis during reexposure to drugs of abuse erases previously learned place preference. *Proc. Natl. Acad. Sci. USA* **2006**, *103*, 2932–2937. [CrossRef]
18. Valjent, E.; Corvol, J.-C.; Trzaskos, J.M.; Girault, J.-A.; Hervé, D. Role of the ERK pathway in psychostimulant-induced locomotor sensitization. *BMC Neurosci.* **2006**, *7*, 20. [CrossRef] [PubMed]
19. Lu, L.; Koya, E.; Zhai, H.; Hope, B.T.; Shaham, Y. Role of ERK in cocaine addiction. *Trends Neurosci.* **2006**, *29*, 695–703. [CrossRef]
20. Ferguson, S.M.; Fasano, S.; Yang, P.; Brambilla, R.; Robinson, T.E. Knockout of ERK1 Enhances Cocaine-Evoked Immediate Early Gene Expression and Behavioral Plasticity. *Neuropsychopharmacology* **2006**, *31*, 2660–2668. [CrossRef]
21. Girault, J.; Valjent, E.; Caboche, J.; Herve, D. ERK2: A logical AND gate critical for drug-induced plasticity? *Curr. Opin. Pharmacol.* **2007**, *7*, 77–85. [CrossRef]

22. Fasano, S.; D'Antoni, A.; Orban, P.C.; Valjent, E.; Putignano, E.; Vara, H.; Pizzorusso, T.; Giustetto, M.; Yoon, B.; Soloway, P.; et al. Ras-Guanine Nucleotide-Releasing Factor 1 (Ras-GRF1) Controls Activation of Extracellular Signal-Regulated Kinase (ERK) Signaling in the Striatum and Long-Term Behavioral Responses to Cocaine. *Biol. Psychiatry* **2009**, *66*, 758–768. [CrossRef] [PubMed]
23. Papale, A.; D'Isa, R.; Menna, E.; Cerovic, M.; Solari, N.; Hardingham, N.; Cambiaghi, M.; Cursi, M.; Barbacid, M.; Leocani, L.; et al. Severe Intellectual Disability and Enhanced Gamma-Aminobutyric Acidergic Synaptogenesis in a Novel Model of Rare RASopathies. *Biol. Psychiatry* **2017**, *81*, 179–192. [CrossRef] [PubMed]
24. Pucilowska, J.; Vithayathil, J.; Pagani, M.; Kelly, C.; Karlo, J.C.; Robol, C.; Morella, I.; Gozzi, A.; Brambilla, R.; Landreth, G.E. Pharmacological Inhibition of ERK Signaling Rescues Pathophysiology and Behavioral Phenotype Associated with 16p11.2 Chromosomal Deletion in Mice. *J. Neurosci.* **2018**, *38*, 6640–6652. [CrossRef] [PubMed]
25. Kyosseva, S.V. Mitogen-Activated Protein Kinase Signaling. *Int. Rev. Neurobiol.* **2004**, *59*, 201–220. [PubMed]
26. Kim, E.K.; Choi, E.-J. Pathological roles of MAPK signaling pathways in human diseases. *Biochim. Biophys. Acta-Mol. Basis Dis.* **2010**, *1802*, 396–405. [CrossRef]
27. Seger, R.; Krebs, E.G. The MAPK signaling cascade. *FASEB J.* **1995**, *9*, 726–735. [CrossRef]
28. Vetter, I.R.; Wittinghofer, A. The Guanine Nucleotide-Binding Switch in Three Dimensions. *Science* **2001**, *294*, 1299–1304. [CrossRef]
29. Mattingly, R.R.; Macara, I.G. Phosphorylation-dependent activation of the Ras-GRF/CDC25Mm exchange factor by muscarinic receptors and G-protein $\beta\gamma$ subunits. *Nature* **1996**, *382*, 268–272. [CrossRef] [PubMed]
30. Baouz, S.; Jacquet, E.; Bernardi, A.; Parmeggiani, A. The N-terminal Moiety of CDC25 Mm, a GDP/GTP Exchange Factor of Ras Proteins, Controls the Activity of the Catalytic Domain. *J. Biol. Chem.* **1997**, *272*, 6671–6676. [CrossRef]
31. Farnsworth, C.L.; Freshney, N.W.; Rosen, L.B.; Ghosh, A.; Greenberg, M.E.; Feig, L.A. Calcium activation of Ras mediated by neuronal exchange factor Ras-GRF. *Nature* **1995**, *376*, 524–527. [CrossRef] [PubMed]
32. Schweighoffer, F.; Faure, M.; Fath, I.; Chevallier-Multon, M.; Apiou, F.; Dutrillaux, B.; Sturani, E.; Jacquet, M.; Tocque, B. Identification of a human guanine nucleotide-releasing factor (H-GRF55) specific for Ras proteins. *Oncogene* **1993**, *8*, 1477–1485. [PubMed]
33. Lenzen, C.; Cool, R.H.; Wittinghofer, A. Analysis of intrinsic and CDC25-stimulated guanine nucleotide exchange of p21ras-nucleotide complexes by fluorescence measurements. *Methods Enzymol.* **1995**, *255*, 95–109. [PubMed]
34. Tian, X.; Gotoh, T.; Tsuji, K.; Lo, E.H.; Huang, S.; Feig, L.A. Developmentally regulated role for Ras-GRFs in coupling NMDA glutamate receptors to Ras, Erk and CREB. *EMBO J.* **2004**, *23*, 1567–1575. [CrossRef] [PubMed]
35. Bar-Sagi, D. The Sos (Son of sevenless) protein. *Trends Endocrinol. Metab.* **1994**, *5*, 165–169. [CrossRef]
36. Tinhofer, I.; Maly, K.; Dietl, P.; Hochholdinger, F.; Mayr, S.; Obermeier, A.; Grunicke, H.H. Differential Ca^{2+} Signaling Induced by Activation of the Epidermal Growth Factor and Nerve Growth Factor Receptors. *J. Biol. Chem.* **1996**, *271*, 30505–30509. [CrossRef] [PubMed]
37. Egan, S.E.; Giddings, B.W.; Brooks, M.W.; Buday, L.; Sizeland, A.M.; Weinberg, R.A. Association of Sos Ras exchange protein with Grb2 is implicated in tyrosine kinase signal transduction and transformation. *Nature* **1993**, *363*, 45–51. [CrossRef] [PubMed]
38. Gale, N.W.; Kaplan, S.; Lowenstein, E.J.; Schlessinger, J.; Bar-Sagi, D. Grb2 mediates the EGF-dependent activation of guanine nucleotide exchange on Ras. *Nature* **1993**, *363*, 88–92. [CrossRef] [PubMed]
39. Li, N.; Batzer, A.; Daly, R.; Yajnik, V.; Skolnik, E.; Chardin, P.; Bar-Sagi, D.; Margolis, B.; Schlessinger, J. Guanine-nucleotide-releasing factor hSos1 binds to Grb2 and links receptor tyrosine kinases to Ras signalling. *Nature* **1993**, *363*, 85–88. [CrossRef] [PubMed]
40. Buday, L.; Downward, J. Epidermal growth factor regulates p21ras through the formation of a complex of receptor, Grb2 adapter protein, and Sos nucleotide exchange factor. *Cell* **1993**, *73*, 611–620. [CrossRef]
41. Lenzen, C.; Cool, R.H.; Prinz, H.; Kuhlmann, J.; Wittinghofer, A. Kinetic Analysis by Fluorescence of the Interaction between Ras and the Catalytic Domain of the Guanine Nucleotide Exchange Factor Cdc25 Mm. *Biochemistry* **1998**, *37*, 7420–7430. [CrossRef] [PubMed]
42. Zarich, N.; Oliva, J.L.; Jorge, R.; Santos, E.; Rojas, J.M. The isoform-specific stretch of hSos1 defines a new Grb2-binding domain. *Oncogene* **2000**, *19*, 5872–5883. [CrossRef]
43. Boriack-Sjodin, P.A.; Margarit, S.M.; Bar-Sagi, D.; Kuriyan, J. The structural basis of the activation of Ras by Sos. *Nature* **1998**, *394*, 337–343. [CrossRef]
44. Chardin, P.; Mattei, M.-G. Chromosomal localization of two genes encoding human ras exchange factors: SOS1 maps to the 2p22 -> p16 region and SOS2 to the 14q21 -> q22 region of the human genome. *Cytogenet. Genome Res.* **1994**, *66*, 68–69. [CrossRef]
45. Boguski, M.S.; McCormick, F. Proteins regulating Ras and its relatives. *Nature* **1993**, *366*, 643–654. [CrossRef]
46. Liu, B.X.; Wei, W.; Broek, D. The catalytic domain of the mouse sos1 gene product activates Ras proteins in vivo and in vitro. *Oncogene* **1993**, *8*, 3081–3084. [PubMed]
47. Margarit, S.M.; Sondermann, H.; Hall, B.E.; Nagar, B.; Hoelz, A.; Pirruccello, M.; Bar-Sagi, D.; Kuriyan, J. Structural Evidence for Feedback Activation by Ras·GTP of the Ras-Specific Nucleotide Exchange Factor SOS. *Cell* **2003**, *112*, 685–695. [CrossRef]
48. Sondermann, H.; Soisson, S.M.; Boykevisch, S.; Yang, S.-S.; Bar-Sagi, D.; Kuriyan, J. Structural Analysis of Autoinhibition in the Ras Activator Son of Sevenless. *Cell* **2004**, *119*, 393–405. [CrossRef] [PubMed]

49. Willumsen, B.M.; Papageorge, A.G.; Kung, H.F.; Bekesi, E.; Robins, T.; Johnsen, M.; Vass, W.C.; Lowy, D.R. Mutational analysis of a ras catalytic domain. *Mol. Cell. Biol.* **1986**, *6*, 2646–2654. [CrossRef] [PubMed]
50. Fasano, O.; Crechet, J.B.; De Vendittis, E.; Zahn, R.; Feger, G.; Vitelli, A.; Parmeggiani, A. Yeast mutants temperature-sensitive for growth after random mutagenesis of the chromosomal RAS2 gene and deletion of the RAS1 gene. *EMBO J.* **1988**, *7*, 3375–3383. [CrossRef] [PubMed]
51. Mistou, M.Y.; Jacquet, E.; Poullet, P.; Rensland, H.; Gideon, P.; Schlichting, I.; Wittinghofer, A.; Parmeggiani, A. Mutations of Ha-ras p21 that define important regions for the molecular mechanism of the SDC25 C-domain, a guanine nucleotide dissociation stimulator. *EMBO J.* **1992**, *11*, 2391–2397. [CrossRef] [PubMed]
52. Howe, L.R.; Marshall, C.J. Identification of amino acids in p21ras involved in exchange factor interaction. *Oncogene* **1993**, *8*, 2583–2590. [PubMed]
53. Segal, M.; Willumsen, B.M.; Levitzki, A. Residues crucial for Ras interaction with GDP-GTP exchangers. *Proc. Natl. Acad. Sci. USA* **1993**, *90*, 5564–5568. [CrossRef] [PubMed]
54. Mosteller, R.D.; Han, J.; Broek, D. Identification of residues of the H-ras protein critical for functional interaction with guanine nucleotide exchange factors. *Mol. Cell. Biol.* **1994**, *14*, 1104–1112. [CrossRef] [PubMed]
55. Park, W.; Mosteller, R.D.; Broek, D. Amino acid residues in the CDC25 guanine nucleotide exchange factor critical for interaction with Ras. *Mol. Cell. Biol.* **1994**, *14*, 8117–8122. [CrossRef] [PubMed]
56. Quilliam, L.A.; Kato, K.; Rabun, K.M.; Hisaka, M.M.; Huff, S.Y.; Campbell-Burk, S.; Der, C.J. Identification of residues critical for Ras(17N) growth-inhibitory phenotype and for Ras interaction with guanine nucleotide exchange factors. *Mol. Cell. Biol.* **1994**, *14*, 1113–1121. [CrossRef] [PubMed]
57. Quilliam, L.A.; Hisaka, M.M.; Zhong, S.; Lowry, A.; Mosteller, R.D.; Han, J.; Drugan, J.K.; Broek, D.; Campbell, S.L.; Der, C.J. Involvement of the Switch 2 Domain of Ras in Its Interaction with Guanine Nucleotide Exchange Factors. *J. Biol. Chem.* **1996**, *271*, 11076–11082. [CrossRef]
58. Day, G.-J.; Mosteller, R.D.; Broek, D. Distinct Subclasses of Small GTPases Interact with Guanine Nucleotide Exchange Factors in a Similar Manner. *Mol. Cell. Biol.* **1998**, *18*, 7444–7454. [CrossRef]
59. Freedman, T.S.; Sondermann, H.; Friedland, G.D.; Kortemme, T.; Bar-Sagi, D.; Marqusee, S.; Kuriyan, J. A Ras-induced conformational switch in the Ras activator Son of sevenless. *Proc. Natl. Acad. Sci. USA* **2006**, *103*, 16692–16697. [CrossRef]
60. Protein Data Bank. Available online: https://pdb101.rcsb.org (accessed on 21 May 2020).
61. Hall, B.E.; Yang, S.S.; Boriack-Sjodin, P.A.; Kuriyan, J.; Bar-Sagi, D. Structure-based Mutagenesis Reveals Distinct Functions for Ras Switch 1 and Switch 2 in Sos-catalyzed Guanine Nucleotide Exchange. *J. Biol. Chem.* **2001**, *276*, 27629–27637. [CrossRef] [PubMed]
62. O'Bryan, J.P. Pharmacological targeting of RAS: Recent success with direct inhibitors. *Pharmacol. Res.* **2019**, *139*, 503–511. [CrossRef] [PubMed]
63. Papale, A.; Morella, I.M.; Indrigo, M.T.; Bernardi, R.E.; Marrone, L.; Marchisella, F.; Brancale, A.; Spanagel, R.; Brambilla, R.; Fasano, S. Impairment of cocaine-mediated behaviours in mice by clinically relevant Ras-ERK inhibitors. *eLife* **2016**, *5*, e17111. [CrossRef] [PubMed]
64. Brambilla, R.; Papale, A.; Fasano, S. Transcription factor modulating terpene biosynthesis. U.S. Patent WO 2012/016963 Al 2012, 13 December 2012.
65. Ramsey, J.D.; Flynn, N.H. Cell-penetrating peptides transport therapeutics into cells. *Pharmacol. Ther.* **2015**, *154*, 78–86. [CrossRef] [PubMed]
66. Raucher, D.; Ryu, J.S. Cell-penetrating peptides: Strategies for anticancer treatment. *Trends Mol. Med.* **2015**, *21*, 560–570. [CrossRef] [PubMed]
67. Brambilla, R.; Papale, A.; Fasano, S. Peptides for the Treatment of Brain Diseases. U.S. Patent WO/2012/016963, 9 February 2012.
68. Gump, J.M.; Dowdy, S.F. TAT transduction: The molecular mechanism and therapeutic prospects. *Trends Mol. Med.* **2007**, *13*, 443–448. [CrossRef] [PubMed]
69. Santini, E.; Valjent, E.; Usiello, A.; Carta, M.; Borgkvist, A.; Girault, J.-A.; Herve, D.; Greengard, P.; Fisone, G. Critical Involvement of cAMP/DARPP-32 and Extracellular Signal-Regulated Protein Kinase Signaling in L-DOPA-Induced Dyskinesia. *J. Neurosci.* **2007**, *27*, 6995–7005. [CrossRef]
70. Santini, E.; Alcacer, C.; Cacciatore, S.; Heiman, M.; Hervé, D.; Greengard, P.; Girault, J.-A.; Valjent, E.; Fisone, G. l-DOPA activates ERK signaling and phosphorylates histone H3 in the striatonigral medium spiny neurons of hemiparkinsonian mice. *J. Neurochem.* **2009**, *108*, 621–633. [CrossRef]
71. Darmopil, S.; Martín, A.B.; De Diego, I.R.; Ares, S.; Moratalla, R. Genetic Inactivation of Dopamine D1 but Not D2 Receptors Inhibits L-DOPA–Induced Dyskinesia and Histone Activation. *Biol. Psychiatry* **2009**, *66*, 603–613. [CrossRef] [PubMed]
72. Pal, S.; Banerjee, S.; Kumar, A.; Prabhakaran, E.N. H-Bond Surrogate-Stabilized Shortest Single-Turn α-Helices: Sp 2 Constraints and Residue Preferences for the Highest α-Helicities. *ACS Omega* **2020**, *5*, 13902–13912. [CrossRef]
73. Patgiri, A.; Jochim, A.L.; Arora, P.S. A Hydrogen Bond Surrogate Approach for Stabilization of Short Peptide Sequences in α-Helical Conformation. *Acc. Chem. Res.* **2008**, *41*, 1289–1300. [CrossRef] [PubMed]
74. Davis, J.M.; Tsou, L.K.; Hamilton, A.D. Synthetic non-peptide mimetics of α-helices. *Chem. Soc. Rev.* **2007**, *36*, 326–334. [CrossRef] [PubMed]

75. Cheng, R.P.; Gellman, S.H.; DeGrado, W.F. β-Peptides: From Structure to Function. *Chem. Rev.* **2001**, *101*, 3219–3232. [CrossRef] [PubMed]
76. Bautista, A.D.; Craig, C.J.; Harker, E.A.; Schepartz, A. Sophistication of foldamer form and function in vitro and in vivo. *Curr. Opin. Chem. Biol.* **2007**, *11*, 685–692. [CrossRef] [PubMed]
77. Garner, J.; Harding, M.M. Design and synthesis of α-helical peptides and mimetics. *Org. Biomol. Chem.* **2007**, *5*, 3577. [CrossRef] [PubMed]
78. Goodman, C.M.; Choi, S.; Shandler, S.; DeGrado, W.F. Foldamers as versatile frameworks for the design and evolution of function. *Nat. Chem. Biol.* **2007**, *3*, 252–262. [CrossRef] [PubMed]
79. Murray, J.K.; Gellman, S.H. Targeting protein–protein interactions: Lessons from p53/MDM2. *Biopolymers* **2007**, *88*, 657–686. [CrossRef]
80. Siedlecka, M.; Goch, G.; Ejchart, A.; Sticht, H.; Bierzynski, A. α-Helix nucleation by a calcium-binding peptide loop. *Proc. Natl. Acad. Sci. USA* **1999**, *96*, 903–908. [CrossRef] [PubMed]
81. Yang, J.; Zhao, K.; Gong, Y.; Vologodskii, A.; Kallenbach, N.R. α-Helix Nucleation Constant in Copolypeptides of Alanine and Ornithine or Lysine. *J. Am. Chem. Soc.* **1998**, *120*, 10646–10652. [CrossRef]
82. Wang, D.; Chen, K.; Kulp, J.L.; Arora, P.S. Evaluation of Biologically Relevant Short α-Helices Stabilized by a Main-Chain Hydrogen-Bond Surrogate. *J. Am. Chem. Soc.* **2006**, *128*, 9248–9256. [CrossRef]
83. Kemp, D.S.; Curran, T.P.; Boyd, J.G.; Allen, T.J. Studies of N-terminal templates for.alpha.-helix formation. Synthesis and conformational analysis of peptide conjugates of (2S,5S,8S,11S)-1-acetyl-1,4-diaza-3-keto-5-carboxy-10-thiatricyclo[2.8.1.04,8]tridecane (Ac-Hel1-OH). *J. Org. Chem.* **1991**, *56*, 6683–6697. [CrossRef]
84. Maurer, T.; Garrenton, L.S.; Oh, A.; Pitts, K.; Anderson, D.J.; Skelton, N.J.; Fauber, B.P.; Pan, B.; Malek, S.; Stokoe, D.; et al. Small-molecule ligands bind to a distinct pocket in Ras and inhibit SOS-mediated nucleotide exchange activity. *Proc. Natl. Acad. Sci. USA* **2012**, *109*, 5299–5304. [CrossRef]
85. Cabezas, E.; Satterthwait, A.C. The Hydrogen Bond Mimic Approach: Solid-Phase Synthesis of a Peptide Stabilized as an α-Helix with a Hydrazone Link. *J. Am. Chem. Soc.* **1999**, *121*, 3862–3875. [CrossRef]
86. Pal, S.; Prabhakaran, E.N. Hydrogen bond surrogate stabilized water soluble 310-helix from a disordered pentapeptide containing coded α-amino acids. *Tetrahedron Lett.* **2018**, *59*, 2515–2519. [CrossRef]
87. Kortemme, T.; Kim, D.E.; Baker, D. Computational Alanine Scanning of Protein-Protein Interfaces. *Sci. Signal.* **2004**, *2004*, pl2. [CrossRef]
88. Kortemme, T.; Baker, D. A simple physical model for binding energy hot spots in protein-protein complexes. *Proc. Natl. Acad. Sci. USA* **2002**, *99*, 14116–14121. [CrossRef]
89. Camacho, C.; Coulouris, G.; Avagyan, V.; Ma, N.; Papadopoulos, J.; Bealer, K.; Madden, T.L. BLAST+: Architecture and applications. *BMC Bioinform.* **2009**, *10*, 421. [CrossRef] [PubMed]
90. Protein BLAST Sequence Alignment. Available online: https://blast.ncbi.nlm.nih.gov/Blast.cgi?PROGRAM=blastp&PAGE_TYPE=BlastSearch&LINK_LOC=blasthome (accessed on 25 August 2020).
91. Bowers, K.J.; Chow, E.; Xu, H.; Dror, R.O.; Eastwood, M.P.; Gregersen, B.A.; Klepeis, J.L.; Kolossvary, I.; Moraes, M.A.; Sacerdoti, F.D.; et al. Scalable Algorithms for Molecular Dynamics Simulations on Commodity Clusters. In Proceedings of the SC '06: 2006 ACM/IEEE Conference on Supercomputing, Tampa, FL, USA, 11–17 November 2006; Association for Computing Machinery: Tampa, FL, USA, 2006.
92. Beard, H.; Cholleti, A.; Pearlman, D.; Sherman, W.; Loving, K.A. Applying Physics-Based Scoring to Calculate Free Energies of Binding for Single Amino Acid Mutations in Protein-Protein Complexes. *PLoS ONE* **2013**, *8*, e82849. [CrossRef] [PubMed]
93. Madhavi Sastry, G.; Adzhigirey, M.; Day, T.; Annabhimoju, R.; Sherman, W. Protein and ligand preparation: Parameters, protocols, and influence on virtual screening enrichments. *J. Comput. Aided. Mol. Des.* **2013**, *27*, 221–234. [CrossRef] [PubMed]
94. Greenwood, J.R.; Calkins, D.; Sullivan, A.P.; Shelley, J.C. Towards the comprehensive, rapid, and accurate prediction of the favorable tautomeric states of drug-like molecules in aqueous solution. *J. Comput. Aided. Mol. Des.* **2010**, *24*, 591–604. [CrossRef]
95. Olsson, M.H.M.; Søndergaard, C.R.; Rostkowski, M.; Jensen, J.H. PROPKA3: Consistent Treatment of Internal and Surface Residues in Empirical p K a Predictions. *J. Chem. Theory Comput.* **2011**, *7*, 525–537. [CrossRef] [PubMed]
96. Mekni, N.; De Rosa, M.; Cipollina, C.; Gulotta, M.R.; De Simone, G.; Lombino, J.; Padova, A.; Perricone, U. In Silico Insights towards the Identification of NLRP3 Druggable Hot Spots. *Int. J. Mol. Sci.* **2019**, *20*, 4974. [CrossRef]
97. Perricone, U.; Gulotta, M.R.; Lombino, J.; Parrino, B.; Cascioferro, S.; Diana, P.; Cirrincione, G.; Padova, A. An overview of recent molecular dynamics applications as medicinal chemistry tools for the undruggable site challenge. *MedChemComm* **2018**, *9*, 920–936. [CrossRef] [PubMed]
98. Gulotta, M.R.; Lombino, J.; Perricone, U.; De Simone, G.; Mekni, N.; De Rosa, M.; Diana, P.; Padova, A. Targeting SARS-CoV-2 RBD Interface: A Supervised Computational Data-Driven Approach to Identify Potential Modulators. *ChemMedChem* **2020**, *15*, 1921–1931. [CrossRef] [PubMed]
99. Gulotta, M.R.; De Simone, G.; John, J.; Perricone, U.; Brancale, A. A Computer-Based Methodology to Design Non-Standard Peptides Potentially Able to Prevent HOX-PBX1-Associated Cancer Diseases. *Int. J. Mol. Sci.* **2021**, *22*, 5670. [CrossRef] [PubMed]
100. Mark, P.; Nilsson, L. Structure and Dynamics of the TIP3P, SPC, and SPC/E Water Models at 298 K. *J. Phys. Chem. A* **2001**, *105*, 9954–9960. [CrossRef]

101. Roos, K.; Wu, C.; Damm, W.; Reboul, M.; Stevenson, J.M.; Lu, C.; Dahlgren, M.K.; Mondal, S.; Chen, W.; Wang, L.; et al. OPLS3e: Extending Force Field Coverage for Drug-Like Small Molecules. *J. Chem. Theory Comput.* **2019**, *15*, 1863–1874. [CrossRef]
102. Jacobson, M.P.; Friesner, R.A.; Xiang, Z.; Honig, B. On the Role of the Crystal Environment in Determining Protein Side-chain Conformations. *J. Mol. Biol.* **2002**, *320*, 597–608. [CrossRef]
103. Jacobson, M.P.; Pincus, D.L.; Rapp, C.S.; Day, T.J.F.; Honig, B.; Shaw, D.E.; Friesner, R.A. A hierarchical approach to all-atom protein loop prediction. *Proteins Struct. Funct. Bioinform.* **2004**, *55*, 351–367. [CrossRef] [PubMed]

pharmaceuticals

MDPI

Review

Mechanistic Understanding from Molecular Dynamics in Pharmaceutical Research 2: Lipid Membrane in Drug Design

Tomasz Róg [1,*], Mykhailo Girych [1] and Alex Bunker [2]

1 Department of Physics, University of Helsinki, 00014 Helsinki, Finland; mykhailo.girych@helsinki.fi
2 Drug Research Program, Division of Pharmaceutical Biosciences, Faculty of Pharmacy, University of Helsinki, 00014 Helsinki, Finland; alex.bunker@helsinki.fi
* Correspondence: tomasz.rog@helsinki.fi

Abstract: We review the use of molecular dynamics (MD) simulation as a drug design tool in the context of the role that the lipid membrane can play in drug action, i.e., the interaction between candidate drug molecules and lipid membranes. In the standard "lock and key" paradigm, only the interaction between the drug and a specific active site of a specific protein is considered; the environment in which the drug acts is, from a biophysical perspective, far more complex than this. The possible mechanisms though which a drug can be designed to tinker with physiological processes are significantly broader than merely fitting to a single active site of a single protein. In this paper, we focus on the role of the lipid membrane, arguably the most important element outside the proteins themselves, as a case study. We discuss work that has been carried out, using MD simulation, concerning the transfection of drugs through membranes that act as biological barriers in the path of the drugs, the behavior of drug molecules within membranes, how their collective behavior can affect the structure and properties of the membrane and, finally, the role lipid membranes, to which the vast majority of drug target proteins are associated, can play in mediating the interaction between drug and target protein. This review paper is the second in a two-part series covering MD simulation as a tool in pharmaceutical research; both are designed as pedagogical review papers aimed at both pharmaceutical scientists interested in exploring how the tool of MD simulation can be applied to their research and computational scientists interested in exploring the possibility of a pharmaceutical context for their research.

Keywords: molecular modeling; permeability; membrane disruption; membrane proteins; drugs; antimicrobial peptides

Citation: Róg, T.; Girych, M.; Bunker, A. Mechanistic Understanding from Molecular Dynamics in Pharmaceutical Research 2: Lipid Membrane in Drug Design. *Pharmaceuticals* **2021**, *14*, 1062. https://doi.org/10.3390/ph14101062

Academic Editor: Osvaldo Andrade Santos-Filho

Received: 20 September 2021
Accepted: 15 October 2021
Published: 19 October 2021

1. Introduction

In the most breathtaking giant leap forward in life science since the determination of the double helix structure of DNA, the general structure from the sequence problem has now been solved for the case of an individual protein domain [1]. Additionally, in 2020, the Human Proteome project, after ten years of work, reported that their complete high-stringency blueprint of the human proteome is 90.4% complete [2]; thus, an accurate sequence of every human protein and the most common variants is in sight. Together, these developments mean that we can now foresee being in possession of accurate structures for the active sites of all human proteins and most common variants; with predicted advances in computational power and the development of better algorithms, it is no longer fantasizing to speculate that, in the near future, it could be possible to obtain a sufficiently accurate estimate of the binding free energy for any given drug candidate molecule for every single possible human protein active site it may encounter. This may represent a Holy Grail of drug design; however, it does not mean the problem of computational drug design will have become a solved problem—it leaves out the rest of the biophysical landscape within which drug action takes place. This review paper explores the role that computational modeling, using the toolkit of molecular dynamics (MD) simulation, can play regarding drug design outside of this "lock and key" paradigm, focusing on one fundamentally important aspect: the lipid membrane.

In our previous review paper [3], part 1 of this series, we presented many examples of how MD simulation has been used as a tool to provide mechanistic insight relevant to drug delivery and how this insight has been used, in concrete practical terms; we now continue the discussion of the role MD simulation has and will continue to play in pharmaceutical research, focusing, in this review paper, on its role in drug design, specifically covering its ability to elucidate a central element left out of the conventional drug design paradigm: lipid membranes. As with part 1, this is a pedagogical review, with two separate target audiences, pharmaceutical researchers interested in understanding the increasing role MD simulation can play in their research, and computational researchers interested in the possibility of developing a pharmaceutical context for their research.

In part 1, we reviewed what MD simulation is and the limitations of both the aforementioned conventional "lock and key" approach to drug design [4,5] and the absorption, distribution, metabolism, and excretion (ADME) approach to drug delivery [6–8] that has led to the diminishing returns known as "Eroom's law" [9]. We showed how MD simulation can provide mechanistic insight needed for the development of advanced drug delivery mechanisms. We argued that research has been hamstrung by the limited paradigm used and that MD simulation has the power to bring into consideration the broader biophysical context within which drug delivery occurs; we now proceed to argue the same for the case of drug design. As discussed in part 1, drug design has been carried out within a limited paradigm that only considered a compromise between the drug interaction with the active site of a specific target protein and its solubility; increasingly sophisticated techniques are being used to approximate the relative binding free energies of different drugs, in each case a balance being reached between maximizing accuracy and minimizing the computational resources used [10]. Although techniques have recently been developed to consider the importance of binding kinetics [10–14], in addition to thermodynamics, this still does not take the broader biophysical context in which the drug interaction with the protein occurs into consideration, i.e., the environment beyond the immediate drug protein interaction; additionally, it is possible for drugs to have an effect that does not even involve interaction with a protein, i.e., a mode of action entirely external to the "lock and key" paradigm.

The elucidation of all aspects of the biophysical context of drug action is currently beyond reach and even all aspects that MD simulation is capable of elucidating are beyond the scope of a single review paper; we thus focus on an important element involved in drug action left out of the "lock and key" paradigm: lipid membranes. Biomembranes, complex fluid structures formed primarily from bilayers of phospholipids, are one of the primary building blocks of life [15–18]. In all cases, drug access to its target and action involves, in some fashion, interaction with biomembranes. Drug molecules must traverse membranes that form biological barriers. The majority of proteins that are drug targets are associated with biomembranes and the membrane plays a role in the interaction with substrates, thus potential drug molecules; interactions of both target proteins and drugs, with the membrane to which the protein is associated, play a role in the drug–target protein interaction. Finally, there are cases where the mode of action of the drug does not even involve interaction with a protein; the drug acts directly on a specific biomembrane rather than with a protein. In all of these cases, MD simulation, a mature tool for the study of biomembranes [19–27], can provide a window on the role the lipid membrane plays in drug action; this review paper describes how MD provides mechanistic insight and includes many examples where it has been successfully applied. We will first discuss the behavior of drug molecules in the membrane, then how drugs transfect through membranes that form biological barriers and how drugs can, collectively, at sufficient concentration, affect the properties of the membrane. Finally, we will discuss the role the membrane plays in the selection of substrates, thus potential drug molecules, for membrane associated proteins. In all these areas, MD simulation has acted as a unique window capable of adding mechanistic insight that can be applied in drug design; we describe many case studies where this has been used effectively.

While previous review papers have shown how MD simulation has helped elucidate the role the lipid membrane plays in substrate and thus drug selection for membrane proteins [28–32], drug membrane interactions [33–41], drug delivery [3,42–45], antimicrobial peptides [46–54], and methodologies [28,55–60], this is the first review paper, that we are aware of, focusing on the entirety of the use of MD simulation to incorporate the role played by interactions with lipid membranes in drug design. This can be seen, in turn, as a case study of the potential for MD simulation to expand the paradigm of drug design to all aspects of the broader biophysical environment within which drug action occurs.

We now refer the reader to our discussion of the basics of the MD simulation method in our previous review paper, i.e., "part 1" [3], or an equivalent discussion found in Braun et al. [61], where its ability to provide an effective visualization of the system studied with all atom resolution (also reviewed in [62–65]) and how coarse grained (CG) potential sets can be used to effectively zoom out to study larger length and time scales (also reviewed in [66–70]) are covered. However, the application of MD simulation to the study of the more complex systems involved in drug action rather than drug delivery, that we cover in this review, requires advanced MD simulation related methodologies not discussed in the aforementioned references; these will now be described and examples of their use will be encountered later, throughout the rest of the paper. As an aside, it is appropriate that we now draw attention to the fact that the chemical structures of the lipids discussed in this manuscript are shown in Figure 1.

2. Advanced Simulation Methods

In its pure form, MD simulation provides a window into the system, with all atom resolutions, at a timescale of up to 1–2 μs and a box size of up to 15–20 nm, significantly greater with CG models [3]. In our previous review paper [3], we discussed many examples where this has been used in issues related to drug delivery, and how it is a valuable tool when used its in pure form; however, significant limitations are encountered when one addresses issues related to drug design rather than delivery.

When expanding what we consider in drug design the oversimplified "lock and key" paradigm to the broader context of all the relevant biophysics, there are many challenges that result from the added complexity. Within the context of biophysics, drug design can be studied through the paradigm of the interaction of four different basic varieties of entities, each of which present their own challenges: (1) small drug molecules, which, while simple in structure, are often chemically/structurally novel as they are often synthetically created molecules that do not naturally exist, thus in many cases new parameter sets must be developed and extra challenges are encountered in attempting the development of CG models; (2) specifically structured large biomolecules, e.g., proteins and nucleic acids, that have a highly specific structure defined by a very rigid, steep, and complex energy landscape that molecules that interact with them must negotiate; (3) large unstructured molecules, e.g., polymers that, while without specific structure but with an uncomplicated energy landscape governing their interactions, exhibit complex behavior that is difficult to model due to topological effects that arise spontaneously due to their size and flexibility; (4) lipid membranes, that are flexible, complex, and diverse entities with very complex interactions with other elements. Clearly, one must adopt more advanced methodologies rooted in MD simulation to explore this complex landscape and these will now be introduced. Discussing this will, however, require the presentation of some mathematical and physical (thermodynamic) constructs.

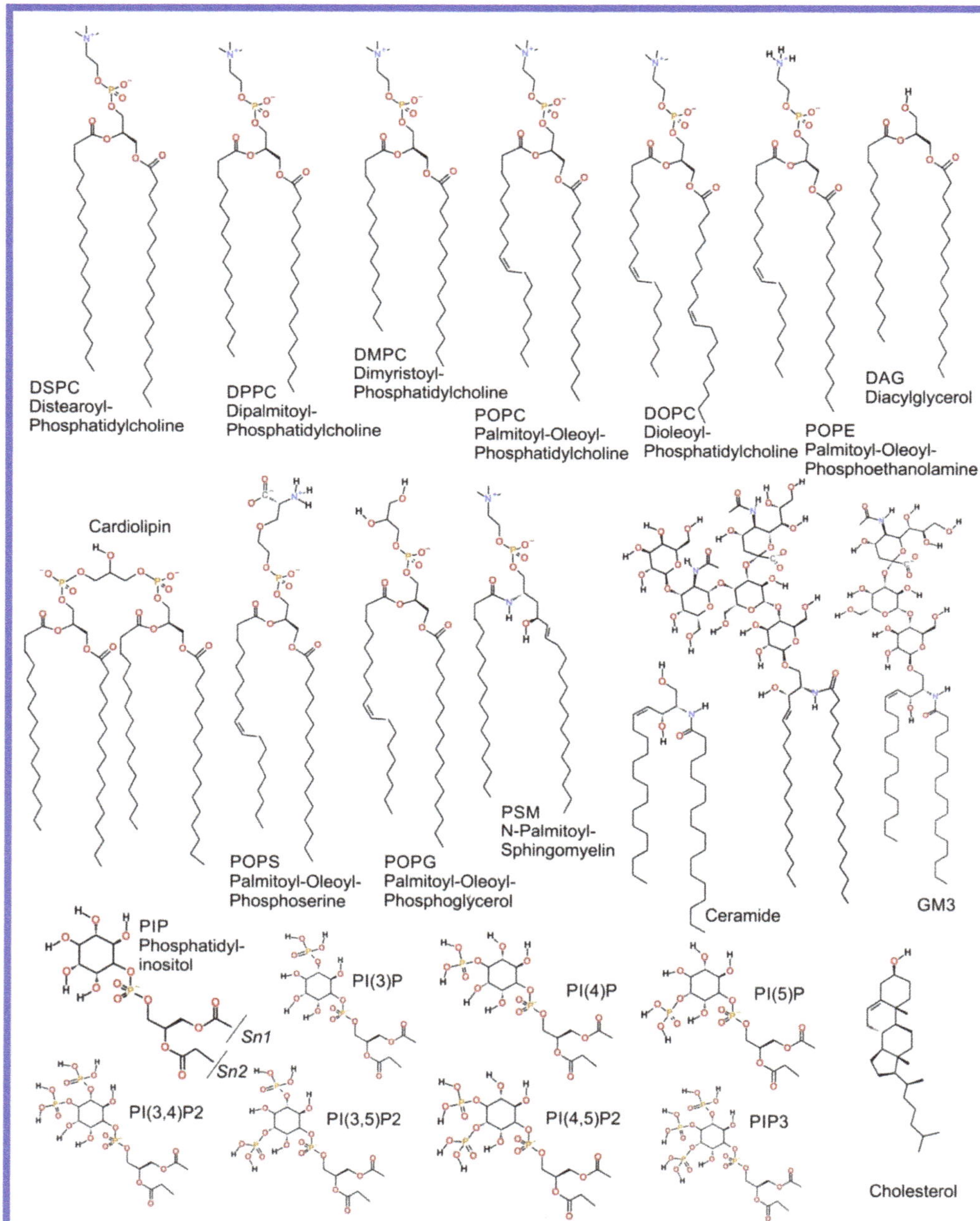

Figure 1. Chemical structure of lipids mentioned in this paper.

Let us consider our window into a given physical system that is provided by MD simulation: a set of molecules with periodic boundary conditions being simulated at temperature T, e.g., a section of lipid membrane, protein, or other macromolecule or molecular complex in solvent. Technically, this can be seen as a set N particles governed by a potential that is a function of the position of all particles: $U(\vec{r}^N)$; $\vec{r}^N$ is the position of all particles, which can in turn be seen as a point in a $3N$ dimensional space with $\{\vec{r}^N\}$ representing the entirety of this space, i.e., the set of all possible particle positions, known as the *conformation space*, i.e., the system of N particles governed by potential $U(\vec{r}^N)$ can be said to inhabit the space $\{\vec{r}^N\}$. If we begin the simulation at a certain point in this space $\vec{r}^N_0$ and simulate, with a thermostat holding the system at constant temperature T, using the MD simulation method described in our previous review paper "part 1" [3], then the system will move around in this space following what can be called a *trajectory*. In any real simulation there will be enough particles and $U(\vec{r}^N)$ will be sufficiently non-trivial so that we can assume what is known as the ergodic hypothesis: given infinite time, the system will eventually pass through all possible points in $\{\vec{r}^N\}$. The relative amount of time spent within a given $3N$ dimensional differential element $d\vec{r}^N$ will be equivalent to the probability of the system being within that element that we will signify as $P(\vec{r}^N, T)d\vec{r}^N$. For a system at constant temperature, i.e., a *canonical ensemble* [71],

$$P(\vec{r}^N, T) = \frac{e^{-\gamma}}{Z_u(T)} \quad \gamma = \frac{U(\vec{r}^N)}{T} \tag{1}$$

where $Z_u(T)$ is a normalization factor known as the *partition function* that is, for any but the most trivial systems, impossible to determine analytically; in this equation, we have assumed temperature to be in units that match $U(\vec{r}^N)$, thus have not included the Boltzmann constant normally seen in this equation. A clever way around the impossible to determine partition function makes use of the principle of detailed balance: given two points in the conformation space $\vec{r}^N_1$ and $\vec{r}^N_2$, the ratio of the transition probabilities between these two points, $W(\vec{r}^N_1 \rightarrow \vec{r}^N_2, T)$ and $W(\vec{r}^N_2 \rightarrow \vec{r}^N_1, T)$ is equal to the ratio of the probabilities of being at the two points:

$$\frac{W(\vec{r}^N_2 \rightarrow \vec{r}^N_1, T)}{W(\vec{r}^N_1 \rightarrow \vec{r}^N_2, T)} = \frac{P(\vec{r}^N_1, T)}{P(\vec{r}^N_2, T)} \tag{2}$$

Given

$$\Delta\gamma = \frac{U(\vec{r}^N_2)}{T} - \frac{U(\vec{r}^N_1)}{T}, \tag{3}$$

an algorithm that satisfies all preceding relations, is: for a system at $\vec{r}^N_1$ considering a transition to $\vec{r}^N_2$, if $\Delta\gamma \leq 0$ the system moves to $\vec{r}^N_2$ otherwise the transition occurs with probability $e^{-\Delta\gamma}$. This can be continued indefinitely, following what is known as a *Markov chain*, moving through conformation space sampling a set of states that will have a distribution of $P(\vec{r}^N, T)$ in the limit of infinite steps. The result of carrying this out for a finite number of steps is thus an approximation of $P(\vec{r}^N, T)$, that we will refer to as $\overline{P(\vec{r}^N, T)}$; as the number of steps in the Markov chain increases, the longer the trajectory, the greater the accuracy of our approximation. The simulation of a system in this fashion is known as a *Monte Carlo (MC) simulation* [72].

If one is able to concisely calculate $P(\vec{r}^N, T)$ over all $\{\vec{r}^N\}$ for any system, then one will know everything that is to be known about that system and any property of that system can be calculated; this is, however, impossible for all but the most trivial systems. Yet, both MC and MD simulation are able to provide an incomplete estimate of this: the above mentioned $\overline{P(\vec{r}^N, T)}$; the longer the trajectory the more information, for the case of

MD as well as MC simulation. Depending on how the algorithms are constructed, each have their relative strengths and weaknesses and can be hybridized, particularly since MD simulation has been shown to be superior at relaxing the local degrees of freedom, while MC simulation, if designed properly, can more effectively relax the more global degrees of freedom [73–76]. While MD simulation, if carried out on its own, can also provide information related to dynamics, this information is usually of secondary importance; we will only consider MC and MD simulation as means to provide a result for $\overline{P(\vec{r}^{N}, T)}$ here.

The problem with both MC and MD simulation, or even the two hybridized, in their basic forms, is that the approximation of $P(\vec{r}^{N}, T)$ ($\overline{P(\vec{r}^{N}, T)}$) will provide the most information in the regions of the conformation space of the system where $P(\vec{r}^{N}, T)$ is greatest. For many cases, for example, the aforementioned systems related to drug delivery [3], this may be sufficient, i.e., the answer to the question "what does the system normally do?" may be all we seek. There are many cases where this will not be sufficient, for example, when calculating the free energy to cross certain barriers from one region of conformation space to another. A useful schematic is to express $\vec{r}^{N}$ as a single dimension x rather than $3N$ dimensions and plot $U(\vec{r}^{N})$ as $U(x)$, as shown in Figure 2. The energy landscape is very rough with many peaks and valleys; with either MC or MD, in their basic form, crossing a very high energy barrier will be an extremely unlikely event. If you have managed to determine the global energy minimum, then you will only obtain results for $\overline{P(\vec{r}^{N}, T)}$ in the local valley of the global minimum. Even worse, usually, you cannot even be certain you have found the global minimum and thus will only be exploring the vicinity of a local minimum. In general, the primary concern is the region of $\{\vec{r}^{N}\}$ where you need to obtain information regarding $P(\vec{r}^{N}, T)$. If you wish to calculate the free energy difference, between two different local minima, then you will need to obtain a result for $\overline{P(\vec{r}^{N}, T)}$ in the region of conformation space along the path that connects them. For example, for the affinity of a drug for a protein, we need to determine the free energy difference between the drug in solution and the drug bound to the specific binding site of the protein that is being targeted. Moreover, in many cases, what is of interest in the simulation is what is known as a "rare event"; this corresponds to a transition through a region of conformation space with low $P(\vec{r}^{N}, T)$. We will now discuss how approximate values of such free energies can be calculated and rare events can be sampled more effectively, using advanced simulation methods.

The most direct way to increase the region of space where $\overline{P(\vec{r}^{N}, T)}$ is obtained, and to ensure the rare events that we wish to observe are sampled, is to globally accelerate the sampling. The simplest way to achieve this is to just artificially raise the concentration of the molecules that would trigger the event. This is known as a *flooding simulation* [77]. Another simple method is to perform an MD simulation at an artificially raised temperature, to move the system through conformation space more quickly and through greater thermal excitation push the system through energy barriers that would otherwise not be crossed. Obviously, just simply raising the temperature will often be problematic as the alterations to the system, e.g., passing through phase transitions, that happen in the real system with elevated temperature, will often occur in the model, producing a false result. A way around this is to anticipate the unphysical changes to the system the temperature rise will invoke and add a bias potential to $U(\vec{r}^{N})$ to block this from occurring while raising the temperature; this method is known as temperature accelerated molecular dynamics (TAMD) [78]. While TAMD has been used effectively in many cases, it suffers from the problem that the bias potential may not completely alleviate the undesired temperature effects. A safer but more complex method to achieve the same acceleration, but with a guarantee of obtaining an unbiased result, is Replica Exchange.

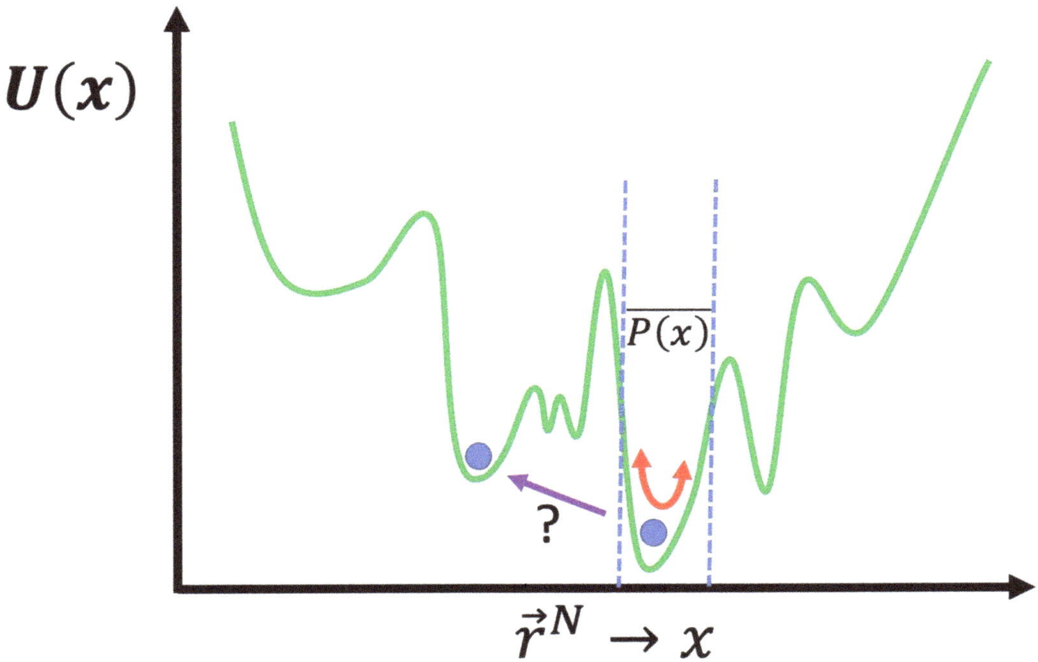

Figure 2. Schematic of the energy landscape of a system; with basic unbiased MD or MC simulation, if performed below a certain temperature, only the region of the local minimum will be explored, thus a result for $\overline{P(\vec{r}^N, T)}$ will only be obtained here. Finding the free energy change to another region of conformation space, where the energy barrier must be crossed and $\overline{P(\vec{r}^N, T)}$ determined along the path, is not practically possible without the advanced biasing schemes we discuss.

In replica exchange [79–81], originally described as *parallel tempering* in the seminal literature, the system of N particles governed by potential $U(\vec{r}^N)$ that inhabits the space $\{\vec{r}^N\}$ being simulated at temperature T, using either MD or MC, can be simulated in parallel with a set of other systems with the same set of particles, however, with other parameters altered. The set of systems can be simulated as a single extended ensemble; this can be seen as a metaverse of parallel universes, a concept that a broader segment of the audience of this paper can understand intuitively now, due to the popularity of recent movies and television shows that have featured such plot elements. Within this new extended ensemble, switching the parameters between two, so to speak, universes within the multiverse that we have created, can be seen as an MC step that can be made with probability $e^{-\Delta\gamma}$ where γ is as above, however, now rather than alteration of particle positions, i.e., a change in $\vec{r}^N$, the change in γ, $\Delta\gamma$, results from temperatures and/or potential functions that governs the systems switching; a schematic of this algorithm is found in Figure 3A. It can be demonstrated mathematically that not only does the collective metaverse that we have created move to equilibrium, but each individual system, separately, moves to equilibrium, thus systems with parameter sets that move more slowly through conformation space are effectively pulled along by those that move more quickly. Initially, this was performed with multiple systems that differed in thermodynamic parameters of the system, like temperature and pressure [82]. Then, Bunker and Dünweg realized that one could more precisely accelerate the dynamics by having the systems differ not in a thermodynamic parameter, but rather a term in the interaction potential $U(\vec{r}^N)$; specifically, they proposed eroding the repulsive core of the Lennard–Jones potentials, allowing for a finite acceptance of MC pivot moves hybridized with MD simulation in the backbones of polymer chains [76] and referred to this as parallel excluded volume tempering. Fukushini et al., then generalized this and applied it to protein structure determination and coined the term by which this procedure is known today: Hamiltonian replica exchange [83].

The aforementioned techniques globally accelerate the motion through conformation space, thus the efficiency with which the quality of $\overline{P(\vec{r}^N, T)}$ as an approximation of $P(\vec{r}^N, T)$ is improved. There are, however, other techniques capable of focusing more specifically on the local region of the conformation space where the system is located—specifically allowing the system to escape the local minimum within which it is trapped. For a system on a discrete space, that is where $\vec{r}^N$ is a set of specific points, or states, i.e., $\{\vec{r}^N\} \rightarrow x_{i=1,N}$, Wang and Landau developed an algorithm [84] where an MC simulation of a system on the discrete space is performed and the number of times the system samples a certain state is recorded and periodically a bias is added to the potential, proportional to the number of times a state has been sampled. Metaphorically, this can be seen as filling up the energy wells that the system has already explored with sand, pushing the system over energy barriers into new energy wells, and then filling them up and so on. This algorithm was adapted to continuum systems, on which MD simulation can be performed, as Statistical Temperature Molecular Dynamics (STMD) [85] and this has been formally shown to be mathematically equivalent [86] to the better-known technique of metadynamics [87–91]. An example of metadynamics at work is shown in Figure 4. An alternative to metadynamics is the application of a specific alteration to the potential to push the system out of a specific local minimum; this is possible when the form of the local minimum can be approximated by an analytical function that can be cancelled out. This technique is known as the addition of a *flooding potential* [92].

We have now described methods to globally accelerate the exploration of conformation space and to, more specifically, escape from the local minima that constrain the system; this, however, still often leaves a conformation space too large to explore to obtain a sufficiently accurate result for $\overline{P(\vec{r}^N, T)}$ in the region of conformation space that we are specifically interested in. Often, this is the transition between two specific local minima, in particular, calculating the free energy difference between them. A specific example of this is a ligand in solution vs. the same ligand docked to a specific active site of a specific protein. The most direct way to achieve this is to push the system through a path in conformation space between the two local minima. There are two means to achieve this: (1) umbrella sampling [93] and (2) steered MD [94,95].

In umbrella sampling, a set of what we refer to as *windows* are created along a path in conformation space that connect the two local minima. This is achieved through the introduction of a biasing force that is in the form of a harmonic interaction, i.e., a spring, centered on a certain distance along the path in conformation space that connects the two local minima. Histograms of the distribution in position along the path in conformation space are determined for each window; a schematic of umbrella sampling is shown in Figure 5. The free energy along any path in conformation space, known as the Potential of Mean Force (PMF), can be determined from these histograms, if the overlap between their tails is sufficient, through a technique known as Weighted Histogram Analysis Method (WHAM) [96]. WHAM is itself an extension of a technique developed by Ferrenberg and Swendsen [97,98] primarily for spin models [99], to specifically adapt it to systems governed by a molecular mechanics potential. A specific example that elucidates the use of umbrella sampling is the study by Nandy et al. [100], where it was used to study the binding of PAMAM dendrimers of different generations to strands of ds-DNA; in the supplementary information of this paper the overlapping set of histograms is shown. The efficiency of the umbrella sampling algorithm can, in many cases, be significantly improved through hybridization with the replica exchange algorithm [101]; the set of all windows can be treated as a single extended ensemble where exchanges of the force biases between neighboring windows can be made through the aforementioned MC moves.

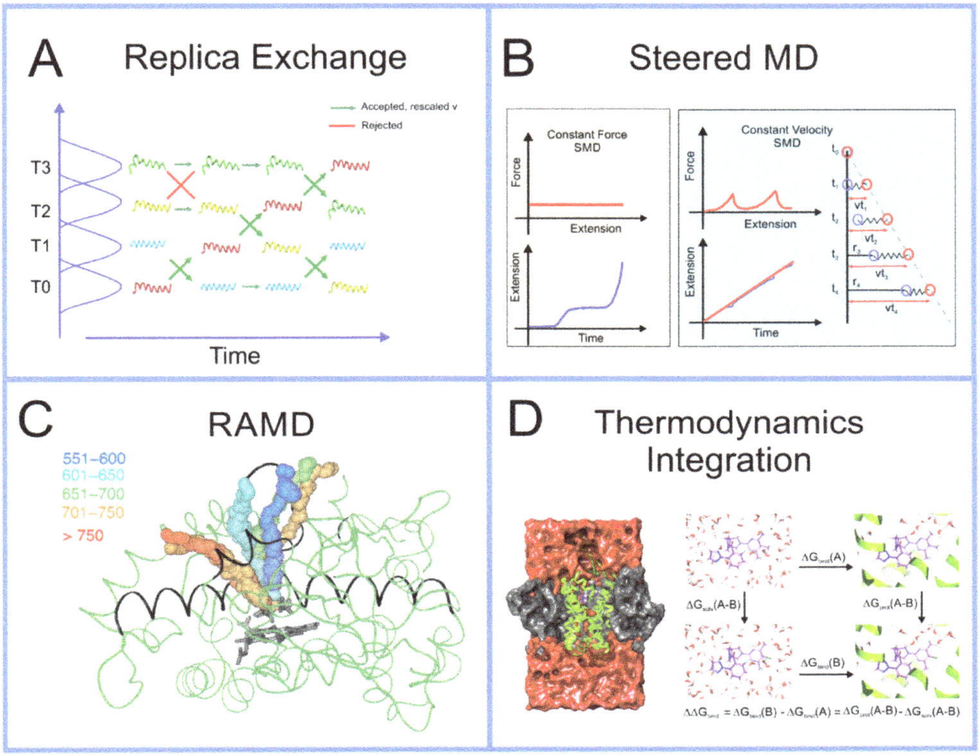

Figure 3. (**A**) Schematic representation of replica exchange (based on ref. [28]); (**B**) force bias/Jarzynsky, reproduced with permission from ref. [94]; (**C**) RAMD, reproduced with permission from ref. [102]; (**D**) thermodynamics integration, reproduced with permission from ref. [103].

Steered MD is another technique capable of determining the free energy change along a path in conformation space that, in many cases, is significantly more computationally efficient than umbrella sampling. It is based on an astounding, counterintuitive, piece of theoretical statistical mechanics proposed by by Jarzynski in 1997, almost 20 years before the computational power to apply this algorithm effectively became available; the relation he derived [104,105], known as the *Jarzynski equality*, can be expressed as

$$\langle e^{\frac{-W}{T}} \rangle = e^{\frac{-\Delta F}{T}} \quad (4)$$

where $\langle\ \rangle$ signifies the average over infinite samples, W is the work carried out along the path in conformation space, i.e., the integral of the force along the path, and ΔF is the difference in free energy between the two ends of the path. The free energy difference between two points in conformation space, a property defined only for a system in equilibrium, can actually be approximated from multiple samples of the work carried out pulling the system from one to the other, a driven system, i.e., a measurement of the system out of equilibrium. Steered MD involves simulating the system while pulling the system along a path in conformation space to determine the work carried out along this path; it is performed multiple times, each time a measurement of W is made. There are two fashions in which this pulling can be performed [94]: constant force, where the velocity is measured along the path, or constant velocity, where the force is measured along the path; this is shown as a schematic in Figure 3B. This algorithm was initially thought not to be practical as, in its early use, it obtained very poor results for the free energy; however, more recently, it was found that if you perform a much larger number of samples than previously feasible, one is able to obtain a result for the free energy difference that, in many cases, is significantly more accurate than that obtained using umbrella sampling using the same computational resources. This algorithm is increasingly being used in drug design [95].

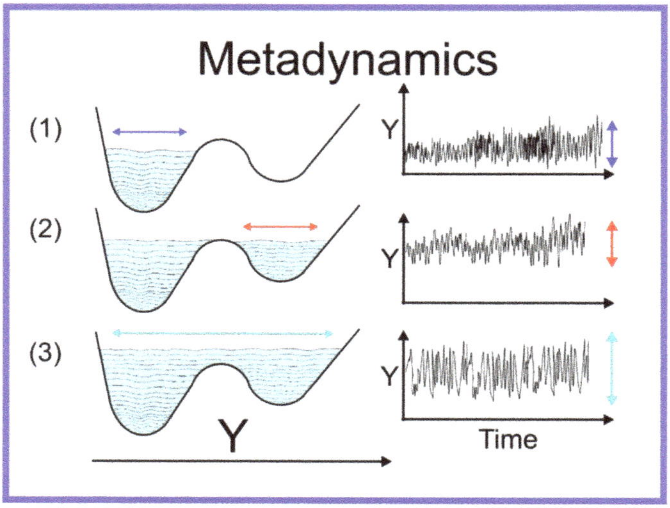

Figure 4. Schematic representation of metadynamics.

The above methods presuppose that the path in conformation space that the system will traverse is known; however, this is not always the case. Often, the active site of a protein is within an internal cavity and the path through channels and mobile loops of the protein that a ligand takes to reach the active site, is unknown. In this case, a technique to not only find the free energy along a path in conformation space must be found, but the path itself must also be found. A technique capable of achieving this is Randomly Accelerated Molecular Dynamics (RAMD) [106]; this involves starting the ligand in its docked position, moving it in a random direction until it gets stuck, then picking another direction and repeating until the ligand has left the protein, bouncing back and forth until it wiggles out of the box it is in; an example of this is shown in Figure 3C. A modified version of RAMD, known as τRAMD allows for the study of the residence time of ligands in the binding pocket [107]. Two additional methods have been developed to find the optimal pathway in complex multidimensional space that bear mentioning: the first is based on the combined use of metadynamics and a path-searching algorithm [108] and the second is based on what is known as a "string method" involving a swarm of trajectories [109,110].

All of the above methods to determine the free energy between two regions of conformation space, usually two different local minima, involved moving the system through a path in conformation space. While accurate, this is not always the most efficient method if all you are interested in is a single quantitative approximation for the free energy difference between the end points of the path and not the free energy along the path, i.e., the PMF. While this information is often useful, as it provides insight into the kinetics in addition to the thermodynamics of the system [10], it does not come without a price; if you is only interested in the free energy difference between the end points of the path, there are more efficient means to obtain an approximation of this. Instead of charting a path through conformation space, you can instead move through a space composed of different possible forms of the interaction potentials, $U(\vec{r}^N)$, itself to determine this; if you start with, for example a ligand bound to the active site of a protein, and that same ligand free in solution, in each case you can gradually dissolve the interactions around the molecules to find the free energy difference to the molecule in empty space: subtracting these from one another determines the free energy difference between them. There are several different related methods that follow this scheme, each with different advantages and disadvantages, including Thermodynamics Integration (TI) [111], Free Energy Perturbation (FEP) [112–114], and Bennett Acceptance Ratio (BAR) [115,116]. If one is also only interested in the difference of the binding affinities of two different molecules and the absolute free energy of binding is not important, then one can perform what is known as *molecular alchemy*, calculating the free energy change along the path of metamorphosis from one molecule to the other, both in solution and at the binding site and subtracting these two from one another, as shown in the schematic in Figure 3D. These techniques in the context of drug design are discussed in detail in a review paper by Limongelli et al. [10].

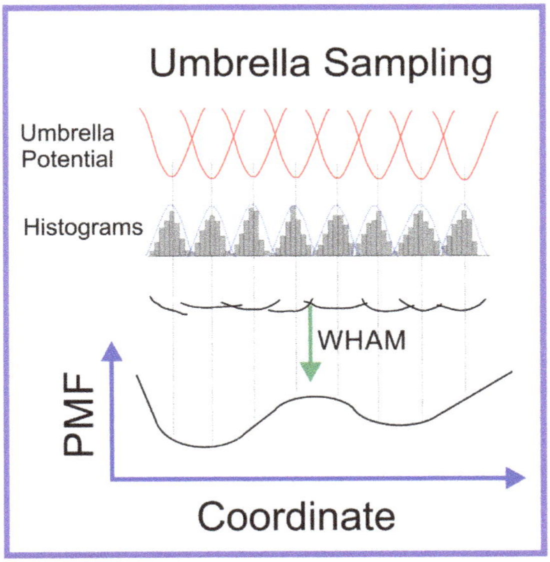

Figure 5. Schematic representation of umbrella sampling algorithm.

Finally, it bears mentioning that, as in other fields of computational science, an emergent trend is the incorporation of the toolkit of novel computational tools widely known as Machine Learning (ML) into hybrid MD algorithms; for a recent review (2020) of achievements in the hybridization of MD with ML, see Noé et al. [117]. Recently, a hybrid FEP + ML algorithm was found to provide a more accurate result, given the same expenditure of computational resources, than the use of FEP alone, for the prediction of hydration free energies [118]; a hybrid MD + ML algorithm was used to predict self-solvation free energies and limiting activity coefficients [119].

3. Location and Orientation of Drug Molecules in the Lipid Bilayer

The beginning of the story of the role of lipid membranes in drug design is a discussion of what individual drugs do when they initially interact with a lipid membrane, where in the membrane they locate to and how they orient within the membrane; this is clearly a result of both the nature of the lipid membrane, i.e., what particular phospholipids and other amphiphilic molecules make up the membrane formulation and the structure of the drug molecule itself, i.e., location and relative dominance of polar, charged, and non–polar regions of the molecule and the flexibility/rigidity of the molecule (Figure 6).

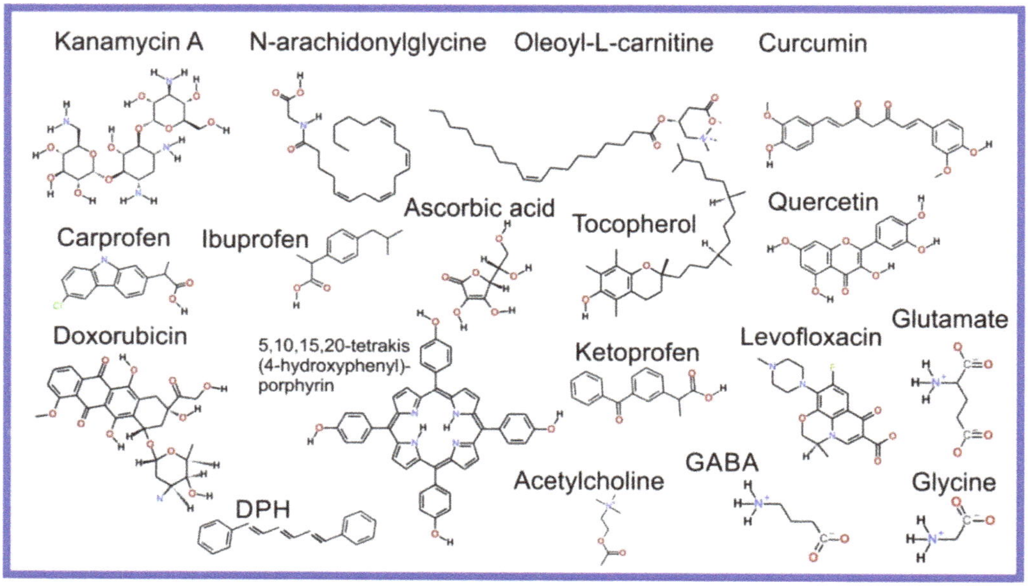

Figure 6. Chemical structure of drugs introduced in Section 3.

The partitioning of small molecules, including proposed drug candidates (see Table 1) but also natural molecules (see Table 2) and other xenobiotic molecules (see Table 3), into lipid bilayers has been extensively studied via a combination of experimental and computational methods. How molecules interact with the membrane, i.e., how they orient and the different regions within the membrane that they locate to, is determined by their structure; MD simulation can provide significant insight into this specific selection. Through simulations carried out on many different drug molecules, a wide range of drug behavior in the membrane, i.e., location and orientation, has been observed.

Berendsen and coworkers [120,121] developed a classification scheme for the behavior of molecules within the membrane according to the region of the membrane that they locate to; they defined four separate regions, as shown in Figure 7: region (1) at the interface between the bulk solvent phase and the lipid headgroups, i.e., the region of the headgroups and the first shells of water adjacent to the membrane, region (2) just below the lipid headgroups, region (3) at the position of the hydrophobic lipid tails, and region (4) at the very center of the membrane core, between the two leaves of the bilayer. Through MD simulations, it has been demonstrated that small hydrophobic molecules e.g., benzene or toluene [122,123], and gases like xenon, O_2, NO, CO, and CO_2 [124–129] locate to region 4; larger hydrophobic molecules, e.g., porphyrins, locate to region 3 [130,131]; amphiphilic molecules, e.g., the majority of drug molecules, our primary interest in this review paper, locate to region 2, their polar components interacting with the polar groups of the lipids and water at the membrane surface and their hydrophobic components located among the hydrocarbon chains of the lipids, as shown in a study by Paloncýová et al., of drug molecules, natural compounds, and other xenobiotics [132]. Mostly polar molecules, including some drug molecules, locate to region 2. Finally, kanamycin A, a highly polar molecule with potential application as an antibiotic, locates to region 1 [133]; antibacterial peptides and saponins [134–136] also locate to this region prior to pore formation. It is possible for drugs to locate to the membrane in a fashion that spans more than one of these regions; examples of this case are particularly interesting as they include several lipid molecules with therapeutic potential. For example, N-arachidonylglycine and oleoyl-L-carnitine are glycine transporter GlyT2 inhibitors that span over regions 2 to 4 [137]. Nevertheless, even molecules that do not directly interact with the membrane can have a long–range membrane association. For example, the concentration of polar molecules relative to the bulk concentration may increase or decrease in the ~1 nm layer of water adjacent to the lipid bilayer; also, acetylcholine is attracted to bilayers that contain negatively charged lipids [138–140] and repulsed by bilayers composed of zwitterionic lipids, as determined through both the MD simulation and experimental study [139]. The zwitterionic neurotransmitters GABA and glycine are attracted to bilayers that contain anionic lipids but are, however, not affected by zwitterionic lipids [139]. Glutamate, another polar, anionic, neurotransmitter, is repulsed from the vicinity of negatively charged lipids [139].

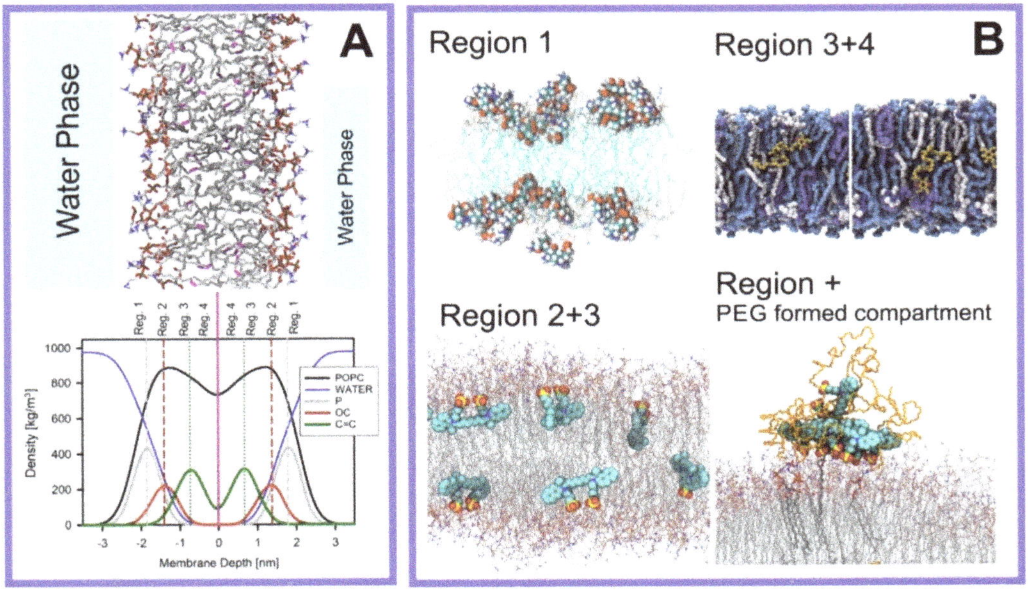

Figure 7. Location of the drugs and small molecules in four regions of a lipid bilayer. (**A**) Top panel: Snapshot of lipid bilayer composed of POPC; Lower panel: corresponding density profiles showing location of lipids, water, phosphate atoms, carbonyl atom (C35), and atoms of double bond of oleoyl chain (C9=C10) of POPC (see Figure 1). Data from 1000 ns simulation of hydrated POPC bilayer with our OPLSaa lipid force field [141–143]. (**B**) Snapshots showing location of small molecules in different regions of the bilayer: kanamycin A locates to region 1 (reproduced with permission from [133]), indocyanine green locates to region 2 and 4, and entangled in PEG corona (reproduced with permission from [144]), ubiquinone locates to region 3 and 4 (reproduced with permission from [145]).

Since drugs and lipids are generally small molecules without the structural complexity often found in biomolecules, studies of drug molecule–lipid bilayer (membrane) interactions are usually relatively straightforward to carry out, even given limited computational resources; the systems studied, lipid membranes with small drug molecules, equilibrate relatively quickly and can be studied effectively using relatively small systems. It is thus not surprising that interactions of proposed drug molecules with lipid bilayers were among the first topics to be studied using MD simulations of lipid membranes [19], for example the studies by Tu et al. [146], Pasenkiewicz-Gierula et al. [147] and Bemporad et al. [148,149] carried out in 1998, 2003, and 2005, respectively. More recently, a particularly noteworthy study by Abdiche and Myszka measured the liposome partitioning of 86 drugs and observed an astounding affinity range of ~1000 fold [150]. In another impressive study, Natesan et al., proposed a theoretical method based on drug structure that allowed for the prediction of the location of drug molecules within the bilayer [151]; this work was performed using experimental results of 107 separate small molecules interacting with lipid membranes. An extensive database was compiled that contains over 3600 cases of compound–membrane interactions gathered from both experimental and theoretical studies, known as the "Molecules on Membranes Database" (MolMeDB), [152]; MolMeDB provides data concerning drug–membrane partitioning, penetration, and positioning.

As is the case for all phenomena studied through MD simulation, the precise values for the parameters of the potential set used are of critical importance, thus the testing and validation of the model are crucial [153–162]. Partition coefficients of the molecule (log K) provide an important test of the potential set that can be directly correlated to experimental measurements. For membrane partitioning of small molecules, comparative studies have demonstrated that the best models predict the partition coefficients (log K) with an accuracy of 0.5–0.8 log units [163]. This result thus provides us with a certain degree of confidence in the accuracy with which MD simulation is capable of effectively modeling the behavior of molecules in the membrane; the partition coefficient plays a dominant role in the drug–membrane interaction.

Simulation studies using MD have demonstrated that the location of the drug molecule is dependent on the hydration level or lipid composition; this relationship has also been studied using MD simulation: a reduced hydration level can be simulated by reducing the thickness of the solvent phase of the simulation box. For example, in a hydrated bilayer, curcumin has been found to locate below the water–membrane interface and orient parallel to the bilayer normal [164]. Interestingly, curcumin, in bilayers with low hydration, locates outside the bilayer and adopts an orientation parallel to the membrane surface, forming a carpet-like structure. Another MD simulation study determined that the distribution of carprofen derivatives along the bilayer normal is bimodal, with the first density maximum located at the position of the lipid headgroup and a second deeper below the membrane–water interface [165]. When the bilayer is in the liquid disordered phase, the second position has been found to be more frequent than in the liquid-ordered phase. The location of ibuprofen is sensitive to cholesterol [166], thus also to the membrane phase. In the DPPC bilayer with 25 mol% of cholesterol, ibuprofen locates slightly closer to the water–membrane interface in comparison to the case of the pure DMPC bilayer (0.81 and 0.95 nm below the position of the phosphate group, respectively); in the bilayer with 50 mol% of cholesterol, ibuprofen, however, is found below the lipid headgroups, within the hydrophobic bilayer core (regions 3 and 4).

Extra complexity to the drug molecule–bilayer interaction is added when a lipid membrane with polymers conjugated to a set of the lipid headgroups is considered [167]. For example, lipids functionalized with poly(ethylene–glycol) (PEG) are most frequently used to fabricate so-called stealth liposomes applied as drug carriers in drug delivery [168]; PEG forms a polymer mesh on the top of the membrane surface, the PEG corona covering the liposome, where hydrophobic and amphipathic molecules may locate instead of within the bilayer. Here, they are shielded, by the polymer, from unfavorable contact with the polar solvent (water), in the same fashion as they would be if located within the membrane if the PEG were not present, however, with a reduced free energy penalty to their normal location within the membrane, leading them to locate instead within the PEG corona [144,168–170]; this can thus be seen as a potential additional compartment for small molecules.

The importance of lipid affinity and exact location in various membrane compartments has also been demonstrated for antioxidants that protect lipids from peroxidation. Two MD simulation studies have found evidence that that the functionalization of antioxidants with lipophilic groups, incapable of free–radical scavenging, decreases the extent of lipid peroxidation [171,172]. This effect results from the increased concentration of functionalized antioxidants in the hydrocarbon phase (regions 3 and 4). Another study, combining MD simulation with experiments, elucidated the mechanism of the effect of flavonoids on the antioxidant activity of tocopherol and ascorbic acid in lipid bilayers [173]; flavonoids, quercetin in this case, synergistically increase the antioxidant activity of tocopherol and ascorbic acid. Through MD simulation, it was demonstrated that the orientation and location within the lipid bilayer of the three antioxidants differ: tocopherol locates below the lipid headgroups (region 2) and is thus capable of translocating through the bilayer, while ascorbic acid locates among the lipid headgroups (region 1), and quercetin prefers an intermediate position (regions 2 and 3). Moreover, these three antioxidants can form non-covalent complexes: quercetin–tocopherol, quercetin–ascorbic acid, tocopherol–ascorbic acid, and tocopherol–tocopherol. The formation of these complexes was observed in MD simulations and subsequently confirmed through explicit quantum mechanical calculations; the formation of quercetin–tocopherol complexes was then also confirmed experimentally, via fluorescence spectroscopy [173]. This formation of non–covalent complexes of the molecules provides a rational explanation for the synergistic effect of using a mixture of antioxidants: (1) the regeneration of tocopherol (a reaction transforming a tocopherol radical back to its native form) is facilitated and (2) quercetin locates deeper within the hydrocarbon phase when complexed with tocopherol.

Biomembranes provide a variety of local environments with physicochemical properties that vary considerably, dependent on the lipid composition; this allows for the optimization of membranes for different roles [174–176]. Even within single biomembrane domains, the lipid composition and properties may vary [177,178]. Here, MD simulation of drug molecules in different membranes can be used as a tool to investigate how drug molecules will interact with different biomembranes encountered in the body or even different lipid domains. For example, Alves et al. [179] studied the well-known chemotherapy agent doxorubicin in both a cholesterol rich, ordered, environment and in a liquid-disordered cholesterol poor environment using a combination of experimental analysis and MD simulation. They found evidence that the presence of cholesterol reduces the effect on membrane fluidity, thus possibly increasing the density of doxorubicin in cholesterol rich membrane domains, where the efflux P-gP protein is found, thus providing a possible explanation of the observed heightened vulnerability to efflux proteins of doxorubicin. On the contrary, amantadine [180] and chlorzoxazone [181] are less soluble in bilayers containing cholesterol.

Drug molecules can be functionalized to polymers to improve their bioavailability and achieve passive targeting. A common choice is direct covalent conjugation to a PEG polymer; however, other polymers have also been considered [43,182]. Conjugation to a polymer will clearly alter the interaction between drug molecules and lipid membranes; this can be studied through MD simulation. Tetraphenyl–porphyrin is a photosensitizer used in photodynamic therapy for cancer treatment. In MD simulations, we observed that tetraphenyl-porphyrin locates to regions 1 and 2 and orients within the lipid bilayer such that the two hydroxyl groups that it possesses are located at the water–membrane interface; PEGylated tetraphenyl–porphyrin, however, remains in the water phase. This result has been validated through MD simulations performed with its initial position within the membrane; it was seen to leave the membrane as the system equilibrated [183].

As we discussed above, for the case of tetraphenyl porphyrin, in addition to location in the lipid bilayer, the orientation of the molecule with respect to the membrane normal will also characterize its behavior. The antifungal drug itraconazole is a rigid and long molecule with weakly polar groups distributed along its backbone (long axis of the molecule); as a result of this particular structure, it adopts an orientation parallel to the membrane surface and locates to the region of the upper segments of the lipid acyl tails (region 3), close to the lipid headgroups (Figure 8) [184]. Due to the rigidity of the itraconazole molecule, its presence can affect the orientation of other molecules in the bilayer. For example, the fluorescent probe 1,6-Diphenyl-1,3,5-hexatriene (DPH) alters its orientation from parallel to the lipid chains to parallel to the itraconazole molecules within the membrane [186]; this change could lead to an incorrect interpretation of steady–state fluorescence anisotropy and fluorescence lifetime measurements. Finally, in bilayers containing cholesterol, itraconazole molecules prefer bilayer regions depleted of cholesterol due to the incompatible orientation of the cholesterol molecules parallel to the membrane normal [187]. For this reason, cholesterol, typically present in liposome formulations used in drug delivery [188,189], is not useful as a component of a vesicle used as a delivery mechanism for itraconazole. Conversely, there are also drug molecules that are sufficiently lipophilic to locate within the membrane that, however, do not adopt a specific orientation when there, i.e., their orientation in the membrane is isotropic. For example, there are many tautomers of the drug molecule piroxicam: six are uncharged (PxA, PxB, PxC, PxD, PxE, and PxF) [190] in addition to zwitterionic, cationic, and anionic tautomers (see Figure 8C). Although, PxA and zwitterionic tautomers are dominant, in vacuum and water solutions respectively, the probability of occurrence of all possible tautomers, when in the environment of the lipid headgroups (regions 2 and 3), is not known; MD simulation studies of four piroxicam tautomers demonstrated that the orientation of the molecules differs significantly between tautomers and, for most cases with the exception of the cationic tautomer, there are no strong preferences for a specific orientation in the bilayer (Figure 8D) [185].

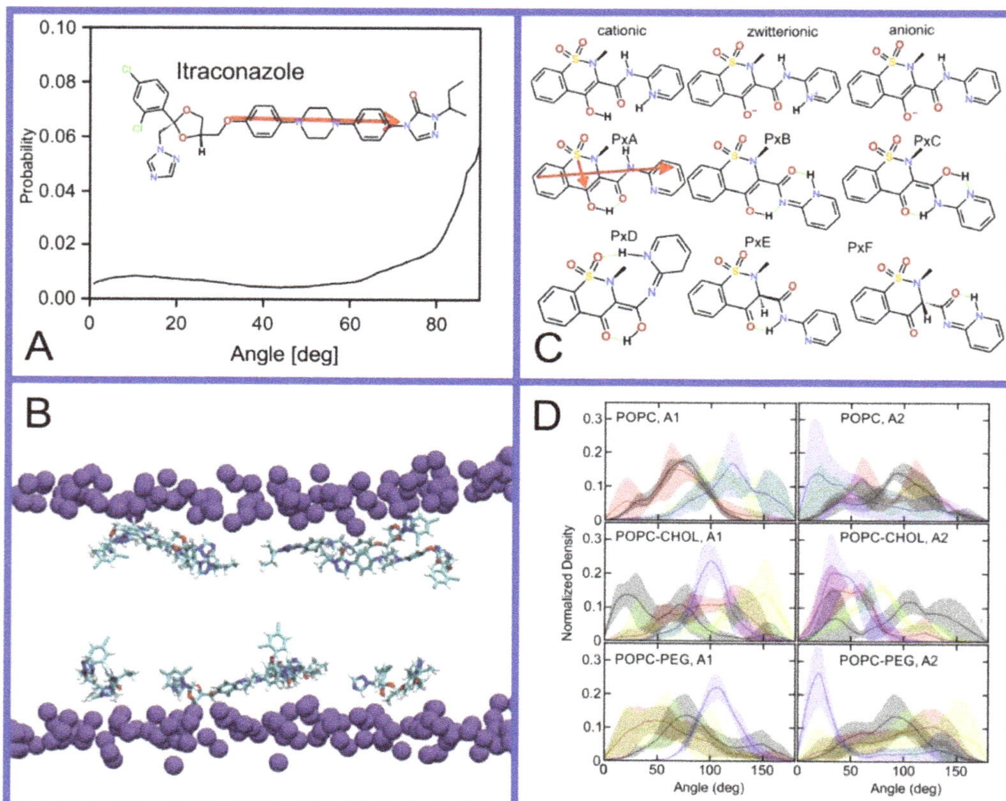

Figure 8. (**A**) Distribution of values of the angle between the vector representing the itraconazole long axis (red arrow at the chemical structure of itraconazole) and the bilayer normal [184]. (**B**) Snapshot showing itraconazole molecules in a lipid bilayer, purple spheres are phosphate groups of the POPC molecules [184]. (**C**) Chemical structures of piroxicam tautomers. (**D**) Distribution of angles between the vector representing the piroxicam long and short axes (red arrows at the chemical structure of PxA) and bilayer normal; PxA—black line, PxE—read line, zwitterionic—green line, cationic—blue line [185].

Table 1. List of recent studies of drug–membrane interactions.

Application and Target	Drugs and Pharmaceutics
High blood pressure treatment, Angiotensin II AT1 receptor	Losartan [191,192], Candesartan [193]
High blood pressure treatment, β–adrenergic receptors, GPCR	Acebutolol [194], Alprenolol [148,195,196], AS408 [197], Atenolol [148,196,198,199], Carazolol [200], Formoterol [201], Idacaterol and its analogs [201], Metoprolol [196], Nadolol [196], Oxprenolol [194], Pindolol [148,196], Propranolol [194,196,202], Salbutamol [199], Salmeterol [201]
High blood pressure treatment	Amlodipine [198,203], Lisinopril [198], Debrisoquine [132]
Anticancer drug	Tamoxifen [204], Cytarabine [205], 5-Fluorouracil [206,207], Daunorubicin [208,209], β-Lapachone [210], Minerval [211], Miltefosine [212], Tofacitinib [213], Edelfosine [214], Miltefosine [214], Perifosine [214], Camptothecin [215,216], Pirarubicin, Ellipticine [217], Perillyl alcohol [218], Cisplatin [219,220], Doxorubicin [179,217,221], 5-fluorouracil [206]; Previous reviews [222,223], Chlorambucil [199], Camptothecin [224], Ohmline [225]
Photosensitizer used in cancer treatment	Tetra–phenylporphyrin [169,183], Hematoporphyrin [130], 1-BODIPY (6,7-dibromo-2-ethyl-1,3-dimethyl-4,4-difluoro-4-bora-3a,4a-diaza-s-indacene) [226], Indocyanine green [144,170]
Potential anticancer drug	Curcumin [164,227–229], Aplysiatoxin [230], Bryostatin [231], Phorbol [231], 12,13-dibutyrate [231], Prostratin [231]
Antibiotics	Imipenem [232], Doripenem [232], Ertapenem [232], Meropenem [232], Ciprofloxacin [233,234], Ciprofloxacin ternary copper complex [235], Daunorubicin [209], Idarubicin [209], Levofloxacin [236–238], Clarithromycin [236], Isoniazid N′-acylated derivatives [239], Rifampicin [234,240], Mangostin [241], Trimethoprim [242], Negamycin [243]
Potential antibiotic	Kanamycin A [133], nTZDpa and its derivatives [244], Cholic acid derived amphiphiles [245], γ-terpineol [246], Bithionol [247]
Antimicrobial compound	Chlorhexidine [248–250], Triclosan [251], Octenidine [250]
Antiparasitic	Praziquantel [252]
Antiviral drugs	Darunavir [253], Amantadine [254–256], Spiro[pyrrolidine-2,2′-adamantane] [254,255], 20,30-dideoxyadenosine (Didanosine) [242], Saffron [257]
Antifungal drug	Itraconazole, [184,186,187,258], Nystatin [259], Amphotericin B [260]
Rheumatoid arthritis	Lapatinib [213]
Nonsteroidal antiinflammatory drugs, inhibitor of cyclooxygenase-1 and -2	Ketoprofen [261–264], Aspirin [199,229,261,265–271], Piroxicam [185,261], Ibuprofen [132,166,199,203,265,270,272–277], Indomethacin [277], Diclofenac [132,270], Xanthone derivatives (KS1, KS2, KS3) [278], Indomethacin [279], Carane derivatives [147], Carprofen [165], Phenylbutazone [199]
Steroids	Danazol [280], Hydrocortisone [281]
Antiinflammatory drugs	Colchicine [282],
Pain medication	Paracetamol [283–285]
Pain medication, opioid receptors	Morphine [132], Fentanyl [132], Fentanyl and its analogues [286], Codeine [287]
Local anesthetics	Benzocaine [288–290], KP-23 [147], Dibucaine [291], Lidocaine [289,292,293], Articaine [289], Tetracaine [294,295], Prilocaine [296], Dyclonine, Butamben [290]
General anesthetic	Xenon [124,125], Chloroform [292,297–301], Halothane [146,298,302,303], Isoflurane [297,299,304,305], Phenyl-ethanol [306], Desflurane [305,307], Sevoflurane [305,308], Propofol [305,309,310], Diethyl ether [298,308], Enflurane [298], Ketamine [311]
Antihistamine	Cetirizine [199], Cimetidine [199], Doxylamine [199], Icotidine [199]
Fibrotic skin disorders	p-aminobenzoic acid [132,290]
Statins	Atorvastatin, Cerivastatin, Fluvastatin, Rosuvastatin, Lovastatin, Pravastatin, Simvastatin [312–317]

Table 1. *Cont.*

Application and Target	Drugs and Pharmaceutics
Antidepressant	Amitriptyline [318], Fluoxetine [319,320], Thioridazine [321], Sertraline [199], Bupropion [199], Imipramine [199]
Antipsychotic	Clozapine [318,322], Haloperidol [322], Promazine [199], Chlorpromazine [199], Olanzapine [199], Alprazolam [199],
Neuroleptics	Trifluoperazine, Haloperidol decanoate, Clozapine, Quetiapine, Olanzapine, Aripiprazole, Amisulpride [323]
Alzheimer disease	Pregnanolone sulfate, Pregnanolone glutamate [324], Carbazoles [325]
Anticonvulsant and muscle relaxant	Carbamazepine [326–328], Nordazepam [199], Lamotrigine [199], Chlorzoxazone [132]
Cardiac arrhythmias	Dronedarone [312]
P2Y1 antagonist	BPTU [329]
Urea cycle disorders	4-phenylbutyrate
Immunosuppressant	Cyclosporine A and E [330]
Cardiac Ca^{2+} pump inhibitors	CDN1163, CP-154526, Ro 41-0960 [331]
Eye drops components	Cetalkonium chloride, Poloxamer 188 [332]
Vaccine adjuvant	Cobalt porphyrin phospholipid [333], Lipidated nicotine [334]
Other potential drugs	Baicalin [282], Emodin [282], Siramesine [335], HMI and HMI-1a3 [336], Peptide mimicking GM1 [337], AMG3 [338], 1,8-naphthyridine derivatives [339], Protein kinase inhibitors [340], Bile salt export pump inhibitors [341]

Pulmonary surfactants form a complex structure on the inner lung surfaces, the alveoli, including the only monolayer in the human body at the boundary between the pulmonary liquids and air. For drugs designed to treat lung conditions that are delivered through pulmonary administration, e.g., corticosteroid and salbutamol inhalers for the treatment of asthma, this monolayer is the first barrier that they encounter. Pulmonary surfactant monolayers are composed predominately of DPPC (85%), and the remaining components are POPG (11%) and cholesterol (4%). A study by Hu et al., comprised a set of MD simulations of a lung surfactant monolayer models at five different surface tensions, representing various stages of monolayer expansion and compression, demonstrated that the nonsteroidal anti-inflammatory drug ketoprofen changes its location in the monolayer depending on the degree of monolayer compression [263]. In expanded monolayers with a surface area per lipid of 0.9 nm^2, ketoprofen locates to the water–membrane interface; in the condensed monolayer, with a surface area per lipid of 0.52 nm^2, ketoprofen locates to the hydrocarbon phase, beneath the headgroups of the monolayer. In other studies that were performed on monolayers mimicking pulmonary surfactants at surface pressures of 55 and 43 mNm^{-1}, the antibiotic levofloxacin located to the water–membrane interface with a tendency to locate deeper within the monolayer when the surface pressure was increased [238]. Moreover, levofloxacin aggregated in the hydrocarbon phase of the monolayer.

Table 2. List of recent studies of natural compound–membrane interactions.

Function	Compounds
Antioxidants	Quercetin [132,173,282,342–348], Biochanin [183], Argenteane [132,171], α-Tocopherol [173,349–352], Ascorbic acid [173], Carbazoles [172], Anthocyanin derivatives (Hemiketal, Chalcone, Pyranoanthocyanin, Aglycone, A4, A5, A7, A-4′7) [353], Trolox [354], PBN [354], Quinones [145,355], Menaquinone [356,357], Lutein [358], Glutathione [359], Flavonoids [360–370], Liponitroxides [371]
Amino acids	L-phenylalanine [372–375], L-Tyrosine [374], L-Phenylglycine, Phenylacetic acid [374,376], Tryptophan [376–378], Glycine [139,284], Glutamate [139], Aginine [379], Alanine [379], 5-aminolevulinic acid and its esters [380], L-dopa [138,199,381,382]
Nucleotides	ATP [383], UMP [384], DNA [385], ADOMET [381]
Sugars and carbohydrates	Trehalose [386], Gastrodin [387], Mannitol [199], 1,3,7-trimethyluric acid [388]
Neurotransmitters	Dopamine [138,389–397], Serotonin [138,378,389,396,398–402], Adenosine [138], Melatonin [138,229,378,389,403–405], Epinephrine [138], Norepinephrine [138], Trace amines (Tyramine and phenethylamine) [406], Acetylcholine [139], GABA [139], Histamine [138,393,407]
Hormones	Testosterone [132,408], Levothyroxine [409], Resolvins [410], Progesterone [326,327]
Vitamins	D2, D3 [411,412]
Alcohols and product of fermentation	Methanol [274,413,414], Ethanol [149,242,284,387,414–420], Propanol [414,421], Isopropanol [284], Buthanol [414,417,422], Caprate [423], Glycerol [424], Isopropanol [416], Thymol [425]
Natural polymers	Lignin [426–428], Polyphenols [429], Cellulose [430,431], Polysialic acid [432]
Gabaergic ketones	Carvone, Menthone, Pulegone, Dihydrocarvone, Thujone [433]
Taste and aroma	Menthol [342,434], Terpenoids [435], Coumarin [132,284,436,437], Limonene [132], 4-ethylphenol (wine/beer aroma) [406], Tannins (wine) [438], Catechin [282]
Caffeine and its derivatives	Caffeine [132,439], Rosmarinic acid [440–442], Caffeic acid [441,443], Chlorogenic acid [441], Paraxanthine [132], Caffeic acid derivatives [444]
Pigments	Violacein [445,446], Marennine [447]
Bile salts	[280,423,448]
Steroids	Betulin [449], Saponins [450,451], Glycyrrhizic acid (saponin) [252,452,453], Withaferin-A and Withanone [454]
Lipids	N-arachidonylglycine and oleoyl-L-carnitine [137], sn-2-arachidonoylglycerol [455], Triolein [456]
Osmolyte in Extremophiles	Trimethylamine-N-oxide [457]
Toxin	Veratridine [458]
Oxidation product	4-hydroxynonenal [459]
Metabolites	5-phenylvaleric acid [203], Ligustrazine [282], Ferulaic acid [282], Imperatorin [282],
Phenolic compounds	Artepillin C [460], Chlorogenic acid and Isochlorogenic acid [461], Proanthocyanidins [462,463], Oleuropein aglycone [464], Other [465–469]

The orientation and location of drug molecules in lipid membranes is clearly only the beginning of our story. Once molecules enter a biomembrane they can do three different things: (1) pass out of the membrane again, possibly on the other side, the membrane merely forming a biological barrier on their way to their eventual destination, (2) act collectively to instigate large scale alteration or even disruption of the membrane structure, or (3) interact with proteins that are associated with the membrane. These three phenomena are all of clear relevance to molecules designed to act as drugs. In the rest of this review article, we will discuss the use of MD simulation to elucidate each of these in the context of drug design.

Table 3. List of recent studies of xenobiotic–membrane interactions.

Application	Xenobiotic
Antiseptic	Picloxydine, Octenidine, Miramistin [470], Polyhexamethylene Biguanide [471]
Insecticide	Parathione [132], Fipronil [472], Dibutyl succinate [203]
Former Drugs	d-sotalol, cisapride [473], piracetam (status varies among countries) [474], ORG-12962 [199]
Toxic xenobiotic	Polybrominated-diphenyl-ethers [475], Bisphenol [476], Perfluoroalkyls [477], nitroaromatic explosives (TNT,2A, and 24DA) [478–481], 1,4-Dioxane [482], Benzo[a]pyrene [483]
Nanomaterials	Graphene [484–487], Carbon Dots [488], Phosphorene Oxide Nanosheets [489], Gold Nanoparticles [490–492], Titanium Dioxide Nanoparticles [493], Generic Nanoparticles (coarse grained) [494], Fullerene [495–498], Previous reviews [499]
Polymers	Poly(ethyleneoxide)-Poly-(propylene oxide) [500], polyethylenimine [501], Poloxamer [502,503], Pluronics [504,505], poly(ethyleneglycol)-desferrioxamine/ gallium [506], PEG functionalized with carbochydrates [507] and peptides [508], poly(2-methyloxazoline) [509], Polyethylenimine and Polylysine [510]
Ionic liquid	Choline-glycine [511], Cholinium-phenylalaninate [512], Imidazolium-IL [bmim][Cl] [513]
Fluorescent labels	[514–529]
Fragrance	Musk xylene [132]
	2-aminoethoxydiphenyl borate (inhibitor of IP_3 receptors and TRP channels) [530]
Organic solvents	Pentanol [422], Hexanol [422], Heptanol [422], Acetic acid [149,415,417], Tolune, Phenol [284,417], Styrene [417], Ethylbenzene [417], Benzaldehyde [531], Benzene [149,415,417], Hexane [415]
Other	Lauryl Ether Sulfate [532], Dodecyl Sulfate [533], CyMe4-BTPhen [534], Acetone [420], DMSO [417,420,535], bis-(3-hydroxy-4-pyridinonato) zinc(II) complex [536], calix[4], resorcinarenes [537], dihydropyrimidine analogues [538], Choline carboxylates [539], Synthetic xanthophylls [540], Triton X-100 [541,542], Benzoic acid [284,287,387], Methane [379], Borneol [282,543], Osthole [282,543], Isopulegol [544], Benzylpiperidine [545], Benzimidazole derivatives [546], Aldehydes [547]
Inorganic	Water [149,284,379,417,548–555], Ammonia [274,284,416,417,549], Urea [284,287,417,549], Na^+ [379,556], Dithionite [550]
Gases	Gases [557], Oxygen [417,557,558], Ozone [558], Carbon dioxide [242,284,416], Propane [284], Fluoromethane [284], Ethylene [415], NO_2 [558], SO_2 [558], Butadiene [285], Gas bubbles [559]

4. Translocation through the Membrane

For all drugs, there is a ubiquitous membrane interaction they need to perform in every case: transfection, or translocation, through biomembranes that form biological barriers that need to be crossed in order to reach the target site for their action (Figure 9). This process has been studied intensively using MD simulations; for previous extensive reviews, see references [34,560–563]. Unsurprisingly, the permeation of small molecules through the lipid bilayer was among the first membrane-related topics studied through MD simulation, e.g., in 2004, Bemporad et al. [149] studied permeation of small organic molecules like benzene or ethanol, and in older studies, Marrink and Berendsen (1994) studied permeation of water [564]. A significant amount of work has been performed to predict the permeability of small molecules through lipid bilayers using various molecular modeling methods and theoretical tools [565–574]; this includes new computational methodologies, developed specifically for the study of membrane permeability [575–577]. A web server and database PerMM is dedicated to gathering experimental and computational data related to small molecule membrane partitioning and translocation [578]. For a recent review of the development of experimental methods used for studying passive diffusion through membranes, see reference [579].

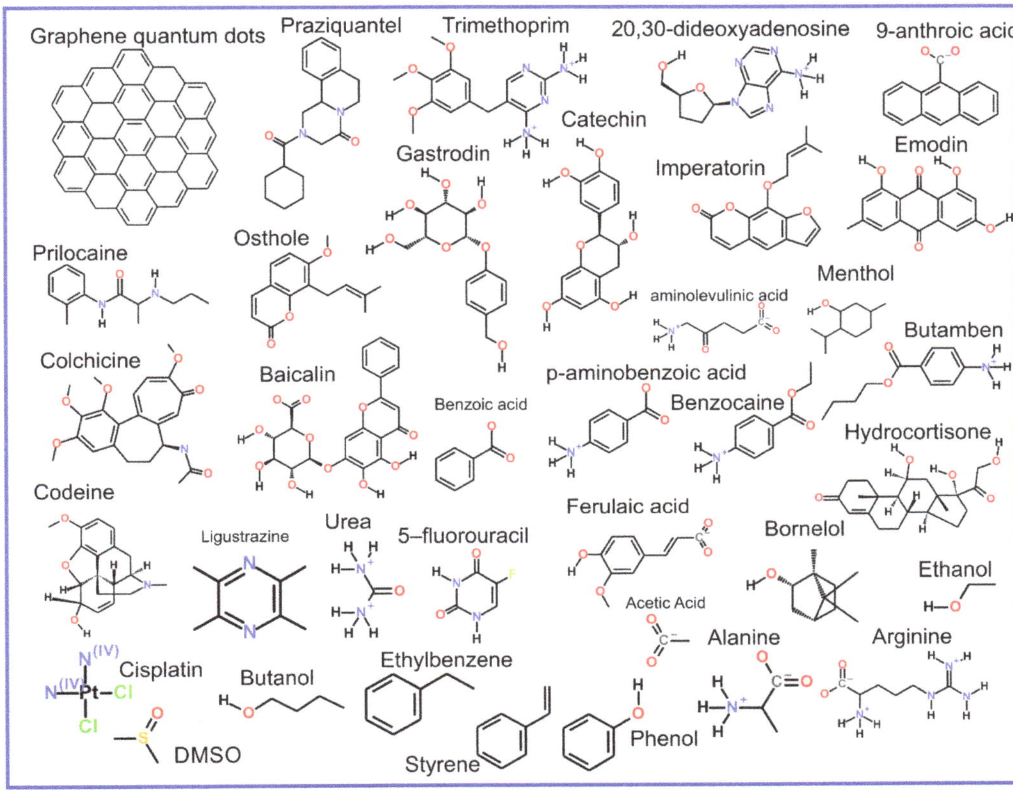

Figure 9. Chemical structure of the chemical compounds introduced in Section 4.

Regarding the study of drug translocation through the lipid bilayer, the main limitation is the time scale that is possible to reach with MD simulations with all atom resolution; this typically is not sufficient to allow for the observation of the entire translocation process without some form of force bias. Translocation in MD simulations can be observed for tiny molecules, e.g., gases [557] or water [548,552,555] in numbers allowing for the observation of a sufficient number of events to allow for a statistically significant result; for larger molecules, only single cases of translocation can be observed, e.g., [550,580–585]. Membrane transfection represents a transition through an energy barrier, as shown in Figure 10; the force biased methods discussed earlier in this review are thus the tools needed to effectively study this. The transition rate will be directly proportional to the height of the energy barrier and force biased methods are an effective means to calculate this. For the case of membrane translocation, the umbrella sampling method [93,586,587] is the most frequent choice to perform this calculation; umbrella sampling calculations show a profile of the potential of mean force (PMF) along selected transition pathways, which, for the case of membrane permeability, is normal to the bilayer surface (Figure 10). The recent review by Lee and Kuczera provides insight into methods used for the calculation of free energies of translocation through lipid bilayers [57].

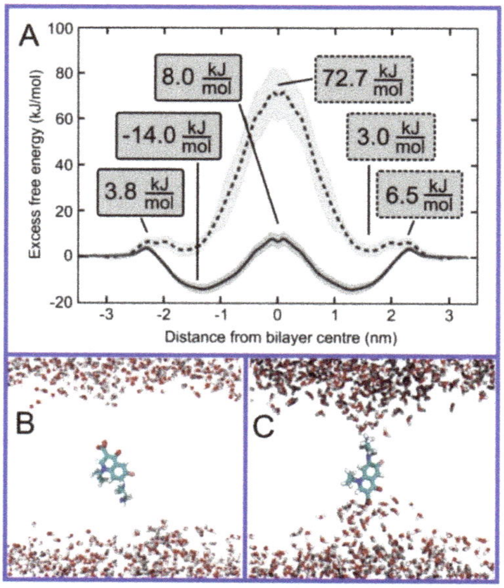

Figure 10. (**A**) Free energy profiles along the bilayer normal of zwitterionic (dashed line) and neutral (full line) ciprofloxacin molecules; the membrane center is at z = 0. Snapshots of ciprofloxacin molecule in the bilayer center: (**B**) uncharged, (**C**) zwitterionic form. Lipids are not shown for clarity. Reproduced with permission from ref. [233].

As discussed previously, the computational cost of an umbrella sampling calculation is relatively high, but through clever tweaks to the algorithm this cost can be reduced; membrane transfection can be seen as a near perfect testbed for the comparison of variants of umbrella sampling and other algorithms for the study of transitions through energy barriers. Nitschke et al., developed a number of shortcuts regarding the calculation of the energy barrier to membrane transfection using umbrella sampling, including decreasing the size of the bilayer, parallel use of multiple solutes, and decreasing the cutoff radius for the Lennard–Jones interactions; this did not significantly affect the quantitative results of the calculations while reducing the computational resources required by up to a factor of 40 [274]. Other methodological studies have determined that adding the so-called flooding potential [92] to the force field allows for improved conformational sampling of the solute before umbrella sampling, thus improving the accuracy of the calculation of the free energy barrier [203]; this was discussed earlier in the paper. A comparison of the four methods used to obtain the free energy profiles (umbrella sampling, replica-exchange umbrella sampling, adaptive biasing force, and multiple-walker adaptive biasing force) for three solutes (urea, benzoic acid, and codeine) found no benefit in implementing the more advanced algorithms, i.e., no improvement in the quantitative accuracy of the results for a given expenditure of computational resources [287]. In another study, three methods were compared: metadynamics, umbrella sampling, and replica-exchange umbrella sampling [379]. Comparisons were performed for six compounds: arginine, sodium ion, side-chain analog of alanine (methane), alanine with neutral termini, zwitterionic alanine, and water. In partial disagreement with the previous result, this study found a significant deviation in the free energy profiles for the case of charged molecules: arginine, sodium ions, and zwitterionic alanine, while for neutral molecules such as methane and zwitterionic alanine, no significant differences were observed [379]. The reason for the discrepancy observed for charged molecules was the slow relaxation of electrostatic interactions between lipid headgroups and the solute. The only method available that allowed for sufficient sampling was replica-exchange umbrella sampling. Recently, Bennett et al., combined MD simulations with ML to study transfer free energies, i.e., free energy difference between two environments [571]. They calculated free energies of transfer from water to cyclohexane for 15,000 small molecules using MD simulations and next used obtained data to train the ML algorithm. The mean absolute error of the obtained prediction in comparison to MD data was only ~4 kJ/mol.

A qualitative insight into the mechanism of drug translocation through a lipid bilayer, i.e., following what the molecule actually does in a physical sense as it passes through the membrane, can also be obtained through MD simulation. For example, Chipot and Comer demonstrated subdiffusive behavior in small molecules translocating through the membrane, with a mean squared displacement proportional to time t as $t^{0.7}$ [413] rather than the expected linear relationship. Cramariuc et al., proposed that the translocation of ciprofloxacin, a fluoroquinolone antibiotic, is facilitated through the collective entrance into the membrane of dimers, or even larger column-like stacks of ciprofloxacin molecules (Figure 11A,B) [233]. The column-like stacks of ciprofloxacin molecules have also been observed by Li et al. [343]. Complexed to form dimers, or larger aggregates, negatively and positively charged groups of ciprofloxacin neutralize each other and thus provide an easy avenue for proton translocation; this leads to the collective transformation of all the ciprofloxacin molecules to their uncharged form. Interestingly, in studies of the antibiotic mangostin (Figure 11C), the formation of a transmembrane aggregate of 16 molecules of the drug was observed [241]; MD simulations can find evidence of general trends connecting drug structure to permeability. For example, performing simulations of 49 compounds, Dickson et al., derived a simple correlation between passive permeation and the number of hydrogen bonds between solute and the surrounding molecules, i.e., water and lipids, with a correlation coefficient of 0.63 [588,589].

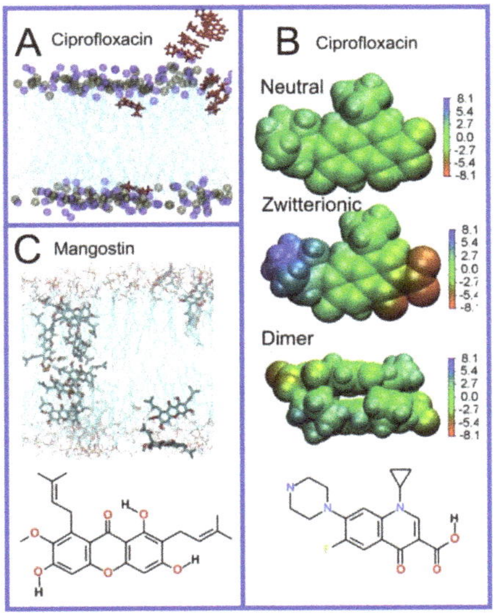

Figure 11. (**A**) Snapshots of MD simulation showing a stack of neutral ciprofloxacin entering the lipid bilayer. (**B**) Electrostatic potential maps at the molecular van der Waals surface in a dielectric continuum corresponding to the water phase calculated using the DFT method and chemical structure of ciprofloxacin. (**C**) Snapshots of MD simulation showing transmembrane arrangement of mangostin molecules and its chemical structure. A and B reproduced with permission from ref. [233]; C reproduced with permission from ref. [241].

The translocation of the drug molecules through lipid bilayers may be facilitated using additional molecules that assist the translocation of the drug through the membrane. Well known examples of such molecules include ionophores facilitating the translocation of ions, e.g., K^+ [590], K^+ and Mg^{2+} [591], Cl^- [592–594] and positively charged doxorubicin [221]. Other examples are so-called molecular umbrellas, capable of transporting hydrophilic cargo through lipid bilayers [595–597] or hydrophobic cargo through aqueous solution [598]. In a similar spirit, the use of conjugated antioxidants with antiretroviral drugs has been proposed to increase drug penetration into the central nervous system [599]. Additionally, peptides, including antimicrobial peptides, were proposed as an effective enhancer [600,601]. Recent MD simulations demonstrated that glycyrrhizic acid enhanced the translocation of the antiparasitic drug praziquantel through a lipid bilayer by lowering the free energy barrier associated with the hydrophobic center of the membrane along with a rearrangement of the lipid headgroups [252]. Similarly, studies of menthol, as an enhancer of translocation, found a large decrease in the free energy barrier in the bilayer center for the translocation of quercetin [342]. Additionally, graphene quantum dots have also been found to decrease the free energy barrier against the translocation of doxorubicin and deoxyadenosine [484]. Interestingly, carbon dioxide increases the permeability of ethanol, 20,30-dideoxyadenosine, and trimethoprim through the POPC bilayer [242]. Recently, cyclic peptides have been proposed as potential enhancers of drug permeation through lipid bilayers [602]. The cyclic peptide (Trp-D-Leu)4-Gln-D-Leu has the ability to assemble into tube-like structures in lipid bilayers; this has been demonstrated to possibly be capable of acting as an enhancer for the antitumor drug 5-fluorouracil [206]—the drug is believed to pass the bilayer through the tube created by the peptide as free energy calculations indicate the presence of only a small 5 kJ/mol barrier against such a translocation. In coarse-grained simulations of lidocaine translocation through a lipid bilayer, two enhancers, ethanol and linoleic acid, were shown to have a synergistic effect on lidocaine permeability [603]. Finally, Gupta et al. [604] performed extensive screening of possible enhancers through a massively parallel array of umbrella sampling calculations using the coarse-grained MARTINI model [605,606] to obtain approximate results for the free energy barriers to translocation for each case (Figure 12) [604].

The effect of the lipid composition of the membrane on its permeability to a broad range of molecules has also been studied though MD simulation. The presence of cholesterol, a major component of the cell membrane, is known to reduce the permeability of the membrane to various solutes [607–609]; this phenomenon has been examined through MD simulation. For example, in POPC bilayers, the addition of 33 mol% of cholesterol has been found to reduce the permeability of the membrane to 9-anthroic acid and 2′,3′-dideoxyadenosine by a factor of ten; however, the permeability to hydrocortisone is reduced by a remarkable factor of 600 [281]. In a lipid bilayer mimicking the cell membrane, with an asymmetric distribution of phospholipid types, i.e., the formulation of the two leaves of the membrane differed, the permeability was found to be lower by 5–6 orders of magnitude in comparison to that of a pure DOPC bilayer [219]. The permeability of this lipid bilayer was further reduced by an order of magnitude when 33 mol% of cholesterol was added to both leaflets [219]. In cancer cells, the cell membrane asymmetry frequently vanishes; thus, comparison of symmetric and asymmetric models of the cell membrane, are of significant interest. A comparison of the permeability to cisplatin of symmetric and asymmetric bilayers found a decrease in permeability in a membrane designed as a model of a cancer cell membrane by a factor of 11. It has also been shown through MD simulation studies that the addition of DOPE, representing a lipid type that does not form a lamellar structure, to a DOPC bilayer, reduces the permeability regarding small molecules (molecular weight less than 100 Da); however, for larger molecules the effect is the opposite [284]. Simulations of lipid bilayers containing products of lipid oxidations have found a decrease in permeability for the case of oxysterols [550] and tail oxidized phosphatidylcholine [481].

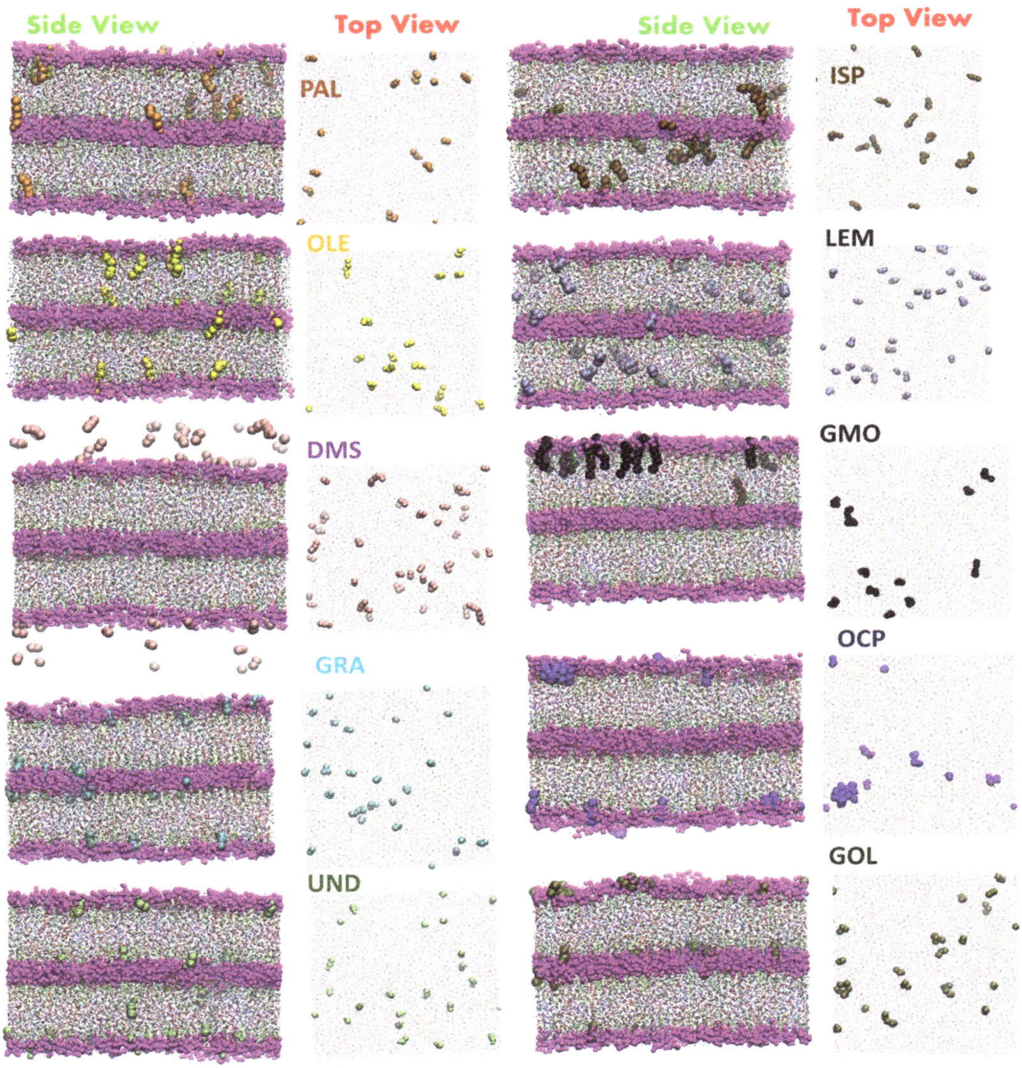

Figure 12. Snapshots of the *stratum corneum* model with selected enhancers: Oleic Acid (OLE), Palmitic Acid (PLA), Geranic Acid (GRA), Undecanoic acid (UND), DMSO (DMS), Geraniol (GOL), Glycerylmonooleate (GMO), Isopropyl palmiate (ISP), Limonene (LEM), and Octyl pyrrolidone (OCP). Reproduced from ref. [604].

From the standpoint of pharmaceutical research, the most interesting are studies of membranes that form a boundary with an extracellular environment, including bacterial membranes [415,610–616], the *stratum corneum*, i.e., the most external layer of the skin [617–626], membranes present in the eyes [557,627–631], and the ocular mucous membrane [632], or lung surfactant monolayers [263,558,633–638]. Specifically, MD simulations have been used in studies of enhancer effects on the permeability of the *stratum corneum* (e.g., [544]). For example, studies of the effects of the terpene derivative borneol on the enhancement of *stratum corneum* permeability for osthole [543] and gastrodin, catechin, quercetin, emodin, imperatorin, ligustrazine, ferulaic acid, colchicine, and baicalin found that borneol facilitates drugs permeation via a destabilization of the condensed and ordered arrangement of ceramides and free fatty acids [282]. Another study found evidence that the destruction of the *stratum corneum*, caused by ethanol, leads to the extraction of lipids from the membrane and subsequently the formation of the pore–like structures that allow for benzoic acid to translocate through the membrane [387]. Next, extensive studies, using umbrella sampling methods, of the permeability of the *stratum corneum* for water, oxygen, ethanol, acetic acid, urea, butanol, benzene, dimethyl sulfoxide (DMSO), toluene, phenol, styrene, and ethylbenzene identified the locations of the free energy barriers to transit through the *stratum corneum* for these compounds [417]. The umbrella sampling method has also used been used for studies of the permeation of p–aminobenzoic acid, benzocaine, and butamben through a lipid bilayer in the gel phase composed of ceramide, one of the main components of the *stratum corneum* [290].

In recent studies, Liu et al., calculated the time of entry of 79 drugs into the lipid bilayer, mimicking the lipid composition of the COVID-19 envelope with and without the spike protein and five bilayers mimicking the lipid composition of the: (1) plasma membrane, (2) lysosome, (3) endoplasmic reticulum, (4) Golgi apparatus, and (5) mitochondrial membranes [639]. The set of 79 drugs was selected from the currently approved drugs as potential antiviral therapeutics [640]. These calculations demonstrated that the presence of the spike protein significantly reduces the time required for drugs to enter the lipid bilayer.

Important membrane-based systems that form barriers that, for the treatment of many conditions, drugs must pass, include the blood–brain barrier and the membrane lining the gastrointestinal tract. Intestinal permeability is essential for pharmacokinetics and is widely studied through both experimental and theoretical methods [641–644]. The blood–brain barrier is another significant intraorganismal barrier considered in treating numerous diseases, e.g., Parkinson's disease [645,646] and even in screening potential drugs against SARS-CoV-2, capable of infecting brain tissue [647,648]. Steered MD simulations have found a correlation between experimental parameters that describe drug permeability through the blood–brain barrier and both the maximum force needed for pulling molecules through it and the overall non-equilibrium work performed during the pulling simulation [199]. Studies have been performed for 26 compounds in simple DOPC and DOPC–Cholesterol bilayers. In another study, unconstrained MD simulations were performed at elevated temperature to observe the spontaneous translocations of drug molecules through a multicomponent asymmetric lipid bilayer [416]. These studies produced results in agreement with the experimental data. Additionally, propionylated amylose has been used as a carrier for hydrophobic drugs designed to cross the blood–brain barrier. Amylose forms a helical structure that captures hydrophobic drugs and transports them through hydrophilic environments; however, when the drug-loaded amylose helix enters the membrane–water interface (region 1) the drugs are released [649]. Lipid membranes are, however, only one component of the structure of the blood–brain barrier; in fact, the most important elements are tight junctions controlling the entrance to the paracellular compartments. The main proteins forming these junctions belong to the claudin family. Since these junctions are large and complex, relatively few MD simulation studies of them have been performed; one example is a recent study of Claudin-5 [650].

It is commonly assumed that small molecules transform into their uncharged (unionized) form when they translocate through lipid bilayers, due to the prohibitively high free energy barriers for transporting charged species through a membrane (Figure 10). This assumption can be justified by, e.g., QM calculations performed in a polarizable continuum that demonstrates that proton transfer from the NH^{3+} to the COO^{-} group in the zwitterionic drug molecule will occur, so long as the dielectric constant is lower than 20 [233]; thus, molecules become neutral in the lipid headgroup region when the dielectric constant drops from 78.4 (water phase) to 12–18 (water–membrane interface) [651]. In order to understand the translocation process, one should thus perform calculations using both the uncharged and charged forms of the molecule. In recent studies, Yue et al., performed free energy calculations for uncharged and charged states of drugs and compared them with simulations where dynamic protonation was applied [202]. These calculations demonstrated that the free energy profile obtained with a more realistic dynamic protonation approach cannot be modeled as a simple superposition of the two other profiles; free energy barriers do not directly correspond to those observed in the simulation of the uncharged/charged form of the molecule; this assumption is thus an oversimplification.

Another methodological issue related to translocation and partitioning of small molecules into the lipid bilayer is the absence of explicit polarizability in the majority of the force fields commonly used for the simulation of biomolecules, i.e., potential sets used in the model. Jämbeck and Lyubartsev proposed a scheme to calculate free energy profiles through simulations with the partial charges in the potential set derived from QM calculations performed in a polarizable continuum; the calculations were performed twice with the dielectric constant set to 78.4 and 2.04, in order to mimic both water and hexane, respectively [292]. Based on these calculations, the authors define polarization correction terms for calculations of free energy differences between water and the environment of the membrane core.

A combination of atomistic and coarse-grained (CG) simulations have been applied to study the permeability of both planar lipid bilayers and a model of a small liposome with a radius of 10.1 nm, to 5-aminolevulinic acid and its esters [380]. In the first step, the free energy profile of solute translocation through a planar lipid bilayer was calculated for both coarse-grained and atomistic models. These calculations found a qualitative agreement between both models. In the second step, free energy profiles were calculated for the coarse-grained model of a liposome and compared with a coarse-grained model of a flat bilayer, demonstrating significant differences in the free energy barrier against translocation. In another coarse-grained study of liposomes, encapsulation and translocation between the outer and inner liposome leaflets, for the local anesthetic prilocaine, was observed [296]. Coarse-grained simulations have also been successfully used in the study of nanoparticles partitioning into lipid bilayers, e.g., [652,653] or where large-scale screening is performed for hundreds of drugs [654–658]. It should be noted that the MARTINI model was recently reparametrized (MARTINI 3) [659] to fix problems related to the imbalance of interactions between beads of various sizes leading to unrealistically strong interactions, e.g., protein–protein interactions [660–662].

5. Effect of Drug Molecules on Membrane Properties

5.1. Drug Molecules Can Do More in the Membrane than Merely Locate, Orient or Pass Through

In many cases, once drug molecules locate to the membrane, they gather in sufficient numbers to alter the structure of the membrane itself; designing drugs to affect the function of membrane proteins via an indirect modification of the properties of the membrane environment of the protein has been proposed. This mechanism is clearly theoretically possible as it is well known that the function of membrane proteins is modulated by their membrane environment [21,663–667]. Additionally, drugs can have a mode of action that involves solely the disruption of specific membranes; the desired activity of the drug does not, in any fashion, involve affecting the behavior of proteins. Regarding this tantalizing possible drug design strategy, it must, however, be determined whether this kind of affect can be induced with a realistic concentration of the drug molecule; the same question is relevant when alteration of a membrane structure is considered as an unwanted side effect (Figure 13).

This question was first addressed, through experimental studies of the anesthetic isoflurane in physiologically relevant concentrations of 1 and 5 mM in 4 membrane types, using multiple methods including fluorescence microscopy, fluorescence recovery after photobleaching, and patch-clamp measurements, among others. The results of these studies indicated that isoflurane, at this concentration, significantly decreases the extent of lipid ordering [304]. In erythrocyte ghosts, i.e., erythrocytes with their contents removed, the effect of the presence of a 1 mM concentration of isoflurane was found to be more substantial than that of 52.2 mM of ethanol. In another experimental study, the anesthetic phenyl-ethanol was shown to affect the properties of hippocampal membranes at a drug/membrane-volume ratio as low as 0.008% [306]; this indicates that the modification of membrane properties as a mechanism of drug action could actually be feasible. Finally, some drugs accumulate in specific cellular organelles, e.g., cationic amphiphilic drugs accumulate in lysosomes, organelles with an internal pH of ~4–5, perturbing the lysosomal membrane [668,669], thus decreasing cellular viability [670]. Among these drugs are numerous psychotropic drugs, which have shown potency as anticancer therapeutics [671,672].

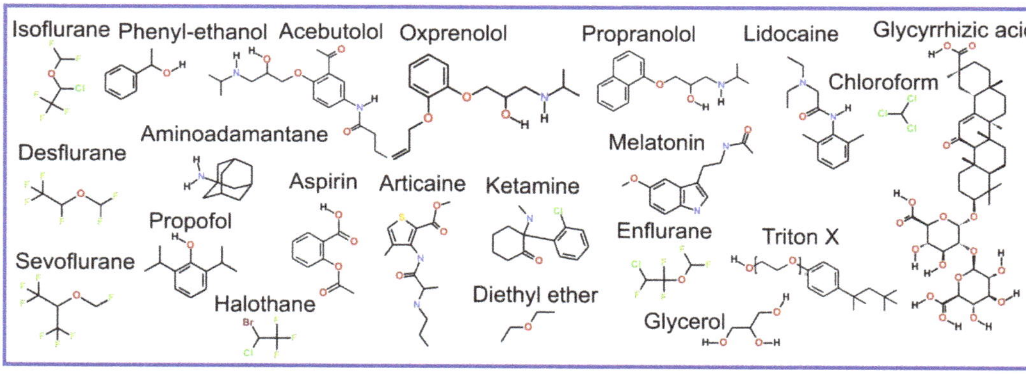

Figure 13. Chemical structure of drugs introduced in Section 5.

From what has been discussed so far in this review paper, regarding the use of MD simulation to study the behavior of drug molecules in lipid membranes, it should be clear that MD simulation can also act as a tool to study the effect on membrane properties of drug molecules that have entered the membrane; MD can model a small microcosm of the large scale global structural changes being made to the membrane. Through MD, it is also possible to measure changes to global properties of the membrane due to the presence of specific new foreign molecules; how this is determined through analysis of the MD trajectory is described in the following section.

5.2. Relevant Aside: Membrane Properties That Can Be Measured in MD Simulations

When studying the effect that drug molecules can have on lipid membranes, MD simulations can provide insight into numerous global structural, elastic, and dynamical properties of lipid bilayers [673,674]; however, in the context of drug–membrane interactions, one usually only calculates a few specific parameters. The results for the surface area per lipid molecule and membrane thickness provide information regarding the lipid bilayer size. The surface area per lipid molecule is easily calculated from MD simulations by dividing the simulation box size in the membrane plane by the number of lipids in a single leaflet of the bilayer. There is no unique definition of bilayer thickness; however, thickness can be estimated from the so-called P–P distance, the distance between the average positions along the membrane normal of the phosphorus atoms of the phosphate groups in opposite leaflets. Both of these parameters, the area per lipid and P–P distance, can be obtained from both X-ray and neutron scattering experiments [675–677]. Order parameters can be defined and calculated to describe the extent of ordering in the hydrocarbon chains; the most frequently used is the S_{CD} deuterium order parameter (Figure 14) that can also be measured experimentally through NMR spectroscopy [678,679]. Thickness and surface area are both global parameters, i.e., they represent the large-scale structure of the membrane; thus, their values will usually not be significantly affected by the presence of drug molecules at low concentration. Nevertheless, through MD simulations, these parameters can be calculated for the local region of the membrane around a specific drug molecule, i.e., by looking at a tiny microcosm of the membrane we can study the effect of a high concentration of many drug molecules entering the membrane.

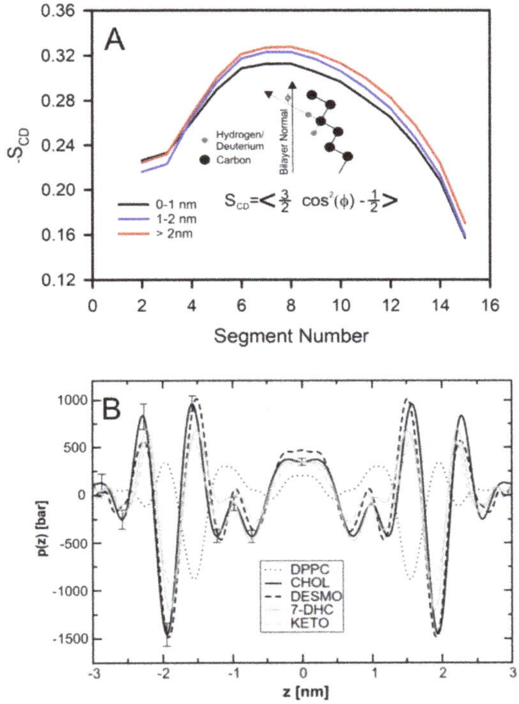

Figure 14. (**A**) Profile of the order parameter S_{CD} for lipids located in three zones: distances 0–1, 1–2, >2 nm from a drug molecule (reproduced with permission from ref. [187]). (**B**) Profile of the lateral pressure in bilayers composed of DPPC, DPPC and cholesterol and DPPC and other steroids (reproduced with permission from ref. [680]).

One more useful parameter is the profile of the lateral pressure (pressure in the direction parallel to the membrane surface) along the bilayer normal [680,681]. It has been hypothesized by Cantor (1997) [682–684] that changes in the lateral pressure profile of the bilayer may affect the structure of membrane proteins, affecting their functionality. The local pressure inside a lipid bilayer can reach a value of as high as 1000 bar (Figure 14); it is thus clearly plausible that the lateral pressure from the membrane can affect protein structure. Finally, MD simulations can provide information that describes the properties of the water–membrane interface. For example, increased membrane hydration due to the presence of nonsteroidal anti-inflammatory drugs has been suggested as a possible cause of some of the side effects of these drugs [261,278]. Moreover, it has been shown that changes in the orientation of the lipid headgroups, involved in signaling, can affect the binding behavior of peripheral membrane proteins [685,686]; the design of drugs to alter the orientation of lipid headgroups can thus be seen as a drug design strategy to alter their signaling and thereby the related metabolic pathways.

5.3. Unwanted Side Effects of Drugs Due to Their Alteration of Membrane Properties

While the possibility of drugs designed to affect membrane properties is indeed an attainable goal, where MD simulation has been brought to bear as a design tool, a more common issue remains the undesired effects that drug molecules can have on the biomembranes they encounter, i.e., drug toxicity (aka side effects); MD simulation has also played a role in elucidating such phenomena. The most frequent effect that drugs have been found to have on biomembranes is a local decrease of the extent of ordering in the acyl tails of the lipids. Examples of such drugs include, e.g., acebutolol, oxprenolol propranolol [194], and aminoadamantane [255]. A less frequent effect is an increase in the extent of lipid ordering; for example, the drug itraconazole increases the ordering of the acyl tails in the upper part of the chain, close to the water–membrane interface (regions 2 and 3) [186].

In most cases, for example, the aforementioned itraconazole, the mechanism of action of the drug is related to the inhibition of enzymes, channels, or receptors rather than their effect on a specific lipid membrane; alterations of the membrane properties caused by the drug are thus not relevant or even possibly an unwanted side effect. For example, glycyrrhizic acid is a saponin found in licorice root that is proposed as a potential component of drug delivery formulations, due to its ability to form complexes with a wide range of hydrophobic molecules. Using MD simulations, it has been demonstrated that glycyrrhizic acid locates inside the lipid bilayer (region 1 and 2) and significantly decreases the extent of lipid tail ordering, even at low concentration (Figure 15) [452,453]; this phenomenon could limit the pharmaceutical applications of this compound. Moreover, the gastrointestinal toxicity that has been observed in many nonsteroidal anti-inflammatory drugs, designed primarily as inhibitors of prostaglandin–endoperoxide synthase, is, at least in part, the result of the effect the drug has on membranes [687–689]. Furthermore, the cardiotoxicity of nonsteroidal anti-inflammatory drugs is in part induced by drug–lipid interactions [690] In addition to demonstrating that certain molecules have unwanted effects on lipid membranes, as described above, MD simulation has found evidence of innocence on the part of several drug molecules; for example, lipid-like potential drugs N-arachidonylglycine and oleoyl-L-carnitine have been shown not to affect membrane properties [137].

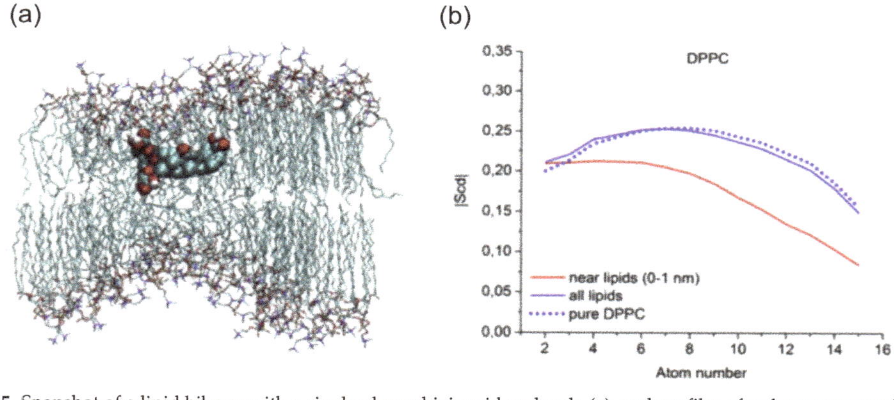

Figure 15. Snapshot of a lipid bilayer with a single glycyrrhizic acid molecule (**a**), and profiles of order parameter for lipids near and far from glycyrrhizic acid molecule (**b**). Reproduced with permission from ref. [453].

5.4. Drug Membrane Interaction Can Play a Role in the Mechanism of Drug Action—Case of Anesthetics

Now, we address the possibility that drugs could influence the membrane structure in a fashion that is desirable, i.e., an element of a drug's mechanism of action could be a direct alteration of the membrane's properties; MD simulation can be used in the same fashion to elucidate such positive effects in addition to the negative effects described in the previous section. The very first instance of the proposal of a mechanism of drug action that solely involved an interaction with the lipid membrane, rather than the active site of a protein, was the case of the theorized mechanism of action of general anesthetics. This hypothesis originates from the correlation between the efficacy of different anesthetics and their respective oil–water partition coefficients (the Meyer–Overton correlation [691,692]); it was later found that their efficacy has an even stronger correlation with their membrane–water partition coefficients [693]. Thus, unsurprisingly, several MD simulation studies of the interaction between general anesthetics and lipids have been undertaken [694]. For example, results obtained from MD simulations of chloroform in DOPC and DSPC–cholesterol bilayers, representing liquid disordered and liquid-ordered phases respectively, have demonstrated a difference in the fashion with which the addition of chloroform affects their properties [695]. In the DOPC bilayer, chloroform induced a small increase in the extent of tail ordering, while, in the DSPC–cholesterol bilayer, it was seen to have the opposite effect, inducing a pronounced reduction in the extent of tail ordering; it is hypothesized that the preference for chloroform to interact with flexible acyl chains and not with rigid cholesterol molecules leads to this effect. As a result, the number of direct cholesterol–cholesterol contacts increased while the number of cholesterol–DSPC contacts decreased.

In MD simulation studies, four anesthetics, desflurane, isoflurane, sevoflurane, and propofol, were shown to have negligible influence on bilayer properties when present in a POPC bilayer [305]. Additionally, chloroform, halothane, diethyl ether, and enflurane in a DPPC membrane, at a temperature of 310 K, were shown to have a negligible effect on the extent of acyl tail ordering, with the exception of the case of diethyl ether, where a small increase in the extent of lipid ordering was observed [298]. The presence of diethyl ether and sevoflurane in the membrane leads to a decrease in the extent of ordering of the acyl tails for the case of both DPPC and PSM bilayers; this effect is more pronounced for the case of bilayers that contain ~50 mol% of cholesterol [308]. Interestingly, evidence has been found that aspirin, one of the most frequently used analgesics, can also disrupt liquid-ordered domains or prevent their formation altogether [271]. The results of MD simulations have indicated that aspirin molecules affect the structure of the acyl tails of the lipids up to a depth of 1 nm into the bilayer with 30 mol% of cholesterol; coherent inelastic neutron scattering experiments have demonstrated liquid-ordered domain disruption, i.e., transition from the liquid ordered to the liquid disordered phase [266]. The local anesthetics lidocaine and articaine have also been found to decrease the extent of ordering of the acyl tails when in their charged (ionized) form; the results, however, indicate that, in their neutral form, their effect on the membrane structure is negligible [289].

Several experimental studies have been carried out that support the conclusions of the above MD simulations. For example, it has been demonstrated that the addition of chloroform loosens the structure of membranes in both gel and liquid-ordered phases [696]. Recent studies performed using multiple experimental techniques (Super–Resolution Microscopy dSTORM, Patch–Clamp, Fluorescence Resonance Energy Transfer) have demonstrated that both chloroform and isoflurane disrupt lipid domains (rafts) that contain the ganglioside GM1 [299]. Another anesthetic, propofol, at concentrations in the range 1 μM to 5 μM, has also been found to destabilize nanodomains in cellular membranes via Binned Imaging Fluorescence Correlation Spectroscopy [309]. Thus, the significant perturbations of the structure of bilayers in the liquid ordered phase, observed in MD simulation studies [271,308], are in agreement with experimental observations.

The aforementioned studies mainly focused on the effect of anesthetic molecules on the properties of the lipids related to the ordering behavior of the hydrocarbon chains of the lipids, i.e., order parameter, phase behavior, bilayer thickness, and surface area per lipid; this is, however, not the entire story. In 1997, Cantor proposed that general anesthesia is related to an alteration of the lateral pressure profile [683], a parameter not easily measured experimentally but relatively easy to calculate from MD simulations. An MD simulation study of ketamine, in a POPC bilayer, found evidence that the presence of the drug molecule could possibly give rise to a significant alteration to the lateral pressure profile with only a very limited alteration to the membrane structure, e.g., the global properties of the membrane discussed previously: membrane thickness, surface area, or the extent of ordering of the acyl chains [311]. Another MD simulation demonstrated that two other anesthetics, diethyl ether and sevoflurane in (1) DPPC, (2) DPPC–cholesterol 50 mol% (3) PSM, and (4) PSM–cholesterol 50 mol% bilayers, were found to significantly affect the lateral pressure profile [308]. It has also been demonstrated, through MD simulation, that the anesthetic chloroform ($CHCl_3$) and the relatively similar molecule carbon tetrachloride (CCl_4), a non–anesthetic, affect the membranes in strikingly different fashions, as measured by the effect on the lateral pressure and electrostatic potential profiles of the presence of one or the other of these two molecules in the membrane [300]. Experimental studies have also been carried out that provide evidence of the activation of transmembrane proteins as a result of alterations to the lipid composition, e.g., using the mild detergent Triton X-100 [541,542], the relationship between lateral pressure profile and lipid composition was investigated both experimentally [697] and through MD simulation [698]. A few MD simulation studies found specific effects due to direct lipid interaction on protein behavior e.g., [699–705]; in most cases, the cholesterol molecules in the membrane were, however, most frequently shown to play the role of modulating the behavior of membrane proteins [706–710].

The entry of certain molecules into the biomembrane can affect its properties in a more complex fashion than just altering the aforementioned parameters: it can affect the extent to which undulations are present in the membrane structure. In MD simulation studies of lipid bilayers using the coarse-grained MARTINI potential, it was found that the addition of chloroform can decrease the degree to which undulations are present in a membrane that contains ordered and disordered domains [301]. In the bilayer free of the anesthetic, the ordered domains in opposite leaflets were not registered, i.e., they were not across from one another. In this case, the bilayer was characterized by clearly visible undulations; the addition of chloroform led to the rearrangement of the bilayer, and ordered domains became registered and the bilayer thus became flat.

Although the above discussed computational and experimental studies demonstrate the possible membrane–mediated mechanisms of action of molecules designed as general anesthetics, namely the disruption of ordered lipid domains, such drug–membrane interactions cannot explain the sensitivity of the potency of anesthetic molecules to drug stereochemistry or single point mutations on the proteins involved in anesthesia [711]. Moreover, binding sites for anesthetics have been found from crystal structures of the membrane proteins [712–714], docking calculations [715], and MD simulation [307]. For these reasons the membrane mediated mechanism of anesthesia is frequently questioned [711], however, the above discussed studies provide clear evidence of anesthetic induced effects on membrane properties; additionally, evidence that the properties of the membrane influence protein functionality exist. Thus, a membrane-associated mechanism of action for general anesthetics cannot be discarded as one of the mechanisms involved in what is, admittedly, a complex process. Nevertheless, the interpretation of the Meyer–Overton correlation as an indication of a membrane-mediated mechanism is incorrect; we return to this issue later, in Section 6.2.1; this point will become clearer to the reader when they have read this section.

5.5. Can Drugs Prevent Amyloid Formation via the Modification of Membrane Properties?

The formation of amyloid plaques deposited on the extracellular membranes of neurons is one of the primary features of Alzheimer's disease [716]. This phenomenon is affected by specific lipids including cholesterol, sphingomyelin, and gangliosides [717,718]: lipid types typically present in the outer leaflet of the cell membrane. Amyloid fibers at a membrane surface have thus been frequently studied using MD simulations, e.g., [719–730], however, a surprisingly small fraction of this work has been performed in the context of drug design [731,732]. Khondker et al., proposed designing drugs with a mode of action that involved modulating membrane properties to affect the aggregation of amyloid-β25-35 at the bilayer surface [229]. They wished to study the modulation of the membrane thickness, ordering, and other properties, as possible modes of drug action; thus, they selected three molecules to study: curcumin, acetylsalicylic acid, and melatonin. Using MD simulations, they demonstrated that curcumin decreases membrane thickness, decreasing the extent of membrane ordering and rigidity; however, acetylsalicylic acid increases membrane thickness, thereby increasing membrane ordering and rigidity while melatonin does not affect the membrane properties at all; it was thus verified that these three molecules represent the needed set of examples of molecules that affect membranes in different ways. It was then determined experimentally that the decrease in the volume fraction of the cross-β sheets was ~70% for the case of curcumin in the membrane; evidence was thus found that decreasing membrane thickness in the vicinity of the amyloid-β25-35 molecules could possibly be a mechanism of drug action for the treatment of Alzheimer's disease.

5.6. A Clear Case of Drug Membrane Interaction as Mechanism of Action—Antimicrobial Agents

Antimicrobial agents represent a clear case of an established therapy where the global alteration of the properties of specific membranes is the clear mechanism of drug action. In general, biomembranes have a high degree of stability under physiological conditions and possess the capacity to adapt to extreme changes in their environment via changes in the lipid composition, e.g., [733–736]; evolution has provided biomembranes with several tools to preserve themselves over a wide range of conditions. They are, however, not completely invulnerable: numerous chemical agents and certain external conditions can disrupt their structure. The lipid bilayer structure emerges from weak, nonspecific, interactions and, additionally, the structure of biomembranes is formed by the cell, in driven processes and can include lipids that do not spontaneously form bilayers; it is thus unsurprising that they have vulnerabilities to several sources of disruption. The structure of a lipid bilayer can be compromised through the formation of pores that perforate the membrane, due to the presence specific molecules or physical stimuli, e.g., electric field [737], ultrasound [738,739], and charge imbalance [740,741]. Finally, a lipid bilayer can be dissolved completely at the molecular level by, e.g., detergents [742,743] or organic solvents [744].

Procaryotic (bacterial) and eurkaryotic (animal, i.e., patient) membranes differ substantially regarding the lipids of which they are composed. The extracellular leaflet of a eukaryotic cell membrane is comprised of cholesterol, saturated phospholipids, and sphingolipids, while procaryotic membranes contain mainly phosphatidylethanolamines, phosphatidylglycerols, and cardiolipin. This substantial difference, combined with the fact that some molecules can disrupt a cell membrane catastrophically enough to lead to cell death, opens the door to a tantalizing opportunity: the design of molecules that severely disrupt the structure of bacterial membranes while leaving eukaryotic membranes, i.e., the membranes of the cells of the patient being treated, relatively intact: they act as an antibiotic. The bacterial membrane is, however, not the only possible target for peptides designed to destroy specific lipid membranes. A recent development is the emergence of a second important target: cancer cells. The overall lipid composition of the cancer cell resembles that of normal cells, however, the asymmetric distribution of lipid classes between the inner and outer leaflets, normally found in eukaryotic cell membranes [745], is lost; they instead display a substantial concentration of phosphatidylserine in the outer leaflet. The selective disruption of lipid membranes rich in phosphatidylserine becomes a possible mode of action for cancer therapy: anticancer peptides [746,747] or drugs affecting the membranes of cancer cells [748].

Peptides that selectively compromise bacterial but not eukaryotic (host/patient) membranes, are a large and diverse group of potential drugs with a long history of research [749]. Currently, the term "antimicrobial peptides" is used as an umbrella term for peptides that display a wide range of different activities against different pathogens. For example, the APD3 database (2016) of natural antimicrobial peptides includes 2169 antibacterial, 172 antiviral, 961 antifungal, 185 anticancer, 307 hemolytic, 80 antiparasitic, 11 spermicidal, 27 insecticidal, and four anti-protist peptides [750]. The current number of antimicrobial peptide sequences deposited in "DBAASP v3: the database of antimicrobial/cytotoxic peptides" is 16,633 (01.02.2021); this number includes over 12,000 synthetic peptides [751]. Interestingly, over 3200 peptides have been the subject of MD simulations. Finally, dbAMP database contains over 12,000 entries [752]. There are at least six other databases dedicated to antimicrobial peptides [753–758] (for review, see [759,760]). Surprisingly, the number of clinical studies of antimicrobial peptides is, as of yet, relatively low (only 76) and the majority of these have ended in failure [761]; so far, only seven peptides have been approved for clinical use by the FDA [762]. However, the literature concerning antimicrobial peptides is extensive; prior comprehensive reviews of various aspects of antimicrobial and anticancer peptides have been published [763–785], including reviews focused specifically on computational studies [46–54]; we provide only a brief overview of this topic. Table 4 includes all antimicrobial peptides discussed in this paragraph.

Molecular dynamics simulations are frequently used to provide information regarding (1) peptide conformation (e.g., % of helicity) [786–798], (2) peptide location (at the membrane interface or inserted into the bilayer core), and (3) orientation in the membrane [783,787–790,792–794,796,799–806]. As we stated previously, simulations can also provide information regarding the effects of the peptides on membrane properties, including (1) the extent of ordering in the acyl tails, (2) the overall membrane thickness, and (3) curvature [793,794,799,800,807] as well as the formation of membrane defects [794] MD simulations and other computational methods, combined with complementary experimental methods, can be used to design more effective antimicrobial [783,798,808–811] and anticancer peptides [747,789,812–814]. For designing new peptides, an understanding of the interactions between peptides and lipids is of particular interest. The results of MD simulations can provide explicit information concerning, for example, (1) hydrogen bonds, (2) hydrophobic contacts, and (3) electrostatic and Van der Waals interaction energies [792–794,799,800,815]. For example, studies of pardaxin in the membrane have demonstrated the importance of cationic residues and phenylalanine residues on peptide association with lipids [806]. Finally, MD simulations allow for the study of the effect of chemical modification on the peptides (e.g., amidation) [787] and the effect of helical kink on peptide insertion into the bilayer [816,817].

The above discussed studies considered only peptides statically located at a membrane; the main mechanism through which antimicrobial peptides kill cells is, however, the formation of transmembrane pores. Simulating pore formation is computationally expensive; thus in a few older studies, to avoid long simulations, antimicrobial peptides were initially placed in the lipid bilayer core [818–820] or simulations were performed using the coarse-grained MARTINI model [821–825]. A few studies set out to elucidate the entire process of pore formation; however, the protocol of the MD simulations was altered e.g., by running simulations at an artificially high temperature or through a biased selection of the initial configuration. For example, Sun et al., modeled the formation of transmembrane pores, created by melittin, by initializing the simulated membrane with artificially created defects already in place [826,827]. The N-terminus of the peptide stabilized these defects, resulting in their transformation into small pores following the recruitment of two additional peptides. Wang et al., performed MD simulation at temperatures in the range 80–120 °C; this allowed for the observation of pore formation by the peptide maculatin [828]. Interestingly, they observed the formation of every variety of possible oligomers, from dimers to octamers. In simulations of the antimicrobial peptide pleurocidin, using a model with all atom resolution, the formation of a small pore composed of two helices was observed; however, in much longer coarse-grained simulations a larger number of helices were seen to be recruited to form a single pore [829].

Unbiased MD simulations of transmembrane pore formation were used to design a new 14 residue long peptide, LDKL, which was then modified to include input from the analysis of known antimicrobial peptides [830]. The final peptide, LDKA, contained only four amino acid types: (1) leucine, (2) aspartic acid, (3) lysine, and (4) alanine. Large pores formed by the LDKA peptide consisted of two overlapping pores formed separately in both membrane monolayers and occurred at low peptide/lipid ratios (1:1000). The ability of the peptide to kill both Gram-positive and Gram-negative bacteria without harming erythrocytes has been confirmed experimentally [830].

The results of MD simulations of magainin 2 in its native form and its covalently bound dimer, provided evidence for the formation of a disordered toroidal pore. The concentration of the peptide necessary for pore formation was substantially lower for the dimeric than the native form of magainin [831].

Calculations of the free energy of collective pore formation using umbrella sampling (Figure 16A) found that six melittin molecules can stabilize a pore; formation is associated with a small free energy (activation) barrier of ~10 kJ/mol. For seven peptide molecules, the barrier is absent; however, after pore formation, one molecule was seen to be diffusing away from the pore. When the number of melittin molecules is lower than six, the free energy barrier becomes significant, but five peptide molecules were also able to form a stable pore [832]. In another study, the free energy for the insertion of a single melittin molecule into a bilayer containing 0 to 6 peptide molecules was calculated (Figure 16B,C), a pore composed of three or more peptide molecules was seen to form [833]. The free energy barrier is reduced when a larger number of peptides is present in the bilayer and almost disappears, i.e., is close to 0 kJ/mol, when six peptides are present in the membrane. Atomistic MD simulation studies have also found that synthetic polycations [834], itraconazole [258], and DMSO [258] induce a decrease in the free energy barrier against pore nucleation.

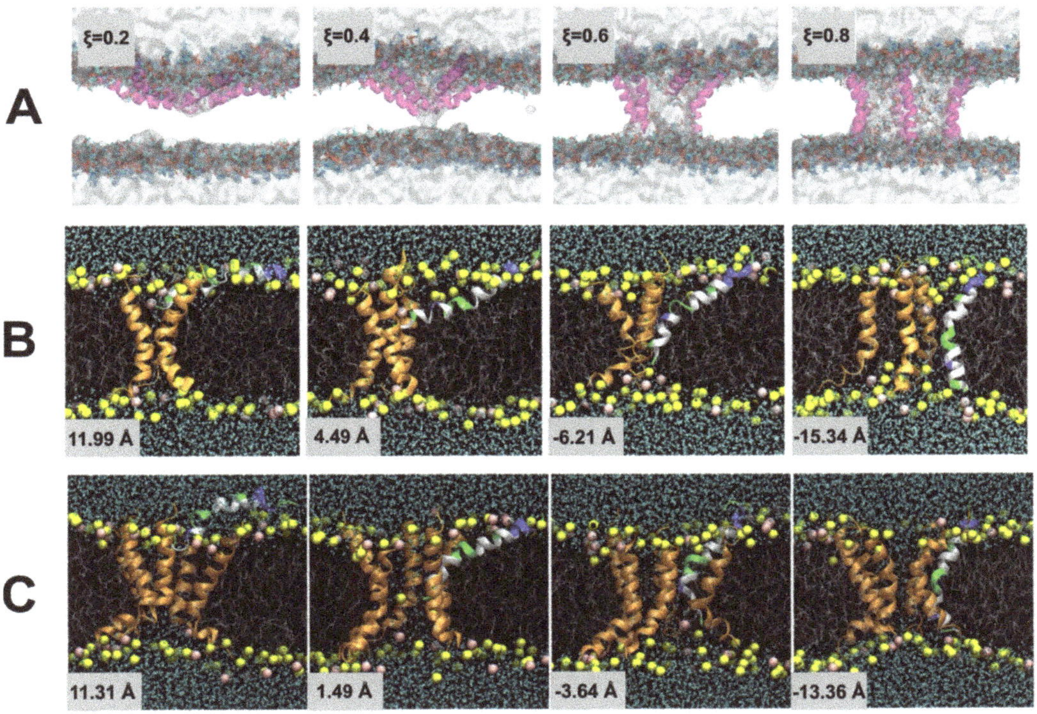

Figure 16. (**A**) Snapshots of stages of pore formation along the collective variable ξ. Reproduced with permission from ref [832]. Snapshot demonstrating the insertion of a single helix into the membrane (colored by residue polarity) where pores formed of (**B**) 3 and (**C**) 5 helices are present. Reproduced with permission from ref [833].

It is worth noting that the results of calculations of the free energy of pore formation are strongly dependent on the force field used [258,835]; other methodological issues related to the simulation of membrane active peptides are (1) the size of the simulation box,

(2) electrostatic interaction treatment, (3) initial conditions, and (4) the simulation protocol used [836].

Peptoids, N-substituted glycine oligomers, are a possible alternative class of molecules to antimicrobial peptides with the advantage of increased flexibility in functionalization via the presence of an amide bond [837]. Peptoids have not been studied with theoretical methods in the context of their membrane activity, but rather in the context of their applications in nanotechnology, e.g., the study by Jin et al., in 2016 [838]. Recently, a coarse-grained force-field created within the MARTINI framework [605] for peptoids was developed [839]. Nevertheless, the interactions between peptoids and membranes have been investigated experimentally [840]. These studies have found that antimicrobial peptoids increase the permeability of bacterial membranes; this effect is increased via cyclization [841]. Moreover, peptoids have recently been found to be potent antiviral agents and have been successfully tested for activity against the SARS-CoV-2 virus [842].

Another class of drug molecules derived from peptides that has been proposed for use as an antimicrobial agent are the $\beta^{2,2}$-amino acid derivatives. In a simulation study carried out by Koivuniemi et al., MD simulations of these derivatives interacting with both prokaryotic and eukaryotic model membranes found evidence of important differences in their behavior in the two membrane types [843]. Additionally, antimicrobial peptides can have their desired properties enhanced through the introduction of non–natural amino acids, e.g., the azoALY peptide derived from ALY (full sequence: ALYLAIRKR) by functionalization of the sole tyrosine residue present with an azobenzene group [844]. Both MD simulations and experimental studies have found evidence that this modification results in a peptide with an enhanced interaction with lipid bilayers. Finally, peptides conjugated with dendrimers have been proposed as a novel form of potential antimicrobial compound; MD simulations have demonstrated the presence of strong interactions between these molecules and bilayers composed of POPG [802].

In the above discussed studies, the bacterial membranes were modeled as simple mixtures of either PC or PE with PG lipids, in spite of the fact that lipopolysaccharides (LPS) are known to be present in bacterial membranes; aspects of the membrane structure, behavior, and interactions with other molecules resulting from the presence of LPS in the membrane were not explored. The reason for this is that when LPS molecules are included in the membranes, the size of the system and timescale needed for system equilibration becomes too large for the system to be tractable for MD simulation with a model with all atom resolution. Theoretical studies have, however, been carried out that indicate LPS plays a protective role against antibacterial peptides, e.g., magainin [845].

Antimicrobial peptides are not the only group of chemical compounds capable of selectively disrupting the bacterial membrane; for example, recent studies of potential antibiotics kanamycin A [133] and bithionol [247], provide evidence that these drugs have an affinity towards model membranes that mimic the bacterial membrane and either do not interact with, or only weakly affect, model membranes designed to mimic eukaryotic membranes. Another set of potential antimicrobial compounds were synthetized on the basis of cholic acid esterified with three glycine and an aliphatic alcohol of length 1, 6, or 12 carbons; MD simulations found evidence of the presence of strong interactions between these compounds and bilayers composed of lipopolysaccharides from Gramm–negative bacteria [846]. The strongest effects on bilayer properties were observed for the compound with the six-carbon long alcohol. Membrane perturbation by antibiotics (e.g., fluoroquinolones and aminoglycosides) was proposed as an additional bactericidal mechanism for these drugs [847]; recent studies of aminoglycosides, macrolides, and fluoroquinolones determined that these antibiotics have a disordering effect on bacterial membranes; however, they found no evidence of large-scale membrane disruption or pore formation [848]. Interestingly, colchicine, a drug frequently used in chemotherapy, is capable of inducing pore formation in lipid bilayers [849].

5.7. Other Effects on Lipid Layers—Pulmonary Surfactants and Indirect Effect on Membrane Proteins

Drug molecules have also been shown to affect the properties of lipid monolayers, e.g., disrupting lung surfactants [264]. To condense pulmonary surfactant monolayers doped with ketoprofen, higher surface pressures were necessary in comparison to the case of the pure monolayer [263]. The difference was found to increase with decreasing surface area per lipid. This observation was in qualitative agreement with data obtained from Langmuir–Blodgett monolayer experiments. A similar result was obtained for pulmonary surfactant monolayers doped with levofloxacin [238]. The increase was more significant when the model was simulated with an elevated value for surface pressure. Additionally, the presence of levofloxacin in the membrane had a disordering effect on the acyl tails; again, the effect was more substantial for the model simulated with a higher surface pressure. Glycerol is often used in the formulation of pulmonary drugs and the liquid medium in electronic cigarettes. It has been demonstrated, both experimentally and through MD simulation, that glycerol affects lipid monolayers and bilayers; its presence leads to significant monolayer expansion, even at the low w/w concentration level of 1% [424].

Table 4. Antimicrobial peptides.

Peptide	Source	Refs.
Alamethicin	Fungus, Trichoderma viride	[818]
Aurein	Frog, Litoria aurea	[787,791]
azoALY	Synthetic with non–natural amino acids	[844]
Bombinins	Toad, Bombina variegata	[783,850,851]
Cathelicidins	Innate immunological system	[792,808,852]
Clavanin A	Tunicate, Styela clava	[799]
Crabrolin	Wasp, Vespa crabro	[786,798]
Daptomycin	Actinobacteria, Streptomyces roseosporus	[853–855]
Dermcidin	Human sweat	[801]
Designed peptides	Synthetic	[795–797,856–866]
Esculentin 2	Frog, Glandirana emeljanovi	[867]
Gramicidins	Gram–Positive bacteria, Bacillus brevis	[853,868]
Kalata B1	Cyclotide from Oldenlandia affinis (plant)	[869]
LDKL, LDKA	Synthetic	[830]
LL-3	Human	[793]
Maculatin	Frog, Litoria aurea	[828]
Magainin 2	African clawed frog Xenopus laevis	[822,831,870,871]
Melittin	Honeybee, Apis mellifera	[807,818–820,822,824–827,832,872–876]
MSI-103	Synthetic	[796]
Nisin	Lactic acid bacteria	[877]
Pardaxin	Fish, Pardachirus marmoratus	[800,806]

Table 4. *Cont.*

Peptide	Source	Refs.
PGLa	African clawed frog Xenopus laevis	[788,796]
Pleurocidin	Fish, Pleuronectes americanus	[871]
Polymyxins	Gram–positive bacteria e.g., Paenibacillus polymyxa	[853,878]
Thanatins	Insect defense peptides	[815]
Trichogin	Fungus, Trichoderma longibrachiatum	[879]
β-Defensin	Innate immunological system	[794]
Cecropin	Moth Hyalophora cecropia	[789]
Peptoids	Synthetic	[837–841]

6. Role of Membrane in Substrate (Drug) Selection of Membrane Proteins

6.1. Membrane Proteins: The Majority of Drug Targets

In addition to direct drug–membrane interactions, lipid membranes also play a role in the interaction between substrates and membrane–associated proteins, with both substrate–membrane and protein–membrane interactions playing roles in the substrate, and thus the drug selection mechanism of membrane-associated proteins. Since membrane–associated proteins are, in fact, the majority of drug targets [880,881], this issue should be central to drug design. However, it can be argued that, so far, it has not received the attention it deserves (Figure 17).

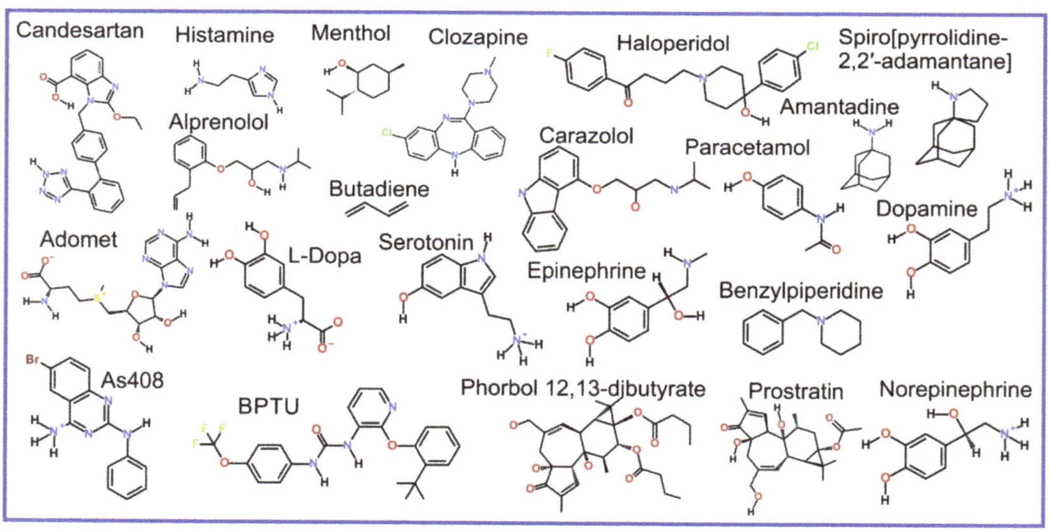

Figure 17. Chemical structure of drugs introduced in Section 6.

Membrane associated proteins can be subdivided into three categories: (1) multi–pass (integral) membrane proteins, where the ligand/substrate binding site is frequently within the membrane core (39% of membrane proteins [882]), (2) bitopic (single-pass) membrane proteins with one or more domains outside the membrane but anchored to the membrane through a single trans-membrane helix, with the functional domain, thus the active site, located outside the membrane (36% of membrane proteins [882]), and (3) peripheral membrane proteins, with no permanent association with the membrane (16% of membrane proteins [882]); however, for catalytic activity that involves interaction with a membrane, catalysis occurs at the membrane surface.

There is what can arguably be described as a fourth variety of membrane associated proteins that we, however, do not discuss in this review paper as they have not been studied to as significant an extent: 9% of membrane proteins are covalently bound with lipids; a common example is a glycosylphosphatidylinositol (GPI) molecule bound to the C terminus of the protein, known as a GPI-anchor [882]. As is the case with bitopic membrane proteins, the functional domain of the protein is located completely outside the membrane but is bound to a lipid membrane through an anchor.

The term "multi-pass" to describe integral membrane proteins refers to the structure of the trans-membrane domain, composed of several (up to 14 [883]) α-helices as the protein threads back and forth through the membrane; another class of integral membrane protein exists with a β–barrel rather than a set of α-helices as the trans-membrane domain. However, such proteins are not common [884] and have not been used as drug targets, thus they are not discussed in this review; yet, it should be mentioned that β-barrel membrane proteins are predominately found in bacterial membranes, e.g., the outer membrane of gram negative bacteria (in eukaryotic cells only in mitochondria and chloroplasts), thus could possibly in the future be potential targets for antibiotics, though, as far as we are aware, this is not yet the case.

A mechanistic understanding of the role the lipid plays in the substrate selection of membrane proteins is a key element of the design of drugs that target them, and MD simulation has a central role to play in obtaining this; we now discuss examples where MD simulation has obtained insight relevant to drug design, for all three varieties of membrane associated proteins.

In contrast to multi-pass (integral) membrane proteins, where considerable work has been performed, in particular the GPCR class of membrane proteins e.g., [885–899] (for review see references: [31,900–903]), that are a very hot topic, peripheral and bitopic (single pass) membrane proteins, which constitute 43–45% of transmembrane proteins [883], are underrepresented in MD simulation studies.

One of the reasons for this is that obtaining experimental insight into the nature of the membrane–protein interaction for weakly membrane associated proteins is extremely challenging. Obtaining structures from x-ray crystallography or cryo-EM, while less straightforward than for the case of water-soluble proteins, is still possible for integral membrane proteins within membrane-like nanodiscs [904–906] or a detergent environment [907–909]; obtaining such information for the more weakly associated proteins directly from experiment is challenging and rarely achieved. The rare cases of success in this regard represent a Herculean effort: one must work with incomplete structures combining fragments originating from several PDB entries and, frequently, the assistance of theoretical methods is necessary (e.g., homology modeling [910–912] and modeling of short loops [913]). Moreover, extracellular domains of bitopic receptors are heavily glycosylated and the precise sequences of these complex carbohydrate branches have, in most cases, not been determined. The few MD simulation studies of glycosylated receptor proteins that have been carried out have demonstrated that glycosylation determines the behavior of these receptors [914–916]. Interactions of these latter two classes of membrane proteins with lipids differ significantly in comparison to multi-pass (integral) membrane proteins since interactions with the lipid headgroups become dominant over interactions with the membrane core. As mentioned in the beginning of this review, the solution of the structure from sequence problem by the Alphafold project [1] completely changes the game; initial results show promise for even the structure of bitopic membrane proteins, so there may soon be rapid progress in this area.

6.2. Multi-Pass (Integral) Membrane Proteins

6.2.1. Our Discussion Follows the Framework of Vauquelin

Multi pass membrane proteins are the class of membrane proteins that have been experimentally and computationally studied the most in their context as drug targets, primarily due to their functions as receptors (40% of multi pass membrane proteins), channels and transporters (another 24%), and enzymes (yet another 16%). The importance of this group of proteins may be exemplified by the Nobel prizes awarded for the study of various aspects of an important family of 901 (in human) integral membrane proteins [917], the G coupled receptors, including Nobel prizes in Medicine and Physiology: 1967 (studies of rhodopsin), 1988 (discovery of β-blockers), 1994 (discovery of G-protein), 2004 (odorant receptors), and even a Nobel prize in Chemistry: 2012 (3D structure of GPCRs) (GPCR) [918–922]. Issues relating to the design of drugs to target integral membrane proteins are covered in several already published reviews [923–926].

In describing the role played by MD simulation in the study of multi-pass membrane proteins, in their context as drug targets, we will follow the categorization scheme developed by Vauquelin, presented in ref [927], shown as a schematic in Figure 18, i.e., we draw attention to the contribution that MD simulations and related methods have made towards understanding drug–membrane–target protein relationships using their classification scheme, as a framework for our discussion. The scheme is summarized (see Figure 18) as: (1) the effective increase in both the kinetics and affinity due to drug accumulation in the membrane and the resultant reduced dimensionality of drug diffusion (Figure 18A–C); (2) how the membrane affects the entry of the ligand into the binding site (Figure 18D); (3) the role the membrane plays in the ligand interaction with the protein (Figure 18E); and (4) the possible design of hybrid drugs connecting orthosteric and allosteric pockets (Figure 18F). Our discussion will now follow this framework in order.

(1) The accumulation of drug molecules in membranes significantly increases the local concentration of the drug molecule in the vicinity of the targeted membrane proteins in comparison to bulk solution, thus increasing the apparent affinity of the drug for the active site and making the drug kinetics more favorable (Figure 18A).

Due to the high affinity of drugs for the lipid membrane, the release of the drug from the membrane environment is slow and the local concentration of the drug remains enhanced in relation to its bulk concentration in the solvent medium. This results in drug molecules being predominantly confined to the two-dimensional environment of the membrane that the protein is associated with, rather than the three-dimensional environment of the bulk solution around the protein. Thus, as a result of geometry alone, diffusion confined to two dimensions is significantly more limited in comparison to diffusion in three dimensions; the drug is more likely to remain in the vicinity of the protein with an increased chance of binding again as a result of locating preferentially to the lipid membrane as opposed to being randomly distributed in the bulk solution. This phenomenon is known as "rebinding" and has been documented experimentally [928] and considered in models of drug kinetics [929]. In order to take this into account, micro–pharmacokinetic models, which consider local drug concentration, have been proposed.

Extensive studies of ligands of the β2-adrenergic receptor have demonstrated that lipophilic drugs that accumulate on the lipid bilayer are characterized by a higher rate of drug—target protein association (K_{on}) in comparison to the more hydrophilic drugs with the same pharmacophore [930]. On the other hand, the dissociation rate (K_{off}) was not found to be dependent on drug lipophilicity [930], as lipids do not affect protein–drug interactions inside the binding site. Subsequent studies that used fluorescently labeled propranolol found an accelerated accumulation of the drug on the cell membrane and suggested that the actual affinity of propranolol for the β2-adrenergic receptor was significantly less than previously anticipated, based on a standard measurement assuming a uniform distribution of the drug in the volume of a sample [931].

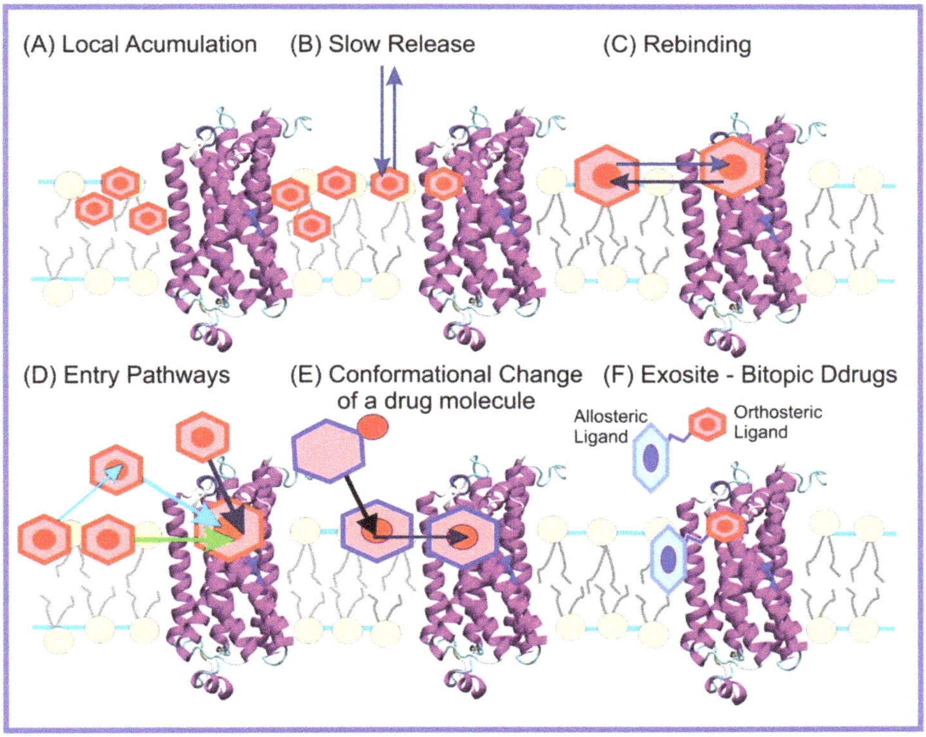

Figure 18. Accumulation of drugs in the membrane and its consequences for drug–protein interactions. Based on Figure 2 from ref. [927].

In addition to the kinetics of binding, this phenomenon will affect the effective affinity, of the binding site, for the ligand; it will be a factor that is missed by conventional docking and scoring studies that do not take the membrane into account. While this will not affect the enthalpic term of the binding affinity, it will have a marked effect on the entropic component; bias of drug molecules to confinement to a two-dimensional plane rather than the three-dimensional bulk medium lowers the entropic penalty of binding. Techniques that use MD simulation with a force bias, that we discussed previously, can be used to obtain a quantitative estimation of this effect. For example, a deconvolution of the membrane and protein binding contributions, i.e., separating the contributions to affinity due to the membrane and the binding site, performed for β2 adrenergic receptor ligands, improved the accuracy of the results of a structure–activity relationship analysis [932].

We can now, in light of the discussion of the activity of membrane proteins, return to our discussion of the mechanism of action of anesthetics. The aforementioned Meyer–Overton correlation is the result that more lipophilic anesthetics have a tendency to produce stronger effects. The correlation can be most easily explained through a micropharmacokinetic model. However, this interpretation, while the most elegant, does not support a membrane mediated mechanism for the action of anesthetics but rather suggests the involvement of membrane proteins; nevertheless, the possibility that modification of the membrane properties plays some role in a more complex mechanism of action for anesthetics is not excluded.

(2) The accumulation of drugs in the membrane will affect the entry pathway of a ligand into the binding site as this will create a bias, increasing the likelihood that drugs approach the protein from within the lipid membrane (Figure 18D).

As discussed previously, the accumulation of ligand molecules in the membrane will increase both the entrance frequency and apparent affinity of ligands for the active site; this is, however, not the only effect of the preferential location of ligands to the membrane: the path taken to enter the protein will also be affected, resulting in further inaccuracy in the standard "lock and key" paradigm that does not take the membrane into account. In many cases, the active site is entirely within the membrane core, with entry being made from the lipid phase into an opening between trans-membrane helices. In fact, the direct entry of a ligand from a membrane into a receptor can be anticipated based on the crystal structure of the receptor. For example, for the case of the sphingosine 1–phosphate receptor 1 the extracellular opening is blocked by the N–terminus and extracellular loops [933]; the entry location for ligands is rather from within the membrane core to a receptor deep within the lipid phase of the membrane between trans membrane (TM) helices TMI and TMVII. For the protein Opsin, the retinal binding site opens directly into the membrane core at two points between TM1–TM7 and TM5–TM6 [934]. The two openings and the central cavity, constitute a channel through the protein, with a length of 7 nm and a width of 1.16–0.32 nm The entry of a ligand into the binding pocket has been studied via MD simulations, in some cases using force bias methods and these will be discussed in detail later in this section. Membrane mediated ligand entry/exit pathways to the binding pocket have been discussed in previously published review articles for the case of GPCRs [935,936], but also for the larger group of membrane proteins that includes GPCRs, ion channels, and transporters [41].

(3) Drug partitioning into the membrane can alter the conformation of the drug molecule, thus affecting its interaction with the binding site of the target protein.

When immersed in the hydrophobic environment of the membrane core, the situation is roughly equivalent to immersion in a non-polar solvent. Many molecules exist that are soluble in both polar and non-polar solvents and achieve this through changing their conformation; it is thus possible for a molecule to exist that first enters the membrane, then alters its conformation within the membrane core and, only at this point, with its new conformation adopted within the hydrophobic environment of the membrane core, has a structure with a high affinity for a specific binding site of a membrane protein (Figure 18E). Through MD simulations, we can directly observe such behavior, for example, the candesartan antagonist of the GPCR AT1 receptor changes conformation after entry into the membrane [193]. Another example is the cannabinoid analog AMG3. This molecule is in possession of six flexible bonds, thus allowing for significant conformational change; MD simulations of AMG3 in a lipid bilayer were used to find the optimal conformation for binding to both the CB1 and CB2 receptors [338].

(4) The exosite model (Figure 18F) assumes that the drug molecule is composed of two linked component ligands: the first binding to the orthosteric pocket and the second to the allosteric site [937].

The allosteric sites are frequently located at the protein–lipid interphase and allow for increased specificity in comparison to a drug that targets only the orthosteric (binding) pocket. Due to the highly conserved structure of orthosteric pockets, e.g., among GPCRs, it is difficult to find a highly selective ligand based on this criterion alone; an inclusion of the allosteric site into the computational drug design approach allows for the necessary targeting specificity. The use of the allosteric site in addition to the orthosteric pocket in drug design has been referred to as the "exosite model" and "the design of bitopic ligands/drugs" by two separate research communities [938,939]. Modeling methods, including MD simulations, are one of the tools used in the design of bitopic drugs [900,940,941]; however, in these studies lipids are only considered as a passive component and their complete role in substrate selection is not fully elucidated.

6.2.2. Exploring the Complex Pathways to the Active Sites of Integral Membrane Proteins

The time scale that can be investigated through MD simulations is a limiting factor for a direct observation of ligand entry into the binding site of receptors or enzymes; only a few studies have thus addressed this problem with unbiased MD simulations. A study of histamine entry into the H4 receptor found evidence of two possible entry pathways [407], one of which overlaps with the previously determined Na^+ entry pathway [556]. In extensive simulations of alprenolol, an inhibitor of the β2 adrenergic receptor, the entrance of the drug into the binding pocket of the receptor was observed 12 times; entry, however, occurred from the water phase despite strong preferences observed for the drug molecule to locate to the lipid phase and remain there for the majority of the simulation [195]; in this case, the membrane acts as a drug reservoir, and its mechanism described in Figure 18A. The ligand entrance into the protein binding site, directly from within the lipid core of the membrane, was demonstrated for the example of the cannabinoid sn-2-arachidonoylglycerol (2-AG) and the CB2 receptors [455]. The entrance gate for the ligand locates between TM6 and TM7. The entry of the ligand into the sphingosine-1-phosphate receptor-1 was characterized using multiple, microsecond long simulations [942]. The entry path began in the vestibule at the top of TM7, then preceded to enter the protein between TM7 and TM1. A similar MD study of the binding and activation of Orexin–A was also carried out [943]. In studies of the dopamine D3 receptor, a set of 1000 short 20 ns simulations of systems, where dopamine was initially located in the water phase, found only 22 cases of direct entrance of dopamine into the binding pocket of the receptor [394]. In 736 cases, the dopamine molecule located to the membrane, settling among the lipids but not in contact with the protein; in another 180 cases, it located to the protein–lipid interface and in the remaining 62 cases located to the protein surface exposed to the water phase. These numbers closely correspond to the surface area of the membrane occupied by lipids and protein in the studied model; thus, this provides evidence that the protein has no inherent properties that attract the ligand, i.e., the relative number of binding events correspond to the relative surface areas, an unexpected result.

Flooding simulation was used to study the interaction between the *Gloeobacter violaceus* ligand-gated ion channel and the general anesthetic desflurane [307]. These studies demonstrated that the desflurane molecule enters a binding site, with a structure known from X-ray crystallography [712], via a membrane-mediated pathway. Moreover, simulations revealed an additional binding site not anticipated in previous studies. In this case, desflurane entered the binding site directly from the lipid core (Figure 19). In another flooding simulation study, menthol, a small compound extracted from mint that acts as a local anesthetic, bound to the α4β2 nicotinic acetylcholine receptor, to a binding site located at the lipid–protein interface via a membrane–mediated pathway [434]. In other flooding simulations of two anesthetics, chloroform and isoflurane, the molecules first entered the lipid bilayer and then subsequently diffused to the allosteric binding sites of the vanilloid-1 receptor (TRPV1) [297]. These studies identified five binding sites for chloroform and three for isoflurane, in spite of the fact that the overall affinity of the aforementioned drug molecules toward TRPV1 was relatively small.

In some cases, MD simulations determined only a fragment of the drug entry pathway or merely demonstrated the accumulation of the drug in the vicinity of possible entry points. For example, multiple 500 ns MD simulations of the drugs clozapine and haloperidol, acting as ligands of the dopamine D2 and D3 receptors, determined the pathway between the binding site and the receptor vestibule, where drugs were placed into the initial structure; however, the pathway between the vestibule and membrane remains unknown [322]. Amantadine is a drug used to treat influenza. At the molecular level, amantadine inhibits the M2 transmembrane proton channel, preventing virus budding. Through MD simulation, it has been demonstrated that the more hydrophobic derivative of amantadine, spiro[pyrrolidine2,2′-adamantane], has a tendency to aggregate around the M2 channel to a greater extent than amantadine; this could be the mechanism behind the experimentally observed higher binding affinity of spiro[pyrrolidine2,2′-adamantane] for the M2 protein in comparison to the case for amantadine [254]. Simulations of candesartan, an antagonist of the GPCR AT1 receptor, an integral membrane protein, found evidence that that the drug approaches the opening between helices 4 and 5 from where entry into the binding site has a high probability [193]. This study then made the important observation that the two-dimensional diffusion coefficient of the drug, in the plane of the membrane, calculated from the MD simulation trajectories, was in excellent agreement with the diffusion coefficient measured experimentally using liposomes as a membrane model. This result further supports the 2D model of drug diffusion when approaching the previously discussed receptor. Finally, Kiriakidi et al., suggest that lipids affect the conformation of the candesartan molecule, potentially affecting the affinity of the drug for the binding site. Yet, for two lipid-like drugs, N-arachidonylglycine, and oleoyl-L-carnitine, the only possible pathway to access the binding site is from within the membrane. Extensive MD simulations of the glycine transporter GlyT2 embedded into the lipid bilayer found evidence for numerous possible drug interactions with the protein; unfortunately, this study was unable to determine the specific binding site responsible for receptor inhibition [137].

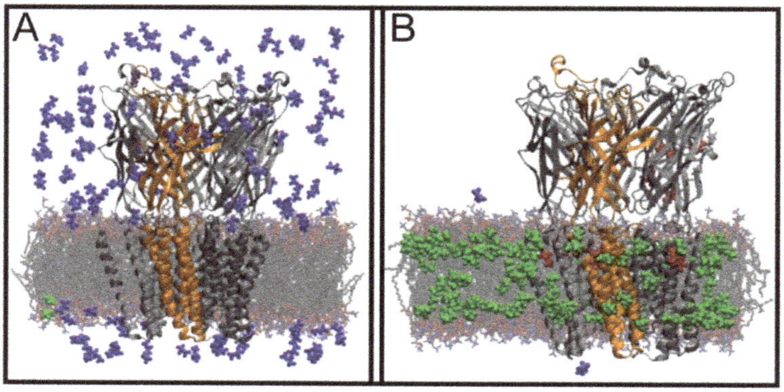

Figure 19. Partitioning of desflurane into the membrane and Gloeobacter violaceus ligand-gated ion channel studied using a flooding simulation. Snapshots of the simulated model at the (**A**) beginning and (**B**) end of the simulation. Desflurane molecules were colored according to their location: blue—water phase, green—lipid bilayer, red—ion channel. Reproduced with permission from ref. [307].

As stated above, the timescales involved limit the extent to which unbiased MD simulation can elucidate the interaction between potential ligands and integral membrane proteins. As a result, several groups have made use of a variety of force bias, and other enhanced sampling techniques to gain further insight; the situation is similar to that regarding membrane translocation discussed earlier, though the specific methods that are optimal differ. Studies of the β-adrenergic receptor using RAMD found five possible exit pathways of the receptor antagonist carazolol [200]. The most frequent entry/exit pathway was passing through the extracellular opening, i.e., the opening exposed to the solvent, at the top of the receptor; however, in 30% of runs, carazolol exited the binding pocket through clefts between the transmembrane helices. The most frequently utilized alternate pathway was the cleft between the TM4 and TM5 helices (TM4–TM5); other pathways pass between helices: TM5–TM6, TM1–TM2, TM1–TM7, and TM6–TM7 (see Figure 20). For the case of dopamine, D3 receptor RAMD simulations revealed an alternative pathway that passed through a lateral gate between helices TM5 and TM6 [394]. Subsequent free energy calculation using the umbrella sampling algorithm [93] demonstrated that there is no energy barrier along this pathway. Temperature accelerated molecular dynamics simulation was applied to the study of protease-activated receptor-1, a GPCR activated by the binding of a peptide; it was determined that an exit/entry patch of a ligand from the binding pocket directly faces into the membrane hydrocarbon core [944]. The two observed exit/entry points were located between helices TM4, TM5, TM6, and TM7. These simulations also found evidence for a third possible entry/exit pathway located between the extracellular loops of the receptor and the water phase.

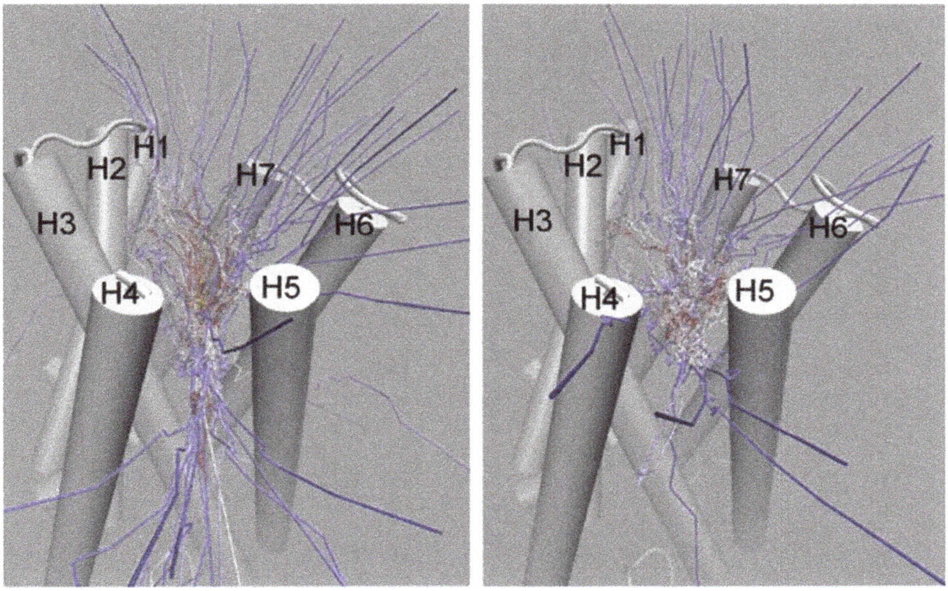

Figure 20. Entry/exit pathways of carazolol observed in the RAMD simulations. Left and right panels show sets of simulations with different acceleration magnitudes. The color scale is from yellow at the beginning of the simulation to blue at the end of the simulation. The starting conformation of the receptor is shown in a cartoon representation. Reproduced with permission from ref. [200].

Most drugs bind to the orthosteric binding pockets of proteins where their natural ligands bind; however, it is possible for proteins to be modulated by a drug binding to an allosteric site, e.g., for the GPCR family, 7 allosteric pockets facing into the membrane hydrocarbon core have been found in 12 GPCRs [945]. Yet, the most recent studies of M5 muscarinic acetylcholine receptor revealed the presence of three allosteric sites including one novel site [946]. Recent studies provide an example of such an allosteric modulator of the β2-adrenergic receptor: compound AS408 was shown to bind between transmembrane helices TM3 and TM5 at the surface, directly facing the membrane core, thus stabilizing the inactive conformation of the receptor [197]. In MD simulations, Yuan et al., demonstrated the binding of the P2Y1 receptor antagonist, BPTU, to the extra-helical site between helices 1 and 3 [329]. The binding took place via the lipid bilayer in three steps: first, BPTU enters the water–membrane interface from the water phase; next, BPTU forms an initial set of interactions with the extracellular loop 2 of the receptor; finally, the drug translocates to the binding site. Similarly, the binding site for ZM241385 in adenosine receptor type 2A was identified at the protein–lipid interface [947]; in this case, lipids stabilized the binding pose of the ligand.

6.3. Bitopic Membrane Proteins

6.3.1. Proteins with a Tenuous, but Permanent Connection to a Specific Lipid Bilayer

As described above, for the case of bitopic proteins, the protein is tethered to the membrane through a single transmembrane helix, but with the functional domain/domains, thus active site/sites, located outside the membrane; there is, however, considerable evidence that the lipid membrane plays a role in substrate selection [381]. Monk et al., [948] in the very first complete structure of a bitopic protein to be determined, already found evidence that the trans–membrane helix and linker segment controls the orientation of the catalytic domain relative to the membrane, thus indicating a role for the membrane in catalysis; bitopic proteins cannot be thought of as merely a catalytic domain loosely attached to the membrane like a balloon with the linker segment as a piece of string attaching it to a the trans membrane helix acting like a pin in a cork board: the linker segment and trans-membrane helix play an active role in positioning the catalytic domain relative to the membrane.

We will now focus on four cases where MD simulation has seen considerable success in elucidating the role the membrane plays in substrate selection (thus drug affinity) for bitopic membrane proteins: (1) cytochrome P450, (2) the membrane bound isoform of catechol-o-methyltransferase (MB–COMT), (3) monoamine oxidase, and (4) tropomyosin receptor kinase B. In many cases, for example MB–COMT, these are proteins with water-soluble in addition to bitopic, membrane bound, isoforms.

6.3.2. Cytochrome P450

Cytochrome P450 (CYP) is a family of 41 (in humans) bitopic membrane enzymes responsible for both the catabolism (synthesis) and anabolism (degradation) of a variety of small molecules [949]. For example, the synthesis of cholesterol, steroid hormones, bile acids, vitamin D3, and second messengers derived from polyunsaturated lipids is performed by CYPs. CYPs are also responsible for the degradation of small molecules, e.g., neurotransmitters, and various xenobiotics, including about 50% of all approved drugs [950–954]. A review of MD simulation studies of CYPs is given in ref. [955].

The catalytic domains of proteins belonging to the cytochrome P450 family have been studied extensively, in a water environment without the trans-membrane helix present, using MD simulation and related molecular modeling methodologies in the context of both drug design (e.g., [956,957]) and their mechanism of catalysis (e.g., [958]). It has been argued that these studies can elucidate the catalytic mechanism of membrane bound proteins, since the catalytic site is placed in an internal pocket of the protein and does not interact directly with the membrane. An analysis of the conformation of the active site of CYP 3A4 in both membrane bound and water-soluble forms reveals a lack of significant difference, the volume of the binding site was, however, larger in the water-soluble simulations [959].

The majority of known crystal structures of CYP P450 are only partial structures, containing only the catalytic domain. The only complete protein structure (including linker, transmembrane helix, and attached membrane) belonging to this family is yeast lanosterol 14α-demethylase [948]. The structure of lanosterol 14α-demethylase suggests that the transmembrane helix affects the orientation of the catalytic domain towards the lipid bilayer. Unsurprisingly, numerous MD simulation studies have been dedicated to elucidating the orientation of the catalytic domain relative to the membrane surface and its specific interactions with lipids: for example, this was achieved for CYP 2C9 [960]; CYP 17A1 [961]; CYP1A2, 2A6, 2C9, 2D6, 2E1, and 3A4 [326,962,963] through MD simulations, then subsequently validated experimentally. Interestingly, the orientation of the catalytic domains of CYP 2C9 and CYP 2C19 were found to differ from each other significantly, in spite of the relatively high extent of sequence similarity; through MD simulation it was determined that the difference was induced by only three residues located at the membrane–protein interface [964]. Interestingly, truncation of the transmembrane helix in CYP 19A1 and 17A1 did not change the orientation of the catalytic domain significantly; however, mutations in the transmembrane helix of CYP 17A1 destabilized the interaction between the membrane and catalytic domain of the protein [965]. MD simulations also demonstrated that lipid composition, e.g., the addition of cholesterol [966] or charged lipids [967], affects the orientation of the extra-membrane domain with respect to the membrane surface. Additionally, the choice of force field (parameters set) may have a measurable, but not significant, effect on the orientation of the domains of the protein that are outside the membrane [968].

The active site of CYP enzymes is located inside the protein, thus substrates and products enter/exit the active site through numerous possible channels [969] (Figure 21). Such channels have been observed in crystal structures [969], MD simulations [969], RAMD calculations [970,971], and steered MD simulations [972]. The channels found can be subdivided into seven classes: channel 1, channel 2, channel 3, channel 4, channel 5, the solvent channel and the water channel; in turn, channel 2 has 7 subclasses. The aforementioned channels open towards the membrane core, membrane–water interface, and directly into the solvent phase (water) (Figure 21).

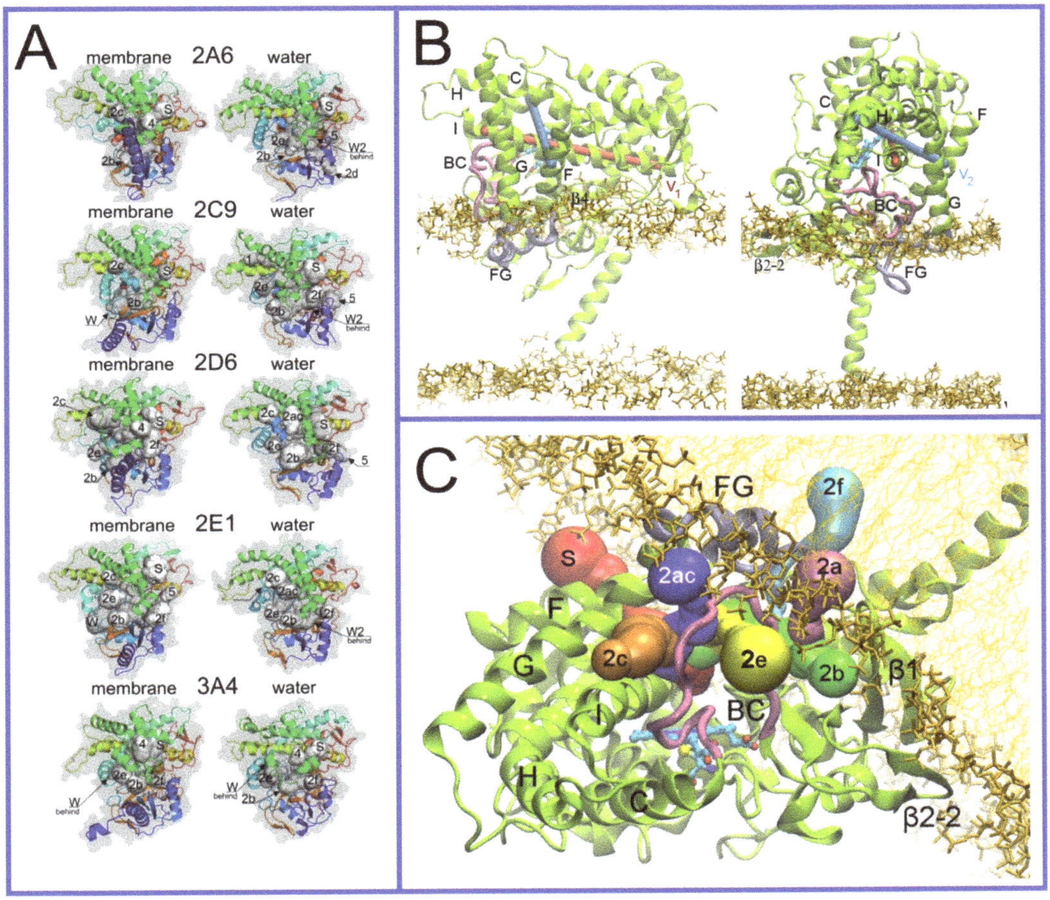

Figure 21. (**A**) Snapshots of five CYP enzymes simulated attached to the membrane (left) and simulated in water (right) with open (minimum radius 1.5 Å) channels shown. Reproduced with permission from ref. [962]. (**B**) Snapshots of the models of membrane-bound CYP 2C9 and (**C**) visualization of the channels observed in MD simulations of these models. Reproduced with permission from ref. [960].

Free energy calculations have demonstrated that the substrate may enter/exit via various channels; however, the free energy barriers encountered traversing the channels, i.e., largest barrier along the pathway for each case, differ by up to 8 kJ/mol [388]. An MD simulation study that compared the aforementioned channels in the human and human parasite *Trypanosoma brucei* versions of CYP51s provided evidence that subtle differences in structure exist which could possibly be taken advantage of to design a drug to specifically target the parasite enzyme [973], i.e., design drugs based on transit through the channels, selecting a drug that has a lower free energy barrier for traversing the channels of the form of the enzyme in the parasite than that present for the host.

The interactions of CYPs with lipids affects the behavior of the entry channels significantly. In studies of CYP 1A2, the authors demonstrated that the probability of the opening of a specific channel is dependent on contact with the membrane, with the radius of the channel regulated through interactions with lipids in the membrane [974]; through very subtle conformational change in the protein, the membrane facing channels 2b, 2d, and 4 are enlarged, i.e., "opened", when the protein is in contact with the membrane while the water facing channel 2c is enlarged when the protein is in the water phase. For the case of the protein CYP 2B4, free energy calculations have determined that the transition from the open to the closed state is associated with a free energy change of 10 Kcal/mol for the membrane-bound protein and 25 Kcal/mol for the protein in solution [975]. Moreover, for the case of CYP 17A1, the membrane facilitates the opening of the entry channels [961]. This opening of channels or catalytic pockets is also observed in peripheral membrane proteins (discussed in more detail in the following section) due to interactions with the lipid membrane, e.g., simulations have observed this occurring for the phospholipase A2 [976,977], dihydroorotate dehydrogenase [978], monoglycosyltransferase [979], and other proteins that we will later discuss.

Combined experimental and simulation studies of CYP 2B4 reveal the presence of a sphingomyelin binding region on the protein and a protein-induced increase in the level of cholesterol and sphingomyelin in nanodiscs incubated with micelles containing lipids [980]. Putting these together, the authors concluded that CYP 2B4 induces the formation of ordered raft-like domains in its environment as lipids are exchanged between the micelles and the nanodisks. In turn, at the ordered membrane, the thermal stability of CYP 2B4 is significantly increased. The lipid environment also affected the affinity of hydrophobic substrates for CYP 2B4: highest in the raft-like environment and lowest in water solution. The behavior of CYPs may also be modulated due to the formation of heterodimers with cytochrome b5 or cytochrome P450 reductase [981,982].

The results of older MD simulation studies have provided evidence that the location and membrane orientation of the entry channels of CYP 2C9 correspond well with possible substrate positions [272]. In recent unbiased MD simulations, spontaneous events of the entry into the catalytic pocket of CYP 2D6, by substrates paracetamol and butadiene, from the water–membrane interface, were seen [285]. In eight observed events of paracetamol entry into the catalytic pocket, three possible channels were used; thus, there is no specificity for the entry pathway for this compound. For butadiene, only two events of entry occurred, both through channel 2c. Using a combination of extensive, unbiased MD simulations and RAMD, the entrance pathway from the membrane to the binding site was determined for testosterone [408]; umbrella sampling calculations along this pathway revealed the free energy landscape.

Through MD simulations, the effect of point mutations on the enzymatic activity of CYP 2C19 was analyzed, providing evidence for a possible mechanism responsible for the reduction of the affinity of the enzyme for the substrate, e.g., local deformation of the secondary structure of the protein results in a change in the shape and the dynamics of the catalytic pocket that, in turn, gives rise to the formation of a new stable network of hydrogen bonds [983]. A study of CYP 1A1 found that point mutations may facilitate the interactions of organic pollutants with the protein [984], while CYP 2D6 is characterized by a high degree of genetic polymorphism that leads to several possible phenotypes [985]. The results of MD simulations of a few variants of CYP 2D6 indicated that a decrease, or even a complete loss, of enzymatic activity may arise from a decrease in the frequency of channel openings, decreased minimal diameters of channels, or decreased catalytic site volume [986]. On the other hand, an increase of active site volume facilitates enzyme activity. MD simulations have been used to design mutations of CYP 3A4, designed to enhance the rate with which it epoxides carbamazepine [328]. Finally, interactions of the drugs progesterone and carbamazepine [326,327] and atorvastatin and dronedarone [312] have been studied using a combination of experimental methods and MD simulations.

6.3.3. Catechol-O-methyltransferase

The enzyme catechol-O-methyltransferase (COMT) is an exciting example of a protein that has two isoforms: a water–soluble form (S–COMT) that is generally thought to perform its catalysis in solution but with the capacity to act also as a peripheral membrane protein and a membrane–bound isoform (MB–COMT), a bitopic protein [987]. The difference between S–COMT and MB–COMT is a 26 residue long transmembrane α–helix and a 24-residue long linker segment connecting the catalytic domain with the transmembrane segment. The function of COMT is the catabolism of catechols (Figure 22), including the neurotransmitters dopamine, epinephrine, and norepinephrine. Inhibitors for COMT are thus used to treat Parkinson's disease together with the dopamine precursor L–DOPA [645,646]; the goal is to prevent dopamine deficiency in neurons, and the role of COMT inhibitors is to avoid L–DOPA degradation before it is converted to dopamine. Importantly, in the central nervous system, MB–COMT is the dominant form of the enzyme; thus, selective inhibition could possibly be profitable for patients. In our studies of MB–COMT, we found evidence, through MD simulation, that a group of inhibitors specific for MB–COMT is characterized by a clear orientation, when in the lipid membrane, with the catechol group oriented outwards and towards the water phase (Figure 22) [381]. The catalytic activity of COMT first involves the binding of the S-adenosyl methionine (ADOMET) cofactor, then an Mg^{++} ion is bound to form the binding pocket (Figure 22). As part of the same study, a simulation of the entire MB–COMT in the lipid membrane in both holo- and apo- (with and without ADOMET cofactor bound) states was performed and it was determined that the binding of ADOMET leads, i.e., orients, the catalytic surface towards the lipid headgroups, through the creation of a membrane binding patch similar to that found in peripheral membrane proteins, where the substrates are methylated at the membrane–water interface. Through MD simulation, the catalytic mechanism, unique to the membrane bound isoform of COMT, has been determined, presenting the tantalizing possibility of designing drugs that selectively target MB–COMT over S–COMT. Through datamining, other examples of proteins where the same mechanism can be exploited have been found.

6.3.4. Monoamine Oxidase

Monoamine oxidase (MAO) A and B are bitopic proteins involved in the degradation of monoamines, particularly monoamine neurotransmitters: dopamine, serotonin, epinephrine, norepinephrine, histamine, and trace amines, as well as the catabolism of xenobiotics. As a result of this role, they are a drug target for inhibition in the treatment of Parkinson's and Alzheimer's disease and major depressive disorder [988–990]. Not surprisingly, MAO inhibitors are frequently studied using computational modeling methods including docking calculations, free energy calculations, and hybrid quantum mechanics/molecular mechanics (QM–MM) simulations, e.g., [991–993]. A recent example is the study of MAO–A and MAO–B inhibition by naturally occurring flavonoids that originate from medicinal plants [994]. Quantum mechanics/molecular mechanics simulations have also been used to elucidate the mechanism of enzymatic reaction catalyzed by MAO–A (e.g., [995]) and MOA–B (e.g., [996,997]); for a review of this topic, see ref. [998].

Simulations of MAO–A at the membrane—water interface provided evidence of the opening of a channel for the substrate and the reaction products that was not seen to occur in simulations performed without the lipid membrane, i.e., the channel remained closed [999]. For the case of MAO–B, the lipid bilayer was found to control the behavior of the two loops at the entrance of the active site, allowing for the opening of a channel [1000]. The other channel-facing membrane was observed in simulations of the MOA–B dimer [1001]. These studies also found evidence of changes in protein dynamics induced by the membrane, potentially affecting MOA–B activity.

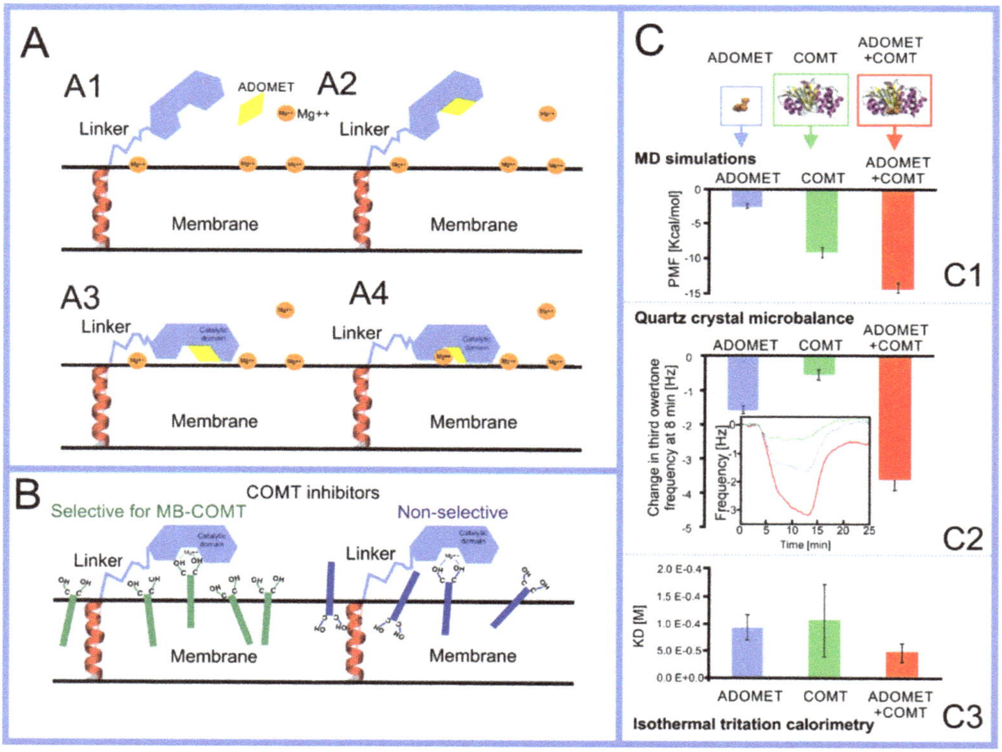

Figure 22. (**A**) Schematic of the catalytic mechanism of MB–COMT. (**B**) The behavior of MB–COMT selective vs. non–selective inhibitors in the membrane. (**C**) Quantitative experimental and computational results for the interactions of the ADOMET and catalytic domain of COMT in complex and separately with lipids: (**C1**) the free energy changes calculated computationally with umbrella sampling methods; (**C2**) quartz crystal microbalance (QCM) frequency changes during interaction of COMT with the lipid bilayer; (**C3**) dissociation constant from liposomes determined by isothermal calorimetry. Reproduced with permission from ref. [381]. Copyright 2018 the Royal Society of Chemistry.

It has been attempted, through experimental mutagenesis studies, to engineer MAOs from *Aspergillus niger* to act on larger substrates like benzyl-piperidine, thus transforming it into a device to synthesize chiral pharmaceuticals based on the benzo-piperidine scaffold; simulations were carried out to assist this endeavor [545] and residues in the channels leading to the catalytic pocket and residues inside the pocket were mutated in silico. The MD simulations demonstrated that increased hydrophobicity of the entrance channel and alteration of shape and size of the binding pocket provided the most efficient version of the enzyme.

6.3.5. Tropomyosin Receptor Kinase B

The tropomyosin receptor kinase B (TRKB) belongs to the tyrosine kinase receptor family of proteins: a set of bitopic membrane proteins that operate as dimers with their trans–membrane α-helices paired in a crisscross orientation (see Figures 23 and 24); their main function is to pass signals through the cell membrane [1002,1003]. The specific tyrosine kinase receptor TRKB is the main receptor of brain-derived neurotrophic factor (BDNF) and plays an important role both in neuron survival and the growth and differentiation of new neurons and synapses; it can thus be seen, on the scale of overall brain function, as an agent that promotes neuron plasticity, the increase of which, through a combination of drug and talk therapies, is currently seen as one of the most promising routes, following a mechanistic biophysical paradigm, for the treatment of clinical depression. Thus, combating the inhibition of TRKB activation by BDNF is a possible strategy for drug therapy [1004].

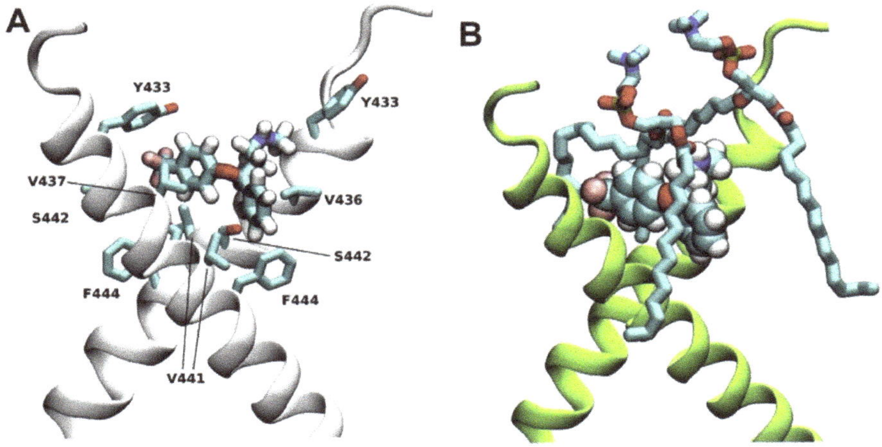

Figure 23. Transmembrane domain of TRKB dimer formed by the crisscross oriented helices forms a pocket for antidepressant binding. (**A**) Antidepressant fluoxetine is embedded in the crevice between the two helices of the TRKB transmembrane domain. Protein backbone shown in white cartoon and protein residues and fluoxetine in licorice representation. (**B**) Binding site for antidepressants at the outer opening of the crossed dimer is stabilized by the phospholipids. Protein backbone shown as green cartoon, the phospholipids in licorice and fluoxetine in vdW representations.

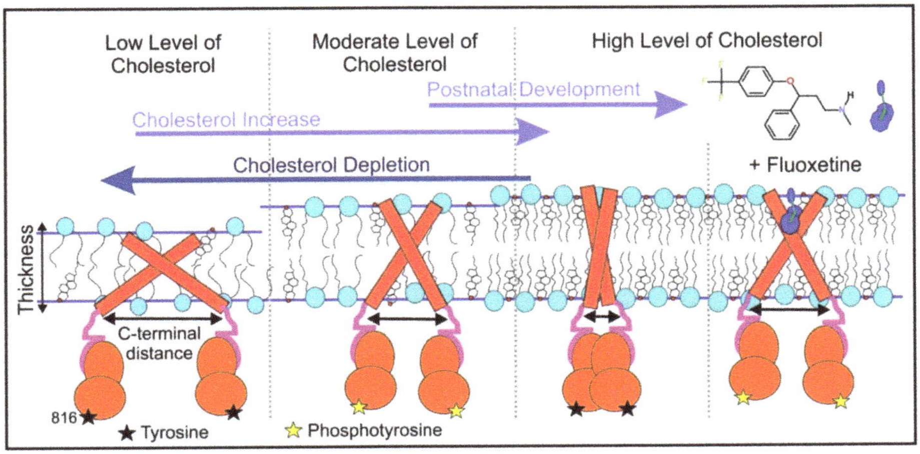

Figure 24. Schematic representation of how cholesterol and antidepressants regulate the activity of TRKB receptors through driving the orientation of its transmembrane helices. The rise of cholesterol content in the membrane increases its thickness. This forces the transition of TRKB transmembrane dimers towards the states with shorter C-terminal distances between the ends of the helixes (red rectangles). In turn, the C-terminal distances determine the arrangement of TRKB kinase domains (shown in orange) and the phosphorylation states of tyrosine 816 (black and yellow stars for native and phosphorylated states, respectively). The antidepressant fluoxetine (shown in blue), when bound to the pocket, preserves the stable transmembrane dimer conformation in a similar fashion to that observed at moderate cholesterol level and optimal for receptor activation.

A recent study of TRKB by Casarotto et al., that utilized numerous experimental and computational methods demonstrated a possible mechanism through which the antidepressant fluoxetine can increase the extent to which TRKB is activated by BDNF, resulting in the desired increase in neuronal plasticity [320]. The angle between the two alpha helices of the TRKB dimer, arranged in the crisscross orientation mentioned above (see Figure 23), is determined by the thickness of the hydrophobic core of the lipid membrane; the two identical alpha helices each have the same fixed hydrophobic length and cholesterol is known to affect the thickness of a lipid membrane, thus the level of cholesterol in the lipid membrane will alter this angle. The angle between the helices determines the distance between the intracellular ends of the helices that, in turn, controls the positioning of the intracellular domains of the proteins; this mechanism switches the protein between the active or inactive states. Through a combination of experimental methodologies, Casarotto et al., found that TRKB activation is affected by the level of cholesterol in the neuronal membranes where the TRKB receptors reside; the study reveals a bell-shaped dependence between the level of cholesterol in the membrane and the extent to which TRKB activation by BDNF occurs: both low and high levels of cholesterol were found to inhibit BDNF receptor activation, while a moderate level of cholesterol was found to be optimal, i.e., the level of TRKB activation had a maximum at a certain level of cholesterol in the membrane. The same bell-shaped dependency was also observed in a direct binding assay of BDNF to TRKB [1005]. It can thus be surmised that BDNF activation is dependent on the angle between the two trans-membrane helices with a certain finite angle being optimal. It was then found that the presence of the antidepressant fluoxetine caused the extent of TRKB activation not to decrease when the cholesterol level in the membrane was raised above the formerly optimal level, i.e., the inhibitory effect of elevated cholesterol level was negated by the presence of fluoxetine.

Next, Casarotto et al., performed MD simulations of a TRKB dimer in a membrane with the antidepressant fluoxetine present; they made a truly startling discovery: a binding site for the fluoxetine molecule was found to exist at the point the two helices crossed; when a fluoxetine molecule was bound to this site, the fluoxetine molecule effectively jammed the two transmembrane helices like a rock in a pair of scissors, as shown in Figure 23. The study thus demonstrates how MD simulation has connected a set of experimental results to provide a complete picture of a hypothesis of the mechanism of action of the antidepressant fluoxetine, shown as a schematic in Figure 24. Mutagenesis experiments were then carried out to verify this; the fluoxetine binding site, found from MD simulation, was removed and the effect of fluoxetine on the cholesterol dependence of TRKB activity was found to disappear, as expected.

This mechanism also explains why antidepressants start activating TRKB only after 2 weeks of postnatal development: data from lipidomics indicates that, at the end of the second week of postnatal development, the level of cholesterol in the synaptic membranes of rodents drastically increases [1006], exactly the time when, in separate studies, antidepressants were found to start to become capable of activating TRKB [1007,1008].

The revolutionary potential of this possible discovery and the key role MD has played in it cannot be understated and already have been widely commented upon in the neuroscience community [1009–1012]; attempts have already been made to find small molecules which directly activate TRKB [1013] or positively stimulate BDNF signaling [1014].

6.4. Peripheral Membrane Proteins

6.4.1. Proteins That Live in the Cytoplasm, but Work at the Membrane Surface

We finally come to the last category of membrane-associated proteins, and arguably the most difficult to study of all: peripheral membrane proteins. While these proteins have no permanent association with the membrane, the activity of the protein takes place at a lipid membrane; interaction with the lipid membrane plays a clear role in its activity. Peripheral membrane proteins are considered as possible drug targets [1015], in particular, the protein domains known to specifically bind lipid headgroups at the membrane surface [1016]; for example, it has been demonstrated that domains that bind phosphatidylinositols could be a possible drug target in cancer therapy [1017,1018].

Peripheral membrane proteins are frequently studied through MD simulations, but frequently without association with the lipid bilayers involved in their activity. For example, galectins, an important class of protein that recognizes carbohydrates, including glycolipids, have been studied in the context of protein–ganglioside carbohydrate headgroup interactions [1019,1020] or in the context of interactions with potential inhibitors [1021,1022]; the lipid bilayer has, however, not been included in any computational studies of galectins.

We will now outline a few examples of peripheral membrane proteins, including domains that recognize phosphatidylinositols and phosphatidylserine, protein toxin, and protein kinase C (PKC) where MD simulation has elucidated key elements of their mechanism of action.

6.4.2. Protein Kinase C

Protein kinase C (PKC) plays many important roles in human physiology and aspects of its activity are thus also involved in several pathologies, including heart failure, cancer, Alzheimer's disease, and diabetes [1023–1025]. The catalytic activity occurs at the surface of a biomembrane, when activated by di-acyl-glycerol (DAG) in the membrane. In many cases moderate activation has been found to be beneficial while prolonged activation detrimental. PKC is thus a drug target for controlled activation and a detailed mechanistic understanding of the factors that modulate its activity and the role the membrane plays in mediating the DAG induced activation is pharmaceutically relevant. For a review of the use of computational methods for the development of ligands of PKC, see Katti and Igumenova (2021) [1026].

A set of MD simulation studies of the C1 and C2 domains of PKC have demonstrated the importance of specific lipids in regard to the docking of the protein to the lipid bilayer; specifically, the importance of anionic lipids has been demonstrated [1027–1030]. In other studies, PKC and its activator aplysiatoxin have been studied using MD simulations of this complex interacting with a lipid bilayer, in order to describe the binding mode of this potential anticancer drug [230]. In another computational study of PKC, the C1B domain was placed at the water–membrane interface and docked to four potential activators bryostatin, a bryostatin analog, phorbol 12,13–dibutyrate, and prostratin [231]; long MD simulations demonstrated that the C1B domain adopted a different orientation and positioning for each of the activators. These differences originated from variation in activator interactions with both water and lipids.

A series of experimental assays were carried out on different DAG mimics based on hydrophobic isophthalic acid derivatives (HMIs) [1031–1034]. Among these, the HMI known as HMI-1a3 (Figure 25) was found to be a particularly effective activator of PKC, however its application is limited due to its low solubility. An analog of HMI-1a3 with a phenyl ring substituted with pyrimidine (PYR-1gP) was synthesized that, unlike HMI-1a3, had an acceptable solubility profile, but this was found in experimental assays not to be effective as a PKC activator. An MD simulation study was carried out by Lautala et al., to determine the cause of this; they found that one of the reasons for this observed low potency to be a drastic change in the orientation of the functional group involved in binding from exposed to the water phase to embedded into the bilayer; this results from the formation of an internal H-bond that increase its effective hydrophobicity [336].

6.4.3. The Binding Domains of PIPs

Phosphatidylinositols (PIPs) are a class of lipid of particular importance in cellular signaling [1035]. There are 8 PIP headgroup types characterized by different behaviors at the membrane surface, e.g., orientation in the membrane [1036]. There are 14 known protein domains that bind PIPs [1037–1039] including: (1) pleckstrin homology (PH), (2) FYVE (the first letter of the first four proteins in which domain was identified), (3) phox homology (PX), (4) epsin N-terminal homology (ENTH), (5) FERM (F stands for 4.1 protein, E for ezrin, R for radixin and M for moesin), (6) PROPPINS (b-propellers that bind polyphospho-inositides), (7) Tubby, and (8) BAR (name from first letter of proteins: Bin, Amphiphysin, Rvs) domains and others not discussed in this paper.

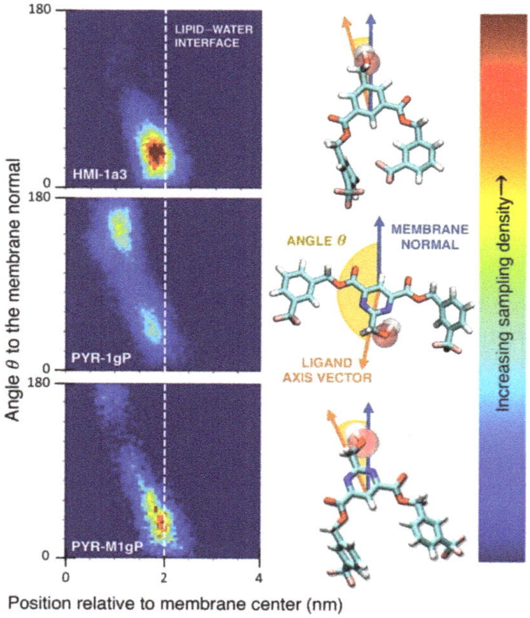

Figure 25. Maps showing orientation-position relations of the hydroxyl groups of HMI-1a3 and PYR-1gP. Reproduced with permission from ref. [336].

The PH domain is the most common PIP binding domain, there are at least 329 different PH domains present in 284 human proteins [1040]. The PH domain is built from 100–150 residues and binds various PIPs. Unsurprisingly, it is the most frequently studied among PIP binding domains. A few MD simulation studies provide insight into PH domain interactions with PIP headgroups and details of interactions with lipids in the bilayer in addition to the orientation of the domain towards the membrane surface [1041–1048] or characterized dynamics of bound domain at the membrane surface [1030]; for example, Yamamoto et al., characterized PH domains originating from 13 different proteins [1049]. Interactions of PH domains with lipid bilayers were also studied through computational free energy calculations. For example, it has been shown that the PH domain from the GRP1 protein has stronger binding to a lipid bilayer with PIP3 than a bilayer with PIP2 [1050]. In another study of the GRP1 PH domain, it was shown that in the canonical binding mode, the free energy difference between the bound and unbound state is about 9 kcal/mol, while in an alternate, non–canonical, binding mode, it is about 7 kcal/mol [1047]. Moreover, it has been shown that the GRP1 PH domain has the ability to bind multiple PIP3 molecules simultaneously, increasing the strength of the binding to the lipid bilayer [1051]. Finally, MD simulations have demonstrated that the binding of the PH domain to the membrane could possibly be facilitated by phosphatidylserine; however, for stable binding, PIP is necessary [1048].

The ACAP1 protein, recently studied with MD simulations, is in possession of two PIP binding domains: the BAR and PH domains [1052]; the orientation of the PH domain at the membrane surface is affected by the BAR domain. The PH domain of ACAP1 has two binding pockets for PIP2 headgroups (pocket 1 and pocket 2); free energy calculations determined that the PIP2 occupancy of pocket 1 decreases the free energy of binding to the membrane by 1 kcl/mol in comparison to when PIP2 is not present, while the occupancy of pocket 2 decreases the free energy of binding by 3.5 kcl/mol.

The over-expression of Grb2-associated binding protein 1 (GAB1) occurs in numerous cancers, thus drugs designed to inhibit the activity of GAB1 are studied, including drugs that target the PH domain. Extensive modeling studies, including virtual screening of five million compounds and MD simulations of the five most promising molecules, have demonstrated that selected molecules strongly bind to the PH domain and induced significant changes to the protein conformation [1053]. Next, it has been shown experimentally that these potential drugs have tumor-specific cytotoxicity against two breast cancer cell lines. The ceramide transfer protein contains both PH and START domains, and dimerization of these domains leads to protein inhibition. Docking calculations, combined with MD simulation, allowed for the selection of a few possible protein inhibitors, which bind to the PH–START domain interface, increasing the strength of the association between these two domains [1054]. The protein AKT1 kinase, also in possession of one or more PH domains, has been studied, using docking calculations and MD simulation, to understand the effect of the cancerous E17K mutation [1055]. It has been observed that inhibitor 7, known to be ineffective for the case of this mutation being present, is characterized by a much lower affinity towards the mutated version of the protein. Moreover, mutation leads to conformational changes in the protein.

The FYVE domain that contains only 70–80 amino acids, has been identified in 30 human proteins. The FYVE domain only binds PIP3 and not the other PIPs, i.e., it is specific for PIP3. The PX domain is present in 49 human proteins and binds several different PIPs [1056]. Studies φf these two domain interactions with lipid bilayers, carried out through MD simulation, have demonstrated that, after binding with a lipid bilayer and PIP3, both domains lose their flexibility that is observed when the domains are in the water phase [1057]. This effect was more pronounced for the FYVE domain. Both domains remained firmly bound to the PIP3 molecule and both domains penetrate the bilayer core, the FYVE domain via the N-terminal hydrophobic loop and the PX domain via two loops: $\alpha1\alpha2$ and $\beta1\beta2$. In another MD simulation study, phospholipase D2 (PLD2) that has both PX and PH domains, was shown to interact with PIP2 predominantly via these specific domains [1058]. Moreover, a second anionic lipid, POPA, was found to participate in the protein-membrane interactions.

The FERM domain was included in a few MD simulation studies of the proteins talin [1059–1061] and focal adhesion kinase (FAK) [1062,1063]. Studies of FAK showed a strong effect of PIP2 on the protein orientation at the membrane surface [1063]. Studies of talin elucidated how talin, in cooperation with PIP2, affects the interaction of dimers of the transmembrane helices of integrins leading to dimer dissociation, the first step in integrin activation [1059,1060]. MD simulation also found a change in the FERM domain conformation [1059]; the FERM domain is composed of four units F0, F1, F2 and F3 which are organized in a linear fashion (Figure 26) as seen in its crystal structure (PBD ID 3IVF) [1064] that is, however, missing loop F1 which was approximated computationally. Due to the presence of the loop F1, the FERM domain became V-shaped (Figure 26). Additionally, a study that combined MD simulations with multiple experimental methods, demonstrated that FERM in talin is more compact and nonlinear [1061] (Figure 26).

The mechanism through which PROPPINS docks to the membrane has been studied using coarse-grained and atomistic MD simulations; the study demonstrated the importance of the loop 6CD for protein binding to the membrane [1065]; a combination of experimental and theoretical studies revealed the presence of two phosphoinositide binding sites in the β-propeller domain [1066]. Coarse-grained MD simulations were used in studies of the aggregation of the ENTH domains at membrane vesicles and membrane tubes, i.e., cylinders formed from lipid membranes [1067]. These studies found evidence that the formation of dimers and larger oligomers occurs within membrane tubes. Finally, MD simulation studies of the tubby domain have demonstrated that it is in possession of two binding sites for PIP2 [1068].

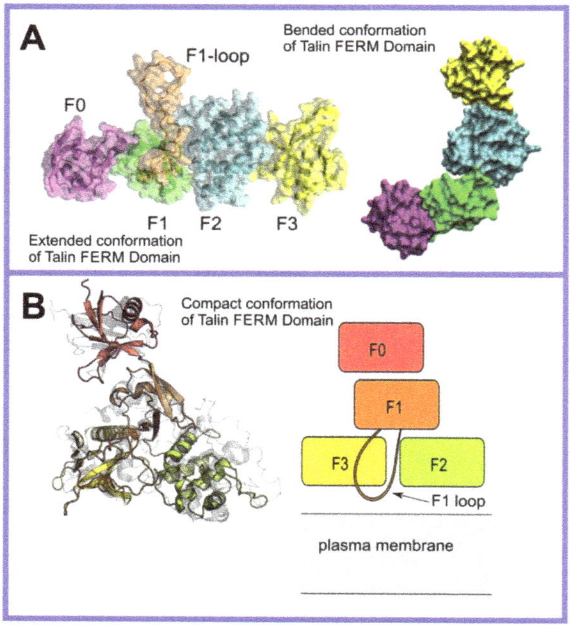

Figure 26. Conformation of talin FERM domain (**A**) extended conformation from crystal structure (PBD ID 3IVF) and after CG simulations [1059], (**B**) compact conformation [1061].

6.4.4. Other Examples

Coagulation factor X is one of several proteins involved in the initiation of the coagulation cascade; its activity is dramatically increased when it binds to a membrane that contains negatively charged lipids, in particular phosphatidylserines. The GLA domain is responsible for the binding of factor X to the lipid bilayers, its characteristic feature is posttranslational modification of glutamic acid residues, which transform the glutamic acid sidechain into γ-carboxyglutamic acid (GLA); GLA is in possession of two carboxylic groups with the ability to strongly bind divalent cations, predominately Ca^{++}. Through MD simulation, evidence has been found that GLA residues with bound Ca^{++} ions bind directly to phosphatidylserine [1069]. Altogether, 7 GLA residues participate in interactions with lipid bilayers and short loops insert three hydrophobic residues directly into the bilayer core.

Protein toxins, including bacterial toxin, have specific requirements to recognize and enter cells [1070], i.e., certain molecules must be present in the membrane. Cholera toxin is a protein, which requires gangliosides, e.g., GM1, to be present in the membrane in order for it to bind and is a potential drug target; for example, peptide mimicking GM1 carbohydrates prevent the binding of toxin to intestinal cells [337]. Through MD simulation, the mechanism of toxin docking to the lipid bilayer has been studied, including its interactions with lipids, in particular GM1 and the effects of the toxin binding on the overall properties of the lipid bilayer [525,1071]. Docking studies have proposed three possible drug candidates with sufficient potency to prevent the binding of the toxin with ganglioside; MD simulations were used next to evaluate the stability of the binding of drug candidates with toxin [1072]. Two compounds, A6225 and A16503, formed a stable complex with the toxin. Cardiotoxin CTII, a component of cobra venom, is known to disrupt mitochondrial membranes. Through MD simulation, the interactions of CTII with a lipid bilayer composed of lipids present in the outer mitochondrial membrane [1073] were elucidated. In particular, residues involved in interactions with cardiolipin were identified.

The enzymes responsible for the metabolism and transportation of lipids, are often peripheral membrane proteins not explored as a drug target although proposed as a target for antiviral therapy against flaviviruses [1074]. Examples of MD simulation studies of enzymes that catalyze the metabolism of lipids include monogalactosyl-diacyl-glycerol synthase 1 [1075], phosphatidylinositol phospholipase Cγ and its cancerous mutation [1076], and lysophosphatidic acid acyltransferase [1077]. Glutathione peroxidase 4 is an enzyme responsible for the removal of lipid hydroperoxides, thus preventing lipid oxidation; MD simulations have recently been used to elucidate the process through which a substrate enters into the active pocket of the enzyme from the membrane surface [1078]. Lipid transporters are proteins that shuttle lipids between two separate membranes, thus acting as peripheral membrane proteins when loading/unloading their cargo and water-soluble proteins when transporting it through the cytoplasm. Lipid transporters studied through MD simulation include the mammalian phosphatidylinositol transfer protein; these studies provided insight into the mechanism and energetics of the loading/unloading of PIPs into the binding cavity of the protein [1079] and studies of the UPS1 protein transporting phosphatidic acid between the inner and outer mitochondrial membrane [1080].

As a large group of peripheral membrane proteins recognize specific lipids, it is also possible to develop drugs that bind to specific lipids, thus preventing the recognition of these lipids by specific peripheral membrane proteins. An example of such a strategy is the study of siramesine, a small compound characterized by its high affinity to phosphatidic acid [335].

7. Conclusions

Through a detailed discussion of how MD simulation can be used to elucidate the roles the interaction with lipid membranes play in drug action, we hope we have provided the reader with an intuitive understanding of the broader landscape within which drug molecules act, beyond the limiting paradigm of ADME and "docking and scoring". Xenobiotics are foreign molecules travelling through the body, uninvited intruders that become involved in the complex melee that is physiology on the molecular length scale. A drug molecule is a xenobiotic with a specific purpose, designed by its maker, like a foreign agent with a mission to perform a specific task travelling across the countryside to reach the city where they must perform it. In the previous review paper, we discussed the role MD simulation can play in providing mechanistic insight relevant to the development of the mechanisms through which this agent can reach their destination; now we have discussed how MD simulation can aid in the design of a more complex set of tasks for the agent than possible within the confines of the "docking and scoring" paradigm. Through MD simulation, (1) drug molecules can be rationally designed to perform more complex tasks than merely fitting to a specific protein and (2) even if the target is the active site of a specific protein, far more is involved in the determination of the effective affinity of a specific drug molecule structure for a specific active site than can be investigated through the "lock and key" paradigm. While there are many possible factors other than the role played by lipid membrane interactions that MD simulation can address, we hope that this provides a case study that expands the intuitive picture the reader has of the scope of computational drug design and the role the specific toolkit of MD simulation can play.

Lipid membranes are fundamental structures with no less complex or important a role in molecular level physiology than proteins; the mechanisms through which small drug molecules can interact with them are equally complex. Drug molecules must cross them, can affect their properties through collective action, and can have their interactions with target proteins mediated by them; a comprehensive inclusion of the role the drug structure plays in its interaction with lipid membranes and the use of MD simulation to model this interaction is clearly a component of the future of drug design.

In the beginning of the paper, we mentioned that we can envision a time in the future when, through the combined solution of the human proteome and the general structure from sequence problem, a program can exist that could input any molecular structure and output its binding affinity for every active site of every protein in the human proteome. Hopefully, when reading this review paper, the reviewer can see that even this fantastic device would merely be one component of the advanced computational toolkit of drug design of the future. This information would form a starting foundation that then would be combined with MD simulation able to investigate the broader context of the protein environment, or possible modes of action of a specific drug molecule that involve different elements of physiology than active sites of proteins. The lipid membrane is an important component of this where we have shown that MD simulation can play a leading role. As in all cases, the computational effort must be matched with complementary experimental techniques that themselves are undergoing revolutionary upgrades as we speak. As recent events have shown, the health challenges to humanity are mounting, but so is our arsenal in combating them and MD simulation as a component of computational drug design will grow in importance, with the increase in computational power and data stored.

Author Contributions: All authors have read and agreed to the published version of the manuscript.

Funding: This research received no external funding.

Institutional Review Board Statement: Not applicable.

Informed Consent Statement: Not applicable.

Data Availability Statement: Not applicable.

Acknowledgments: Open access funding provided by University of Helsinki.

Conflicts of Interest: The authors declare no conflict of interest.

References

1. Jumper, J.; Evans, R.; Pritzel, A.; Green, T.; Figurnov, M.; Ronneberger, O.; Tunyasuvunakool, K.; Bates, R.; Žídek, A.; Potapenko, A.; et al. Highly accurate protein structure prediction with AlphaFold. *Nature* **2021**, *596*, 583–589. [CrossRef]
2. Adhikari, S.; Nice, E.C.; Deutsch, E.W.; Lane, L.; Omenn, G.S.; Pennington, S.R.; Paik, Y.-K.; Overall, C.M.; Corrales, F.J.; Cristea, I.M.; et al. A high-stringency blueprint of the human proteome. *Nat. Commun.* **2020**, *11*, 5301. [CrossRef]
3. Bunker, A.; Róg, T. Mechanistic Understanding From Molecular Dynamics Simulation in Pharmaceutical Research 1: Drug Delivery. *Front. Mol. Biosci.* **2020**, *7*, 604770. [CrossRef]
4. Jorgensen, W.L. Rusting of the lock and key model for protein-ligand binding. *Science* **1991**, *254*, 954–955. [CrossRef]
5. Tutone, M.; Almerico, A.M. The In Silico Fischer Lock-and-Key Model: The Combined Use of Molecular Descriptors and Docking Poses for the Repurposing of Old Drugs BT—Targeting Enzymes for Pharmaceutical Development: Methods and Protocols. In *Targeting Enzymes for Pharmaceutical Development*; Labrou, N.E., Ed.; Springer: New York, NY, USA, 2020; pp. 29–39. ISBN 978-1-0716-0163-1.
6. Balani, S.K.; Miwa, G.T.; Gan, L.-S.; Wu, J.-T.; Lee, F.W. Strategy of Utilizing In Vitro and In Vivo ADME Tools for Lead Optimization and Drug Candidate Selection. *Curr. Top. Med. Chem.* **2005**, *5*, 1033–1038. [CrossRef]
7. Su, C.; Liu, Y.; Li, R.; Wu, W.; Fawcett, J.P.; Gu, J. Absorption, distribution, metabolism and excretion of the biomaterials used in Nanocarrier drug delivery systems. *Adv. Drug Deliv. Rev.* **2019**, *143*, 97–114. [CrossRef]
8. Nirogi, R.; Bhyrapuneni, G.; Muddana, N.R.; Manoharan, A.; Shinde, A.K.; Mohammed, A.R.; Padala, N.P.; Ajjala, D.R.; Subramanian, R.; Palacharla, V.R.C. Absorption, distribution, metabolism, excretion (ADME), drug-drug interaction potential and prediction of human pharmacokinetics of SUVN-G3031, a novel histamine 3 receptor (H3R) inverse agonist in clinical development for the treatment of narcolepsy. *Eur. J. Pharm. Sci.* **2020**, *152*, 105425. [CrossRef] [PubMed]
9. Hall, J.; Matos, S.; Gold, S.; Severino, L.S. The paradox of sustainable innovation: The 'Eroom' effect (Moore's law backwards). *J. Clean. Prod.* **2018**, *172*, 3487–3497. [CrossRef]
10. Limongelli, V. Ligand binding free energy and kinetics calculation in 2020. *Wiley Interdiscip. Rev. Comput. Mol. Sci.* **2020**, *10*, e1455. [CrossRef]
11. Wong, C.F. Molecular simulation of drug-binding kinetics. *Mol. Simul.* **2014**, *40*, 889–903. [CrossRef]
12. Schuetz, D.A.; Bernetti, M.; Bertazzo, M.; Musil, D.; Eggenweiler, H.M.; Recanatini, M.; Masetti, M.; Ecker, G.F.; Cavalli, A. Predicting Residence Time and Drug Unbinding Pathway through Scaled Molecular Dynamics. *J. Chem. Inf. Model.* **2019**, *59*, 535–549. [CrossRef]
13. Bruce, N.J.; Ganotra, G.K.; Richter, S.; Wade, R.C. KBbox: A Toolbox of Computational Methods for Studying the Kinetics of Molecular Binding. *J. Chem. Inf. Model.* **2019**, *59*, 3630–3634. [CrossRef] [PubMed]
14. Ahn, S.H.; Jagger, B.R.; Amaro, R.E. Ranking of ligand binding kinetics using a weighted ensemble approach and comparison with a multiscale milestoning approach. *J. Chem. Inf. Model.* **2020**, *60*, 5340–5352. [CrossRef]

15. Efremov, R.G. Dynamic "molecular portraits" of biomembranes drawn by their lateral nanoscale inhomogeneities. *Int. J. Mol. Sci.* **2021**, *22*, 6250. [CrossRef] [PubMed]
16. Watson, H. Biological membranes. *Essays Biochem.* **2015**, *59*, 43–69. [CrossRef] [PubMed]
17. Luckey, M. *Membrane Structural Biology: With Biochemical and Biophysical Foundations*; Cambridge University Press: Cambridge, UK, 2008.
18. Nicolson, G.L. The Fluid—Mosaic Model of Membrane Structure: Still relevant to understanding the structure, function and dynamics of biological membranes after more than 40 years. *Biochim. Biophys. Acta-Biomembr.* **2014**, *1838*, 1451–1466. [CrossRef]
19. Enkavi, G.; Javanainen, M.; Kulig, W.; Róg, T.; Vattulainen, I. Multiscale Simulations of Biological Membranes: The Challenge to Understand Biological Phenomena in a Living Substance. *Chem. Rev.* **2019**, *119*, 5607–5774. [CrossRef]
20. Friedman, R.; Khalid, S.; Aponte-Santamaría, C.; Arutyunova, E.; Becker, M.; Boyd, K.J.; Christensen, M.; Coimbra, J.T.S.; Concilio, S.; Daday, C.; et al. Understanding Conformational Dynamics of Complex Lipid Mixtures Relevant to Biology. *J. Membr. Biol.* **2018**, *251*, 609–631. [CrossRef]
21. Muller, M.P.; Jiang, T.; Sun, C.; Lihan, M.; Pant, S.; Mahinthichaichan, P.; Trifan, A.; Tajkhorshid, E. Characterization of Lipid-Protein Interactions and Lipid-Mediated Modulation of Membrane Protein Function through Molecular Simulation. *Chem. Rev.* **2019**, *119*, 6086–6161. [CrossRef] [PubMed]
22. Miranda, W.E.; Ngo, V.A.; Perissinotti, L.L.; Noskov, S.Y. Computational membrane biophysics: From ion channel interactions with drugs to cellular function. *Biochim. Biophys. Acta-Proteins Proteomics* **2017**, *1865*, 1643–1653. [CrossRef] [PubMed]
23. Oakes, V.; Domene, C. Chapter 2 Molecular Dynamics Simulations: Principles and Applications for the Study of Membrane Proteins. In *Computational Biophysics of Membrane Proteins*; The Royal Society of Chemistry: London, UK, 2017; pp. 19–58. ISBN 978-1-78262-490-5.
24. Vattulainen, I.; Róg, T. Lipid membranes: Theory and simulations bridged to experiments. *Biochim. Biophys. Acta-Biomembr.* **2016**, *1858*, 2251–2253. [CrossRef] [PubMed]
25. Loschwitz, J.; Olubiyi, O.O.; Hub, J.S.; Strodel, B.; Poojari, C.S. Computer simulations of protein–membrane systems. In *Progress in Molecular Biology and Translational Science*; Elsevier Inc.: Amsterdam, The Netherlands, 2020; Volume 170, pp. 273–403. ISBN 9780128211359.
26. Manna, M.; Róg, T.; Vattulainen, I. The challenges of understanding glycolipid functions: An open outlook based on molecular simulations. *Biochim. Biophys. Acta-Mol. Cell Biol. Lipids* **2014**, *1841*, 1130–1145. [CrossRef] [PubMed]
27. Vattulainen, I.; Róg, T. Lipid simulations: A perspective on lipids in action. *Cold Spring Harb. Perspect. Biol.* **2011**, *3*, 1–13. [CrossRef] [PubMed]
28. Salo-Ahen, O.M.H.; Alanko, I.; Bhadane, R.; Bonvin, A.M.J.J.; Honorato, R.V.; Hossain, S.; Juffer, A.H.; Kabedev, A.; Lahtela-kakkonen, M.; Larsen, A.S.; et al. Molecular Dynamics Simulations in Drug Discovery and Pharmaceutical Development. *Processes* **2021**, *9*, 71. [CrossRef]
29. Zhao, B.; Li, W.; Sun, L.; Fu, W. The Use of Computational Approaches in the Discovery and Mechanism Study of Opioid Analgesics. *Front. Chem.* **2020**, *8*, 335. [CrossRef]
30. Salmaso, V.; Jacobson, K.A. In silico drug design for purinergic gpcrs: Overview on molecular dynamics applied to adenosine and p2y receptors. *Biomolecules* **2020**, *10*, 812. [CrossRef]
31. Zou, Y.; Ewalt, J.; Ng, H.L. Recent insights from molecular dynamics simulations for g protein-coupled receptor drug discovery. *Int. J. Mol. Sci.* **2019**, *20*, 4237. [CrossRef]
32. Yuan, X.; Xu, Y. Recent trends and applications of molecular modeling in GPCR–Ligand recognition and structure-based drug design. *Int. J. Mol. Sci.* **2018**, *19*, 2105. [CrossRef]
33. Mayne, C.G.; Arcario, M.J.; Mahinthichaichan, P.; Baylon, J.L.; Vermaas, J.V.; Navidpour, L.; Wen, P.-C.; Thangapandian, S.; Tajkhorshid, E. The cellular membrane as a mediator for small molecule interaction with membrane proteins. *Biochim. Biophys. Acta-Biomembr.* **2016**, *1858*, 2290–2304. [CrossRef]
34. Di Meo, F.; Fabre, G.; Berka, K.; Ossman, T.; Chantemargue, B.; Paloncýová, M.; Marquet, P.; Otyepka, M.; Trouillas, P. In silico pharmacology: Drug membrane partitioning and crossing. *Pharmacol. Res.* **2016**, *111*, 471–486. [CrossRef]
35. Cramariuc, O.; Rogl, T.; Vattulainen, I. Drug-lipid membrane interaction mechanisms revealed through molecular simulations. *Curr. Phys. Chem.* **2012**, *2*, 379–400. [CrossRef]
36. Lopes, D.; Jakobtorweihen, S.; Nunes, C.; Sarmento, B.; Reis, S. Shedding light on the puzzle of drug-membrane interactions: Experimental techniques and molecular dynamics simulations. *Prog. Lipid Res.* **2017**, *65*, 24–44. [CrossRef] [PubMed]
37. Filipe, H.A.L.; Cardoso, R.M.S.; Loura, L.M.S.; Moreno, M.J. Interaction of Amphiphilic Molecules with Lipid Bilayers: Kinetics of Insertion, Desorption and Translocation. In *Membrane Organization and Dynamics*; Chattopadhyay, A., Ed.; Springer International Publishing: Cham, Switzerland, 2017; pp. 49–89. ISBN 978-3-319-66601-3.
38. Martinotti, C.; Ruiz-Perez, L.; Deplazes, E.; Mancera, R.L. Molecular Dynamics Simulation of Small Molecules Interacting with Biological Membranes. *Chem. Phys. Chem.* **2020**, *21*, 1486–1514. [CrossRef] [PubMed]
39. Seddon, A.M.; Casey, D.; Law, R.V.; Gee, A.; Templer, R.H.; Ces, O. Drug interactions with lipid membranes. *Chem. Soc. Rev.* **2009**, *38*, 2509–2519. [CrossRef]
40. Kopec, W.; Telenius, J.; Khandelia, H. Molecular dynamics simulations of the interactions of medicinal plant extracts and drugs with lipid bilayer membranes. *FEBS J.* **2013**, *280*, 2785–2805. [CrossRef] [PubMed]

41. Payandeh, J.; Volgraf, M. Ligand binding at the protein-lipid interface: Strategic considerations for drug design. *Nat. Rev. Drug Discov.* **2021**, *13*. [CrossRef]
42. Katiyar, R.S.; Jha, P.K. Molecular simulations in drug delivery: Opportunities and challenges. *WIREs Comput. Mol. Sci.* **2018**, *8*, e1358. [CrossRef]
43. Lee, H. Molecular simulations of PEGylated biomolecules, liposomes, and nanoparticles for drug delivery applications. *Pharmaceutics* **2020**, *12*, 533. [CrossRef]
44. Casalini, T. Not only in silico drug discovery: Molecular modeling towards in silico drug delivery formulations. *J. Control. Release* **2021**, *332*, 390–417. [CrossRef] [PubMed]
45. Shariatinia, Z. Chapter 10—Molecular Dynamics Simulations on Drug Delivery Systems. In *Modeling and Control of Drug Delivery Systems*; Ahmad Taher Azar, Ed.; Academic Press: Cambridge, MA, USA, 2021; pp. 153–182. ISBN 978-0-12-821185-4.
46. Mondal, J. A brief appraisal of computational modeling of antimicrobial peptides' activity. *Drug Dev. Res.* **2019**, *80*, 28–32. [CrossRef]
47. De Paula, V.S.; Valente, A.P. A dynamic overview of antimicrobial peptides and their complexes. *Molecules* **2018**, *23*, 2040. [CrossRef] [PubMed]
48. Lipkin, R.; Lazaridis, T. Computational studies of peptide-induced membrane pore formation. *Philos. Trans. R. Soc. B Biol. Sci.* **2017**, *372*, 20160219. [CrossRef] [PubMed]
49. Chen, C.H.; Melo, M.C.; Berglund, N.; Khan, A.; de la Fuente, C.; Ulmschneider, J.P.; Ulmschneider, M.B. Understanding and modelling the interactions of peptides with membranes: From partitioning to self-assembly. *Curr. Opin. Struct. Biol.* **2020**, *61*, 160–166. [CrossRef] [PubMed]
50. Bertrand, B.; Garduño-Juárez, R.; Munoz-Garay, C. Estimation of pore dimensions in lipid membranes induced by peptides and other biomolecules: A review. *Biochim. Biophys. Acta-Biomembr.* **2021**, *1863*, 183551. [CrossRef] [PubMed]
51. Der Torossian Torres, M.; De La Fuente-Nunez, C. Reprogramming biological peptides to combat infectious diseases. *Chem. Commun.* **2019**, *55*, 15020–15032. [CrossRef]
52. Cardoso, M.H.; Orozco, R.Q.; Rezende, S.B.; Rodrigues, G.; Oshiro, K.G.N.; Cândido, E.S.; Franco, O.L. Computer-Aided Design of Antimicrobial Peptides: Are We Generating Effective Drug Candidates? *Front. Microbiol.* **2020**, *10*, 3097. [CrossRef]
53. Palmer, N.; Maasch, J.R.M.A.; Torres, M.D.T.; de la Fuente-Nunez, C. Molecular Dynamics for Antimicrobial Peptide Discovery. *Infect. Immun.* **2021**, *89*, e00703-20. [CrossRef]
54. Aronica, P.G.A.; Reid, L.M.; Desai, N.; Li, J.; Fox, S.J.; Yadahalli, S.; Essex, J.W.; Verma, C.S. Computational Methods and Tools in Antimicrobial Peptide Research. *J. Chem. Inf. Model.* **2021**, *61*, 3172–3196. [CrossRef]
55. Lin, X.; Li, X.; Lin, X. A review on applications of computational methods in drug screening and design. *Molecules* **2020**, *25*, 1375. [CrossRef]
56. Li, J.; Fu, A.; Zhang, L. An Overview of Scoring Functions Used for Protein–Ligand Interactions in Molecular Docking. *Interdiscip. Sci. Comput. Life Sci.* **2019**, *11*, 320–328. [CrossRef]
57. Lee, B.L.; Kuczera, K. Simulating the free energy of passive membrane permeation for small molecules. *Mol. Simul.* **2018**, *44*, 1147–1157. [CrossRef]
58. Armacost, K.A.; Riniker, S.; Cournia, Z. Exploring Novel Directions in Free Energy Calculations. *J. Chem. Inf. Model.* **2020**, *60*, 5283–5286. [CrossRef]
59. Boittier, E.D.; Tang, Y.Y.; Buckley, M.E.; Schuurs, Z.P.; Richard, D.J.; Gandhi, N.S. Assessing molecular docking tools to guide targeted drug discovery of cd38 inhibitors. *Int. J. Mol. Sci.* **2020**, *21*, 5183. [CrossRef]
60. Lee, T.-S.; Allen, B.K.; Giese, T.J.; Guo, Z.; Li, P.; Lin, C.; McGee, T.D.; Pearlman, D.A.; Radak, B.K.; Tao, Y.; et al. Alchemical Binding Free Energy Calculations in AMBER20: Advances and Best Practices for Drug Discovery. *J. Chem. Inf. Model.* **2020**, *60*, 5595–5623. [CrossRef]
61. Braun, E.; Gilmer, J.; Mayes, H.B.; Mobley, D.L.; Monroe, J.I.; Prasad, S.; Zuckerman, D.M. Best Practices for Foundations in Molecular Simulations [Article v1.0]. *Living J. Comput. Mol. Sci.* **2019**, *1*, 5957. [CrossRef]
62. Hollingsworth, S.A.; Dror, R.O. Molecular Dynamics Simulation for All. *Neuron* **2018**, *99*, 1129–1143. [CrossRef]
63. Lazim, R.; Suh, D.; Choi, S. Advances in molecular dynamics simulations and enhanced sampling methods for the study of protein systems. *Int. J. Mol. Sci.* **2020**, *21*, 6339. [CrossRef] [PubMed]
64. Childers, M.C.; Daggett, V. Insights from molecular dynamics simulations for computational protein design. *Mol. Syst. Des. Eng.* **2017**, *2*, 9–33. [CrossRef] [PubMed]
65. Hospital, A.; Goñi, J.R.; Orozco, M.; Gelpí, J.L. Molecular dynamics simulations: Advances and applications. *Adv. Appl. Bioinform. Chem.* **2015**, *8*, 37–47. [CrossRef] [PubMed]
66. Pak, A.J.; Voth, G.A. Advances in coarse-grained modeling of macromolecular complexes. *Curr. Opin. Struct. Biol.* **2018**, *52*, 119–126. [CrossRef]
67. Kmiecik, S.; Gront, D.; Kolinski, M.; Wieteska, L.; Dawid, A.E.; Kolinski, A. Coarse-Grained Protein Models and Their Applications. *Chem. Rev.* **2016**, *116*, 7898–7936. [CrossRef] [PubMed]
68. Singh, N.; Li, W. Recent Advances in Coarse-Grained Models for Biomolecules and Their Applications. *Int. J. Mol. Sci.* **2019**, *20*, 3774. [CrossRef] [PubMed]
69. Joshi, S.Y.; Deshmukh, S.A. A review of advancements in coarse-grained molecular dynamics simulations. *Mol. Simul.* **2020**, *2020*, 1–18. [CrossRef]

70. Arnarez, C.; Uusitalo, J.J.; Masman, M.F.; Ingólfsson, H.I.; De Jong, D.H.; Melo, M.N.; Periole, X.; De Vries, A.H.; Marrink, S.J. Dry martini, a coarse-grained force field for lipid membrane simulations with implicit solvent. *J. Chem. Theory Comput.* **2015**, *11*, 260–275. [CrossRef]
71. Huang, K. *Introduction to Statistical Physics*; CRC Press: Boca Raton, FL, USA, 2001; ISBN 9780748409426.
72. Landau, D.P.; Binder, K. *A Guide to Monte Carlo Simulations in Statistical Physics*; Cambridge University Press: Cambridge, UK, 2014; ISBN 9781108780346.
73. Paquet, E.; Viktor, H.L. Molecular dynamics, monte carlo simulations, and langevin dynamics: A computational review. *Biomed. Res. Int.* **2015**, *2015*, 183918. [CrossRef]
74. Chen, J. The Development and Comparison of Molecular Dynamics Simulation and Monte Carlo Simulation. *IOP Conf. Ser. Earth Environ. Sci.* **2018**, *128*, 012110. [CrossRef]
75. Binder, K. *Monte Carlo and Molecular Dynamics Simulations in Polymer Science*; Oxford University Press: Oxford, UK, 1995; ISBN 0-19-509438-7.
76. Bunker, A.; Dünweg, B. Parallel excluded volume tempering for polymer melts. *Phys. Rev. E Stat. Nonlin Soft Matter Phys.* **2001**, *63*, 016701. [CrossRef]
77. Gray, G.M.; Ma, N.; Wagner, C.E.; van der Vaart, A. Molecular dynamics simulations and molecular flooding studies of the retinoid X-receptor ligand binding domain. *J. Mol. Model.* **2017**, *23*, 98. [CrossRef]
78. Maragliano, L.; Vanden-Eijnden, E. A temperature accelerated method for sampling free energy and determining reaction pathways in rare events simulations. *Chem. Phys. Lett.* **2006**, *426*, 168–175. [CrossRef]
79. Oshima, H.; Re, S.; Sugita, Y. Replica-Exchange Umbrella Sampling Combined with Gaussian Accelerated Molecular Dynamics for Free-Energy Calculation of Biomolecules. *J. Chem. Theory Comput.* **2019**, *15*, 5199–5208. [CrossRef]
80. Sugita, Y.; Okamoto, Y. Replica exchange molecular dynamics method for protein folding simulation. *Chem. Phys. Lett.* **1999**, *314*, 141–151. [CrossRef]
81. Swendsen, R.H.; Wang, J.-S. Replica Monte Carlo Simulation of Spin-Glasses. *Phys. Rev. Lett.* **1986**, *57*, 2607–2609. [CrossRef]
82. Yan, Q.; de Pablo, J.J. Hyper-parallel tempering Monte Carlo: Application to the Lennard-Jones fluid and the restricted primitive model. *J. Chem. Phys.* **1999**, *111*, 9509–9516. [CrossRef]
83. Fukunishi, H.; Watanabe, O.; Takada, S. On the Hamiltonian replica exchange method for efficient sampling of biomolecular systems: Application to protein structure prediction. *J. Chem. Phys.* **2002**, *116*, 9058–9067. [CrossRef]
84. Wang, F.; Landau, D.P. Efficient, Multiple-Range Random Walk Algorithm to Calculate the Density of States. *Phys. Rev. Lett* **2001**, *86*, 2050. [CrossRef] [PubMed]
85. Kim, J.; Straub, J.E.; Keyes, T. Statistical-Temperature Monte Carlo and Molecular Dynamics Algorithms. *Phys. Rev. Lett.* **2006**, *97*, 050601. [CrossRef]
86. Junghans, C.; Perez, D.; Vogel, T. Molecular Dynamics in the Multicanonical Ensemble: Equivalence of Wang–Landau Sampling, Statistical Temperature Molecular Dynamics, and Metadynamics. *J. Chem. Theory Comput.* **2014**, *10*, 1843–1847. [CrossRef]
87. Bussi, G.; Laio, A. Using metadynamics to explore complex free-energy landscapes. *Nat. Rev. Phys.* **2020**, *2*, 200–212. [CrossRef]
88. Laio, A.; Parrinello, M. Escaping free-energy minima. *Proc. Natl. Acad. Sci. USA* **2002**, *99*, 12562–12566. [CrossRef]
89. Valsson, O.; Tiwary, P.; Parrinello, M. Enhancing Important Fluctuations: Rare Events and Metadynamics from a Conceptual Viewpoint. *Annu. Rev. Phys. Chem.* **2016**, *67*, 159–184. [CrossRef]
90. Invernizzi, M.; Parrinello, M. Rethinking Metadynamics: From Bias Potentials to Probability Distributions. *J. Phys. Chem. Lett.* **2020**, *11*, 2731–2736. [CrossRef]
91. Bussi, G.; Laio, A.; Tiwary, P. Metadynamics: A Unified Framework for Accelerating Rare Events and Sampling Thermodynamics and Kinetics BT. In *Handbook of Materials Modeling: Methods: Theory and Modeling*; Andreoni, W., Yip, S., Eds.; Springer International Publishing: Cham, Switzerland, 2018; pp. 1–31. ISBN 978-3-319-42913-7.
92. Lange, O.E.; Schafer, L.V.; Grubmuller, H. Flooding in GROMACS: Accelerated barrier crossings in molecular dynamics. *J. Comput. Chem.* **2006**, *27*, 1693–1702. [CrossRef]
93. Kästner, J. Umbrella sampling: Umbrella sampling. *Wiley Interdiscip. Rev. Comput. Mol. Sci.* **2011**, *1*, 932–942. [CrossRef]
94. Sotomayor, M. Computational exploration of single-protein mechanics by steered molecular dynamics. *AIP Conf. Proc.* **2015**, *1703*, 030001. [CrossRef]
95. Do, P.C.; Lee, E.H.; Le, L. Steered Molecular Dynamics Simulation in Rational Drug Design. *J. Chem. Inf. Model.* **2018**, *58*, 1473–1482. [CrossRef]
96. Kumar, S.; Rosenberg, J.M.; Bouzida, D.; Swendsen, R.H.; Kollman, P.A. THE weighted histogram analysis method for free-energy calculations on biomolecules. I. The method. *J. Comput. Chem.* **1992**, *13*, 1011–1021. [CrossRef]
97. Ferrenberg, A.M.; Swendsen, R.H. Optimized Monte Carlo data analysis. *Phys. Rev. Lett.* **1989**, *63*, 1195–1198. [CrossRef]
98. Ferrenberg, A.M.; Swendsen, R.H. New Monte Carlo technique for studying phase transitions. *Phys. Rev. Lett.* **1988**, *61*, 2635–2638. [CrossRef] [PubMed]
99. Bunker, A.; Gaulin, B.D.; Kallin, C. Multiple-histogram Monte Carlo study of the Ising antiferromagnet on a stacked triangular lattice. *Phys. Rev. B* **1993**, *48*, 15861–15872. [CrossRef] [PubMed]
100. Nandy, B.; Maiti, P.K.; Bunker, A. Force Biased Molecular Dynamics Simulation Study of Effect of Dendrimer Generation on Interaction with DNA. *J. Chem. Theory Comput.* **2013**, *9*, 722–729. [CrossRef] [PubMed]

101. Park, S.; Kim, T.; Im, W. Transmembrane helix assembly by window exchange umbrella sampling. *Phys. Rev. Lett.* **2012**, *108*, 1–4 [CrossRef] [PubMed]
102. Lüdemann, S.K.; Lounnas, V.; Wade, R.C. How do substrates enter and products exit the buried active site of cytochrome P450cam? 2. Steered molecular dynamics and adiabatic mapping of substrate pathways11Edited by J. Thornton. *J. Mol. Biol.* **2000**, *303*, 813–830. [CrossRef]
103. Deflorian, F.; Perez-Benito, L.; Lenselink, E.B.; Congreve, M.; van Vlijmen, H.W.T.; Mason, J.S.; Graaf, C.D.; Tresadern, G. Accurate Prediction of GPCR Ligand Binding Affinity with Free Energy Perturbation. *J. Chem. Inf. Model.* **2020**, *60*, 5563–5579. [CrossRef]
104. Jarzynski, C. Nonequilibrium equality for free energy differences. *Phys. Rev. Lett.* **1997**, *78*, 2690–2693. [CrossRef]
105. Hartmann, C.; Schütte, C.; Zhang, W. Jarzynski's Equality, Fluctuation Theorems, and Variance Reduction: Mathematical Analysis and Numerical Algorithms. *J. Stat. Phys.* **2019**, *175*, 1214–1261. [CrossRef]
106. Lüdemann, S.K.; Lounnas, V.; Wade, R.C. How do substrates enter and products exit the buried active site of cytochrome P450cam? 1. Random expulsion molecular dynamics investigation of ligand access channels and mechanisms. *J. Mol. Biol.* **2000**, *303*, 797–811. [CrossRef]
107. Kokh, D.B.; Amaral, M.; Bomke, J.; Grädler, U.; Musil, D.; Buchstaller, H.P.; Dreyer, M.K.; Frech, M.; Lowinski, M.; Vallee, F.; et al. Estimation of drug-target residence times by τ-random acceleration molecular dynamics simulations. *J. Chem. Theory Comput.* **2018**, *14*, 3859–3869. [CrossRef]
108. Fu, H.; Chen, H.; Wang, X.; Chai, H.; Shao, X.; Cai, W.; Chipot, C. Finding an optimal pathway on a multidimensional free-energy landscape. *J. Chem. Inf. Model.* **2020**, *60*, 5366–5374. [CrossRef] [PubMed]
109. Lev, B.; Allen, T.W. Simulating ion channel activation mechanisms using swarms of trajectories. *J. Comput. Chem.* **2020**, *41*, 387–401. [CrossRef]
110. Patel, S.J.; Van Lehn, R.C. Analysis of Charged Peptide Loop-Flipping across a Lipid Bilayer Using the String Method with Swarms of Trajectories. *J. Phys. Chem. B* **2021**, *125*, 5862–5873. [CrossRef]
111. Kirkwood, J.G. Statistical Mechanics of Fluid Mixtures. *J. Chem. Phys.* **1935**, *3*, 300–313. [CrossRef]
112. Zwanzig, R.W. High-Temperature Equation of State by a Perturbation Method. I. Nonpolar Gases. *J. Chem. Phys.* **1954**, *22*, 1420–1426. [CrossRef]
113. Song, L.F.; Merz, K.M. Evolution of Alchemical Free Energy Methods in Drug Discovery. *J. Chem. Inf. Model.* **2020**, *60*, 5308–5318. [CrossRef] [PubMed]
114. Schindler, C.E.M.; Baumann, H.; Blum, A.; Böse, D.; Buchstaller, H.-P.; Burgdorf, L.; Cappel, D.; Chekler, E.; Czodrowski, P.; Dorsch, D.; et al. Large-Scale Assessment of Binding Free Energy Calculations in Active Drug Discovery Projects. *J. Chem. Inf. Model.* **2020**, *60*, 5457–5474. [CrossRef] [PubMed]
115. Bennett, C.H. Efficient estimation of free energy differences from Monte Carlo data. *J. Comput. Phys.* **1976**, *22*, 245–268. [CrossRef]
116. Shirts, M.R.; Chodera, J.D. Statistically optimal analysis of samples from multiple equilibrium states. *J. Chem. Phys.* **2008**, *129*, 124105. [CrossRef]
117. Noé, F.; Tkatchenko, A.; Müller, K.R.; Clementi, C. Machine learning for molecular simulation. *Annu. Rev. Phys. Chem.* **2020**, *71*, 361–390. [CrossRef]
118. Scheen, J.; Wu, W.; Mey, A.S.J.S.; Tosco, P.; Mackey, M.; Michel, J. Hybrid alchemical free Energy/Machine-Learning methodology for the computation of hydration free energies. *J. Chem. Inf. Model.* **2020**, *60*, 5331–5339. [CrossRef]
119. Gebhardt, J.; Kiesel, M.; Riniker, S.; Hansen, N. Combining molecular dynamics and machine learning to predict self-solvation free energies and limiting activity coefficients. *J. Chem. Inf. Model.* **2020**, *60*, 5319–5330. [CrossRef]
120. MacCallum, J.L.; Tieleman, D.P. Chapter 8 Interactions between Small Molecules and Lipid Bilayers. *Curr. Top. Membr.* **2008**, *60*, 227–256. [CrossRef]
121. Marrink, S.J.; Berendsen, H.J. Permeation process of small molecules across lipid mem- branes studied by molecular dynamics simulations. *J. Phys. Chem.* **1996**, *100*, 16729–16738. [CrossRef]
122. Odinokov, A.; Ostroumov, D. Structural Degradation and Swelling of Lipid Bilayer under the Action of Benzene. *J. Phys. Chem. B* **2015**, *119*, 15006–15013. [CrossRef]
123. Gupta, R.; Dwadasi, B.S.; Rai, B. Molecular Dynamics Simulation of Skin Lipids: Effect of Ceramide Chain Lengths on Bilayer Properties. *J. Phys. Chem. B* **2016**, *120*, 12536–12546. [CrossRef]
124. Stimson, L.M.; Vattulainen, I.; Róg, T.; Karttunen, M. Exploring the effect of xenon on biomembranes. *Cell. Mol. Biol. Lett.* **2005**, *10*, 563–569.
125. Booker, R.D.; Sum, A.K. Biophysical changes induced by xenon on phospholipid bilayers. *Biochim. Biophys. Acta-Biomembr.* **2013**, *1828*, 1347–1356. [CrossRef]
126. Jedlovszky, P.; Mezei, M. Calculation of the Free Energy Profile of H_2O, O_2, CO, CO_2, NO, and $CHCl_3$ in a Lipid Bilayer with a Cavity Insertion Variant of the Widom Method. *J. Am. Chem. Soc.* **2000**, *122*, 5125–5131. [CrossRef]
127. Wang, Y.; Tajkhorshid, E. Nitric Oxide Conduction by the Brain Aquaporin AQP4 Yi. *Proteins Struct. Funct. Genet.* **2010**, *78*, 661–670. [CrossRef] [PubMed]
128. Bacellar, I.O.L.; Cordeiro, R.M.; Mahling, P.; Baptista, M.S.; Röder, B.; Hackbarth, S. Oxygen distribution in the fluid/gel phases of lipid membranes. *Biochim. Biophys. Acta-Biomembr.* **2019**, *1861*, 879–886. [CrossRef]
129. Dotson, R.J.; Smith, C.R.; Bueche, K.; Angles, G.; Pias, S.C. Influence of Cholesterol on the Oxygen Permeability of Membranes: Insight from Atomistic Simulations. *Biophys. J.* **2017**, *112*, 2336–2347. [CrossRef] [PubMed]

130. Stepniewski, M.; Kepczynski, M.; Jamróz, D.; Nowakowska, M.; Rissanen, S.; Vattulainen, I.; Róg, T. Interaction of hematoporphyrin with lipid membranes. *J. Phys. Chem. B* **2012**, *116*, 4889–4897. [CrossRef] [PubMed]
131. Magarkar, A.; Stepniewski, M.; Karakas, E.; Róg, T.; Yliperttula, M.; Urtti, A.; Bunker, A. Molecular modeling of the PEGylated bilayer as a model for the PEGylated liposome surface in the bloodstream. *NSTI-Nanotech* **2012**, *3*, 293–295.
132. Paloncýová, M.; Devane, R.; Murch, B.; Berka, K.; Otyepka, M. Amphiphilic drug-like molecules accumulate in a membrane below the head group region. *J. Phys. Chem. B* **2014**, *118*, 1030–1039. [CrossRef]
133. John, T.; Thomas, T.; Abel, B.; Wood, B.R.; Chalmers, D.K.; Martin, L.L. How kanamycin A interacts with bacterial and mammalian mimetic membranes. *Biochim. Biophys. Acta-Biomembr.* **2017**, *1859*, 2242–2252. [CrossRef]
134. Lorent, J.H.; Quetin-Leclercq, J.; Mingeot-Leclercq, M.P. The amphiphilic nature of saponins and their effects on artificial and biological membranes and potential consequences for red blood and cancer cells. *Org. Biomol. Chem.* **2014**, *12*, 8803–8822. [CrossRef]
135. Sudji, I.R.; Subburaj, Y.; Frenkel, N.; García-Sáez, A.J.; Wink, M. Membrane disintegration caused by the steroid saponin digitonin is related to the presence of cholesterol. *Molecules* **2015**, *20*, 20146–20160. [CrossRef]
136. Sreij, R.; Dargel, C.; Schweins, R.; Prévost, S.; Dattani, R.; Hellweg, T. Aescin-Cholesterol Complexes in DMPC Model Membranes: A DSC and Temperature-Dependent Scattering Study. *Sci. Rep.* **2019**, *9*, 5542. [CrossRef] [PubMed]
137. Schumann-Gillett, A.; Mara, M.L.O. Lipid-Based Inhibitors Act Directly on GlyT2. *ACS Chem. Biol.* **2019**, *10*, 1668–1678. [CrossRef] [PubMed]
138. Postila, P.A.; Vattulainen, I.; Róg, T. Selective effect of cell membrane on synaptic neurotransmission. *Sci. Rep.* **2016**, *6*, 19345. [CrossRef] [PubMed]
139. Wang, C.; Ye, F.; Valardez, G.F.; Peters, G.H.; Westh, P. Affinity of four polar neurotransmitters for lipid bilayer membranes. *J. Phys. Chem. B* **2011**, *115*, 196–203. [CrossRef] [PubMed]
140. Pérez-Isidoro, R.; Ruiz-Suárez, J.C. Calcium and protons affect the interaction of neurotransmitters and anesthetics with anionic lipid membranes. *Biochim. Biophys. Acta-Biomembr.* **2016**, *1858*, 2215–2222. [CrossRef]
141. Kulig, W.; Pasenkiewicz-Gierula, M.; Róg, T. Topologies, structures and parameter files for lipid simulations in GROMACS with the OPLS-aa force field: DPPC, POPC, DOPC, PEPC, and cholesterol. *Data Br.* **2015**, *5*, 333–336. [CrossRef]
142. Kulig, W.; Pasenkiewicz-Gierula, M.; Róg, T.; Róg, T. Cis and trans unsaturated phosphatidylcholine bilayers: A molecular dynamics simulation study. *Chem. Phys. Lipids* **2016**, *195*, 12–20. [CrossRef]
143. Maciejewski, A.; Pasenkiewicz-Gierula, M.; Cramariuc, O.; Vattulainen, I.; Róg, T. Refined OPLS-AA Force Field for Saturated Phosphatidylcholine Bilayers at Full Hydration. *J. Phys. Chem. B* **2014**, *118*, 4571–4581. [CrossRef]
144. Lajunen, T.; Kontturi, L.S.; Viitala, L.; Manna, M.; Cramariuc, O.; Róg, T.; Bunker, A.; Laaksonen, T.; Viitala, T.; Murtomäki, L.; et al. Indocyanine green loaded liposomes for light triggered drug release. *Mol. Pharm.* **2016**, *13*, 2095–2107. [CrossRef]
145. Kaurola, P.; Sharma, V.; Vonk, A.; Vattulainen, I.; Róg, T. Distribution and dynamics of quinones in the lipid bilayer mimicking the inner membrane of mitochondria. *Biochim. Biophys. Acta-Biomembr.* **2016**, *1858*, 2116–2122. [CrossRef]
146. Tu, K.; Tarek, M.; Klein, M.L.; Scharf, D. Effects of anesthetics on the structure of a phospholipid bilayer: Molecular dynamics investigation of halothane in the hydrated liquid crystal phase of dipalmitoylphosphatidylcholine. *Biophys. J.* **1998**, *75*, 2123–2134. [CrossRef]
147. Pasenkiewicz-Gierula, M.; Róg, T.; Grochowski, J.; Serda, P.; Czarnecki, R.; Librowski, T.; Lochynski, S. Effects of carane derivative local anesthetic on a phospholipid bilayer studied by molecular dynamics simulation. *Biophys. J.* **2003**, *85*, 1248–1258. [CrossRef]
148. Bemporad, D.; Luttmann, C.; Essex, J.W. Behaviour of small solutes and large drugs in a lipid bilayer from computer simulations. *Biochim. Biophys. Acta-Biomembr.* **2005**, *1718*, 1–21. [CrossRef] [PubMed]
149. Bemporad, D.; Luttmann, C.; Essex, J.W. Computer simulation of small moleculle permeation across a lipid bilayer: Dependence on bilayer properties and solute volume, size, and cross-sectional area. *Biophys. J.* **2004**, *87*, 1–13. [CrossRef] [PubMed]
150. Abdiche, Y.N.; Myszka, D.G. Probing the mechanism of drug/lipid membrane interactions using Biacore. *Anal. Biochem.* **2004**, *328*, 233–243. [CrossRef] [PubMed]
151. Natesan, S.; Lukacova, V.; Peng, M.; Subramaniam, R.; Lynch, S.; Wang, Z.; Tandlich, R.; Balaz, S. Structure-Based Prediction of Drug Distribution Across the Headgroup and Core Strata of a Phospholipid Bilayer Using Surrogate Phases. *Mol. Pharm.* **2014**, *11*, 3577–3595. [CrossRef]
152. Juračka, J.; Šrejber, M.; Melíková, M.; Bazgier, V.; Berka, K. MolMeDB: Molecules on Membranes Database. *Database* **2019**, *2019*, baz07. [CrossRef]
153. Ollila, O.H.S.; Pabst, G. Atomistic resolution structure and dynamics of lipid bilayers in simulations and experiments. *Biochim. Biophys. Acta-Biomembr.* **2016**, *1858*, 2512–2528. [CrossRef]
154. Botan, A.; Favela-Rosales, F.; Fuchs, P.F.J.; Javanainen, M.; Kanduč, M.; Kulig, W.; Lamberg, A.; Loison, C.; Lyubartsev, A.; Miettinen, M.S.; et al. Toward atomistic resolution structure of phosphatidylcholine headgroup and glycerol backbone at different ambient conditions. *J. Phys. Chem. B* **2015**, *119*, 15075–15088. [CrossRef]
155. Catte, A.; Girych, M.; Javanainen, M.; Loison, C.; Melcr, J.; Miettinen, M.S.; Monticelli, L.; Määttä, J.; Oganesyan, V.S.; Ollila, O.H.S.; et al. Molecular electrometer and binding of cations to phospholipid bilayers. *Phys. Chem. Chem. Phys.* **2016**, *18*, 32560–32569. [CrossRef]

156. Antila, H.; Buslaev, P.; Favela-Rosales, F.; Ferreira, T.M.; Gushchin, I.; Javanainen, M.; Kav, B.; Madsen, J.J.; Melcr, J.; Miettinen, M.S.; et al. Headgroup Structure and Cation Binding in Phosphatidylserine Lipid Bilayers. *J. Phys. Chem. B* **2019**, *123*, 9066–9079. [CrossRef]
157. Owen, M.C.; Karner, A.; Šachl, R.; Preiner, J.; Amaro, M.; Vácha, R. Force Field Comparison of GM1 in a DOPC Bilayer Validated with AFM and FRET Experiments. *J. Phys. Chem. B* **2019**, *123*, 7504–7517. [CrossRef] [PubMed]
158. Klauda, J.B. Considerations of Recent All-Atom Lipid Force Field Development. *J. Phys. Chem. B* **2021**, *125*, 5676–5682. [CrossRef] [PubMed]
159. Shih, A.Y.; Hack, M.; Mirzadegan, T. Impact of Protein Preparation on Resulting Accuracy of FEP Calculations. *J. Chem. Inf. Model.* **2020**, *60*, 5287–5289. [CrossRef]
160. Tsai, H.-C.; Tao, Y.; Lee, T.-S.; Merz, K.M.; York, D.M. Validation of Free Energy Methods in AMBER. *J. Chem. Inf. Model.* **2020**, *60*, 5296–5300. [CrossRef] [PubMed]
161. Capelli, R.; Gardin, A.; Empereur-mot, C.; Doni, G.; Pavan, G.M. A Data-Driven Dimensionality Reduction Approach to Compare and Classify Lipid Force Fields. *J. Phys. Chem. B* **2021**, *125*, 7785–7796. [CrossRef]
162. Bratek, M.; Wójcik-Augustyn, A.; Kania, A.; Majta, J.; Murzyn, K. Condensed phase properties of n-pentadecane emerging from application of biomolecular force fields. *Acta Biochim. Pol.* **2020**, *67*, 309–318. [CrossRef]
163. Paloncýova, M.; Fabre, G.; Devane, R.H.; Trouillas, P.; Berka, K.; Otyepka, M. Benchmarking of Force Fields for Molecule—Membrane Interactions. *J. Chem. Theory Comput.* **2014**, *10*, 4143–4151. [CrossRef]
164. Alsop, R.J.; Dhaliwal, A.; Rheinstädter, M.C. Curcumin Protects Membranes through a Carpet or Insertion Model Depending on Hydration. *Langmuir* **2017**, *33*, 8516–8524. [CrossRef]
165. Salnikov, E.; Drung, B.; Fabre, G.; Itkin, A.; Otyepka, M.; Dencher, N.A.; Schmidt, B.; Hauß, T.; Trouillas, P.; Bechinger, B. Lipid bilayer position and orientation of novel carprofens, modulators of γ-secretase in Alzheimer's disease. *Biochim. Biophys. Acta-Biomembr.* **2018**, *1860*, 2224–2233. [CrossRef]
166. Khajeh, A.; Modarress, H. The influence of cholesterol on interactions and dynamics of ibuprofen in a lipid bilayer. *Biochim. Biophys. Acta-Biomembr.* **2014**, *1838*, 2431–2438. [CrossRef] [PubMed]
167. Wong, W.C.; Juo, J.Y.; Lin, C.H.; Liao, Y.H.; Cheng, C.Y.; Hsieh, C.L. Characterization of Single-Protein Dynamics in Polymer-Cushioned Lipid Bilayers Derived from Cell Plasma Membranes. *J. Phys. Chem. B* **2019**, *123*, 6492–6504. [CrossRef] [PubMed]
168. Bunker, A.; Magarkar, A.; Viitala, T. Rational design of liposomal drug delivery systems, a review: Combined experimental and computational studies of lipid membranes, liposomes and their PEGylation. *Biochim. Biophys. Acta-Biomembr.* **2016**, *1858*, 2334–2352. [CrossRef] [PubMed]
169. Dzieciuch, M.; Rissanen, S.; Szydłowska, N.; Bunker, A.; Kumorek, M.; Jamróz, D.; Vattulainen, I.; Nowakowska, M.; Róg, T.; Kepczynski, M.; et al. Pegylated liposomes as carriers of hydrophobic porphyrins. *J. Phys. Chem. B* **2015**, *119*, 6646–6657. [CrossRef]
170. Lajunen, T.; Nurmi, R.; Wilbie, D.; Ruoslahti, T.; Johansson, N.G.; Korhonen, O.; Róg, T.; Bunker, A.; Ruponen, M.; Urtti, A. The effect of light sensitizer localization on the stability of indocyanine green liposomes. *J. Control. Release* **2018**, *284*, 213–223. [CrossRef] [PubMed]
171. Podloucká, P.; Berka, K.; Fabre, G.; Paloncýová, M.; Duroux, J.L.; Otyepka, M.; Trouillas, P. Lipid bilayer membrane affinity rationalizes inhibition of lipid peroxidation by a natural lignan antioxidant. *J. Phys. Chem. B* **2013**, *117*, 5043–5049. [CrossRef] [PubMed]
172. Fabre, G.; Hänchen, A.; Calliste, C.A.; Berka, K.; Banala, S.; Otyepka, M.; Süssmuth, R.D.; Trouillas, P. Lipocarbazole, an efficient lipid peroxidation inhibitor anchored in the membrane. *Bioorganic Med. Chem.* **2015**, *23*, 4866–4870. [CrossRef]
173. Fabre, G.; Bayach, I.; Berka, K.; Paloncýová, M.; Starok, M.; Rossi, C.; Duroux, J.L.; Otyepka, M.; Trouillas, P. Synergism of antioxidant action of vitamins E, C and quercetin is related to formation of molecular associations in biomembranes. *Chem. Commun.* **2015**, *51*, 7713–7716. [CrossRef]
174. Yang, Y.; Lee, M.; Fairn, G.D. Phospholipid subcellular localization and dynamics. *J. Biol. Chem.* **2018**, *293*, 6230–6240. [CrossRef]
175. Van Meer, G.; Voelker, D.R.; Feigenson, G.W. Membrane lipids: Where they are and how they behave. *Nat. Rev. Mol. Cell Biol.* **2008**, *9*, 112–124. [CrossRef]
176. Menon, A.K.; Levine, T.P. The cellular lipid landscape. *Biochim. Biophys. Acta-Mol. Cell Biol. Lipids* **2016**, *1861*, 755–756. [CrossRef]
177. Lingwood, D.; Kaiser, H.-J.H.-J.; Levental, I.; Simons, K. Lipid rafts as functional heterogeneity in cell membranes. *Biochem. Soc. Trans.* **2009**, *37*, 955–960. [CrossRef]
178. Lingwood, D.; Simons, K. Lipid Rafts As a Membrane-Organizing Principle. *Science* **2012**, *327*, 46–50. [CrossRef] [PubMed]
179. Alves, A.C.; Magarkar, A.; Horta, M.; Lima, J.L.F.C.; Bunker, A.; Nunes, C.; Reis, S. Influence of doxorubicin on model cell membrane properties: Insights from in vitro and in silico studies. *Sci. Rep.* **2017**, *7*, 6343. [CrossRef] [PubMed]
180. Yang, Y.; Dong, H.; Zhou, H.X. Effects of Cholesterol on the Partitioning of a Drug Molecule in Lipid Bilayers. *J. Phys. Chem. B* **2021**, *125*, 5338–5345. [CrossRef] [PubMed]
181. Yuan, J.; Meng, F. Effects of cholesterol on chlorzoxazone translocation across POPC bilayer. *J. Mol. Model.* **2021**, *27*. [CrossRef]
182. Li, Y.-C.; Rissanen, S.; Stepniewski, M.; Cramariuc, O.; Róg, T.; Mirza, S.; Xhaard, H.; Wytrwal, M.; Kepczynski, M.; Bunker, A. Study of interaction between PEG carrier and three relevant drug molecules: Piroxicam, paclitaxel, and hematoporphyrin. *J. Phys. Chem. B* **2012**, *116*, 7334–7341. [CrossRef]

183. Rissanen, S.; Kumorek, M.; Martinez-Seara, H.; Li, Y.C.; Jamróz, D.; Bunker, A.; Nowakowska, M.; Vattulainen, I.; Kepczynski, M.; Róg, T. Effect of PEGylation on drug entry into lipid bilayer. *J. Phys. Chem. B* **2014**, *118*, 144–151. [CrossRef]
184. Dzieciuch-Rojek, M.; Poojari, C.; Bednar, J.; Bunker, A.; Kozik, B.; Nowakowska, M.; Vattulainen, I.; Wydro, P.P.; Kepczynski, M.; Róg, T. Effects of membrane PEGylation on entry and location of antifungal drug itraconazole and their pharmacological implications. *Mol. Pharmacol.* **2017**, *14*, 1057–1070. [CrossRef]
185. Wilkosz, N.; Rissanen, S.; Cyza, M.; Szybka, R.; Nowakowska, M.; Bunker, A.; Róg, T.; Kepczynski, M. Effect of piroxicam on lipid membranes: Drug encapsulation and gastric toxicity aspects. *Eur. J. Pharm. Sci.* **2017**, *100*, 116–125. [CrossRef] [PubMed]
186. Poojari, C.; Wilkosz, N.; Lira, R.B.; Dimova, R.; Jurkiewicz, P.; Petka, R.; Kepczynski, M.; Róg, T. Behavior of the DPH fluorescence probe in membranes perturbed by drugs. *Chem. Phys. Lipids* **2019**, *223*, 104784. [CrossRef]
187. Poojari, C.; Zak, A.; Dzieciuch-Rojek, M.; Bunker, A.; Kepczynski, M.; Róg, T. Cholesterol Reduces Partitioning of Antifungal Drug Itraconazole into Lipid Bilayers. *J. Phys. Chem. B* **2020**, *124*, 2139–2148. [CrossRef] [PubMed]
188. Bulbake, U.; Doppalapudi, S.; Kommineni, N.; Khan, W. Liposomal formulations in clinical use: An updated review. *Pharmaceutics* **2017**, *9*, 12. [CrossRef] [PubMed]
189. Juszkiewicz, K.; Sikorski, A.F.; Czogalla, A. Building blocks to design liposomal delivery systems. *Int. J. Mol. Sci.* **2020**, *21*, 9559. [CrossRef]
190. Ivanova, D.; Deneva, V.; Nedeltcheva, D.; Kamounah, F.S.; Gergov, G.; Hansen, P.E.; Kawauchi, S.; Antonov, L. Tautomeric transformations of piroxicam in solution: A combined experimental and theoretical study. *RSC Adv.* **2015**, *5*, 31852–31860. [CrossRef]
191. Lamprakis, C.; Stocker, A.; Cascella, M. Mechanisms of recognition and binding of α-TTP to the plasma membrane by multi-scale molecular dynamics simulations. *Front. Mol. Biosci.* **2015**, *2*, 36. [CrossRef]
192. Fotakis, C.; Christodouleas, D.; Zoumpoulakis, P.; Kritsi, E.; Benetis, N.P.; Mavromoustakos, T.; Reis, H.; Gili, A.; Papadopoulos, M.G.; Zervou, M. Comparative biophysical studies of sartan class drug molecules losartan and candesartan (CV-11974) with membrane bilayers. *J. Phys. Chem. B* **2011**, *115*, 6180–6192. [CrossRef]
193. Kiriakidi, S.; Chatzigiannis, C.; Papaemmanouil, C.; Tzakos, A.G.; Mavromoustakos, T. Exploring the role of the membrane bilayer in the recognition of candesartan by its GPCR AT1 receptor. *Biochim. Biophys. Acta-Biomembr.* **2020**, *1862*, 183142. [CrossRef] [PubMed]
194. Först, G.; Cwiklik, L.; Jurkiewicz, P.; Schubert, R.; Hof, M. Interactions of beta-blockers with model lipid membranes: Molecular view of the interaction of acebutolol, oxprenolol, and propranolol with phosphatidylcholine vesicles by time-dependent fluorescence shift and molecular dynamics simulations. *Eur. J. Pharm. Biopharm.* **2014**, *87*, 559–569. [CrossRef]
195. Dror, R.O.; Pan, A.C.; Arlow, D.H.; Borhani, D.W.; Maragakis, P.; Shan, Y.; Xu, H.; Shaw, D.E. Pathway and mechanism of drug binding to G-protein-coupled receptors. *Proc. Natl. Acad. Sci. USA* **2011**, *108*, 13118–13123. [CrossRef] [PubMed]
196. Wang, H.; Ren, X.; Meng, F. Molecular dynamics simulation of six β-blocker drugs passing across POPC bilayer. *Mol. Simul.* **2016**, *42*, 56–63. [CrossRef]
197. Liu, X.; Kaindl, J.; Korczynska, M.; Stößel, A.; Dengler, D.; Stanek, M.; Hübner, H.; Clark, M.J.; Mahoney, J.; Matt, R.A.; et al. An allosteric modulator binds to a conformational hub in the β2 adrenergic receptor. *Nat. Chem. Biol.* **2020**, *16*, 749–755. [CrossRef]
198. Yousefpour, A.; Modarress, H.; Goharpey, F.; Amjad-Iranagh, S. Interaction of PEGylated anti-hypertensive drugs, amlodipine, atenolol and lisinopril with lipid bilayer membrane: A molecular dynamics simulation study. *Biochim. Biophys. Acta-Biomembr.* **2015**, *1848*, 1687–1698. [CrossRef]
199. Thai, N.Q.; Theodorakis, P.E.; Li, M.S. Fast Estimation of the Blood-Brain Barrier Permeability by Pulling a Ligand through a Lipid Membrane. *J. Chem. Inf. Model.* **2020**, *60*, 3057–3067. [CrossRef]
200. Wang, T.; Duan, Y. Ligand Entry and Exit Pathways in the β2-Adrenergic Receptor. *J. Mol. Biol.* **2009**, *392*, 1102–1115. [CrossRef]
201. Yan, S.; Shaw, D.E.; Yang, L.; Sandham, D.A.; Healy, M.P.; Reilly, J.; Wang, B. Interactions between β2-Adrenoceptor Ligands and Membrane: Atomic-Level Insights from Magic-Angle Spinning NMR. *J. Med. Chem.* **2017**, *60*, 6867–6879. [CrossRef]
202. Yue, Z.; Li, C.; Voth, G.A.; Swanson, J.M.J. Dynamic Protonation Dramatically Affects the Membrane Permeability of Drug-like Molecules. *J. Am. Chem. Soc.* **2019**, *141*, 13421–13433. [CrossRef] [PubMed]
203. Coimbra, J.T.S.; Fernandes, P.A.; Ramos, M.J. Revisiting Partition in Hydrated Bilayer Systems. *J. Chem. Theory Comput.* **2017**, *13*, 2290–2299. [CrossRef] [PubMed]
204. Khadka, N.K.; Cheng, X.; Ho, C.S.; Katsaras, J.; Pan, J. Interactions of the Anticancer Drug Tamoxifen with Lipid Membranes. *Biophys. J.* **2015**, *108*, 2492–2501. [CrossRef] [PubMed]
205. Karami, L.; Jalili, S. Effects of cholesterol concentration on the interaction of cytarabine with lipid membranes: A molecular dynamics simulation study. *J. Biomol. Struct. Dyn.* **2015**, *33*, 1254–1268. [CrossRef]
206. Liu, H.; Chen, J.; Shen, Q.; Fu, W.; Wu, W. Molecular insights on the cyclic peptide nanotube-mediated transportation of antitumor drug 5-fluorouracil. *Mol. Pharm.* **2010**, *7*, 1985–1994. [CrossRef] [PubMed]
207. Khajeh, A.; Modarress, H. Effect of cholesterol on behavior of 5-fluorouracil (5-FU) in a DMPC lipid bilayer, a molecular dynamics study. *Biophys. Chem.* **2014**, *187–188*, 43–50. [CrossRef]
208. Alves, A.C.; Ribeiro, D.; Horta, M.; Lima, J.L.F.C.; Nunes, C.; Reis, S. The daunorubicin interplay with mimetic model membranes of cancer cells: A biophysical interpretation. *Biochim. Biophys. Acta-Biomembr.* **2017**, *1859*, 941–948. [CrossRef]
209. Matyszewska, D. The influence of charge and lipophilicity of daunorubicin and idarubicin on their penetration of model biological membranes—Langmuir monolayer and electrochemical studies. *Biochim. Biophys. Acta-Biomembr.* **2020**, *1862*, 183104. [CrossRef]

210. Wu, X.; Chantemargue, B.; Di Meo, F.; Bourgaux, C.; Chapron, D.; Trouillas, P.; Rosilio, V. Deciphering the Peculiar Behavior of β-Lapachone in Lipid Monolayers and Bilayers. *Langmuir* **2019**, *35*, 14603–14615. [CrossRef]
211. Węder, K.; Mach, M.; Hąc-Wydro, K.; Wydro, P. Studies on the interactions of anticancer drug—Minerval—with membrane lipids in binary and ternary Langmuir monolayers. *Biochim. Biophys. Acta-Biomembr.* **2018**, *1860*, 2329–2336. [CrossRef]
212. Petit, K.; Suwalsky, M.; Colina, J.R.; Aguilar, L.F.; Jemiola-Rzeminska, M.; Strzalka, K. In vitro effects of the antitumor drug miltefosine on human erythrocytes and molecular models of its membrane. *Biochim. Biophys. Acta-Biomembr.* **2019**, *1861*, 17–25. [CrossRef]
213. Haralampieva, I.; de Armiño, D.J.A.; Luck, M.; Fischer, M.; Abel, T.; Huster, D.; Di Lella, S.; Scheidt, H.A.; Müller, P. Interaction of the small-molecule kinase inhibitors tofacitinib and lapatinib with membranes. *Biochim. Biophys. Acta-Biomembr.* **2020**, *1862*, 183414. [CrossRef]
214. Mahadeo, M.; Prenner, E.J. Differential impact of synthetic antitumor lipid drugs on the membrane organization of phosphatidic acid and diacylglycerol monolayers. *Chem. Phys. Lipids* **2020**, *229*, 104896. [CrossRef] [PubMed]
215. Tang, P.K.; Chakraborty, K.; Hu, W.; Kang, M.; Loverde, S.M. Interaction of Camptothecin with Model Cellular Membranes. *J. Chem. Theory Comput.* **2020**, *16*, 3373–3384. [CrossRef] [PubMed]
216. Tang, P.K.; Manandhar, A.; Hu, W.; Kang, M.; Loverde, S.M. The interaction of supramolecular anticancer drug amphiphiles with phospholipid membranes. *Nanoscale Adv.* **2021**, *3*, 370–382. [CrossRef] [PubMed]
217. Zhang, L.; Bennett, W.F.D.; Zheng, T.; Ouyang, P.-K.; Ouyang, X.; Qiu, X.; Luo, A.; Karttunen, M.; Chen, P. Effect of Cholesterol on Cellular Uptake of Cancer Drugs Pirarubicin and Ellipticine. *J. Phys. Chem. B* **2016**, *120*, 3148–3156. [CrossRef] [PubMed]
218. Da Fonseca, C.; Khandelia, H.; Salazar, M.; Schönthal, A.; Meireles, O.; Quirico-Santos, T. Perillyl alcohol: Dynamic interactions with the lipid bilayer and implications for long-term inhalational chemotherapy for gliomas. *Surg. Neurol. Int.* **2016**, *7*, 1. [CrossRef] [PubMed]
219. Rivel, T.; Ramseyer, C.; Yesylevskyy, S. The asymmetry of plasma membranes and their cholesterol content influence the uptake of cisplatin. *Sci. Rep.* **2019**, *9*, 5627. [CrossRef]
220. Yesylevskyy, S.; Cardey, B.; Kraszewski, S.; Foley, S.; Enescu, M.; da Silva, A.M.; Santos, H.F.D.; Ramseyer, C. Empirical force field for cisplatin based on quantum dynamics data: Case study of new parameterization scheme for coordination compounds. *J. Mol. Model.* **2015**, *21*, 268. [CrossRef]
221. Chakraborty, K.; Dutta, C.; Mukherjee, S.; Biswas, A.; Gayen, P.; George, G.; Raghothama, S.; Ghosh, S.; Dey, S.; Bhattacharyya, D.; et al. Engineering Ionophore Gramicidin-Inspired Self-Assembled Peptides for Drug Delivery and Cancer Nanotherapeutics. *Adv. Ther.* **2018**, *1*, 1800018. [CrossRef]
222. Alves, A.C.; Ribeiro, D.; Nunes, C.; Reis, S. Biophysics in cancer: The relevance of drug-membrane interaction studies. *Biochim. Biophys. Acta-Biomembr.* **2016**, *1858*, 2231–2244. [CrossRef] [PubMed]
223. Bourgaux, C.; Couvreur, P. Interactions of anticancer drugs with biomembranes: What can we learn from model membranes? *J. Control. Release* **2014**, *190*, 127–138. [CrossRef] [PubMed]
224. Almeida, A.; Fernandes, E.; Sarmento, B.; Lúcio, M. A biophysical insight of camptothecin biodistribution: Towards a molecular understanding of its pharmacokinetic issues. *Pharmaceutics* **2021**, *13*, 869. [CrossRef]
225. Herrera, F.E.; Sevrain, C.M.; Jaffrès, P.-A.; Couthon, H.; Grélard, A.; Dufourc, E.J.; Chantôme, A.; Potier-Cartereau, M.; Vandier, C.; Bouchet, A.M. Singular Interaction between an Antimetastatic Agent and the Lipid Bilayer: The Ohmline Case. *ACS Omega* **2017**, *2*, 6361–6370. [CrossRef] [PubMed]
226. Pederzoli, M.; Wasif Baig, M.; Kývala, M.; Pittner, J.; Cwiklik, L. Photophysics of BODIPY-Based Photosensitizer for Photodynamic Therapy: Surface Hopping and Classical Molecular Dynamics. *J. Chem. Theory Comput.* **2019**, *15*, 5046–5057. [CrossRef]
227. Leite, N.B.; Martins, D.B.; Fazani, V.E.; Vieira, M.R.; dos Santos Cabrera, M.P. Cholesterol modulates curcumin partitioning and membrane effects. *Biochim. Biophys. Acta-Biomembr.* **2018**, *1860*, 2320–2328. [CrossRef]
228. Lyu, Y.; Xiang, N.; Mondal, J.; Zhu, X.; Narsimhan, G. Characterization of Interactions between Curcumin and Different Types of Lipid Bilayers by Molecular Dynamics Simulation. *J. Phys. Chem. B* **2018**, *122*, 2341–2354. [CrossRef]
229. Khondker, A.; Alsop, R.J.; Himbert, S.; Tang, J.; Shi, A.C.; Hitchcock, A.P.; Rheinstädter, M.C. Membrane-Modulating Drugs can Affect the Size of Amyloid-β 25–35 Aggregates in Anionic Membranes. *Sci. Rep.* **2018**, *8*, 12367. [CrossRef]
230. Ashida, Y.; Yanagita, R.C.; Takahashi, C.; Kawanami, Y.; Irie, K. Binding mode prediction of aplysiatoxin, a potent agonist of protein kinase C, through molecular simulation and structure–activity study on simplified analogs of the receptor-recognition domain. *Bioorganic Med. Chem.* **2016**, *24*, 4218–4227. [CrossRef]
231. Ryckbosch, S.M.; Wender, P.A.; Pande, V.S. Molecular dynamics simulations reveal ligand-controlled positioning of a peripheral protein complex in membranes. *Nat. Commun.* **2017**, *8*, 6. [CrossRef]
232. Khondker, A.; Malenfant, D.J.; Dhaliwal, A.K.; Rheinstädter, M.C. Carbapenems and Lipid Bilayers: Localization, Partitioning, and Energetics. *ACS Infect. Dis.* **2018**, *4*, 926–935. [CrossRef]
233. Cramariuc, O.; Róg, T.; Javanainen, M.; Monticelli, L.; Polishchuk, A.V.; Vattulainen, I. Mechanism for translocation of fluoroquinolones across lipid membranes. *Biochim. Biophys. Acta-Biomembr.* **2012**, *1818*, 2563–2571. [CrossRef]
234. Cetuk, H.; Anishkin, A.; Scott, A.J.; Rempe, S.B.; Ernst, R.K.; Sukharev, S. Partitioning of Seven Different Classes of Antibiotics into LPS Monolayers Supports Three Different Permeation Mechanisms through the Outer Bacterial Membrane. *Langmuir* **2021**, *37*, 1372–1385. [CrossRef]

235. Sousa, C.F.; Coimbra, J.T.S.; Ferreira, M.; Pereira-Leite, C.; Reis, S.; Ramos, M.J.; Fernandes, P.A.; Gameiro, P. Passive Diffusion of Ciprofloxacin and its Metalloantibiotic: A Computational and Experimental study. *J. Mol. Biol.* **2021**, *433*, 166911. [CrossRef]
236. Ortiz-Collazos, S.; Picciani, P.H.S.; Oliveira, O.N.; Pimentel, A.S.; Edler, K.J. Influence of levofloxacin and clarithromycin on the structure of DPPC monolayers. *Biochim. Biophys. Acta-Biomembr.* **2019**, *1861*, 182994. [CrossRef] [PubMed]
237. Vignoli Muniz, G.S.; Souza, M.C.; Duarte, E.L.; Lamy, M.T. Comparing the interaction of the antibiotic levofloxacin with zwitterionic and anionic membranes: Calorimetry, fluorescence, and spin label studies. *Biochim. Biophys. Acta-Biomembr.* **2021**, *1863*, 183622. [CrossRef]
238. Ortiz-Collazos, S.; Estrada-López, E.D.; Pedreira, A.A.; Picciani, P.H.S.; Oliveira, O.N.; Pimentel, A.S. Interaction of levofloxacin with lung surfactant at the air-water interface. *Colloids Surf. B Biointerfaces* **2017**, *158*, 689–696. [CrossRef] [PubMed]
239. Vila-Viçosa, D.; Victor, B.L.; Ramos, J.; Machado, D.; Viveiros, M.; Switala, J.; Loewen, P.C.; Leitao, R.; Martins, F.; Machuqueiro, M. Insights on the Mechanism of Action of INH-C10 as an Antitubercular Prodrug. *Mol. Pharm.* **2017**, *14*, 4597–4605. [CrossRef] [PubMed]
240. Samelo, J.; Mora, M.J.; Granero, G.E.; Moreno, M.J. Partition of amphiphilic molecules to lipid bilayers by ITC: Low-affinity solutes. *ACS Omega* **2017**, *2*, 6863–6869. [CrossRef]
241. Li, J.; Beuerman, R.W.; Verma, C.S. Molecular Insights into the Membrane Affinities of Model Hydrophobes. *ACS Omega* **2018**, *3*, 2498–2507. [CrossRef]
242. Zhang, H.; Shao, X.; Dehez, F.; Cai, W.; Chipot, C. Modulation of membrane permeability by carbon dioxide. *J. Comput. Chem.* **2020**, *41*, 421–426. [CrossRef]
243. Hörömpöli, D.; Ciglia, C.; Glüsenkamp, K.-H.; Haustedt, O.L.; Falkenstein, H.-P.; Bendas, G.; Berscheid, A.; Brötz-Oesterhelt, H. The Antibiotic Negamycin Crosses the Bacterial Cytoplasmic Membrane by Multiple Routes. *Antimicrob. Agents Chemother.* **2021**, *65*, e00986-20. [CrossRef]
244. Kim, W.; Steele, A.D.; Zhu, W.; Csatary, E.E.; Fricke, N.; Dekarske, M.M.; Jayamani, E.; Pan, W.; Kwon, B.; Sinitsa, I.F.; et al. Discovery and Optimization of nTZDpa as an Antibiotic Effective Against Bacterial Persisters. *ACS Infect. Dis.* **2018**, *4*, 1540–1545. [CrossRef]
245. Kumar, S.; Thakur, J.; Yadav, K.; Mitra, M.; Pal, S.; Ray, A.; Gupta, S.; Medatwal, N.; Gupta, R.; Mishra, D.; et al. Cholic Acid-Derived Amphiphile which Combats Gram-Positive Bacteria-Mediated Infections via Disintegration of Lipid Clusters. *ACS Biomater. Sci. Eng.* **2019**, *5*, 4764–4775. [CrossRef] [PubMed]
246. Jaroque, G.N.; Sartorelli, P.; Caseli, L. The effect of the monocyclic monoterpene tertiary alcohol γ-terpineol on biointerfaces containing cholesterol. *Chem. Phys. Lipids* **2020**, *230*, 104915. [CrossRef] [PubMed]
247. Kim, W.; Zou, G.; Hari, T.P.A.; Wilt, I.K.; Zhu, W.; Galle, N.; Faizi, H.A.; Hendricks, G.L.; Tori, K.; Pan, W.; et al. A selective membrane-targeting repurposed antibiotic with activity against persistent methicillin-resistant Staphylococcus aureus. *Proc. Natl. Acad. Sci. USA* **2019**, *116*, 16529–16534. [CrossRef]
248. Van Oosten, B.; Marquardt, D.; Harroun, T.A. Testing High Concentrations of Membrane Active Antibiotic Chlorhexidine Via Computational Titration and Calorimetry. *J. Phys. Chem. B* **2017**, *121*, 4657–4668. [CrossRef] [PubMed]
249. Van Oosten, B.; Marquardt, D.; Komljenović, I.; Bradshaw, J.P.; Sternin, E.; Harroun, T.A. Small molecule interaction with lipid bilayers: A molecular dynamics study of chlorhexidine. *J. Mol. Graph. Model.* **2014**, *48*, 96–104. [CrossRef]
250. Rzycki, M.; Drabik, D.; Szostak-Paluch, K.; Hanus-Lorenz, B.; Kraszewski, S. Unraveling the mechanism of octenidine and chlorhexidine on membranes: Does electrostatics matter? *Biophys. J.* **2021**, *120*, 3392–3408. [CrossRef]
251. Poger, D.; Mark, A.E. Effect of Triclosan and Chloroxylenol on Bacterial Membranes. *J. Phys. Chem. B* **2019**, *123*, 5291–5301. [CrossRef]
252. Kim, A.V.; Shelepova, E.A.; Selyutina, O.Y.; Meteleva, E.S.; Dushkin, A.V.; Medvedev, N.N.; Polyakov, N.E.; Lyakhov, N.Z. Glycyrrhizin-assisted transport of praziquantel anthelmintic drug through the lipid membrane: An experiment and MD simulation. *Mol. Pharm.* **2019**, *16*, 3188–3198. [CrossRef]
253. Leonis, G.; Czyżnikowska, Ż.; Megariotis, G.; Reis, H.; Papadopoulos, M.G. Computational studies of darunavir into HIV-1 protease and DMPC bilayer: Necessary conditions for effective binding and the role of the flaps. *J. Chem. Inf. Model.* **2012**, *52*, 1542–1558. [CrossRef]
254. Konstantinidi, A.; Chountoulesi, M.; Naziris, N.; Sartori, B.; Amenitsch, H.; Plakantonaki, M.; Triantafyllakou, I.; Tselios, T.; Demetzos, C.; Busath, D.D.; et al. The boundary lipid around DMPC-spanning in fl uenza A M2 transmembrane domain channels: Its structure and potential for drug accommodation. *Biochim. Biophys. Acta-Biomembr.* **2020**, *1862*, 183156. [CrossRef] [PubMed]
255. Konstantinidi, A.; Naziris, N.; Chountoulesi, M.; Kiriakidi, S.; Sartori, B.; Kolokouris, D.; Amentisch, H.; Mali, G.; Ntountaniotis, D.; Demetzos, C.; et al. Comparative Perturbation Effects Exerted by the Influenza A M2 WT Protein Inhibitors Amantadine and the Spiro[pyrrolidine-2,2′-adamantane] Variant AK13 to Membrane Bilayers Studied Using Biophysical Experiments and Molecular Dynamics Simulations. *J. Phys. Chem. B* **2018**, *122*, 9877–9895. [CrossRef] [PubMed]
256. Khurana, E.; Devane, R.H.; Dal Peraro, M.; Klein, M.L. Computational study of drug binding to the membrane-bound tetrameric M2 peptide bundle from influenza A virus. *Biochim. Biophys. Acta-Biomembr.* **2011**, *1808*, 530–537. [CrossRef] [PubMed]
257. Kordzadeh, A.; Ramazani Saadatabadi, A.; Hadi, A. Investigation on penetration of saffron components through lipid bilayer bound to spike protein of SARS-CoV-2 using steered molecular dynamics simulation. *Heliyon* **2020**, *6*, e05681. [CrossRef]
258. Kasparyan, G.; Poojari, C.; Róg, T.; Hub, J.S. Cooperative Effects of an Antifungal Moiety and DMSO on Pore Formation over Lipid Membranes Revealed by Free Energy Calculations. *J. Phys. Chem. B* **2020**, *124*, 8811–8821. [CrossRef]

259. Szomek, M.; Reinholdt, P.; Petersen, D.; Caci, A.; Kongsted, J.; Wüstner, D. Direct observation of nystatin binding to the plasma membrane of living cells. *Biochim. Biophys. Acta-Biomembr.* **2021**, *1863*, 183528. [CrossRef]
260. Grela, E.; Wieczór, M.; Luchowski, R.; Zielinska, J.; Barzycka, A.; Grudzinski, W.; Nowak, K.; Tarkowski, P.; Czub, J.; Gruszecki, W.I. Mechanism of Binding of Antifungal Antibiotic Amphotericin B to Lipid Membranes: An Insight from Combined Single-Membrane Imaging, Microspectroscopy, and Molecular Dynamics. *Mol. Pharm.* **2018**, *15*, 4202–4213. [CrossRef]
261. Markiewicz, M.; Pasenkiewicz-Gierula, M. Comparative model studies of gastric toxicity of nonsteroidal anti-inflammatory drugs. *Langmuir* **2011**, *27*, 6950–6961. [CrossRef]
262. Blasi, P.; Casagrande, S.; Pedretti, A.; Fioretto, D.; Vistoli, G.; Corezzi, S. Ketoprofen poly(lactide-co-glycolide) physical interaction studied by Brillouin spectroscopy and molecular dynamics simulations. *Int. J. Pharm.* **2020**, *580*, 119235. [CrossRef] [PubMed]
263. Hu, J.; Liu, H.H.; Xu, P.; Shang, Y.; Liu, H.H. Investigation of Drug for Pulmonary Administration-Model Pulmonary Surfactant Monolayer Interactions Using Langmuir-Blodgett Monolayer and Molecular Dynamics Simulation: A Case Study of Ketoprofen. *Langmuir* **2019**, *35*, 13452–13460. [CrossRef] [PubMed]
264. Da Silva, E.; Autilio, C.; Hougaard, K.S.; Baun, A.; Cruz, A.; Perez-Gil, J.; Sørli, J.B. Molecular and biophysical basis for the disruption of lung surfactant function by chemicals. *Biochim. Biophys. Acta-Biomembr.* **2021**, *1863*, 183499. [CrossRef] [PubMed]
265. Sodeifian, G.; Razmimanesh, F. Diffusional interaction behavior of NSAIDs in lipid bilayer membrane using molecular dynamics (MD) simulation: Aspirin and Ibuprofen. *J. Biomol. Struct. Dyn.* **2019**, *37*, 1666–1684. [CrossRef]
266. Alsop, R.J.; Himbert, S.; Dhaliwal, A.; Schmalzl, K.; Rheinstädter, M.C. Aspirin locally disrupts the liquid-ordered phase. *R. Soc. Open Sci.* **2018**, *5*, 171710. [CrossRef]
267. Barrett, M.A.; Zheng, S.; Roshankar, G.; Alsop, R.J.; Belanger, R.K.R.; Rheinsta, M.C.; Huynh, C.; Kuc, N. Interaction of Aspirin (Acetylsalicylic Acid) with Lipid Membranes. *PLoS ONE* **2012**, *7*, e34357. [CrossRef]
268. Sharma, V.K.; Mamontov, E.; Ohl, M.; Tyagi, M. Incorporation of aspirin modulates the dynamical and phase behavior of the phospholipid membrane. *Phys. Chem. Chem. Phys.* **2017**, *19*, 2514–2524. [CrossRef]
269. Alsop, R.J.; Barrett, M.A.; Zheng, S. Acetylsalicylic acid (ASA) increases the solubility of cholesterol when incorporated in lipid membranes. *Soft Matter* **2014**, *10*, 4275–4286. [CrossRef] [PubMed]
270. Jämbeck, J.P.M.; Lyubartsev, A.P. Exploring the free energy landscape of solutes embedded in lipid bilayers. *J. Phys. Chem. Lett.* **2013**, *4*, 1781–1787. [CrossRef] [PubMed]
271. Alsop, R.J.; Toppozini, L.; Marquardt, D.; Ku, N.; Harroun, T.A.; Rheinstädter, M.C. Aspirin inhibits formation of cholesterol rafts in fluid lipid membranes. *Biochim. Biophys. Acta-Biomembr.* **2015**, *1848*, 805–812. [CrossRef]
272. Berka, K.; Hendrychová, T.; Anzenbacher, P.; Otyepka, M. Membrane position of ibuprofen agrees with suggested access path entrance to cytochrome P450 2C9 active site. *J. Phys. Chem. A* **2011**, *115*, 11248–11255. [CrossRef]
273. Kremkow, J.; Luck, M.; Huster, D.; Müller, P.; Scheidt, H.A. Membrane Interaction of Ibuprofen with Cholesterol-Containing Lipid Membranes. *Biomolecules* **2020**, *10*, 1384. [CrossRef]
274. Nitschke, N.; Atkovska, K.; Hub, J.S. Accelerating potential of mean force calculations for lipid membrane permeation: System size, reaction coordinate, solute-solute distance, and cutoffs. *J. Chem. Phys.* **2016**, *145*, 125101. [CrossRef]
275. Boggara, M.B.; Mihailescu, M.; Krishnamoorti, R. Structural association of nonsteroidal anti-inflammatory drugs with lipid membranes. *J. Am. Chem. Soc.* **2012**, *134*, 19669–19676. [CrossRef]
276. Rojas-Valencia, N.; Gómez, S.; Montillo, S.; Manrique-Moreno, M.; Cappelli, C.; Hadad, C.; Restrepo, A. Evolution of Bonding during the Insertion of Anionic Ibuprofen into Model Cell Membranes. *J. Phys. Chem. B* **2020**, *124*, 79–90. [CrossRef]
277. Sharma, V.K.; Mamontov, E.; Tyagi, M. Effects of NSAIDs on the nanoscopic dynamics of lipid membrane. *Biochim. Biophys. Acta-Biomembr.* **2020**, *1862*, 183100. [CrossRef]
278. Markiewicz, M.; Librowski, T.; Lipkowska, A.; Serda, P.; Baczynski, K.; Pasenkiewicz-Gierula, M. Assessing gastric toxicity of xanthone derivatives of anti-inflammatory activity using simulation and experimental approaches. *Biophys. Chem.* **2017**, *220*, 20–33. [CrossRef] [PubMed]
279. Fearon, A.D.; Stokes, G.Y. Thermodynamics of Indomethacin Adsorption to Phospholipid Membranes. *J. Phys. Chem. B* **2017**, *121*, 10508–10518. [CrossRef] [PubMed]
280. Kabedev, A.; Hossain, S.; Hubert, M.; Larsson, P.; Bergström, C.A.S. Molecular Dynamics Simulations Reveal Membrane Interactions for Poorly Water-Soluble Drugs: Impact of Bile Solubilization and Drug Aggregation. *J. Pharm. Sci.* **2021**, *110*, 176–185. [CrossRef] [PubMed]
281. Tse, C.H.; Comer, J.; Wang, Y.; Chipot, C. Link between Membrane Composition and Permeability to Drugs. *J. Chem. Theory Comput.* **2018**, *14*, 2895–2909. [CrossRef]
282. Yang, C.; Guo, S.; Wu, X.; Yang, P.; Han, L.; Dai, X.; Shi, X. Multiscale study on the enhancing effect and mechanism of borneolum on transdermal permeation of drugs with different log P values and molecular sizes. *Int. J. Pharm.* **2020**, *580*, 119225. [CrossRef]
283. Nademi, Y.; Amjad Iranagh, S.; Yousefpour, A.; Mousavi, S.Z.; Modarress, H. Molecular dynamics simulations and free energy profile of Paracetamol in DPPC and DMPC lipid bilayers. *J. Chem. Sci.* **2014**, *126*, 637–647. [CrossRef]
284. Palaiokostas, M.; Ding, W.; Shahane, G.; Orsi, M. Effects of lipid composition on membrane permeation. *Soft Matter* **2018**, *14*, 8496–8508. [CrossRef] [PubMed]
285. Fischer, A.; Smieško, M. Spontaneous Ligand Access Events to Membrane-Bound Cytochrome P450 2D6 Sampled at Atomic Resolution. *Sci. Rep.* **2019**, *9*, 16411. [CrossRef] [PubMed]

286. Faulkner, C.; de Leeuw, N.H. Predicting the Membrane Permeability of Fentanyl and Its Analogues by Molecular Dynamics Simulations. *J. Phys. Chem. B* **2021**, *125*, 8443–8449. [CrossRef]
287. Lee, C.T.; Comer, J.; Herndon, C.; Leung, N.; Pavlova, A.; Swift, R.V.; Tung, C.; Rowley, C.N.; Amaro, R.E.; Chipot, C.; et al. Simulation-Based Approaches for Determining Membrane Permeability of Small Compounds. *J. Chem. Inf. Model.* **2016**, *56*, 721–733. [CrossRef]
288. López Cascales, J.J.J.; Oliveira Costa, S.D.D. Effect of the interfacial tension and ionic strength on the thermodynamic barrier associated to the benzocaine insertion into a cell membrane. *Biophys. Chem.* **2013**, *172*, 1–7. [CrossRef]
289. Saeedi, M.; Lyubartsev, A.P.; Jalili, S. Anesthetics mechanism on a DMPC lipid membrane model: Insights from molecular dynamics simulations. *Biophys. Chem.* **2017**, *226*, 1–13. [CrossRef]
290. Paloncyová, M.; Devane, R.H.; Murch, B.P.; Berka, K.; Otyepka, M. Rationalization of reduced penetration of drugs through ceramide gel phase membrane. *Langmuir* **2014**, *30*, 13942–13948. [CrossRef]
291. Lopes, S.C.; Ivanova, G.; de Castro, B.; Gameiro, P. Cardiolipin and phosphatidylethanolamine role in dibucaine interaction with the mitochondrial membrane. *Biochim. Biophys. Acta-Biomembr.* **2019**, *1861*, 1152–1161. [CrossRef]
292. Jambeck, J.P.M.; Lyubartsev, A.P. Implicit inclusion of atomic polarization in modeling of partitioning between water and lipid bilayers. *Phys. Chem. Chem. Phys.* **2013**, *15*, 4677–4686. [CrossRef]
293. Santa-Maria, A.R.; Walter, F.R.; Valkai, S.; Brás, A.R.; Mészáros, M.; Kincses, A.; Klepe, A.; Gaspar, D.; Castanho, M.A.R.B.; Zimányi, L.; et al. Lidocaine turns the surface charge of biological membranes more positive and changes the permeability of blood-brain barrier culture models. *Biochim. Biophys. Acta-Biomembr.* **2019**, *1861*, 1579–1591. [CrossRef]
294. Hu, S.; Zhao, T.; Li, H.; Cheng, D.; Sun, Z. Effect of tetracaine on dynamic reorganization of lipid membranes. *Biochim. Biophys. Acta-Biomembr.* **2020**, *1862*, 183351. [CrossRef]
295. Velez-Saboyá, C.S.; Oropeza-Guzman, E.; Sierra-Valdez, F.J.; Ruiz-Suárez, J.C. Ca2+-mediated enhancement of anesthetic diffusion across phospholipid multilamellar systems. *Biochim. Biophys. Acta-Biomembr.* **2021**, *1863*, 183509. [CrossRef]
296. Pickholz, M.; Giupponi, G. Coarse grained simulations of local anesthetics encapsulated into a liposome. *J. Phys. Chem. B* **2010**, *114*, 7009–7015. [CrossRef]
297. Jorgensen, C.; Domene, C. Location and Character of Volatile General Anesthetics Binding Sites in the Transmembrane Domain of TRPV1. *Mol. Pharm.* **2018**, *15*, 3920–3930. [CrossRef] [PubMed]
298. Fábián, B.; Darvas, M.; Picaud, S.; Sega, M.; Jedlovszky, P. The effect of anaesthetics on the properties of a lipid membrane in the biologically relevant phase: A computer simulation study. *Phys. Chem. Chem. Phys.* **2015**, *17*, 14750–14760. [CrossRef] [PubMed]
299. Pavel, M.A.; Petersen, E.N.; Wang, H.; Lerner, R.A.; Hansen, S.B. Studies on the mechanism of general anesthesia. *Proc. Natl. Acad. Sci. USA* **2020**, *117*, 13757–13766. [CrossRef] [PubMed]
300. Reigada, R. Atomistic Study of Lipid Membranes Containing Chloroform: Looking for a Lipid-Mediated Mechanism of Anesthesia. *PLoS ONE* **2013**, *8*, e52631. [CrossRef] [PubMed]
301. Reigada, R.; Sagues, F. Chloroform alters interleaflet coupling in lipid bilayers: An entropic mechanism. *J. R. Soc. Interface* **2015**, *12*, 20150197. [CrossRef]
302. Chau, P.-L.; Tu, K.M.; Liang, K.K.; Todorov, I.T.; Roser, S.J.; Barker, R.; Matubayasi, N. The effect of pressure on halothane binding to hydrated DMPC bilayers. *Mol. Phys.* **2012**, *110*, 1461–1467. [CrossRef]
303. Tu, K.M.; Matubayasi, N.; Liang, K.K.; Todorov, I.T.; Chan, S.L.; Chau, P.-L. A possible molecular mechanism for the pressure reversal of general anaesthetics: Aggregation of halothane in POPC bilayers at high pressure. *Chem. Phys. Lett.* **2012**, *543*, 148–154. [CrossRef]
304. Patel, J.; Chowdhury, E.A.; Noorani, B.; Bickel, U.; Huang, J. Isoflurane increases cell membrane fluidity significantly at clinical concentrations. *Biochim. Biophys. Acta-Biomembr.* **2020**, *1862*, 183140. [CrossRef] [PubMed]
305. Arcario, M.J.; Mayne, C.G.; Tajkhorshid, E. Atomistic Models of General Anesthetics for Use in in Silico Biological Studies. *J. Phys. Chem. B* **2014**, *118*, 12075–12086. [CrossRef] [PubMed]
306. Rao, B.D.; Shrivastava, S.; Pal, S.; Chattopadhyay, A. Effect of Local Anesthetics on the Organization and Dynamics of Hippocampal Membranes: A Fluorescence Approach. *J. Phys. Chem. B* **2019**, *123*, 639–647. [CrossRef] [PubMed]
307. Arcario, M.J.; Mayne, C.G.; Tajkhorshid, E. A membrane-embedded pathway delivers general anesthetics to two interacting binding sites in the *Gloeobacter violaceus* ion channel. *J. Biol. Chem.* **2017**, *292*, 9480–9492. [CrossRef]
308. Hantal, G.; Fábián, B.; Sega, M.; Jójárt, B.; Jedlovszky, P. Effect of general anesthetics on the properties of lipid membranes of various compositions. *Biochim. Biophys. Acta-Biomembr.* **2019**, *1861*, 594–609. [CrossRef]
309. Jin, W.; Zucker, M.; Pralle, A. Membrane nanodomains homeostasis during propofol anesthesia as function of dosage and temperature. *Biochim. Biophys. Acta-Biomembr.* **2021**, *1863*, 183511. [CrossRef]
310. Hansen, A.H.; Sørensen, K.T.; Mathieu, R.; Serer, A.; Duelund, L.; Khandelia, H.; Hansen, P.L.; Simonsen, A.C. Propofol modulates the lipid phase transition and localizes near the headgroup of membranes. *Chem. Phys. Lipids* **2013**, *175–176*, 84–91. [CrossRef]
311. Jerabek, H.; Pabst, G.; Rappolt, M.; Stockner, T. Membrane-Mediated Effect on Ion Channels Induced by the Anesthetic Drug Ketamine. *J. Am. Chem. Soc.* **2010**, *132*, 7990–7997. [CrossRef] [PubMed]
312. Denisov, I.G.; Baylon, J.L.; Grinkova, Y.V.; Tajkhorshid, E.; Sligar, S.G. Drug-Drug Interactions between Atorvastatin and Dronedarone Mediated by Monomeric CYP3A4. *Biochemistry* **2018**, *57*, 805–816. [CrossRef]
313. Galiullina, L.F.; Scheidt, H.A.; Huster, D.; Aganov, A.; Klochkov, V. Interaction of statins with phospholipid bilayers studied by solid-state NMR spectroscopy. *Biochim. Biophys. Acta-Biomembr.* **2019**, *1861*, 584–593. [CrossRef]

314. Sodero, A.O.; Barrantes, F.J. Pleiotropic effects of statins on brain cells. *Biochim. Biophys. Acta-Biomembr.* **2020**, *1862*, 183340 [CrossRef]
315. Kuba, J.O.; Yu, Y.; Klauda, J.B. Estimating localization of various statins within a POPC bilayer. *Chem. Phys. Lipids* **2021**, *236*, 105074. [CrossRef]
316. Teo, R.D.; Tieleman, D.P. Modulation of Phospholipid Bilayer Properties by Simvastatin. *J. Phys. Chem. B* **2021**, *125*, 8406–8418 [CrossRef]
317. Murphy, C.; Deplazes, E.; Cranfield, C.G.; Garcia, A. The role of structure and biophysical properties in the pleiotropic effects of statins. *Int. J. Mol. Sci.* **2020**, *21*, 8745. [CrossRef]
318. Ma, J.; Domicevica, L.; Schnell, J.R.; Biggin, P.C. Position and orientational preferences of drug-like compounds in lipid membranes: A computational and NMR approach. *Phys. Chem. Chem. Phys.* **2015**, *17*, 19766–19776. [CrossRef]
319. Xie, B.; Hao, C.; Sun, R. Effect of fluoxetine at different concentrations on the adsorption behavior of Langmuir monolayers. *Biochim. Biophys. Acta-Biomembr.* **2020**, *1862*, 183418. [CrossRef] [PubMed]
320. Casarotto, P.C.; Girych, M.; Fred, S.M.; Kovaleva, V.; Moliner, R.; Enkavi, G.; Biojone, C.; Cannarozzo, C.; Sahu, M.P.; Kaurinkoski, K.; et al. Antidepressant drugs act by directly binding to TRKB neurotrophin receptors. *Cell* **2021**, *184*, 1299–1313. [CrossRef] [PubMed]
321. Kopec, W.; Khandelia, H. Reinforcing the membrane-mediated mechanism of action of the anti-tuberculosis candidate drug thioridazine with molecular simulations. *J. Comput. Aided. Mol. Des.* **2014**, *28*, 123–134. [CrossRef]
322. Thomas, T.; Fang, Y.; Yuriev, E.; Chalmers, D.K. Ligand Binding Pathways of Clozapine and Haloperidol in the Dopamine D2 and D3 Receptors. *J. Chem. Inf. Model.* **2016**, *56*, 308–321. [CrossRef] [PubMed]
323. Pérez-Isidoro, R.; Costas, M. The effect of neuroleptic drugs on DPPC/sphingomyelin/cholesterol membranes. *Chem. Phys. Lipids* **2020**, *229*, 104913. [CrossRef] [PubMed]
324. Riedlová, K.; Nekardová, M.; Kačer, P.; Syslová, K.; Vazdar, M.; Jungwirth, P.; Kudová, E.; Cwiklik, L. Distributions of therapeutically promising neurosteroids in cellular membranes. *Chem. Phys. Lipids* **2017**, *203*, 78–86. [CrossRef] [PubMed]
325. Heydari Dokoohaki, M.; Zolghadr, A.R.; Klein, A. Impact of the chemical structure on the distribution of neuroprotective: N -alkyl-9 H -carbazoles at octanol/water interfaces. *New J. Chem.* **2020**, *44*, 1211–1220. [CrossRef]
326. Denisov, I.G.; Grinkova, Y.V.; Baylon, J.L.; Tajkhorshid, E.; Sligar, S.G. Mechanism of Drug-Drug Interactions Mediated by Human Cytochrome P450 CYP3A4 Monomer. *Biochemistry* **2015**, *54*, 2227–2239. [CrossRef] [PubMed]
327. Denisov, I.G.; Grinkova, Y.V.; Nandigrami, P.; Shekhar, M.; Tajkhorshid, E.; Sligar, S.G. Allosteric Interactions in Human Cytochrome P450 CYP3A4: The Role of Phenylalanine 213. *Biochemistry* **2019**, *58*, 1411–1422. [CrossRef]
328. Müller, C.S.; Knehans, T.; Davydov, D.R.; Bounds, P.L.; Von Mandach, U.; Halpert, J.R.; Caflisch, A.; Koppenol, W.H. Concurrent cooperativity and substrate inhibition in the epoxidation of carbamazepine by cytochrome P450 3A4 active site mutants inspired by molecular dynamics simulations. *Biochemistry* **2015**, *54*, 711–721. [CrossRef]
329. Yuan, X.; Raniolo, S.; Limongelli, V.; Xu, Y. The Molecular Mechanism Underlying Ligand Binding to the Membrane-Embedded Site of a G-Protein-Coupled Receptor. *J. Chem. Theory Comput.* **2018**, *14*, 2761–2770. [CrossRef]
330. Witek, J.; Mühlbauer, M.; Keller, B.G.; Blatter, M.; Meissner, A.; Wagner, T.; Riniker, S. Interconversion Rates between Conformational States as Rationale for the Membrane Permeability of Cyclosporines. *Chem. Phys. Chem.* **2017**, *18*, 3309–3314. [CrossRef]
331. Aguayo-Ortiz, R.; Creech, J.; Jiménez-Vázquez, E.N.; Guerrero-Serna, G.; Wang, N.; da Rocha, A.M.; Herron, T.J.; Espinoza-Fonseca, L.M. From atoms to cells: Bridging the gap between potency, efficacy, and safety of small molecules directed at a membrane protein. *bioRxiv* **2021**. [CrossRef]
332. Eftimov, P.; Olżyńska, A.; Melcrová, A.; Georgiev, G.A.; Daull, P.; Garrigue, J.S.; Cwiklik, L. Improving stability of tear film lipid layer via concerted action of two drug molecules: A biophysical view. *Int. J. Mol. Sci.* **2020**, *21*, 9490. [CrossRef] [PubMed]
333. Federizon, J.; Feugmo, C.G.T.; Huang, W.C.; He, X.; Miura, K.; Razi, A.; Ortega, J.; Karttunen, M.; Lovell, J.F. Experimental and computational observations of immunogenic cobalt porphyrin lipid bilayers: Nanodomain-enhanced antigen association. *Pharmaceutics* **2021**, *13*, 98. [CrossRef]
334. Chen, X.Z.; Zhang, R.Y.; Wang, X.F.; Yin, X.G.; Wang, J.; Wang, Y.C.; Liu, X.; Du, J.J.; Liu, Z.; Guo, J. Peptide-free Synthetic Nicotine Vaccine Candidates with α-Galactosylceramide as Adjuvant. *Mol. Pharm.* **2019**, *16*, 1467–1476. [CrossRef]
335. Parry, M.J.; Alakoskela, J.M.I.; Khandelia, H.; Kumar, S.A.; Jäättelä, M.; Mahalka, A.K.; Kinnunen, P.K.J. High-affinity small molecule-phospholipid complex formation: Binding of siramesine to phosphatidic acid. *J. Am. Chem. Soc.* **2008**, *130*, 12953–12960. [CrossRef]
336. Lautala, S.; Provenzani, R.; Koivuniemi, A.; Kulig, W.; Talman, V.; Róg, T.; Tuominen, R.K.; Yli-Kauhaluoma, J.; Bunker, A. Rigorous computational study reveals what docking overlooks: Double trouble from Membrane Association in Protein Kinase C Modulators. *J. Chem. Inf. Model.* **2020**, *60*, 5624–5633. [CrossRef]
337. Yu, R.K.; Usuki, S.; Itokazu, Y.; Wu, H.C. Novel GM1 ganglioside-like peptide mimics prevent the association of cholera toxin to human intestinal epithelial cells in vitro. *Glycobiology* **2015**, *26*, 63–73. [CrossRef]
338. Durdagi, S.; Papadopoulos, M.G.; Mavromoustakos, T. An effort to discover the preferred conformation of the potent AMG3 cannabinoid analog when reaching the active sites of the cannabinoid receptors. *Eur. J. Med. Chem.* **2012**, *47*, 44–51. [CrossRef]
339. Guest, E.E.; Oatley, S.A.; Macdonald, S.J.F.; Hirst, J.D. Molecular simulation of αvβ6 integrin inhibitors. *J. Chem. Inf. Model.* **2020**, *60*, 5487–5498. [CrossRef] [PubMed]

340. Luck, M.; Fischer, M.; Werle, M.; Scheidt, H.A.; Müller, P. Impact of selected small-molecule kinase inhibitors on lipid membranes. *Pharmaceuticals* **2021**, *14*, 746. [CrossRef] [PubMed]
341. Toroz, D.; Khanna, T.; Gould, I.R. Modeling the Effect of BSEP Inhibitors in Lipid Bilayers by Means of All-Atom Molecular Dynamics Simulation. *ACS Omega* **2019**, *4*, 3341–3350. [CrossRef]
342. Huang, C.; Wang, H.; Tang, L.; Meng, F. Penetration enhancement of menthol on quercetin through skin: Insights from atomistic simulation. *J. Mol. Model.* **2019**, *25*, 235. [CrossRef] [PubMed]
343. Sinha, R.; Gadhwal, M.K.; Joshi, U.J.; Srivastava, S.; Govil, G. Interaction of quercetin with DPPC model membrane: Molecular dynamic simulation, DSC and multinuclear NMR studies. *J. Indian Chem. Soc.* **2011**, *88*, 1203–1210.
344. Pawlikowska-Pawlęga, B.; Dziubińska, H.; Król, E.; Trębacz, K.; Jarosz-Wilkołazka, A.; Paduch, R.; Gawron, A.; Gruszecki, W.I. Characteristics of quercetin interactions with liposomal and vacuolar membranes. *Biochim. Biophys. Acta-Biomembr.* **2014**, *1838*, 254–265. [CrossRef] [PubMed]
345. Pawlikowska-Pawlega, B.; Kapral, J.; Gawron, A.; Stochmal, A.; Zuchowski, J.; Pecio, L.; Luchowski, R.; Grudzinski, W.; Gruszecki, W.I. Interaction of a quercetin derivative-lensoside Aβ with liposomal membranes. *Biochim. Biophys. Acta-Biomembr.* **2018**, *1860*, 292–299. [CrossRef] [PubMed]
346. Eid, J.; Jraij, A.; Greige-Gerges, H.; Monticelli, L. Effect of quercetin on lipid membrane rigidity: Assessment by atomic force microscopy and molecular dynamics simulations. *BBA Adv.* **2021**, *1*, 100018. [CrossRef]
347. De Granada-Flor, A.; Sousa, C.; Filipe, H.A.L.; Santos, M.S.C.S.; de Almeida, R.F.M. Quercetin dual interaction at the membrane level. *Chem. Commun.* **2019**, *55*, 1750–1753. [CrossRef]
348. Strugała, P.; Tronina, T.; Huszcza, E.; Gabrielska, J. Bioactivity In Vitro of Quercetin Glycoside Obtained in Beauveria bassiana Culture and Its Interaction with Liposome Membranes. *Molecules* **2017**, *22*, 1520. [CrossRef]
349. Boonnoy, P.; Karttunen, M.; Wong-Ekkabut, J. Does α-Tocopherol Flip-Flop Help to Protect Membranes Against Oxidation? *J. Phys. Chem. B* **2018**, *122*, 10362–10370. [CrossRef]
350. Boonnoy, P.; Karttunen, M.; Wong-Ekkabut, J. Alpha-tocopherol inhibits pore formation in oxidized bilayers. *Phys. Chem. Chem. Phys.* **2017**, *19*, 5699–5704. [CrossRef]
351. DiPasquale, M.; Nguyen, M.H.L.; Rickeard, B.W.; Cesca, N.; Tannous, C.; Castillo, S.R.; Katsaras, J.; Kelley, E.G.; Heberle, F.A.; Marquardt, D. The antioxidant vitamin E as a membrane raft modulator: Tocopherols do not abolish lipid domains. *Biochim. Biophys. Acta-Biomembr.* **2020**, *1862*, 183189. [CrossRef] [PubMed]
352. Neunert, G.; Tomaszewska-Gras, J.; Baj, A.; Gauza-Włodarczyk, M.; Witkowski, S.; Polewski, K. Phase Transitions and Structural Changes in DPPC Liposomes Induced by a 1-Carba-Alpha-Tocopherol Analogue. *Molecules* **2021**, *26*, 2851. [CrossRef] [PubMed]
353. Ossman, T.; Fabre, G.; Trouillas, P. Interaction of wine anthocyanin derivatives with lipid bilayer membranes. *Comput. Theor. Chem.* **2016**, *1077*, 80–86. [CrossRef]
354. Socrier, L.; Rosselin, M.; Gomez Giraldo, A.M.; Chantemargue, B.; Di Meo, F.; Trouillas, P.; Durand, G.; Morandat, S. Nitrone-Trolox conjugate as an inhibitor of lipid oxidation: Towards synergistic antioxidant effects. *Biochim. Biophys. Acta-Biomembr.* **2019**, *1861*, 1489–1501. [CrossRef]
355. Teixeira, M.H.; Arantes, G.M. Effects of lipid composition on membrane distribution and permeability of natural quinones. *RSC Adv.* **2019**, *9*, 16892–16899. [CrossRef]
356. Feng, S.; Wang, R.; Pastor, R.W.; Klauda, J.B.; Im, W. Location and Conformational Ensemble of Menaquinone and Menaquinol, and Protein–Lipid Modulations in Archaeal Membranes. *J. Phys. Chem. B* **2021**, *125*, 4714–4725. [CrossRef]
357. Van Cleave, C.; Murakami, H.A.; Samart, N.; Koehn, J.T.; Maldonado, P.; Kreckel, H.D.; Cope, E.J.; Basile, A.; Crick, D.C.; Crans, D.C. Location of menaquinone and menaquinol headgroups in model membranes. *Can. J. Chem.* **2020**, *98*, 307–317. [CrossRef]
358. Makuch, K.; Markiewicz, M.; Pasenkiewicz-Gierula, M. Asymmetric Spontaneous Intercalation of Lutein into a Phospholipid Bilayer, a Computational Study. *Comput. Struct. Biotechnol. J.* **2019**, *17*, 516–526. [CrossRef]
359. Garcia, A.; Eljack, N.D.; Sani, M.A.; Separovic, F.; Rasmussen, H.H.; Kopec, W.; Khandelia, H.; Cornelius, F.; Clarke, R.J. Membrane accessibility of glutathione. *Biochim. Biophys. Acta-Biomembr.* **2015**, *1848*, 2430–2436. [CrossRef] [PubMed]
360. Selvaraj, S.; Krishnaswamy, S.; Devashya, V.; Sethuraman, S.; Krishnan, U.M. Influence of membrane lipid composition on flavonoid–membrane interactions: Implications on their biological activity. *Prog. Lipid Res.* **2015**, *58*, 1–13. [CrossRef]
361. Saha, S.; Panieri, E.; Suzen, S.; Saso, L. The Interaction of Flavonols with Membrane Components: Potential Effect on Antioxidant Activity. *J. Membr. Biol.* **2020**, *253*, 57–71. [CrossRef] [PubMed]
362. Fernandes, I.; Pérez-Gregorio, R.; Soares, S.; Mateus, N.; De Freitas, V. Wine Flavonoids in Health and Disease Prevention. *Molecules* **2017**, *22*, 292. [CrossRef]
363. Sadžak, A.; Brkljača, Z.; Crnolatac, I.; Baranović, G.; Šegota, S. Flavonol clustering in model lipid membranes: DSC, AFM, force spectroscopy and MD simulations study. *Colloids Surf. B Biointerfaces* **2020**, *193*, 111147. [CrossRef] [PubMed]
364. Nie, R.; Dang, M.; Ge, Z.; Huo, Y.; Yu, B.; Tang, S. Influence of the gallate moiety on the interactions between green tea polyphenols and lipid membranes elucidated by molecular dynamics simulations. *Biophys. Chem.* **2021**, *274*, 106592. [CrossRef] [PubMed]
365. Prates, É.T.; Rodrigues da Silva, G.H.; Souza, T.F.; Skaf, M.S.; Pickholz, M.; de Paula, E. Articaine interaction with phospholipid bilayers. *J. Mol. Struct.* **2020**, *1222*, 128854. [CrossRef]
366. Verstraeten, S.V.; Fraga, C.G.; Oteiza, P.I. Interactions of flavan-3-ols and procyanidins with membranes: Mechanisms and the physiological relevance. *Food Funct.* **2015**, *6*, 32–40. [CrossRef]

367. Chulkov, E.G.; Schagina, L.V.; Ostroumova, O.S. Membrane dipole modifiers modulate single-length nystatin channels via reducing elastic stress in the vicinity of the lipid mouth of a pore. *Biochim. Biophys. Acta-Biomembr.* **2015**, *1848*, 192–199. [CrossRef]
368. Souza, F.R.; Fornasier, F.; Souza, L.M.P.; Peñafiel, M.P.; Nascimento, J.B.; Malfatti-Gasperini, A.A.; Pimentel, A.S. Interaction of naringin and naringenin with DPPC monolayer at the air-water interface. *Colloids Surf. A Physicochem. Eng. Asp.* **2020**, *584*, 124024. [CrossRef]
369. Sadžak, A.; Mravljak, J.; Maltar-Strmečki, N.; Arsov, Z.; Baranović, G.; Erceg, I.; Kriechbaum, M.; Strasser, V.; Přibyl, J.; Šegota, S. The Structural Integrity of the Model Lipid Membrane during Induced Lipid Peroxidation: The Role of Flavonols in the Inhibition of Lipid Peroxidation. *Antioxidants* **2020**, *9*, 430. [CrossRef]
370. Kosina, P.; Paloncýová, M.; Rajnochová Svobodová, A.; Zálešák, B.; Biedermann, D.; Ulrichová, J.; Vostálová, J. Dermal Delivery of Selected Polyphenols from Silybum marianum. Theoretical and Experimental Study. *Molecules* **2019**, *24*, 61. [CrossRef]
371. Laudadio, E.; Galeazzi, R.; Mobbili, G.; Minnelli, C.; Barbon, A.; Bortolus, M.; Stipa, P. Depth Distribution of Spin-Labeled Liponitroxides within Lipid Bilayers: A Combined EPR and Molecular Dynamics Approach. *ACS Omega* **2019**, *4*, 5029–5037. [CrossRef]
372. Griffith, E.C.; Perkins, R.J.; Telesford, D.M.; Adams, E.M.; Cwiklik, L.; Allen, H.C.; Roeselová, M.; Vaida, V. Interaction of L-Phenylalanine with a Phospholipid Monolayer at the Water-Air Interface. *J. Phys. Chem. B* **2015**, *119*, 9038–9048. [CrossRef]
373. Perkins, R.; Vaida, V. Phenylalanine Increases Membrane Permeability. *J. Am. Chem. Soc.* **2017**, *139*, 14388–14391. [CrossRef]
374. 3Perkins, R.J.; Kukharchuk, A.; Delcroix, P.; Shoemaker, R.K.; Roeselová, M.; Cwiklik, L.; Vaida, V. The Partitioning of Small Aromatic Molecules to Air-Water and Phospholipid Interfaces Mediated by Non-Hydrophobic Interactions. *J. Phys. Chem. B* **2016**, *120*, 7408–7422. [CrossRef]
375. Nandi, S.; Ghosh, B.; Ghosh, M.; Layek, S.; Nandi, P.K.; Sarkar, N. Phenylalanine Interacts with Oleic Acid-Based Vesicle Membrane. Understanding the Molecular Role of Fibril–Vesicle Interaction under the Context of Phenylketonuria. *J. Phys. Chem. B* **2021**, *125*, 9776–9793. [CrossRef]
376. MacCallum, J.L.; Bennett, W.F.D.; Tieleman, D.P. Distribution of Amino Acids in a Lipid Bilayer from Computer Simulations. *Biophys. J.* **2008**, *94*, 3393–3404. [CrossRef]
377. Cardenas, A.E.; Anderson, C.M.; Elber, R.; Webb, L.J. Partition of Positively and Negatively Charged Tryptophan Ions in Membranes with Inverted Phospholipid Heads: Simulations and Experiments. *J. Phys. Chem. B* **2019**, *123*, 3272–3281. [CrossRef]
378. Robinson, M.; Turnbull, S.; Lee, B.Y.; Leonenko, Z. The effects of melatonin, serotonin, tryptophan and NAS on the biophysical properties of DPPC monolayers. *Biochim. Biophys. Acta-Biomembr.* **2020**, *1862*, 183363. [CrossRef] [PubMed]
379. Pokhrel, N.; Maibaum, L. Free Energy Calculations of Membrane Permeation: Challenges Due to Strong Headgroup-Solute Interactions. *J. Chem. Theory Comput.* **2018**, *14*, 1762–1771. [CrossRef] [PubMed]
380. Genheden, S.; Eriksson, L.A. Estimation of Liposome Penetration Barriers of Drug Molecules with All-Atom and Coarse-Grained Models. *J. Chem. Theory Comput.* **2016**, *12*, 4651–4661. [CrossRef] [PubMed]
381. Magarkar, A.; Parkkila, P.; Viitala, T.; Lajunen, T.; Mobarak, E.; Licari, G.; Cramariuc, O.; Vauthey, E.; Róg, T.; Bunker, A. Membrane bound COMT isoform is an interfacial enzyme: General mechanism and new drug design paradigm. *Chem. Commun.* **2018**, *54*, 3440–3443. [CrossRef] [PubMed]
382. Megariotis, G.; Romanos, N.; Avramopoulos, A.; Mikaelian, G.; Theodorou, D.N. In silico study of levodopa in hydrated lipid bilayers at the atomistic level. *J. Mol. Graph. Model.* **2021**, *107*, 107972. [CrossRef] [PubMed]
383. Garcia, A.; Pochinda, S.; Elgaard-Jørgensen, P.N.; Khandelia, H.; Clarke, R.J. Evidence for ATP Interaction with Phosphatidylcholine Bilayers. *Langmuir* **2019**, *35*, 9944–9953. [CrossRef]
384. Sasidharan, S.; Pochinda, S.; Elgaard-Jørgensen, P.N.; Rajamani, S.; Khandelia, H.; Raghunathan, V.A. Interaction of the mononucleotide UMP with a fluid phospholipid bilayer. *Soft Matter* **2019**, *15*, 8129–8136. [CrossRef] [PubMed]
385. Kato, A.; Tsuji, A.; Yanagisawa, M.; Saeki, D.; Juni, K.; Morimoto, Y.; Yoshikawa, K. Phase separation on a phospholipid membrane inducing a characteristic localization of DNA accompanied by its structural transition. *J. Phys. Chem. Lett.* **2010**, *1*, 3391–3395. [CrossRef]
386. Link, K.A.; Spurzem, G.N.; Tuladhar, A.; Chase, Z.; Wang, Z.; Wang, H.; Walker, R.A. Cooperative Adsorption of Trehalose to DPPC Monolayers at the Water-Air Interface Studied with Vibrational Sum Frequency Generation. *J. Phys. Chem. B* **2019**, *123*, 8931–8938. [CrossRef]
387. Gupta, R.; Badhe, Y.; Rai, B.; Mitragotri, S. Molecular mechanism of the skin permeation enhancing effect of ethanol: A molecular dynamics study. *RSC Adv.* **2020**, *10*, 12234–12248. [CrossRef]
388. Paloncýová, M.; Navrátilová, V.; Berka, K.; Laio, A.; Otyepka, M. Role of Enzyme Flexibility in Ligand Access and Egress to Active Site: Bias-Exchange Metadynamics Study of 1,3,7-Trimethyluric Acid in Cytochrome P450 3A4. *J. Chem. Theory Comput.* **2016**, *12*, 2101–2109. [CrossRef]
389. Postila, P.A.; Róg, T. A perspective: Active role of lipids in neurotransmitter dynamics. *Mol. Neurobiol.* **2020**, *57*, 910–925. [CrossRef]
390. Orłowski, A.; Grzybek, M.; Bunker, A.; Pasenkiewicz-Gierula, M.; Vattulainen, I.; Männistö, P.T.; Róg, T. Strong preferences of dopamine and l -dopa towards lipid head group: Importance of lipid composition and implication for neurotransmitter metabolism. *J. Neurochem.* **2012**, *122*, 681–690. [CrossRef]
391. Shen, C.; Xue, M.; Qiu, H.; Guo, W. Insertion of Neurotransmitters into a Lipid Bilayer Membrane and Its Implication on Membrane Stability: A Molecular Dynamics Study. *Chem. Phys. Chem.* **2017**, *18*, 626–633. [CrossRef] [PubMed]

392. Mokkila, S.; Postila, P.A.; Rissanen, S.; Juhola, H.; Vattulainen, I.; Róg, T. Calcium Assists Dopamine Release by Preventing Aggregation on the Inner Leaflet of Presynaptic Vesicles. *ACS Chem. Neurosci.* **2017**, *8*, 1242–1250. [CrossRef] [PubMed]
393. Juhola, H.; Postila, P.A.; Rissanen, S.; Lolicato, F.; Vattulainen, I.; Róg, T. Negatively Charged Gangliosides Promote Membrane Association of Amphipathic Neurotransmitters. *Neuroscience* **2018**, *384*, 214–223. [CrossRef] [PubMed]
394. Lolicato, F.; Juhola, H.; Zak, A.; Postila, P.A.; Saukko, A.; Rissanen, S.; Enkavi, G.; Vattulainen, I.; Kepczynski, M.; Róg, T. Membrane-Dependent Binding and Entry Mechanism of Dopamine into Its Receptor. *ACS Chem. Neurosci.* **2020**, *11*, 1914–1924. [CrossRef] [PubMed]
395. Parkkila, P.; Viitala, T. Partitioning of Catechol Derivatives in Lipid Membranes: Implications for Substrate Specificity to Catechol-O-methyltransferase. *ACS Chem. Neurosci.* **2020**, *11*, 969–978. [CrossRef] [PubMed]
396. Biswas, B.; Singh, P.C. Restructuring of Membrane Water and Phospholipids in Direct Interaction of Neurotransmitters with Model Membranes Associated with Synaptic Signaling: Interface-Selective Vibrational Sum Frequency Generation Study. *J. Phys. Chem. Lett.* **2021**, *12*, 2871–2879. [CrossRef]
397. Megariotis, G.; Romanos, N.A.; Theodorou, D.N. Molecular simulations of dopamine in a lipid bilayer. *AIP Conf. Proc.* **2021**, *2343*, 130007.
398. Peters, G.H.; Wang, C.; Cruys-Bagger, N.; Velardez, G.F.; Madsen, J.J.; Westh, P. Binding of serotonin to lipid membranes. *J. Am. Chem. Soc.* **2013**, *135*, 2164–2171. [CrossRef]
399. Josey, B.P.; Heinrich, F.; Silin, V.; Lösche, M. Association of Model Neurotransmitters with Lipid Bilayer Membranes. *Biophys. J.* **2020**, *118*, 1044–1057. [CrossRef]
400. Dey, S.; Surendran, D.; Enberg, O.; Gupta, A.; Fanibunda, S.E.; Das, A.; Maity, B.K.; Dey, A.; Visvakarma, V.; Kallianpur, M.; et al. Altered Membrane Mechanics Provides a Receptor-Independent Pathway for Serotonin Action. *Chem.—A Eur. J.* **2021**, *27*, 1–10. [CrossRef]
401. 4Bochicchio, A.; Brandner, A.F.; Engberg, O.; Huster, D.; Böckmann, R.A. Spontaneous Membrane Nanodomain Formation in the Absence or Presence of the Neurotransmitter Serotonin. *Front. Cell Dev. Biol.* **2020**, *8*, 601145. [CrossRef]
402. Engberg, O.; Bochicchio, A.; Brandner, A.F.; Gupta, A.; Dey, S.; Böckmann, R.A.; Maiti, S.; Huster, D. Serotonin Alters the Phase Equilibrium of a Ternary Mixture of Phospholipids and Cholesterol. *Front. Physiol.* **2020**, *11*, 578868. [CrossRef]
403. Choi, Y.; Attwood, S.J.; Hoopes, M.I.; Drolle, E.; Karttunen, M.; Leonenko, Z. Melatonin directly interacts with cholesterol and alleviates cholesterol effects in dipalmitoylphosphatidylcholine monolayers. *Soft Matter* **2014**, *10*, 206–213. [CrossRef]
404. Drolle, E.; Kučerka, N.; Hoopes, M.I.; Choi, Y.; Katsaras, J.; Karttunen, M.; Leonenko, Z. Effect of melatonin and cholesterol on the structure of DOPC and DPPC membranes. *Biochim. Biophys. Acta-Biomembr.* **2013**, *1828*, 2247–2254. [CrossRef]
405. Kondela, T.; Dushanov, E.; Vorobyeva, M.; Mamatkulov, K.; Drolle, E.; Soloviov, D.; Hrubovčák, P.; Kholmurodov, K.; Arzumanyan, G.; Leonenko, Z.; et al. Investigating the competitive effects of cholesterol and melatonin in model lipid membranes. *Biochim. Biophys. Acta-Biomembr.* **2021**, *1863*, 183651. [CrossRef]
406. Tejwani, R.W.; Davis, M.E.; Anderson, B.D.; Stouch, T.R. An atomic and molecular view of the depth dependence of the free energies of solute transfer from water into lipid bilayers. *Mol. Pharm.* **2011**, *8*, 2204–2215. [CrossRef]
407. Wittmann, H.J.; Strasser, A. Binding pathway of histamine to the hH4R, observed by unconstrained molecular dynamics. *Bioorganic Med. Chem. Lett.* **2015**, *25*, 1259–1268. [CrossRef]
408. Hackett, J.C. Membrane-embedded substrate recognition by cytochrome P450 3A4. *J. Biol. Chem.* **2018**, *293*, 4037–4046. [CrossRef] [PubMed]
409. Aleskndrany, A.; Sahin, I. The effects of Levothyroxine on the structure and dynamics of DPPC liposome: FTIR and DSC studies. *Biochim. Biophys. Acta-Biomembr.* **2020**, *1862*, 183245. [CrossRef] [PubMed]
410. Gc, J.B.; Szlenk, C.T.; Gao, J.; Dong, X.; Wang, Z.; Natesan, S. Molecular Dynamics Simulations Provide Insight into the Loading Efficiency of Proresolving Lipid Mediators Resolvin D1 and D2 in Cell Membrane-Derived Nanovesicles. *Mol. Pharm.* **2020**, *17*, 2155–2164. [CrossRef] [PubMed]
411. Devarajan, A.; Kim, Y.C.; Isakovic, A.F.; Gater, D.L. Effect of cholecalciferol on unsaturated model membranes. *Chem. Phys. Lipids* **2021**, *235*, 105058. [CrossRef]
412. Sofferman, D.L.; Konar, A.; Mastron, J.N.; Spears, K.G.; Cisneros, C.; Smith, A.C.; Tapavicza, E.; Sension, R.J. Probing the Formation and Conformational Relaxation of Previtamin D3and Analogues in Solution and in Lipid Bilayers. *J. Phys. Chem. B* **2021**, *125*, 10085–10096. [CrossRef]
413. Chipot, C.; Comer, J. Subdiffusion in Membrane Permeation of Small Molecules. *Sci. Rep.* **2016**, *6*, 35913. [CrossRef] [PubMed]
414. Comer, J.; Schulten, K.; Chipot, C. Permeability of a Fluid Lipid Bilayer to Short-Chain Alcohols from First Principles. *J. Chem. Theory Comput.* **2017**, *13*, 2523–2532. [CrossRef] [PubMed]
415. Carpenter, T.S.; Parkin, J.; Khalid, S. The Free Energy of Small Solute Permeation through the Escherichia coli Outer Membrane Has a Distinctly Asymmetric Profile. *J. Phys. Chem. Lett.* **2016**, *7*, 3446–3451. [CrossRef] [PubMed]
416. Wang, Y.; Gallagher, E.; Jorgensen, C.; Troendle, E.P.; Hu, D.; Searson, P.C.; Ulmschneider, M.B. An experimentally validated approach to calculate the blood-brain barrier permeability of small molecules. *Sci. Rep.* **2019**, *9*, 6117. [CrossRef] [PubMed]
417. Gupta, R.; Sridhar, D.B.; Rai, B. Molecular Dynamics Simulation Study of Permeation of Molecules through Skin Lipid Bilayer. *J. Phys. Chem. B* **2016**, *120*, 8987–8996. [CrossRef]
418. Kumari, P.; Kumari, M.; Kashyap, H.K. Counter-effects of Ethanol and Cholesterol on the Heterogeneous PSM-POPC Lipid Membrane: A Molecular Dynamics Simulation Study. *J. Phys. Chem. B* **2019**, *123*, 9616–9628. [CrossRef]

419. Eslami, H.; Das, S.; Zhou, T.; Müller-Plathe, F. How Alcoholic Disinfectants Affect Coronavirus Model Membranes: Membrane Fluidity, Permeability, and Disintegration. *J. Phys. Chem. B* **2020**, *124*, 10374–10385. [CrossRef]
420. Kumari, P.; Kaur, S.; Sharma, S.; Kashyap, H.K. Impact of amphiphilic molecules on the structure and stability of homogeneous sphingomyelin bilayer: Insights from atomistic simulations. *J. Chem. Phys.* **2018**, *148*, 165102. [CrossRef]
421. Menichetti, R.; Kremer, K.; Bereau, T. Efficient potential of mean force calculation from multiscale simulations: Solute insertion in a lipid membrane. *Biochem. Biophys. Res. Commun.* **2018**, *498*, 282–287. [CrossRef]
422. Algaba, J.; Míguez, J.M.; Gómez-Álvarez, P.; Mejía, A.; Blas, F.J. Preferential Orientations and Anomalous Interfacial Tensions in Aqueous Solutions of Alcohols. *J. Phys. Chem. B* **2020**, *124*, 8388–8401. [CrossRef]
423. Hossain, S.; Joyce, P.; Parrow, A.; Jõemetsa, S.; Höök, F.; Larsson, P.; Bergström, C.A.S. Influence of Bile Composition on Membrane Incorporation of Transient Permeability Enhancers. *Mol. Pharm.* **2020**, *17*, 4226–4240. [CrossRef]
424. Terakosolphan, W.; Trick, J.L.; Royall, P.G.; Rogers, S.E.; Lamberti, O.; Lorenz, C.D.; Forbes, B.; Harvey, R.D. Glycerol Solvates DPPC Headgroups and Localizes in the Interfacial Regions of Model Pulmonary Interfaces Altering Bilayer Structure. *Langmuir* **2018**, *34*, 6941–6954. [CrossRef] [PubMed]
425. Ferreira, J.V.N.; Capello, T.M.; Siqueira, L.J.A.; Lago, J.H.G.; Caseli, L. Mechanism of Action of Thymol on Cell Membranes Investigated through Lipid Langmuir Monolayers at the Air–Water Interface and Molecular Simulation. *Langmuir* **2016**, *32*, 3234–3241. [CrossRef] [PubMed]
426. Tong, X.; Moradipour, M.; Novak, B.; Kamali, P.; Asare, S.O.; Knutson, B.L.; Rankin, S.E.; Lynn, B.C.; Moldovan, D. Experimental and Molecular Dynamics Simulation Study of the Effects of Lignin Dimers on the Gel-to-Fluid Phase Transition in DPPC Bilayers. *J. Phys. Chem. B* **2019**, *123*, 8247–8260. [CrossRef] [PubMed]
427. Vermaas, J.V.; Dixon, R.A.; Chen, F.; Mansfield, S.D.; Boerjan, W.; Ralph, J.; Crowley, M.F.; Beckham, G.T. Passive membrane transport of lignin-related compounds. *Proc. Natl. Acad. Sci. USA.* **2019**, *116*, 23117–23123. [CrossRef]
428. Moradipour, M.; Tong, X.; Novak, B.; Kamali, P.; Asare, S.O.; Lynn, B.C.; Moldovan, D.; Rankin, S.E.; Knutson, B.L. Interaction of lignin dimers with model cell membranes: A quartz crystal microbalance and molecular dynamics simulation study. *Biointerphases* **2021**, *16*, 41003. [CrossRef]
429. Reis, A.; Soares, S.; Sousa, C.F.; Dias, R.; Gameiro, P.; Soares, S.; de Freitas, V. Interaction of polyphenols with model membranes: Putative implications to mouthfeel perception. *Biochim. Biophys. Acta-Biomembr.* **2020**, *1862*, 183133. [CrossRef]
430. Gurtovenko, A.A.; Mukhamadiarov, E.I.; Kostritskii, A.Y.; Karttunen, M. Phospholipid-Cellulose Interactions: Insight from Atomistic Computer Simulations for Understanding the Impact of Cellulose-Based Materials on Plasma Membranes. *J. Phys. Chem. B* **2018**, *122*, 9973–9981. [CrossRef]
431. Gurtovenko, A.A.; Karttunen, M. Controlled On-Off Switching of Tight-Binding Hydrogen Bonds between Model Cell Membranes and Acetylated Cellulose Surfaces. *Langmuir* **2019**, *35*, 13753–13760. [CrossRef]
432. Sapoń, K.; Janas, T.; Sikorski, A.F.; Janas, T. Polysialic acid chains exhibit enhanced affinity for ordered regions of membranes. *Biochim. Biophys. Acta-Biomembr.* **2019**, *1861*, 245–255. [CrossRef]
433. Miguel, V.; Sánchez-Borzone, M.E.; García, D.A. Interaction of gabaergic ketones with model membranes: A molecular dynamics and experimental approach. *Biochim. Biophys. Acta-Biomembr.* **2018**, *1860*, 1563–1570. [CrossRef]
434. Shahoei, R.; Tajkhorshid, E. Menthol Binding to the Human α4β2 Nicotinic Acetylcholine Receptor Facilitated by Its Strong Partitioning in the Membrane. *J. Phys. Chem. B* **2020**, *124*, 1866–1880. [CrossRef]
435. Vermaas, J.V.; Bentley, G.J.; Beckham, G.T.; Crowley, M.F. Membrane Permeability of Terpenoids Explored with Molecular Simulation. *J. Phys. Chem. B* **2018**, *122*, 10349–10361. [CrossRef]
436. Paloncýová, M.; Berka, K.; Otyepka, M. Convergence of free energy profile of coumarin in lipid bilayer. *J. Chem. Theory Comput.* **2012**, *8*, 1200–1211. [CrossRef] [PubMed]
437. Duncan, K.M.; Casey, A.; Gobrogge, C.A.; Trousdale, R.C.; Piontek, S.M.; Cook, M.J.; Steel, W.H.; Walker, R.A. Coumarin Partitioning in Model Biological Membranes: Limitations of log P as a Predictor. *J. Phys. Chem. B* **2020**, *124*, 8299–8308. [CrossRef] [PubMed]
438. Dufourc, E.J. Wine tannins, saliva proteins and membrane lipids. *Biochim. Biophys. Acta-Biomembr.* **2021**, *1863*, 183670. [CrossRef]
439. Tavagnacco, L.; Corucci, G.; Gerelli, Y. Interaction of Caffeine with Model Lipid Membranes. *J. Phys. Chem. B* **2021**, *125*, 10174–10181. [CrossRef] [PubMed]
440. Sherratt, S.C.R.; Villeneuve, P.; Durand, E.; Mason, R.P. Rosmarinic acid and its esters inhibit membrane cholesterol domain formation through an antioxidant mechanism based, in nonlinear fashion, on alkyl chain length. *Biochim. Biophys. Acta-Biomembr.* **2019**, *1861*, 550–555. [CrossRef] [PubMed]
441. Filipe, H.A.L.; Sousa, C.; Marquês, J.T.; Vila-Viçosa, D.; de Granada-Flor, A.; Viana, A.S.; Santos, M.S.C.S.; Machuqueiro, M.; de Almeida, R.F.M. Differential targeting of membrane lipid domains by caffeic acid and its ester derivatives. *Free Radic. Biol. Med.* **2018**, *115*, 232–245. [CrossRef] [PubMed]
442. Huang, J.; Chen, P.X.; Rogers, M.A.; Wettig, S.D. Investigating the phospholipid effect on the bioaccessibility of rosmarinic acid-phospholipid complex through a dynamic gastrointestinal in vitro model. *Pharmaceutics* **2019**, *11*, 156. [CrossRef] [PubMed]
443. Colina, J.R.; Suwalsky, M.; Manrique-Moreno, M.; Petit, K.; Aguilar, L.F.; Jemiola-Rzeminska, M.; Strzalka, K. An in vitro study of the protective effect of caffeic acid on human erythrocytes. *Arch. Biochem. Biophys.* **2019**, *662*, 75–82. [CrossRef]

444. Lopes, R.; Costa, M.; Ferreira, M.; Gameiro, P.; Fernandes, S.; Catarino, C.; Santos-Silva, A.; Paiva-Martins, F. Caffeic acid phenolipids in the protection of cell membranes from oxidative injuries. Interaction with the membrane phospholipid bilayer. *Biochim. Biophys. Acta-Biomembr.* **2021**, *1863*, 183727. [CrossRef]
445. Gupta, R.; Mitra, S.; Chowdhury, S.; Das, G.; Priyadarshini, R. Discerning perturbed assembly of lipids in a model membrane in presence of violacein. *Biochim. Biophys. Acta-Biomembr.* **2021**, *1863*, 183647. [CrossRef]
446. Cauz, A.C.G.; Carretero, G.P.B.; Saraiva, G.K.V.; Park, P.; Mortara, L.; Cuccovia, I.M.; Brocchi, M.; Gueiros-Filho, F.J. Violacein Targets the Cytoplasmic Membrane of Bacteria. *ACS Infect. Dis.* **2019**, *5*, 539–549. [CrossRef]
447. Bouhlel, Z.; Arnold, A.A.; Deschênes, J.-S.; Mouget, J.-L.; Warschawski, D.E.; Tremblay, R.; Marcotte, I. Investigating the action of the microalgal pigment marennine on Vibrio splendidus by in vivo 2H and 31P solid-state NMR. *Biochim. Biophys. Acta-Biomembr.* **2021**, *1863*, 183642. [CrossRef]
448. Neves, M.C.; Filipe, H.A.L.; Reis, R.L.; Ramalho, J.P.P.; Coreta-Gomes, F.; Moreno, M.J.; Loura, L.M.S. Interaction of bile salts with lipid bilayers: An atomistic molecular dynamics study. *Front. Physiol.* **2019**, *10*, 393. [CrossRef]
449. Dubinin, M.V.; Semenova, A.A.; Ilzorkina, A.I.; Mikheeva, I.B.; Yashin, V.A.; Penkov, N.V.; Vydrina, V.A.; Ishmuratov, G.Y.; Sharapov, V.A.; Khoroshavina, E.I.; et al. Effect of betulin and betulonic acid on isolated rat liver mitochondria and liposomes. *Biochim. Biophys. Acta-Biomembr.* **2020**, *1862*, 183383. [CrossRef]
450. Jurek, I.; Góral, I.; Mierzyńska, Z.; Moniuszko-Szajwaj, B.; Wojciechowski, K. Effect of synthetic surfactants and soapwort (*Saponaria officinalis* L.) extract on skin-mimetic model lipid monolayers. *Biochim. Biophys. Acta-Biomembr.* **2019**, *1861*, 556–564. [CrossRef] [PubMed]
451. Geisler, R.; Dargel, C.; Hellweg, T. The biosurfactant β-aescin: A review on the physico-chemical properties and its interaction with lipid model membranes and langmuir monolayers. *Molecules* **2020**, *25*, 117. [CrossRef] [PubMed]
452. Selyutina, O.Y.; Apanasenko, I.E.; Kim, A.V.; Shelepova, E.A.; Khalikov, S.S.; Polyakov, N.E. Spectroscopic and molecular dynamics characterization of glycyrrhizin membrane-modifying activity. *Colloids Surf. B Biointerfaces* **2016**, *147*, 459–466. [CrossRef] [PubMed]
453. Selyutina, O.Y.; Shelepova, E.A.; Paramonova, E.D.; Kichigina, L.A.; Khalikov, S.S.; Polyakov, N.E. Glycyrrhizin-induced changes in phospholipid dynamics studied by 1H NMR and MD simulation. *Arch. Biochem. Biophys.* **2020**, *686*, 108368. [CrossRef] [PubMed]
454. Wadhwa, R.; Yadav, N.S.; Katiyar, S.P.; Yaguchi, T.; Lee, C.; Ahn, H.; Yun, C.-O.; Kaul, S.C.; Sundar, D. Molecular dynamics simulations and experimental studies reveal differential permeability of withaferin-A and withanone across the model cell membrane. *Sci. Rep.* **2021**, *11*, 2352. [CrossRef] [PubMed]
455. Hurst, D.P.; Grossfield, A.; Lynch, D.L.; Feller, S.; Romo, T.D.; Gawrisch, K.; Pitman, M.C.; Reggio, P.H. A lipid pathway for ligand binding is necessary for a cannabinoid G protein-coupled receptor. *J. Biol. Chem.* **2010**, *285*, 17954–17964. [CrossRef]
456. Kim, S.; Voth, G.A. Physical Characterization of Triolein and Implications for Its Role in Lipid Droplet Biogenesis. *J. Phys. Chem. B* **2021**, *125*, 6874–6888. [CrossRef]
457. Maiti, A.; Daschakraborty, S. Effect of TMAO on the Structure and Phase Transition of Lipid Membranes: Potential Role of TMAO in Stabilizing Cell Membranes under Osmotic Stress. *J. Phys. Chem. B* **2021**, *125*, 1167–1180. [CrossRef]
458. Craig, R.A.; Garrison, C.E.; Nguyen, P.T.; Yarov-Yarovoy, V.; Du Bois, J. Veratridine: A Janus-Faced Modulator of Voltage-Gated Sodium Ion Channels. *ACS Chem. Neurosci.* **2020**, *11*, 418–426. [CrossRef]
459. Vazdar, M.; Jurkiewicz, P.; Hof, M.; Jungwirth, P.; Cwiklik, L. Behavior of 4-hydroxynonenal in phospholipid membranes. *J. Phys. Chem. B* **2012**, *116*, 6411–6415. [CrossRef]
460. Pazin, W.M.; da Silva Olivier, D.; Vilanova, N.; Ramos, A.P.; Voets, I.K.; Soares, A.E.E.; Ito, A.S. Interaction of Artepillin C with model membranes. *Eur. Biophys. J.* **2017**, *46*, 383–393. [CrossRef]
461. Nie, R.; Dang, M.; Ge, Z.; Huo, Y.; Yu, B.; Tang, S. Interactions of chlorogenic acid and isochlorogenic acid A with model lipid bilayer membranes: Insights from molecular dynamics simulations. *Chem. Phys. Lipids* **2021**, *240*, 105136. [CrossRef] [PubMed]
462. Zhu, W.; Xiong, L.; Peng, J.; Deng, X.; Gao, J.; Li, C. Molecular Insight into Affinities of Gallated and Nongallated Proanthocyanidins Dimers to Lipid Bilayers. *Sci. Rep.* **2016**, *6*, 37680. [CrossRef] [PubMed]
463. Zhu, W.; Khalifa, I.; Peng, J.; Li, C. Position and orientation of gallated proanthocyanidins in lipid bilayer membranes: Influence of polymerization degree and linkage type. *J. Biomol. Struct. Dyn.* **2018**, *36*, 2862–2875. [CrossRef] [PubMed]
464. Galiano, V.; Villalaín, J. Oleuropein aglycone in lipid bilayer membranes. A molecular dynamics study. *Biochim. Biophys. Acta-Biomembr.* **2015**, *1848*, 2849–2858. [CrossRef]
465. Hossain, S.I.; Saha, S.C.; Deplazes, E. Phenolic compounds alter the ion permeability of phospholipid bilayers via specific lipid interactions. *Phys. Chem. Chem. Phys.* **2021**, *23*, 22352–222366. [CrossRef]
466. Wang, R.; Zhu, W.; Peng, J.; Li, K.; Li, C. Lipid rafts as potential mechanistic targets underlying the pleiotropic actions of polyphenols. *Crit. Rev. Food Sci. Nutr.* **2020**, 1–14. [CrossRef]
467. Reis, A.; Perez-Gregorio, R.; Mateus, N.; de Freitas, V. Interactions of dietary polyphenols with epithelial lipids: Advances from membrane and cell models in the study of polyphenol absorption, transport and delivery to the epithelium. *Crit. Rev. Food Sci. Nutr.* **2021**, *61*, 3007–3030. [CrossRef]
468. Šturm, L.; Poklar Ulrih, N. Basic Methods for Preparation of Liposomes and Studying Their Interactions with Different Compounds, with the Emphasis on Polyphenols. *Int. J. Mol. Sci.* **2021**, *22*, 6547. [CrossRef]

469. Reis, A.; de Freitas, V. When polyphenols meet lipids: Challenges in membrane biophysics and opportunities in epithelial lipidomics. *Food Chem.* **2020**, *333*, 127509. [CrossRef]
470. Kholina, E.G.; Kovalenko, I.B.; Bozdaganyan, M.E.; Strakhovskaya, M.G.; Orekhov, P.S. Cationic Antiseptics Facilitate Pore Formation in Model Bacterial Membranes. *J. Phys. Chem. B* **2020**, *124*, 8593–8600. [CrossRef]
471. Sowlati-Hashjin, S.; Carbone, P.; Karttunen, M. Insights into the Polyhexamethylene Biguanide (PHMB) Mechanism of Action on Bacterial Membrane and DNA: A Molecular Dynamics Study. *J. Phys. Chem. B* **2020**, *124*, 4487–4497. [CrossRef] [PubMed]
472. Felsztyna, I.; Sánchez-Borzone, M.E.; Miguel, V.; García, D.A. The insecticide fipronil affects the physical properties of model membranes: A combined experimental and molecular dynamics simulations study in Langmuir monolayers. *Biochim. Biophys. Acta-Biomembr.* **2020**, *1862*, 183378. [CrossRef]
473. DeMarco, K.R.; Bekker, S.; Clancy, C.E.; Noskov, S.Y.; Vorobyov, I. Digging into lipid membrane permeation for cardiac ion channel blocker d-sotalol with all-atom simulations. *Front. Pharmacol.* **2018**, *9*, 26. [CrossRef] [PubMed]
474. Ribeiro, R.P.; Coimbra, J.T.S.; Ramos, M.J.; Fernandes, P.A. Diffusion of the small, very polar, drug piracetam through a lipid bilayer: An MD simulation study. *Theor. Chem. Acc.* **2017**, *136*, 1–10. [CrossRef]
475. Ermilova, I.; Stenberg, S.; Lyubartsev, A.P. Quantum chemical and molecular dynamics modelling of hydroxylated polybrominated diphenyl ethers. *Phys. Chem. Chem. Phys.* **2017**, *19*, 28263–28274. [CrossRef]
476. Chen, L.; Chen, J.; Zhou, G.; Wang, Y.; Xu, C.; Wang, X. Molecular Dynamics Simulations of the Permeation of Bisphenol A and Pore Formation in a Lipid Membrane. *Sci. Rep.* **2016**, *6*, 33399. [CrossRef]
477. Shen, Z.; Ge, J.; Ye, H.; Tang, S.; Li, Y. Cholesterol-like Condensing Effect of Perfluoroalkyl Substances on a Phospholipid Bilayer. *J. Phys. Chem. B* **2020**, *124*, 5415–5425. [CrossRef]
478. Yang, H.; Li, H.; Liu, L.; Zhou, Y.; Long, X. Molecular Simulation Studies on the Interactions of 2,4,6-Trinitrotoluene and Its Metabolites with Lipid Membranes. *J. Phys. Chem. B* **2019**, *123*, 6481–6491. [CrossRef]
479. Yang, H.; Li, H.; Zhou, M.; Wei, T.; Tang, C.; Liu, L.; Zhou, Y.; Long, X. A relationship between membrane permeation and partitioning of nitroaromatic explosives and their functional groups. A computational study. *Phys. Chem. Chem. Phys.* **2020**, *22*, 8791–8799. [CrossRef]
480. Golius, A.; Gorb, L.; Isayev, O.; Leszczynski, J. Diffusion of energetic compounds through biological membrane: Application of classical MD and COSMOmic approximations. *J. Biomol. Struct. Dyn.* **2019**, *37*, 247–255. [CrossRef]
481. Yang, H.; Zhou, M.; Li, H.; Wei, T.; Tang, C.; Zhou, Y.; Long, X. Effects of Low-level Lipid Peroxidation on the Permeability of Nitroaromatic Molecules across a Membrane: A Computational Study. *ACS Omega* **2020**, *5*, 4798–4806. [CrossRef]
482. Rózsa, Z.B.; Németh, L.J.; Jójárt, B.; Nehéz, K.; Viskolcz, B.; Szöri, M. Molecular Dynamics and Metadynamics Insights of 1,4-Dioxane-Induced Structural Changes of Biomembrane Models. *J. Phys. Chem. B* **2019**, *123*, 7869–7884. [CrossRef] [PubMed]
483. Stachowicz-Kuśnierz, A.; Trojan, S.; Cwiklik, L.; Korchowiec, B.; Korchowiec, J. Modeling Lung Surfactant Interactions with Benzo[a]pyrene. *Chem.—A Eur. J.* **2017**, *23*, 5307–5316. [CrossRef] [PubMed]
484. Xue, Z.; Sun, Q.; Zhang, L.; Kang, Z.; Liang, L.; Wang, Q.; Shen, J.W. Graphene quantum dot assisted translocation of drugs into a cell membrane. *Nanoscale* **2019**, *11*, 4503–4514. [CrossRef]
485. Raczyński, P.; Górny, K.; Bełdowski, P.; Yuvan, S.; Dendzik, Z. Application of graphene as a nanoindenter interacting with phospholipid membranes-computer simulation study. *J. Phys. Chem. B* **2020**, *124*, 6592–6602. [CrossRef] [PubMed]
486. Zhu, X.; Li, N.; Huang, C.; Li, Z.; Fan, J. Membrane Perturbation and Lipid Flip-Flop Mediated by Graphene Nanosheet. *J. Phys. Chem. B* **2020**, *124*, 10632–10640. [CrossRef]
487. Moore, T.C.; Yang, A.H.; Ogungbesan, O.; Hartkamp, R.; Iacovella, C.R.; Zhang, Q.; McCabe, C. Influence of single-stranded DNA Coatings on the Interaction between Graphene Nanoflakes and Lipid Bilayers. *J. Phys. Chem. B* **2019**, *123*, 7711–7721. [CrossRef]
488. Kaminari, A.; Nikoli, E.; Athanasopoulos, A.; Sakellis, E.; Sideratou, Z. Engineering Mitochondriotropic Carbon Dots for Targeting Cancer Cells. *Pharmaceuticals* **2021**, *14*, 932. [CrossRef]
489. Chen, Y.; Zhang, W.; Huang, C.; Feng, M.; Yang, Y.; Gou, Y. Destructive Extraction and Enhanced Diffusion of Phospholipids on Lipid Membranes by Phosphorene Oxide Nanosheets. *J. Phys. Chem. B* **2021**, *125*, 2636–2643. [CrossRef]
490. Ou, L.; Corradi, V.; Tieleman, D.P.; Liang, Q. Atomistic simulations on interactions between amphiphilic Janus nanoparticles and lipid bilayers: Effects of lipid ordering and leaflet asymmetry. *J. Phys. Chem. B* **2020**, *124*, 4466–4475. [CrossRef]
491. Das, M.; Dahal, U.; Mesele, O.; Liang, D.; Cui, Q. Molecular dynamics simulation of interaction between functionalized nanoparticles with lipid membranes: Analysis of coarse-grained models. *J. Phys. Chem. B* **2019**, *123*, 10547–10561. [CrossRef]
492. 4Salassi, S.; Canepa, E.; Ferrando, R.; Rossi, G. Anionic nanoparticle-lipid membrane interactions: The protonation of anionic ligands at the membrane surface reduces membrane disruption. *RSC. Adv.* **2019**, *9*, 13992–13997. [CrossRef]
493. Ivanov, M.; Lyubartsev, A.P. Atomistic Molecular Dynamics Simulations of Lipids Near TiO 2 Nanosurfaces. *J. Phys. Chem. B* **2021**, *125*, 8048–8059. [CrossRef]
494. Zhang, L.; Chen, H.; Xie, J.; Becton, M.; Wang, X. Interplay of Nanoparticle Rigidity and Its Translocation Ability through Cell Membrane. *J. Phys. Chem. B* **2019**, *123*, 8923–8930. [CrossRef]
495. Nalakarn, P.; Boonnoy, P.; Nisoh, N.; Karttunen, M.; Wong-ekkabut, J. Dependence of fullerene aggregation on lipid saturation due to a balance between entropy and enthalpy. *Sci. Rep.* **2019**, *9*, 1037. [CrossRef]
496. Nisoh, N.; Jarerattanachat, V.; Karttunen, M.; Wong-ekkabut, J. Formation of aggregates, icosahedral structures and percolation clusters of fullerenes in lipids bilayers: The key role of lipid saturation. *Biochim. Biophys. Acta-Biomembr.* **2020**, *1862*, 183328. [CrossRef] [PubMed]

497. Nisoh, N.; Karttunen, M.; Monticelli, L.; Wong-Ekkabut, J. Lipid monolayer disruption caused by aggregated carbon nanoparticles. *RSC Adv.* **2015**, *5*, 11676–11685. [CrossRef]
498. Alves, E.D.; Colherinhas, G.; Mendanha, S.A. Assessing the DOPC-cholesterol interactions and their influence on fullerene C60 partitioning in lipid bilayers. *J. Mol. Liq.* **2020**, *315*, 113698. [CrossRef]
499. Jiménez-Jiménez, C.; Manzano, M.; Vallet-Regí, M. Nanoparticles coated with cell membranes for biomedical applications. *Biology* **2020**, *9*, 406. [CrossRef]
500. Zhang, W.; Metzger, J.M.; Hackel, B.J.; Bates, F.S.; Lodge, T.P. Influence of the Headgroup on the Interaction of Poly(ethylene oxide)-Poly(propylene oxide) Block Copolymers with Lipid Bilayers. *J. Phys. Chem. B* **2020**, *124*, 2417–2424. [CrossRef]
501. Gurtovenko, A.A. Molecular-Level Insight into the Interactions of DNA/Polycation Complexes with Model Cell Membranes. *J. Phys. Chem. B* **2019**, *123*, 6505–6514. [CrossRef]
502. Zaki, A.M.; Carbone, P. Amphiphilic copolymers change the nature of the ordered-to-disordered phase transition of lipid membranes from discontinuous to continuous. *Phys. Chem. Chem. Phys.* **2019**, *21*, 13746–13757. [CrossRef]
503. Houang, E.M.; Haman, K.J.; Kim, M.; Zhang, W.; Lowe, D.A.; Sham, Y.Y.; Lodge, T.P.; Hackel, B.J.; Bates, F.S.; Metzger, J.M. Chemical End Group Modified Diblock Copolymers Elucidate Anchor and Chain Mechanism of Membrane Stabilization. *Mol. Pharm.* **2017**, *14*, 2333–2339. [CrossRef]
504. Pérez-Sánchez, G.; Vicente, F.A.; Schaeffer, N.; Cardoso, I.S.; Ventura, S.P.M.; Jorge, M.; Coutinho, J.A.P. Unravelling the interactions between surface-active ionic liquids and triblock copolymers for the design of thermal responsive systems. *J. Phys. Chem. B* **2020**, *124*, 7046–7058. [CrossRef] [PubMed]
505. Ileri Ercan, N.; Stroeve, P.; Tringe, J.W.; Faller, R. Understanding the Interaction of Pluronics L61 and L64 with a DOPC Lipid Bilayer: An Atomistic Molecular Dynamics Study. *Langmuir* **2016**, *32*, 10026–10033. [CrossRef] [PubMed]
506. 5Qiao, J.; Purro, M.; Liu, Z.; Xiong, M.P. Effects of Polyethyelene Glycol-Desferrioxamine:Gallium Conjugates on Pseudomonas aeruginosa Outer Membrane Permeability and Vancomycin Potentiation. *Mol. Pharm.* **2021**, *18*, 735–742. [CrossRef]
507. Martin, A.; Tomasini, M.; Kholodovych, V.; Gu, L.; Sommerfeld, S.; Uhrich, K.; Murthy, N.; Welsh, W.; Moghe, P. Carbohydrate-Derived Amphiphilic Macromolecules: A Biophysical Structural Characterization and Analysis of Binding Behaviors to Model Membranes. *J. Funct. Biomater.* **2015**, *6*, 171–191. [CrossRef] [PubMed]
508. Lehtinen, J.; Magarkar, A.; Stepniewski, M.; Hakola, S.; Bergman, M.; Róg, T.; Yliperttula, M.; Urtti, A.; Bunker, A. Analysis of cause of failure of new targeting peptide in PEGylated liposome: Molecular modeling as rational design tool for nanomedicine. *Eur. J. Pharm. Sci.* **2012**, *46*, 121–130. [CrossRef]
509. Magarkar, A.; Róg, T.; Bunker, A. A computational study suggests that replacing PEG with PMOZ may increase exposure of hydrophobic targeting moiety. *Eur. J. Pharm. Sci.* **2017**, *103*, 128–135. [CrossRef]
510. Jeong, H.; Hwang, J.; Lee, H.; Hammond, P.T.; Choi, J.; Hong, J. In vitro blood cell viability profiling of polymers used in molecular assembly. *Sci. Rep.* **2017**, *7*, 9481. [CrossRef]
511. Kumari, P.; Kashyap, H.K. Sensitivity and Resilience of Phosphatidylcholine and Phosphatidylethanolamine Lipid Membranes against Cholinium Glycinate Biocompatible Ionic Liquid. *J. Phys. Chem. B* **2019**, *123*, 4550–4561. [CrossRef] [PubMed]
512. Kumari, M.; Gupta, A.; Shobhna; Kashyap, H.K. Molecular Dynamics Evaluation of the Effect of Cholinium Phenylalaninate Biocompatible Ionic Liquid on Biomimetic Membranes. *J. Phys. Chem. B* **2020**, *124*, 6748–6762. [CrossRef]
513. Kumari, P.; Faraone, A.; Kelley, E.G.; Benedetto, A. Stiffening Effect of the [Bmim][Cl] Ionic Liquid on the Bending Dynamics of DMPC Lipid Vesicles. *J. Phys. Chem. B* **2021**, *125*, 7241–7250. [CrossRef]
514. Cardoso, R.M.S.; Martins, P.A.T.; Ramos, C.V.; Cordeiro, M.M.; Leote, R.J.B.; Razi Naqvi, K.; Vaz, W.L.C.; Moreno, M.J. Effect of dipole moment on amphiphile solubility and partition into liquid ordered and liquid disordered phases in lipid bilayers. *Biochim. Biophys. Acta-Biomembr.* **2020**, *1862*, 183157. [CrossRef]
515. Kofod, C.S.; Prioli, S.; Hornum, M.; Kongsted, J.; Reinholdt, P. Computational Characterization of Novel Malononitrile Variants of Laurdan with Improved Photophysical Properties for Sensing in Membranes. *J. Phys. Chem. B* **2020**, *124*, 9526–9534. [CrossRef]
516. Do Canto, A.M.T.M.; Robalo, J.R.; Santos, P.D.; Carvalho, A.J.P.; Ramalho, J.P.P.; Loura, L.M.S. Diphenylhexatriene membrane probes DPH and TMA-DPH: A comparative molecular dynamics simulation study. *Biochim. Biophys. Acta-Biomembr.* **2016**, *1858*, 2647–2661. [CrossRef]
517. Filipe, H.A.L.; Santos, L.S.; Prates Ramalho, J.P.; Moreno, M.J.; Loura, L.M.S. Behaviour of NBD-head group labelled phosphatidylethanolamines in POPC bilayers: A molecular dynamics study. *Phys. Chem. Chem. Phys.* **2015**, *17*, 20066–20079. [CrossRef] [PubMed]
518. Filipe, H.A.L.; Pokorná, Š.; Hof, M.; Amaro, M.; Loura, L.M.S. Orientation of nitro-group governs the fluorescence lifetime of nitrobenzoxadiazole (NBD)-labeled lipids in lipid bilayers. *Phys. Chem. Chem. Phys.* **2019**, *21*, 1682–1688. [CrossRef]
519. Kulkarni, R.U.; Yin, H.; Pourmandi, N.; James, F.; Adil, M.M.; Schaffer, D.V.; Wang, Y.; Miller, E.W. A Rationally Designed, General Strategy for Membrane Orientation of Photoinduced Electron Transfer-Based Voltage-Sensitive Dyes. *ACS Chem. Biol.* **2017**, *12*, 407–413. [CrossRef]
520. Chmielińska, A.; Stepien, P.; Bonarek, P.; Girych, M.; Enkavi, G.; Róg, T.; Dziedzicka-Wasylewska, M.; Polit, A. Can di-4-ANEPPDHQ reveal the structural differences between nanodiscs and liposomes? *Biochim. Biophys. Acta-Biomembr.* **2021**, *1863*, 183649. [CrossRef] [PubMed]

521. Bouquiaux, C.; Castet, F.; Champagne, B. Unravelling the Effects of Cholesterol on the Second-Order Nonlinear Optical Responses of Di-8-ANEPPS Dye Embedded in Phosphatidylcholine Lipid Bilayers. *J. Phys. Chem. B* **2021**, *125*, 10195–10212. [CrossRef] [PubMed]
522. Suhaj, A.; Gowland, D.; Bonini, N.; Owen, D.M.; Lorenz, C.D. Laurdan and Di-4-ANEPPDHQ influence the properties of lipid membranes: A classical molecular dynamics and fluorescence study. *J. Phys. Chem. B* **2020**, *124*, 11419–11430. [CrossRef]
523. Filipe, H.A.L.; Moreno, M.J.; Loura, L.M.S. The secret lives of fluorescent membrane probes as revealed by molecular dynamics simulations. *Molecules* **2020**, *25*, 3424. [CrossRef]
524. Thomas, D.; Rubio, V.; Iragavarapu, V.; Guzman, E.; Pelletier, O.B.; Alamgir, S.; Zhang, Q.; Stawikowski, M.J. Solvatochromic and pH-Sensitive Fluorescent Membrane Probes for Imaging of Live Cells. *ACS Chem. Neurosci.* **2021**, *12*, 719–734. [CrossRef] [PubMed]
525. Rissanen, S.; Grzybek, M.; Orłowski, A.; Róg, T.; Cramariuc, O.; Levental, I.; Eggeling, C.; Sezgin, E.; Vattulainen, I. Phase partitioning of GM1 and its bodipy-labeled analog determine their different binding to Cholera Toxin. *Front. Physiol.* **2017**, *8*, 252. [CrossRef]
526. Filipe, H.A.L.; Moreno, M.J.; Róg, T.; Vattulainen, I.; Loura, L.M.S. How to tackle the issues in free energy simulations of long amphiphiles interacting with lipid membranes: Convergence and local membrane deformations. *J. Phys. Chem. B* **2014**, *118*, 3572–3581. [CrossRef] [PubMed]
527. Kepczynski, M.; Kumorek, M.; Stepniewski, M.; Róg, T.; Kozik, B.; Jamróz, D.; Bednar, J.; Nowakowska, M. Behavior of 2,6-Bis(decyloxy)naphthalene inside lipid bilayer. *J. Phys. Chem. B* **2010**, *114*, 15483–15494. [CrossRef]
528. Baig, M.W.; Pederzoli, M.; Jurkiewicz, P.; Cwiklik, L.; Pittner, J. Orientation of Laurdan in phospholipid bilayers influences its fluorescence: Quantum mechanics and classical molecular dynamics study. *Molecules* **2018**, *23*, 1707. [CrossRef] [PubMed]
529. Licari, G.; Cwiklik, L.; Jungwirth, P.; Vauthey, E. Exploring Fluorescent Dyes at Biomimetic Interfaces with Second Harmonic Generation and Molecular Dynamics. *Langmuir* **2017**, *33*, 3373–3383. [CrossRef]
530. Zhu, Q.; Lu, Y.; He, X.; Liu, T.; Chen, H.; Wang, F.; Zheng, D.; Dong, H.; Ma, J. Entropy and Polarity Control the Partition and Transportation of Drug-like Molecules in Biological Membrane. *Sci. Rep.* **2017**, *7*, 17749. [CrossRef]
531. Wen, W.; Luo, J.; Li, P.; Huang, W.; Wang, P.; Xu, S. Benzaldehyde, A New Absorption Promoter, Accelerating Absorption on Low Bioavailability Drugs Through Membrane Permeability. *Front. Pharmacol.* **2021**, *12*, 663743. [CrossRef]
532. Song, Y.; Lee, J.H.; Jung, I.; Seo, B.; Hwang, H. Molecular Dynamics Simulations of Micelle Properties and Behaviors of Sodium Lauryl Ether Sulfate Penetrating Ceramide and Phospholipid Bilayers. *J. Phys. Chem. B* **2020**, *124*, 5919–5929. [CrossRef] [PubMed]
533. Liu, J.; Li, X.; Hou, J.; Liu, F. Electric-Field-Induced Interface Behavior of Dodecyl Sulfate with Large Organic Counterions: A Molecular Dynamics Study. *J. Phys. Chem. B* **2020**, *124*, 5498–5506. [CrossRef] [PubMed]
534. Liu, Z.; Ren, X.; Tan, R.; Chai, Z.; Wang, D. Key Factors Determining Efficiency of Liquid—Liquid Extraction: Implications from Molecular Dynamics Simulations of Biphasic Behaviors of CyMe4-BTPhen and Its Am(III) Complexes. *J. Phys. Chem. B* **2020**, *124*, 1751–1766. [CrossRef]
535. de Ménorval, M.A.; Mir, L.M.; Fernández, M.L.; Reigada, R. Effects of dimethyl sulfoxide in cholesterol-containing lipid membranes: A comparative study of experiments in silico and with cells. *PLoS ONE* **2012**, *7*, e41733. [CrossRef]
536. Coimbra, J.T.S.; Brás, N.F.; Fernandes, P.A.; Rangel, M.; Ramos, M.J. Membrane partition of bis-(3-hydroxy-4-pyridinonato) zinc(ii) complexes revealed by molecular dynamics simulations. *RSC Adv.* **2018**, *8*, 27081–27090. [CrossRef]
537. Zappacosta, R.; Aschi, M.; Ammazzalorso, A.; Di Profio, P.; Fontana, A.; Siani, G. Embedding calix [4] resorcinarenes in liposomes: Experimental and computational investigation of the effect of resorcinarene inclusion on liposome properties and stability. *Biochim. Biophys. Acta-Biomembr.* **2019**, *1861*, 1252–1259. [CrossRef] [PubMed]
538. Sánchez-Borzone, M.E.; Mariani, M.E.; Miguel, V.; Gleiser, R.M.; Odhav, B.; Venugopala, K.N.; García, D.A. Membrane effects of dihydropyrimidine analogues with larvicidal activity. *Colloids Surf. B Biointerfaces* **2017**, *150*, 106–113. [CrossRef]
539. Duša, F.; Chen, W.; Witos, J.; Rantamäki, A.H.; King, A.W.T.; Sklavounos, E.; Roth, M.; Wiedmer, S.K. Immobilization of natural lipid biomembranes and their interactions with choline carboxylates. A nanoplasmonic sensing study. *Biochim. Biophys. Acta-Biomembr.* **2020**, *1862*, 183115. [CrossRef]
540. Lopes, R.; Costa, M.; Ferreira, M.; Gameiro, P.; Paiva-Martins, F. A new family of hydroxytyrosol phenolipids for the antioxidant protection of liposomal systems. *Biochim. Biophys. Acta-Biomembr.* **2021**, *1863*, 183505. [CrossRef]
541. Schmidt, A.; Lenzig, P.; Oslender-Bujotzek, A.; Kusch, J.; Lucas, S.D.; Gründer, S.; Wiemuth, D. The Bile Acid-Sensitive Ion Channel (BASIC) Is activated by alterations of its membrane environment. *PLoS ONE* **2014**, *9*, e111549. [CrossRef] [PubMed]
542. Lundbæk, J.A.; Koeppe, R.E.; Andersen, O.S. Amphiphile regulation of ion channel function by changes in the bilayer spring constant. *Proc. Natl. Acad. Sci. USA* **2010**, *107*, 15427–15430. [CrossRef] [PubMed]
543. Yin, Q.; Wang, R.; Yang, S.; Wu, Z.; Guo, S.; Dai, X.; Qiao, Y.; Shi, X. Influence of temperature on transdermal penetration enhancing mechanism of borneol: A multi-scale study. *Int. J. Mol. Sci.* **2017**, *18*, 195. [CrossRef] [PubMed]
544. Liu, X.; Liu, M.; Liu, C.; Quan, P.; Zhao, Y.; Fang, L. An insight into the molecular mechanism of the temporary enhancement effect of isopulegol decanoate on the skin. *Int. J. Pharm.* **2017**, *529*, 161–167. [CrossRef]
545. Li, G.; Yao, P.; Gong, R.; Li, J.; Liu, P.; Lonsdale, R.; Wu, Q.; Lin, J.; Zhu, D.; Reetz, M.T. Simultaneous engineering of an enzyme's entrance tunnel and active site: The case of monoamine oxidase MAO-N. *Chem. Sci.* **2017**, *8*, 4093–4099. [CrossRef]

546. Aragón-Muriel, A.; Liscano, Y.; Morales-Morales, D.; Polo-Cerón, D.; Oñate-Garzón, J. A study of the interaction of a new benzimidazole schiff base with synthetic and simulated membrane models of bacterial and mammalian membranes. *Membranes* **2021**, *11*, 449. [CrossRef]
547. Bakarić, D.; Carić, D.; Vazdar, K.; Vazdar, M. Vibrational spectroscopy combined with molecular dynamics simulations as a tool for studying behavior of reactive aldehydes inserted in phospholipid bilayers. *Chem. Phys. Lipids* **2019**, *225*, 104793. [CrossRef]
548. Issack, B.B.; Peslherbe, G.H. Accuracy and precision of simulated free energies: Water permeation of hydrated DPPC bilayers as a paradigm. *Mol. Simul.* **2019**, *45*, 466–473. [CrossRef]
549. Hub, J.S.; Winkler, F.K.; Merrick, M.; de Groot, B.L. Potentials of Mean Force and Permeabilities for Carbon Dioxide, Ammonia, and Water Flux across a Rhesus Protein Channel and Lipid Membranes. *J. Am. Chem. Soc.* **2010**, *132*, 13251–13263. [CrossRef]
550. Olzynska, A.; Kulig, W.; Mikkolainen, H.; Czerniak, T.; Jurkiewicz, P.; Cwiklik, L.; Róg, T.; Hof, M.; Jungwirth, P.; Vattulainen, I. Tail-Oxidized Cholesterol Enhances Membrane Permeability for Small Solutes. *Langmuir* **2020**, *36*, 10438–10447. [CrossRef] [PubMed]
551. Bu, B.; Crowe, M.; Diao, J.; Ji, B.; Li, D. Cholesterol suppresses membrane leakage by decreasing water penetrability. *Soft Matter* **2018**, *14*, 5277–5282. [CrossRef]
552. Hong, C.; Tieleman, D.P.; Wang, Y. Microsecond Molecular Dynamics Simulations of Lipid Mixing. *Langmuir* **2014**, *30*, 11993–12001. [CrossRef]
553. Saito, H.; Shinoda, W. Cholesterol effect on water permeability through DPPC and PSM lipid bilayers: A molecular dynamics study. *J. Phys. Chem. B* **2011**, *115*, 15241–15250. [CrossRef] [PubMed]
554. Issack, B.B.; Peslherbe, G.H. Effects of Cholesterol on the Thermodynamics and Kinetics of Passive Transport of Water through Lipid Membranes. *J. Phys. Chem. B* **2015**, *119*, 9391–9400. [CrossRef] [PubMed]
555. Hartkamp, R.; Moore, T.C.; Iacovella, C.R.; Thompson, M.A.; Bulsara, P.A.; Moore, D.J.; McCabe, C. Composition Dependence of Water Permeation Across Multicomponent Gel-Phase Bilayers. *J. Phys. Chem. B* **2018**, *122*, 3113–3123. [CrossRef]
556. Wittmann, H.J.; Seifert, R.; Strasser, A. Sodium binding to hH3R and hH4R—A molecular modeling study. *J. Mol. Model.* **2014**, *20*, 2394. [CrossRef]
557. Plesnar, E.; Szczelina, R.; Subczynski, W.K.; Pasenkiewicz-Gierula, M. Is the cholesterol bilayer domain a barrier to oxygen transport into the eye lens? *Biochim. Biophys. Acta-Biomembr.* **2018**, *1860*, 434–441. [CrossRef]
558. Yuan, Y.; Liu, X.; Liu, T.; Liu, W.; Zhu, Y.; Zhang, H.; Zhao, C. Molecular dynamics exploring of atmosphere components interacting with lung surfactant phospholipid bilayers. *Sci. Total Environ.* **2020**, *743*, 140547. [CrossRef]
559. Man, V.H.; Truong, P.M.; Li, M.S.; Wang, J.; Van-Oanh, N.-T.; Derreumaux, P.; Nguyen, P.H. Molecular Mechanism of the Cell Membrane Pore Formation Induced by Bubble Stable Cavitation. *J. Phys. Chem. B* **2019**, *123*, 71–78. [CrossRef]
560. Venable, R.M.; Krämer, A.; Pastor, R.W. Molecular Dynamics Simulations of Membrane Permeability. *Chem. Rev.* **2019**, *119*, 5954–5997. [CrossRef] [PubMed]
561. Awoonor-Williams, E.; Rowley, C.N. Molecular simulation of nonfacilitated membrane permeation. *Biochim. Biophys. Acta-Biomembr.* **2016**, *1858*, 1672–1687. [CrossRef]
562. Amaro, R.E.; Mulholland, A.J. Multiscale methods in drug design bridge chemical and biological complexity in the search for cures. *Nat. Rev. Chem.* **2018**, *2*, 0148. [CrossRef] [PubMed]
563. Hannesschlaeger, C.; Horner, A.; Pohl, P. Intrinsic Membrane Permeability to Small Molecules. *Chem. Rev.* **2019**, *119*, 5922–5953. [CrossRef] [PubMed]
564. Marrink, S.-J.; Berendsen, H.J.C. Simulation of Water Transport through a Lipid Membrane Siewert-Jan. *J. Phys. Chem.* **1994**, *98*, 4155–4168. [CrossRef]
565. Ingram, T.; Storm, S.; Kloss, L.; Mehling, T.; Jakobtorweihen, S.; Smirnova, I. Prediction of micelle/water and liposome/water partition coefficients based on molecular dynamics simulations, COSMO-RS, and COSMOmic. *Langmuir* **2013**, *29*, 3527–3537. [CrossRef] [PubMed]
566. Schwöbel, J.A.H.; Ebert, A.; Bittermann, K.; Huniar, U.; Goss, K.U.; Klamt, A. COSMO perm: Mechanistic Prediction of Passive Membrane Permeability for Neutral Compounds and Ions and Its pH Dependence. *J. Phys. Chem. B* **2020**, *124*, 3343–3354. [CrossRef]
567. Turchi, M.; Kognole, A.A.; Kumar, A.; Cai, Q.; Lian, G.; Mackerell, A.D. Predicting Partition Coefficients of Neutral and Charged Solutes in the Mixed SLES-Fatty Acid Micellar System. *J. Phys. Chem. B* **2020**, *124*, 1653–1664. [CrossRef]
568. Bennion, B.J.; Be, N.A.; McNerney, M.W.; Lao, V.; Carlson, E.M.; Valdez, C.A.; Malfatti, M.A.; Enright, H.A.; Nguyen, T.H.; Lightstone, F.C.; et al. Predicting a Drug's Membrane Permeability: A Computational Model Validated with in Vitro Permeability Assay Data. *J. Phys. Chem. B* **2017**, *121*, 5228–5237. [CrossRef]
569. Lomize, A.L.; Pogozheva, I.D. Physics-Based Method for Modeling Passive Membrane Permeability and Translocation Pathways of Bioactive Molecules. *J. Chem. Inf. Model.* **2019**, *59*, 3198–3213. [CrossRef]
570. Fukunishi, Y.; Mashimo, T.; Kurosawa, T.; Wakabayashi, Y.; Nakamura, H.K.; Takeuchi, K. Prediction of Passive Membrane Permeability by Semi-Empirical Method Considering Viscous and Inertial Resistances and Different Rates of Conformational Change and Diffusion. *Mol. Inform.* **2020**, *39*, 1900071. [CrossRef]
571. Bennett, D.W.F.; He, S.; Bilodeau, C.L.; Jones, D.; Sun, D.; Kim, H.; Allen, J.E.; Lightstone, F.C.; Ingólfsson, H.I. Predicting small molecule transfer free energies by combining molecular dynamics simulations and deep learning. *J. Chem. Inf. Model.* **2020**, *60*, 5375–5381. [CrossRef]

572. Brocke, S.A.; Degen, A.; Mackerell, A.D.; Dutagaci, B.; Feig, M. Prediction of Membrane Permeation of Drug Molecules by Combining an Implicit Membrane Model with Machine Learning. *J. Chem. Inf. Model.* **2019**, *59*, 1147–1162. [CrossRef]
573. Sun, R.; Han, Y.; Swanson, J.M.J.; Tan, J.S.; Rose, J.P.; Voth, G.A. Molecular transport through membranes: Accurate permeability coefficients from multidimensional potentials of mean force and local diffusion constants. *J. Chem. Phys.* **2018**, *149*, 072310. [CrossRef] [PubMed]
574. Sun, R.; Dama, J.F.; Tan, J.S.; Rose, J.P.; Voth, G.A. Transition-Tempered Metadynamics Is a Promising Tool for Studying the Permeation of Drug-like Molecules through Membranes. *J. Chem. Theory Comput.* **2016**, *12*, 5157–5169. [CrossRef] [PubMed]
575. Tse, C.H.; Comer, J.; Sang Chu, S.K.; Wang, Y.; Chipot, C. Affordable Membrane Permeability Calculations: Permeation of Short-Chain Alcohols through Pure-Lipid Bilayers and a Mammalian Cell Membrane. *J. Chem. Theory Comput.* **2019**, *15*, 2913–2924. [CrossRef]
576. Badaoui, M.; Kells, A.; Molteni, C.; Dickson, C.J.; Hornak, V.; Rosta, E. Calculating Kinetic Rates and Membrane Permeability from Biased Simulations. *J. Phys. Chem. B* **2018**, *122*, 11571–11578. [CrossRef]
577. Votapka, L.W.; Lee, C.T.; Amaro, R.E. Two Relations to Estimate Membrane Permeability Using Milestoning. *J. Phys. Chem. B* **2016**, *120*, 8606–8616. [CrossRef]
578. Lomize, A.L.; Hage, J.M.; Schnitzer, K.; Golobokov, K.; Lafaive, M.B.; Forsyth, A.C.; Pogozheva, I.D. PerMM: A Web Tool and Database for Analysis of Passive Membrane Permeability and Translocation Pathways of Bioactive Molecules. *J. Chem. Inf. Model.* **2019**, *59*, 3094–3099. [CrossRef]
579. Sharifian, G.M. Recent Experimental Developments in Studying Passive Membrane Transport of Drug Molecules. *Mol. Pharm.* **2021**, *18*, 2122–2141. [CrossRef]
580. Neuvonen, M.; Manna, M.; Mokkila, S.; Javanainen, M.; Róg, T.; Liu, Z.; Bittman, R.; Vattulainen, I.; Ikonen, E. Enzymatic oxidation of cholesterol: Properties and functional effects of cholestenone in cell membranes. *PLoS ONE* **2014**, *9*, e103743. [CrossRef] [PubMed]
581. Róg, T.; Stimson, L.M.; Pasenkiewicz-Gierula, M.; Vattulainen, I.; Karttunen, M. Replacing the cholesterol hydroxyl group with the ketone group facilitates sterol flip-flop and promotes membrane fluidity. *J. Phys. Chem. B* **2008**, *112*, 1946–1952. [CrossRef]
582. Kulig, W.; Mikkolainen, H.; Olzyńska, A.; Jurkiewicz, P.; Cwiklik, L.; Hof, M.; Vattulainen, I.; Jungwirth, P.; Róg, T.; Olżyńska, A.; et al. Bobbing of Oxysterols: Molecular Mechanism for Translocation of Tail-Oxidized Sterols through Biological Membranes. *J. Phys. Chem. Lett.* **2018**, *9*, 1118–1123. [CrossRef]
583. Stimson, L.M.; Dong, L.; Karttunen, M.; Wisniewska, A.; Dutka, M.; Róg, T. Stearic acid spin labels in lipid bilayers: Insight through atomistic simulations. *J. Phys. Chem. B* **2007**, *111*, 12447–12453. [CrossRef] [PubMed]
584. Kulig, W.; Olzyńska, A.; Jurkiewicz, P.; Kantola, A.M.; Komulainen, S.; Manna, M.; Pourmousa, M.; Vazdar, M.; Cwiklik, L.; Róg, T.; et al. Cholesterol under oxidative stress—How lipid membranes sense oxidation as cholesterol is being replaced by oxysterols. *Free Radic. Biol. Med.* **2015**, *84*, 30–41. [CrossRef] [PubMed]
585. Yee, S.M.; Lorenz, C.D. On the Structure and Flip-Flop of Free Docosahexaenoic Acid in a Model Human Brain Membrane. *J. Phys. Chem. B* **2021**, *125*, 8038–8047. [CrossRef] [PubMed]
586. Roux, B. The calculation of the potential of mean force using computer simulations. *Comput. Phys. Commun.* **1995**, *91*, 275–282. [CrossRef]
587. Neale, C.; Pomès, R. Sampling errors in free energy simulations of small molecules in lipid bilayers. *Biochim. Biophys. Acta-Biomembr.* **2016**, *1858*, 2539–2548. [CrossRef]
588. Dickson, C.J.; Hornak, V.; Bednarczyk, D.; Duca, J.S. Using Membrane Partitioning Simulations to Predict Permeability of Forty-Nine Drug-Like Molecules. *J. Chem. Inf. Model.* **2019**, *59*, 236–244. [CrossRef]
589. Dickson, C.J.; Hornak, V.; Pearlstein, R.A.; Duca, J.S. Structure–Kinetic Relationships of Passive Membrane Permeation from Multiscale Modeling. *J. Am. Chem. Soc.* **2017**, *139*, 442–452. [CrossRef] [PubMed]
590. Debnath, M.; Chakraborty, S.; Kumar, Y.P.; Chaudhuri, R.; Jana, B.; Dash, J. Ionophore constructed from non-covalent assembly of a G-quadruplex and liponucleoside transports K+-ion across biological membranes. *Nat. Commun.* **2020**, *11*, 469. [CrossRef]
591. Kim, G.; Han, S.; Won, H. Isolation of Microcystin-LR and Its Potential Function of Ionophore. *J. Korean Magn. Reson. Soc.* **2015**, *19*, 67–73. [CrossRef]
592. Marques, I.; Costa, P.M.R.; Miranda, M.Q.; Busschaert, N.; Howe, E.N.W.; Clarke, H.J.; Haynes, C.J.E.; Kirby, I.L.; Rodilla, A.M.; Pérez-Tomás, R.; et al. Full elucidation of the transmembrane anion transport mechanism of squaramides using: In silico investigations. *Phys. Chem. Chem. Phys.* **2018**, *20*, 20796–20811. [CrossRef]
593. Spooner, M.J.; Li, H.; Marques, I.; Costa, P.M.R.; Wu, X.; Howe, E.N.W.; Busschaert, N.; Moore, S.J.; Light, M.E.; Sheppard, D.N.; et al. Fluorinated synthetic anion carriers: Experimental and computational insights into transmembrane chloride transport. *Chem. Sci.* **2019**, *10*, 1976–1985. [CrossRef] [PubMed]
594. Pilato, S.; Aschi, M.; Bazzoni, M.; Bonati, F.C.; Cera, G.; Moffa, S.; Canale, V.; Ciulla, M.; Secchi, A.; Arduini, A.; et al. Calixarene-based artificial ionophores for chloride transport across natural liposomal bilayer: Synthesis, structure-function relationships, and computational study. *Biochim. Biophys. Acta-Biomembr.* **2021**, *1863*, 183667. [CrossRef]
595. Janout, V.; Cline, L.L.; Feuston, B.P.; Klein, L.; O'Brien, A.; Tucker, T.; Yuan, Y.; O'Neill-Davis, L.A.; Peiffer, R.L.; Nerurkar, S.S.; et al. Molecular umbrella conjugate for the ocular delivery of siRNA. *Bioconjugate Chem.* **2014**, *25*, 197–201. [CrossRef]
596. Janout, V.; Regen, S.L. A needle-and-thread approach to bilayer transport: Permeation of a molecular umbrella-oligonucliotide conjugation across a phospholipid membrane. *J. Am. Chem. Soc.* **2005**, *127*, 22–23. [CrossRef]

597. Janout, V.; Regen, S.L. Bioconjugate-based molecular umbrellas. *Bioconjugate Chem.* **2009**, *20*, 183–192. [CrossRef]
598. Chen, A.; Karanastasis, A.; Casey, K.R.; Necelis, M.; Carone, B.R.; Caputo, G.A.; Palermo, E.F. Cationic Molecular Umbrellas as Antibacterial Agents with Remarkable Cell-Type Selectivity. *ACS Appl. Mater. Interfaces* **2020**, *12*, 21270–21282. [CrossRef] [PubMed]
599. Danta, C.C.; Piplani, P. Investigation of Molecular Properties of Antiretroviral Agents to Enhance CNS Penetration Abilities for the Treatment of Cognitive Impairment in HIV-Associated Neurocognitive Disorder. *ACS Chem. Neurosci.* **2020**, *11*, 2034–2038. [CrossRef] [PubMed]
600. Ashrafuzzaman, M. The antimicrobial peptide gramicidin s enhances membrane adsorption and ion pore formation potency of chemotherapy drugs in lipid bilayers. *Membranes* **2021**, *11*, 247. [CrossRef]
601. Pereira, R.; Silva, S.G.; Pinheiro, M.; Reis, S.; Luísa Do Vale, M. Current status of amino acid-based permeation enhancers in transdermal drug delivery. *Membranes* **2021**, *11*, 343. [CrossRef] [PubMed]
602. Park, S.E.; Sajid, M.I.; Parang, K.; Tiwari, R.K. Cyclic cell-penetrating peptides as efficient intracellular drug delivery tools. *Mol. Pharm.* **2019**, *16*, 3727–3743. [CrossRef]
603. Bozdaganyan, M.E.; Orekhov, P.S. Synergistic effect of chemical penetration enhancers on lidocaine permeability revealed by coarse-grained molecular dynamics simulations. *Membranes* **2021**, *11*, 410. [CrossRef] [PubMed]
604. Gupta, R.; Dwadasi, B.S.; Rai, B.; Mitragotri, S. Effect of Chemical Permeation Enhancers on Skin Permeability: In silico screening using Molecular Dynamics simulations. *Sci. Rep.* **2019**, *9*, 1456. [CrossRef]
605. Marrink, S.J.; Risselada, H.J.; Yefimov, S.; Tieleman, D.P.; de Vries, A.H. The MARTINI force field: Coarse grained model for biomolecular simulations. *J. Phys. Chem. B* **2007**, *111*, 7812–7824. [CrossRef]
606. Monticelli, L.; Kandasamy, S.K.; Periole, X.; Larson, R.G.; Tieleman, D.P.; Marrink, S.-J. The MARTINI Coarse-Grained Force Field: Extension to Proteins. *J. Chem. Theory Comput.* **2008**, *4*, 819–834. [CrossRef] [PubMed]
607. Róg, T.; Pasenkiewicz-Gierula, M. Cholesterol-sphingomyelin interactions: A molecular dynamics simulation study. *Biophys. J.* **2006**, *91*, 3756–3767. [CrossRef]
608. Róg, T.; Pasenkiewicz-Gierula, M.; Vattulainen, I.; Karttunen, M. Ordering effects of cholesterol and its analogues. *Biochim. Biophys. Acta-Biomembr.* **2009**, *1788*, 97–121. [CrossRef]
609. Róg, T.; Vattulainen, I. Cholesterol, sphingolipids, and glycolipids: What do we know about their role in raft-like membranes? *Chem. Phys. Lipids* **2014**, *184*, 82–104. [CrossRef] [PubMed]
610. Khalid, S.; Berglund, N.A.; Holdbrook, D.A.; Leung, Y.M.; Parkin, J. The membranes of Gram-negative bacteria: Progress in molecular modelling and simulation. *Biochem. Soc. Trans.* **2015**, *43*, 162–167. [CrossRef]
611. Pavlova, A.; Hwang, H.; Lundquist, K.; Balusek, C.; Gumbart, J.C. Living on the edge: Simulations of bacterial outer-membrane proteins. *Biochim. Biophys. Acta-Biomembr.* **2016**, *1858*, 1753–1759. [CrossRef] [PubMed]
612. Shearer, J.; Marzinek, J.K.; Bond, P.J.; Khalid, S. Molecular dynamics simulations of bacterial outer membrane lipid extraction: Adequate sampling? *J. Chem. Phys.* **2020**, *153*, 044122. [CrossRef] [PubMed]
613. Nickels, J.D.; Chatterjee, S.; Mostofian, B.; Stanley, C.B.; Ohl, M.; Zolnierczuk, P.; Schulz, R.; Myles, D.A.A.; Standaert, R.F.; Elkins, J.G.; et al. Bacillus subtilis Lipid Extract, A Branched-Chain Fatty Acid Model Membrane. *J. Phys. Chem. Lett.* **2017**, *8*, 4214–4217. [CrossRef] [PubMed]
614. Gao, Y.; Lee, J.; Widmalm, G.; Im, W. Modeling and Simulation of Bacterial Outer Membranes with Lipopolysaccharides and Enterobacterial Common Antigen. *J. Phys. Chem. B* **2020**, *124*, 5948–5956. [CrossRef]
615. Pluhackova, K.; Horner, A. Native-like membrane models of E. coli polar lipid extract shed light on the importance of lipid composition complexity. *BMC Biol.* **2021**, *19*, 4. [CrossRef]
616. Mostofian, B.; Zhuang, T.; Cheng, X.; Nickels, J.D. Branched-Chain Fatty Acid Content Modulates Structure, Fluidity, and Phase in Model Microbial Cell Membranes. *J. Phys. Chem. B* **2019**, *123*, 5814–5821. [CrossRef]
617. Gupta, R.; Rai, B. Molecular Dynamics Simulation Study of Skin Lipids: Effects of the Molar Ratio of Individual Components over a Wide Temperature Range. *J. Phys. Chem. B* **2015**, *119*, 11643–11655. [CrossRef]
618. Paloncýová, M.; Vávrová, K.; Sovová, Ž.; DeVane, R.; Otyepka, M.; Berka, K. Structural Changes in Ceramide Bilayers Rationalize Increased Permeation through Stratum Corneum Models with Shorter Acyl Tails. *J. Phys. Chem. B* **2015**, *119*, 9811–9819. [CrossRef]
619. Podewitz, M.; Wang, Y.; Gkeka, P.; Von Grafenstein, S.; Liedl, K.R.; Cournia, Z. Phase Diagram of a Stratum Corneum Lipid Mixture. *J. Phys. Chem. B* **2018**, *122*, 10505–10521. [CrossRef]
620. Badhe, Y.; Gupta, R.; Rai, B. Structural and barrier properties of the skin ceramide lipid bilayer: A molecular dynamics simulation study. *J. Mol. Model.* **2019**, *25*, 140. [CrossRef]
621. Han, S. Effect of Hydration on a Lipid Membrane Composed of Ceramide[NP]24, Lignoceric Acid, and Cholesterol: A Molecular Dynamics Simulation Study. *Bull. Korean Chem. Soc.* **2019**, *40*, 1215–1221. [CrossRef]
622. Wang, E.; Klauda, J.B. Molecular Structure of the Long Periodicity Phase in the Stratum Corneum. *J. Am. Chem. Soc.* **2019**, *141*, 16930–16943. [CrossRef]
623. Wang, E.; Klauda, J.B. Structure and Permeability of Ceramide Bilayers and Multilayers. *J. Phys. Chem. B* **2019**, *123*, 2525–2535. [CrossRef] [PubMed]
624. Otto, D.P.; Combrinck, J.; Otto, A.; Tiedt, L.R.; De Villiers, M.M. Dissipative particle dynamics investigation of the transport of salicylic acid through a simulated in vitro skin permeation model. *Pharmaceuticals* **2018**, *11*, 134. [CrossRef]

625. Gorzelanny, C.; Mess, C.; Schneider, S.W.; Huck, V.; Brandner, J.M. Skin barriers in dermal drug delivery: Which barriers have to be overcome and how can we measure them? *Pharmaceutics* **2020**, *12*, 684. [CrossRef] [PubMed]
626. Neupane, R.; Boddu, S.H.S.; Renukuntla, J.; Babu, R.J.; Tiwari, A.K. Alternatives to biological skin in permeation studies: Current trends and possibilities. *Pharmaceutics* **2020**, *12*, 152. [CrossRef] [PubMed]
627. Paananen, R.O.; Javanainen, M.; Holopainen, J.M.; Vattulainen, I. Crystalline Wax Esters Regulate the Evaporation Resistance of Tear Film Lipid Layers Associated with Dry Eye Syndrome. *J. Phys. Chem. Lett.* **2019**, *10*, 3893–3898. [CrossRef]
628. Mainali, L.; Pasenkiewicz-Gierula, M.; Subczynski, W.K. Formation of cholesterol Bilayer Domains Precedes Formation of Cholesterol Crystals in Membranes Made of the Major Phospholipids of Human Eye Lens Fiber Cell Plasma Membranes. *Curr. Eye Res.* **2020**, *45*, 162–172. [CrossRef]
629. Olżyńska, A.; Delcroix, P.; Dolejšová, T.; Krzaczek, K.; Korchowiec, B.; Czogalla, A.; Cwiklik, L. Properties of Lipid Models of Lung Surfactant Containing Cholesterol and Oxidized Lipids: A Mixed Experimental and Computational Study. *Langmuir* **2020**, *36*, 1023–1033. [CrossRef]
630. Paananen, R.O.; Viitaja, T.; Olżyńska, A.; Ekholm, F.S.; Moilanen, J.; Cwiklik, L. Interactions of polar lipids with cholesteryl ester multilayers elucidate tear film lipid layer structure. *Ocul. Surf.* **2020**, *18*, 545–553. [CrossRef]
631. Cwiklik, L. Tear film lipid layer: A molecular level view. *Biochim. Biophys. Acta-Biomembr.* **2016**, *1858*, 2421–2430. [CrossRef]
632. Pai, R.V.; Monpara, J.D.; Vavia, P.R. Exploring molecular dynamics simulation to predict binding with ocular mucin: An in silico approach for screening mucoadhesive materials for ocular retentive delivery systems. *J. Control. Release* **2019**, *309*, 190–202. [CrossRef] [PubMed]
633. Liekkinen, J.; de Santos Moreno, B.; Paananen, R.O.; Vattulainen, I.; Monticelli, L.; Bernardino de la Serna, J.; Javanainen, M. Understanding the Functional Properties of Lipid Heterogeneity in Pulmonary Surfactant Monolayers at the Atomistic Level. *Front. Cell Dev. Biol.* **2020**, *8*, 581016. [CrossRef]
634. Liekkinen, J.; Enkavi, G.; Javanainen, M.; Olmeda, B.; Pérez-Gil, J.; Vattulainen, I. Pulmonary Surfactant Lipid Reorganization Induced by the Adsorption of the Oligomeric Surfactant Protein B Complex. *J. Mol. Biol.* **2020**, *432*, 3251–3268. [CrossRef] [PubMed]
635. Sou, T.; Bergström, C.A.S. Contemporary Formulation Development for Inhaled Pharmaceuticals. *J. Pharm. Sci.* **2021**, *110*, 66–86. [CrossRef] [PubMed]
636. Sou, T.; Kukavica-Ibrulj, I.; Levesque, R.C.; Friberg, L.E.; Bergström, C.A.S. Model-Informed Drug Development in Pulmonary Delivery: Semimechanistic Pharmacokinetic-Pharmacodynamic Modeling for Evaluation of Treatments against Chronic Pseudomonas aeruginosa Lung Infections. *Mol. Pharm.* **2020**, *17*, 1458–1469. [CrossRef]
637. Sou, T.; Soukarieh, F.; Williams, P.; Stocks, M.J.; Cámara, M.; Bergström, C.A.S. Model-Informed Drug Discovery and Development in Pulmonary Delivery: Biopharmaceutical Pharmacometric Modeling for Formulation Evaluation of Pulmonary Suspensions. *ACS Omega* **2020**, *5*, 25733–25746. [CrossRef] [PubMed]
638. Sou, T.; Kukavica-Ibrulj, I.; Soukarieh, F.; Halliday, N.; Levesque, R.C.; Williams, P.; Stocks, M.; Cámara, M.; Friberg, L.E.; Bergström, C.A.S. Model-Based Drug Development in Pulmonary Delivery: Pharmacokinetic Analysis of Novel Drug Candidates for Treatment of Pseudomonas aeruginosa Lung Infection. *J. Pharm. Sci.* **2019**, *108*, 630–640. [CrossRef]
639. Liu, C.; Elvati, P.; Violi, A. On Drug-Membrane Permeability of Antivirals for SARS-CoV-2. *J. Phys. Chem. Lett.* **2021**, *12*, 1384–1389. [CrossRef] [PubMed]
640. Gordon, D.E.; Jang, G.M.; Bouhaddou, M.; Xu, J.; Obernier, K.; White, K.M.; O'Meara, M.J.; Rezelj, V.V.; Guo, J.Z.; Swaney, D.L.; et al. A SARS-CoV-2 protein interaction map reveals targets for drug repurposing. *Nature* **2020**, *583*, 459–468. [CrossRef] [PubMed]
641. Dahlgren, D.; Lennernäs, H. Intestinal permeability and drug absorption: Predictive experimental, computational and in vivo approaches. *Pharmaceutics* **2019**, *11*, 411. [CrossRef]
642. Hermann, K.F.; Neuhaus, C.S.; Micallef, V.; Wagner, B.; Hatibovic, M.; Aschmann, H.E.; Paech, F.; Alvarez-Sanchez, R.; Krämer, S.D.; Belli, S. Kinetics of lipid bilayer permeation of a series of ionisable drugs and their correlation with human transporter-independent intestinal permeability. *Eur. J. Pharm. Sci.* **2017**, *104*, 150–161. [CrossRef] [PubMed]
643. Fagerberg, J.H.; Karlsson, E.; Ulander, J.; Hanisch, G.; Bergström, C.A.S. Computational prediction of drug solubility in fasted simulated and aspirated human intestinal fluid. *Pharm. Res.* **2015**, *32*, 578–589. [CrossRef]
644. Bergstrom, C.A.S.; Parrow, A.; Larsson, P.; Augustijns, P. Molecular dynamics simulations on interindividual variability of intestinal fluids: Impact on drug solubilization. *Mol. Pharm.* **2020**, *17*, 3837–3844. [CrossRef]
645. Lewitt, P.A. Levodopa therapy for Parkinson's disease: Pharmacokinetics and pharmacodynamics. *Mov. Disord.* **2015**, *30*, 64–72. [CrossRef] [PubMed]
646. Detrait, E.R.; Carr, G.V.; Weinberger, D.R.; Lamberty, Y. Brain catechol-O-methyltransferase (COMT) inhibition by tolcapone counteracts recognition memory deficits in normal and chronic phencyclidine-treated rats and in COMT-Val transgenic mice. *Behav. Pharmacol.* **2016**, *27*, 415–421. [CrossRef]
647. Danta, C.C. CNS Penetration Ability: A Critical Factor for Drugs in the Treatment of SARS-CoV-2 Brain Infection. *ACS Chem. Neurosci.* **2020**, *11*, 2137–2144. [CrossRef] [PubMed]
648. Verma, K.; Amitabh; Prasad, D.N.; Kumar, B.; Kohli, E. Brain and COVID-19 Crosstalk: Pathophysiological and Psychological Manifestations. *ACS Chem. Neurosci.* **2020**, *11*, 3194–3203. [CrossRef] [PubMed]

649. Gao, W.; Liu, Y.; Jing, G.; Li, K.; Zhao, Y.; Sha, B.; Wang, Q.; Wu, D. Rapid and efficient crossing blood-brain barrier: Hydrophobic drug delivery system based on propionylated amylose helix nanoclusters. *Biomaterials* **2017**, *113*, 133–144. [CrossRef]
650. Rajagopal, N.; Irudayanathan, F.J.; Nangia, S. Computational nanoscopy of tight junctions at the blood–brain barrier interface. *Int. J. Mol. Sci.* **2019**, *20*, 5583. [CrossRef]
651. Nymeyer, H.; Zhou, H.X. A method to determine dielectric constants in nonhomogeneous systems: Application to biological membranes. *Biophys. J.* **2008**, *94*, 1185–1193. [CrossRef] [PubMed]
652. Oroskar, P.; Jameson, C.J.; Murad, S. Molecular dynamics simulations reveal how characteristics of surface and permeant affect permeation events at the surface of soft matter. *Mol. Simul.* **2017**, *43*, 439–466. [CrossRef]
653. Smith, D.J.; Leal, L.-G.; Mitragorti, S.; Shell, M.S. Nanoparticle transport across model cellular membranes: When do solubility-diffusion models break down? *J. Phys. D Appl. Phys.* **2018**, *51*, 294004. [CrossRef]
654. Hoffmann, C.; Centi, A.; Menichetti, R.; Bereau, T. Molecular dynamics trajectories for 630 coarse-grained drug-membrane permeations. *Sci. Data* **2020**, *7*, 51. [CrossRef]
655. Menichetti, R.; Kanekal, K.H.; Bereau, T. Drug-Membrane Permeability across Chemical Space. *ACS Cent. Sci.* **2019**, *5*, 290–298. [CrossRef] [PubMed]
656. Menichetti, R.; Kanekal, K.H.; Kremer, K.; Bereau, T. In silico screening of drug-membrane thermodynamics reveals linear relations between bulk partitioning and the potential of mean force. *J. Chem. Phys.* **2017**, *147*, 125101. [CrossRef]
657. Menichetti, R.; Bereau, T. Revisiting the Meyer-Overton rule for drug-membrane permeabilities. *Mol. Phys.* **2019**, *117*, 2900–2909. [CrossRef]
658. Centi, A.; Dutta, A.; Parekh, S.H.; Bereau, T. Inserting Small Molecules across Membrane Mixtures: Insight from the Potential of Mean Force. *Biophys. J.* **2020**, *118*, 1321–1332. [CrossRef]
659. Souza, P.C.T.; Alessandri, R.; Barnoud, J.; Faustino, I.; Grunewald, F.; Patmanidis, I.; Abdizadeh, H.; Bruininks, B.M.H.; Wassenaar, T.A.; Kroon, P.C.; et al. Martini 3: A General Purpose Force Field for Coarse-Grained Molecular Dynamics. *Nat. Methods* **2021**, *18*, 382–388. [CrossRef]
660. Alessandri, R.; Souza, P.C.T.; Thallmair, S.; Melo, M.N.; De Vries, A.H.; Marrink, S.J. Pitfalls of the Martini Model. *J. Chem. Theory Comput.* **2019**, *15*, 5448–5460. [CrossRef]
661. Javanainen, M.; Martinez-Seara, H.; Vattulainen, I. Excessive aggregation of membrane proteins in the Martini model. *PLoS ONE* **2017**, *12*, e0187936. [CrossRef]
662. Jarin, Z.; Newhouse, J.; Voth, G.A. Coarse-Grained Force Fields from the Perspective of Statistical Mechanics: Better Understanding of the Origins of a MARTINI Hangover. *J. Chem. Theory Comput.* **2021**, *17*, 1170–1180. [CrossRef]
663. Cornelius, F.; Habeck, M.; Kanai, R.; Toyoshima, C.; Karlish, S.J.D. General and specific lipid-protein interactions in Na,K-ATPase. *Biochim. Biophys. Acta-Biomembr.* **2015**, *1848*, 1729–1743. [CrossRef]
664. Brown, M.F. Soft Matter in Lipid—Protein Interactions. *Annu. Rev. Biophys.* **2017**, *46*, 379–410. [CrossRef]
665. Gu, R.X.; de Groot, B.L. Lipid-protein interactions modulate the conformational equilibrium of a potassium channel. *Nat. Commun.* **2020**, *11*, 2162. [CrossRef]
666. Corradi, V.; Sejdiu, B.I.; Mesa-Galloso, H.; Abdizadeh, H.; Noskov, S.Y.; Marrink, S.J.; Tieleman, D.P. Emerging Diversity in Lipid-Protein Interactions. *Chem. Rev.* **2019**, *119*, 5775–5848. [CrossRef] [PubMed]
667. Haghighi, F.; Yesylevskyy, S.; Davani, S.; Ramseyer, C. Membrane environment modulates ligand-binding propensity of P2Y12 receptor. *Pharmaceutics* **2021**, *13*, 524. [CrossRef] [PubMed]
668. Schmitt, M.V.; Lienau, P.; Fricker, G.; Reichel, A. Quantitation of lysosomal trapping of basic lipophilic compounds using in vitro assays and in silico predictions based on the determination of the full pH profile of the endo-/lysosomal system in rat hepatocytes. *Drug Metab. Dispos.* **2019**, *47*, 49–57. [CrossRef] [PubMed]
669. Lu, S.; Sung, T.; Lin, N.; Abraham, R.T.; Jessen, B.A. Lysosomal adaptation: How cells respond to lysosomotropic compounds. *PLoS ONE* **2017**, *12*, e0173771. [CrossRef]
670. Villamil Giraldo, A.M.; Appelqvist, H.; Ederth, T.; Öllinger, K. Lysosomotropic agents: Impact on lysosomal membrane permeabilization and cell death. *Biochem. Soc. Trans.* **2014**, *42*, 1460–1464. [CrossRef]
671. Varalda, M.; Antona, A.; Bettio, V.; Roy, K.; Vachamaram, A.; Yellenki, V.; Massarotti, A.; Baldanzi, G.; Capello, D. Psychotropic Drugs Show Anticancer Activity by Disrupting Mitochondrial and Lysosomal Function. *Front. Oncol.* **2020**, *10*, 562196. [CrossRef]
672. Petersen, N.H.T.; Olsen, O.D.; Groth-Pedersen, L.; Ellegaard, A.M.; Bilgin, M.; Redmer, S.; Ostenfeld, M.S.; Ulanet, D.; Dovmark, T.H.; Lønborg, A.; et al. Transformation-Associated Changes in Sphingolipid Metabolism Sensitize Cells to Lysosomal Cell Death Induced by Inhibitors of Acid Sphingomyelinase. *Cancer Cell* **2013**, *24*, 379–393. [CrossRef] [PubMed]
673. Javanainen, M.; Martinez-Seara, H. Efficient preparation and analysis of membrane and membrane protein systems. *Biochim. Biophys. Acta-Biomembr.* **2016**, *1858*, 2468–2482. [CrossRef]
674. Venable, R.M.; Brown, F.L.H.; Pastor, R.W. Mechanical properties of lipid bilayers from molecular dynamics simulation. *Chem. Phys. Lipids* **2015**, *192*, 60–74. [CrossRef] [PubMed]
675. Pan, J.; Heberle, F.A.; Tristram-Nagle, S.; Szymanski, M.; Koepfinger, M.; Katsaras, J.; Kučerka, N. Molecular structures of fluid phase phosphatidylglycerol bilayers as determined by small angle neutron and X-ray scattering. *Biochim. Biophys. Acta-Biomembr.* **2012**, *1818*, 2135–2148. [CrossRef]
676. Nagle, J.F.; Tristram-Nagle, S. Structure of lipid bilayers. *Biochim. Biophys. Acta-Rev. Biomembr.* **2000**, *1469*, 159–195. [CrossRef]

677. Kučerka, N.; Heberle, F.A.; Pan, J.; Katsaras, J. Structural significance of lipid diversity as studied by small angle neutron and X-ray scattering. *Membranes* **2015**, *5*, 454–472. [CrossRef]
678. Vermeer, L.S.; de Groot, B.L.; Réat, V.; Milon, A.; Czaplicki, J. Acyl chain order parameter profiles in phospholipid bilayers: Computation from molecular dynamics simulations and comparison with 2H NMR experiments. *Eur. Biophys. J.* **2007**, *36*, 919–931. [CrossRef] [PubMed]
679. Lafleur, M.; Fine, B.; Sternin, E.; Cullis, P.R.; Bloom, M. Smoothed orientational order profile of lipid bilayers by 2H-nuclear magnetic resonance. *Biophys. J.* **1989**, *56*, 1037–1041. [CrossRef]
680. Ollila, S.O.H.; Róg, T.; Karttunen, M.; Vattulainen, I. Role of sterol type on lateral pressure profiles of lipid membranes affecting membrane protein functionality: Comparison between cholesterol, desmosterol, 7-dehydrocholesterol and ketosterol. *J. Struct. Biol.* **2007**, *159*, 311–323. [CrossRef]
681. Xie, J.Y.; Ding, G.H.; Karttunen, M. Molecular dynamics simulations of lipid membranes with lateral force: Rupture and dynamic properties. *Biochim. Biophys. Acta-Biomembr.* **2014**, *1838*, 994–1002. [CrossRef] [PubMed]
682. Cantor, R.S. Lateral Pressures in Cell Membranes: A Mechanism for Modulation of Protein Function. *J. Phys. Chem. B* **1997**, *101*, 1723–1725. [CrossRef]
683. Cantor, R.S. The lateral pressure profile in membranes: A physical mechanism of general anesthesia. *Biochemistry* **1997**, *36*, 2339–2344. [CrossRef]
684. Cantor, R.S. The influence of membrane lateral pressures on simple geometric models of protein conformational equilibria. *Chem. Phys. Lipids* **1999**, *101*, 45–56. [CrossRef]
685. Lingwood, D.; Binnington, B.; Róg, T.; Vattulainen, I.; Grzybek, M.; Coskun, Ü.; Lingwood, C.A.; Simons, K. Cholesterol modulates glycolipid conformation and receptor activity. *Nat. Chem. Biol.* **2011**, *7*, 260–262. [CrossRef]
686. Bilkova, E.; Pleskot, R.; Rissanen, S.; Sun, S.; Czogalla, A.; Cwiklik, L.; Róg, T.; Vattulainen, I.; Cremer, P.S.; Jungwirth, P.; et al. Calcium Directly Regulates Phosphatidylinositol 4,5-Bisphosphate Headgroup Conformation and Recognition. *J. Am. Chem. Soc.* **2017**, *139*, 4019–4024. [CrossRef]
687. Pereira-Leite, C.; Nunes, C.; Reis, S. Interaction of nonsteroidal anti-inflammatory drugs with membranes: In vitro assessment and relevance for their biological actions. *Prog. Lipid Res.* **2013**, *52*, 571–584. [CrossRef]
688. Lichtenberger, L.M.; Zhou, Y.; Dial, E.J.; Raphael, R.M. NSAID injury to the gastrointestinal tract: Evidence that NSAIDs interact with phospholipids to weaken the hydrophobic surface barrier and induce the formation of unstable pores in membranes. *J. Pharm. Pharmacol.* **2006**, *58*, 1421–1428. [CrossRef] [PubMed]
689. Nunes, C.; Brezesinski, G.; Pereira-Leite, C.; Lima, J.L.F.C.; Reis, S.; Lúcio, M. NSAIDs interactions with membranes: A biophysical approach. *Langmuir* **2011**, *27*, 10847–10858. [CrossRef]
690. Pereira-Leite, C.; Figueiredo, M.; Burdach, K.; Nunes, C.; Reis, S. Unraveling the role of drug-lipid interactions in nsaids-induced cardiotoxicity. *Membranes* **2021**, *11*, 24. [CrossRef]
691. Overton, E. *Studien uber die Narkose Zugleich ein Beitrag zur Allgemeinen Pharmakologie*; Verlag von Gustav Fischer: Jena, Germany, 1901.
692. Meyer, H. Zur theorie der alkoholnarkose. *Naunyn. Schmiedebergs. Arch. Pharmacol.* **1899**, *42*, 109–118. [CrossRef]
693. Janoff, A.S.; Pringle, M.J.; Miller, K.W. Correlation of general anesthetic potency with solubility in membranes. *Biochim. Biophys. Acta* **1981**, *649*, 125–128. [CrossRef]
694. Oakes, V.; Domene, C. Capturing the Molecular Mechanism of Anesthetic Action by Simulation Methods. *Chem. Rev.* **2019**, *119*, 5998–6014. [CrossRef]
695. Reigada, R. Influence of chloroform in liquid-ordered and liquid-disordered phases in lipid membranes. *J. Phys. Chem. B* **2011**, *115*, 2527–2535. [CrossRef] [PubMed]
696. Turkyilmaz, S.; Chen, W.H.; Mitomo, H.; Regen, S.L. Loosening and reorganization of fluid phospholipid bilayers by chloroform. *J. Am. Chem. Soc.* **2009**, *131*, 5068–5069. [CrossRef] [PubMed]
697. De Vlugt, J.E.; Xiao, P.; Munro, R.; Charchoglyan, A.; Brewer, D.; Al-Abdul-Wahid, M.S.; Brown, L.S.; Ladizhansky, V. Identifying lipids tightly bound to an integral membrane protein. *Biochim. Biophys. Acta-Biomembr.* **2020**, *1862*, 183345. [CrossRef]
698. Sharma, V.; Belevich, G.; Gamiz-Hernandez, A.P.; Róg, T.; Vattulainen, I.; Verkhovskaya, M.L.; Wikström, M.; Hummer, G.; Kaila, V.R.I. Redox-induced activation of the proton pump in the respiratory complex I. *Proc. Natl. Acad. Sci. USA* **2015**, *112*, 11571–11576. [CrossRef]
699. Bruzzese, A.; Dalton, J.A.R.; Giraldo, J. Insights into adenosine A2A receptor activation through cooperative modulation of agonist and allosteric lipid interactions. *PLoS Comput. Biol.* **2020**, *16*, e1007818. [CrossRef]
700. Takahashi, H.; Yoshino, M.; Morita, K.; Takagi, T.; Yokoyama, Y.; Kikukawa, T.; Amii, H.; Kanamori, T.; Sonoyama, M. Stability of the two-dimensional lattice of bacteriorhodopsin reconstituted in partially fluorinated phosphatidylcholine bilayers. *Biochim. Biophys. Acta-Biomembr.* **2019**, *1861*, 631–642. [CrossRef]
701. Mao, X.; Yao, S.; Yi, Q.; Xu, Z.M.; Cang, X. Function-related asymmetry of the specific cardiolipin binding sites on the mitochondrial ADP/ATP carrier. *Biochim. Biophys. Acta-Biomembr.* **2021**, *1863*, 183466. [CrossRef]
702. Pöyry, S.; Cramariuc, O.; Postila, P.A.; Kaszuba, K.; Sarewicz, M.; Osyczka, A.; Vattulainen, I.; Róg, T.; Róg, T. Atomistic simulations indicate cardiolipin to have an integral role in the structure of the cytochrome bc1 complex. *Biochim. Biophys. Acta-Bioenerg.* **2013**, *1827*, 769–778. [CrossRef]

703. Škulj, S.; Brkljača, Z.; Vazdar, M. Molecular Dynamics Simulations of the Elusive Matrix-Open State of Mitochondrial ADP/ATP Carrier. *Isr. J. Chem.* **2020**, *60*, 735–743. [CrossRef]
704. Manna, M.; Nieminen, T.; Vattulainen, I. Understanding the Role of Lipids in Signaling Through Atomistic and Multiscale Simulations of Cell Membranes. *Annu. Rev. Biophys.* **2019**, *48*, 421–439. [CrossRef]
705. Jodaitis, L.; van Oene, T.; Martens, C. Assessing the role of lipids in the molecular mechanism of membrane proteins. *Int. J. Mol. Sci.* **2021**, *22*, 7267. [CrossRef] [PubMed]
706. Legler, D.F.; Matti, C.; Laufer, J.M.; Jakobs, B.D.; Purvanov, V.; Uetz-von Allmen, E.; Thelen, M. Modulation of Chemokine Receptor Function by Cholesterol: New Prospects for Pharmacological Intervention. *Mol. Pharmacol.* **2017**, *91*, 331–338. [CrossRef]
707. McGraw, C.; Yang, L.; Levental, I.; Lyman, E.; Robinson, A.S. Membrane cholesterol depletion reduces downstream signaling activity of the adenosine A 2A receptor. *Biochim. Biophys. Acta-Biomembr.* **2019**, *1861*, 760–767. [CrossRef] [PubMed]
708. Manna, M.; Niemelä, M.; Tynkkynen, J.; Javanainen, M.; Kulig, W.; Müller, D.J.; Róg, T.; Vattulainen, I. Mechanism of allosteric regulation of β 2 -adrenergic receptor by cholesterol. *Elife* **2016**, *5*, e18432. [CrossRef]
709. Delle Bovi, R.J.; Kim, J.H.; Suresh, P.; London, E.; Miller, W.T. Sterol structure dependence of insulin receptor and insulin-like growth factor 1 receptor activation. *Biochim. Biophys. Acta-Biomembr.* **2019**, *1861*, 819–826. [CrossRef]
710. Lemel, L.; Nieścierowicz, K.; García-Fernández, M.D.; Darré, L.; Durroux, T.; Busnelli, M.; Pezet, M.; Rébeillé, F.; Jouhet, J.; Mouillac, B.; et al. The ligand-bound state of a G protein-coupled receptor stabilizes the interaction of functional cholesterol molecules. *J. Lipid Res.* **2021**, *62*, 100059. [CrossRef]
711. Bovill, J.G. Mechanisms of anaesthesia: Time to say farewell to the Meyer-Overton rule. *Curr. Opin. Anaesthesiol.* **2000**, *13*, 433–436. [CrossRef]
712. Nury, H.; Van Renterghem, C.; Weng, Y.; Tran, A.; Baaden, M.; Dufresne, V.; Changeux, J.-P.; Sonner, J.M.; Delarue, M.; Corringer, P.-J.; et al. X-ray structures of general anesthetics bound to a pentameric ligand-gated ion channel. *Nature* **2011**, *469*, 428–431. [CrossRef] [PubMed]
713. Pan, J.; Chen, Q.; Willenbring, D.; Mowrey, D.; Kong, X.P.; Cohen, A.; Divito, C.B.; Xu, Y.; Tang, P. Structure of the pentameric ligand-gated ion channel GLIC bound with anesthetic ketamine. *Structure* **2012**, *20*, 1463–1469. [CrossRef] [PubMed]
714. Gamal El-Din, T.M.; Lenaeus, M.J.; Zheng, N.; Catterall, W.A. Fenestrations control resting-state block of a voltage-gated sodium channel. *Proc. Natl. Acad. Sci. USA* **2018**, *115*, 13111–13116. [CrossRef]
715. Liu, R.; Perez-Aguilar, J.M.; Liang, D.; Saven, J.G. Binding site and affinity prediction of general anesthetics to protein targets using docking. *Anesth. Analg.* **2012**, *114*, 947–955. [CrossRef]
716. Selkoe, D.J.; Hardy, J. The amyloid hypothesis of Alzheimer's disease at 25 years. *EMBO Mol. Med.* **2016**, *8*, 595–608. [CrossRef]
717. Scollo, F.; Rosa, C. La Amyloidogenic intrinsically disordered proteins: New insights into their self-assembly and their interaction with membranes. *Life* **2020**, *10*, 144. [CrossRef] [PubMed]
718. Errico, S.; Ramshini, H.; Capitini, C.; Canale, C.; Spaziano, M.; Barbut, D.; Calamai, M.; Zasloff, M.; Oropesa-Nuñez, R.; Vendruscolo, M.; et al. Quantitative Measurement of the Affinity of Toxic and Nontoxic Misfolded Protein Oligomers for Lipid Bilayers and of its Modulation by Lipid Composition and Trodusquemine. *ACS Chem. Neurosci.* **2021**, *12*, 3189–3202. [CrossRef]
719. Banchelli, M.; Cascella, R.; D'Andrea, C.; La Penna, G.; Li, M.S.; Machetti, F.; Matteini, P.; Pizzanelli, S. Probing the Structure of Toxic Amyloid-β Oligomers with Electron Spin Resonance and Molecular Modeling. *ACS Chem. Neurosci.* **2021**, *12*, 1150–1161. [CrossRef]
720. Manna, M.; Murarka, R.K. Polyunsaturated fatty acid modulates membrane-bound monomeric α-synuclein by modulating membrane microenvironment through preferential interactions. *ACS Chem. Neurosci.* **2021**, *12*, 675–688. [CrossRef]
721. Khayat, E.; Lockhart, C.; Delfing, B.M.; Smith, A.K.; Klimov, D.K. Met35 Oxidation Hinders Aβ25-35 Peptide Aggregation within the Dimyristoylphosphatidylcholine Bilayer. *ACS Chem. Neurosci.* **2021**, *12*, 3225–3236. [CrossRef]
722. Yang, Y.; Jalali, S.; Nilsson, B.L.; Dias, C.L. Binding Mechanisms of Amyloid-like Peptides to Lipid Bilayers and Effects of Divalent Cations. *ACS Chem. Neurosci.* **2021**, *12*, 2027–2035. [CrossRef]
723. Khayat, E.; Klimov, D.K.; Smith, A.K. Phosphorylation Promotes Aβ25-35 Peptide Aggregation within the DMPC Bilayer. *ACS Chem. Neurosci.* **2020**, *11*, 3430–3441. [CrossRef] [PubMed]
724. Banerjee, S.; Hashemi, M.; Zagorski, K.; Lyubchenko, Y.L. Cholesterol in membranes facilitates aggregation of amyloid β protein at physiologically relevant concentrations. *ACS Chem. Neurosci.* **2021**, *12*, 506–516. [CrossRef]
725. Owen, M.C.; Kulig, W.; Poojari, C.; Róg, T.; Strodel, B. Physiologically-relevant levels of sphingomyelin, but not GM1, induces a β-sheet-rich structure in the amyloid-β(1-42) monomer. *Biochim. Biophys. Acta-Biomembr.* **2018**, *1860*, 1709–1720. [CrossRef]
726. Dias, C.L.; Jalali, S.; Yang, Y.; Cruz, L. Role of Cholesterol on Binding of Amyloid Fibrils to Lipid Bilayers. *J. Phys. Chem. B* **2020**, *124*, 3036–3042. [CrossRef]
727. Ngo, S.T.; Nguyen, P.H.; Derreumaux, P. Cholesterol Molecules Alter the Energy Landscape of Small Aβ1-42 Oligomers. *J. Phys. Chem. B* **2021**, *125*, 2299–2307. [CrossRef]
728. Ngo, S.T.; Nguyen, P.H.; Derreumaux, P. Impact of the rat R5G, Y10F, and H13R mutations on tetrameric Aβ42 β-barrel in a lipid bilayer membrane model. *J. Phys. Chem. B* **2021**, *125*, 3105–3113. [CrossRef] [PubMed]
729. Kawasaki, T.; Man, V.H.; Sugimoto, Y.; Sugiyama, N.; Yamamoto, H.; Tsukiyama, K.; Wang, J.; Derreumaux, P.; Nguyen, P.H. Infrared Laser-Induced Amyloid Fibril Dissociation: A Joint Experimental/Theoretical Study on the GNNQQNY Peptide. *J. Phys. Chem. B* **2020**, *124*, 6266–6277. [CrossRef] [PubMed]

730. Kurochka, A.S.; Yushchenko, D.A.; Bouř, P.; Shvadchak, V.V. Influence of lipid membranes on α-synuclein aggregation. *ACS Chem. Neurosci.* **2021**, *12*, 825–830. [CrossRef]
731. Doig, A.J.; Derreumaux, P. Inhibition of protein aggregation and amyloid formation by small molecules. *Curr. Opin. Struct. Biol.* **2015**, *30*, 50–56. [CrossRef]
732. Mrdenovic, D.; Zarzycki, P.; Majewska, M.; Pieta, I.S.; Nowakowski, R.; Kutner, W.; Lipkowski, J.; Pieta, P. Inhibition of Amyloid β-Induced Lipid Membrane Permeation and Amyloid β Aggregation by K162. *ACS Chem. Neurosci.* **2021**, *12*, 531–541. [CrossRef] [PubMed]
733. Barrero-Sicilia, C.; Silvestre, S.; Haslam, R.P.; Michaelson, L.V. Lipid remodelling: Unravelling the response to cold stress in Arabidopsis and its extremophile relative Eutrema salsugineum. *Plant Sci.* **2017**, *263*, 194–200. [CrossRef] [PubMed]
734. Hassan, N.; Anesio, A.M.; Rafiq, M.; Holtvoeth, J.; Bull, I.; Haleem, A.; Shah, A.A.; Hasan, F. Temperature Driven Membrane Lipid Adaptation in Glacial Psychrophilic Bacteria. *Front. Microbiol.* **2020**, *11*, 824. [CrossRef]
735. Siliakus, M.F.; van der Oost, J.; Kengen, S.W.M. Adaptations of archaeal and bacterial membranes to variations in temperature, pH and pressure. *Extremophiles* **2017**, *21*, 651–670. [CrossRef]
736. Bejaoui, F.; Salas, J.J.; Nouairi, I.; Smaoui, A.; Abdelly, C.; Martínez-Force, E.; Youssef, N. Ben Changes in chloroplast lipid contents and chloroplast ultrastructure in Sulla carnosa and Sulla coronaria leaves under salt stress. *J. Plant Physiol.* **2016**, *198*, 32–38. [CrossRef] [PubMed]
737. Kotnik, T.; Rems, L.; Tarek, M.; Miklavcic, D. Membrane Electroporation and Electropermeabilization: Mechanisms and Models. *Annu. Rev. Biophys.* **2019**, *48*, 63–91. [CrossRef]
738. Koshiyama, K.; Kodama, T.; Yano, T.; Fujikawa, S. Molecular dynamics simulation of structural changes of lipid bilayers induced by shock waves: Effects of incident angles. *Biochim. Biophys. Acta-Biomembr.* **2008**, *1778*, 1423–1428. [CrossRef]
739. Man, V.H.; Li, M.S.; Wang, J.; Derreumaux, P.; Nguyen, P.H. Interaction mechanism between the focused ultrasound and lipid membrane at the molecular level. *J. Chem. Phys.* **2019**, *150*, 215101. [CrossRef]
740. Gurtovenko, A.A.; Vattulainen, I. Pore formation coupled to ion transport through lipid membranes as induced by transmembrane ionic charge imbalance: Atomistic molecular dynamics study. *J. Am. Chem. Soc.* **2005**, *127*, 17570–17571. [CrossRef]
741. Lin, J.; Dargazany, R.; Alexander-Katz, A. Lipid Flip-Flop and Pore Nucleation on Zwitterionic Bilayers are Asymmetric under Ionic Imbalance. *Small* **2017**, *13*, 1603708. [CrossRef]
742. Lete, M.G.; Monasterio, B.G.; Collado, M.I.; Medina, M.; Sot, J.; Alonso, A.; Goñi, F.M. Fast and slow biomembrane solubilizing detergents: Insights into their mechanism of action. *Colloids Surf. B Biointerfaces* **2019**, *183*, 110430. [CrossRef]
743. Lichtenberg, D.; Ahyayauch, H.; Alonso, A.; Goñi, F.M. Detergent solubilization of lipid bilayers: A balance of driving forces. *Trends Biochem. Sci.* **2013**, *38*, 85–93. [CrossRef] [PubMed]
744. Dyrda, G.; Boniewska-Bernacka, E.; Man, D.; Barchiewicz, K.; Słota, R. The effect of organic solvents on selected microorganisms and model liposome membrane. *Mol. Biol. Rep.* **2019**, *46*, 3225–3232. [CrossRef] [PubMed]
745. Clarke, R.J.; Hossain, K.R.; Cao, K. Physiological roles of transverse lipid asymmetry of animal membranes. *Biochim. Biophys. Acta-Biomembr.* **2020**, *1862*, 183382. [CrossRef] [PubMed]
746. Chang, W.; Fa, H.; Xiao, D.; Wang, J. Targeting phosphatidylserine for Cancer therapy: Prospects and challenges. *Theranostics* **2020**, *10*, 9214–9229. [CrossRef] [PubMed]
747. Ma, R.; Kwok, H.F. New opportunities and challenges of venom-based and bacteria-derived molecules for anticancer targeted therapy. *Semin. Cancer Biol.* **2020**. [CrossRef] [PubMed]
748. Bernardes, N.; Fialho, A.M. Perturbing the dynamics and organization of cell membrane components: A new paradigm for cancer-targeted therapies. *Int. J. Mol. Sci.* **2018**, *19*, 3871. [CrossRef]
749. Nakatsuji, T.; Gallo, R.L. Antimicrobial peptides: Old molecules with new ideas. *J. Invest. Dermatol.* **2012**, *132*, 887–895. [CrossRef]
750. Wang, G.; Li, X.; Wang, Z. APD3: The antimicrobial peptide database as a tool for research and education. *Nucleic Acids Res.* **2016**, *44*, D1087–D1093. [CrossRef]
751. Pirtskhalava, M.; Amstrong, A.A.; Grigolava, M.; Chubinidze, M.; Alimbarashvili, E.; Vishnepolsky, B.; Gabrielian, A.; Rosenthal, A.; Hurt, D.E.; Tartakovsky, M. DBAASP v3: Database of antimicrobial/cytotoxic activity and structure of peptides as a resource for development of new therapeutics. *Nucleic Acids Res.* **2021**, *49*, D288–D297. [CrossRef]
752. Jhong, J.H.; Chi, Y.H.; Li, W.C.; Lin, T.H.; Huang, K.Y.; Lee, T.Y. DbAMP: An integrated resource for exploring antimicrobial peptides with functional activities and physicochemical properties on transcriptome and proteome data. *Nucleic Acids Res.* **2019**, *47*, D285–D297. [CrossRef] [PubMed]
753. Waghu, F.H.; Barai, R.S.; Gurung, P.; Idicula-Thomas, S. CAMPR3: A database on sequences, structures and signatures of antimicrobial peptides. *Nucleic Acids Res.* **2016**, *44*, D1094–D1097. [CrossRef]
754. Zhao, X.; Wu, H.; Lu, H.; Li, G.; Huang, Q. LAMP: A Database Linking Antimicrobial Peptides. *PLoS ONE* **2013**, *8*, e66557. [CrossRef]
755. Seebah, S.; Suresh, A.; Zhuo, S.; Choong, Y.H.; Chua, H.; Chuon, D.; Beuerman, R.; Verma, C. Defensins knowledgebase: A manually curated database and information source focused on the defensins family of antimicrobial peptides. *Nucleic Acids Res.* **2007**, *35*, D265–D268. [CrossRef]
756. Mulvenna, J.P.; Wang, C.; Craik, D.J. CyBase: A database of cyclic protein sequence and structure. *Nucleic Acids Res.* **2006**, *34*, D192–D194. [CrossRef]

757. Hammami, R.; Ben Hamida, J.; Vergoten, G.; Fliss, I. PhytAMP: A database dedicated to antimicrobial plant peptides. *Nucleic Acids Res.* **2009**, *37*, D963–D968. [CrossRef]
758. Das, D.; Jaiswal, M.; Khan, F.N.; Ahamad, S.; Kumar, S. PlantPepDB: A manually curated plant peptide database. *Sci. Rep.* **2020**, *10*, 2194. [CrossRef] [PubMed]
759. Liu, S.; Fan, L.; Sun, J.; Lao, X.; Zheng, H. Computational resources and tools for antimicrobial peptides. *J. Pept. Sci.* **2017**, *23*, 4–12. [CrossRef] [PubMed]
760. Santos-Silva, C.A.D.; Zupin, L.; Oliveira-Lima, M.; Vilela, L.M.B.; Bezerra-Neto, J.P.; Ferreira-Neto, J.R.; Ferreira, J.D.C.; Oliveira-Silva, R.L.; de Pires, C.J.; Aburjaile, F.F.; et al. Plant Antimicrobial Peptides: State of the Art, In Silico Prediction and Perspectives in the Omics Era. *Bioinform. Biol. Insights* **2020**, *14*, 1177932220952739. [CrossRef]
761. Kang, X.; Dong, F.; Shi, C.; Liu, S.; Sun, J.; Chen, J.; Li, H.; Xu, H.; Lao, X.; Zheng, H. DRAMP 2.0, an updated data repository of antimicrobial peptides. *Sci. Data* **2019**, *6*, 148. [CrossRef] [PubMed]
762. Chen, C.H.; Lu, T.K. Development and challenges of antimicrobial peptides for therapeutic applications. *Antibiotics* **2020**, *9*, 24. [CrossRef]
763. Cardoso, P.; Glossop, H.; Meikle, T.G.; Aburto-Medina, A.; Conn, C.E.; Sarojini, V.; Valery, C. Molecular engineering of antimicrobial peptides: Microbial targets, peptide motifs and translation opportunities. *Biophys. Rev.* **2021**, *13*, 1–35. [CrossRef] [PubMed]
764. Lazzaro, B.P.; Zasloff, M.; Rolff, J. Antimicrobial peptides: Application informed by evolution. *Science* **2020**, *368*, eaau5480. [CrossRef] [PubMed]
765. Roncevic, T.; Puizina, J.; Tossi, A. Antimicrobial Peptides as Anti-Infective Agents in Pre-Post-Antibiotic Era? *Int. J. Mol. Sci.* **2019**, *20*, 5713. [CrossRef] [PubMed]
766. Guha, S.; Ghimire, J.; Wu, E.; Wimley, W.C. Mechanistic Landscape of Membrane-Permeabilizing Peptides. *Chem. Rev.* **2019**, *119*, 6040–6085. [CrossRef]
767. Bhandari, D.; Rafiq, S.; Gat, Y.; Gat, P.; Waghmare, R.; Kumar, V. A Review on Bioactive Peptides: Physiological Functions, Bioavailability and Safety. *Int. J. Pept. Res. Ther.* **2020**, *26*, 139–150. [CrossRef]
768. Huan, Y.; Kong, Q.; Mou, H.; Yi, H. Antimicrobial Peptides: Classification, Design, Application and Research Progress in Multiple Fields. *Front. Microbiol.* **2020**, *11*, 582779. [CrossRef]
769. Datta, S.; Roy, A. Antimicrobial Peptides as Potential Therapeutic Agents: A Review. *Int. J. Pept. Res. Ther.* **2021**, *27*, 555–577. [CrossRef]
770. Gan, B.H.; Gaynord, J.; Rowe, S.M.; Deingruber, T.; Spring, D.R. The multifaceted nature of antimicrobial peptides: Current synthetic chemistry approaches and future directions. *Chem. Soc. Rev.* **2021**, 7820–7880. [CrossRef] [PubMed]
771. Li, W.; Separovic, F.; O'Brien-Simpson, N.M.; Wade, J.D. Chemically modified and conjugated antimicrobial peptides against superbugs. *Chem. Soc. Rev.* **2021**, *50*, 4932–4973. [CrossRef] [PubMed]
772. Boparai, J.K.; Sharma, P.K. Mini Review on Antimicrobial Peptides, Sources, Mechanism and Recent Applications. *Protein Pept. Lett.* **2020**, *27*, 4–16. [CrossRef]
773. Wang, J.; Dou, X.; Song, J.; Lyu, Y.; Zhu, X.; Xu, L.; Li, W.; Shan, A. Antimicrobial peptides: Promising alternatives in the post feeding antibiotic era. *Med. Res. Rev.* **2019**, *39*, 831–859. [CrossRef]
774. Pirtskhalava, M.; Vishnepolsky, B.; Grigolava, M.; Managadze, G. Physicochemical features and peculiarities of interaction of amp with the membrane. *Pharmaceuticals* **2021**, *14*, 471. [CrossRef]
775. Felício, M.R.; Silva, O.N.; Gonçalves, S.; Santos, N.C.; Franco, O.L. Peptides with dual antimicrobial and anticancer activities. *Front. Chem.* **2017**, *5*, 5. [CrossRef]
776. Roque-borda, C.A.; da Silva, P.B.; Rodrigues, M.C.; Azevedo, R.B.; Di Filippo, L.; Duarte, J.L.; Chorilli, M.; Vicente, E.F.; Pavan, F.R. Challenge in the discovery of new drugs: Antimicrobial peptides against who-list of critical and high-priority bacteria. *Pharmaceutics* **2021**, *13*, 773. [CrossRef]
777. Gradisteanu Pircalabioru, G.; Popa, L.I.; Marutescu, L.; Gheorghe, I.; Popa, M.; Czobor Barbu, I.; Cristescu, R.; Chifiriuc, M.C. Bacteriocins in the era of antibiotic resistance: Rising to the challenge. *Pharmaceutics* **2021**, *13*, 196. [CrossRef]
778. Stiltner, J.; McCandless, K.; Zahid, M. Cell-penetrating peptides: Applications in tumor diagnosis and therapeutics. *Pharmaceutics* **2021**, *13*, 890. [CrossRef] [PubMed]
779. Gaspar, D.; Salomé Veiga, A.; Castanho, M.A.R.B. From antimicrobial to anticancer peptides. A review. *Front. Microbiol.* **2013**, *4*, 294. [CrossRef] [PubMed]
780. Mahlapuu, M.; Håkansson, J.; Ringstad, L.; Björn, C. Antimicrobial peptides: An emerging category of therapeutic agents. *Front. Cell. Infect. Microbiol.* **2016**, *6*, 194. [CrossRef] [PubMed]
781. Li, J.; Koh, J.J.; Liu, S.; Lakshminarayanan, R.; Verma, C.S.; Beuerman, R.W. Membrane active antimicrobial peptides: Translating mechanistic insights to design. *Front. Neurosci.* **2017**, *11*, 73. [CrossRef] [PubMed]
782. Sani, M.A.; Separovic, F. Antimicrobial Peptide Structures: From Model Membranes to Live Cells. *Chem.—A Eur. J.* **2018**, *24*, 286–291. [CrossRef]
783. Kang, H.K.; Kim, C.; Seo, C.H.; Park, Y. The therapeutic applications of antimicrobial peptides (AMPs): A patent review. *J. Microbiol.* **2017**, *55*, 1–12. [CrossRef]
784. Mookherjee, N.; Anderson, M.A.; Haagsman, H.P.; Davidson, D.J. Antimicrobial host defence peptides: Functions and clinical potential. *Nat. Rev. Drug Discov.* **2020**, *19*, 311–332. [CrossRef] [PubMed]

785. Hammond, K.; Ryadnov, M.G.; Hoogenboom, B.W. Atomic force microscopy to elucidate how peptides disrupt membranes. *Biochim. Biophys. Acta-Biomembr.* **2021**, *1863*, 183447. [CrossRef] [PubMed]
786. Aschi, M.; Bozzi, A.; Luzi, C.; Bouchemal, N.; Sette, M. Crabrolin, a natural antimicrobial peptide: Structural properties. *J. Pept. Sci.* **2017**, *23*, 693–700. [CrossRef] [PubMed]
787. Mura, M.; Wang, J.; Zhou, Y.; Pinna, M.; Zvelindovsky, A.V.; Dennison, S.R.; Phoenix, D.A. The effect of amidation on the behaviour of antimicrobial peptides. *Eur. Biophys. J.* **2016**, *45*, 195–207. [CrossRef]
788. Ulmschneider, J.P.; Smith, J.C.; Ulmschneider, M.B.; Ulrich, A.S.; Strandberg, E. Reorientation and dimerization of the membrane-bound antimicrobial peptide pgla from microsecond all-atom MD simulations. *Biophys. J.* **2012**, *103*, 472–482. [CrossRef]
789. Ramos-Martín, F.; D'Amelio, N. Molecular basis of the anticancer and antibacterial properties of cecropinXJ peptide: An in silico study. *Int. J. Mol. Sci.* **2021**, *22*, 691. [CrossRef]
790. Pourmousa, M.; Karttunen, M. Early stages of interactions of cell-penetrating peptide penetratin with a DPPC bilayer. *Chem. Phys. Lipids* **2013**, *169*, 85–94. [CrossRef]
791. Mura, M.; Dennison, S.R.; Zvelindovsky, A.V.; Phoenix, D.A. Aurein 2.3 functionality is supported by oblique orientated α-helical formation. *Biochim. Biophys. Acta-Biomembr.* **2013**, *1828*, 586–594. [CrossRef] [PubMed]
792. Sahoo, B.R.; Fujiwara, T. Membrane mediated antimicrobial and antitumor activity of cathelicidin 6: Structural insights from molecular dynamics simulation on multi-microsecond scale. *PLoS ONE* **2016**, *11*, e0158702. [CrossRef] [PubMed]
793. Zhao, L.; Cao, Z.; Bian, Y.; Hu, G.; Wang, J.; Zhou, Y. Molecular dynamics simulations of human antimicrobial peptide LL-37 in model POPC and POPG lipid bilayers. *Int. J. Mol. Sci.* **2018**, *19*, 1186. [CrossRef]
794. Zhang, L. Disulfide Bonds Affect the Binding Sites of Human β Defensin Type 3 on Negatively Charged Lipid Membranes. *J. Phys. Chem. B* **2020**, *124*, 2088–2100. [CrossRef] [PubMed]
795. Pandit, G.; Biswas, K.; Ghosh, S.; Debnath, S.; Bidkar, A.P.; Satpati, P.; Bhunia, A.; Chatterjee, S. Rationally designed antimicrobial peptides: Insight into the mechanism of eleven residue peptides against microbial infections. *Biochim. Biophys. Acta-Biomembr.* **2020**, *1862*, 183177. [CrossRef] [PubMed]
796. Reißer, S.; Strandberg, E.; Steinbrecher, T.; Elstner, M.; Ulrich, A.S. Best of Two Worlds? How MD Simulations of Amphiphilic Helical Peptides in Membranes Can Complement Data from Oriented Solid-State NMR. *J. Chem. Theory Comput.* **2018**, *14*, 6002–6014. [CrossRef]
797. Ermondi, G.; Vallaro, M.; Camacho-Leal, M.P.; Potter, T.; Visentin, S.; Caron, G. Charged cyclic hexapeptides: Updating molecular descriptors for permeability purposes. *Eur. J. Pharm. Sci.* **2018**, *122*, 85–93. [CrossRef]
798. Aschi, M.; Perini, N.; Bouchemal, N.; Luzi, C.; Savarin, P.; Migliore, L.; Bozzi, A.; Sette, M. Structural characterization and biological activity of Crabrolin peptide isoforms with different positive charge. *Biochim. Biophys. Acta-Biomembr.* **2020**, *1862*, 183055. [CrossRef]
799. Duay, S.S.; Sharma, G.; Prabhakar, R.; Angeles-Boza, A.M.; May, E.R. Molecular Dynamics Investigation into the Effect of Zinc(II) on the Structure and Membrane Interactions of the Antimicrobial Peptide Clavanin A. *J. Phys. Chem. B* **2019**, *123*, 3163–3176. [CrossRef]
800. Jafari, M.; Mehrnejad, F.; Aghdami, R.; Chaparzadeh, N.; Razaghi Moghadam Kashani, Z.; Doustdar, F. Identification of the Crucial Residues in the Early Insertion of Pardaxin into Different Phospholipid Bilayers. *J. Chem. Inf. Model.* **2017**, *57*, 929–941. [CrossRef]
801. Song, C.; de Groot, B.L.; Sansom, M.S.P. Lipid Bilayer Composition Influences the Activity of the Antimicrobial Peptide Dermcidin Channel. *Biophys. J.* **2019**, *116*, 1658–1666. [CrossRef]
802. Fernandez, J.; Acosta, G.; Pulido, D.; Malý, M.; Copa-Patiño, J.L.; Soliveri, J.; Royo, M.; Gómez, R.; Albericio, F.; Ortega, P.; et al. Carbosilane Dendron-Peptide Nanoconjugates as Antimicrobial Agents. *Mol. Pharm.* **2019**, *16*, 2661–2674. [CrossRef]
803. Grasso, G.; Muscat, S.; Rebella, M.; Morbiducci, U.; Audenino, A.; Danani, A.; Deriu, M.A. Cell penetrating peptide modulation of membrane biomechanics by Molecular dynamics. *J. Biomech.* **2018**, *73*, 137–144. [CrossRef]
804. Irudayam, S.J.; Berkowitz, M.L. Binding and reorientation of melittin in a POPC bilayer: Computer simulations. *Biochim. Biophys. Acta-Biomembr.* **2012**, *1818*, 2975–2981. [CrossRef] [PubMed]
805. Lee, H.; Kim, H.R.; Larson, R.G.; Park, J.C. Effects of the size, shape, and structural transition of thermosensitive polypeptides on the stability of lipid bilayers and liposomes. *Macromolecules* **2012**, *45*, 7304–7312. [CrossRef]
806. Jafari, M.; Mehrnejad, F.; Doustdar, F. Insight into the interactions, residue snorkeling, and membrane disordering potency of a single antimicrobial peptide into different lipid bilayers. *PLoS ONE* **2017**, *12*, e0187216. [CrossRef]
807. Liu, J.; Xiao, S.; Li, J.; Yuan, B.; Yang, K.; Ma, Y. Molecular details on the intermediate states of melittin action on a cell membrane. *Biochim. Biophys. Acta-Biomembr.* **2018**, *1860*, 2234–2241. [CrossRef]
808. Waghu, F.H.; Joseph, S.; Ghawali, S.; Martis, E.A.; Madan, T.; Venkatesh, K.V.; Idicula-Thomas, S. Designing antibacterial peptides with enhanced killing kinetics. *Front. Microbiol.* **2018**, *9*, 325. [CrossRef]
809. Ashrafuzzaman, M.; Tseng, C.Y.; Tuszynski, J.A. Charge-based interactions of antimicrobial peptides and general drugs with lipid bilayers. *J. Mol. Graph. Model.* **2020**, *95*, 107502. [CrossRef]
810. Cao, Z.; Liu, L.; Hu, G.; Bian, Y.; Li, H.; Wang, J.; Zhou, Y. Interplay of hydrophobic and hydrophilic interactions in sequence-dependent cell penetration of spontaneous membrane-translocating peptides revealed by bias-exchange metadynamics simulations. *Biochim. Biophys. Acta-Biomembr.* **2020**, *1862*, 183402. [CrossRef] [PubMed]

811. Walrant, A.; Bauzá, A.; Girardet, C.; Alves, I.D.; Lecomte, S.; Illien, F.; Cardon, S.; Chaianantakul, N.; Pallerla, M.; Burlina, F.; et al. Ionpair-π interactions favor cell penetration of arginine/tryptophan-rich cell-penetrating peptides. *Biochim. Biophys. Acta-Biomembr.* **2020**, *1862*, 183098. [CrossRef] [PubMed]
812. Capozzi, E.; Aureli, S.; Minicozzi, V.; Rossi, G.C.; Stellato, F.; Morante, S. Designing effective anticancer-radiopeptides. A Molecular Dynamics study of their interaction with model tumor and healthy cell membranes. *Biochim. Biophys. Acta-Biomembr.* **2018**, *1860*, 2348–2355. [CrossRef]
813. Ma, R.; Wong, S.W.; Ge, L.; Shaw, C.; Siu, S.W.I.; Kwok, H.F. In Vitro and MD Simulation Study to Explore Physicochemical Parameters for Antibacterial Peptide to Become Potent Anticancer Peptide. *Mol. Ther.-Oncolytics* **2020**, *16*, 7–19. [CrossRef]
814. Song, J.; Zhang, W.; Kai, M.; Chen, J.; Liang, R.; Zheng, X.; Li, G.; Zhang, B.; Wang, K.; Zhang, Y.; et al. Design of an acid-activated antimicrobial peptide for tumor therapy. *Mol. Pharm.* **2013**, *10*, 2934–2941. [CrossRef] [PubMed]
815. Sinha, S.; Zheng, L.; Mu, Y.; Ng, W.J.; Bhattacharjya, S. Structure and interactions of a host defense antimicrobial peptide thanatin in lipopolysaccharide micelles reveal mechanism of bacterial cell agglutination. *Sci. Rep.* **2017**, *7*, 17795. [CrossRef]
816. Brožek, R.; Kabelka, I.; Vácha, R. Effect of Helical Kink on Peptide Translocation across Phospholipid Membranes. *J. Phys. Chem. B* **2020**, *124*, 5940–5947. [CrossRef] [PubMed]
817. Tuerkova, A.; Kabelka, I.; Králová, T.; Sukeník, L.; Pokorná, Š.; Hof, M.; Vácha, R. Effect of Helical Kink in Antimicrobial Peptides on Membrane Pore Formation. *Elife* **2020**, *9*, e47946. [CrossRef] [PubMed]
818. Mihajlovic, M.; Lazaridis, T. Antimicrobial peptides in toroidal and cylindrical pores. *Biochim. Biophys. Acta-Biomembr.* **2010**, *1798*, 1485–1493. [CrossRef]
819. Mihajlovic, M.; Lazaridis, T. Charge distribution and imperfect amphipathicity affect pore formation by antimicrobial peptides. *Biochim. Biophys. Acta-Biomembr.* **2012**, *1818*, 1274–1283. [CrossRef]
820. Lyu, Y.; Zhu, X.; Xiang, N.; Narsimhan, G. Molecular Dynamics Study of Pore Formation by Melittin in a 1,2-Dioleoyl-sn-glycero-3-phosphocholine and 1,2-Di(9Z-octadecenoyl)-sn-glycero-3-phospho-(1′-rac-glycerol) Mixed Lipid Bilayer. *Ind. Eng. Chem. Res.* **2015**, *54*, 10275–10283. [CrossRef]
821. Sun, D.; Forsman, J.; Woodward, C.E. Amphipathic membrane-active peptides recognize and stabilize ruptured membrane pores: Exploring cause and effect with coarse-grained simulations. *Langmuir* **2015**, *31*, 752–761. [CrossRef]
822. Santo, K.P.; Berkowitz, M.L. Difference between magainin-2 and melittin assemblies in phosphatidylcholine bilayers: Results from coarse-grained simulations. *J. Phys. Chem. B* **2012**, *116*, 3021–3030. [CrossRef]
823. Hu, Y.; Sinha, S.K.; Patel, S. Investigating Hydrophilic Pores in Model Lipid Bilayers Using Molecular Simulations: Correlating Bilayer Properties with Pore-Formation Thermodynamics. *Langmuir* **2015**, *31*, 6615–6631. [CrossRef] [PubMed]
824. Santo, K.P.; Irudayam, S.J.; Berkowitz, M.L. Melittin creates transient pores in a lipid bilayer: Results from computer simulations. *J. Phys. Chem. B* **2013**, *117*, 5031–5042. [CrossRef] [PubMed]
825. Li, J.; Lu, X.; Ma, W.; Chen, Z.; Sun, S.; Wang, Q.; Yuan, B.; Yang, K. Cholesterols Work as a Molecular Regulator of the Antimicrobial Peptide-Membrane Interactions. *Front. Mol. Biosci.* **2021**, *8*, 638988. [CrossRef]
826. Sun, D.; Forsman, J.; Woodward, C.E. Multistep Molecular Dynamics Simulations Identify the Highly Cooperative Activity of Melittin in Recognizing and Stabilizing Membrane Pores. *Langmuir* **2015**, *31*, 9388–9401. [CrossRef] [PubMed]
827. Sun, D.; Forsman, J.; Woodward, C.E. Molecular Simulations of Melittin-Induced Membrane Pores. *J. Phys. Chem. B* **2017**, *121*, 10209–10214. [CrossRef]
828. Wang, Y.; Chen, C.H.; Hu, D.; Ulmschneider, M.B.; Ulmschneider, J.P. Spontaneous formation of structurally diverse membrane channel architectures from a single antimicrobial peptide. *Nat. Commun.* **2016**, *7*, 13535. [CrossRef]
829. Talandashti, R.; Mehrnejad, F.; Rostamipour, K.; Doustdar, F.; Lavasanifar, A. Molecular Insights into Pore Formation Mechanism, Membrane Perturbation, and Water Permeation by the Antimicrobial Peptide Pleurocidin: A Combined All-Atom and Coarse-Grained Molecular Dynamics Simulation Study. *J. Phys. Chem. B* **2021**, *125*, 7163–7176. [CrossRef]
830. Chen, C.H.; Starr, C.G.; Troendle, E.; Wiedman, G.; Wimley, W.C.; Ulmschneider, J.P.; Ulmschneider, M.B. Simulation-Guided Rational de Novo Design of a Small Pore-Forming Antimicrobial Peptide. *J. Am. Chem. Soc.* **2019**, *141*, 4839–4848. [CrossRef]
831. Lorenzón, E.N.; Nobre, T.M.; Caseli, L.; Cilli, E.M.; da Hora, G.C.A.; Soares, T.A.; Oliveira, O.N. The "pre-assembled state" of magainin 2 lysine-linked dimer determines its enhanced antimicrobial activity. *Colloids Surf. B Biointerfaces* **2018**, *167*, 432–440. [CrossRef]
832. Miyazaki, Y.; Okazaki, S.; Shinoda, W. Free energy analysis of membrane pore formation process in the presence of multiple melittin peptides. *Biochim. Biophys. Acta-Biomembr.* **2019**, *1861*, 1409–1419. [CrossRef]
833. Lyu, Y.; Xiang, N.; Zhu, X.; Narsimhan, G. Potential of mean force for insertion of antimicrobial peptide melittin into a pore in mixed DOPC/DOPG lipid bilayer by molecular dynamics simulation. *J. Chem. Phys.* **2017**, *146*, 155101. [CrossRef] [PubMed]
834. Awasthi, N.; Kopec, W.; Wilkosz, N.; Jamróz, D.; Hub, J.S.; Zatorska, M.; Petka, R.; Nowakowska, M.; Kepczynski, M. Molecular Mechanism of Polycation-Induced Pore Formation in Biomembranes. *ACS Biomater. Sci. Eng.* **2019**, *5*, 780–794. [CrossRef]
835. Bennett, W.F.D.; Hong, C.K.; Wang, Y.; Tieleman, D.P. Antimicrobial Peptide Simulations and the Influence of Force Field on the Free Energy for Pore Formation in Lipid Bilayers. *J. Chem. Theory Comput.* **2016**, *12*, 4524–4533. [CrossRef] [PubMed]
836. Yesylevskyy, S.; Marrink, S.; Mark, A.E. Alternative Mechanisms for the Interaction of the Cell-Penetrating Peptides Penetratin and the TAT Peptide with Lipid Bilayers. *Biophysj* **2009**, *97*, 40–49. [CrossRef]
837. Simon, R.J.; Kania, R.S.; Zuckermann, R.N.; Huebner, V.D.; Jewell, D.A.; Banville, S.; Ng, S.; Wang, L.; Rosenberg, S.; Marlowe, C.K.; et al. Peptoids: A modular approach to drug discovery. *Proc. Natl. Acad. Sci. USA* **1992**, *89*, 9367–9371. [CrossRef]

838. Jin, H.; Jiao, F.; Daily, M.D.; Chen, Y.; Yan, F.; Ding, Y.H.; Zhang, X.; Robertson, E.J.; Baer, M.D.; Chen, C.-L. Highly stable and self-repairing membrane-mimetic 2D nanomaterials assembled from lipid-like peptoids. *Nat. Commun.* **2016**, *7*, 12252. [CrossRef] [PubMed]
839. Zhao, M.; Sampath, J.; Alamdari, S.; Shen, G.; Chen, C.L.; Mundy, C.J.; Pfaendtner, J.; Ferguson, A.L. MARTINI-Compatible Coarse-Grained Model for the Mesoscale Simulation of Peptoids. *J. Phys. Chem. B* **2020**, *124*, 7745–7764. [CrossRef]
840. Landry, M.R.; Rangel, J.L.; Dao, V.P.; Mackenzie, M.A.; Gutierrez, F.L.; Dowell, K.M.; Calkins, A.L.; Fuller, A.A.; Stokes, G.Y. Length and Charge of Water-Soluble Peptoids Impact Binding to Phospholipid Membranes. *J. Phys. Chem. B* **2019**, *123*, 5822–5831. [CrossRef]
841. Andreev, K.; Martynowycz, M.W.; Ivankin, A.; Huang, M.L.; Kuzmenko, I.; Meron, M.; Lin, B.; Kirshenbaum, K.; Gidalevitz, D. Cyclization Improves Membrane Permeation by Antimicrobial Peptoids. *Langmuir* **2016**, *32*, 12905–12913. [CrossRef]
842. Diamond, G.; Molchanova, N.; Herlan, C.; Fortkort, J.A.; Lin, J.S.; Figgins, E.; Bopp, N.; Ryan, L.K.; Chung, D.; Adcock, R.S.; et al. Potent antiviral activity against HSV-1 and SARS-CoV-2 by antimicrobial peptoids. *Pharmaceuticals* **2021**, *14*, 304. [CrossRef] [PubMed]
843. Koivuniemi, A.; Fallarero, A.; Bunker, A. Insight into the antimicrobial mechanism of action of β2,2-amino acid derivatives from molecular dynamics simulation: Dancing the can-can at the membrane surface. *Biochim. Biophys. Acta-Biomembr.* **2019**, *1861*, 183028. [CrossRef]
844. Sessa, L.; Concilio, S.; Walde, P.; Robinson, T.; Dittrich, P.S.; Porta, A.; Panunzi, B.; Caruso, U.; Piotto, S. Study of the interaction of a novel semi-synthetic peptide with model lipid membranes. *Membranes* **2020**, *10*, 294. [CrossRef]
845. Nourbakhsh, S.; Yu, L.; Ha, B.Y. Modeling the Protective Role of Bacterial Lipopolysaccharides against Membrane-Rupturing Peptides. *J. Phys. Chem. B* **2021**, *125*, 8839–8854. [CrossRef]
846. Mitra, M.; Asad, M.; Kumar, S.; Yadav, K.; Chaudhary, S.; Bhavesh, N.S.; Khalid, S.; Thukral, L.; Bajaj, A. Distinct intramolecular hydrogen bonding dictates antimicrobial action of membrane-targeting amphiphiles. *J. Phys. Chem. Lett.* **2019**, *10*, 754–760. [CrossRef] [PubMed]
847. Dalhoff, A.A. Membrane Interactions of Antibacterial Agents. *Trends Clin. Microbiol.* **2018**, *1*, 4–48.
848. Khondker, A.; Bider, R.C.; Passos-Gastaldo, I.; Wright, G.D.; Rheinstädter, M.C. Membrane interactions of non-membrane targeting antibiotics: The case of aminoglycosides, macrolides, and fluoroquinolones. *Biochim. Biophys. Acta-Biomembr.* **2021**, *1863*, 183448. [CrossRef] [PubMed]
849. Ashrafuzzaman, M.; Khan, Z.; Alqarni, A.; Alanazi, M.; Alam, M.S. Cell surface binding and lipid interactions behind chemotherapy-drug-induced ion pore formation in membranes. *Membranes* **2021**, *11*, 501. [CrossRef]
850. Annaval, T.; Ramos-Martin, F.; Herrera-Leon, C.; Adelaide, M.; Antonietti, V.; Buchoux, S.; Sonnet, P.; Sarazin, C.; D'Amelio, N. Antimicrobial Bombinin-like Peptide 3 Selectively Recognizes and Inserts into Bacterial Biomimetic Bilayers in Multiple Steps. *J. Med. Chem.* **2021**, *64*, 5185–5197. [CrossRef]
851. Petkov, P.; Lilkova, E.; Ilieva, N.; Litov, L. Self-association of antimicrobial peptides: A molecular dynamics simulation study on bombinin. *Int. J. Mol. Sci.* **2019**, *20*, 5450. [CrossRef]
852. Savini, F.; Loffredo, M.R.; Troiano, C.; Bobone, S.; Malanovic, N.; Eichmann, T.O.; Caprio, L.; Canale, V.C.; Park, Y.; Mangoni, M.L.; et al. Binding of an antimicrobial peptide to bacterial cells: Interaction with different species, strains and cellular components. *Biochim. Biophys. Acta-Biomembr.* **2020**, *1862*, 183291. [CrossRef] [PubMed]
853. Huang, H.W. DAPTOMYCIN, its membrane-active mechanism vs. that of other antimicrobial peptides. *Biochim. Biophys. Acta-Biomembr.* **2020**, *1862*, 183395. [CrossRef]
854. Mescola, A.; Ragazzini, G.; Alessandrini, A. Daptomycin Strongly Affects the Phase Behavior of Model Lipid Bilayers. *J. Phys. Chem. B* **2020**, *124*, 8562–8571. [CrossRef] [PubMed]
855. Liu, B.; Karttunen, M. Lipopeptide daptomycin: Interactions with bacterial and phospholipid membranes, stability of membrane aggregates and micellation in solution. *Biochim. Biophys. Acta-Biomembr.* **2018**, *1860*, 1949–1954. [CrossRef] [PubMed]
856. Ramos-Martín, F.; Herrera-León, C.; Antonietti, V.; Sonnet, P.; Sarazin, C.; D'amelio, N. Antimicrobial peptide k11 selectively recognizes bacterial biomimetic membranes and acts by twisting their bilayers. *Pharmaceuticals* **2021**, *14*, 1. [CrossRef]
857. Grishin, S.Y.; Domnin, P.A.; Kravchenko, S.V.; Azev, V.N.; Mustaeva, L.G.; Gorbunova, E.Y.; Kobyakova, M.I.; Surin, A.K.; Makarova, M.A.; Kurpe, S.R.; et al. Is It Possible to Create Antimicrobial Peptides Based on the Amyloidogenic Sequence of Ribosomal S1 Protein of P. aeruginosa? *Int. J. Mol. Sci.* **2021**, *22*, 9776. [CrossRef]
858. Shi, J.; Chen, C.; Wang, D.; Tong, Z.; Wang, Z.; Liu, Y. Amphipathic peptide antibiotics with potent activity against multidrug-resistant pathogens. *Pharmaceutics* **2021**, *13*, 438. [CrossRef]
859. Aguiar, L.; Pinheiro, M.; Neves, A.R.; Vale, N.; Defaus, S.; Andreu, D.; Reis, S.; Gomes, P. Insights into the membranolytic activity of antimalarial drug-cell penetrating peptide conjugates. *Membranes* **2021**, *11*, 4. [CrossRef]
860. Ohgita, T.; Takechi-Haraya, Y.; Okada, K.; Matsui, S.; Takeuchi, M.; Saito, C.; Nishitsuji, K.; Uchimura, K.; Kawano, R.; Hasegawa, K.; et al. Enhancement of direct membrane penetration of arginine-rich peptides by polyproline II helix structure. *Biochim. Biophys. Acta-Biomembr.* **2020**, *1862*, 183403. [CrossRef]
861. Strandberg, E.; Bentz, D.; Wadhwani, P.; Bürck, J.; Ulrich, A.S. Terminal charges modulate the pore forming activity of cationic amphipathic helices. *Biochim. Biophys. Acta-Biomembr.* **2020**, *1862*, 183243. [CrossRef]
862. Wu, E.; Jenschke, R.M.; Hristova, K.; Wimley, W.C. Rational Modulation of pH-Triggered Macromolecular Poration by Peptide Acylation and Dimerization. *J. Phys. Chem. B* **2020**, *124*, 8835–8843. [CrossRef] [PubMed]

863. Bansal, S.; Su, W.C.; Budamagunta, M.; Xiao, W.; Ajena, Y.; Liu, R.; Voss, J.C.; Carney, R.P.; Parikh, A.N.; Lam, K.S. Discovery and mechanistic characterization of a structurally-unique membrane active peptide. *Biochim. Biophys. Acta-Biomembr.* **2020**, *1862*, 183394. [CrossRef] [PubMed]
864. Lima, B.; Ricci, M.; Garro, A.; Juhász, T.; Szigyártó, I.C.; Papp, Z.I.; Feresin, G.; Garcia de la Torre, J.; Lopez Cascales, J.; Fülöp, L.; et al. New short cationic antibacterial peptides. Synthesis, biological activity and mechanism of action. *Biochim. Biophys. Acta-Biomembr.* **2021**, *1863*, 183665. [CrossRef] [PubMed]
865. Das, P.; Sercu, T.; Wadhawan, K.; Padhi, I.; Gehrmann, S.; Cipcigan, F.; Chenthamarakshan, V.; Strobelt, H.; dos Santos, C.; Chen, P.Y.; et al. Accelerated antimicrobial discovery via deep generative models and molecular dynamics simulations. *Nat. Biomed. Eng.* **2021**, *5*, 613–623. [CrossRef]
866. Chakraborty, A.; Kobzev, E.; Chan, J.; De Zoysa, G.H.; Sarojini, V.; Piggot, T.J.; Allison, J.R. Molecular Dynamics Simulation of the Interaction of Two Linear Battacin Analogs with Model Gram-Positive and Gram-Negative Bacterial Cell Membranes. *ACS Omega* **2021**, *6*, 388–400. [CrossRef]
867. Malik, E.; Phoenix, D.A.; Badiani, K.; Snape, T.J.; Harris, F.; Singh, J.; Morton, L.H.G.; Dennison, S.R. Biophysical studies on the antimicrobial activity of linearized esculentin 2EM. *Biochim. Biophys. Acta-Biomembr.* **2020**, *1862*, 183141. [CrossRef] [PubMed]
868. Abel, S.; Marchi, M. Deciphering the structure of the gramicidin A channel in the presence of AOT reverse micelles in pentane using molecular dynamics simulations. *J. Phys. Chem. B* **2021**, *124*, 11802–11818. [CrossRef]
869. Nawae, W.; Hannongbua, S.; Ruengjitchatchawalya, M. Defining the membrane disruption mechanism of kalata B1 via coarse-grained molecular dynamics simulations. *Sci. Rep.* **2014**, *4*, 3933. [CrossRef]
870. Rashid, M.M.O.; Moghal, M.M.R.; Billah, M.M.; Hasan, M.; Yamazaki, M. Effect of membrane potential on pore formation by the antimicrobial peptide magainin 2 in lipid bilayers. *Biochim. Biophys. Acta-Biomembr.* **2020**, *1862*, 183381. [CrossRef]
871. Amos, S.B.T.A.; Vermeer, L.S.; Ferguson, P.M.; Kozlowska, J.; Davy, M.; Bui, T.T.; Drake, A.F.; Lorenz, C.D.; Mason, A.J. Antimicrobial Peptide Potency is Facilitated by Greater Conformational Flexibility when Binding to Gram-negative Bacterial Inner Membranes. *Sci. Rep.* **2016**, *6*, 37639. [CrossRef]
872. Hong, J.; Lu, X.; Deng, Z.; Xiao, S.; Yuan, B.; Yang, K. How Melittin Inserts into Cell Membrane: And Disturbance on the Membrane. *Molecules* **2019**, *24*, 1775. [CrossRef]
873. Irudayam, S.J.; Pobandt, T.; Berkowitz, M.L. Free energy barrier for melittin reorientation from a membrane-bound state to a transmembrane state. *J. Phys. Chem. B* **2013**, *117*, 13457–13463. [CrossRef]
874. Manna, M.; Mukhopadhyay, C. Cause and effect of melittin-induced pore formation: A computational approach. *Langmuir* **2009**, *25*, 12235–12242. [CrossRef]
875. Leveritt, J.M.; Pino-Angeles, A.; Lazaridis, T. The structure of a melittin-stabilized pore. *Biophys. J.* **2015**, *108*, 2424–2426. [CrossRef] [PubMed]
876. Pal, S.; Chakraborty, H.; Chattopadhyay, A. Lipid Headgroup Charge Controls Melittin Oligomerization in Membranes: Implications in Membrane Lysis. *J. Phys. Chem. B* **2021**, *125*, 8450–8459. [CrossRef]
877. Koch, D.C.; Schmidt, T.H.; Sahl, H.G.; Kubitscheck, U.; Kandt, C. Structural dynamics of the cell wall precursor lipid II in the presence and absence of the lantibiotic nisin. *Biochim. Biophys. Acta-Biomembr.* **2014**, *1838*, 3061–3068. [CrossRef] [PubMed]
878. Jefferies, D.; Hsu, P.C.; Khalid, S. Through the Lipopolysaccharide Glass: A Potent Antimicrobial Peptide Induces Phase Changes in Membranes. *Biochemistry* **2017**, *56*, 1672–1679. [CrossRef] [PubMed]
879. Afanasyeva, E.F.; Syryamina, V.N.; De Zotti, M.; Formaggio, F.; Toniolo, C.; Dzuba, S.A. Peptide antibiotic trichogin in model membranes: Self-association and capture of fatty acids. *Biochim. Biophys. Acta-Biomembr.* **2019**, *1861*, 524–531. [CrossRef]
880. Arinaminpathy, Y.; Khurana, E.; Engelman, D.M.; Gerstein, M.B. Computational analysis of membrane proteins: The largest class of drug targets. *Drug Discov. Today* **2009**, *14*, 1130–1135. [CrossRef]
881. Yin, H.; Flynn, A.D. Drugging Membrane Protein Interactions. *Annu. Rev. Biomed. Eng.* **2016**, *18*, 51–76. [CrossRef]
882. Alballa, M.; Butler, G. Integrative approach for detecting membrane proteins. *BMC Bioinform.* **2020**, *21*, 575. [CrossRef] [PubMed]
883. Dobson, L.L.; Remenyi, I.; Tusnady, G.E.; Reményi, I.; Tusnády, G.E. The human transmembrane proteome. *Biol. Direct* **2015**, *10*, 31. [CrossRef]
884. Garrow, A.G.; Agnes, A.; Westhead, D.R.; Agnew, A.; Westhead, D.R. TMB-Hunt: An amino acid composition based method to screen proteomes for beta-barrel transmembrane proteins. *BMC Bioinform.* **2005**, *6*, 56. [CrossRef] [PubMed]
885. Potterton, A.; Husseini, F.S.; Southey, M.W.Y.; Bodkin, M.J.; Heifetz, A.; Coveney, P.V.; Townsend-Nicholson, A. Ensemble-Based Steered Molecular Dynamics Predicts Relative Residence Time of A 2A Receptor Binders. *J. Chem. Theory Comput.* **2019**, *15*, 3316–3330. [CrossRef]
886. Zhang, X.; Sun, H.; Wen, X.; Yuan, H. A Selectivity Study of FFAR4/FFAR1 Agonists by Molecular Modeling. *J. Chem. Inf. Model.* **2019**, *59*, 4467–4474. [CrossRef] [PubMed]
887. Perez-Aguilar, J.M.; Kang, S.G.; Zhang, L.; Zhou, R. Modeling and Structural Characterization of the Sweet Taste Receptor Heterodimer. *ACS Chem. Neurosci.* **2019**, *10*, 4579–4592. [CrossRef] [PubMed]
888. Bellucci, L.; Felline, A.; Fanelli, F. Dynamics and structural communication in the ternary complex of fully phosphorylated V2 vasopressin receptor, vasopressin, and β-arrestin 1. *Biochim. Biophys. Acta-Biomembr.* **2020**, *1862*, 183355. [CrossRef] [PubMed]
889. Azhagiya Singam, E.R.; Tachachartvanich, P.; La Merrill, M.A.; Smith, M.T.; Durkin, K.A. Structural Dynamics of Agonist and Antagonist Binding to the Androgen Receptor. *J. Phys. Chem. B* **2019**, *123*, 7657–7666. [CrossRef]

890. An, X.; Bai, Q.; Bing, Z.; Liu, H.; Zhang, Q.; Liu, H.; Yao, X. Revealing the Positive Binding Cooperativity Mechanism between the Orthosteric and the Allosteric Antagonists of CCR2 by Metadynamics and Gaussian Accelerated Molecular Dynamics Simulations. *ACS Chem. Neurosci.* **2020**, *11*, 628–637. [CrossRef]
891. Lei, T.; Hu, Z.; Ding, R.; Chen, J.; Li, S.; Zhang, F.; Pu, X.; Zhao, N. Exploring the Activation Mechanism of a Metabotropic Glutamate Receptor Homodimer via Molecular Dynamics Simulation. *ACS Chem. Neurosci.* **2020**, *11*, 133–145. [CrossRef]
892. Yang, J.F.; Williams, A.H.; Penthala, N.R.; Prather, P.L.; Crooks, P.A.; Zhan, C.G. Binding Modes and Selectivity of Cannabinoid 1 (CB1) and Cannabinoid 2 (CB2) Receptor Ligands. *ACS Chem. Neurosci.* **2020**, *11*, 3455–3463. [CrossRef]
893. Reis, M.H.; Antunes, D.; Santos, L.H.S.; Guimarães, A.C.R.; Caffarena, E.R. Shared Binding Mode of Perrottetinene and Tetrahydrocannabinol Diastereomers inside the CB1 Receptor May Incentivize Novel Medicinal Drug Design: Findings from an in Silico Assay. *ACS Chem. Neurosci.* **2020**, *11*, 4289–4300. [CrossRef] [PubMed]
894. Ji, B.; Liu, S.; He, X.; Man, V.H.; Xie, X.Q.; Wang, J. Prediction of the Binding Affinities and Selectivity for CB1 and CB2 Ligands Using Homology Modeling, Molecular Docking, Molecular Dynamics Simulations, and MM-PBSA Binding Free Energy Calculations. *ACS Chem. Neurosci.* **2020**, *11*, 1139–1158. [CrossRef]
895. Poudel, H.; Leitner, D.M. Activation-Induced Reorganization of Energy Transport Networks in the β 2 Adrenergic Receptor. *J. Phys. Chem. B* **2021**, *125*, 6522–6531. [CrossRef]
896. Shang, Y.; Yeatman, H.R.; Provasi, D.; Alt, A.; Christopoulos, A.; Canals, M.; Filizola, M. Proposed Mode of Binding and Action of Positive Allosteric Modulators at Opioid Receptors. *ACS Chem. Biol.* **2016**, *11*, 1220–1229. [CrossRef]
897. Bortolato, A.; Deflorian, F.; Weiss, D.R.; Mason, J.S. Decoding the Role of Water Dynamics in Ligand-Protein Unbinding: CRF1R as a Test Case. *J. Chem. Inf. Model.* **2015**, *55*, 1857–1866. [CrossRef] [PubMed]
898. Provasi, D.; Bortolato, A.; Filizola, M. Exploring molecular mechanisms of ligand recognition by opioid receptors with metadynamics. *Biochemistry* **2009**, *48*, 10020–10029. [CrossRef]
899. Kaszuba, K.; Róg, T.; Bryl, K.; Vattulainen, I.; Karttunen, M. Molecular dynamics simulations reveal fundamental role of water as factor determining affinity of binding of β-blocker nebivolol to β-adrenergic receptor. *J. Phys. Chem. B* **2010**, *114*, 8374–8386. [CrossRef]
900. Ribeiro, J.M.L.; Filizola, M. Insights From Molecular Dynamics Simulations of a Number of G-Protein Coupled Receptor Targets for the Treatment of Pain and Opioid Use Disorders. *Front. Mol. Neurosci.* **2019**, *12*, 207. [CrossRef] [PubMed]
901. Yang, D.; Zhou, Q.; Labroska, V.; Qin, S.; Darbalaei, S.; Wu, Y.; Yuliantie, E.; Xie, L.; Tao, H.; Cheng, J.; et al. G protein-coupled receptors: Structure- and function-based drug discovery. *Signal Transduct. Target. Ther.* **2021**, *6*, 7. [CrossRef] [PubMed]
902. Tautermann, C.S.; Seeliger, D.; Kriegl, J.M. What can we learn from molecular dynamics simulations for GPCR drug design? *Comput. Struct. Biotechnol. J.* **2015**, *13*, 111–121. [CrossRef]
903. Odoemelam, C.S.; Percival, B.; Wallis, H.; Chang, M.W.; Ahmad, Z.; Scholey, D.; Burton, E.; Williams, I.H.; Kamerlin, C.L.; Wilson, P.B. G-Protein coupled receptors: Structure and function in drug discovery. *RSC Adv.* **2020**, *10*, 36337–36348. [CrossRef]
904. Denisov, I.G.; Sligar, S.G. Nanodiscs in membrane biochemistry and biophysics. *Chem. Rev.* **2017**, *117*, 4669–4713. [CrossRef]
905. Denisov, I.G.; Sligar, S.G. Nanodiscs for structural and functional studies of membrane proteins. *Nat. Struct. Mol. Biol.* **2016**, *23*, 481–486. [CrossRef]
906. Pollock, N.L.; Lee, S.C.; Patel, J.H.; Gulamhussein, A.A.; Rothnie, A.J. Structure and function of membrane proteins encapsulated in a polymer-bound lipid bilayer. *Biochim. Biophys. Acta-Biomembr.* **2018**, *1860*, 809–817. [CrossRef]
907. Loll, P.J. Membrane proteins, detergents and crystals: What is the state of the art? *Acta Crystallogr. Sect. FStructural Biol. Commun.* **2014**, *70*, 1576–1583. [CrossRef]
908. 9Stetsenko, A.; Guskov, A. An Overview of the Top Ten Detergents Used for Membrane Protein Crystallization. *Crystals* **2017**, *7*, 197. [CrossRef]
909. Caffrey, M. A comprehensive review of the lipid cubic phase or in meso method for crystallizing membrane and soluble proteins and complexes. *Acta Crystallogr. Sect. F Struct. Biol. Commun.* **2015**, *71*, 3–18. [CrossRef]
910. Hameduh, T.; Haddad, Y.; Adam, V.; Heger, Z. Homology modeling in the time of collective and artificial intelligence. *Comput. Struct. Biotechnol. J.* **2020**, *18*, 3494–3506. [CrossRef]
911. Haddad, Y.; Adam, V.; Heger, Z. Ten quick tips for homology modeling of high-resolution protein 3D structures. *PLOS Comput. Biol.* **2020**, *16*, e1007449. [CrossRef]
912. Muhammed, M.T.; Aki-Yalcin, E. Homology modeling in drug discovery: Overview, current applications, and future perspectives. *Chem. Biol. Drug Des.* **2019**, *93*, 12–20. [CrossRef]
913. Barozet, A.; Bianciotto, M.; Vaisset, M.; Siméon, T.; Minoux, H.; Cortés, J. Protein loops with multiple meta-stable conformations: A challenge for sampling and scoring methods. *Proteins Struct. Funct. Bioinform.* **2021**, *89*, 218–231. [CrossRef]
914. Kaszuba, K.; Grzybek, M.; Orłowski, A.; Danne, R.; Róg, T.; Simons, K.; Coskun, Ü.; Vattulainen, I. N-Glycosylation as determinant of epidermal growth factor receptor conformation in membranes. *Proc. Natl. Acad. Sci. USA* **2015**, *112*, 4334–4339. [CrossRef]
915. Polley, A.; Orłowski, A.; Danne, R.; Gurtovenko, A.A.; Bernardino de La Serna, J.; Eggeling, C.; Davis, S.J.; Róg, T.; Vattulainen, I. Glycosylation and Lipids Working in Concert Direct CD2 Ectodomain Orientation and Presentation. *J. Phys. Chem. Lett.* **2017**, *8*, 1060–1066. [CrossRef]
916. Mobarak, E.; Håversen, L.; Manna, M.; Rutberg, M.; Levin, M.; Perkins, R.; Róg, T.; Vattulainen, I.; Borén, J. Glucosylceramide modifies the LPS-induced inflammatory response in macrophages and the orientation of the LPS/TLR4 complex in silico. *Sci. Rep.* **2018**, *8*, 13600. [CrossRef]

917. Almén, M.S.; Nordström, K.J.V.; Fredriksson, R.; Schiöth, H.B. Mapping the human membrane proteome: A majority of the human membrane proteins can be classified according to function and evolutionary origin. *BMC Biol.* **2009**, *7*, 50. [CrossRef]
918. Lefkowitz, R.J.; Kobilka, B.K. *The Nobel Prize in Chemistry 2012*; Royal Swedish Academy of Sciences: Stockholm, Sweden, 2012.
919. Royal Swedish Academy of Sciences. The Nobel Prize in Physiology or Medicine 1967 Ragnar Granit, Haldan Keffer Hartline and George Wald for Their Discoveries Concerning the Primary Physiological and Chemical Visual Processes in the Eye. Available online: https://www.nobelprize.org/prizes/medicine/1967/ (accessed on 18 October 2021).
920. Royal Swedish Academy of Sciences. The Nobel Prize in Physiology or Medicine 1988 Sir James W. Black, Gertrude B. Elion and George H. Hitchings for Their Discoveries of Important Principles for Drug Treatment. Available online: https://www.nobelprize.org/prizes/medicine/1988/ (accessed on 18 October 2021).
921. Royal Swedish Academy of Sciences. The Nobel Prize in Physiology or Medicine 1994 Alfred G. Gilman and Martin Rodbell for Their Discovery of G-proteins and the Role of These Proteins in Signal Transduction in Cells. Available online: https://www.nobelprize.org/prizes/medicine/1994/ (accessed on 18 October 2021).
922. Axel, R.; Buck, L.B. *The Nobel Prize in Physiology or Medicine 2004*; Alberta Aromatherapy Institute: Edmonton, AB, Canada, 2004.
923. Vauquelin, G.; Packeu, A. Ligands, their receptors and ... plasma membranes. *Mol. Cell. Endocrinol.* **2009**, *311*, 1–10. [CrossRef]
924. Vauquelin, G. Cell membranes ... and how long drugs may exert beneficial pharmacological activity in vivo. *Br. J. Clin. Pharmacol.* **2016**, 673–682. [CrossRef]
925. Vauquelin, G. Rebinding: Or why drugs may act longer in vivo than expected from their in vitro target residence time. *Expert Opin. Drug Discov.* **2010**, *5*, 927–941. [CrossRef]
926. Lappano, R.; Maggiolini, M. G protein-coupled receptors: Novel targets for drug discovery in cancer. *Nat. Rev. Drug Discov.* **2011**, *10*, 47–60. [CrossRef]
927. Vauquelin, G. On the 'micro'-pharmacodynamic and pharmacokinetic mechanisms that contribute to long-lasting drug action. *Expert Opin. Drug Discov.* **2015**, *10*, 1085–1098. [CrossRef]
928. Vauquelin, G.; Charlton, S.J. Long-lasting target binding and rebinding as mechanisms to prolong in vivo drug action. *Br. J. Pharmacol.* **2010**, *161*, 488–508. [CrossRef]
929. Erbaş, A.; Olvera de la Cruz, M.; Marko, J.F. Receptor-Ligand Rebinding Kinetics in Confinement. *Biophys. J.* **2019**, *116*, 1609–1624. [CrossRef]
930. Sykes, D.A.; Parry, C.; Reilly, J.; Wright, P.; Fairhurst, R.A.; Charlton, S.J. Observed Drug-Receptor Association Rates Are Governed by Membrane Affinity: The Importance of Establishing "Micro-Pharmacokinetic/Pharmacodynamic Relationships" at the β2 -Adrenoceptors. *Mol. Pharmacol.* **2014**, *85*, 608–617. [CrossRef]
931. Gherbi, K.; Briddon, S.J.; Charlton, S.J. Micro-pharmacokinetics: Quantifying local drug concentration at live cell membranes. *Sci. Rep.* **2018**, *8*, 3479. [CrossRef]
932. Dickson, C.J.; Hornak, V.; Velez-Vega, C.; McKay, D.J.J.; Reilly, J.; Sandham, D.A.; Shaw, D.; Fairhurst, R.A.; Charlton, S.J.; Sykes, D.A.; et al. Uncoupling the Structure-Activity Relationships of β2 Adrenergic Receptor Ligands from Membrane Binding. *J. Med. Chem.* **2016**, *59*, 5780–5789. [CrossRef]
933. Sanna, M.G.; Cahalan, S.M.; Han, G.W.; Schuerer, S.C.; Kuhn, P.; Stevens, R.C.; Desale, H.; Scott, F.L.; Clemons, B.; Griffith, M.T.; et al. Crystal Structure of a Lipid G Protein-Coupled Receptor. *Science* **2012**, *335*, 851–855. [CrossRef]
934. Hildebrand, P.W.; Scheerer, P.; Park, J.H.; Choe, H.W.; Piechnick, R.; Ernst, O.P.; Hofmann, K.P.; Heck, M. A ligand channel through the G protein coupled receptor opsin. *PLoS ONE* **2009**, *4*, e4382. [CrossRef]
935. Strasser, A.; Wittmann, H.J.; Seifert, R. Binding Kinetics and Pathways of Ligands to GPCRs. *Trends Pharmacol. Sci.* **2017**, *38*, 717–732. [CrossRef]
936. Szlenk, C.T.; Gc, J.B.; Natesan, S. Does the lipid bilayer orchestrate access and binding of ligands to transmembrane orthosteric/allosteric sites of G protein-coupled receptors? *Mol. Pharmacol.* **2019**, *96*, 527–541. [CrossRef]
937. Clark, R.B.; Allal, C.; Friedman, J.; Johnson, M.; Barber, R. Stable activation and desensitization of β2-adrenergic receptor stimulation of adenylyl cyclase by salmeterol: Evidence for quasi-irreversible binding to an exosite. *Mol. Pharmacol.* **1996**, *49*, 182–189.
938. Fronik, P.; Gaiser, B.I.; Sejer Pedersen, D. Bitopic Ligands and Metastable Binding Sites: Opportunities for G Protein-Coupled Receptor (GPCR) Medicinal Chemistry. *J. Med. Chem.* **2017**, *60*, 4126–4134. [CrossRef]
939. Volpato, D.; Kauk, M.; Messerer, R.; Bermudez, M.; Wolber, G.; Bock, A.; Hoffmann, C.; Holzgrabe, U. The Role of Orthosteric Building Blocks of Bitopic Ligands for Muscarinic M1 Receptors. *ACS Omega* **2020**, *5*, 31706–31715. [CrossRef]
940. Feng, Z.; Hu, G.; Ma, S.; Xie, X.Q. Computational Advances for the Development of Allosteric Modulators and Bitopic Ligands in G Protein-Coupled Receptors. *AAPS J.* **2015**, *17*, 1080–1095. [CrossRef]
941. Wang, H.; Reinecke, B.A.; Zhang, Y. Computational insights into the molecular mechanisms of differentiated allosteric modulation at the mu opioid receptor by structurally similar bitopic modulators. *J. Comput. Aided. Mol. Des.* **2020**, *34*, 879–895. [CrossRef]
942. Stanley, N.; Pardo, L.; Fabritiis, G. De The pathway of ligand entry from the membrane bilayer to a lipid G protein-coupled receptor. *Sci. Rep.* **2016**, *6*, 22639. [CrossRef]
943. Karhu, L.; Magarkar, A.; Bunker, A.; Xhaard, H. Determinants of Orexin Receptor Binding and Activation—A Molecular Dynamics Study. *J. Phys. Chem. B* **2019**, *123*, 2609–2622. [CrossRef]

944. Bokoch, M.P.; Jo, H.; Valcourt, J.R.; Srinivasan, Y.; Pan, A.C.; Capponi, S.; Grabe, M.; Dror, R.O.; Shaw, D.E.; Degrado, W.F.; et al. Entry from the Lipid Bilayer: A Possible Pathway for Inhibition of a Peptide G Protein-Coupled Receptor by a Lipophilic Small Molecule. *Biochemistry* **2018**, *57*, 5748–5758. [CrossRef]
945. Feng, Z.; Liang, T.; Wang, S.; Chen, M.; Hou, T.; Zhao, J.; Chen, H.; Zhou, Y.; Xie, X.Q. Binding Characterization of GPCRs-Modulator by Molecular Complex Characterizing System (MCCS). *ACS Chem. Neurosci.* **2020**, *11*, 3333–3345. [CrossRef]
946. Burger, W.A.C.; Gentry, P.R.; Berizzi, A.E.; Vuckovic, Z.; van der Westhuizen, E.T.; Thompson, G.; Yeasmin, M.; Lindsley, C.W.; Sexton, P.M.; Langmead, C.J.; et al. Identification of a Novel Allosteric Site at the M 5 Muscarinic Acetylcholine Receptor. *ACS Chem. Neurosci.* **2021**, *12*, 3112–3123. [CrossRef]
947. Cao, R.; Giorgetti, A.; Bauer, A.; Neumaier, B.; Rossetti, G.; Carloni, P. Role of extracellular loops and membrane lipids for ligand recognition in the neuronal adenosine receptor type 2A: An enhanced sampling simulation study. *Molecules* **2018**, *23*, 2616. [CrossRef]
948. Monk, B.C.; Tomasiak, T.M.; Keniya, M.V.; Huschmann, F.U.; Tyndall, J.D.A.; O'Connell, J.D.; Cannon, R.D.; McDonald, J.G.; Rodriguez, A.; Finer-Moore, J.S.; et al. Architecture of a single membrane spanning cytochrome P450 suggests constraints that orient the catalytic domain relative to a bilayer. *Proc. Natl. Acad. Sci. USA* **2014**, *111*, 3865–3870. [CrossRef]
949. Manikandan, P.; Nagini, S. Cytochrome P450 Structure, Function and Clinical Significance: A Review. *Curr. Drug Targets* **2018**, *19*, 38–54. [CrossRef]
950. Hasler, J.A.; Estabrook, R.; Murray, M.; Pikuleva, I.; Waterman, M.; Capdevila, J.; Holla, V.; Helvig, C.; Falck, J.R.; Farrell, G.; et al. Human cytochromes P450. *Mol. Aspects Med.* **1999**, *20*, 1–137. [CrossRef]
951. Burkina, V.; Rasmussen, M.K.; Pilipenko, N.; Zamaratskaia, G. Comparison of xenobiotic-metabolising human, porcine, rodent, and piscine cytochrome P450. *Toxicology* **2016**, *375*, 10–27. [CrossRef]
952. Shalan, H.; Kato, M.; Cheruzel, L. Keeping the spotlight on cytochrome P450. *Biochim. Biophys. Acta-Proteins Proteomics* **2018**, *1866*, 80–87. [CrossRef]
953. Zanger, U.M.; Schwab, M. Cytochrome P450 enzymes in drug metabolism: Regulation of gene expression, enzyme activities, and impact of genetic variation. *Pharmacol. Ther.* **2013**, *138*, 103–141. [CrossRef]
954. Backman, J.T.; Filppula, A.M.; Niemi, M.; Neuvonen, P.J. Role of Cytochrome P450 2C8 in Drug Metabolism and Interactions. *Pharmacol. Rev.* **2015**, *68*, 168–241. [CrossRef]
955. Šrejber, M.; Navrátilová, V.; Paloncýová, M.; Bazgier, V.; Berka, K.; Anzenbacher, P.; Otyepka, M. Membrane-attached mammalian cytochromes P450: An overview of the membrane's effects on structure, drug binding, and interactions with redox partners. *J. Inorg. Biochem.* **2018**, *183*, 117–136. [CrossRef]
956. Neves Cruz, J.; Santana De Oliveira, M.; Gomes Silva, S.; Pedro Da Silva Souza Filho, A.; Santiago Pereira, D.; Lima E Lima, A.H.; De Aguiar Andrade, E.H. Insight into the Interaction Mechanism of Nicotine, NNK, and NNN with Cytochrome P450 2A13 Based on Molecular Dynamics Simulation. *J. Chem. Inf. Model.* **2020**, *60*, 766–776. [CrossRef]
957. Yousefpour, A.; Modarress, H.; Goharpey, F.; Amjad-Iranagh, S. Interaction of drugs amlodipine and paroxetine with the metabolizing enzyme CYP2B4: A molecular dynamics simulation study. *J. Mol. Model.* **2018**, *24*, 67. [CrossRef]
958. Spinello, A.; Ritacco, I.; Magistrato, A. The catalytic mechanism of steroidogenic cytochromes P450 from all-atom simulations: Entwinement with membrane environment, redox partners, and post-transcriptional regulation. *Catalysts* **2019**, *9*, 81. [CrossRef]
959. Lonsdale, R.; Rouse, S.L.; Sansom, M.S.P.; Mulholland, A.J. A Multiscale Approach to Modelling Drug Metabolism by Membrane-Bound Cytochrome P450 Enzymes. *PLoS Comput. Biol.* **2014**, *10*, e1003714. [CrossRef]
960. Cojocaru, V.; Balali-Mood, K.; Sansom, M.S.P.; Wade, R.C. Structure and dynamics of the membrane-bound cytochrome P450 2C9. *PLoS Comput. Biol.* **2011**, *7*, e1002152. [CrossRef] [PubMed]
961. Cui, Y.-L.L.; Xue, Q.; Zheng, Q.-C.C.; Zhang, J.-L.L.; Kong, C.-P.P.; Fan, J.-R.R.; Zhang, H.-X.X. Structural features and dynamic investigations of the membrane-bound cytochrome P450 17A1. *Biochim. Biophys. Acta-Biomembr.* **2015**, *1848*, 2013–2021. [CrossRef] [PubMed]
962. Berka, K.; Paloncýová, M.; Anzenbacher, P.; Otyepka, M. Behavior of human cytochromes P450 on lipid membranes. *J. Phys. Chem. B* **2013**, *117*, 11556–11564. [CrossRef]
963. Baylon, J.L.; Lenov, I.L.; Sligar, S.G.; Tajkhorshid, E. Characterizing the membrane-bound state of cytochrome P450 3A4: Structure, depth of insertion, and orientation. *J. Am. Chem. Soc.* **2013**, *135*, 8542–8551. [CrossRef]
964. Mustafa, G.; Nandekar, P.P.; Bruce, N.J.; Wade, R.C. Differing membrane interactions of two highly similar drug-metabolizing cytochrome P450 isoforms: CYP 2C9 and CYP 2C19. *Int. J. Mol. Sci.* **2019**, *20*, 4328. [CrossRef]
965. Mustafa, G.; Nandekar, P.P.; Camp, T.J.; Bruce, N.J.; Gregory, M.C.; Sligar, S.G.; Wade, R.C. Influence of Transmembrane Helix Mutations on Cytochrome P450-Membrane Interactions and Function. *Biophys. J.* **2019**, *116*, 419–432. [CrossRef]
966. Navrátilová, V.; Paloncýová, M.; Kajšová, M.; Berka, K.; Otyepka, M. Effect of cholesterol on the structure of membrane-attached cytochrome P450 3A4. *J. Chem. Inf. Model.* **2015**, *55*, 628–635. [CrossRef]
967. Navrátilová, V.; Paloncýová, M.; Berka, K.; Otyepka, M. Effect of Lipid Charge on Membrane Immersion of Cytochrome P450 3A4. *J. Phys. Chem. B* **2016**, *120*, 11205–11213. [CrossRef] [PubMed]
968. Mustafa, G.; Nandekar, P.P.; Mukherjee, G.; Bruce, N.J.; Wade, R.C. The Effect of Force-Field Parameters on Cytochrome P450-Membrane Interactions: Structure and Dynamics. *Sci. Rep.* **2020**, *10*, 7284. [CrossRef] [PubMed]
969. Cojocaru, V.; Winn, P.J.; Wade, R.C. The ins and outs of cytochrome P450s. *Biochim. Biophys. Acta-Gen. Subj.* **2007**, *1770*, 390–401. [CrossRef]

970. Li, W.; Shen, J.; Liu, G.; Tang, Y.; Hoshino, T. Exploring coumarin egress channels in human cytochrome p450 2a6 by random acceleration and steered molecular dynamics simulations. *Proteins Struct. Funct. Bioinform.* **2011**, *79*, 271–281. [CrossRef]
971. Shen, Z.; Cheng, F.; Xu, Y.; Fu, J.; Xiao, W.; Shen, J.; Liu, G.; Li, W.; Tang, Y. Investigation of indazole unbinding pathways in CYP2E1 by molecular dynamics simulations. *PLoS ONE* **2012**, *7*, e33500. [CrossRef]
972. Fishelovitch, D.; Shaik, S.; Wolfson, H.J.; Nussinov, R. Theoretical characterization of substrate access/exit channels in the human cytochrome P450 3A4 enzyme: Involvement of phenylalanine residues in the gating mechanism. *J. Phys. Chem. B* **2009**, *113*, 13018–13025. [CrossRef]
973. Yu, X.; Nandekar, P.; Mustafa, G.; Cojocaru, V.; Lepesheva, G.I.; Wade, R.C. Ligand tunnels in T. brucei and human CYP51: Insights for parasite-specific drug design. *Biochim. Biophys. Acta-Gen. Subj.* **2016**, *1860*, 67–78. [CrossRef]
974. Jeřábek, P.; Florián, J.; Martínek, V. Lipid molecules can induce an opening of membrane-facing tunnels in cytochrome P450 1A2. *Phys. Chem. Chem. Phys.* **2016**, *18*, 30344–30356. [CrossRef] [PubMed]
975. Li, J.; Zhou, Y.; Tang, Y.; Li, W.; Tu, Y. Dissecting the structural plasticity and dynamics of cytochrome P450 2B4 by molecular dynamics simulations. *J. Chem. Inf. Model.* **2020**, *60*, 5026–5035. [CrossRef] [PubMed]
976. Mouchlis, V.D.; Bucher, D.; McCammon, J.A.; Dennis, E.A. Membranes serve as allosteric activators of phospholipase A 2, enabling it to extract, bind, and hydrolyze phospholipid substrates. *Proc. Natl. Acad. Sci. USA* **2015**, *112*, E516–E525. [CrossRef] [PubMed]
977. Mouchlis, V.D.; Chen, Y.; Andrew McCammon, J.; Dennis, E.A. Membrane Allostery and Unique Hydrophobic Sites Promote Enzyme Substrate Specificity. *J. Am. Chem. Soc.* **2018**, *140*, 3285–3291. [CrossRef] [PubMed]
978. Costeira-Paulo, J.; Gault, J.; Popova, G.; Ladds, M.J.G.W.; van Leeuwen, I.M.M.; Sarr, M.; Olsson, A.; Lane, D.P.; Laín, S.; Marklund, E.G.; et al. Lipids Shape the Electron Acceptor-Binding Site of the Peripheral Membrane Protein Dihydroorotate Dehydrogenase. *Cell Chem. Biol.* **2018**, *25*, 309–317. [CrossRef] [PubMed]
979. Goossens, K.; Neves, R.P.P.; Fernandes, P.A.; De Winter, H. A computational and modeling study of the reaction mechanism of Staphylococcus aureus monoglycosyltransferase reveals new insights on the GT51 family of Enzymes. *J. Chem. Inf. Model.* **2020**, *60*, 5513–5528. [CrossRef]
980. Barnaba, C.; Sahoo, B.R.; Ravula, T.; Medina-Meza, I.G.; Im, S.C.; Anantharamaiah, G.M.; Waskell, L.; Ramamoorthy, A. Cytochrome-P450-Induced Ordering of Microsomal Membranes Modulates Affinity for Drugs. *Angew. Chemie-Int. Ed.* **2018**, *57*, 3391–3395. [CrossRef]
981. Jeřábek, P.; Florián, J.; Martínek, V. Membrane-Anchored Cytochrome P450 1A2–Cytochrome b_5 Complex Features an X-Shaped Contact between Antiparallel Transmembrane Helices. *Chem. Res. Toxicol.* **2016**, *29*, 626–636. [CrossRef]
982. Sellner, M.; Fischer, A.; Don, C.G.; Smieško, M. Conformational landscape of cytochrome P450 reductase interactions. *Int. J. Mol. Sci.* **2021**, *22*, 1023. [CrossRef]
983. Cui, Y.-L.; Wu, R.-L. Molecular dynamics investigations of membrane-bound CYP2C19 polymorphisms reveal distinct mechanisms for peripheral variants by long-range effects on the enzymatic activity. *Mol. Biosyst.* **2017**, *13*, 1070–1079. [CrossRef]
984. Navrátilová, V.; Paloncýová, M.; Berka, K.; Mise, S.; Haga, Y.; Matsumura, C.; Sakaki, T.; Inui, H.; Otyepka, M. Molecular insights into the role of a distal F240A mutation that alters CYP1A1 activity towards persistent organic pollutants. *Biochim. Biophys. Acta-Gen. Subj.* **2017**, *1861*, 2852–2860. [CrossRef]
985. Caudle, K.E.; Dunnenberger, H.M.; Freimuth, R.R.; Peterson, J.F.; Burlison, J.D.; Whirl-Carrillo, M.; Scott, S.A.; Rehm, H.L.; Williams, M.S.; Klein, T.E.; et al. Standardizing Terms for Clinical Pharmacogenetic Test Results: Consensus Terms from the Clinical Pharmacogenetics Implementa- tion Consortium (CPIC). *Genet. Med.* **2017**, *19*, 215–223. [CrossRef] [PubMed]
986. Fischer, A.; Don, C.G.; Smieško, M. Molecular Dynamics Simulations Reveal Structural Differences among Allelic Variants of Membrane-Anchored Cytochrome P450 2D6. *J. Chem. Inf. Model.* **2018**, *58*, 1962–1975. [CrossRef] [PubMed]
987. Bastos, P.; Gomes, T.; Ribeiro, L. Catechol-O-Methyltransferase (COMT): An Update on Its Role in Cancer, Neurological and Cardiovascular Diseases. *Rev. Physiol. Biochem. Pharmacol.* **2017**, *173*, 1–40. [CrossRef] [PubMed]
988. Ramsay, R.R.; Albreht, A. Kinetics, mechanism, and inhibition of monoamine oxidase. *J. Neural Transm.* **2018**, *125*, 1659–1683. [CrossRef]
989. Ramsay, R.R. Molecular aspects of monoamine oxidase B. *Prog. Neuro-Psychopharmacology Biol. Psychiatry* **2016**, *69*, 81–89. [CrossRef]
990. Fišar, Z. Drugs related to monoamine oxidase activity. *Prog. Neuro-Psychopharmacology Biol. Psychiatry* **2016**, *69*, 112–124. [CrossRef]
991. Kumar, B.; Dwivedi, A.R.; Sarkar, B.; Gupta, S.K.; Krishnamurthy, S.; Mantha, A.K.; Parkash, J.; Kumar, V. 4,6-Diphenylpyrimidine Derivatives as Dual Inhibitors of Monoamine Oxidase and Acetylcholinesterase for the Treatment of Alzheimer's Disease. *ACS Chem. Neurosci.* **2019**, *10*, 252–265. [CrossRef]
992. Mangiatordi, G.F.; Alberga, D.; Pisani, L.; Gadaleta, D.; Trisciuzzi, D.; Farina, R.; Carotti, A.; Lattanzi, G.; Catto, M.; Nicolotti, O. A rational approach to elucidate human monoamine oxidase molecular selectivity. *Eur. J. Pharm. Sci.* **2017**, *101*, 90–99. [CrossRef] [PubMed]
993. Ahmad, S.; Zaib, S.; Jalil, S.; Shafiq, M.; Ahmad, M.; Sultan, S.; Iqbal, M.; Aslam, S.; Iqbal, J. Synthesis, characterization, monoamine oxidase inhibition, molecular docking and dynamic simulations of novel 2,1-benzothiazine-2,2-dioxide derivatives. *Bioorg. Chem.* **2018**, *80*, 498–510. [CrossRef] [PubMed]

994. Larit, F.; Elokely, K.M.; Chaurasiya, N.D.; Benyahia, S.; Nael, M.A.; León, F.; Abu-Darwish, M.S.; Efferth, T.; Wang, Y.H.; Belouahem-Abed, D.; et al. Inhibition of human monoamine oxidase A and B by flavonoids isolated from two Algerian medicinal plants. *Phytomedicine* **2018**, *40*, 27–36. [CrossRef] [PubMed]
995. Prah, A.; Purg, M.; Stare, J.; Vianello, R.; Mavri, J. How Monoamine Oxidase A Decomposes Serotonin: An Empirical Valence Bond Simulation of the Reactive Step. *J. Phys. Chem. B* **2020**, *124*, 8259–8265. [CrossRef] [PubMed]
996. Abad, E.; Zenn, R.K.; Kästner, J. Reaction Mechanism of Monoamine Oxidase from QM/MM Calculations. *J. Phys. Chem. B* **2013**, *117*, 14238–14246. [CrossRef] [PubMed]
997. Maršavelski, A.; Vianello, R. What a Difference a Methyl Group Makes: The Selectivity of Monoamine Oxidase B Towards Histamine and N-Methylhistamine. *Chem.—A Eur. J.* **2017**, *23*, 2915–2925. [CrossRef]
998. Vianello, R.; Domene, C.; Mavri, J. The Use of Multiscale Molecular Simulations in Understanding a Relationship between the Structure and Function of Biological Systems of the Brain: The Application to Monoamine Oxidase Enzymes. *Front. Neurosci.* **2016**, *10*, 327. [CrossRef]
999. Apostolov, R.; Yonezawa, Y.; Standley, D.M.; Kikugawa, G.; Takano, Y.; Nakamura, H. Membrane attachment facilitates ligand access to the active site in monoamine oxidase A. *Biochemistry* **2009**, *48*, 5864–5873. [CrossRef]
1000. Allen, W.J.; Bevan, D.R. Steered molecular dynamics simulations reveal important mechanisms in reversible monoamine oxidase B inhibition. *Biochemistry* **2011**, *50*, 6441–6454. [CrossRef]
1001. Jones, H.B.L.; Crean, R.M.; Mullen, A.; Kendrick, E.G.; Bull, S.D.; Wells, S.A.; Carbery, D.R.; Macmillan, F.; Van Der Kamp, M.W.; Pudney, C.R. Exposing the Interplay between Enzyme Turnover, Protein Dynamics, and the Membrane Environment in Monoamine Oxidase B. *Biochemistry* **2019**, *58*, 2362–2372. [CrossRef]
1002. Karpov, O.A.; Fearnley, G.W.; Smith, G.A.; Kankanala, J.; McPherson, M.J.; Tomlinson, D.C.; Harrison, M.A.; Ponnambalam, S. Receptor tyrosine kinase structure and function in health and disease. *AIMS Biophys.* **2015**, *2*, 476–502. [CrossRef]
1003. Karl, K.; Paul, M.D.; Pasquale, E.B.; Hristova, K. Ligand bias in receptor tyrosine kinase signaling. *J. Biol. Chem.* **2020**, *295*, 18494–18507. [CrossRef] [PubMed]
1004. Castrén, E.; Monteggia, L. Brain-Derived Neurotrophic Factor Signaling in Depression and Antidepressant Action. *Biol. Psychiatry* **2021**, *90*, 128–136. [CrossRef] [PubMed]
1005. Cannarozzo, C.; Fred, S.M.; Girych, M.; Biojone, C.; Enkavi, G.; Róg, T.; Vattulainen, I.; Casarotto, P.C.; Castrén, E. Cholesterol-recognition motifs in the transmembrane domain of the tyrosine kinase receptor family: The case of TRKB. *Eur. J. Neurosci.* **2021**, *53*, 3311–3322. [CrossRef] [PubMed]
1006. Tulodziecka, K.; Diaz-Rohrer, B.B.; Farley, M.M.; Chan, R.B.; Di Paolo, G.; Levental, K.R.; Waxham, M.N.; Levental, I. Remodeling of the postsynaptic plasma membrane during neural development. *Mol. Biol. Cell* **2016**, *27*, 3480–3489. [CrossRef]
1007. Rantamäki, T. TrkB neurotrophin receptor at the core of antidepressant effects, but how? *Cell Tissue Res.* **2019**, *377*, 115–124. [CrossRef]
1008. Lieto, A.; Rantamäki, T.; Vesa, L.; Yanpallewar, S.; Antila, H.; Lindholm, J.; Rios, M.; Tessarollo, L.; Castrén, E. The responsiveness of trkb to bdnf and antidepressant drugs is differentially regulated during mouse development. *PLoS ONE* **2012**, *7*, e32869. [CrossRef]
1009. Conroy, J.N.; Jhaveri, D.J.; Coulson, E.J. Fast-Trk(B)ing the mechanism of antidepressants. *Neuron* **2021**, *109*, 1593–1595. [CrossRef]
1010. Slattery, D.A.; Cryan, J.F. Membrane molecules for mood. *Trends Neurosci.* **2021**, *44*, 602–604. [CrossRef]
1011. Ateaque, S.; Barde, Y.A. A new molecular target for antidepressants. *Cell Res.* **2021**, *31*, 489–490. [CrossRef]
1012. Kornhuber, J.; Gulbins, E. New Molecular Targets for Antidepressant Drugs. *Pharmaceuticals* **2021**, *14*, 894. [CrossRef]
1013. Pankiewicz, P.; Szybiński, M.; Kisielewska, K.; Gołębiowski, F.; Krzemiński, P.; Rutkowska-Włodarczyk, I.; Moszczyński-Pętkowski, R.; Gurba-Bryśkiewicz, L.; Delis, M.; Mulewski, K.; et al. Do small molecules activate the TrkB receptor in the same manner as BDNF? Limitations of published TrkB low molecular agonists and screening for novel TrkB orthosteric agonists. *Pharmaceuticals* **2021**, *14*, 704. [CrossRef] [PubMed]
1014. Dahlström, M.; Madjid, N.; Nordvall, G.; Halldin, M.M.; Vazquez-Juarez, E.; Lindskog, M.; Sandin, J.; Winblad, B.; Eriksdotter, M.; Forsell, P. Identification of Novel Positive Allosteric Modulators of Neurotrophin Receptors for the Treatment of Cognitive Dysfunction. *Cells* **2021**, *10*, 1871. [CrossRef] [PubMed]
1015. Boes, D.M.; Godoy-Hernandez, A.; McMillan, D.G.G. Peripheral Membrane Proteins: Promising Therapeutic Targets across Domains of Life. *Membranes* **2021**, *11*, 346. [CrossRef] [PubMed]
1016. Sudhahar, C.G.; Haney, R.M.; Xue, Y.; Stahelin, R.V. Cellular Membranes and Lipid-Binding Domains as Attractive Targets for Drug Development. *Curr Drug Targets* **2008**, *9*, 603–613. [CrossRef] [PubMed]
1017. Meuillet, E.J.; Mahadevan, D.; Vankayalapati, H.; Berggren, M.; Williams, R.; Coon, A.; Kozikowski, A.P.; Powis, G. Specific inhibition of the akt1 pleckstrin homology domain by D-3-deoxy-phosphatidyl-myo-inositol analogues. *Mol. Cancer Ther.* **2003**, *2*, 389–399. [PubMed]
1018. Indarte, M.; Puentes, R.; Maruggi, M.; Ihle, N.T.; Grandjean, G.; Scott, M.; Ahmed, Z.; Meuillet, E.J.; Zang, S.; Lemos, R.; et al. An inhibitor of the pleckstrin homology domain of CNK1 selectively blocks the growth of mutant KRAS cells and tumors. *Cancer Res.* **2019**, *79*, 3100–3111. [CrossRef] [PubMed]
1019. Bertuzzi, S.; Gimeno, A.; Núñez-Franco, R.; Bernardo-Seisdedos, G.; Delgado, S.; Jiménez-Osés, G.; Millet, O.; Jiménez-Barbero, J.; Ardá, A. Unravelling the Time Scale of Conformational Plasticity and Allostery in Glycan Recognition by Human Galectin-1. *Chem.—A Eur. J.* **2020**, *26*, 15643–15653. [CrossRef]

1020. Parasuraman, P.; Murugan, V.; Selvin, J.F.A.; Gromiha, M.M.; Fukui, K.; Veluraja, K. Theoretical investigation on the glycan-binding specificity of Agrocybe cylindracea galectin using molecular modeling and molecular dynamics simulation studies. *J. Mol. Recognit.* **2015**, *28*, 528–538. [CrossRef] [PubMed]
1021. Jayakody, R.S.; Wijewardhane, P.; Herath, C.; Perera, S. Bergenin: A computationally proven promising scaffold for novel galectin-3 inhibitors. *J. Mol. Model.* **2018**, *24*, 302. [CrossRef] [PubMed]
1022. Miller, M.C.; Cai, C.; Wichapong, K.; Bhaduri, S.; Pohl, N.L.B.; Linhardt, R.J.; Gabius, H.J.; Mayo, K.H. Structural insight into the binding of human galectins to corneal keratan sulfate, its desulfated form and related saccharides. *Sci. Rep.* **2020**, *10*, 15708. [CrossRef]
1023. Newton, A.C.; Brognard, J. Reversing the Paradigm: Protein Kinase C as a Tumor Suppressor. *Trends Pharmacol. Sci.* **2017**, *38*, 438–447. [CrossRef]
1024. Newton, A.C. Protein kinase C: Perfectly balanced. *Crit. Rev. Biochem. Mol. Biol.* **2018**, *53*, 208–230. [CrossRef]
1025. 1Talman, V.; Pascale, A.; Jäntti, M.; Amadio, M.; Tuominen, R.K. Protein Kinase C Activation as a Potential Therapeutic Strategy in Alzheimer's Disease: Is there a Role for Embryonic Lethal Abnormal Vision-like Proteins? *Basic Clin. Pharmacol. Toxicol.* **2016**, *119*, 149–160. [CrossRef]
1026. Katti, S.; Igumenova, T.I. Structural insights into C1-ligand interactions: Filling the gaps by in silico methods. *Adv. Biol. Regul.* **2021**, *79*, 100784. [CrossRef]
1027. Alwarawrah, M.; Wereszczynski, J. Investigation of the effect of bilayer composition on PKCα-C2 domain docking using molecular dynamics simulations. *J. Phys. Chem. B* **2017**, *121*, 78–88. [CrossRef] [PubMed]
1028. Li, J.; Ziemba, B.P.; Falke, J.J.; Voth, G.A. Interactions of Protein Kinase C-α C1A and C1B Domains with Membranes: A Combined Computational and Experimental Study. *J. Am. Chem. Soc.* **2014**, *136*, 11757–11766. [CrossRef] [PubMed]
1029. Lai, C.L.; Landgraf, K.E.; Voth, G.A.; Falke, J.J. Membrane docking geometry and target lipid stoichiometry of membrane-bound PKCα C2 domain: A combined molecular dynamics and experimental study. *J. Mol. Biol.* **2010**, *402*, 301–310. [CrossRef] [PubMed]
1030. Geragotelis, A.D.; Freites, J.A.; Tobias, D.J. Anomalous Diffusion of Peripheral Membrane Signaling Proteins from All-Atom Molecular Dynamics Simulations. *J. Phys. Chem. B* **2021**, *125*, 9990–9998. [CrossRef]
1031. Boije af Gennäs, G.; Talman, V.; Aitio, O.; Ekokoski, E.; Finel, M.; Tuominen, R.K.; Yli-Kauhaluoma, J. Design, Synthesis, and Biological Activity of Isophthalic Acid Derivatives Targeted to the C1 Domain of Protein Kinase C. *J. Med. Chem.* **2009**, *52*, 3969–3981. [CrossRef]
1032. Provenzani, R.; Tarvainen, I.; Brandoli, G.; Lempinen, A.; Artes, S.; Turku, A.; Jäntti, M.H.; Talman, V.; Yli-Kauhaluoma, J.; Tuominen, R.K.; et al. Scaffold hopping from (5- hydroxymethyl) isophthalates to multisubstituted pyrimidines diminishes binding affinity to the C1 domain of protein kinase C. *PLoS ONE* **2018**, *13*, e0195668. [CrossRef] [PubMed]
1033. Talman, V.; Tuominen, R.K.; Boije af Gennäs, G.; Yli- Kauhaluoma, J.; Ekokoski, E. C1 Domain-targeted isophthalate derivatives induce cell elongation and cell cycle arrest in HeLa cells. *PLoS ONE* **2011**, *6*, e20053. [CrossRef]
1034. Jäntti, M.H.; Talman, V.; Räsänen, K.; Tarvainen, I.; Koistinen, H.; Tuominen, R.K. Anticancer activity of the protein kinase C modulator HMI-1a3 in 2D and 3D cell culture models of androgenresponsive and androgen-unresponsive prostate cancer. *FEBS Open Bio* **2018**, *8*, 817–828. [CrossRef]
1035. Dickson, E.J.; Hille, B. Understanding phosphoinositides: Rare, dynamic, and essential membrane phospholipids. *Biochem. J.* **2019**, *476*, 1–23. [CrossRef]
1036. Wu, E.L.; Qi, Y.; Song, K.C.; Klauda, J.B.; Im, W. Preferred orientations of phosphoinositides in bilayers and their implications in protein recognition mechanisms. *J. Phys. Chem. B* **2014**, *118*, 4315–4325. [CrossRef]
1037. Stahelin, R.V.; Scott, J.L.; Frick, C.T. Cellular and molecular interactions of phosphoinositides and peripheral proteins. *Chem. Phys. Lipids* **2014**, *182*, 3–18. [CrossRef]
1038. Moravcevic, K.; Oxley, C.L.L.; Lemmon, M.A.A. Conditional peripheral membrane proteins: Facing up to limited specificity. *Structure* **2012**, *20*, 15–27. [CrossRef] [PubMed]
1039. Hammond, G.R.V.; Balla, T. Polyphosphoinositide binding domains: Key to inositol lipid biology. *Biochim. Biophys. Acta-Mol. Cell Biol. Lipids* **2015**, *1851*, 746–758. [CrossRef] [PubMed]
1040. Letunic, I.; Khedkar, S.; Bork, P. SMART: Recent updates, new developments and status in 2020. *Nucleic Acids Res.* **2021**, *49*, D458–D460. [CrossRef] [PubMed]
1041. Kuang, G.; Bulone, V.; Tu, Y. Computational studies of the binding profile of phosphoinositide PtdIns (3,4,5) P3 with the pleckstrin homology domain of an oomycete cellulose synthase. *Sci. Rep.* **2016**, *6*, 20555. [CrossRef] [PubMed]
1042. Rosen, S.A.J.; Gaffney, P.R.J.; Spiess, B.; Gould, I.R. Understanding the relative affinity and specificity of the pleckstrin homology domain of protein kinase B for inositol phosphates. *Phys. Chem. Chem. Phys.* **2012**, *14*, 929–936. [CrossRef]
1043. Rai, S.; Mohanty, P.; Bhatnagar, S. Modeling, dynamics and phosphoinositide binding of the pleckstrin homology domain of two novel PLCs: η1 and η2. *J. Mol. Graph. Model.* **2018**, *85*, 130–144. [CrossRef]
1044. Lumb, C.N.; He, J.; Xue, Y.; Stansfeld, P.J.; Stahelin, R.V.; Kutateladze, T.G.; Sansom, M.S.P. Biophysical and computational studies of membrane penetration by the GRP1 pleckstrin homology domain. *Structure* **2011**, *19*, 1338–1346. [CrossRef]
1045. Psachoulia, E.; Sansom, M.S.P. Interactions of the pleckstrin homology domain with phosphatidylinositol phosphate and membranes: Characterization via molecular dynamics simulations. *Biochemistry* **2008**, *47*, 4211–4220. [CrossRef]
1046. Buyan, A.; Kalli, A.C.; Sansom, M.S.P. Multiscale Simulations Suggest a Mechanism for the Association of the Dok7 PH Domain with PIP-Containing Membranes. *PLoS Comput. Biol.* **2016**, *12*, e1005028. [CrossRef]

1047. Pant, S.; Tajkhorshid, E. Microscopic Characterization of GRP1 PH Domain Interaction with Anionic Membranes. *J. Comput. Chem.* **2020**, *41*, 489–499. [CrossRef]
1048. Lai, C.-L.; Srivastava, A.; Pilling, C.; Chase, A.R.; Falke, J.J.; Voth, G.A. Molecular Mechanism of Membrane Binding of the GRP1 PH Domain. *J. Mol. Biol.* **2013**, *425*, 3073–3090. [CrossRef] [PubMed]
1049. Yamamoto, E.; Kalli, A.C.C.; Yasuoka, K.; Sansom, M.S.P.S.P. Interactions of Pleckstrin Homology Domains with Membranes: Adding Back the Bilayer via High-Throughput Molecular Dynamics. *Structure* **2016**, *24*, 1421–1431. [CrossRef] [PubMed]
1050. Naughton, F.B.; Kalli, A.C.; Sansom, M.S.P. Association of Peripheral Membrane Proteins with Membranes: Free Energy of Binding of GRP1 PH Domain with Phosphatidylinositol Phosphate-Containing Model Bilayers. *J. Phys. Chem. Lett.* **2016**, *7*, 1219–1224. [CrossRef]
1051. Yamamoto, E.; Domański, J.; Naughton, F.B.; Best, R.B.; Kalli, A.C.; Stansfeld, P.J.; Sansom, M.S.P. Multiple lipid binding sites determine the affinity of PH domains for phosphoinositide-containing membranes. *Sci. Adv.* **2020**, *6*, eaay5736. [CrossRef]
1052. Chan, K.C.; Lu, L.; Sun, F.; Fan, J. Molecular Details of the PH Domain of ACAP1BAR-PH Protein Binding to PIP-Containing Membrane. *J. Phys. Chem. B* **2017**, *121*, 3586–3596. [CrossRef]
1053. Chen, L.; Du-Cuny, L.; Moses, S.; Dumas, S.; Song, Z.; Rezaeian, A.H.; Lin, H.K.; Meuillet, E.J.; Zhang, S. Novel Inhibitors Induce Large Conformational Changes of GAB1 Pleckstrin Homology Domain and Kill Breast Cancer Cells. *PLoS Comput. Biol.* **2015**, *11*, e1004021. [CrossRef]
1054. Ghoula, M.; Le Marec, A.; Magnan, C.; Le Stunff, H.; Taboureau, O. Identification of the Interactions Interference Between the PH and START Domain of CERT by Limonoid and HPA Inhibitors. *Front. Mol. Biosci.* **2020**, *7*, 603983. [CrossRef] [PubMed]
1055. Kumar, A.; Purohit, R. Cancer Associated E17K Mutation Causes Rapid Conformational Drift in AKT1 Pleckstrin Homology (PH) Domain. *PLoS ONE* **2013**, *8*, e64364. [CrossRef] [PubMed]
1056. Chandra, M.; Chin, Y.K.Y.; Mas, C.; Feathers, J.R.; Paul, B.; Datta, S.; Chen, K.E.; Jia, X.; Yang, Z.; Norwood, S.J.; et al. Classification of the human phox homology (PX) domains based on their phosphoinositide binding specificities. *Nat. Commun.* **2019**, *10*, 1528. [CrossRef] [PubMed]
1057. Psachoulia, E.; Sansom, M.S.P. PX- and FYVE-mediated interactions with membranes: Simulation studies. *Biochemistry* **2009**, *48*, 5090–5095. [CrossRef]
1058. Han, K.; Pastor, R.W.; Fenollar–Ferrer, C. PLD2–PI(4,5)P2 interactions in fluid phase membranes: Structural modeling and molecular dynamics simulations. *PLoS ONE* **2020**, *15*, e0236201. [CrossRef] [PubMed]
1059. Kalli, A.C.; Campbell, I.D.; Sansom, M.S.P. Conformational Changes in Talin on Binding to Anionic Phospholipid Membranes Facilitate Signaling by Integrin Transmembrane Helices. *PLoS Comput. Biol.* **2013**, *9*, e1003316. [CrossRef]
1060. Orłowski, A.; Kukkurainen, S.; Pöyry, A.; Rissanen, S.; Vattulainen, I.; Hytönen, V.P.; Róg, T. PIP2 and Talin Join Forces to Activate Integrin. *J. Phys. Chem. B* **2015**, *119*, 12381–12389. [CrossRef] [PubMed]
1061. Kukkurainen, S.; Azizi, L.; Zhang, P.; Jacquier, M.-C.; Baikoghli, M.; von Essen, M.; Tuukkanen, A.; Laitaoja, M.; Liu, X.; Rahikainen, R.; et al. The F1 loop of the talin head domain acts as a gatekeeper in integrin activation and clustering. *J. Cell Sci.* **2020**, *133*, jcs239202. [CrossRef] [PubMed]
1062. Zhou, J.; Aponte-Santamaría, C.; Sturm, S.; Bullerjahn, J.T.; Bronowska, A.; Gräter, F. Mechanism of Focal Adhesion Kinase Mechanosensing. *PLoS Comput. Biol.* **2015**, *11*, e1004593. [CrossRef] [PubMed]
1063. Herzog, F.A.; Braun, L.; Schoen, I.; Vogel, V. Structural Insights How PIP2 Imposes Preferred Binding Orientations of FAK at Lipid Membranes. *J. Phys. Chem. B* **2017**, *121*, 3523–3535. [CrossRef] [PubMed]
1064. Elliott, P.R.; Goult, B.T.; Kopp, P.M.; Bate, N.; Grossmann, J.G.; Roberts, G.C.K.; Critchley, D.R.; Barsukov, I.L. The structure of the talin head reveals a novel extended conformation of the FERM domain. *Structure* **2010**, *18*, 1289–1299. [CrossRef]
1065. Busse, R.A.A.; Scacioc, A.; Krick, R.; Pérez-Lara, Á.; Thumm, M.; Kühnel, K. Characterization of PROPPIN-phosphoinositide binding and role of loop 6CD in PROPPIN-membrane binding. *Biophys. J.* **2015**, *108*, 2223–2234. [CrossRef]
1066. Krick, R.; Busse, R.A.; Scacioc, A.; Stephan, M.; Janshoff, A.; Thumm, M.; Kühnel, K. Structural and functional characterization of the two phosphoinositide binding sites of PROPPINs, a β-propeller protein family. *Proc. Natl. Acad. Sci. USA* **2012**, *109*, E2042–E2049. [CrossRef]
1067. Lai, C.-L.; Jao, C.C.; Lyman, E.; Gallop, J.L.; Peter, B.J.; McMahon, H.T.; Langen, R.; Voth, G.A. Membrane Binding and Self-Association of the Epsin N-Terminal Homology Domain. *J. Mol. Biol.* **2012**, *423*, 800–817. [CrossRef]
1068. Thallmair, V.; Schultz, L.; Marrink, S.J.; Oliver, D.; Thallmair, S. A second PI (4, 5) P2 binding site determines PI (4, 5) P2 sensitivity of the tubby domain. *bioRxiv* **2020**. [CrossRef]
1069. Muller, M.P.; Wang, Y.; Morrissey, J.H.; Tajkhorshid, E. Lipid specificity of the membrane binding domain of coagulation factor X. *J. Thromb. Haemost.* **2017**, *15*, 2005–2016. [CrossRef] [PubMed]
1070. Sandvig, K.; Bergan, J.; Kavaliauskiene, S.; Skotland, T. Lipid requirements for entry of protein toxins into cells. *Prog. Lipid Res.* **2014**, *54*, 1–13. [CrossRef] [PubMed]
1071. Basu, I.; Mukhopadhyay, C. Insights into Binding of Cholera Toxin to GM1 Containing Membrane. *Langmuir* **2014**, *30*, 15244–15252. [CrossRef] [PubMed]
1072. Gangopadhyay, A.; Chakraborty, H.J.; Datta, A. Employing virtual screening and molecular dynamics simulations for identifying hits against the active cholera toxin. *Toxicon* **2019**, *170*, 1–9. [CrossRef] [PubMed]
1073. 1Li, F.; Shrivastava, I.H.; Hanlon, P.; Dagda, R.K.; Gasanoff, E.S. Molecular mechanism by which cobra venom cardiotoxins interact with the outer mitochondrial membrane. *Toxins* **2020**, *12*, 425. [CrossRef]

1074. Martín-Acebes, M.A.; de Oya, N.J.; Saiz, J.C. Lipid metabolism as a source of druggable targets for antiviral discovery against zika and other flaviviruses. *Pharmaceuticals* **2019**, *12*, 97. [CrossRef]
1075. Nitenberg, M.; Makshakova, O.; Rocha, J.; Perez, S.; Maréchal, E.; Block, M.A.; Girard-Egrot, A.; Breton, C. Mechanism of activation of plant monogalactosyldiacylglycerol synthase 1 (MGD1) by phosphatidylglycerol. *Glycobiology* **2020**, *30*, 396–406. [CrossRef]
1076. Koss, H.; Bunney, T.D.; Esposito, D.; Martins, M.; Katan, M.; Driscoll, P.C. Dynamic Allostery in PLCγ1 and Its Modulation by a Cancer Mutation Revealed by MD Simulation and NMR. *Biophys. J.* **2018**, *115*, 31–45. [CrossRef]
1077. Robertson, R.M.; Yao, J.; Gajewski, S.; Kumar, G.; Martin, E.W.; Rock, C.O.; White, S.W. A two-helix motif positions the active site of lysophosphatidic acid acyltransferase for catalysis within the membrane bilayer Rosanna. *Nat. Struct. Mol. Biol.* **2017**, *24*, 666–671. [CrossRef] [PubMed]
1078. Cozza, G.; Rossetto, M.; Bosello-Travain, V.; Maiorino, M.; Roveri, A.; Toppo, S.; Zaccarin, M.; Zennaro, L.; Ursini, F. Glutathione peroxidase 4-catalyzed reduction of lipid hydroperoxides in membranes: The polar head of membrane phospholipids binds the enzyme and addresses the fatty acid hydroperoxide group toward the redox center. *Free Radic. Biol. Med.* **2017**, *112*, 1–11. [CrossRef] [PubMed]
1079. Grabon, A.; Orłowski, A.; Tripathi, A.; Vuorio, J.; Javanainen, M.; Róg, T.; Lönnfors, M.; McDermott, M.I.M.I.; Siebert, G.; Somerharju, P.; et al. Dynamics and energetics of the mammalian phosphatidylinositol transfer protein phospholipid exchange cycle. *J. Biol. Chem.* **2017**, *292*, 14438–14455. [CrossRef]
1080. Lu, J.; Chan, C.; Yu, L.; Fan, J.; Sun, F.; Zhai, Y. Molecular mechanism of mitochondrial phosphatidate transfer by Ups1. *Commun. Biol.* **2020**, *3*, 468. [CrossRef] [PubMed]

pharmaceuticals

Article

In Silico Studies of Potential Selective Inhibitors of Thymidylate Kinase from *Variola virus*

Danielle R. Garcia [1], Felipe R. Souza [2], Ana P. Guimarães [3], Martin Valis [4], Zbyšek Pavelek [4], Kamil Kuca [5,6,*], Teodorico C. Ramalho [5,7] and Tanos C. C. França [1,5,*]

1 Laboratory of Molecular Modeling Applied to Chemical and Biological Defense, Military Institute of Engineering, Praça General Tiburcio 80, Urca, Rio de Janeiro 22290-270, Brazil; danielle.ime@gmail.com
2 Department of Chemistry, Pontifical Catholic University of Rio de Janeiro, Rio de Janeiro 22541-041, Brazil; feliperodsouza@gmail.com
3 Department of Chemistry, Federal University of Viçosa, Avenida P. H. Rolfs, s/n, Centro, Viçosa 36570-000, Brazil; ana.paula.guimaraesime@gmail.com
4 Department of Neurology of the Medical Faculty of Charles University and University Hospital in Hradec Kralove, Sokolska 581, 50005 Hradec Kralove, Czech Republic; martin.valis@fnhk.cz (M.V.); zbysekpavelek@email.cz (Z.P.)
5 Department of Chemistry, Faculty of Science, University of Hradec Kralove, Rokitanskeho 62, 50003 Hradec Kralove, Czech Republic; teo@dqi.ufla.br
6 Biomedical Research Center, University Hospital in Hradec Kralove, Sokolska 581, 50005 Hradec Kralove, Czech Republic
7 Laboratory of Computational Chemistry, Department of Chemistry, UFLA, Lavras 37200-000, Brazil
* Correspondence: kamil.kuca@uhk.cz (K.K.); tanos@ime.eb.br (T.C.C.F.)

Citation: Garcia, D.R.; Souza, F.R.; Guimarães, A.P.; Valis, M.; Pavelek, Z.; Kuca, K.; Ramalho, T.C.; França, T.C.C. In Silico Studies of Potential Selective Inhibitors of Thymidylate Kinase from *Variola virus*. *Pharmaceuticals* **2021**, *14*, 1027. https://doi.org/10.3390/ph14101027

Academic Editors: Osvaldo Andrade Santos-Filho and Eynde Jean Jacques Vanden

Received: 11 August 2021
Accepted: 30 September 2021
Published: 9 October 2021

Publisher's Note: MDPI stays neutral with regard to jurisdictional claims in published maps and institutional affiliations.

Abstract: Continuing the work developed by our research group, in the present manuscript, we performed a theoretical study of 10 new structures derived from the antivirals cidofovir and ribavirin, as inhibitor prototypes for the enzyme thymidylate kinase from *Variola virus* (*Var*TMPK). The proposed structures were subjected to docking calculations, molecular dynamics simulations, and free energy calculations, using the molecular mechanics Poisson-Boltzmann surface area (MM-PBSA) method, inside the active sites of *Var*TMPK and human TMPK (*Hss*TMPK). The docking and molecular dynamic studies pointed to structures 2, 3, 4, 6, and 9 as more selective towards *Var*TMPK. In addition, the free energy data calculated through the MM-PBSA method, corroborated these results. This suggests that these compounds are potential selective inhibitors of *Var*TMPK and, thus, can be considered as template molecules to be synthesized and experimentally evaluated against smallpox.

Keywords: *Variola virus*; thymidylate kinase; smallpox; docking; molecular dynamics

1. Introduction

Despite the declaration of the World Health Organization (WHO) that the *Variola virus* was eradicated from the world by the 1980s, smallpox is still a matter of concern. Moreover, many studies on the development of drugs against this disease have been reported in the literature [1–16]. This is due to the fact that *Variola virus* strains may have been stored in clandestine sites around the world, and their potential use for bioterrorist purposes cannot be ignored [17,18]. Furthermore, the recreation of this kind of virus has proven to be easy to carry out, considering the current technologies [19]. As viruses can survive long periods in nature, there is no guarantee that smallpox will never return as a natural pandemic [20,21]. It is also important to mention that since the 1980s the public vaccination campaigns against smallpox do not exist anymore [4,7,9], a fact that makes all of the world's population under 40 years of age particularly vulnerable.

Currently, there is only one drug approved by the Food and Drug Administration (FDA) of the United States for the treatment of smallpox. This drug, named tecovirimat (Figure 1), acts as an inhibitor of the protein complex needed for the survival of extracellular viruses, and thereby prevents its spread throughout the body from the infected cells [1,2,10] However, despite the fact that it was approved by the FDA, tecovirimat is still in phase II of clinical trials and has not been tested in humans yet, due to the lack of patients with smallpox. It has been effective in laboratory tests to protect animals against monkeypox and rabbitpox as well as presented low toxicity to humans [1,2,10,22,23].

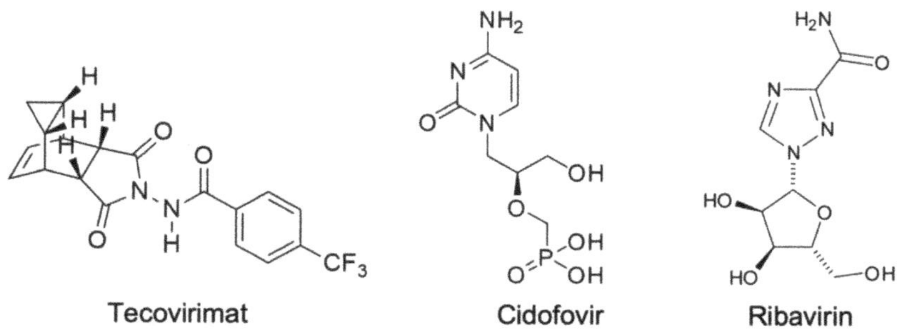

Figure 1. Structures of tecovirimat, cidofovir, and ribavirin.

The risk of smallpox resurgence either, as a natural pandemic or consequence of a terrorist attack, combined with the huge number of non-immunized people in the world, and the scarcity of drugs to combat this disease, highlight the importance of the search for new drugs against it.

It is known from the literature that the Variola virus belongs to the genus Orthopoxvirus, which, similar to all poxviruses, are capable of encoding their own thymidine and thymidylate kinases (TK and TMPK) [24]. Caillat et al. [24] have detailed the sequence alignment of TMPKs from different Orthopoxviruses (vaccinia virus, smallpox, cowpox, camelpox, and monkeypox) and showed that those enzymes present highly similar amino acid sequencing, which are practically identical, except for a few residues. The majority of the different residues among the viral enzymes belong to the protein loops [24]. Therefore, the crystallographic structure of the Vaccinia virus TMPK (VaccTMPK) can be used as a template for modeling the structure of the Variola virus TMPK (VarTMPK), which is not available yet in the protein data bank (PDB) (https://www.rcsb.org/).

Moreover, the study by Caillat et al. [24] included data on practical experiments using compounds such as brivudine monophosphate to test their inhibition of VaccTMPK and human TMPK (HssTMPK). HssTMPK and VaccTMPK are only 42% similar in their amino acid sequence alignments and the dimer interface arrangements of both enzymes are different, as well as their active site geometry [24–26]. Due to these differences, as stated by the authors, VaccTMPK is able to accommodate more voluminous compounds, such as brivudine monophosphate, which stabilizes the enzyme and is phosphorylated. The specificity of the bond with brivudine monophosphate shows that selective antipox agents can be developed based on this finding. Therefore, these antivirals can also be investigated for their use in the treatment of TMPK-related diseases from other viruses of the Orthopoxvirus genus [24].

According to the literature, TMPK is responsible for the synthesis of thymidine 5′-triphosphate (TTP) based on the phosphorylation of thymidine 5′-monophosphate (TMP) [27,28]. TTP participates in DNA synthesis (as a building block) and its levels are controlled during the different phases of the cell cycle. Since TMPK is important for the biosynthesis of TTP, the enzyme is considered a molecular target for the development of antiviral drugs against many diseases, and the interruption of the metabolism of TTP can be used to stop the development of said illnesses. In addition to its direct effect on the metabolism of TTP, TMPK also interacts directly with the DNA synthesis process, since it plays an important role in the activation of DNA precursor nucleoside analogues. As a result, its inhibition directly affects the synthesis of genetic material, thus provoking the deactivation (death) of the virus [25,29,30].

Previously, we proposed VarTMPK as a potential target to the design of potential selective inhibitors and studied the behavior of known antivirals inside it, thus pointing to the relevant residues to be targeted in the drug design [7]. Next, we proposed the structures of 10 potential VarTMPK inhibitors based on theoretical studies of another series of antivirals [4,8,24,26]. The best ranked compounds after docking and MD simulations studies were, then, selected to design a new series of compounds based on alterations of their structural features, having in mind the synthetic viability and selectivity towards VarTMPK [9]. A few compounds of this new series presented promising theoretical results [9].

In the present work, we performed the theoretical study of 10 new compounds whose design was based on structural modifications of the antivirals cidofovir and ribavirin (Figure 1), seeking the application of these new compounds against the Variola virus. Cidofovir and ribavirin were chosen to serve as templates for this study, since they have already been extensively studied and validated for diseases caused by Orthopoxviruses. Therefore, they have much data available in specialized databanks [31,32].

Maintaining the main idea of our previous studies [4,7,9], the objective of this work was to minimize the structural complexity of the template compounds, in order to make the synthesis of these structures more feasible and less cumbersome.

To analyze the binding modes and selectivity of the proposed compounds inside *Var*TMPK and *Hss*TMPK, the molecular docking method was used [33,34]. In order to assess their dynamical behavior and corroborate the docking achievements, molecular dynamics (MD) simulations rounds were performed on the best poses obtained from docking. Finally, free energy calculations, applying the molecular mechanics Poisson-Boltzmann surface area (MM-PBSA) method, were performed on the most promising compounds to verify the effectiveness, reliability, and selectivity of their binding inside each enzyme [35–45].

2. Results

2.1. Docking Calculations

Table 1 lists the active site residues of *Var*TMPK and *Hss*TMPK. It is possible to see that seven of these 14 residues are different. This 50% difference highlights the possibility of designing selective inhibitors for *Var*TMPK.

Table 1. Active site residues of VarTMPK and HssTMPK. The non-matching amino acids are shown in red.

VarTMPK	Asp13, Lys14, Ser15, Lys17, Thr18, Arg41, Leu53, Asn65, Phe68, Cys69, Arg72, Arg93, Tyr101, Ala102
HssTMPK	Asp15, Arg16, Ala17, Lys19, Ser20, Arg45, Leu57, His69, Phe72, Ser73, Arg76, Arg97, Phe105, Thr106

Similar to our previous works [4,9], the ionization states of the compounds used in this study corresponded to the predominant microspecies at physiological conditions (pH = 7.4). According to the chemicalize server (www.chemicalize.com), our compounds except compound 1, are 100% in the neutral form at pH 7.4. The dominant microspecies for compound 1 predicted by chemicalize (www.chemicalize.com) is the one negatively charged in the phosphate group, with 74% of prevalence at pH 7.4. Moreover, according to the chemicalize server (www.chemicalize.com), all of our compounds meet the Lipinski's criterion of drug likeness [46], as shown in Table 2.

Table 2. Calculated values of acute toxicity, carcinogenicity (in mouse), and Lipinski's rule of the compounds and antivirals.

Structure	Acute Toxicity (Algae)	Carcinogenicity (Mouse)	Meets Lipinski's Rule?
1	1.10	negative	Yes
2	0.30	positive	Yes
3	0.15	positive	Yes
4	0.22	positive	Yes
5	0.51	positive	Yes
6	0.25	positive	Yes
7	0.38	positive	Yes
8	0.31	positive	Yes
9	0.37	positive	Yes
10	0.60	positive	Yes
Cidofovir	1.19	Positive	Yes
Ribavirin	0.54	negative	Yes

The docking studies were meant to identify the compounds with better interactions and higher selectivity towards *Var*TMPK. The best poses for each compound were selected in accordance with the best (more negative) interaction energies inside *Var*TMPK and *Hss*TMPK (intermolecular and hydrogen bond) and the best superposition onto TDP. As shown in Figure 2, the poses selected in the docking studies present an optimal superposition onto TDP for both *Var*TMPK and *Hss*TMPK. These poses were analyzed according to: Their interaction energy values with the enzymes ($E_{interaction}$) and the cofactor ($E_{cofactor}$); the H-bond energies between the compounds and the enzymes (H_{bond}); and, finally, the amino acids involved in the interactions with the compounds in both enzymes. The results obtained for those parameters are summarized in Table 3. Figure 3a–j shows the interactions observed between the proposed compounds inside *Var*TMPK and *Hss*TMPK. The active site residues of both enzymes are shown in red and the red spheres represent water molecules.

2.2. Molecular Dynamics Simulations

The best poses of compounds **2**, **3**, **4**, **5**, **6**, **8**, and **9** were selected for additional rounds of MD simulations, since they were pointed as more selective towards *Var*TMPK by the docking studies. The results are shown in the plots of root-mean-square deviation (RMSD) and number of H-bonds formed during the MD simulations, for their complexes inside *Var*TMPK and *Hss*TMPK, shown in Figures 4 and 5, respectively.

In order to validate our MD protocol, we performed three rounds of MD simulations for the complexes of compound **2** with both enzymes. The obtained plots of RMSD are shown in Figures S1–S6 of the Supplementary Material.

2.3. MM-PBSA Calculations

According to the literature, one of the limitations of docking studies lies in determining the affinities of ligand-protein complexes using calculations based solely on the poses generated for these complexes. In this regard, the MM-PBSA method tends to improve the results related to the binding energy, which is due to the fact that MM-PBSA provides more accurate results when the affinities between the ligand and protein are determined. Moreover, this is achieved by calculating the free binding energy associated with the formation of ligand-protein complexes [47] and decomposing it in the contributing components, as proposed before by Bren et al. [44,45]. Table 4 shows the average binding energy values calculated for compounds **2**, **3**, **4**, **6**, and **9** complexed with *Var*TMPK and *Hss*TMPK, while Figure 6 illustrates the favorable and unfavorable energy contributions of compounds **3** and **6** inside *Var*TMPK.

Table 3. Docking results for the compounds studied and TDP inside *Var*TMPK and *Hss*TMPK active sites.

#	$E_{interaction}$ (kcal.mol^{-1})		$E_{cofactor}$ (kcal.mol^{-1})		H-Bond Energy (kcal.mol^{-1})		H-Bond Interactions		$\Delta E_{int.}$ (kcal.mol^{-1})
	*Var*TMPK	*Hss*TMPK	*Var*TMPK	*Hss*TMPK	*Var*TMPK	*Hss*TMPK	*Var*TMPK	*Hss*TMPK	
1	−100.00	−128.35	−25.04	−4.13	−14.74	−15.18	Asn37 (2.91Å) Lys17 (2.08Å; 2.98Å) Phe38 (3.23Å) Arg93 (2.87Å) Tyr101 (3.06Å) Ser97 (3.36Å) H_2O (2.67Å; 3.20Å)	Asp15 (3.10Å; 2.97Å; 2.97Å) Arg97 (2.60Å; 2.60Å; 3.05Å) Ser101 (2.93Å) H_2O (3.21Å; 2.49Å; 2.52Å; 2.96Å; 2.94Å; 2.87Å; 3.33Å)	+28.35
2	−95.43	−32.58	−0.24	−0.19	−7.93	−2.50	Pro39 (3.06Å) Arg93 (2.88Å; 3.10Å) Arg41 (2.76Å)	Asp15 (3.10Å)H_2O (3.38Å)	−62.85
3	−110.95	−75.54	−2.45	−0.34	−6.44	−1.58	Tyr94 (3.11Å) Arg93 (3.10Å) Arg41 (2.61Å)	Arg97 (2.65Å) H_2O (2.84Å)	−35.41
4	−89.18	−50.61	−0.61	−0.53	−4.84	−2.73	Arg93 (3.10Å) Tyr101 (3.13Å)	Arg97 (2.6Å; 2.85Å) Ser101 (2.49Å) H_2O (2.46Å; 3.43Å; 3.38Å)	−38.57
5	−90.77	−35.37	−1.47	−0.21	−3.86	−2.58	Arg41 (3.09Å) Arg93 (3.10Å)	Asp15 (3.10Å) H_2O (2.45Å; 3.02Å; 3.09Å)	−55.40
6	−112.24	−84.39	−2.64	−0.17	−3.32	−2.50	Tyr94 (3.32Å) Arg41(2.69Å)	Pro43 (2.64Å) H_2O (2.93Å; 3.33Å)	−27.85
7	−41.11	−58.87	−1.33	−0.47	−4.22	−3.70	Arg93 (3.11Å) Tyr101 (2.63Å)	Arg97 (3.10Å; 3.12Å) H_2O (3.27Å)	+17.76
8	−106.20	−94.88	−0.63	−0.28	−12.93	−7.79	Phe38 (3.17Å) Arg41 (3.06Å)Glu142 (3.10Å) Asp13 (3.10Å)Glu145 (2.65Å) H_2O (3.05Å)	Asp15 (2.72Å; 3.10Å; 3.10Å) H_2O (3.28Å; 2.77Å; 3.21Å; 2.94Å; 3.33Å; 3.25Å)	−11.32
9	−120.94	−75.04	−1.23	−0.08	−12.33	−10.00	Arg72 (2.70Å) Phe38 (2.90Å) Arg41 (2.98Å) Asp13 (3.10Å) Glu145 (3.10Å)	Arg76 (2.60Å) Asp15 (3.10Å; 3.00Å; 3.00Å) H_2O (2.67Å; 3.30Å; 2.73Å; 3.04Å)	−45.90
10	−44.85	−101.15	−0.80	−0.64	−8.63	−7.40	Arg72 (2.75Å; 2.88Å; 3.19Å) Arg93 (3.10Å) Tyr101 (3.10Å)Asp13 (3.10Å) H_2O (2.84Å)	Pro43 (3.28Å) Arg97 (3.24Å; 2.67Å) Ser101 (3.24Å) H_2O (3.36Å)	56.30
TDP	228.18	−195.60	−50.38	−18.13	−3.82	−13.97	Asp13, Lys17, Asn37, Arg41, Arg72, Arg93	Asp15, Arg45, Arg76, Arg97, H_2O	

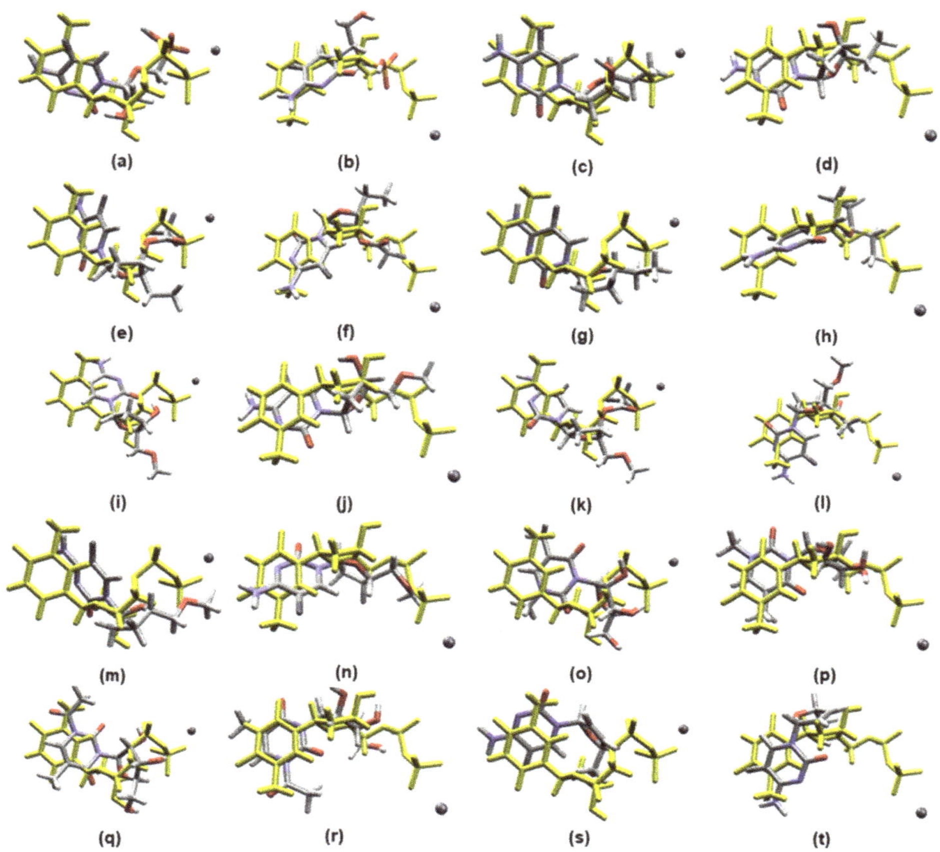

Figure 2. Best molecular docking poses for the prototypes inside *Var*TMPK and *Hss*TMPK: (**a**) *Var*TMPK/compound **1**, (**b**) *Hss*TMPK/compound **1**, (**c**) *Var*TMPK/compound **2**, (**d**) *Hss*TMPK/compound **2**, (**e**) *Var*TMPK/compound **3**, (**f**) *Hss*TMPK/compound **3**, (**g**) *Var*TMPK/compound **4**, (**h**) *Hss*TMPK/compound **4**, (**i**) *Var*TMPK/compound **5**, (**j**) *Hss*TMPK/compound **5**, (**k**) *Var*TMPK/compound **6**, (**l**) *Hss*TMPK/compound **6**, (**m**) *Var*TMPK/compound **7**, (**n**) *Hss*TMPK/compound **7**, (**o**) *Var*TMPK/compound **8**, (**p**) *Hss*TMPK/compound **8**, (**q**) *Var*TMPK/compound **9**, (**r**) *Hss*TMPK/compound **9**, (**s**) *Var*TMPK/compound **10**, (**t**) *Hss*TMPK/compound **10**.

Table 4. MM-PBSA results for compounds **2**, **3**, **4**, **6**, and **9**.

	Binding Energies kJ.mol^{-1}	
Compound	***Var*TMPK**	***Hss*TMPK**
2	−133.69 ± 6.92	−36.60 ± 3.71
3	−189.90 ± 3.05	−90.79 ± 3.56
4	−59.50 ± 4.37	−33.50 ± 4.41
6	−206.04 ± 12.98	−100.85 ± 2.24
9	−81.72 ± 2.58	−43.16 ± 4.36

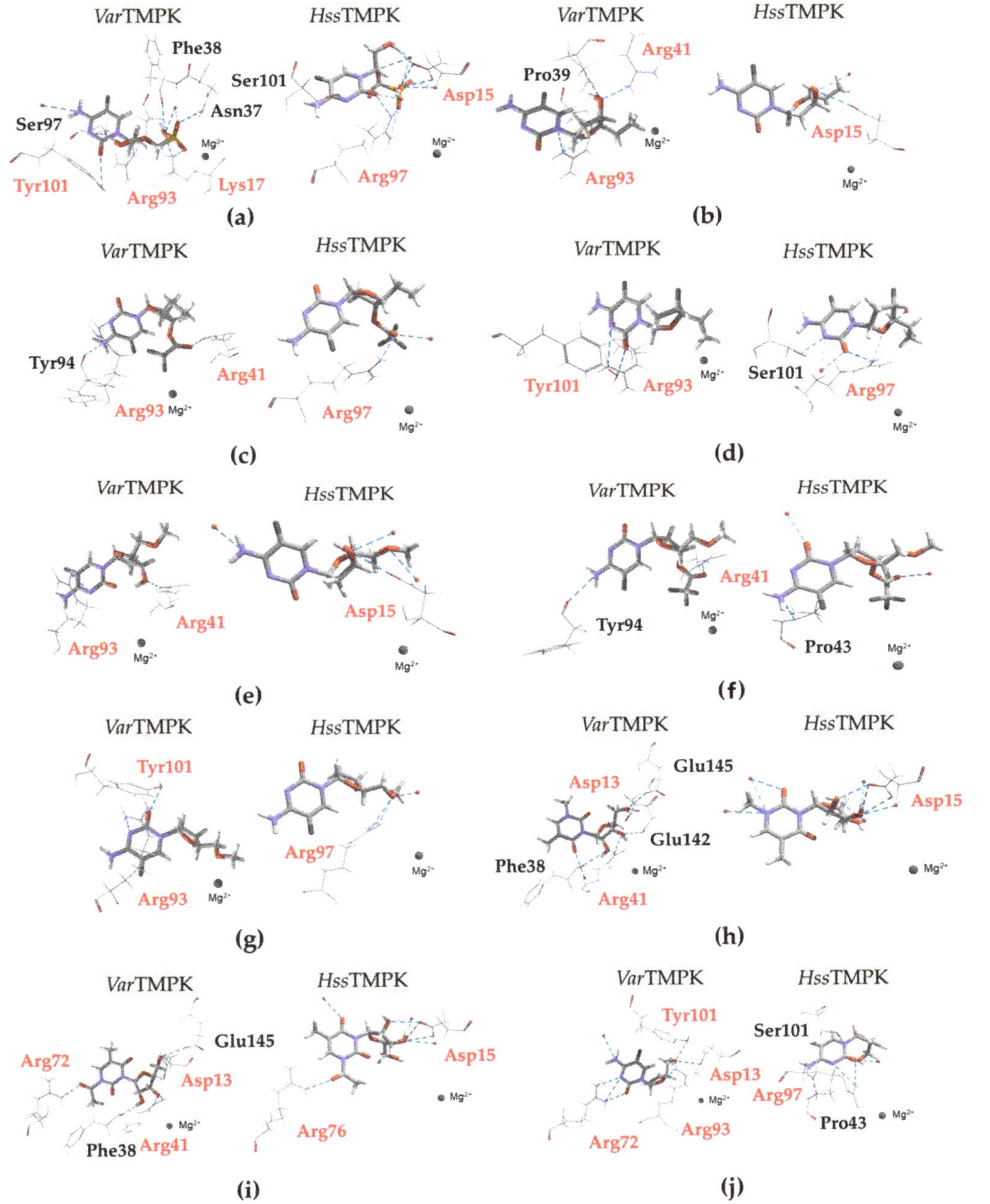

Figure 3. Interactions observed for the best poses obtained inside the *Var*TMPK and *Hss*TMPK active sites: (**a**) Compound **1**, (**b**) compound **2**, (**c**) compound **3**, (**d**) compound **4**, (**e**) compound **5**, (**f**) compound **6**, (**g**) compound **7**, (**h**) compound **8**, (**i**) compound **9**, (**j**) compound **10**.

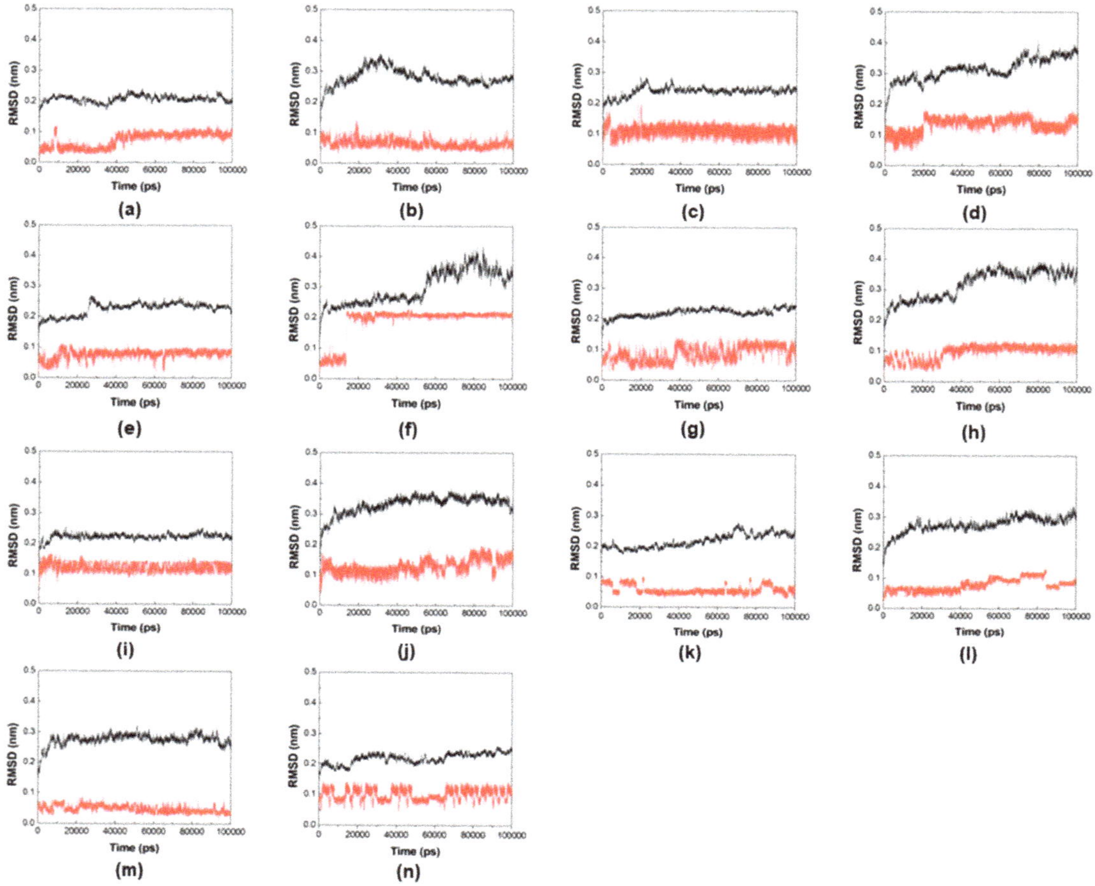

Figure 4. RMSD of the systems formed by the enzymes (in black) and compounds (in red): (**a**) *Var*TMPK/compound **2**, (**b**) *Hss*TMPK/compound **2**, (**c**) *Var*TMPK/compound **3**, (**d**) *Hss*TMPK/compound **3**, (**e**) *Var*TMPK/compound **4**, (**f**) *Hss*TMPK/compound **4**, (**g**) *Var*TMPK/compound **5**, (**h**) *Hss*TMPK/compound **5**, (**i**) *Var*TMPK/compound **6**, (**j**) *Hss*TMPK/compound **6**, (**k**) *Var*TMPK/compound **8**, (**l**) *Hss*TMPK/compound **8**, (**m**) *Var*TMPK/compound **9**, (**n**) *Hss*TMPK/compound **9**.

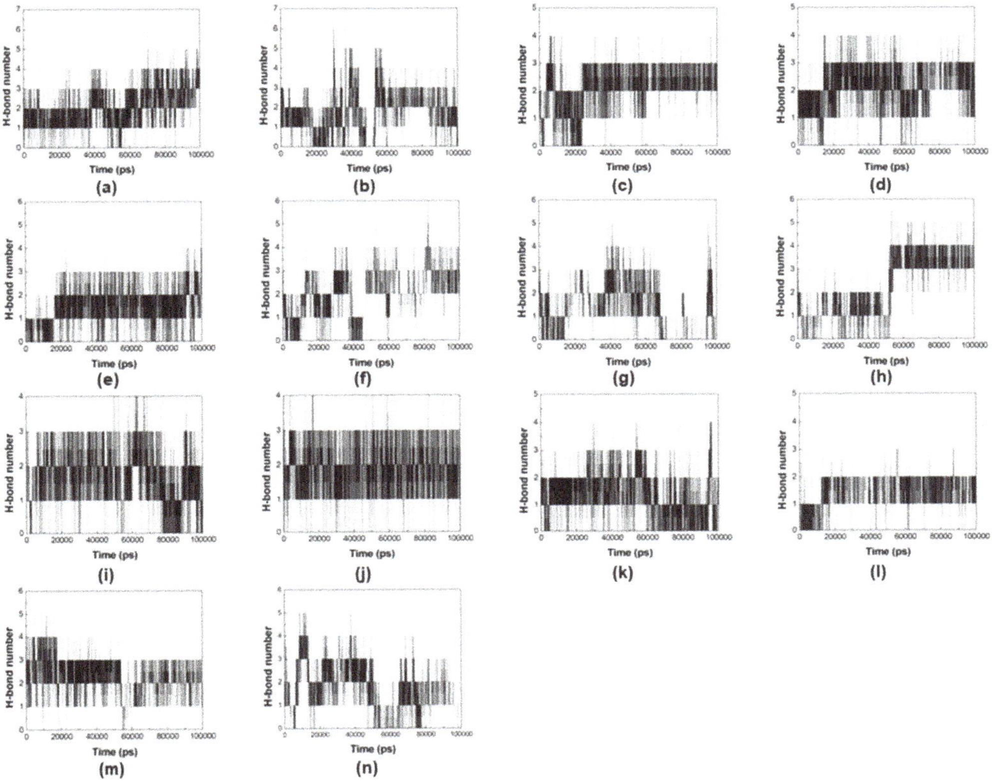

Figure 5. H-bonds between (**a**) VarTMPK/compound **2**, (**b**) HssTMPK/compound **2**, (**c**) VarTMPK/compound **3**, (**d**) HssTMPK/compound **3**, (**e**) VarTMPK/compound **4**, (**f**) HssTMPK/compound **4**, (**g**) VarTMPK/compound **5**, (**h**) HssTMPK/compound **5**, (**i**) VarTMPK/compound **6**, (**j**) HssTMPK/compound **6**, (**k**) VarTMPK/compound **8**, (**l**) HssTMPK/compound **8**, (**m**) VarTMPK/compound **9**, (**n**) HssTMPK/compound **9**.

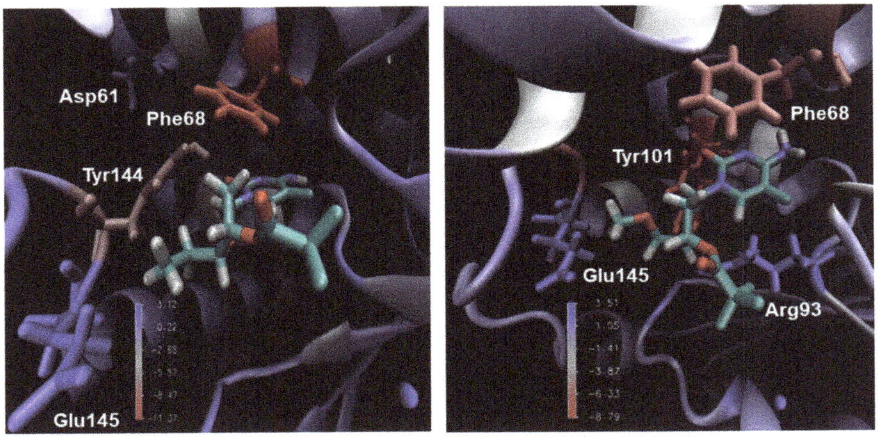

Figure 6. Main interactions of the complexes *Var*TMPK/compound **3** (**left**) and *Var*TMPK/compound **6** (**right**) calculated by MM-PBSA.

3. Discussion

As can be seen, Table 2 shows the toxicity and mouse carcinogenicity values of the investigated structures and the antivirals used as precursors. In short, with respect to the proposed compounds, it is important to point out that the acute toxicity values in algae calculated for all the structures were lower than the value found for cidofovir (1.19), which is not toxic. Furthermore, except for compounds **1** and **10**, all the structures had lower toxicity values in comparison with those of ribavirin (0.54).

According to the literature, the cavity of *Hss*TMPK acquired through the software Molegro virtual docker (MVD)®, presents a volume of 90.112 Å^3, which is greater than the value of 76.288 Å^3 observed for the cavity of *Var*TMPK. It is important to point out that the *Hss*TMPK cavity is more outspread and narrower. Therefore, it is expected to have issues in the entrance and/or permanence of larger inhibitors in the binding site [7].

The results in Table 3 show that all the compounds are capable of binding to the active sites of both enzymes. This is reflected by the negative values of $E_{interaction}$ observed for all of them. Comparing the docking results obtained, we can state that compounds **2**, **3**, **4**, **5**, **6**, **8**, and **9** form more stable complexes with VarTMPK. This enables us to infer that they might show higher affinity for the active site of this enzyme, since the systems formed among these compounds and the viral enzyme presented lower values of $E_{interaction}$, $E_{cofactor}$, and H-bond energy. Regarding the $\Delta E_{interaction}$ values, determined based on the difference between $E_{interaction}$ inside *Var*TMPK (lower value) and *Hss*TMPK, the compounds listed above ranked: **2** (−62.85 kcal.mol^{-1}) < **5** (−55.40 kcal.mol^{-1}) < **9** (−45.90 kcal.mol^{-1}) < **4** (−38.57 kcal.mol^{-1}) < **3** (−35.41 kcal.mol^{-1}) < **6** (−27.85 kcal.mol^{-1}) < **8** (−11.32 kcal.mol^{-1}).

The best pose of compound 1 interacts with three active site residues of *Var*TMPK and two active site residues of *Hss*TMPK, as shown in Figure 3a. Among these residues, Arg93 from *Var*TMPK and Arg97 from *Hss*TMPK are equivalent between both enzymes.

Regarding compound **2** (Figure 3b), we observed interactions with three residues from *Var*TMPK, of which two belong to the active site, while for *Hss*TMPK, an interaction with only one residue was observed, which also belongs to the active site.

Compounds **3** (Figure 3c) and **4** (Figure 3d) interact with the same number of residues inside both enzymes. However, for *Var*TMPK, two interacting residues belong to the active site versus only one for *Hss*TMPK. Residues Arg93 from *Var*TMPK and Arg97 from *Hss*TMPK are the only equivalent interacting residues observed.

Figure 3e shows that compound 5 interacts with two active site residues from *Var*TMPK and one from *Hss*TMPK. No matching interacting residues were observed.

According to Figure 3f, compound 6 interacts solely with one active site residue from *Var*TMPK and has no interaction with the *Hss*TMPK active site residues. On the other hand, for compound **7**, Figure 3g shows interactions with two active site residues from *Var*TMPK and one from *Hss*TMPK. Arg93 from *Var*TMPK and Arg97 from *Hss*TMPK were the only equivalent interacting residues observed.

Regarding the complexes formed with compound **8** (shown in Figure 3h), we can see interactions with two active site residues from *Var*TMPK and one from *Hss*TMPK. In this case, Asp13 from *Var*TMPK and Asp15 from *Hss*TMPK are the equivalent interacting residues observed.

Figure 3i shows that compound **9** interacts with three active site residues from *Var*TMPK, and two from *Hss*TMPK. The equivalent interacting residues observed are: Asp13 (*Var*TMPK) and Asp15 (*Hss*TMPK), and Arg72 (*Var*TMPK) and Arg76 (*Hss*TMPK).

Finally, Figure 3j shows that compound **10** interacts with four active site residues from *Var*TMPK, and only one from *Hss*TMPK. The equivalent residues observed are Arg93 from *Var*TMPK and Arg97 from *Hss*TMPK.

The RMSD plots for the multiple MD simulations, performed for the systems enzyme/compound 2 (Figures S1–S6), showed the same behavior for all dynamics, with no variation above 0.1 nm. This validates our MD simulations protocol for the systems under study.

Comparing the RMSD plots in Figure 4 for both enzymes, it is possible to see that for all the systems, the RMSD values never passed 0.4 nm for the enzyme (black lines) and 0.2 nm for the ligands (red lines) during the simulated time. However, for most of the systems, both the enzyme and compounds presented more fluctuations inside *Hss*TMPK. Inside *Var*TMPK, this fluctuation never passed 0.05 nm for compounds **2**, **3**, **4**, **6**, and **9**.

Compounds **5** and **8** were the only ones showing a similar or more instable behavior inside *Var*TMPK compared to *Hss*TMPK (see Figure 4g,h,k,l). This does not corroborate with the docking results and suggests that these compounds are not selective towards *Var*TMPK.

In addition, we analyzed the number of H-bonds formed during the MD simulations for the complexes inside *Var*TMPK and *Hss*TMPK (Figure 5). The H-bonds profiles of the complexes with compounds **2** (Figure 5a,b), **3** (Figure 5c,d), **4** (Figure 5e,f), **6** (Figure 5i,j), and **9** (Figure 5m,n) show that these compounds were capable of keeping at least three H-bonds with *Var*TMPK during the whole simulated time, presenting a profile better or similar to *Hss*TMPK. Conversely, the H-bond graphs of the complexes with compounds **5** (Figure 5g,h) and 8 (Figure 5k,l) show a more unstable behavior with the prevalence of no more than two H-bonds during the whole simulation, presenting a worse (compound **5**) or similar (compound **8**) profile compared to *Hss*TMPK.

The results regarding the formation of H-bonds can be correlated to the RMSD observed during the MD simulations, and point to compounds **2**, **3**, **4**, **6**, and **9** as more selective towards *Var*TMPK. For this reason, these compounds were selected for the determination of their binding energies inside *Var*TMPK and *Hss*TMPK based on the MM-PBSA calculations.

Regarding the MM-PBSA calculations, the results in Table 4 show that for all compounds, the mean binding energy values of the complexes formed with *Var*TMPK were lower than the values determined for the complexes formed with *Hss*TMPK. These data confirm the results obtained by the docking and MD simulations, which suggested the selectivity of these compounds towards *Var*TMPK.

Moreover, the results in Table 4 show that compounds **3** and **6** stand out among the others in terms of binding energy with *Var*TMPK, which are the most stable ones. Furthermore, the difference related to *Hss*TMPK was higher than 90 KJ/mol in both cases, suggesting a high selectivity towards *Var*TMPK.

A possible explanation for the high free energy values of the complexes between *Var*TMPK and compounds **3** and **6**, is the presence of the trifluoroacetate group (–$COOCF_3$) attached to the tetrahydrofuran ring. The presence of three fluorine atoms—a chemical element with high electronegativity and with isolated and free electron pairs on its structure—likely favors the selective interactions inside *Var*TMPK. Therefore, these interactions can help in maintaining the complexes formed between *Var*TMPK and compounds **3** and **6**—thus contributing to the higher stability of these systems.

4. Materials and Methods

4.1. Compounds Studied

The 2D structures of the compounds studied in this work are shown in Figure 7. As mentioned above, they are all derivatives from the antivirals cidofovir and ribavirin, designed to better explore the potential selective interactions with residues of the active site of *Var*TMPK.

The ionization states of each compound in Figure 7 at physiological pH (7.4)—as well as the drug likeness criteria established according to the Lipinski's rule of five [48]—were calculated with the aid of the Chemicalize databank (https://chemicalize.com) [46]. Their toxicity and carcinogenicity in mice were calculated with the online program PreADMET (https://preadmet.bmdrc.kr/adme-prediction/).

The tridimensional structures of these compounds, and the calculation of their atomic charges, were done through the Recife model 1 (RM1) semiempirical model [49,50], using the Spartan 08® Suite software.

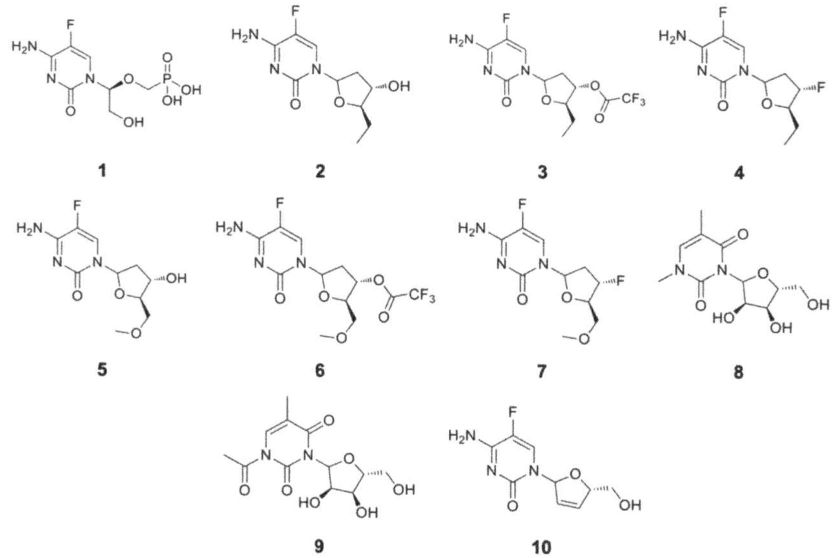

Figure 7. Structures of the studied compounds.

4.2. Applied Protocols

In previous works [4,7,9], the tridimensional structures of *Var*TMPK and *Hss*TMPK that were used for our studies include, respectively, the homology model complexed with TDP and the Mg^{2+} cofactor, constructed by Guimarães et al. [7], and the crystallographic structure of *Hss*TMPK complexed with TDP and Mg^{2+}, available in the protein data bank (PDB) under the code 1E2G [51]. According to Guimarães et al. [7], the Ramachandran plot of the homology model showed that 99.5% of the residues were situated in the most favored regions.

The docking protocol used, as well as its validation by re-docking studies, was the same as employed by Guimarães et al. [7]. The MolDock algorithm [52] from the Molegro virtual docker (MVD®) was used to perform the energy calculations of the ligands inside VarTMPK and *Hss*TMPK. The binding site was restricted to spheres with radii of 6 and 10 Å, respectively, around TDP, and all the residues inside these spheres were set to be flexible. The coordinates were centered on x = 8.95, y = 22.41, and z = 0.69 for VarTMPK, and x = 13.92, y = 75.19, and z = 25.05 for *Hss*TMPK [7]. The best poses for each ligand in the viral and human enzymes were selected for further MD simulations.

The protocol comprising the application of MD simulations rounds to the best poses selected from the docking studies was based on our most recent work [9]. Each ligand was parameterized in order to be recognized by the OPLS-AA force field [53]. The enzyme/ligand complexes were put inside cubic boxes of 450 nm^3 containing around 13,000 Tip4P type water molecules under periodic boundary conditions (PBCs), using the GROMACS 5.1.4 software [54]. The energy minimization steps used were: (1) Steepest descent with position restraint (PR) of the ligand; (2) steepest descent without PR; (3) conjugate gradients; and, lastly, (4) quasi Newton Broyden–Fletcher–Goldfarb–Shanno (L-BFGS) algorithm [55], with a minimal energy of 1 kcal.mol^{-1}. Thereafter, the systems were submitted to temperature (NVT) and pressure (NPT) balancing phases in order to attain equilibrium. The equilibrated systems were, then, submitted to 500 ps of MD at 310 K with a PR for the entire system, except for water molecules, in order to ensure the equilibrium of solvent molecules, and finally, 100,000 ps of free MD simulations at 310 K without PR, with 2 fs of integration time, and a cutting radius of 10 Å for long-distance interactions [9]. All the Glu and Asp residues were assigned with negative charges, and the Lys and Arg residues were assigned with positive charges. As mentioned above, the visual molecular dynamics (VMD) software [56] was used to analyze the MD results of the systems. In order to validate our MD simulations protocol, three MD simulations were performed for the systems VarTMPK/compound 2 and *Hss*TMPK/compound 2.

The MM-PBSA method was employed to predict the free binding energies of the ligands inside the VarTMPK and *Hss*TMPK. This study allows us to infer whether the binding process is spontaneous (freeing energy) or nonspontaneous (requiring energy), thus enabling us to point to the prototype that is more interesting and promising regarding the selective inhibition of VarTMPK. The determination of the free energy of formation of the complexes, in association with the MD simulations, take into consideration three energetic terms in the calculation of binding energy: (1) Changes in the potential energy of the system in a vacuum; (2) polar and apolar solvation of the different species; and (3) the entropy related to the formation of the complexes during the gaseous phase [9,36,37,44,45]. For all the enzyme/ligand complexes, MM-PBSA calculations were performed using the g_mmpbsa tool [37] from the GROMACS package. In order to consider non-correlated frames, the structures for the free energy calculations were obtained at 500 ps each after the stabilization of the systems [9].

The parameters used for the docking, MD simulations, and MM-PBSA calculations performed in this work are summarized in Table 5.

Table 5. Parameters used in the docking and MD studies.

<table>
<tr><td rowspan="2">Docking</td><td>Software Used in Energy Calculations</td><td>Algorithm Used in Energy Calculations</td><td>Radius of the Anchoring Area</td><td colspan="2">Enzyme Site Coordinates</td><td>No. of Repetitions</td><td>No. of Poses</td></tr>
<tr><td>Molegro virtual docker (MVD®)</td><td>MolDock [52]</td><td>6–10 Å</td><td>HssTMPK
x = 8.95
y = 22.41
z = 0.69</td><td>VarTMPK
x = 13.92
y = 75.19
z = 25.05</td><td>10</td><td>30</td></tr>
<tr><td rowspan="2">Molecular Dynamics</td><td>Force Field</td><td>Software Used in Coordinate Parameters and Topologies</td><td>Software Used in Construction of Cubic Boxes *</td><td colspan="2">Simulation Stage Parameters</td><td colspan="2">Software Used to Analyze MD Results</td></tr>
<tr><td>OPLS-AA [53]</td><td>AnteChamber PYthon Parser InterfacE (AcPype) [57]</td><td>GROMACS 5.1.4 [54]</td><td>1st
t = 500 ps
T = 310 K
w/ position restriction</td><td>2nd
t = 100.000 ps
T = 310 K</td><td colspan="2">Visual molecular dynamics (VMD) [56]</td></tr>
</table>

* Parameters of cubic boxes: 450 nm^3/1300 H_2O/Tip4P molecules.

5. Conclusions

According to the docking studies, it was found that only compounds **1**, **7**, and **10** did not demonstrate selectivity towards *Var*TMPK. The MD simulations studies corroborated the docking results for compounds **2**, **3**, **4**, **6**, and **9**, implying that the complexes formed between each of them and *Var*TMPK are more stable when compared to the same complexes with *Hss*TMPK. This was also observed in the further MM-PBSA calculations of the binding energies that showed lower binding values for these compounds inside *Var*TMPK than inside *Hss*TMPK. Moreover, the MM-PBSA studies pointed to compounds **3** and **6** as the most promising selective inhibitors of *Var*TMPK with the higher difference in binding energies. This is probably due to the presence of the—$COOCF_3$ group on these compounds that could be favoring their stabilization inside *Var*TMPK.

In conclusion, our results suggest that five of the 10 proposed compounds, derived from the antivirals cidofovir and ribavirin, can be excellent alternatives for the development of new drugs against smallpox. Since TMPK is highly conserved amongst other Orthopoxviruses, similar to the vaccinia and monkeypox viruses, the same theoretical approach used here can be done with the TMPKs of those viruses as a proof of concept. Furthermore, the experimental evaluation of these compounds should be first performed against those viruses as a primarily model to check their potential in vitro. This would help in confirming the activity of those compounds before moving to the more complicated evaluation against the Variola virus, which will demand both an authorized laboratory and a stricter safety protocol.

Supplementary Materials: The following are available online at https://www.mdpi.com/article/10.3390/ph14101027/s1, Figure S1: RMSD of the first MD simulation for the system HssTMPK/Compound 2, Figure S2: RMSD of the second MD simulation for the system HssTMPK/Compound 2, Figure S3: RMSD of the third MD simulation for the system HssTMPK/Compound 2, Figure S4: RMSD of the first MD simulation for the system VarTMPK/Compound 2, Figure S5: RMSD of the second MD simulation for the system VarTMPK/Compound 2, Figure S6: RMSD of the third MD simulation for the system VarTMPK/Compound 2.

Author Contributions: Conceptualization, T.C.C.F., A.P.G. and D.R.G.; methodology, D.R.G. and F.R.S.; software, T.C.R. and T.C.C.F.; validation, T.C.C.F. and D.R.G.; formal analysis, T.C.C.F. and D.R.G.; investigation, D.R.G. and F.R.S.; resources, T.C.C.F., Z.P., K.K. and M.V.; data curation, T.C.C.F. and T.C.R.; writing—original draft preparation, D.R.G.; writing—review and editing, D.R.G., T.C.C.F., M.V., Z.P. and K.K.; visualization, D.R.G.; supervision, A.P.G., T.C.R. and T.C.C.F.; project administration, T.C.C.F. and K.K.; funding acquisition, T.C.C.F., M.V., Z.P. and K.K. All authors have read and agreed to the published version of the manuscript.

Funding: This research was funded by the Brazilian agencies Conselho Nacional de Pesquisa (CNPq), grant no. 308225/2018–0; Fundação de Amparo a Pesquisa do Estado do Rio de Janeiro (FAPERJ), grant no. E-02/202.961/2017; and the *Excelence project PřF* UHK 2011/2021-2022. This study was also partially supported by grants from the Ministry of Health of the Czech Republic (FN HK 00179906) and Charles University in Prague, Czech Republic (PROGRES Q40).

Institutional Review Board Statement: Not applicable.

Informed Consent Statement: Not applicable.

Data Availability Statement: Data is contained within the article and supplementary material.

Acknowledgments: The authors are grateful to the Military Institute of Engineering, Federal University of Lavras, Federal University of Viçosa and University of Hradec Kralové for the infrastructure.

Conflicts of Interest: The authors declare no conflict of interest.

References

1. Russo, A.T.; Berhanu, A.; Bigger, C.B.; Prigge, J.; Silvera, P.M.; Grosenbach, D.W.; Hruby, D. Co-administration of tecovirimat and ACAM2000™ in non-human primates: Effect of tecovirimat treatment on ACAM2000 immunogenicity and efficacy versus lethal monkeypox virus challenge. *Vaccine* **2020**, *38*, 644–654. [CrossRef]
2. Chan-Tack, K.M.; Harrington, P.R.; Choi, S.-Y.; Myers, L.; O'Rear, J.; Seo, S.; McMillan, D.; Ghantous, H.; Birnkrant, D.; Sherwat, A.I. Assessing a drug for an eradicated human disease: US Food and Drug Administration review of tecovirimat for the treatment of smallpox. *Lancet Infect. Dis.* **2019**, *19*, e221–e224. [CrossRef]
3. Bastos, L.D.C.; De Souza, F.R.; Guimarães, A.P.; Sirouspour, M.; Guizado, T.R.C.; Forgione, P.; Ramalho, T.C.; França, T.C.C. Virtual screening, docking, and dynamics of potential new inhibitors of dihydrofolate reductase from Yersinia pestis. *J. Biomol. Struct. Dyn.* **2016**, *34*, 2184–2198. [CrossRef] [PubMed]
4. Guimarães, A.P.; de Souza, F.R.; Oliveira, A.A.; Gonçalves, A.S.; de Alencastro, R.B.; Ramalho, T.C.; França, T.C.C. Design of inhibitors of thymidylate kinase from Variola virus as new selective drugs against smallpox. *Eur. J. Med. Chem.* **2015**, *91*, 72–90. [CrossRef] [PubMed]
5. Trost, L.C.; Rose, M.L.; Khouri, J.; Keilholz, L.; Long, J.; Godin, S.J.; Foster, S.A. The efficacy and pharmacokinetics of brincidofovir for the treatment of lethal rabbitpox virus infection: A model of smallpox disease. *Antivir. Res.* **2015**, *117*, 115–121. [CrossRef] [PubMed]
6. Damon, I.K.; Damaso, C.R.; McFadden, G. Are We There Yet? The Smallpox Research Agenda Using Variola Virus. *PLoS Pathog.* **2014**, *10*, e1004108. [CrossRef] [PubMed]
7. Guimarães, A.P.; Ramalho, T.C.; França, T.C.C. Preventing the return of smallpox: Molecular modeling studies on thymidylate kinase fromVariola virus. *J. Biomol. Struct. Dyn.* **2014**, *32*, 1601–1612. [CrossRef] [PubMed]
8. Prichard, M.N.; Kern, E.R. Orthopoxvirus targets for the development of new antiviral agents. *Antivir. Res.* **2012**, *94*, 111–125. [CrossRef]
9. Garcia, D.R.; De Souza, F.R.; Guimarães, A.P.; Ramalho, T.C.; De Aguiar, A.P.; França, T.C.C. Design of inhibitors of thymidylate kinase from Variola virus as new selective drugs against smallpox: Part II. *J. Biomol. Struct. Dyn.* **2019**, *37*, 4569–4579. [CrossRef]

10. Merchlinsky, M.; Albright, A.; Olson, V.; Schiltz, H.; Merkeley, T.; Hughes, C.; Petersen, B.; Challberg, M. The development and approval of tecoviromat (TPOXX®), the first antiviral against smallpox. *Antivir. Res.* **2019**, *168*, 168–174. [CrossRef]
11. Nuth, M.; Guan, H.; Xiao, Y.; Kulp, J.L., III; Parker, M.H.; Strobel, E.D.; Isaacs, S.N.; Scott, R.W.; Reitz, A.B.; Ricciardi, R.P. Mutation and structure guided discovery of an antiviral small molecule that mimics an essential C-Terminal tripeptide of the vaccinia D4 processivity factor. *Antivir. Res.* **2018**, *162*, 178–185. [CrossRef]
12. Chaudhuri, S.; Symons, J.A.; Deval, J. Innovation and trends in the development and approval of antiviral medicines: 1987–2017 and beyond. *Antivir. Res.* **2018**, *155*, 76–88. [CrossRef]
13. Noyce, R.S.; Lederman, S.; Evans, D.H. Construction of an infectious horsepox virus vaccine from chemically synthesized DNA fragments. *PLoS ONE* **2018**, *13*, e0188453. [CrossRef]
14. Chittick, G.; Morrison, M.; Brundage, T.; Nichols, W.G. Short-term clinical safety profile of brincidofovir: A favorable benefit–risk proposition in the treatment of smallpox. *Antivir. Res.* **2017**, *143*, 269–277. [CrossRef] [PubMed]
15. Crump, R.; Korom, M.; Buller, R.M.; Parker, S. Buccal viral DNA as a trigger for brincidofovir therapy in the mousepox model of smallpox. *Antivir. Res.* **2017**, *139*, 112–116. [CrossRef] [PubMed]
16. Grossi, I.M.; Foster, S.A.; Gainey, M.R.; Krile, R.T.; Dunn, J.A.; Brundage, T.; Khouri, J.M. Efficacy of delayed brincidofovir treatment against a lethal rabbitpox virus challenge in New Zealand White rabbits. *Antivir. Res.* **2017**, *143*, 278–286. [CrossRef] [PubMed]
17. Arita, I. Discovery of forgotten variola specimens at the National Institutes of Health in the USA. *Expert Rev. Anti-Infect. Ther.* **2014**, *12*, 1419–1421. [CrossRef]
18. Gómez-Tatay, L.; Hernández-Andreu, J.M. Biosafety and biosecurity in synthetic biology: A review. *Crit. Rev. Environ. Sci. Technol.* **2019**, *49*, 1587–1621. [CrossRef]
19. Esparza, J.; Schrick, L.; Damaso, C.R.; Nitsche, A. Equination (inoculation of horsepox): An early alternative to vaccination (inoculation of cowpox) and the potential role of horsepox virus in the origin of the smallpox vaccine. *Vaccine* **2017**, *35*, 7222–7230. [CrossRef]
20. Schoepp, R.J.; Morin, M.D.; Martinez, M.J.; Kulesh, D.A.; Hensley, L.; Geisbert, T.W.; Brady, D.R.; Jahrling, P.B. Detection and identification of Variola virus in fixed human tissue after prolonged archival storage. *Lab. Investig.* **2004**, *84*, 41–48. [CrossRef]
21. Berche, P. The threat of smallpox and bioterrorism. *Trends Microbiol.* **2001**, *9*, 15–18. [CrossRef]
22. Chen, D.; Qi, E.Y. Innovative highlights of clinical drug trial design. *Transl. Res.* **2020**, *224*, 71–77. [CrossRef] [PubMed]
23. Mucker, E.M.; Goff, A.J.; Shamblin, J.D.; Grosenbach, D.W.; Damon, I.K.; Mehal, J.M.; Holman, R.C.; Carroll, D.; Gallardo, N.; Olson, V.A.; et al. Efficacy of Tecovirimat (ST-246) in Nonhuman Primates Infected with Variola Virus (Smallpox). *Antimicrob. Agents Chemother.* **2013**, *57*, 6246–6253. [CrossRef] [PubMed]
24. Caillat, C.; Topalis, D.; Agrofoglio, L.A.; Pochet, S.; Balzarini, J.; Deville-Bonne, D.; Meyer, P. Crystal structure of poxvirus thymidylate kinase: An unexpected dimerization has implications for antiviral therapy. *Proc. Natl. Acad. Sci. USA* **2008**, *105*, 16900–16905. [CrossRef]
25. Auvynet, C.; Topalis, D.; Caillat, C.; Munier-Lehmann, H.; Seclaman, E.; Balzarini, J.; Agrofoglio, L.A.; Kaminski, P.A.; Meyer, P.R.; Deville-Bonne, D.; et al. Phosphorylation of dGMP analogs by vaccinia virus TMP kinase and human GMP kinase. *Biochem. Biophys. Res. Commun.* **2009**, *388*, 6–11. [CrossRef]
26. Topalis, D.; Collinet, B.; Gasse, C.; Dugué, L.; Balzarini, J.; Pochet, S.; Deville-Bonne, D. Substrate specificity of vaccinia virus thymidylate kinase. *FEBS J.* **2005**, *272*, 6254–6265. [CrossRef]
27. Cui, Q.; Shin, W.S.; Luo, Y.; Tian, J.; Cui, H.; Yin, D. Thymidylate Kinase: An Old Topic Brings New Perspectives. *Curr. Med. Chem.* **2013**, *20*, 1286–1305. [CrossRef]
28. Irwin, C.R.; Hitt, M.M.; Evans, D.H. Targeting Nucleotide Biosynthesis: A Strategy for Improving the Oncolytic Potential of DNA Viruses. *Front. Oncol.* **2017**, *7*, 229. [CrossRef]
29. El Omari, K.; Solaroli, N.; Karlsson, A.; Balzarini, J.; Stammers, D.K. Structure of vaccinia virus thymidine kinase in complex with dTTP: Insights for drug design. *BMC Struct. Biol.* **2006**, *6*, 22. [CrossRef]
30. Solaroli, N.; Johansson, M.; Persoons, L.; Balzarini, J.; Karlsson, A. Substrate specificity of feline and canine herpesvirus thymidine kinase. *Antivir. Res.* **2008**, *79*, 128–132. [CrossRef]
31. Baker, R.O.; Bray, M.; Huggins, J.W. Potential antiviral therapeutics for smallpox, monkeypox and other orthopoxvirus infections. *Antivir. Res.* **2003**, *57*, 13–23. [CrossRef]
32. Bray, M. Pathogenesis and potential antiviral therapy of complications of smallpox vaccination. *Antivir. Res.* **2003**, *58*, 101–114. [CrossRef]
33. Bursulaya, B.D.; Totrov, M.; Abagyan, R.; Brooks, C.L., III. Comparative study of several algorithms for flexible ligand docking. *J. Comput. Aided Mol. Des.* **2003**, *17*, 755–763. [CrossRef]
34. Huang, S.-Y.; Zou, X. Advances and Challenges in Protein-Ligand Docking. *Int. J. Mol. Sci.* **2010**, *11*, 3016–3034. [CrossRef] [PubMed]
35. Wang, C.; Greene, D.A.; Xiao, L.; Qi, R.; Luo, R. Recent Developments and Applications of the MMPBSA Method. *Front. Mol. Biosci.* **2018**, *4*, 87. [CrossRef]
36. Genheden, S.; Kuhn, O.; Mikulskis, P.; Hoffmann, D.; Ryde, U. The normal-mode entropy in the MM/GBSA method: Effect of system truncation, buffer region, and dielectric constant. *J. Chem. Inf. Model.* **2012**, *52*, 2079–2088. [CrossRef]

37. Kumari, R.; Kumar, R.; Lynn, A.; Open Source Drug Discovery Consortium. G-mmpbsa -A GROMACS tool for high-throughput MM-PBSA calculations. *J. Chem. Inf. Model.* **2014**, *54*, 1951–1962. [CrossRef]
38. Kar, P.; Lipowsky, R.; Knecht, V. Importance of Polar Solvation and Configurational Entropy for Design of Antiretroviral Drugs Targeting HIV-1 Protease. *J. Phys. Chem. B* **2013**, *117*, 5793–5805. [CrossRef]
39. Evertts, A.G.; Zee, B.M.; Garcia, B.A. Modern approaches for investigating epigenetic signaling pathways. *J. Appl. Physiol.* **2010**, *109*, 927–933. [CrossRef]
40. Norambuena, T.; Melo, F. The Protein-DNA Interface database. *BMC Bioinform.* **2010**, *11*, 1–12. [CrossRef]
41. Shao, Y.; Molnar, L.F.; Jung, Y.; Kussmann, J.; Ochsenfeld, C.; Brown, S.T.; Gilbert, A.T.; Slipchenko, L.V.; Levchenko, S.V.; O'Neill, D.P.; et al. Advances in methods and algorithms in a modern quantum chemistry program package. *Phys. Chem. Chem. Phys.* **2006**, *8*, 3172–3191. [CrossRef] [PubMed]
42. Luscombe, N.M.; Austin, S.E.; Berman, H.M.; Thornton, J.M. An overview of the structures of protein-DNA complexes. *Genome Biol.* **2000**, *1*, REVIEWS001. [CrossRef] [PubMed]
43. Jayaram, B.; Sprous, D.; Young, M.; Beveridge, D.L. Free Energy Analysis of the Conformational Preferences of A and B Forms of DNA in Solution. *J. Am. Chem. Soc.* **1998**, *120*, 10629–10633. [CrossRef]
44. Bren, U.; Martínek, V.; Florián, J. Decomposition of the Solvation Free Energies of Deoxyribonucleoside Triphosphates Using the Free Energy Perturbation Method. *J. Phys. Chem. B* **2006**, *110*, 12782–12788. [CrossRef] [PubMed]
45. Bren, M.; Florián, J.; Mavri, J.; Bren, U. Do all pieces make a whole? Thiele cumulants and the free energy decomposition. *Theor. Chem. Acc.* **2007**, *117*, 535–540. [CrossRef]
46. Swain, M. chemicalize.org. *J. Chem. Inf. Model.* **2012**, *52*, 613–615. [CrossRef]
47. Poli, G.; Granchi, C.; Rizzolio, F.; Tuccinardi, T. Application of MM-PBSA Methods in Virtual Screening. *Molecules* **2020**, *25*, 1971. [CrossRef] [PubMed]
48. Lipinski, C.A. Lead- and drug-like compounds: The rule-of-five revolution. *Drug Discov. Today Technol.* **2004**, *1*, 337–341. [CrossRef]
49. Rocha, G.B.; Freire, R.O.; Simas, A.M.; Stewart, J.J.P. RM1: A reparameterization of AM1 for H, C, N, O, P, S, F, Cl, Br, and I. *J. Comput. Chem.* **2006**, *27*, 1101–1111. [CrossRef]
50. Gonçalves, A.D.S.; França, T.C.C.; Figueroa-Villar, J.D.; Pascutti, P.G. Conformational Analysis of Toxogonine, TMB-4 and HI-6 using PM6 and RM1 methods. *J. Braz. Chem. Soc.* **2010**, *21*, 179–184. [CrossRef]
51. Berman, H.M.; Westbrook, J.; Feng, Z.; Gilliland, G.; Bhat, T.N.; Weissig, H.; Shindyalov, I.N.; Bourne, P.E. The Protein Data Bank. *Nucleic Acids Res.* **2000**, *28*, 235–242. [CrossRef]
52. Thomsen, R.; Christensen, M.H. MolDock: A New Technique for High-Accuracy Molecular Docking. *J. Med. Chem.* **2006**, *49*, 3315–3321. [CrossRef]
53. Kaminski, G.A.; Friesner, R.A.; Tirado-Rives, J.; Jorgensen, W.L. Evaluation and Reparametrization of the OPLS-AA Force Field for Proteins via Comparison with Accurate Quantum Chemical Calculations on Peptides†. *J. Phys. Chem. B* **2001**, *105*, 6474–6487. [CrossRef]
54. Abraham, M.J.; Murtola, T.; Schulz, R.; Páll, S.; Smith, J.C.; Hess, B.; Lindahl, E. –GROMACS: High performance molecular simulations through multi-level parallelism from laptops to supercomputers. *SoftwareX* **2015**, *1–2*, 19–25. [CrossRef]
55. Byrd, R.H.; Lu, P.; Nocedal, J.; Zhu, C. A Limited Memory Algorithm for Bound Constrained Optimization. *SIAM J. Sci. Comput.* **1995**, *16*, 1190–1208. [CrossRef]
56. Humphrey, W.; Dalke, A.; Schulten, K. VMD: Visual molecular dynamics. *J. Mol. Graph.* **1996**, *14*, 33–38. [CrossRef]
57. Da Silva, A.W.S.; Vranken, W.F. ACPYPE-Antechamber python parser interface. *BMC Res. Notes* **2012**, *5*, 367. [CrossRef]

pharmaceuticals

MDPI

Article

Deep Modeling of Regulating Effects of Small Molecules on Longevity-Associated Genes

Jiaying You, Michael Hsing and Artem Cherkasov *

Vancouver Prostate Centre, Department of Urologic Sciences, Faculty of Medicine, University of British Columbia, Vancouver, BC V6H 3Z6, Canada; jyou@prostatecentre.com (J.Y.); mhsing@prostatecentre.com (M.H.)
* Correspondence: acherkasov@prostatecentre.com

Abstract: Aging is considered an inevitable process that causes deleterious effects in the functioning and appearance of cells, tissues, and organs. Recent emergence of large-scale gene expression datasets and significant advances in machine learning techniques have enabled drug repurposing efforts in promoting longevity. In this work, we further developed our previous approach—DeepCOP, a quantitative chemogenomic model that predicts gene regulating effects, and extended its application across multiple cell lines presented in LINCS to predict aging gene regulating effects induced by small molecules. As a result, a quantitative chemogenomic Deep Model was trained using gene ontology labels, molecular fingerprints, and cell line descriptors to predict gene expression responses to chemical perturbations. Other state-of-the-art machine learning approaches were also evaluated as benchmarks. Among those, the deep neural network (DNN) classifier has top-ranked known drugs with beneficial effects on aging genes, and some of these drugs were previously shown to promote longevity, illustrating the potential utility of this methodology. These results further demonstrate the capability of "hybrid" chemogenomic models, incorporating quantitative descriptors from biomarkers to capture cell specific drug–gene interactions. Such models can therefore be used for discovering drugs with desired gene regulatory effects associated with longevity.

Keywords: library of integrated network-based cellular signatures (LINCS); longevity; gene regulating effects; gene descriptors; molecular fingerprints; machine learning; deep neural network; drug repurposing

Citation: You, J.; Hsing, M.; Cherkasov, A. Deep Modeling of Regulating Effects of Small Molecules on Longevity-Associated Genes. *Pharmaceuticals* **2021**, *14*, 948. https://doi.org/10.3390/ph14100948

Academic Editor: Osvaldo Andrade Santos-Filho

Received: 25 August 2021
Accepted: 18 September 2021
Published: 22 September 2021

1. Introduction

Aging is an ultimate, intrinsic risk factor for all degenerative conditions, and the incidence of age-associated diseases, such as Alzheimer's, Parkinson's, dementia, and osteoporosis (among many others), increases dramatically as we age. Moreover, humans are likely to suffer from conditions, such as vision impairment, chronic diseases, and cancers in older ages, all of which can greatly reduce the quality of life. Numerous studies were conducted in recent years to reverse the biological aging clock in animals, and a recent work has successfully demonstrated restored vision in mice by switching certain cells to a "younger" state [1]; thus, promising the possibility to regenerate tissues and organs in mammals, and encouraging researchers to explore longevity beyond laboratory animals. For example, mTOR inhibitors marked a milestone in anti-aging drug discovery and produced an FDA-approved drug, rapamycin, which extended the life spans of several model organisms. Rapamycin succeeded in increasing the lifespans by nearly three-fold in mice [2] and was proven to prolong life in yeast, worms, and flies [3]. However, there are objections to rapamycin, including warnings that such an immunosuppressive drug could lead to the development of malignancies, such as skin cancer (noted in an FDA statement). Moreover, irreversible side effects, such as diabetes [4], are also main concerns that have prevented the use of rapamycin at a larger scale. In recent years, a variety of similar studies have proposed geroprotector candidates that could potentially promote life spans [5–7].

For example, acarbose [8], initially used to treat diabetes, showed significant effects in improving the health and life spans of mice.

Recent developments in genomics and transcriptomics have led to a vast collection of large-scale gene expression datasets. Connectivity Map (CMap) [9], introduced in 2006, is aimed to link connections among genes, drugs, and diseases, by comparing gene signatures with reference perturbations; thus, it is a great resource when developing drug candidates with desired efficacies. CMap data have greatly been used in the bioinformatics field, especially in drug discovery applications, to retrieve novel chemicals that share similar regulatory effects on gene expressions with known perturbations. The NIH Library of Integrated Network-based Cellular Signatures (LINCS), inspired by the success of CMap, was funded as a next generation platform, using a more advanced approach at a lower cost, producing high-throughput gene expression profiles that have outpaced CMap. LINCS, with data stored in NCBI Gene Expression Omnibus (GEO), describes over 1 M gene perturbations, inflicted by thousands of small molecules at a variety of conditions and across multiple cell lines. With the increasing availability in gene expression profiles, we now have the opportunity to study how small molecules affect genes in human cells and to utilize the available gene expression data to predict drug responses, offering tremendous value for drug discovery and repurposing. For example, the limited biological knowledge on the recent COVID-19 outbreak made it difficult to choose appropriate treatments; however, querying differentially expressed genes in similar diseases (SARS-CoV-2) against CMap, to detect similarly behaved drug candidates without any prior knowledge, was shown to be an efficient therapeutic strategy [10]. In addition, rapidly emerging machine learning technologies provide powerful computational tools to discover the underlying biological mechanisms in a variety of domains. Thus, our previous study, DeepCOP, has proven the capacity of deep learning models in predicting gene expression regulating effects using LINCS perturbation datasets [11].

In this work, we propose repurposed anti-aging drug candidates by analyzing their regulation effects on the expression of pro-longevity and anti-longevity genes from the LINCS dataset. While simply querying LINCS is still a valid method to repurpose the existing drugs, this approach is limited to a very small portion of the chemical space with only about 5000 compounds. Moreover, most of the experiments described in the CMap/LINCS depository were designed to measure perturbation responses in cancer cell lines; thus, making it challenging to study longevity effects of drugs in normal, non-tumorous cell lines. Thus, it is essential to build more general machine learning models that can harness the existing data from LINCS and apply to larger chemical space and non-cancer cell lines.

Herein, we hypothesize that deep neural network (DNN) could learn from high dimensional features, including gene ontology terms, small molecule descriptors, cell line mutation, and methylation data to produce reliable predictions on drug–gene regulation effects across multiple cell lines. To build testable computational models to predict regulating effects on unknown data, we applied assorted classification approaches, including DNN, random forest (RF), Naïve Bayes, and logistic regression. We tested the drug (D)–gene (G) regulation effects on external normal cell lines using the pre-trained DNN models. We identified 13 small molecules from the LINCS dataset that demonstrated potential ability to regulate aging gene expressions with the desired effects. We further demonstrated that the efficacy of these repurposed drugs on longevity is supported by some examples from the literature.

2. Results and Discussion

2.1. Sample Distributions

We have labeled the upregulated and downregulated D–G–C interactions with the top/bottom 5% Z-score cut-off in LINCS for each cell line. This results in a comparably much smaller proportion in positive samples then the negatives. In addition, LINCS experiments are not distributed evenly across cell lines, so that the sample size differs from different cell lines. For example, cell line A375 contains 73,610 unique D–G–Cs, labeled as positive samples with top 5% threshold, while the remaining 1.2 million D–G–Cs with unknown regulating effects form the negative set. Table 1 demonstrates the unique drugs and genes in each cell line for the upregulated models.

Table 1. Sample distribution for each cell line in upregulated models; positive samples are defined as the top 5% gene signatures, while negative samples are the remaining 95%. Unique numbers of drugs and aging genes are summarized below. For example, cell line A375 contains 73,610 unique D–G–Cs as positive samples with the top 5% threshold, while the remaining 1.2 million D–G–Cs with unknown regulating effects form the negatives. (#: Counts.)

Cell Lines	A375	A549	HUH7	PC3	VCAP	HL60	U266	NOMO1
Positive samples	73,610	196,027	See supplementary data	See supplementary data	See supplementary data	2138	735	1145
Negative samples	1.2M	3.4M				27,022	19,677	11,248
# Unique genes	729	729				729	729	729
# Unique drugs	1731	4875				40	28	17

2.2. CMAP LINCS Dataset Querying Results

By diving into the positive samples from the model 1 dataset labeled as upregulated D–G–C pairs, we ranked compounds that interact with the most pro-longevity genes across all LINCS cell lines. For each small molecule in the positive samples of model 1, we built a pool of (drug)–(pro-longevity gene)–(cell line) pairs and selected the molecules with the most interactions. To avoid chemicals that only upregulated pro-longevity genes within a small range of cell lines, or chemicals that only interacted with a few certain genes, we calculated the unique number of pro-longevity genes and cell lines to ensure the diversity and robustness of the selected chemicals. Only pairs that covered above 100 pro-longevity genes and more than five cell lines were included for the final ranking. Table 2 shows the top 10 small molecules that upregulate the most pro-longevity genes across all LINCS cell lines.

Table 2. Top-ranked 10 small molecules that upregulate the most pro-longevity genes across all cell lines in LINCS. (#: Counts.)

Rank	Drug	# Interactions	# Unique Pro-Longevity Genes	# Unique Cell Lines
1	Trichostatin-a	926	218	10
2	AT 7519	871	226	7
3	CGP-60474	843	200	6
4	Alvocidib	743	218	6
5	PHA-793887	730	244	7
6	Emetine	714	225	6
7	Narciclasine	711	239	6
8	Zibotentan	700	218	7
9	Oxetane	673	214	6
10	Mitoxantrone	632	201	6

Conversely, positive samples in model 2 indicate downregulated D–G–C interactions for anti-longevity genes. We ranked small molecules that downregulated the most anti-longevity genes in model 2, using the same filter as Table 2, and obtained the 10 top-ranked chemicals, as shown in Table 3.

Table 3. Top-ranked 10 small molecules that downregulate the most anti-longevity genes across all cell lines in LINCS. (#: Counts.)

Rank	Drug	# Interactions	# Unique Anti-Longevity Genes	# Unique Cell Lines
1	AT-7519	585	201	7
2	BI-2536	536	207	9
3	Emetine	520	205	6
4	Narciclasine	510	212	6
5	CGP-60474	497	177	6
6	Oxetane	494	177	7
7	Trichostatin-a	454	198	6
8	Alvocidib	445	174	6
9	LSM-3353	433	215	6
10	BMS-345541	426	176	6

We observed seven identical drugs AT 7519, CGP-60474, trichostatin-a, alvocidib, narciclasine, oxetane, emetine in both tables, which showed not only upregulation effects with pro-longevity genes, but also downregulation effects with anti-longevity genes across multiple cancer cell lines in LINCS. In addition, PHA-793887, zibotentan, and mitoxantrone showed potential in upregulating pro-longevity gene expression, while chemical BI-2536, LSM-3353, and BMS-345541 showed downregulated expressions on anti-longevity genes. In total, we can repurpose 13 unique small molecules in LINCS perturbations for longevity purpose.

Figure 1 shows the top 10 ranked small molecules with D–G (pro-longevity genes)–C interactions from model 1, and Figure 2 illustrates D–G (anti-longevity genes)–C interactions on the top 10 ranked small molecules from model 2. The color indicates the occurrence on different cell lines. From green to blue, the line connecting longevity genes with repurposed chemicals demonstrates a higher occurrence on different LINCS cell lines. For example, drug BI-2536 connects with anti-longevity gene RAD51 with downregulating effects in 9 cancer cell lines, while drug trichostatin-a promotes pro-longevity gene expressions (*GDI1*, *ZNF224*, *MAP3K13*, *EPHB1*, *ZNF500*, *PPFIA3*) in 10 cancer cell lines.

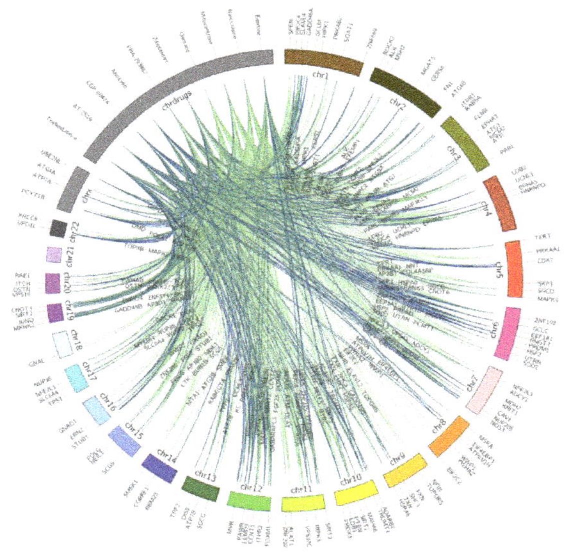

Figure 1. Top 10 small molecules that upregulate pro-longevity genes across all LINCS cell lines. Pro-longevity genes are shown on chromosomes bands, repurposed chemicals are shown on the drug band. Colors of interactions indicate the relationship occurrence on different cell lines. Green D–G (pro-longevity genes) links indicate the interactions were captured in less than six cell lines; pairs found in above five cell lines are labeled in blue.

2.3. Model Performance

We estimated the accuracy parameter, AUC score, precision, and recall values for each model, as shown in Table 4. A skewed class distribution in models 3–8 failed accuracy on evaluation of the model performance. Another commonly used interpretation metric, ROC curve, was employed in binary classification problems [12] to diagnose the trade-off between sensitivity and specificity, and a higher ROC value indicates the trained model is better in distinguishing between categories. However, area under the ROC curve could be misleading when the one class significantly outweighs the other [13]. AUC score and ROC visualization could be deceptively appealing in this scenario. Instead, precision and recall provide a straightforward evaluation, focusing on the comparably small positive class based on the imbalanced dataset [13], given the concept of the precision-recall curve (PRC) being the indictor of true positives in all positive predictions. Our results demonstrate that DNN outperformed the other benchmark approaches including RF, Naïve Bayes, and ridge regression for every model, despite the selected features in terms of the APR score with an acceptable drop in AUC and accuracy. We also found that by concatenating the cell line methylation beta values and binarized mutation status, the deep neural network is more capable at extracting useful features from high-dimensional feature sets through the learning process and results in better performance than learning with single cell line annotation resource. Deep neural network models (model 1–2) have outstanding APR scores and, thus, encourage making reliable predictions in further investigations on unknown datasets. ROC and precision recall curves are shown in Figure 3 for model 1 and model 2, and curves for the rest of the DNN models are provided in the supplementary figures.

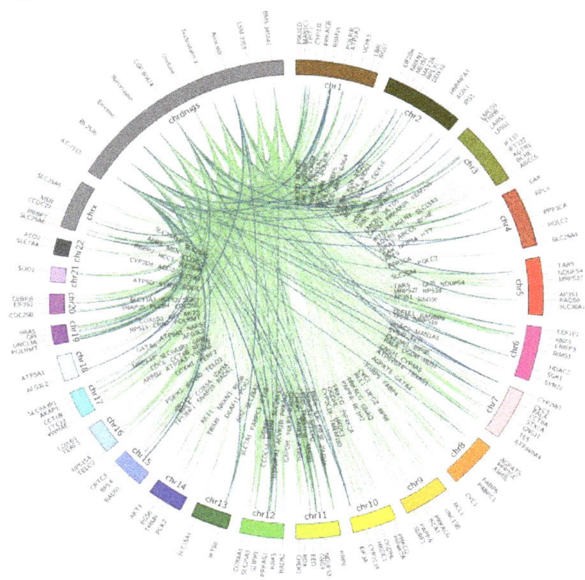

Figure 2. Top 10 small molecules that downregulate anti-longevity genes across all LINCS cell lines. Anti-longevity genes are shown on chromosomes bands, repurposed chemicals are shown on the drug band. Colors of interactions indicate the relationship occurrence on different cell lines. Green D–G (anti-longevity genes) links indicate the interactions were captured in less than six cell lines; pairs found in above five are labeled in blue.

Table 4. Model performance on overall accuracy, Area under the ROC curve (AUC), and area under the precision-recall curve (PRC) for the positive class on deep neural network(DNN), random forest, naïve bayes and logistic regression models.

Model	Evaluation	DNN	Random Forest	Naïve Bayes	Logistic Regression
1	Accuracy	0.73	0.71	0.54	0.62
	AUC	0.82	0.71	0.54	0.62
	APR	0.82	0.78	0.55	0.68
2	Accuracy	0.73	0.66	0.54	0.59
	AUC	0.8	0.66	0.54	0.59
	APR	0.78	0.71	0.54	0.64
3	Accuracy	0.95	0.94	0.6	0.95
	AUC	0.89	0.64	0.76	0.63
	APR	0.46	0.39	0.12	0.44

Table 4. *Cont.*

Model	Evaluation	DNN	Random Forest	Naïve Bayes	Logistic Regression
4	Accuracy	0.95	0.95	0.59	0.95
	AUC	0.84	0.58	0.74	0.56
	APR	0.4	0.29	0.1	0.33
5	Accuracy	0.95	0.94	0.68	0.95
	AUC	0.85	0.64	0.78	0.65
	APR	0.46	0.4	0.14	0.46
6	Accuracy	0.95	0.95	0.54	0.95
	AUC	0.81	0.58	0.72	0.57
	APR	0.39	0.29	0.09	0.35
7	Accuracy	0.95	0.95	0.58	0.95
	AUC	0.88	0.64	0.75	0.64
	APR	0.46	0.4	0.11	0.45
8	Accuracy	0.95	0.95	0.58	0.95
	AUC	0.84	0.58	0.74	0.56
	APR	0.4	0.3	0.1	0.54

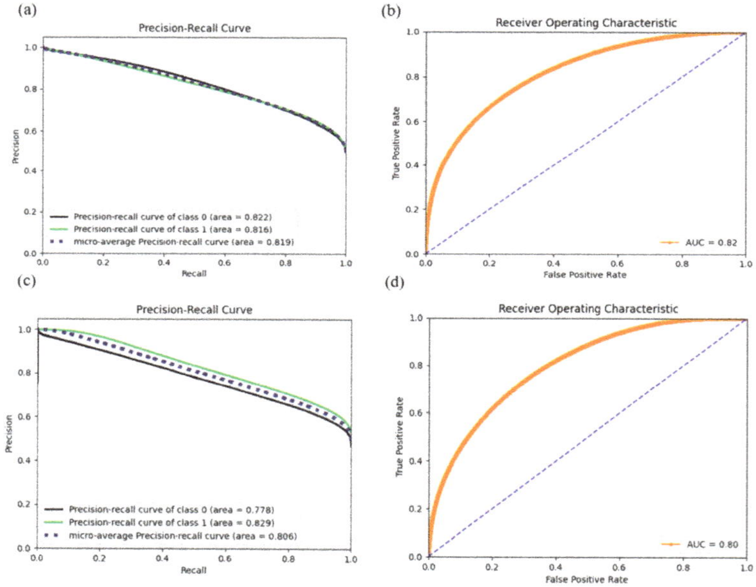

Figure 3. ROC and precision curves for model 1 ((**a**): PRC, (**b**): ROC) and model 2 ((**c**): PRC, (**d**): ROC). While the AUC score dropped compared with models 3–8, the dramatic increase in the APR score (positive class) gained confidence in predicting the positives in further exploration.

2.4. Prediction on Normal Cell Lines

Newly generated pairs with top-ranked repurposed chemicals and longevity genes were predicted with our best-performed models—model 1 to predict upregulating effects and model 2 for downregulating the effects on normal cell lines, NHBEC and HGEC6B. In each drug candidate pool (Equation (1)), we generated D (drug candidate)–G (longevity genes)–C (normal cell line) connections as input for the pre-trained deep neural network models, and explored the positive predictions with desired regulation effects, respectively. We summarized the total positive predictions along with the number of corresponding aging genes for each drug candidate in model 1 and model 2, respectively, in Figure 4. The prediction results confirmed the efficacy of the potential desired aging gene regulation effects on normal cell lines.

$$\text{Overall samples of D(i)} = \text{Pool(D(i))} = \text{D(i)} - \text{G(Aging gene)} - \text{C(Normal cell line)} \quad (1)$$

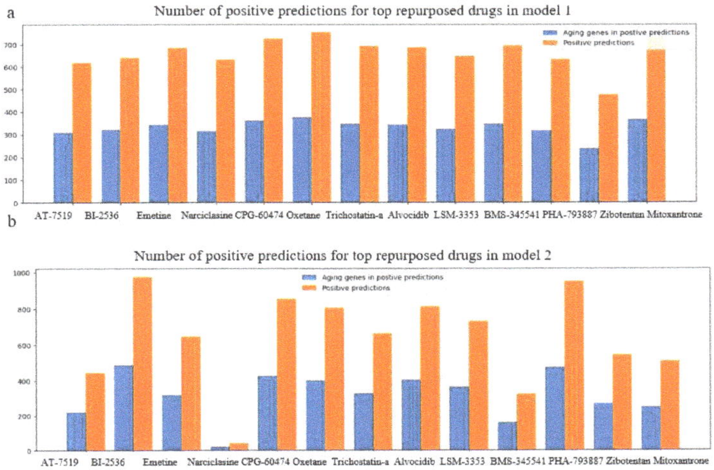

Figure 4. Bar charts on positive predictions for repurposed drugs in CMAP LINCS dataset, for normal cell lines, NHBEC and HCEC6B, using model 1(**a**) and model 2(**b**). Orange bars demonstrate the total number of positive predictions for each drug candidate, and blue bars illustrate the number of unique aging genes among positive predictions.

Table 5 shows the proportion of positive predictions against the D–G–C pool for each promising drug candidate. We observed an above 80% positive prediction rate for drugs "BI-2536", "CGP-60474", "oxetane", "alvocidib" and "PHA-793887" in both model 1 and model 2, demonstrating their great potential to upregulate pro-longevity gene expression and downregulate anti-longevity gene expression in normal cells. All of the D–G–C connections in BI-2536 pool were predicted positive in model 2, meaning that 'BI-2536' downregulated all of the anti-longevity genes we collected from GenAge.

Table 5. Percentage of positively predicted D (drug candidates)–G (aging genes)–C (normal cell line) pairs for each promising drug candidate in model 1 and model 2. Highlighted repurposed drugs showed great potential in regulating aging gene expressions on normal cell lines in both models. Drugs in bold achieved high positive rate (above 80%) on both models.

Drug	Model 1 Positive Rate	Model 2 Positive Rate
AT 7519	78%	45%
BI-2536	81%	100%
Emetine	87%	66%
Narciclasine	80%	4%
CGP-60474	92%	87%
Oxetane	95%	82%
Trichostatin-a	88%	68%
Alvocidib	87%	83%
LSM-3353	82%	75%
BMS-345541	88%	33%
PHA-793887	80%	97%
Zibotentan	60%	56%
Mitoxantrone	92%	52%

2.5. Repurposed Drugs

We finally identified 13 molecules that helped to promote pro-longevity gene expressions, inhibit anti-longevity gene expressions, or act in both desired ways. Structures of repurposed molecules are shown in Figure 5. While performing experimental validations on these 13 molecules in longevity studies in model organisms is out of the scope for this paper, previous research has uncovered a number of relevant traits of those chemicals with our repurposed objectives. Table 6 summarizes the evidence that supports our findings.

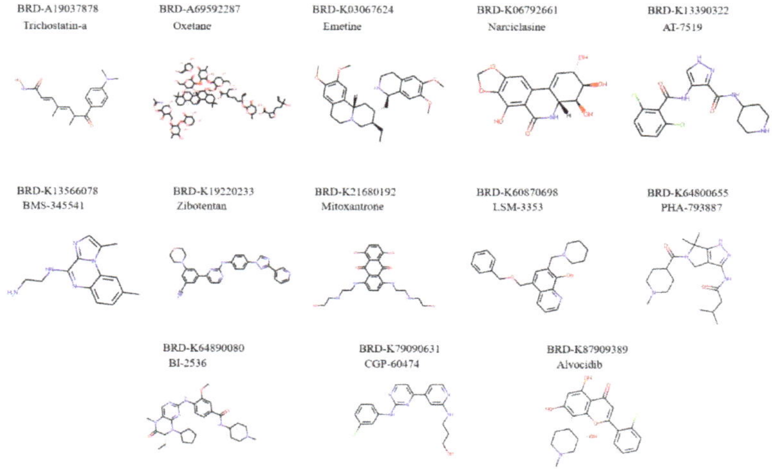

Figure 5. Molecular structures of repurposed drug candidates for longevity purpose.

Among 13 discovered longevity-promoting chemicals, four (AT 7519, alvocidib, CGP-60474, and PHA-793887) are indicated as cyclin-dependent kinase (CDK) inhibitors. Interestingly, previous studies have shown inhibition on CDK-2 resulted in tolerance towards environmental stress and promoted anti-aging in *Caenorhabditis elegans* [14,15]. Moreover, "BI-2536" inhibits tumor growth in vivo by inducing apoptosis on cancer cells as an inhibitor of polo-like kinase 1 [16]. Experiments have found the effectiveness in anti-aging on emetine dihydrochloride treated to leukemic mice [17]. In addition, narciclasine was proven to attenuate diet-induced obesity by promoting oxidative metabolism [18] while trichostatin-a, a histone deacetylase (HDAC) inhibitor, was proven to increase lifespans by promoting hsp22 gene expression on *Drosophila melanogaster* [19]. Zibotentan was designed and tested on castration-resistant prostate cancer patients as an endothelin A receptor antagonist [20], it is also proven to prevent hypertension and maintains cerebral perfusion [21]. A study conducted among 42 women with breast cancer showed great potential in mitoxantrone as a treatment for advanced breast cancer with mild side effects compared to traditional treatments, such as chemotherapy [22].

Table 6. Summary of previous research findings for repurposed pro-longevity drugs.

Repurposed Drug	Traits	Evidence
AT 7519	Inhibitor of CDKs	/
BI-2536	Inhibits tumor growth	[16]
Emetine	Increases lifespan of leukemic mice	[17]
Narciclasine	Attenuates diet-induced obesity	[18]
CGP-60474	Inhibitor of CDKs	/
Oxetane	/	/
Trichostatin-a	Increases lifespan by promoting hsp22 gene expression	[19]
Alvocidib	Inhibits metastasis of human osteosarcoma cells	[23]
LSM-3353	/	/

Table 6. *Cont.*

Repurposed Drug	Traits	Evidence
BMS-345541	Inhibitor of kB-kinase (IKK)	/
PHA-793887	Inhibitor of pan-CDK	/
Zibotentan	Inhibits blood vessel growth	[21]
Mitoxantrone	Treatment of advanced breast cancer	[22]

3. Materials and Methods

3.1. Datasets

Connectivity map (CMap) is a pilot project that aims to characterize cellular responses under pharmacologic perturbagens, thus, fulfilling the underdeveloped space in disease-associated gene functions, and contributing toward drug development by estimating off-target activities and eliminating unfit candidates at early stages. To date, the CMap LINCS dataset encompasses more than 1.5 million gene expression signatures related to up to 5000 small molecules and more than 10,000 genes across a total of 77 cancer cell lines [9]. Such a vast amount of gene expression information enables computational approaches, such as the deep neural network, to learn data patterns, to predict gene regulation effects [11], and drug side effects [24]. In this work, we collected L1000 high-throughput gene expression data from LINCS phase I dataset; the dataset contains perturbation data points on gene expression level under small molecular treatments at different conditions, such as dosages, cell line cultures, and time points. To reduce the data size and to maintain consistency across multiple cell lines, only perturbations with 24-h treatment were kept, and samples with molecular dose units other than "μM" were excluded.

Aging-related genes were downloaded from the GenAge (the Aging Gene Database) source, which labels pro- and anti-longevity genes in various model organisms, including (but not limited to) *Caenorhabditis elegans*, *Drosophila melanogaster*, and *Zaprionus paravittiger*. GenAge has been developed through manual curation by experts and several collaborated associations. In this work, we collected a total of 2205 genes from GenAge that are considered to have either pro- or anti-longevity effects in 10 different model organisms, including *Caenorhabditis elegans*, *Mus musculus*, *Saccharomyces cerevisiae*, *Drosophila melanogaster*, *Mesocricetus auratus*, *Podospora anserina*, *Schizosaccharomyces pombe*, *Danio rerio*, and *Caenorhabditis briggsae*. These aging-related genes identified from the model organisms were mapped to 889 human genes in total, where 397 were labeled with pro-longevity effects and 492 with anti-longevity effects, respectively (these datasets are downloadable online through https://genomics.senescence.info/download.html (accessed on 17 September 2021)). Out of a total of 889 collected aging genes, 729 were successfully mapped to the LINCS dataset and were further investigated in our models.

Only filtered LINCS perturbations that contained 729 aging-related genes were kept for further machine learning modeling and prediction. To label gene expression regulations, we used the left–right percentile method on the Z-score with a threshold of 5% for each cell line. Only the top 5% of gene expression values were considered as upregulation samples in the upregulation models, and the bottom 5% of gene expression values were marked as downregulated in the downregulation models, while the remaining 95% samples were treated with 'unknown' effects (Figure 6). In the training models that predicted upregulation effects, the above defined upregulation samples were treated as positive samples, while the remaining 95% were treated as negative samples. In the training models that predicted downregulation effects, the above defined downregulation samples were treated as positive-, while the remaining 95% were treated as negative samples. Figure 7 features gene expression Z-score distribution and data sampling in upregulation and downregulation models.

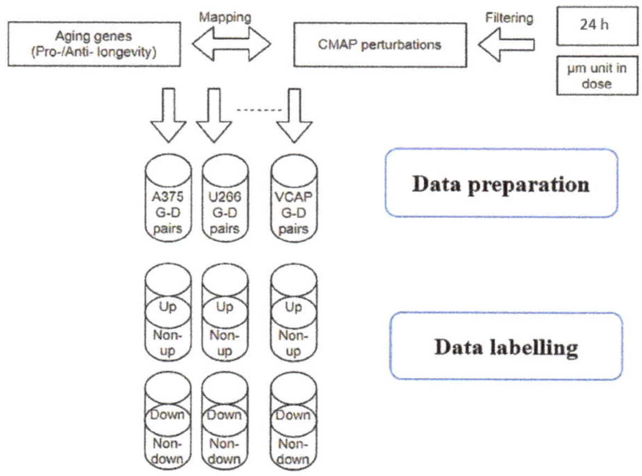

Figure 6. Data pipeline in collecting and labelling LINCS perturbations. Only perturbations include aging genes were kept for further analysis. The left–right percentile method was applied to label upregulation and downregulation effects with 5% threshold on the Z-score for each cell line.

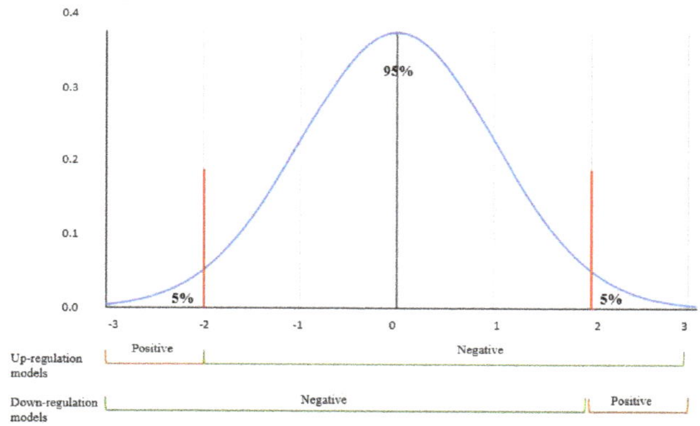

Figure 7. Z-score normal distribution. Positive samples were selected from the top 5% gene expressions perturbations for each cell lines in models predicting up/non-upregulation effects. Similarly, the bottom 5% perturbations were identified as the positives in models predicting down/non-downregulation effects.

3.2. Gene Descriptors

Gene ontology (GO) terms have been commonly used for gene annotations in recent drug discovery applications [25,26]. The GO terms consist of a set of categories that describe the gene functions as in cellular components, biological processes, and molecular functions. R package "ontologySimliarity" was built for comparing gene semantic similarity as encapsulated by the GO annotations, including nearly 20,000 terms that relate to all branches of gene ontology. The gene ontology descriptors for the 729 aging related human genes in LINCS were generated to a list of binary integers using one-hot encoding with R package "ontologySimliarity". Only GO terms that shared with at least three age-related gene domains were selected to reduce the feature size, which resulted in 946 GO features in the final standard dataset of aging-related genes. Our previous works [11,27] already illustrated the efficacy of using GO terms as gene descriptors in machine learning models, especially with deep learning architectures.

3.3. Molecular Fingerprints

The molecular fingerprints were encoded into 0 | 1 binary vectors to encode chemical structures, where 1 indicated a specific substructure was found in a given molecule. In this paper, Morgan fingerprints [28] were generated for small molecules in the LINCS phase I dataset using the python library "RDKIT". The Morgan fingerprints were calculated by counting the path through each atom in the chemical given a specific radius and a bit number. By increasing the radius, more fragments can be included in the Morgan fingerprint computations and can output a larger chemical feature space. We set the radius to 2 in this work and generated 2048 Morgan fingerprints for each molecular using canonical SMILES.

3.4. Cell Line Features

Gene mutations play an important role in cancer genetics and can be utilized to represent cell line functionalities, as previous studies have demonstrated significant performance of mutation features in machine learning approaches [29,30]. We collected copy number alternations and coding variants in "pan-cancer" from the Genomics of Drug Sensitivity in Cancer public platform, and a total of 735 mutation markers were labeled for each cell line. The mutation annotation dataset for pan-cancer is freely downloadable at https://www.cancerrxgene.org/downloads (accessed on 17 September 2021).

Besides mutation markers, DNA methylation levels also contributed to drug response prediction applications [31,32]. Its impact in regulating gene expression determines organ functionalities and may cause severe diseases, such as cancer. The 450K BeadChip array provides high-throughput methylation data at more than 450K CpG sites, at a low cost, making it feasible for machine-learning algorithms to learn and extract informative features. We collected methylation profiling from the NCBI gene expression omnibus (GEO) series GSE68379, where a total of 1028 cell lines were tested with the methylation level for each CpG island. Ranging from 0 to 1, beta value was calculated as a ratio of methylated intensity verses the sum of methylated and unmethylated intensity at the probe level. The formular of beta value B at the specific j CpG site is defined as Equation (2):

$$B(j) = \frac{\max\left(y_{j,methylated}, 0\right)}{\max\left(y_{j,methylated}, 0\right) + \max\left(y_{j,unmethylated}, 0\right) + \alpha} \tag{2}$$

where $y_{j,q}$ stands for j_{th} probe intensities in q status. α is the added in denominator to avoid computational error. As recommended by Illumina [33], beta value is used in this work to represent the methylation level for cell lines. We used R package "FCBF" to select limited informative methylation beta values from 450 K CpG sites. The fast correlation based filter (FCBF) algorithm [34] selected the most relevant features towards histology sites of LINCS cancer cell line. Figure 8 shows the corresponding number of selected variables under a variety of (cell line)–(cancer histology sites) correlations. By choosing a correlation cut-off at 0.6, we obtained 1183 subset methylation levels for each cell line.

3.5. Querying Camp LINCS Dataset

To retrieve aging-related drug (D)-gene and (G)-cell line (C) combinations, we queried perturbations with the aging-related genes in the LINCS phase I dataset. Samples were consequently labeled through 5% left–right percentiles as upregulation effects and downregulation effects, respectively. Human pro-/anti-longevity genes extracted from the GenAge platform were used as input samples to query against CMAP LINCS dataset signatures. Drugs that upregulated pro-longevity gene expression or downregulate anti-longevity gene expression across multiple cell lines were identified and could be repurposed for promoting longevity. Top chemicals, ranked by the number of D–G–C interactions, showed great potential in increasing lifespans in humans, as supported by previous studies.

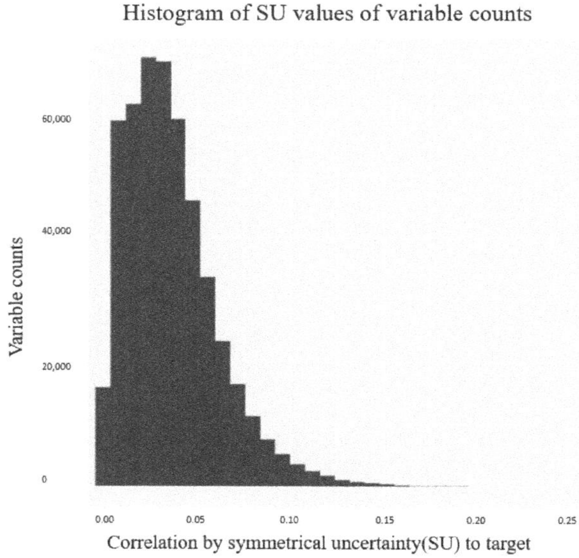

Figure 8. Histogram of correlation values and the corresponding variable counts using FCBF. Correlations were calculated between CpG sites and cancer histology categories.

3.6. Machine Learning Models and Deep Neural Network

Machine learning (ML) models have demonstrated unprecedented performance in recent computational biology applications [35–37]. ML approaches are programmed without explicit knowledge to self-extract informative features by learning the parameters, such as weights, and illustrate patterns towards the output. The pervasive applications in ML have changed our day-to-day lives, e.g., via object recognition applied in auto-driving cars, recommender systems on social media, and in-depth understanding on drug behavior. The capable solutions that trained models can learn are generally divided into regression and classification problems, where a regression model predicts the true numeric value given a set of features, and a classification model gives a category the input sample belongs. Commonly deployed classification algorithms include logistic regression, random forest (RF), and neural network (NN), each with pros and cons. It is notable that in the family of ML, deep learning (DL) plays an important part and is capable of learning more complex patterns with neurons, just as human brains. The advantage of DNN lies in absorbing datasets with high dimensions and recognizing nonlinearity; thus, providing solutions to a vast range of practical problems.

To better illustrate D–G–C relationships and have a clear evaluation on the feature power, here we differentiated the sample size and feature sets, respective to up- and downregulation effects predictions, and designed the following eight models. The selected feature set in each model is: model 1, model 2, model 3, and model 4: gene descriptor, drug descriptor, cell line mutation status, cell line methylations; model 5 and model 6: gene descriptor, drug descriptor, cell line mutation status; model 7 and model 8: gene descriptor, drug descriptor, cell line methylations.

Due to the harsh filter on the sample selection process of determining up- or downregulation effects, only the top 5% samples were labeled as positive samples from LINCS for each model. Such severe imbalanced datasets challenged the ML approaches and could be difficult in measuring model performance for future predictions. To avoid models from being heavily influenced only by the majority class, we randomly selected the same number of negative and positive samples in model 1 and model 2. We used samples across all the cell lines in LINCS for models (1–2), and compared them with the remaining models (3–8) that used the imbalanced dataset extracted from two cell lines "U266" and "NOMO1", which contained less data points and, thus, were easier for traditional machine learning benchmarks to train (details are provided in Table 7).

Table 7. Detailed model layouts on predictive labels, sample cell lines, used feature set, and whether the negative class is being downsampled. For example, model 3 was trained with gene ontology term, drug descriptors, both cell line mutation status, and methylation values on perturbation responses on cell lines "U266" and "NOMO1". The positive samples from model 3 were D–G–C interactions with the top 5% upregulated gene expression signatures, whereas the negative samples were the remaining 95% perturbation data.

Model Predictive Direction	Cultured Cell Lines	If Balanced Sample Feature
1 Up/Non-upregulation	Includes all cell lines	True, Type 1
2 Down/Non-downregulation	Includes all cell lines	True, Type 1
3 Up/Non-upregulation	U266, NOMO1	False, Type 1
4 Down/Non-downregulation	U266, NOMO1	False, Type 1
5 Up/Non-upregulation	U266, NOMO1	False, Type 2
6 Down/Non-downregulation	U266, NOMO1	False, Type 2
7 Up/Non-upregulation	U266, NOMO1	False, Type 3
8 Down/Non-downregulation	U266, NOMO1	False, Type 3

Feature definitions: Type 1: gene ontology descriptors + drug fingerprints + cell line mutational status + cell line methylation levels. Type 2: gene ontology descriptors + drug fingerprints + cell line mutational status. Type 3: gene ontology descriptors + drug fingerprints + cell line methylation levels.

We then compared DNN model performance with commonly used classification solving algorithms including RF, Naïve Bayes, and logistic regression. Due to the large feature size, L2 norm(ridge) regulation was applied in logistic regression models to avoid coverage failure and overfitting, by taking the squared value of trained weighs as the penalty term in the cost function. DNN was constructed with four layers (one input layer, two hidden layers, and one output layer), and the information was randomly dropped by 50% in forward propagation. Selu and Rule activation functions were used for the internal hidden layers, adding complexity and non-linearity to the model, followed by a SoftMax activation for the final output layer, to transfer values into possibilities. The neural numbers of the hidden layers were identical as those from the initial input feature list. Figure 9 illustrates the DNN structure with the number of neurons and activation functions for model 1 and model 2. For more robust evaluation results, early stopping and three-fold cross validation (CV) were applied in the DNN model to avoid overfitting. We initiated the model with hyperparameters, such as layer numbers identical with our previous studies that demonstrate decent performance, and slightly revised them by watching validation results in such a manner where model complexity must decrease when overfitting and increase when underfitting.

3.7. Model Evaluation

To evaluate the performance on the developed models, we computed the overall accuracy score, area under the ROC curve (AUC) parameter, as well as precision and recall values for each model. Accuracy is simply calculated as the correct prediction proportion on the whole dataset, whereas the receiver operating characteristic curve (ROC) visualizes the model performance at all classification thresholds by comparing true positive rate (TPR) versus the false positive rate (FPR). Accuracy and AUC score are commonly used in evaluating machine-learning models and offer fairly accurate insight on model performance. However, both values are easily dominated by the majority group in the imbalanced datasets and could achieve misleading high scores. To address this issue, we introduced precision and recall as supplementary evaluations. Precision (Equation (3)), also known as positive predictive value, signifies the proportion of positive samples that are predicted positive. Recall (Equation (4)), also referred as true positive rate or sensitivity, evaluates the proportion of true positives out of all predicted positive samples. Overall, precision and recall estimate the prediction power on the positives, which is highly important in our case, given that future repurposed drug candidates are based on the positive predictions and a false positive is more disastrous and costly than a false negative. As an alternative visualization of ROC curve on imbalanced datasets, the precision-recall curve (PRC) illustrates the trade-off on precision and sensitivity on every possible cut-off. A reasonable PRC curve should be above the diagonal line, with the area under the curve more than 0.5.

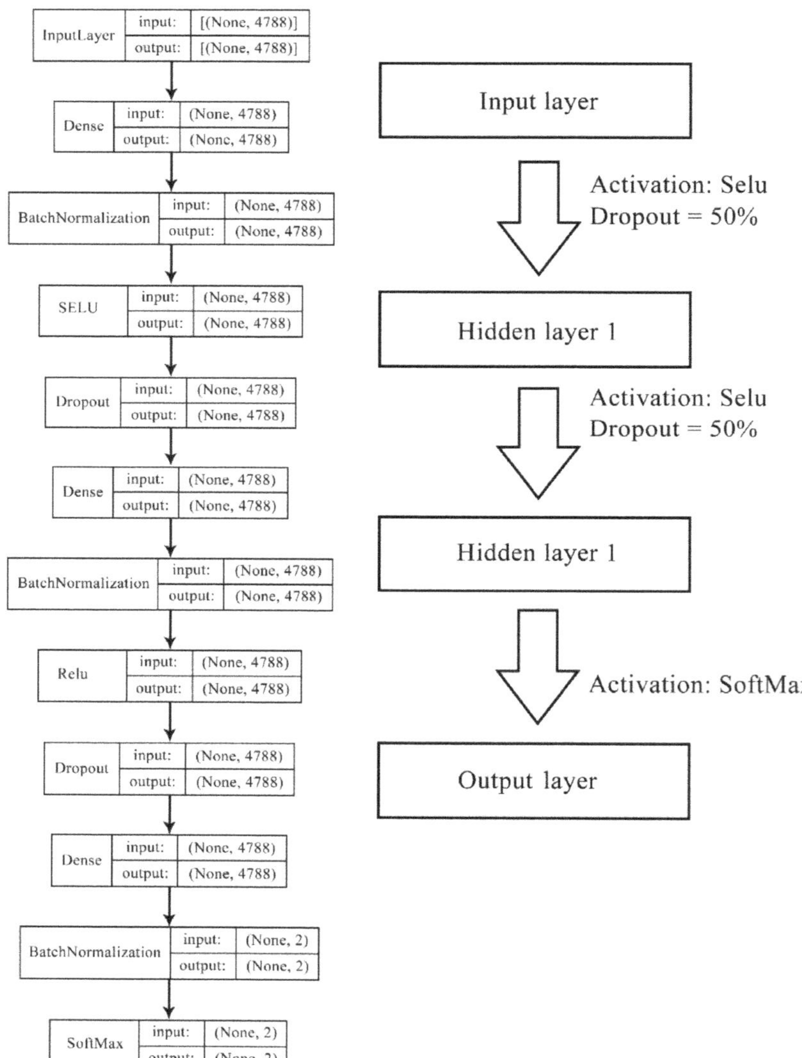

Figure 9. Deep neural network structure for model 1 and model 2. Features of models 1–2 were contributed by gene ontology terms (946 bits), molecular fingerprints (2048 bits), cell line mutation status (735 bits), and cell line methylation beta level (1183 bits), forming the length of 4788 bits in total.

$$\text{Precision} = \text{true positive}/(\text{true positive} + \text{false positive}) \quad (3)$$

$$\text{Recall} = \text{true positive}/(\text{true positive} + \text{false negative}) \quad (4)$$

3.8. Prediction on Normal Cell Lines

Given the fact that all data in LINCS are for cancer cell lines, it is essential to run computational predictions for repurposing drugs with expected pro-longevity effects in normal, non-cancerous cells. The determining factor in choosing normal cell lines for prediction is the availability of features that are identical with our trained models. Two normal cell lines "NHBEC" and "HGEC6B" were tested for methylations in beta values using the same technology—Illumina 450K BeadChip arrays—and were annotated with identical CpG sites, as in GSE92843 and GSM2438425, respectively. As for the mutational status, these two normal cell lines were simply annotated as having 'none' in the prediction models.

We tested the regulation effects on the top 10 ranked promising drugs that we previously queried from LINCS on these two normal cell lines, "NHBEC" and "HGEC6B", with our best performed models, and provided the probabilities on desired regulating effects with pro-/anti-longevity genes. These 10 potential pro-longevity chemicals were paired with age genes under two normal cell lines, forming in total 7940 D–G–C pairs to be tested with up/non-upregulating (Equation (5)) and 9840 D–G–C down/non-down (Equation (6)), respectively. Figure 10 illustrates a flowchart for applying the longevity prediction models to these two normal cell lines. The mutational profiling for normal cell lines was labeled "0" in feature representation, and the methylation beta levels were collected from the Gene Expression Omnibus (GEO) "GSE92843" and "GSM2438425".

$$10\ (\text{promising drugs}) \times 397\ (\text{pro}-\text{longevity genes}) \times 2\ (\text{cell lines}) = 7940 \quad (5)$$

$$10\ (\text{promising drugs}) \times 492\ (\text{anti}-\text{longevity genes}) \times 2\ (\text{cell lines}) = 9840 \quad (6)$$

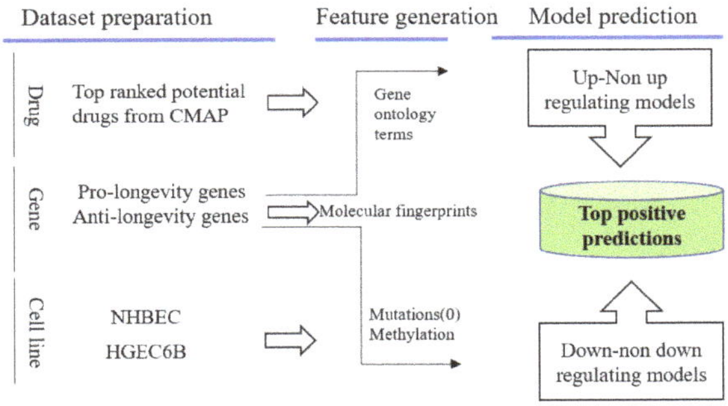

Figure 10. Predictions on normal cell lines with aging related genes and promising drug candidates queried from LINCS. Positive predictions will be of interest with desired regulating effects towards pro-/anti-longevity genes.

4. Conclusions

It is estimated that the anti-aging global market value was over 60 billion US dollars annually in 2020 [38]. Machine learning tools can utilize substantial transcriptional perturbation data from resources, such as CMap and LINCS, and transfer them into predictive models and actionable knowledge on modulation of longevity genes. In this study, we labeled gene expression changes using the left–right percentile at a 5% threshold for each drug–gene–cell perturbation in the LINCS datasets and analyzed the labeled samples with known human aging-related genes. We created several machine-learning models to classify the direction of gene expression changes by using combined descriptive features of small molecules and genes along with information on cell line mutations and methylation levels. The deep neural network models outperformed the other K-machine learning methods and demonstrated promising accuracy in predicting up- or down-gene-regulating effects on perturbations beyond the scope of the original LINCS dataset. In addition, we demonstrated that the longevity models, while trained from cancer cell lines, are applicable to normal cell lines, and the models predicted a list of drug candidates that could have potential to be repurposed as pro-longevity agents. Quantitative predictions on all possible combinations of D (repurposed drug)–G (aging gene)–C (normal cell line) demonstrated the desired regulating effects on normal cells for the repurposed drugs with high positive rates. As a result, we identified 13 repurposing drug candidates that could potentially promote longevity by regulating aging-related gene expressions towards the desired direction, either upregulating pro-longevity genes, downregulating anti-longevity genes, or both. Interestingly, some of the proposed drug candidates were previously reported with aging-related functionalities in a number of model organisms. For example, one of the repositioned drug candidates, trichostatin-a, was found efficient at promoting anti-aging gene expression among fruit flies [19].

Our study utilized knowledge transferring from high-throughput gene expression profiling to testable data models, and achieved accurate performance in validating regulation effects, despite the severe imbalance of the data classes. In comparison to our previous model, DeepCOP [11], which is limited to only drug and gene descriptors, our current model has incorporated additional cell line descriptors that allow knowledge to be transferred from one set of cells (for example, cancer cells) to another set of cells (such as normal cells) using a single unified DNN. This task would not have been possible with DeepCOP models, where separate, disconnected DNN models were built for each individual cell line.

The limitations of this study include the possible improved methodologies in NN schemes and the lack of experimental validation of repurposed chemicals. One noticeable NN scheme—the graph convolutional neural network (GCN)—was presented in various studies, from drug discovery [39] to gene interactions [40]. In bioinformatics applications, two major types of graph structures were applied [41]: molecular structures and interaction networks. A multi-relational interaction network could be explored in GCN models using our preprocessed dataset that contains three domains—cells, genes, and drugs. Experimental validations should also be considered in future studies, in conjunction with docking simulations and ADMET estimations (a work in progress) using our in-house drug development platforms [42].

Supplementary Materials: The following are available online at https://www.mdpi.com/article/10.3390/ph14100948/s1, Figure S1: Model 3 AUC curve, Figure S2: Model 3 PR curve, Figure S3: Model 4 AUC curve, Figure S4: Model 4 PR curve, Figure S5: Model 5 AUC curve, Figure S6: Model 5 PR curve, Figure S7: Model 6 AUC curve, Figure S8: Model 6 PR curve, Figure S9: Model 7 AUC curve. Figure S10: Model 7 PR curve, Figure S11: Model 8 AUC curve, Figure S12: Model 8 PR curve, Table S1: Sample distribution in down-regulated models, Table S2: Sample distribution in up-regulated models.

Author Contributions: Conceptualization, J.Y., M.H. and A.C.; methodology, J.Y., M.H. and A.C.; software, J.Y.; validation, J.Y., M.H. and A.C.; formal analysis, J.Y., M.H. and A.C.; investigation, J.Y., M.H. and A.C.; resources, J.Y., M.H. and A.C.; data curation, J.Y., M.H. and A.C.; writing—original draft preparation, J.Y.; writing—review and editing, J.Y., M.H. and A.C.; visualization, J.Y.; supervision, M.H. and A.C.; project administration, A.C.; funding acquisition, A.C. All authors have read and agreed to the published version of the manuscript.

Funding: This research was funded by the Canadian Institutes of Health Research (CIHR), grant number 20R34369.

Institutional Review Board Statement: Not applicable.

Informed Consent Statement: Not applicable.

Data Availability Statement: Data are contained within the article or Supplementary Material.

Conflicts of Interest: The authors declare no conflict of interest.

Abbreviations

APR	area under precision recall curve
AUC	area under the roc curve
CDK	cyclin-dependent kinase
CMAP	connectivity map
CV	cross validation
FPR	false positive rate
GEO	gene expression omnibus
GO	gene ontology
LINCS	library of integrated network-based cellular signature
NN	neural networks
PRC	precision recall curve
RF	random forest
ROC	receiver operating characteristic curve
TPR	true positive rate

References

1. Ledford, H. Reversal of biological clock restores vision in old mice. *Nat. Cell Biol.* **2020**, *588*, 209. [CrossRef]
2. Johnson, S.C.; Yanos, M.E.; Kayser, E.-B.; Quintana, A.; Sangesland, M.; Castanza, A.; Uhde, L.; Hui, J.; Wall, V.Z.; Gagnidze, A.; et al. mTOR Inhibition Alleviates Mitochondrial Disease in a Mouse Model of Leigh Syndrome. *Science* **2013**, *342*, 1524–1528. [CrossRef] [PubMed]
3. Blagosklonny, M.V. Rapamycin for longevity: Opinion article. *Aging* **2019**, *11*, 8048–8067. [CrossRef] [PubMed]
4. Blagosklonny, M.V. Fasting and rapamycin: Diabetes versus benevolent glucose intolerance. *Cell Death Dis.* **2019**, *10*, 607. [CrossRef] [PubMed]
5. Trendelenburg, A.; Scheuren, A.; Potter, P.; Müller, R.; Bellantuono, I. Geroprotectors: A role in the treatment of frailty. *Mech. Ageing Dev.* **2019**, *180*, 11–20. [CrossRef] [PubMed]
6. Schubert, D.; Currais, A.; Goldberg, J.; Finley, K.; Petrascheck, M.; Maher, P. Geroneuroprotectors: Effective Geroprotectors for the Brain. *Trends Pharmacol. Sci.* **2018**, *39*, 1004–1007. [CrossRef] [PubMed]
7. Mallikarjun, V.; Swift, J. Therapeutic Manipulation of Ageing: Repurposing Old Dogs and Discovering New Tricks. *EBioMedicine* **2016**, *14*, 24–31. [CrossRef] [PubMed]
8. Harrison, D.E.; Strong, R.; Alavez, S.; Astle, C.M.; DiGiovanni, J.; Fernandez, E.; Flurkey, K.; Garratt, M.; Gelfond, J.A.L.; Javors, M.A.; et al. Acarbose improves health and lifespan in aging HET3 mice. *Aging Cell* **2019**, *18*, e12898. [CrossRef]
9. Lamb, J.; Crawford, E.D.; Peck, D.; Modell, J.W.; Blat, I.C.; Wrobel, M.J.; Lerner, J.; Brunet, J.-P.; Subramanian, A.; Ross, K.N.; et al. The Connectivity Map: Using Gene-Expression Signatures to Connect Small Molecules, Genes, and Disease. *Science* **2006**, *313*, 1929–1935. [CrossRef]
10. Mousavi, S.Z.; Rahmanian, M.; Sami, A. A connectivity map-based drug repurposing study and integrative analysis of transcriptomic profiling of SARS-CoV-2 infection. *Infect. Genet. Evol.* **2020**, *86*, 104610. [CrossRef] [PubMed]
11. Woo, G.; Fernandez, M.; Hsing, M.; Lack, N.A.; Cavga, A.D.; Cherkasov, A. DeepCOP—Deep Learning-Based Approach to Predict Gene Regulating Effects of Small Molecules. *Bioinformatics* **2019**, *36*, 813–818. [CrossRef] [PubMed]
12. Nellore, S.B. Various Performance Measures in Binary Classification-An Overview of ROC Study. *IJISET-Int. J. Innov. Sci. Eng. Technol.* **2015**, *2*, 596–605.
13. Saito, T.; Rehmsmeier, M. The Precision-Recall Plot Is More Informative than the ROC Plot When Evaluating Binary Classifiers on Imbalanced Datasets. *PLoS ONE* **2015**, *10*, e0118432. [CrossRef] [PubMed]
14. Dottermusch, M.; Lakner, T.; Peyman, T.; Klein, M.; Walz, G.; Neumann-Haefelin, E. Cell cycle controls stress response and longevity in C. elegans. *Aging* **2016**, *8*, 2100–2126. [CrossRef] [PubMed]
15. Richter, A.; Schoenwaelder, N.; Sender, S.; Junghanss, C.; Maletzki, C. Cyclin-Dependent Kinase Inhibitors in Hematological Malignancies—Current Understanding, (Pre-)Clinical Application and Promising Approaches. *Cancers* **2021**, *13*, 2497. [CrossRef] [PubMed]
16. Steegmaier, M.; Hoffmann, M.; Baum, A.; Lenart, P.; Petronczki, M.; Krššák, M.; Gürtler, U.; Garin-Chesa, P.; Lieb, S.; Quant, J.; et al. BI 2536, a Potent and Selective Inhibitor of Polo-like Kinase 1, Inhibits Tumor Growth In Vivo. *Curr. Biol.* **2007**, *17*, 316–322. [CrossRef]
17. Jondorf, W.; Abbott, B.; Greenberg, N.; Mead, J. Increased Lifespan of Leukemic Mice Treated with Drugs Related to (–)-Emetine. *Chemotherapy* **1971**, *16*, 109–129. [CrossRef]
18. Narciclasine Attenuates Diet-Induced Obesity by Promoting Oxidative Metabolism in Skeletal Muscle. Available online: https://journals.plos.org/plosbiology/article?id=10.1371/journal.pbio.1002597 (accessed on 15 September 2021).

19. Tao, D.; Lu, J.; Sun, H.; Zhao, Y.-M.; Yuan, Z.-G.; Li, X.-X.; Huang, B.-Q. Trichostatin A Extends the Lifespan of Drosophila melanogaster by Elevating hsp22 Expression. *Acta Biochim. Biophys. Sin.* **2004**, *36*, 618–622. [CrossRef]
20. Clarkson-Jones, J.; Kenyon, A.; Tomkinson, H. The disposition and metabolism of zibotentan (ZD4054): An oral-specific endothelin A receptor antagonist in mice, rats and dogs. *Xenobiotica* **2011**, *41*, 784–796. [CrossRef]
21. Palmer, J.C.; Tayler, H.M.; Dyer, L.; Kehoe, P.G.; Paton, J.F.; Love, S. Zibotentan, an Endothelin A Receptor Antagonist, Prevents Amyloid-β-Induced Hypertension and Maintains Cerebral Perfusion. *J. Alzheimer Dis.* **2020**, *73*, 1185–1199. [CrossRef]
22. Landys, K.; Borgström, S.; Andersson, T.; Noppa, H. Mitoxantrone as a first-line treatment of advanced breast cancer. *Investig. New Drugs* **1985**, *3*, 133–137. [CrossRef] [PubMed]
23. Zocchi, L.; Wu, S.C.; Wu, J.; Hayama, K.L.; Benavente, C.A. The cyclin-dependent kinase inhibitor flavopiridol (alvocidib) inhibits metastasis of human osteosarcoma cells. *Oncotarget* **2018**, *9*, 23505–23518. [CrossRef]
24. Chen, Y.W.; Arneson, D.; Diamente, G.; Garcia, J.; Zaghari, N.; Patel, P.; Allard, P.; Yang, X.C. PharmOmics: A species- and tissue-specific drug signature database and online tool for toxicity prediction and drug repurposing. *bioRxiv* **2019**, 837773. Available online: https://www.biorxiv.org/content/10.1101/837773v1 (accessed on 17 September 2021).
25. Zdrazil, B.; Richter, L.; Brown, N.; Guha, R. Moving targets in drug discovery. *Sci. Rep.* **2020**, *10*, 20213. [CrossRef] [PubMed]
26. Mutowo, P.; Bento, A.P.; Dedman, N.; Gaulton, A.; Hersey, A.; Lomax, J.; Overington, J.P. A drug target slim: Using gene ontology and gene ontology annotations to navigate protein-ligand target space in ChEMBL. *J. Biomed. Semant.* **2016**, *7*, 59. [CrossRef] [PubMed]
27. Hsing, M.; Byler, K.G.; Cherkasov, A. The use of Gene Ontology terms for predicting highly-connected 'hub' nodes in protein-protein interaction networks. *BMC Syst. Biol.* **2008**, *2*, 80. [CrossRef]
28. Morgan, H.L. The Generation of a Unique Machine Description for Chemical Structures-A Technique Developed at Chemical Abstracts Service. *J. Chem. Doc.* **2002**, *5*, 107–113. [CrossRef]
29. Wood, D.E.; White, J.R.; Georgiadis, A.; Van Emburgh, B.; Parpart-Li, S.; Mitchell, J.; Anagnostou, V.; Niknafs, N.; Karchin, R.; Papp, E.; et al. A machine learning approach for somatic mutation discovery. *Sci. Transl. Med.* **2018**, *10*, eaar7939. [CrossRef]
30. Way, G.P.; Sanchez-Vega, F.; La, K.; Armenia, J.; Chatila, W.K.; Luna, A.; Sander, C.; Cherniack, A.D.; Mina, M.; Ciriello, G.; et al. Machine Learning Detects Pan-cancer Ras Pathway Activation in The Cancer Genome Atlas. *Cell Rep.* **2018**, *23*, 172–180. [CrossRef] [PubMed]
31. Miranda, S.P.; Baião, F.A.; Fleck, J.L.; Piccolo, S.R. Predicting drug sensitivity of cancer cells based on DNA methylation levels. *bioRxiv* **2020**. Available online: https://www.biorxiv.org/content/10.1101/2020.08.25.266049v1 (accessed on 17 September 2021).
32. Yuan, R.; Chen, S.; Wang, Y. Computational Prediction of Drug Responses in Cancer Cell Lines From Cancer Omics and Detection of Drug Effectiveness Related Methylation Sites. *Front. Genet.* **2020**, *11*, 917. [CrossRef]
33. Bibikova, M.; Fan, J.-B. GoldenGate® Assay for DNA Methylation Profiling. *Stem Cells Aging* **2009**, *507*, 149–163. [CrossRef]
34. Yu, L.; Liu, H. Feature Selection for High-Dimensional Data: A Fast Correlation-Based Filter Solution. In Proceedings of the 20th Iinternational Conference on Machine Learning, Fort Lauderdale, FL, USA, 1 November 2003; pp. 856–863.
35. Raja, K.; Patrick, M.; Elder, J.T.; Tsoi, L.C. Machine learning workflow to enhance predictions of Adverse Drug Reactions (ADRs) through drug-gene interactions: Application to drugs for cutaneous diseases. *Sci. Rep.* **2017**, *7*, 1–11. [CrossRef]
36. You, J.; McLeod, R.D.; Hu, P. Predicting drug-target interaction network using deep learning model. *Comput. Biol. Chem.* **2019**, *80*, 90–101. [CrossRef] [PubMed]
37. Adam, G.; Rampášek, L.; Safikhani, Z.; Smirnov, P.; Haibe-Kains, B.; Goldenberg, A. Machine learning approaches to drug response prediction: Challenges and recent progress. *NPJ Precis. Oncol.* **2020**, *4*, 1–10. [CrossRef]
38. Ltd, R.; Globa, M. Anti-Aging Market Report and Forecast (2021–2026). Available online: https://www.researchandmarkets.com/reports/5264056/global-anti-aging-market-report-and-forecast (accessed on 24 August 2021).
39. Lim, J.; Ryu, S.; Park, K.; Choe, Y.J.; Ham, J.; Kim, W.Y. Predicting Drug–Target Interaction Using a Novel Graph Neural Network with 3D Structure-Embedded Graph Representation. *J. Chem. Inf. Model.* **2019**, *59*, 3981–3988. [CrossRef] [PubMed]
40. Yuan, Y.; Bar-Joseph, Z. GCNG: Graph convolutional networks for inferring gene interaction from spatial transcriptomics data. *Genome Biol.* **2020**, *21*, 300. [CrossRef] [PubMed]
41. Zhang, X.-M.; Liang, L.; Liu, L.; Tang, M.-J. Graph Neural Networks and Their Current Applications in Bioinformatics. *Front. Genet.* **2021**, *12*, 1073. [CrossRef]
42. Gentile, F.; Agrawal, V.; Hsing, M.; Ton, A.-T.; Ban, F.; Norinder, U.; Gleave, M.E.; Cherkasov, A. Deep Docking: A Deep Learning Platform for Augmentation of Structure Based Drug Discovery. *ACS Central Sci.* **2020**, *6*, 939–949. [CrossRef] [PubMed]

pharmaceuticals

MDPI

Article

High-Throughput Screening and Molecular Dynamics Simulation of Natural Product-like Compounds against Alzheimer's Disease through Multitarget Approach

Danish Iqbal [1,*], Md Tabish Rehman [2], Abdulaziz Bin Dukhyil [1], Syed Mohd Danish Rizvi [3], Mohamed F. Al Ajmi [2], Bader Mohammed Alshehri [1], Saeed Banawas [1,4,5], M. Salman Khan [6], Wael Alturaiki [1] and Mohammed Alsaweed [1]

1 Department of Medical Laboratory Sciences, College of Applied Medical Sciences, Majmaah University, Majmaah 11952, Saudi Arabia; a.dukhyil@mu.edu.sa (A.B.D.); b.alshehri@mu.edu.sa (B.M.A.); s.banawas@mu.edu.sa (S.B.); w.alturaiki@mu.edu.sa (W.A.); m.alsaweed@mu.edu.sa (M.A.)
2 Department of Pharmacognosy, College of Pharmacy, King Saud University, Riyadh 11451, Saudi Arabia; mrehman@ksu.edu.sa (M.T.R.); malajmii@ksu.edu.sa (M.F.A.A.)
3 Department of Pharmaceutics, College of Pharmacy, University of Hail, Hail 81442, Saudi Arabia; sm.danish@uoh.edu.sa
4 Health and Basic Sciences Research Center, Majmaah University, Majmaah 15341, Saudi Arabia
5 Department of Biomedical Sciences, Oregon State University, Corvallis, OR 97331, USA
6 Clinical Biochemistry & Natural Product Research Laboratory, Department of Biosciences, Integral University, Lucknow 226026, India; contactskhan@gmail.com
* Correspondence: da.mohammed@mu.edu.sa

Citation: Iqbal, D.; Rehman, M.T.; Bin Dukhyil, A.; Rizvi, S.M.D.; Al Ajmi, M.F.; Alshehri, B.M.; Banawas, S.; Khan, M.S.; Alturaiki, W.; Alsaweed, M. High-Throughput Screening and Molecular Dynamics Simulation of Natural Product-like Compounds against Alzheimer's Disease through Multitarget Approach. *Pharmaceuticals* **2021**, *14*, 937. https://doi.org/10.3390/ph14090937

Academic Editor: Osvaldo Andrade Santos-Filho

Received: 23 August 2021
Accepted: 16 September 2021
Published: 18 September 2021

Publisher's Note: MDPI stays neutral with regard to jurisdictional claims in published maps and institutional affiliations.

Abstract: Alzheimer's disease (AD) is a progressive neurological disorder that affects 50 million people. Despite this, only two classes of medication have been approved by the FDA. Therefore, we have planned to develop therapeutics by multitarget approach. We have explored the library of 2029 natural product-like compounds for their multi-targeting potential against AD by inhibiting AChE, BChE (cholinergic pathway) MAO-A, and MOA-B (oxidative stress pathway) through in silico high-throughput screening and molecular dynamics simulation. Based on the binding energy of these target enzymes, approximately 189 compounds exhibited a score of less than −10 kcal/mol against all targets. However, none of the control inhibitors exhibited a binding affinity of less than −10 kcal/mol. Among these, the top 10 hits of compounds against all four targets were selected for ADME-T analysis. As a result, only F0850-4777 exhibited an acceptable range of physicochemical properties, drug-likeness, pharmacokinetics, and suitability for BBB permeation with high GI-A and non-toxic effects. The molecular dynamics study confirmed that F0850-4777 remained inside the binding cavity of targets in a stable conformation throughout the simulation and Prime-MM/GBSA study revealed that van der Waals' energy (ΔG_{vdW}) and non-polar solvation or lipophilic energy (ΔG_{Sol_Lipo}) contribute favorably towards the formation of a stable protein–ligand complex. Thus, F0850-4777 could be a potential candidate against multiple targets of two pathophysiological pathways of AD and opens the doors for further confirmation through in vitro and in vivo systems.

Keywords: Alzheimer's disease; multitarget; molecular dynamics simulations; natural-like compounds; virtual screening

1. Introduction

Neurological disorders including Alzheimer's disease (AD) have a significant negative impact on the mental, psychological, physical, and economic health of patients and their caregivers [1,2]. Almost 50 million people are affected globally from Alzheimer and other dementias [2]. AD is the second leading cause of death among high-income countries, and the seventh leading cause of death worldwide, ranking sixth in Saudi Arabia (currently over 130,000 cases) [3,4]. Patients with AD exhibit memory loss, agitation, dysphoria, apathy, aberrant motor behavior, problems with speaking or writing, and cognitive impairments [1].

Alzheimer's disease has a very intricate etiology, and several reports have hypothesized that the four major pathophysiological pathways (oxidative stress, amyloid-beta pathway, tau pathway, and cholinergic pathway) are responsible for the progression of AD [5–11]. These pathways include the formation of senile plaques through amyloid-beta (Aβ) plaque deposition [8], the agglomeration of neurofibrillary tangles after tau neurofibrillary degeneration [12], the disruption of cholinergic activity [11], and oxidative stress [10,13].

Oxidative stress is promoted by an increased production of hydrogen peroxide through the catalytic action of monoamine oxidases (MAO-A and MAO-B) on the primary amine deamination of major neurotransmitters [13], which results in tissue damage, especially in brain cell and disrupts the blood–brain barrier, which could lead to AD [10]. It has also been well established that during AD, there is deterioration of cholinergic neuron-rich regions, resulting in the decline of acetylcholine (ACh) levels, which are believed to be associated with memory loss, agitation, and apathy [11,14]. Moreover, cholinesterase enzymes such as acetylcholinesterase (AChE) and butyrylcholinesterase (BChE), have been found to further decrease the concentration of acetylcholine (ACh) by hydrolyzing it [8,9].

Until now, the US Food and Drug Administration (FDA) has approved two classes of medications to treat AD: (1) cholinesterase inhibitors (donepezil, galantamine, and rivastigmine) and (2) an NDMA receptor antagonist (memantine). However, although these drugs relieve some symptoms and have beneficial effects on cognition and function, they do not treat neuropsychiatric symptoms and do not slowdown or stop the progression of the disease. Moreover, these medications have several side effects including nausea, vomiting, loss of appetite, headache, constipation, confusion, and dizziness [15,16].

At present, there is a lack of disease-modifying medications or a complete cure for AD. The enzymes that promote the pathways responsible for the progression of AD include AChE, BChE, MAO-A, and MOA-B, which would need to be targeted individually or in combination [5,6,17–21]. Advances in computing have recently allowed for the development of various cheminformatics approaches for the faster screening and optimization of bioactive compounds through enzyme inhibition [22–27].

Since nature has an endless resource of bioactive compounds, it would be economical and safe to obtain bioactive moieties to produce novel multitarget agents against Alzheimer's disease [18,28]. Due to the popularity and therapeutic potential of natural products and their derivatives, Life Chemicals Inc. have recently developed proprietary of synthetic compounds, namely, natural product-like compounds, based on cheminformatics and substructure searches (www.lifechemicals.com). However, a "one disease, one target, one drug" strategy is limited by its inability to completely cure complex diseases, such as neurodegenerative diseases or mood disorders [29,30]. These limitations have driven us to explore the development of therapeutics using multiple targeted approaches aimed at several different pathological cascades of AD simultaneously.

In the present study, we explored a library of natural product-like compounds for their multi-targeting (AChE, BChE, MAO-A, MOA-B) potential against AD through in silico high-throughput screening and ADME-T analysis. Furthermore, the validation of the best hit via molecular dynamics simulation was also conducted. To the best of our knowledge, this study is the first to explore this library of natural product-like compounds for multi-targeting against AD.

2. Results and Discussion

2.1. Virtual Screening Analysis

Although the process of drug discovery is time-consuming and expensive, new drugs are needed to fulfill unmet clinical needs [31]. The number of drug or lead-like molecules available in different databases is estimated to be as high as 1×10^{24}. Moreover, the structures of potential drug target molecules are increasingly being added to the Protein Data Bank on a regular basis. Thus, to deal with such a large number of molecules and to assist in the drug discovery process, computer-aided drug discovery techniques, such as in silico virtual screening, play a significant role owing to their faster speed and lower cost compared to in vitro high-throughput screening [32]. In the present study, we employed in silico virtual screening, molecular docking, and molecular dynamics simulation to identify a novel inhibitor against multiple targets of Alzheimer's disease such as AChE, BChE, MAO-A, and MAO-B.

All natural-like compounds in the library and three control inhibitors (Tacrine, Harmine, and Safinamide) against the target proteins (AChE, BChE, MOA-A, and MOA-B) were subjected to docking analysis, generating 10 binding combinations. Based on the binding energy (ΔG), 189 out of 2029 compounds exhibited binding energy score of −10 to −12.9 kcal/mol, −10 to −12.6 kcal/mol, and −10 to −13.6 kcal/mol against AChE, BChE, and monoaminoxidases, respectively. The control inhibitors, such as Tacrine, exhibited a binding affinity of −8.5 kcal/mol and −8.4 kcal/mol against AChE and BChE, respectively. Harmine got binding affinity of −8.7 kcal/mol for MOA-A and Safinamide showed −9.5 kcal/mol of binding affinity against MOA-B. Among these 189 compounds, the top 10 hits of compounds against all four targets were selected (Table 1) for further analysis.

Table 1. Molecular docking scores of best hit natural product-like compounds against AChE, BChE, MAO-A and MAO-B.

S. No.	ID Number	Targets/ Formula	Docking Energy (kcal/mol)			
			AChE (1acj)	BChE (4bds)	MAO-A (2z5x)	MAO-B (2v5z)
1	F0870-0001	$C_{24}H_{15}NO_6$	−12.9	−12.6	−11.5	−13.6
2	F1094-0205	$C_{26}H_{23}NO_4$	−12.9	−11	−10.8	−12.6
3	F3293-0320	$C_{22}H_{13}NO_7$	−12.4	−11.1	−12.3	−13.4
4	F1094-0201	$C_{26}H_{19}NO_4$	−12.3	−11.2	−12.3	−11.5
5	F0850-4777	$C_{24}H_{18}O_5$	−12.2	−10.7	−13.6	−12.5
6	F3385-6048	$C_{27}H_{21}NO_8$	−12.2	−11.1	−13.2	−12.6
7	F1094-0200	$C_{25}H_{17}NO_4$	−12.1	−11.2	−11	−13.2
8	F1865-0198	$C_{23}H_{15}NO_6$	−12	−10.9	−12.6	−13.3
9	F3139-1101	$C_{24}H_{16}O_4$	−12	−10.3	−12.4	−13.6
10	F3139-1218	$C_{26}H_{18}O_6$	−11.8	−10.4	−12.9	−13.3
11	Tacrine	$C_{13}H_{14}N_2$	−8.5	−8.4	ND	ND
12	Harmine	$C_{13}H_{12}N_2O$	ND	ND	−8.7	ND
13	Safinamide	$C_{17}H_{19}FN_2O_2$	ND	ND	ND	−9.5

ND: Not determined.

2.2. Prediction of Physicochemical, Pharmacokinetics Properties, Drug-Likeness, and Toxicity Potentials

Natural product-like compounds' physicochemical properties drug-likeness and pharmacokinetics were evaluated using the SwissADME tool [33]. Among the top 10 hits analyzed against targets of Alzheimer's disease (AChE, BChE, MOAA, and MOAB), five compounds (F0870-0001, F3293-0320, F3385-6048, F1865-0198, and F3139-1218) were found to be unsuitable for BBB permeation. However, all of the compounds had a molecular mass of less than 500 g/mol, showed high gastrointestinal absorption, and showed zero violation of Lipinski's rule. Moreover, five other compounds (F1094-0205, F1094-0201, F0850-4777, F1094-0200, and F3139-1101) were found to be suitable for BBB permeation including the acceptable range of other parameters (Table 2). Considering the analyzed physicochemical properties and absorption potential, further toxicological investigation was carried out and found that only three compounds (F0850-4777, F3293-0320, and F3385-6048) exhibited no toxicity for all the tested parameters (Table 3). The results showed that F0850-4777 (3-(2-methoxyphenyl)-4-oxo-4H-chromen-7-yl 4-methylbenzoate) has a higher affinity towards all the target proteins and found acceptable range of physicochemical properties, drug-likeness, and pharmacokinetics (Figure S1). This confirmed its amelioration of Alzheimer's disease and was selected for molecular docking and molecular dynamics simulation analysis.

Table 2. Physicochemical properties, drug-likeness, and pharmacokinetics of best hit natural product-like compounds.

		Pharmacokinetics		Physicochemical Properties						Drug-Likeness	
S. No.	**ID Number**	**BBB-P**	**GI-A**	**MW**	**Clog-P**	**HBA**	**HBD**	**RB**	**TPSA**	**L-V**	**FSP^3**
1	F0870-0001	NO	High	413.37	3.29	7	2	3	113.77	0	0.04
2	F1094-0205	YES	High	413.47	6.32	5	0	3	59.75	0	0.3
3	F3293-0320	NO	High	403.34	3.25	7	0	6	119.4	0	0.04
4	F1094-0201	YES	High	409.43	5.79	5	0	2	59.75	0	0.15
5	F0850-4777	YES	High	386.39	4.51	5	0	5	65.74	0	0.08
6	F3385-6048	NO	High	487.46	4.99	9	0	6	96.67	0	0.18
7	F1094-0200	YES	High	395.4	5.48	5	0	2	59.75	0	0.12
8	F1865-0198	NO	High	401.37	5.34	6	0	5	102.37	0	0.04
9	F3139-1101	YES	High	368.38	5.12	4	0	5	56.51	0	0
10	F3139-1218	NO	High	426.42	4.45	6	0	5	78.88	0	0.07

Molecular weight (MW), number of hydrogen bond donors (HBD), number of hydrogen bond acceptors (HBA), rotatable bonds (RB), cLogP value (clogP), topological polar surface area (TPSA), Lipinski's rule violation (L-V), human gastrointestinal absorption (GI-A), blood–brain barrier permeation (BBB-P) and fraction Csp3 (FSP^3).

Table 3. Toxicity potential of 10 hits compounds.

S. No.	Compound	Mutagenic	Tumorigenic	Reproductive Effect	Irritant
1	F0850-4777	None	None	None	None
2	F0870-0001	None	None	Low	None
3	F1094-0200	None	None	High	None
4	F1094-0201	None	None	High	None
5	F1094-0205	None	None	High	None
6	F1865-0198	None	None	High	None
7	F3139-1101	None	None	None	High
8	F3139-1218	None	None	High	None
9	F3293-0320	None	None	None	None
10	F3385-6048	None	None	None	None

Toxicity assessment has been performed by DataWarrior tool.

2.3. Molecular Docking Analysis

Based on the virtual screening against a library of natural product-like compounds, F0850-4777 has been identified as the most potent inhibitor against multiple targets (AChE, BChE, MAO-A, and MAO-B) of AD. Further analysis by molecular docking between F0850-4777 and target proteins enabled us to closely examine the amino acid residues and the nature of interactions responsible for the formation of a stable protein–inhibitor complex. The interactions of F0850-4777 with the active site of AChE, BChE, MAO-A and MAO-B are shown in Figures 1–4, respectively.

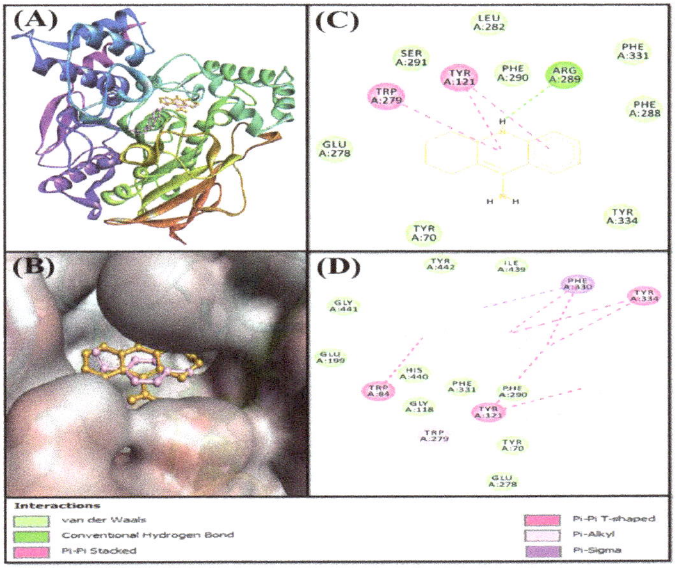

Figure 1. Interaction of target protein, AChE with F0850-4777 and their respective control ligands. (**A**) Position of F0850-4777 and Tacrine in AChE. (**B**) Interactions between AChE and Tacrine. (**C**) Superimposed image of F0850-4777 and Tacrine in AChE. (**D**) Interactions between AChE and F0850-4777.

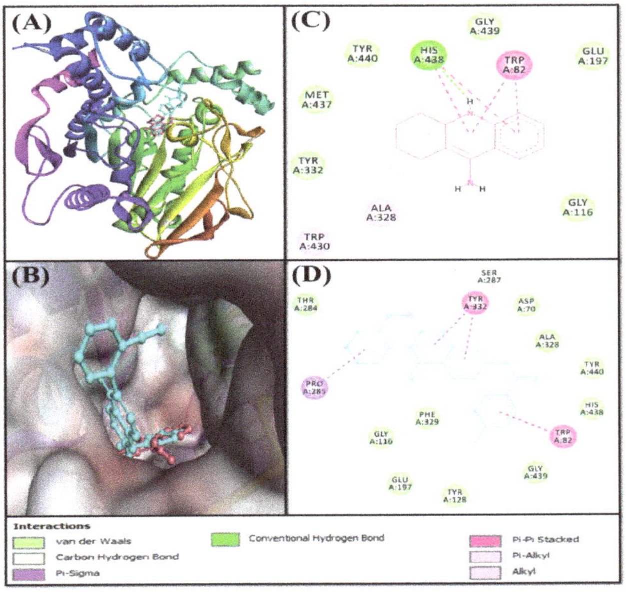

Figure 2. Interaction of target protein, BChE with F0850-4777 and their respective control ligands. (**A**) Position of F0850-4777 and Tacrine in BChE. (**B**) Interactions between BChE and Tacrine (**C**). Superimposed image of F0850-4777 and Tacrine in BChE. (**D**) Interactions between BChE and F0850-4777.

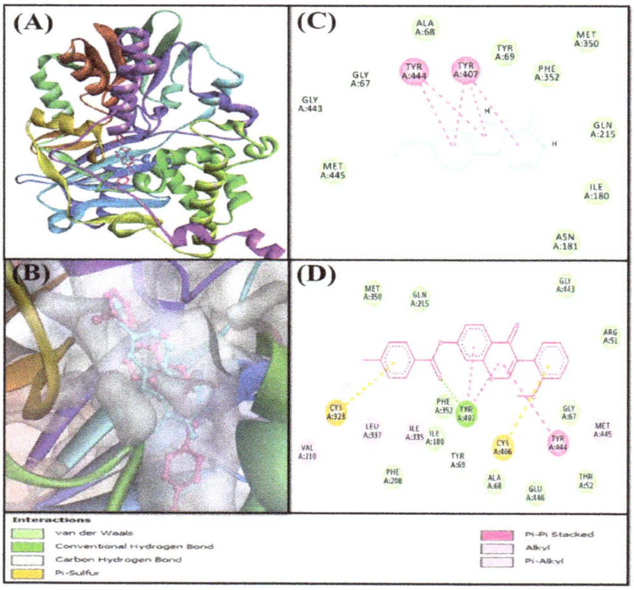

Figure 3. Interaction of target protein, MAO-A with F0850-4777 and their respective control ligands. (**A**) Position of F0850-4777 and Harmine in MAO-A. (**B**) Interactions between MAO-A and Harmine. (**C**) Superimposed image of F0850-4777 and Harmine in MAO-A. (**D**) Interactions between MAO-A and F0850-4777.

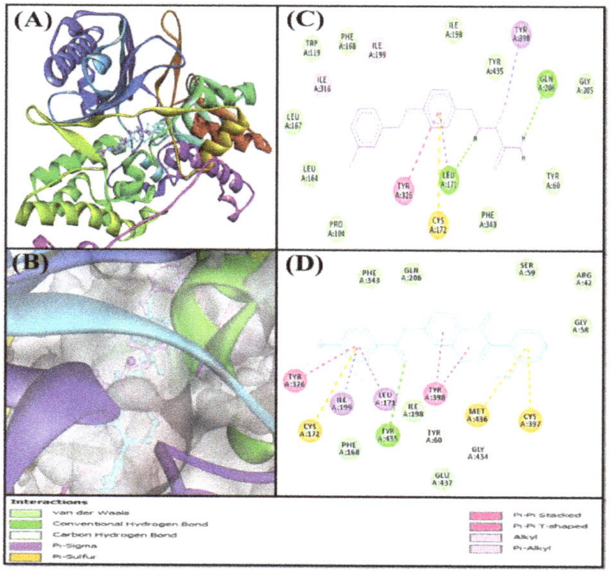

Figure 4. Interaction of target protein, MAO-B with F0850-4777 and their respective control ligands. (**A**) Position of F0850-4777 and Safinamide in MAO-B. (**B**) Interactions between MAO-B and Safinamide. (**C**) Superimposed image of F0850-4777 and Safinamide in MAO-B. (**D**) Interactions between MAO-B and F0850-4777.

2.3.1. Analysis of the Interaction between AChE and F0850-4777

Acetylcholinesterase (AChE) is an essential enzyme that catalyzes the hydrolysis of acetylcholine, which is critical for memory and cognition [34]. The inhibition of AChE activity is a major therapeutic intervention in the treatment of Alzheimer's disease (AD), which is characterized by cholinergic deficiency. The majority of the drugs approved for the treatment of AD, such as Tacrine, donepezil, and rivastigmine, are AChE inhibitors [15,16,35]. The inhibitors of AChE activity bind to its catalytic active site (CAS), characterized by the presence of a long, narrow, and hydrophobic gorge, harboring a catalytic triad of Ser200, Glu327, and His440 [36]. The residues Trp84 and Phe330 play a significant role in stabilizing the transition state during the catalytic reaction. Furthermore, it has been recently demonstrated that a secondary noncholinergic function of AChE, associated with the peripheral anionic site (PAS), is involved in the pathogenesis of AD. PAS is formed by aromatic amino acid residues such as Tyr70, Asp72, Tyr121, Trp279, and Tyr334 lining the rim of the gorge [37]. Through its PAS, AChE co-localizes with Aβ peptide deposits in patients with AD and forms a stable Aβ-AChE complex, which in turn promotes fibrillogenesis and aggregation [38,39]. Thus, these observations suggest that both the CAS and PAS of AChE can be targeted as therapeutic interventions for AD.

In the present study, molecular docking analysis between AChE and F0850-4777 revealed that the ligand was bound to the central active site cavity of AChE (Figure 1). The binding pose of F0850-4777 at the active site of AChE was further compared with the binding mode of a control ligand, that is, Tacrine. Both F0850-4777 and Tacrine were found to occupy the same site located in the deep cavity of AChE (Figure 1A,B). The AChE-Tacrine complex was stabilized by one conventional hydrogen bond between the Lig:NH and Arg289:O atoms. In addition, five hydrophobic interactions (with Tyr121 and Trp279) and eight van der Waals' interactions (Tyr70, Glu278, Leu282, Phe288, Phe290, Ser291, Phe331, and Tyr334) further stabilized the AChE-Tacrine complex (Figure 1C). Conversely, the AChE-F0580-4777 complex was mainly stabilized by hydrophobic interactions. F0850-4777 formed one Pi-Sigma interaction with Phe330, three Pi-Pi stacked interactions with Trp84 and Tyr121, five Pi-Pi T-shaped interactions with Tyr121, Phe330 and Tyr334, and two Pi-alkyl interactions with Tyr121 and Trp279 (Figure 1D and Table S1). In addition, several amino acid residues, such as Tyr70, Gly118, Glu199, Glu278, Phe290, Phe331, His440, Gly441, Ile439, and Tyr442 formed van der Waals' interactions. It should be noted that F0850-4777 interacts with many CAS residues of AChE, including Trp84, Phe330, and His440, and PAS residues of AChE, such as Tyr121, Trp279, and Tyr334. Interestingly, the amino acid residues of AChE commonly interact with F0850-4777 as well as Tacrine includes Tyr121, Glu278, Trp279, Phe290, and Phe331. Moreover, the docking energy and the corresponding binding affinity were estimated to be -8.5 kcal mol^{-1} and 1.72×10^6 M^{-1} for the AChE-Tacrine interaction, respectively, and -12.2 kcal mol^{-1} and 8.87×10^8 M^{-1} for the AChE-F0850-4777 interaction, respectively. The binding affinity of F0850-4777 for AChE was approximately 515.7-fold higher than that of the control inhibitor Tacrine and RMSD value between best pose of Tacrine and F0850-4777 was found to be 1.345 Å.

2.3.2. Analysis of the Interaction between BChE and F0850-4777

Butyrylcholinesterase (BChE), also known as pseudocholinesterase, is responsible for the hydrolysis of choline esters (e.g., butyrylcholine, succinylcholine, and acetylcholine) and non-choline esters (e.g., cocaine, acetylsalicylic acid, and heroin) [40,41]. BChE is a multifaceted enzyme expressed in different regions of neurons; it co-regulates cholinergic neurotransmission and is also partially involved in the development of the nervous system [42–46]. The fact that the biochemical properties of BChE are altered in AD makes it a potential target for use in therapeutic interventions [47–50]. Structurally and functionally, BChE is similar to AChE, which has a catalytic serine buried in a deep gorge. The catalytic triad of BChE is formed by Ser226, His438 and Glu352 [51]. The anionic site of BChE contains Trp82, which interacts with the cationic quaternary nitrogen of choline [52]. In addition, Asp70 and Tyr332 guide the positively charged substrates such as butyrylcholine to the active site located at the bottom of the gorge [53]. Furthermore, Leu286 and Val288, which line the acyl pocket within the active site gorge, hold the acyl group of choline in place during catalysis [52]. The acyl pocket of BChE is larger due to the presence of amino acid residues with smaller site chains (Leu286 and Val288) compared to the AChE acyl pocket lining Phe330.

Evaluating the interaction between BChE and F0850-4777 along with the control inhibitor (Tacrine) confirmed that both ligands occupied a similar position inside the binding cavity of BChE (Figure 2A,B). The BChE-Tacrine complex was stabilized by one conventional hydrogen bond between Lig:NH and the active site residue His438:O atoms. In addition, Tacrine formed four Pi-Pi stacked hydrophobic interactions with Trp82, and two Pi-Pi stacked interactions with His438. In addition, there were two Pi-alkyl (with Trp82 and Trp430) and one alkyl hydrophobic interaction with Ala328. Furthermore, the BChE and Tacrine complex was stabilized by six van der Waals interactions with Gly116, Glu197, Tyr332, Gly439, Tyr440, and Met437 (Figure 2C). Conversely, the BChE and F0850-4777 complex was stabilized by one carbon hydrogen bond with the Ser287:O atom, and seven hydrophobic interactions with Trp82, Pro285, and Tyr332 (Figure 2D and Table S2). In addition, several amino acid residues such as Asp70, Gly116, Tyr128, Glu197, Thr284, Ser287, Ala328, Phe329, His438, Gly439, and Tyr440 formed van der Waals' interactions. It is worth noting that F0850-4777 interacts with some of the important amino acid residues of BChE such as Asp70, Trp82, and His438. Interestingly, the amino acid residues of BChE commonly engaged in interactions with F0850-4777 and Tacrine includes Trp82, Gly116, Glu197, Ala328, His438, Gly439, and Tyr440. Moreover, the docking energy and the corresponding binding affinity were estimated to be -8.4 kcal mol^{-1} and 1.45×10^6 M^{-1} for the BChE-Tacrine interaction, respectively, and -10.7 kcal mol^{-1} and 7.04×10^7 M^{-1} for the BChE-F0850-4777 interaction, respectively. We found that the binding affinity of F0850-4777 for BChE was approximately 48.6-fold higher than that of the control inhibitor Tacrine and RMSD value between best pose of Tacrine and F0850-4777 was found to be 1.401 Å.

2.3.3. Analysis of the Interaction between Monoamine Oxidases and F0850-4777

Monoamine oxidases A and B (MAO-A and MAO-B) are located on the outer membrane of mitochondria. They catalyze the oxidation of amines to imines, which are then hydrolyzed non-enzymatically to the corresponding aldehydes or ketones [54]. MAO-A metabolizes serotonin, dopamine, and norepinephrine, whereas MAO-B oxidizes dopamine, benzylamine, and phenylethylamine [55,56]. MAO-B has also been reported to form a neurotoxin (1-methyl-4-phenyl-pyridinium), which causes Parkinson's disease, from 1-methyl-4-phenyl-1,2,3,6-tetrahydropyridine [57]. Thus, monoamine oxidases are excellent targets for the development of novel therapeutics against Parkinson's, Alzheimer's, and other neurodegenerative diseases.

Structurally, MAO-A and MAO-B share 70% identical amino acid sequences, and both contain an FAD-binding domain, a substrate-binding domain, and a membrane-binding domain [58,59]. The catalytic sites of both monoamine oxidases are mainly hydrophobic and are lined with aromatic and aliphatic amino acid residues. A conserved lysine residue (Lys305 in MAO-A and Lys296 in MAO-B) interacts with a water molecule, which is attached to the N5-atom of the flavin co-factor [60]. The amino acid residues Tyr407 and Tyr444 in MAO-A, and Tyr398 and Tyr435 in MAO-B are conserved in all MAOs and are located on opposite sides of the covalently bound substrates and inhibitors [61,62]. It has been shown that these tyrosine residues orient the substrate for oxidation, or enhance the nucleophilicity of the amine [63].The selectivity of these enzymes in substrate binding sites is defined by the presence of Ile335 in MAO-A and Tyr326 in MAO-B [64]. Another difference between the two enzymes is the size of the substrate-binding site. In MAO-A, the volume of the substrate-binding site is 400 Å^3, whereas in MAO-B, there is a smaller hydrophobic "entrance cavity" positioned between the surface and main substrate-binding site. Depending on the substrate, the two cavities in MAO-B are fused together because of the rotation in Ile199 to form a larger cavity of 400 Å^3 [60].

Analysis of the Interaction between MAO-A and F0850-4777

Molecular docking analysis between MAO-A and F0850-4777 revealed that the ligand was bound to the central active site cavity of MAO-A (Figure 3). The binding pose of F0850-4777 at the active site of MAO-A was further compared with the binding mode of a control ligand, that is, Harmine. Both F0850-4777 and Harmine were found to occupy the same site located in the deep cavity of MAO-A (Figure 3A,B). The MAO-A-Harmine complex was stabilized by two carbon hydrogen bonds (Gly67:CA-Lig:O and Lig:C-Gly443:O), and five hydrophobic interactions with Tyr407 and Tyr444. In addition, Harmine formed eight van der Waals' interactions with Ala68, Tyr69, Ile180, Asn181, Gln215, Met350, Phe352, and Met445 to further stabilize the MAO-A-Harmine complex (Figure 3C). Conversely, the MAO-A and F0850-4777 complex was stabilized by one conventional hydrogen bond (Tyr407:HH-Lig:O) and one carbon hydrogen bond (Lig:C-Tyr69:O). In addition, F0850-4777 formed three Pi-Pi stacks (Tyr407 and Tyr444), and seven Pi-alkyl hydrophobic interactions (with Val210, Cys323, Ile335, Leu337, and Met445). In addition, F0850-4777 formed two Pi-Sulfur interactions with Cys323 and Cys406 (Figure 3D and Table S3). Furthermore, the MAO-A-F0850-4777 complex was stabilized by van der Waals' interactions with several amino acid residues such as Arg51, Thr52, Gly67, Ala68, Ile180, Phe208, Gln215, Met350, Phe352, Gly443, and Glu446. Interestingly, the amino acid residues of MAO-A commonly interacted with F0850-4777 and Harmine with Gly67, Ala68, Tyr69, Ile180, Gln215, Met350, Phe352, Tyr407, Gly443, and Tyr444. Moreover, the docking energy and the corresponding binding affinity were estimated to be -8.7 kcal mol^{-1} and 2.40×10^6 M^{-1} for the MAO-A-Harmine interaction, respectively, and -13.6 kcal mol^{-1} and 9.44×10^9 M^{-1} for the MAO-A-F0850-4777 interaction, respectively. The binding affinity of F0850-4777 for MAO-A was approximately 3933.33-fold higher than that of the control inhibitor Harmine and RMSD value between best pose of Harmine and F0850-4777 was found to be 1.840 Å.

Analysis of the Interaction between MAO-B and F0850-4777

An insight into the interaction between MAO-B and F0850-4777 along with the control inhibitor (Sulfinamide) confirmed that both the ligands occupied a similar pose inside the binding cavity of MAO-B (Figure 4A,B). The MAO-B-Sulfinamide complex was stabilized by two conventional hydrogen bonds (Lig:H-Leu171:O, and Lig:H-Gln206:OE1). In addition, Sulfinamide formed two Pi-Sigma hydrophobic interactions with Leu171:CD2, and Tyr398 along with one Pi-Pi T-shaped interaction with Tyr326, and two Pi-alkyl interactions with Ile199 and Ile316. In addition, there was one Pi-Sulfur interaction with Cys172:SG. Furthermore, the MAO-B and Sulfinamide complex was stabilized by ten van der Waals' interactions with Tyr60, Pro104, Trp119, Leu164, Leu167, Phe168, Ile198, Gly205, Phe343, and Tyr435 (Figure 4C). Conversely, the MAO-B and F0850-4777 complex was stabilized by one conventional hydrogen bond with Tyr435, and two carbon hydrogen bonds with Tyr60, and Gly434 (Figure 4D and Table S4). In addition, F0850-4777 formed two Pi-Sigma hydrophobic interactions (with Leu171:CD2 and Ile199:CA), two Pi-Pi-stacked interactions with Tyr398, one Pi-Pi T-shaped interaction with Tyr326, two Pi-Pi stacked interactions with Tyr398, one Pi-alkyl interaction with Tyr326, and two alkyl interactions with Leu171 and Ile199. Moreover, F0850-4777 also formed three Pi-Sulfur interactions with Cys172:SG, Cys397:SG, and Met436:SD residues. Several amino acid residues, such as Arg42, Gly58, Ser59, Phe168, Ile198, Gln206, Phe343, and Glu437, were found to form van der Waals' interactions. Interestingly, the amino acid residues of MAO-B commonly engaged in the interaction with F0850-4777 as well as Sulfinamide were Tyr60, Phe168, Leu171, Cys172, Ile198, Ile199, Gln206, Tyr326, Phe343, Tyr398, and Tyr435. Moreover, the docking energy and the corresponding binding affinity were estimated to be -9.5 kcal mol^{-1} and 9.28×10^6 M^{-1} for the MAO-B-Sulfinamide interaction, respectively, and -12.5 kcal mol^{-1} and 1.47×10^9 M^{-1} for the MAO-B-F0850-4777 interaction, respectively. We found that the binding affinity of F0850-4777 for MAO-B was approximately 158.41-fold higher than the control inhibitor Sulfinamide and RMSD value between best pose of Sulfinamide and F0850-4777 was found to be 2.880 Å.

2.4. Analysis of Molecular Dynamics Simulation

2.4.1. Root Mean Square Deviation (RMSD) Analysis

In molecular dynamics simulations, the measurement of RMSD provides an estimate of the stability and dynamic nature of the protein–ligand complex. RMSD is measured as the deviation in the structure of a protein or protein–ligand complex from its initial pose, which eventually gives an insight into the stability of protein–ligand complex during simulation. Here, we report the behavior of RMSD of AChE, BChE, MAO-A, and MAO-B alone or in complex with F0850-4777 during molecular dynamics simulation under physiological conditions (Figure 5). The RMSD of AChE and BChE in the absence of F0850-4777 increased sharply for the initial 2 ns, and then stayed consistent for the rest of simulation, while the RMSDs of AChE-F0850-4777 and BChE-F0850-4777 complexes fluctuated within the acceptable limits throughout the simulation (Figure 5A,B). Moreover, the RMSD of MAO-A and MAO-B in the absence of F0850-4777 fluctuated slightly during 0–15 ns, and thereafter remained constant for the remaining simulation time, while the RMSDs of MAO-A and MAO-B in the presence of F0850-4777 followed a consistent path throughout the simulation (Figure 5C,D). The average RMSD values of AChE, BChE, MAO-A, and MAO-B in the absence and presence of F0850-4777 estimated during 20–100 ns were 2.33 ± 0.16 Å, 2.08 ± 0.12 Å, 1.70 ± 0.09 Å, 1.98 ± 0.10 Å, 2.15 ± 0.11 Å, 2.06 ± 0.07 Å, 5.81 ± 0.34 Å, and 5.33 ± 0.41 Å, respectively. It is worth noting that none of the fluctuations in RMSD were more than the acceptable limit of 2.0 Å. These results suggest that the overall structures of target enzymes (AChE, BChE, MAO-A, and MAO-B) did not change significantly due to the binding of F0850-4777, and the protein–ligand complexes remained stable throughout the simulation.

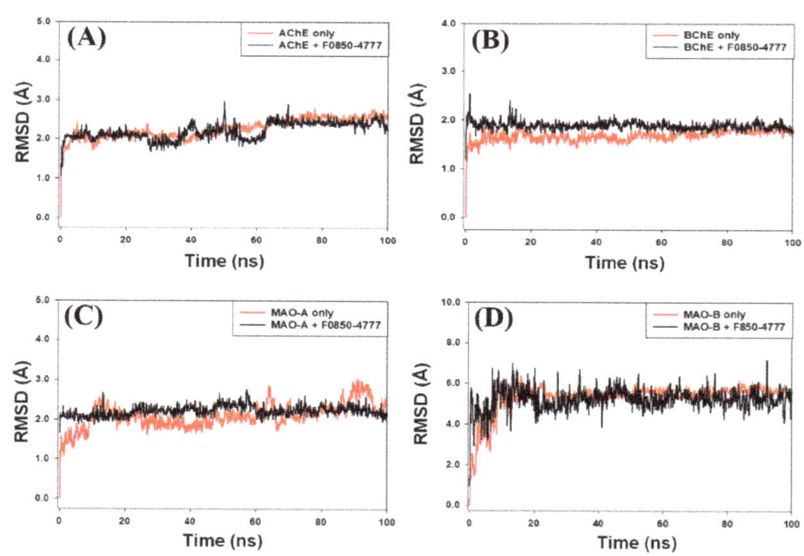

Figure 5. Behavior of root mean square deviation (RMSD) of (**A**) AChE, (**B**) BChE, (**C**) MAO-A, and (**D**) MAO-B alone or in complex with F0850-4777.

2.4.2. Root Mean Square Fluctuation (RMSF) Analysis

During molecular dynamics simulation, the measurement of protein RMSF is significant to access the local conformational changes in the side chains of a protein occurred due to ligand binding. In this study, we monitored the RMSF of F0850-4777 bound with AChE, BChE, MAO-A, and MAO-B (Figure 6A). It is generally observed that the residues at the N and C-terminal or loop regions display higher fluctuations. The average RMSF values of AChE, BChE, MAO-A, and MAO-B in the presence of F0850-4777 were 0.98 ± 0.06 Å, 0.79 ± 0.04 Å, 1.04 ± 0.09 Å, and 1.16 ± 0.11 Å, respectively. These results indicate that the RMSF of AChE, BChE, MAO-A, and MAO-B did not deviate significantly in the presence of F0850-4777 and the average values remained within the acceptable limits, thereby indicating that the overall conformation of target proteins was conserved.

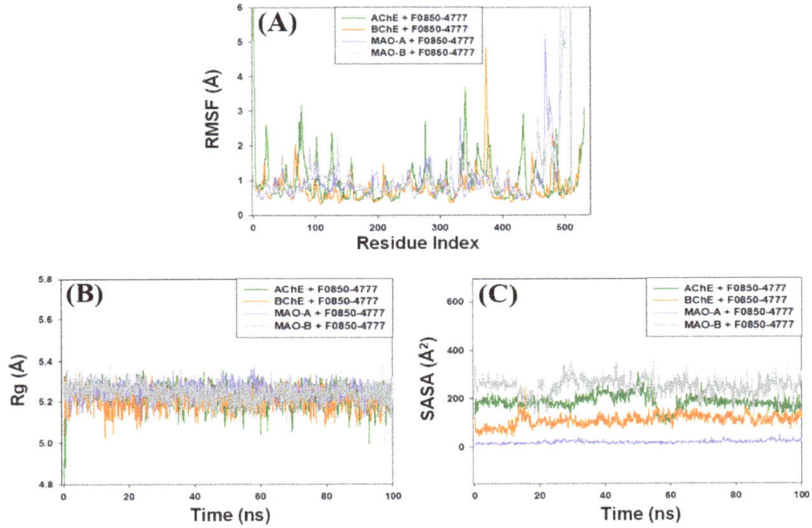

Figure 6. (**A**) Average root mean square fluctuation (RMSF) values of AChE, BChE, MAO-A, and MAO-B in the presence of F0850-4777; (**B**) the variation in Rg of F0850-4777 bound with different proteins (AChE, BChE, MAO-A, and MAO-B); (**C**) SASA of target proteins AChE, BChE, MAO-A, and MAO-B bound to F0850-4777.

2.4.3. Analysis of Radius of Gyration (Rg) and Solvent Accessible Surface Area (SASA)

The dependency of radius of gyration (Rg) and solvent accessible surface area (SASA) of a ligand on simulation time give information about the behavior of the ligand inside the binding pocket of the enzyme. The Rg values describe the RMSD of an atom's width from the common center of mass. The Rg may also be used to determine whether the complex remains folded during the MD simulation. The variation in Rg of F0850-4777 bound with different proteins (AChE, BChE, MAO-A, and MAO-B) as a function of simulation time is presented in Figure 6B. The results show that the Rg values of different protein–ligand systems fluctuated within the acceptable limit throughout the simulation. The average Rg values of AChE, BChE, MAO-A, and MAO-B bound with F0850-4777 were estimated as 5.23 ± 0.28 Å, 5.21 ± 0.24 Å, 5.25 ± 0.19 Å, and 5.24 ± 0.27 Å, respectively.

The solvent accessible surface area (SASA) measures the exposure of a protein to the solvent, thereby indicating if the protein is in native conformation upon the binding of a ligand. Here, we measured SASA of target proteins AChE, BChE, MAO-A, and MAO-B bound to F0850-4777 (Figure 6C). It is evident that the SASA of AChE-F0850-4777, BChE-F0850-4777, MAO-A-F0850-4777, and MAO-B-F0850-4777 complexes varied slightly with the acceptable limits. The average SASA values of F0850-4777 bound with AChE, BChE, MAO-A, and MAO-B were 185.4 ± 5.63 $Å^2$, 110.0 ± 4.39 $Å^2$, 19.6 ± 1.01 $Å^2$, and 250.7 ± 4.73 $Å^2$, respectively. These results suggest that F0850-4777 remained inside the binding cavity of AChE, BChE, MAO-A, and MAO-B in a stable conformation.

2.4.4. Secondary Structure Analysis

The interaction between a ligand and protein often leads to changes in the protein's secondary structural elements (SSE). Thus, evaluating the variation in SSE during simulation is critical to verify the establishment of a stable complex between the ligand and protein. In this study, we monitored the variation in the total SSE (α-helix + β-sheet) of AChE, BChE, MAO-A, and MAO-B in the presence of F0850-4777 during the simulation (Figure 7: Panel I). We found that the total SSE of AChE, BChE, MAO-A, and MAO-B in complex with F0850-4777 was 40.09 ± 2.62 % (α-helix: 26.92 ± 2.41 % and β-sheets: 13.17 ± 1.03 %), 38.71 ± 3.43 % (α-helix: 26.57 ± 2.76 % and β-sheets: 12.14 ± 2.04 %), 42.33 ± 3.12 % (α-helix: 25.81 ± 2.59 % and β-sheets: 16.52 ± 1.74 %), and 40.87 ± 2.63 % (α-helix: 25.94 ± 2.12 % and β-sheets: 14.93 ± 1.55 %), respectively. It is worth noting that the SSE of all the targeted proteins in combination with F0850-4777 remained consistent throughout the simulation, suggesting a stable interaction between proteins and ligand.

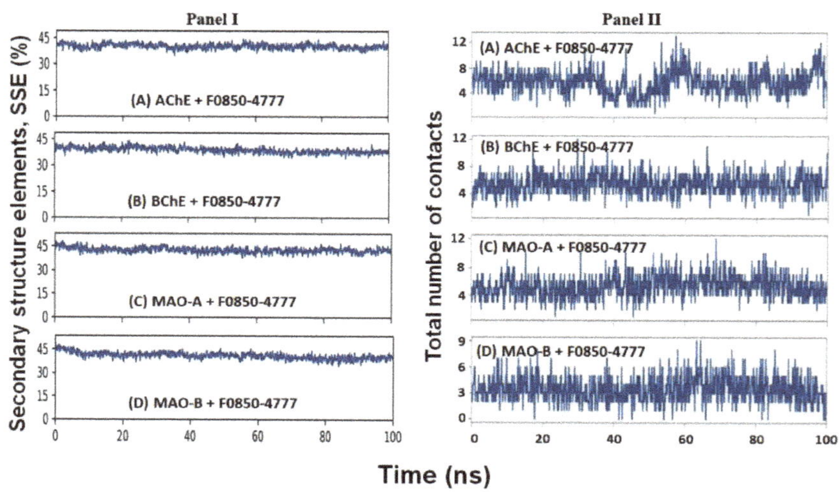

Figure 7. (Panel I) Variation in total secondary structural elements (α-helix + β-sheet) of AChE, BChE, MAO-A and MAO-B in the presence of F0850-4777 during simulation. (Panel II) Total number of contacts formed between F0850-4777 and (**A**) AChE, (**B**) BChE, (**C**) MAO-A, and (**D**) MAO-B during simulation.

2.4.5. Contact between F0850-4777 and Target Proteins

The formation of a stable protein and ligand complex was established by determining the total number of contacts formed between them during the simulation (Figure 7: Panel II). It is clear that during simulation, the total number of contacts between F0850-4777 and AChE, BChE, MAO-A, and MAO-B varied between 2–13, 2–13, 1–12, and 0–9, respectively. On average, AChE, BChE, MAO-A, and MAO-B formed 7, 6, 6, and 4 contacts with F0850-4777 respectively. These results confirmed that F0850-4777 remained in the binding pockets of target proteins throughout the simulation.

The overall interaction between target proteins and F0850-4777 over the simulation was also determined and represented in Figure 8. We found that the interaction between AChE and F0850-4777 through amino acid residues such as Tyr70, Asp72, Tyr121, Trp279, Phe290, Phe330, Phe331, and Tyr334 remained consistent throughout the MD simulation (Figure 8A). Similarly, the interaction between BChE and F0850-4777 through Met81, Trp82, Leu286, Phe329, Tyr332, and His438 remain intact during the MD simulation (Figure 8B). The amino acid residues of MAO-A forming a stable contact with F850-4777 during MD simulation were Tyr407, Tyr444, and Lys520 (Figure 8C). Furthermore, the interaction between MAO-B and F850-4777 through amino acid residues such as Leu171, Tyr188,

Ile198, Gln206, Lys296, Tyr326, Tyr398, and Tyr435 remain stable throughout the MD simulation (Figure 8D). Furthermore, the stability of ligand inside the binding pocket of their respective protein targets was evaluated by monitoring RMSF of the ligand, as shown in Figure S2. It was observed that none of the RMSF values exceeded 2 Å, confirming the stability of the protein–ligand complexes.

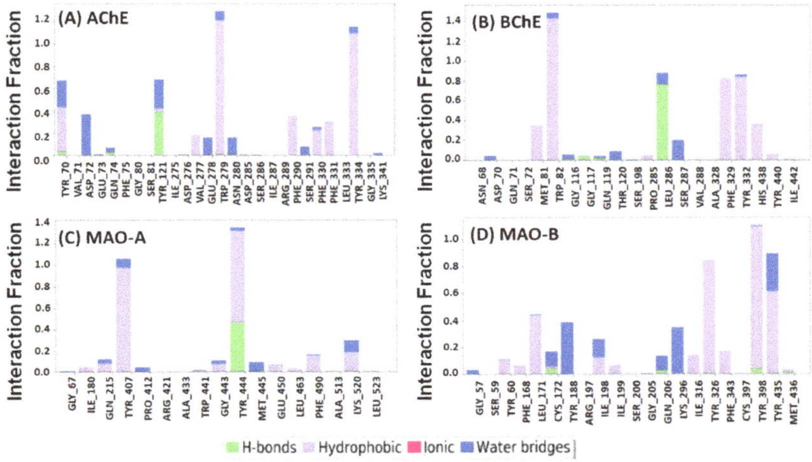

Figure 8. Interactions of F0850-4777 with (**A**) AChE, (**B**) BChE, (**C**) MAO-A, and (**D**) MAO-B.

2.4.6. Analysis of Free Energy (Prime-MM/GBSA) Calculations

Free energy calculation by Prime-MM/GBSA is an accurate method to evaluate protein–ligand stability in the presence of a solvent. In this study, the Prime-MM/GBSA of targeted proteins and F0850-4777 was calculated and the results are presented in Table 4. As evident from Table 4, AChE has the lowest ΔG_{Bind} energy (-30.35 ± 3.28 kcal mol^{-1}), followed by MAO-B (-29.38 ± 2.99 kcal mol^{-1}), BChE (-23.39 ± 3.07 kcal mol^{-1}), and MAO-A (-20.64 ± 2.93 kcal mol^{-1}). Principally, van der Waals' energy (ΔG_{vdW}) and non-polar solvation or lipophilic energy (ΔG_{Sol_Lipo}) contribute favorably towards the formation of a stable protein–ligand complex, while covalent ($\Delta G_{Covalent}$) and polar solvation energies (ΔG_{Solv} or ΔG_{SolGB}) oppose the formation of a stable protein–ligand complex.

Table 4. Free energy calculation of targeted proteins and F0850-4777 complexes using Prime/MM-GBSA.

Proteins	$\Delta G_{Coulomb}$	ΔE_{MM} ΔG_{vdW}	$\Delta G_{Covalent}$	ΔG_{Solv} or ΔG_{SolGB}	$\Delta G_{Self\text{-}contact}$	$\Delta G_{H\text{-}bond}$	ΔG_{SA} or ΔG_{Sol_Lipo}	$\Delta G_{Packing}$	ΔG or ΔG_{Bind}
AChE	1.25 ± 0.87	-19.24 ± 1.52	0.65 ± 0.05	6.18 ± 0.54	0	-0.16 ± 0.04	-15.81 ± 1.22	-3.22 ± 0.28	-30.35 ± 3.28
BChE	-0.54 ± 0.04	-20.17 ± 1.41	1.16 ± 0.06	9.65 ± 0.69	0	0	-13.49 ± 1.07	0	-23.39 ± 3.07
MAO-A	-6.14 ± 0.39	-17.21 ± 1.19	3.79 ± 0.06	12.71 ± 1.06	0	-1.20 ± 0.03	-11.65 ± 0.08	-0.94 ± 0.03	-20.64 ± 2.93
MAO-B	-3.97 ± 0.23	-17.80 ± 1.14	-0.05 ± 0.01	9.39 ± 0.57	0	−0.18 v	-16.28 ± 1.09	-0.49 ± 0.02	-29.38 ± 2.99

All the energies are in kcal mol^{-1}. ΔE_{MM}, $\Delta G_{Coulomb}$, ΔG_{vdW}, $\Delta G_{Covalent}$, ΔG_{Solv} or ΔG_{SolGB}, $\Delta G_{Self\text{-}contact}$, $\Delta G_{H\text{-}bond}$, ΔG_{SA} or ΔG_{Sol_Lipo}, and ΔG or ΔG_{Bind} stands for minimized molecular mechanics energy, coulomb energy, van der Waals' energy, covalent binding energy, solvation energy, energy due to self contact, energy due to H-bonds, lipophilic energy, and binding energy, respectively.

3. Materials and Methods

3.1. Hardware and Software Used

The three-dimensional coordinates of the target enzymes (AChE, BChE, MAO-A and MAO-B) were downloaded from the PDB database (http://www.rcsb.org/pdb/). PyRx-Python Prescription 0.8 [65] using Autodock-Vina [66] with the Lamarckian genetic algorithm as a scoring function was used for molecular docking. Molecular interactions for the best scoring ligand were separately analyzed by Discovery Studio 2020 (BIOVIA) software package. Molecular dynamics was performed on an Intel Xenon workstation-E3-1245-8C, 3.50 GHz processor with 28 GB RAM. The workstation was powered by a NVIDIA Quadro P5000 GPU card. Desmond (Shchrodinger-2020, LLC, NY, USA) was employed to conduct molecular dynamics simulation.

3.2. Ligands Preparation

The natural product-like compound library from Life Chemicals (www.lifechemicals.com) was screened to identify novel inhibitors of the targeted enzymes. The library contains 2029 compounds (accessed November 2020). The ligands were downloaded in sdf format and converted to Autodock suitable pdbqt format along with density function theory (DFT) optimization of the minimum energy conformer using the inbuilt function in PyRx. The energy of all the ligands was minimized in PyRx using universal force field (UFF).

3.3. Protein Target Preparation

The three-dimensional coordinates of AChE (PDB Id: 1ACJ), BChE (PDB Id: 4BDS), MAO-A (PDB Id: 2Z5X), and MAO-B (PDB Id: 2V5Z) were downloaded from the PDB database (http://www.rcsb.org/pdb/). The target proteins were prepared for molecular docking by native ligand and non-essential water molecules, assigning hydrogen polarities, calculating Gasteiger charges to protein structures, and converting protein structures from the pdb file format to pdbqt format. Energy minimization and geometry optimization of all structures were performed using a built-in tool in PyRx. Subsequently, the targeted proteins were exploited for the binding pockets from crystal structures and were further evaluated using the Uniprot.

3.4. Molecular Docking

Molecular docking was performed using the PyRx-Python 0.8 virtual screening tool coupled with AutoDock 4.2, employing the Lamarckian genetic algorithm method [67,68]. All of the ligands were individually docked with each of the targeted enzymes as separate docking runs. The grid dimensions for AChE were selected through discovery studio visualizer (BIOVIA) from the attributes of docked ligand (control inhibitor) in its specific target protein and set to 60 × 60 × 60 Å centered at 4.6 × 70.1 × 65.9 Å, whereas grid dimensions for BChE, MAO-A, and MAO-B were set to 33 × 33 × 33 Å centered at 140.1 × 122.2 × 38.9 Å, 126 × 126 × 126 Å centered at 30.9 × 28.8 × 14.9 Å, and 126 × 126 × 126 Å centered at 53.5 × 147.8 × 24.4 Å, respectively, as discussed in previous reports [69,70]. The results were clustered according to the root-mean-square deviation (RMSD) criterion and in the current study we selected the ligands with lower than 3Å RMSD modes between the best docked pose of natural product-like compound and reference inhibitor. The docking was performed with the "exhaustiveness" set to 8. All other docking parameters were set to the default values of the software. The binding affinity (K_d) of ligands for the target enzyme was calculated from the binding energy (ΔG) using the following relation [71,72]:

$$\Delta G = -RT \ln K_d \quad (1)$$

where R and T were the Boltzmann's gas constant and temperature respectfully.

The ligands with the minimum binding energy were selected for further analysis. The best pose of each "protein–ligand complex" was generated and analyzed using Discovery Studio 2020 (BIOVIA).

3.5. Prediction of Physicochemical, Pharmacokinetics Properties, Drug-Likeness, and Toxicity Potentials

About the 10 top best hits from the total 2029 compounds were analyzed against cholinesterases and monoamine oxidases were assessed for their physicochemical properties, drug-likeness, and pharmacokinetics using the SwissADME (http://www.swissadme.ch)

web-based tool. The tool was used to assess the molecular weight, the number of hydrogen bond donors and acceptors, rotatable bonds, cLogP value, topological polar surface area, Lipinski's rule violation, human gastrointestinal absorption (HIA), and blood–brain barrier (BBB) permeation to finalize the bioactive compound for further computational analysis [33]. The fraction of sp^3 carbon atoms (Fsp^3), a key factor for drug-likeness, was also analyzed through SwissADME [73]. Moreover, various aspects and effects of the toxicity, including the tumorigenicity, mutagenicity, and irritability of the selected compounds, were also tested using the Orisis Datawarrior tool [74]. In the Orisis Datawarrior tool's analysis, the predicted toxicity values were depended on comparing the precalculated investigated molecules with the tested molecule's structures.

3.6. Molecular Dynamics (MD) Simulation

MD simulation of the best scoring ligand was performed in complex with their respective targeted enzymes (AChE, BChE, MAO-A, and MAO-B) in triplicates using "Desmond (Schrodinger-2020, LLC, NY, USA)" as described earlier [26,75]. The protein–ligand complex obtained in the AutoDock Vina is imported to the Maestro interface of the Schrodinger's software. Prior to MD simulation, the protein–ligand complex was optimized by adding missing hydrogen atoms, assigning proper protonation state of the ligand and other parameters using Protein preparation wizard. The protein–ligand complex was placed at the center of an orthorhombic box, keeping a distance of at least 10 Å from the sides of the box. TIP3P water molecules were added to solvate the simulation box, and proper counterions were also added to neutralize the system. The physiological conditions were mimicked by adding 150 mM NaCl. The energy of the whole system was minimized with 2000 iteration and convergence criteria of 1 kcal/mol/Å, using OPLS3e forcefield. The production MD simulation run was performed for 100 ns employing NPT ensemble at 298 K and 1 bar. Temperature and pressure were maintained with the help of Nose-Hoover Chain thermostat and Matrtyna–Tobias–Klein barostate [76,77]. A 2 fs time step was fixed, and at every 10 ps, energies and structures were documented in the trajectory. The parameters such as root mean square deviation (RMSD), root mean square fluctuation (RMSF), radius of gyration (Rg), solvent accessible surface area (SASA), secondary structure analysis, and protein–ligand interactions were analyzed to establish the stability of protein–ligand complexes. The results are presented as mean $\pm$ standard deviation of the three independent experiments.

3.7. Free Energy (Prime-MM/GBSA) Calculations

The binding free energy of each protein–ligand complex was estimated using Prime module (Schrodinger, LLC, NY, USA) employing the MM-GBSA approach, as described previously [75,78]. In this approach, free energy was computed on the final 10 ns MD simulation trajectories, once equilibration had been reached. Briefly, first, the docked complexes were subjected to local optimization through molecular mechanics (MM) in Prime, and then their energies were minimized with OPLS-AA (2005) force field with the generalized Born surface area (GBSA) continuum solvent model. The binding free energy (ΔG_{Bind}) is estimated as:

$$\Delta G_{Bind} = \Delta E_{MM} + \Delta G_{Solv\_GB} + \Delta G_{SA} \tag{2}$$

$$\Delta E_{MM} = E_{Complex} - \left(E_{Protein} + E_{Ligand}\right) \tag{3}$$

where $E_{Complex}$, $E_{Protein}$, and E_{Ligand} are the respective values of minimized energies of protein–ligand complex, protein, and ligand.

$$\Delta G_{Solv\_GB} = G_{Solv\_GB\ (Complex)} - \left(G_{Solv\_GB\ (Protein)} + G_{Solv\_GB\ (Ligand)}\right) \tag{4}$$

where $G_{Solv\_GB\ (Complex)}$, $G_{Solv\_GB\ (Protein)}$, and $G_{Solv\_GB\ (Ligand)}$ are the respective values of free energies of solvation of protein–ligand complex, protein, and ligand.

$$\Delta G_{SA} = G_{SA\ (Complex)} - \left(G_{SA\ (Protein)} - G_{SA(Ligand)}\right) \quad (5)$$

where $G_{SA\ (Complex)}$, $G_{SA\ (Protein)}$, and $G_{SA\ (Ligand)}$ are the respective values of surface area energies of protein–ligand complex, protein, and ligand.

In the Prime-MM/GBSA method, the free energy is calculated as:

$$\Delta G_{Bind} = \Delta G_{Coulomb} + \Delta G_{vdW} + \Delta G_{Covalent} + \Delta G_{H-bond} + \Delta G_{Sol\_Lipo} + \Delta G_{Solv\_GB} + \Delta G_{Packing} + \Delta G_{Self-contact} \quad (6)$$

4. Conclusions

Using high-throughput screening and the molecular dynamics simulation study, we concluded that the F0850-4777 compound, out of 2029 natural product-like compounds, showed the best binding affinity against all the four targets and exhibited the finest drug-likeness, pharmacokinetics and physiological properties which can cross the BBB as well as high absorption through GI tract with non-toxic potential. The findings of this study suggest that the F0850-4777 can be a potential candidate against multiple-targets of two pathophysiological pathways pertaining to AD. In this study, neuroprotective potentials of candidate drug were explored only via in silico approaches and open the window for confirmation of its therapeutic efficacy through in vitro and in vivo systems.

Supplementary Materials: The following are available online at https://www.mdpi.com/article/10.3390/ph14090937/s1, Table S1: Molecular docking parameters for the interaction of target protein, acetylcholinesterase with F0850-4777 and their respective control ligands; Table S2: Molecular docking parameters for the interaction of target protein, butyrylcholinesterase with F0850-4777 and their respective control ligands; Table S3: Molecular docking parameters for the interaction of target protein, monoamine oxidase-A with F0850-4777 and their respective control ligands; Table S4: Molecular docking parameters for the interaction of target protein, monoamine oxidase-B with F0850-4777 and their respective control ligands; Figure S1: (A) structure of F0850-4777 (3-(2-methoxyphenyl)-4-oxo-4H-chromen-7-yl 4-methylbenzoate), (B) acceptable range (pink color region) for pharmacokinetics properties of F0850-4777, (C) description of BOILED-Egg image for F0850-4777 to predict gastrointestinal absorption (HIA) and brain penetration (BBB); Figure S2. RMSF of ligand (F0850-4777) inside the binding pocket of their respective protein targets.

Author Contributions: Conceptualization, D.I. and M.T.R.; methodology, M.T.R. and S.M.D.R.; software, M.F.A.A.; validation, M.T.R. and A.B.D.; formal analysis, D.I. and B.M.A.; investigation, M.T.R.; resources, D.I.; data curation, M.F.A.A.; writing—original draft preparation, D.I. and M.T.R.; writing—review and editing, D.I., M.T.R., M.F.A.A. and M.S.K.; visualization, S.B., M.A. and W.A.; supervision, D.I.; project administration, D.I.; funding acquisition, D.I. and B.M.A. All authors have read and agreed to the published version of the manuscript.

Funding: This research was funded by deputyship for Research & lnnovation, Ministry of Education in Saudi Arabia, grant number lFP-2020-32.

Institutional Review Board Statement: Not applicable.

Informed Consent Statement: Not applicable.

Data Availability Statement: Not applicable.

Acknowledgments: We are thankful to the deputyship for Research & lnnovation, Ministry of Education in Saudi Arabia for funding this research work through grant number lFP-2020-32.

Conflicts of Interest: The authors declare no conflict of interest. The funders had no role in the design of the study; in the collection, analyses, or interpretation of data; in the writing of the manuscript, or in the decision to publish the results.

References

1. Kim, B.; Noh, G.O.; Kim, K. Behavioural and Psychological Symptoms of Dementia in Patients with Alzheimer's Disease and Family Caregiver Burden: A Path Analysis. *BMC Geriatr.* **2021**, *21*, 160. [CrossRef]
2. Dementia. Available online: https://www.who.int/news-room/fact-sheets/detail/dementia (accessed on 18 August 2021).

3. The Top 10 Causes of Death. Available online: https://www.who.int/news-room/fact-sheets/detail/the-top-10-causes-of-death (accessed on 18 August 2021).
4. Health Days 2020—World Alzheimer's Day. Available online: https://www.moh.gov.sa/en/HealthAwareness/healthDay/2020/Pages/HealthDay-2020-09-21.aspx (accessed on 18 August 2021).
5. Abeysinghe, A.A.D.T.; Deshapriya, R.D.U.S.; Udawatte, C. Alzheimer's Disease: A Review of the Pathophysiological Basis and Therapeutic Interventions. *Life Sci.* **2020**, *256*, 117996. [CrossRef]
6. Sayeed Ahmad, S.; Akhtar, S.; Mohammad Sajid Jamal, Q.; Mohd Danish Rizvi, S.A.; Kamal, M.; Kalim, A.; Khan, M.; Haris Siddiqui, M. Multiple Targets for the Management of Alzheimer's Disease. *CNS Neurol. Disord.—Drug Targets—CNS Neurol. Disord.* **2016**, *15*, 1279–1289. [CrossRef] [PubMed]
7. Calabrò, M.; Rinaldi, C.; Santoro, G.; Crisafulli, C. The Biological Pathways of Alzheimer Disease: A Review. *AIMS Neurosci.* **2020**, *8*, 86–132. [CrossRef] [PubMed]
8. Turner, P.R.; O'Connor, K.; Tate, W.P.; Abraham, W.C. Roles of Amyloid Precursor Protein and Its Fragments in Regulating Neural Activity, Plasticity and Memory. *Prog. Neurobiol.* **2003**, *70*, 1–32. [CrossRef]
9. Reid, G.A.; Chilukuri, N.; Darvesh, S. Butyrylcholinesterase and the Cholinergic System. *Neuroscience* **2013**, *234*, 53–68. [CrossRef] [PubMed]
10. Song, K.; Li, Y.; Zhang, H.; An, N.; Wei, Y.; Wang, L.; Tian, C.; Yuan, M.; Sun, Y.; Xing, Y.; et al. Oxidative Stress-Mediated Blood-Brain Barrier (BBB) Disruption in Neurological Diseases. *Oxid. Med. Cell. Longev.* **2020**, *2020*, e4356386. [CrossRef]
11. Whitehouse, P.J.; Price, D.L.; Clark, A.W.; Coyle, J.T.; DeLong, M.R. Alzheimer Disease: Evidence for Selective Loss of Cholinergic Neurons in the Nucleus Basalis. *Ann. Neurol.* **1981**, *10*, 122–126. [CrossRef]
12. Goedert, M.; Spillantini, M.G.; Crowther, R.A. Tau Proteins and neurofibrillary Degeneration. *Brain Pathol. Zur. Switz.* **1991**, *1*, 279–286. [CrossRef]
13. Strolin Benedetti, M.; Dostert, P. Monoamine oxidase, Brain Ageing and Degenerative Diseases. *Biochem. Pharmacol.* **1989**, *38*, 555–561. [CrossRef]
14. Rosenberg, P.B.; Nowrangi, M.A.; Lyketsos, C.G. Neuropsychiatric Symptoms in Alzheimer's Disease: What Might be Associated Brain Circuits? *Mol. Asp. Med.* **2015**, *43–44*, 25–37. [CrossRef]
15. Dou, K.-X.; Tan, M.-S.; Tan, C.-C.; Cao, X.-P.; Hou, X.-H.; Guo, Q.-H.; Tan, L.; Mok, V.; Yu, J.-T. Comparative Safety and Effectiveness of Cholinesterase Inhibitors and Memantine for Alzheimer's Disease: A Network Meta-Analysis of 41 Randomized Controlled Trials. *Alzheimers Res. Ther.* **2018**, *10*, 126. [CrossRef]
16. Huang, L.-K.; Chao, S.-P.; Hu, C.-J. Clinical Trials of New Drugs for Alzheimer Disease. *J. Biomed. Sci.* **2020**, *27*, 18. [CrossRef] [PubMed]
17. Benek, O.; Korabecny, J.; Soukup, O. A Perspective on Multi-Target Drugs for Alzheimer's Disease. *Trends Pharmacol. Sci.* **2020**, *41*, 434–445. [CrossRef]
18. Grewal, A.S.; Singh, S.; Sharma, N.; Grover, R. In Silico Docking Studies of Some Flavonoids Against Multiple Targets of Alzheimer's Disease. *Plant Arch.* **2020**, *20*, 3271–3278.
19. Khatoon, A.; Khan, F.; Ahmad, N.; Shaikh, S.; Rizvi, S.M.D.; Shakil, S.; Al-Qahtani, M.H.; Abuzenadah, A.M.; Tabrez, S.; Ahmed, A.B.F.; et al. Silver Nanoparticles from Leaf Extract of *Mentha piperita*: Eco-Friendly Synthesis and Effect on Acetylcholinesterase Activity. *Life Sci.* **2018**, *209*, 430–434. [CrossRef]
20. Maramai, S.; Benchekroun, M.; Gabr, M.T.; Yahiaoui, S. Multitarget Therapeutic Strategies for Alzheimer's Disease: Review on Emerging Target Combinations. *BioMed Res. Int.* **2020**, *2020*, e5120230. [CrossRef]
21. Shamsi, A.; Anwar, S.; Mohammad, T.; Alajmi, M.F.; Hussain, A.; Rehman, M.d.T.; Hasan, G.M.; Islam, A.; Hassan, M.d.I. MARK4 Inhibited by AChE Inhibitors, Donepezil and Rivastigmine Tartrate: Insights into Alzheimer's Disease Therapy. *Biomolecules* **2020**, *10*, 789. [CrossRef]
22. Ahmad, S.S.; Khan, H.; Danish Rizvi, S.M.; Ansari, S.A.; Ullah, R.; Rastrelli, L.; Mahmood, H.M.; Siddiqui, M.H. Computational Study of Natural Compounds for the Clearance of Amyloid-Beta: A Potential Therapeutic Management Strategy for Alzheimer's Disease. *Molecules* **2019**, *24*, 3233. [CrossRef] [PubMed]
23. Alvi, S.S.; Iqbal, D.; Ahmad, S.; Khan, M.S. Molecular Rationale Delineating the Role of Lycopene as a Potent HMG-CoA Reductase Inhibitor: In Vitro and In Silico Study. *Nat. Prod. Res.* **2016**, *30*, 2111–2114. [CrossRef]
24. Iqbal, D.; Khan, M.S.; Khan, M.S.; Ahmad, S.; Srivastava, A.K. An In Vitro and Molecular Informatics Study to Evaluate the Antioxidative and β-hydroxy-β-methylglutaryl-CoA Reductase Inhibitory Property of Ficus Virens Ait. *Phytother. Res. PTR* **2014**, *28*, 899–908. [CrossRef]
25. Jabir, N.R.; Shakil, S.; Tabrez, S.; Khan, M.S.; Rehman, M.T.; Ahmed, B.A. In Silico Screening of Glycogen Synthase kinase-3β Targeted Ligands against Acetylcholinesterase and Its Probable Relevance to Alzheimer's Disease. *J. Biomol. Struct. Dyn.* **2021**, *39*, 5083–5092. [CrossRef]
26. Rehman, M.T.; AlAjmi, M.F.; Hussain, A.; Rather, G.M.; Khan, M.A. High-Throughput Virtual Screening, Molecular Dynamics Simulation, and Enzyme Kinetics Identified ZINC84525623 as a Potential Inhibitor of NDM-1. *Int. J. Mol. Sci.* **2019**, *20*, 819. [CrossRef]
27. Shamsi, A.; Mohammad, T.; Khan, M.S.; Shahwan, M.; Husain, F.M.; Rehman, M.T.; Hassan, M.I.; Ahmad, F.; Islam, A. Unraveling Binding Mechanism of Alzheimer's Drug Rivastigmine Tartrate with Human Transferrin: Molecular Docking and Multi-Spectroscopic Approach towards Neurodegenerative Diseases. *Biomolecules* **2019**, *9*, 495. [CrossRef] [PubMed]

28. Atanasov, A.G.; Zotchev, S.B.; Dirsch, V.M.; Supuran, C.T. Natural Products in Drug Discovery: Advances and Opportunities. *Nat. Rev. Drug Discov.* **2021**, *20*, 200–216. [CrossRef]
29. Ramsay, R.R.; Popovic-Nikolic, M.R.; Nikolic, K.; Uliassi, E.; Bolognesi, M.L. A perspective on multi-target drug discovery and design for complex diseases. *Clin. Transl. Med.* **2018**, *7*, 3. [CrossRef]
30. Talevi, A. Multi-target pharmacology: Possibilities and limitations of the "skeleton key approach" from a medicinal chemist perspective. *Front. Pharmacol.* **2015**, *6*, 205. [CrossRef]
31. DiMasi, J.A.; Hansen, R.W.; Grabowski, H.G. The price of innovation: New estimates of drug development costs. *J. Health Econ.* **2003**, *22*, 151–185. [CrossRef]
32. Walters, W.P.; Stahl, M.T.; Murcko, M.A. Virtual screening—An overview. *Drug Discov. Today* **1998**, *4*, 160–178. [CrossRef]
33. Daina, A.; Michielin, O.; Zoete, V. SwissADME: A free web tool to evaluate pharmacokinetics, drug-likeness and medicinal chemistry friendliness of small molecules. *Sci. Rep.* **2017**, *7*, 42717. [CrossRef]
34. Muñoz-Muriedas, J.; Lopez, J.M.; Orozco, M.; Luque, F.J. Molecular modelling approaches to the design of acetylcholinesterase inhibitors: New challenges for the treatment of Alzheimer's disease. *Curr. Pharm. Des.* **2004**, *10*, 3131–3140. [CrossRef]
35. Crismon, M.L. Tacrine: First drug approved for Alzheimer's disease. *Ann. Pharmacother.* **1994**, *28*, 744–751. [CrossRef]
36. Sussman, J.L.; Harel, M.; Frolow, F.; Oefner, C.; Goldman, A.; Toker, L.; Silman, I. Atomic structure of acetylcholinesterase from Torpedo californica: A prototypic acetylcholine-binding protein. *Science* **1991**, *253*, 872–879. [CrossRef] [PubMed]
37. Barak, D.; Kronman, C.; Ordentlich, A.; Ariel, N.; Bromberg, A.; Marcus, D.; Lazar, A.; Velan, B.; Shafferman, A. Acetylcholinesterase peripheral anionic site degeneracy conferred by amino acid arrays sharing a common core. *J. Biol. Chem.* **1994**, *269*, 6296–6305. [CrossRef]
38. Inestrosa, N.C.; Alvarez, A.; Pérez, C.A.; Moreno, R.D.; Vicente, M.; Linker, C.; Casanueva, O.I.; Soto, C.; Garrido, J. Acetylcholinesterase accelerates assembly of amyloid-beta-peptides into Alzheimer's fibrils: Possible role of the peripheral site of the enzyme. *Neuron* **1996**, *16*, 881–891. [CrossRef]
39. Inestrosa, N.C.; Dinamarca, M.C.; Alvarez, A. Amyloid-cholinesterase interactions. Implications for Alzheimer's disease. *FEBS J.* **2008**, *275*, 625–632. [CrossRef]
40. Alles, G.A.; Hawes, R.C. Cholinesterases in the Blood of Man. *J. Biol. Chem.* **1940**, *133*, 375–390. [CrossRef]
41. Mendel, B.; Rudney, H. On the Type of Cholinesterase Present in Brain Tissue. *Science* **1943**, *98*, 201–202. [CrossRef]
42. Darvesh, S.; Grantham, D.L.; Hopkins, D.A. Distribution of butyrylcholinesterase in the human amygdala and hippocampal formation. *J. Comp. Neurol.* **1998**, *393*, 374–390. [CrossRef]
43. Tago, H.; Maeda, T.; McGeer, P.L.; Kimura, H. Butyrylcholinesterase-rich neurons in rat brain demonstrated by a sensitive histochemical method. *J. Comp. Neurol.* **1992**, *325*, 301–312. [CrossRef] [PubMed]
44. Mesulam, M.-M.; Guillozet, A.; Shaw, P.; Levey, A.; Duysen, E.G.; Lockridge, O. Acetylcholinesterase knockouts establish central cholinergic pathways and can use butyrylcholinesterase to hydrolyze acetylcholine. *Neuroscience* **2002**, *110*, 627–639. [CrossRef]
45. Layer, P.G. Cholinesterases during development of the avian nervous system. *Cell. Mol. Neurobiol.* **1991**, *11*, 7–33. [CrossRef]
46. Dubovy, P.; Haninec, P. Non-specific cholinesterase activity of the developing peripheral nerves and its possible function in cells in intimate contact with growing axons of chick embryo. *Int. J. Dev. Neurosci. Off. J. Int. Soc. Dev. Neurosci.* **1990**, *8*, 589–602. [CrossRef]
47. Geula, C.; Mesulam, M. Special properties of cholinesterases in the cerebral cortex of Alzheimer's disease. *Brain Res.* **1989**, *498*, 185–189. [CrossRef]
48. Geula, C.; Mesulam, M.M. Cholinesterases and the pathology of Alzheimer disease. *Alzheimer Dis. Assoc. Disord.* **1995**, *9* (Suppl. 2), 23–28. [CrossRef]
49. Arendt, T.; Brückner, M.K.; Lange, M.; Bigl, V. Changes in acetylcholinesterase and butyrylcholinesterase in Alzheimer's disease resemble embryonic development—A study of molecular forms. *Neurochem. Int.* **1992**, *21*, 381–396. [CrossRef]
50. Wright, C.I.; Geula, C.; Mesulam, M.M. Neurological cholinesterases in the normal brain and in Alzheimer's disease: Relationship to plaques, tangles, and patterns of selective vulnerability. *Ann. Neurol.* **1993**, *34*, 373–384. [CrossRef]
51. Lockridge, O.; Bartels, C.F.; Vaughan, T.A.; Wong, C.K.; Norton, S.E.; Johnson, L.L. Complete amino acid sequence of human serum cholinesterase. *J. Biol. Chem.* **1987**, *262*, 549–557. [CrossRef]
52. Vellom, D.C.; Radić, Z.; Li, Y.; Pickering, N.A.; Camp, S.; Taylor, P. Amino acid residues controlling acetylcholinesterase and butyrylcholinesterase specificity. *Biochemistry* **1993**, *32*, 12–17. [CrossRef]
53. Masson, P.; Xie, W.; Froment, M.T.; Levitsky, V.; Fortier, P.L.; Albaret, C.; Lockridge, O. Interaction between the peripheral site residues of human butyrylcholinesterase, D70 and Y332, in binding and hydrolysis of substrates. *Biochim. Biophys. Acta* **1999**, *1433*, 281–293. [CrossRef]
54. Edmondson, D.E.; Bhattacharyya, A.K.; Walker, M.C. Spectral and kinetic studies of imine product formation in the oxidation of p-(N,N-dimethylamino)benzylamine analogues by monoamine oxidase B. *Biochemistry* **1993**, *32*, 5196–5202. [CrossRef] [PubMed]
55. Fowler, C.J.; Benedetti, M.S. The metabolism of dopamine by both forms of monoamine oxidase in the rat brain and its inhibition by cimoxatone. *J. Neurochem.* **1983**, *40*, 1534–1541. [CrossRef] [PubMed]
56. Hall, D.W.; Logan, B.W.; Parsons, G.H. Further studies on the inhibition of monoamine oxidase by M and B 9302 (clorgyline). I. Substrate specificity in various mammalian species. *Biochem. Pharmacol.* **1969**, *18*, 1447–1454. [CrossRef]
57. Chiba, K.; Trevor, A.; Castagnoli, N. Metabolism of the neurotoxic tertiary amine, MPTP, by brain monoamine oxidase. *Biochem. Biophys. Res. Commun.* **1984**, *120*, 574–578. [CrossRef]

58. Ma, J.; Yoshimura, M.; Yamashita, E.; Nakagawa, A.; Ito, A.; Tsukihara, T. Structure of rat monoamine oxidase A and its specific recognitions for substrates and inhibitors. *J. Mol. Biol.* **2004**, *338*, 103–114. [CrossRef]
59. Binda, C.; Newton-Vinson, P.; Hubálek, F.; Edmondson, D.E.; Mattevi, A. Structure of human monoamine oxidase B, a drug target for the treatment of neurological disorders. *Nat. Struct. Biol.* **2002**, *9*, 22–26. [CrossRef]
60. Binda, C.; Li, M.; Hubalek, F.; Restelli, N.; Edmondson, D.E.; Mattevi, A. Insights into the mode of inhibition of human mitochondrial monoamine oxidase B from high-resolution crystal structures. *Proc. Natl. Acad. Sci. USA* **2003**, *100*, 9750–9755. [CrossRef]
61. Nandigama, R.K.; Miller, J.R.; Edmondson, D.E. Loss of serotonin oxidation as a component of the altered substrate specificity in the Y444F mutant of recombinant human liver MAO A. *Biochemistry* **2001**, *40*, 14839–14846. [CrossRef]
62. Geha, R.M.; Chen, K.; Wouters, J.; Ooms, F.; Shih, J.C. Analysis of Conserved Active Site Residues in Monoamine Oxidase A and B and Their Three-dimensional Molecular Modeling. *J. Biol. Chem.* **2002**, *277*, 17209–17216. [CrossRef]
63. Li, M.; Binda, C.; Mattevi, A.; Edmondson, D.E. Functional role of the "aromatic cage" in human monoamine oxidase B: Structures and catalytic properties of Tyr435 mutant proteins. *Biochemistry* **2006**, *45*, 4775–4784. [CrossRef]
64. Son, S.-Y.; Ma, J.; Kondou, Y.; Yoshimura, M.; Yamashita, E.; Tsukihara, T. Structure of human monoamine oxidase A at 2.2-A resolution: The control of opening the entry for substrates/inhibitors. *Proc. Natl. Acad. Sci. USA* **2008**, *105*, 5739–5744. [CrossRef]
65. Nastasă, C.; Tamaian, R.; Oniga, O.; Tiperciuc, B. 5-Arylidene(chromenyl-methylene)-thiazolidinediones: Potential New Agents against Mutant Oncoproteins K-Ras, N-Ras and B-Raf in Colorectal Cancer and Melanoma. *Med. Kaunas Lith.* **2019**, *55*, 85. [CrossRef]
66. Trott, O.; Olson, A.J. AutoDock Vina: Improving the speed and accuracy of docking with a new scoring function, efficient optimization and multithreading. *J. Comput. Chem.* **2010**, *31*, 455–461. [CrossRef]
67. Rizvi, S.M.D.; Shaikh, S.; Naaz, D.; Shakil, S.; Ahmad, A.; Haneef, M.; Abuzenadah, A.M. Kinetics and Molecular Docking Study of an Anti-diabetic Drug Glimepiride as Acetylcholinesterase Inhibitor: Implication for Alzheimer's Disease-Diabetes Dual Therapy. *Neurochem. Res.* **2016**, *41*, 1475–1482. [CrossRef]
68. Shaker, B.; Yu, M.-S.; Lee, J.; Lee, Y.; Jung, C.; Na, D. User guide for the discovery of potential drugs via protein structure prediction and ligand docking simulation. *J. Microbiol. Seoul Korea* **2020**, *58*, 235–244. [CrossRef]
69. Svobodova, B.; Mezeiova, E.; Hepnarova, V.; Hrabinova, M.; Muckova, L.; Kobrlova, T.; Jun, D.; Soukup, O.; Jimeno, M.L.; Marco-Contelles, J.; et al. Exploring Structure-Activity Relationship in Tacrine-Squaramide Derivatives as Potent Cholinesterase Inhibitors. *Biomolecules* **2019**, *9*, 379. [CrossRef]
70. Jung, H.A.; Roy, A.; Choi, J.S. In vitro monoamine oxidase A and B inhibitory activity and molecular docking simulations of fucoxanthin. *Fish. Sci.* **2016**, *1*, 123–132. [CrossRef]
71. Rabbani, N.; Tabrez, S.; Islam, B.U.; Rehman, M.T.; Alsenaidy, A.M.; AlAjmi, M.F.; Khan, R.A.; Alsenaidy, M.A.; Khan, M.S. Characterization of colchicine binding with normal and glycated albumin: In vitro and molecular docking analysis. *J. Biomol. Struct. Dyn.* **2018**, *36*, 3453–3462. [CrossRef]
72. Rehman, M.T.; Shamsi, H.; Khan, A.U. Insight into the binding mechanism of imipenem to human serum albumin by spectroscopic and computational approaches. *Mol. Pharm.* **2014**, *11*, 1785–1797. [CrossRef] [PubMed]
73. Wei, W.; Cherukupalli, S.; Jing, L.; Liu, X.; Zhan, P. Fsp3: A new parameter for drug-likeness. *Drug Discov. Today* **2020**, *25*, 1839–1845. [CrossRef] [PubMed]
74. Openmolecules.org. Available online: http://www.openmolecules.org/datawarrior/download.html (accessed on 7 December 2020).
75. AlAjmi, M.F.; Rehman, M.T.; Hussain, A.; Rather, G.M. Pharmacoinformatics approach for the identification of Polo-like kinase-1 inhibitors from natural sources as anti-cancer agents. *Int. J. Biol. Macromol.* **2018**, *116*, 173–181. [CrossRef] [PubMed]
76. Brańka, A.C. Nosé-Hoover chain method for nonequilibrium molecular dynamics simulation. *Phys. Rev. E* **2000**, *61*, 4769–4773. [CrossRef] [PubMed]
77. Martyna, G.J.; Tobias, D.J.; Klein, M.L. Constant pressure molecular dynamics algorithms. *J. Chem. Phys.* **1994**, *101*, 4177–4189. [CrossRef]
78. Tripathi, S.K.; Muttineni, R.; Singh, S.K. Extra precision docking, free energy calculation and molecular dynamics simulation studies of CDK2 inhibitors. *J. Theor. Biol.* **2013**, *334*, 87–100. [CrossRef] [PubMed]

pharmaceuticals

Article

In Silico Prediction of Novel Inhibitors of SARS-CoV-2 Main Protease through Structure-Based Virtual Screening and Molecular Dynamic Simulation

Sobia Ahsan Halim [1,*], Muhammad Waqas [1,2], Ajmal Khan [1] and Ahmed Al-Harrasi [1,*]

1 Natural and Medical Sciences Research Center, University of Nizwa, Nizwa 616, Oman; waqastakkar@gmail.com (M.W.); ajmalkhan@unizwa.edu.om (A.K.)
2 Department of Biotechnology and Genetic Engineering, Hazara University Mansehra, Dhodial 21120, Pakistan
* Correspondence: sobia_halim@unizwa.edu.om (S.A.H.); aharrasi@unizwa.edu.om (A.A.-H.)

Abstract: The unprecedented pandemic of severe acute respiratory syndrome coronavirus 2 (SARS-CoV-2) is threatening global health. SARS-CoV-2 has caused severe disease with significant mortality since December 2019. The enzyme chymotrypsin-like protease (3CLpro) or main protease (M^{pro}) of the virus is considered to be a promising drug target due to its crucial role in viral replication and its genomic dissimilarity to human proteases. In this study, we implemented a structure-based virtual screening (VS) protocol in search of compounds that could inhibit the viral M^{pro}. A library of >eight hundred compounds was screened by molecular docking into multiple structures of M^{pro}, and the result was analyzed by consensus strategy. Those compounds that were ranked mutually in the 'Top-100' position in at least 50% of the structures were selected and their analogous binding modes predicted simultaneously in all the structures were considered as bioactive poses. Subsequently, based on the predicted physiological and pharmacokinetic behavior and interaction analysis, eleven compounds were identified as 'Hits' against SARS-CoV-2 M^{pro}. Those eleven compounds, along with the apo form of M^{pro} and one reference inhibitor (**X77**), were subjected to molecular dynamic simulation to explore the ligand-induced structural and dynamic behavior of M^{pro}. The MM-GBSA calculations reflect that eight out of eleven compounds specifically possess high to good binding affinities for M^{pro}. This study provides valuable insights to design more potent and selective inhibitors of SARS-CoV-2 M^{pro}.

Keywords: SARS coronavirus; SARS-CoV-2 main protease; structure-based virtual screening; molecular dynamic simulation; hit identification

Citation: Halim, S.A.; Waqas, M.; Khan, A.; Al-Harrasi, A. In Silico Prediction of Novel Inhibitors of SARS-CoV-2 Main Protease through Structure-Based Virtual Screening and Molecular Dynamic Simulation. *Pharmaceuticals* **2021**, *14*, 896. https://doi.org/10.3390/ph14090896

Academic Editor: Osvaldo Andrade Santos-Filho

Received: 14 July 2021
Accepted: 11 August 2021
Published: 3 September 2021

1. Introduction

The current global pandemic, so called COVID-19 (COronaVIrus Disease 2019), has spread rapidly since it initially emerged in Wuhan in China, in late 2019 [1–4]. The virus called 'severe acute respiratory syndrome coronavirus 2 (SARS-CoV-2)' is responsible for the outbreak of this pandemic [5]. SARS-CoV-2 belongs to the β coronavirus subgroup of the Coronaviridae family and was found to be related to acute respiratory syndrome coronavirus (SARS-CoV) [6], which previously emerged in China in February 2003 and caused an outbreak in China and spread to several other countries [5,6]. SARS-CoV-2 specifically infects humans by causing an atypical pneumonia, which possesses specific mild to severe symptoms including dry cough, fatigue, fever, shortness of breath, severe progressive pneumonia, multiorgan failure, and eventually death [1]. The World Health Organization (WHO) has declared a state of global health emergency since the outbreak of SARS-CoV-2. According to the World Health Organization (WHO) Coronavirus (COVID-19) dashboard (https://covid19.who.int/, accessed on 30 June 2021), there have been 181,344,224 confirmed cases of COVID-19 globally, including 3,934,252 deaths worldwide, reported to the WHO [7]. Moreover, during the summer of 2020 and spring of 2021, a huge spike was seen in COVID-19 cases [8,9].

SARS-CoV-2 is a positive-sense single-stranded RNA (+ssRNA) virus, with a single linear RNA sequence with ~30,000 nucleotides [10–12]. The SARS-CoV-2 virion is 50–200 nanometers in diameter [6], comprising four structural proteins, known as the S (spike), E (envelope), M (membrane), and N (nucleocapsid) proteins, which are encoded by the 3′ end, whereas two viral replicase polyproteins, called pp1a and pp1b, are encoded by the 5′ end of the genome. The N protein holds the RNA genome, while the viral envelope is composed of S, E, and M proteins. S proteins are glycoproteins that are divided into two functional parts (S1 and S2), which are involved in viral attachment and fusion with the membrane of a host cell. pp1a and pp1b proteolytically cleave into 16 non-structural proteins (nsp1 to nsp16) by the main protease and the papain-like protease. nsp5, also called chymotrypsin-like protease (3CLpro) or main protease (M^{pro}) located in the pp1a, is essential in the replication and maturation of coronavirus, while the papain-like protease is a deubiquitinase [13–20].

At present, specific antiviral or targeted therapies against SARS-CoV-2 do not exist. However, supportive care, which is augmented by the combination of broad-spectrum antibiotics, antivirals, corticosteroids, and convalescent plasma, is the main treatment approach for COVID-19 [18,19]. The scientific community is involved in extensive research worldwide to formulate suitable therapeutics to control the effects of SARS-CoV-2. Many efforts have been applied to screen existing drugs as potential treatments to eradicate this infection. Since the beginning of the pandemic, several antiviral drugs have been tested in clinical trials against COVID-19, including remdesivir (which was originally designed for the Ebola virus [21]), anti-malarial drugs including chloroquine and hydroxychloroquine [22,23], anti-rheumatoid arthritis drug 'tocilizumab' [24,25], and anti-HIV drugs lopinavir/ritonavir [26], among others [27,28]. Nevertheless, the efficacy of some drugs remains controversial. This is the case with a clinical trial involving lopinavir/ritonavir, which reported that no benefits were observed with this treatment compared to standard care [26].

Vaccines against COVID-19 are now available to control the infection [29]; however, there is still an urgent need to discover specific drugs that can target SARS-CoV-2 in patients suffering from COVID-19 due to various emerging variants of the virus. The important targets of SARS-CoV-2 have been identified [30,31] that may be exploited to develop novel therapeutics. Since M^{pro} is one of the key targets of coronavirus, therefore M^{pro} can be targeted to develop antiviral agents. M^{pro} cleaves polyproteins to produce non-structural proteins that are part of the replicase–transcriptase complex. The advantages of targeting M^{pro} are that it specifically exists in the virus and not in humans, it has high sequence identity (i.e., >96%) with SARS-CoV, and it is highly conserved among related viruses [32–35].

M^{pro} is composed of three domains. The domains I and II are composed of 8–101 and 102–184 residues, respectively. These domains acquire a β-barrel shape and resemble chymotrypsin, while domain III (201-306 residues) mainly comprises α-helices. The cleft of domain I and II constitutes the substrate binding region, which consists of the conserved His41 and Cys145 catalytic dyad, where Cys and His act as a nucleophile and a proton acceptor, respectively. Additionally, two deeply buried subsites, called S1 and S2, and three shallow subsites (S3–S5) are also present in the structure. The S1 subsite consists of Phe140, Gly143, Cys145, His163, Glu166, and His172, while S2 consists of Thr25, His41, and Cys145. These residues are mainly involved in hydrophobic and electrostatic interactions. The shallow subsites (S3–S5) are composed of His41, Met49, Met165, Glu166, and Gln189. Despite the high genomic similarity of SARS-CoV-2 with the other members of the coronavirus family, their binding sites have differences in shape and size, which gives us an opportunity to explore more diverse chemical scaffolds by enhanced sampling [32–36]. The three-dimensional (3D-) structure of M^{pro} is depicted in Figure 1a. Herein, we have applied target-specific virtual screening of our in-house compound database with the aim to obtain structurally diverse and potential inhibitors of SARS-CoV-2. Several compounds were identified with high inhibitory potential for M^{pro}, and subsequently, could be tested as a treatment against COVID-19.

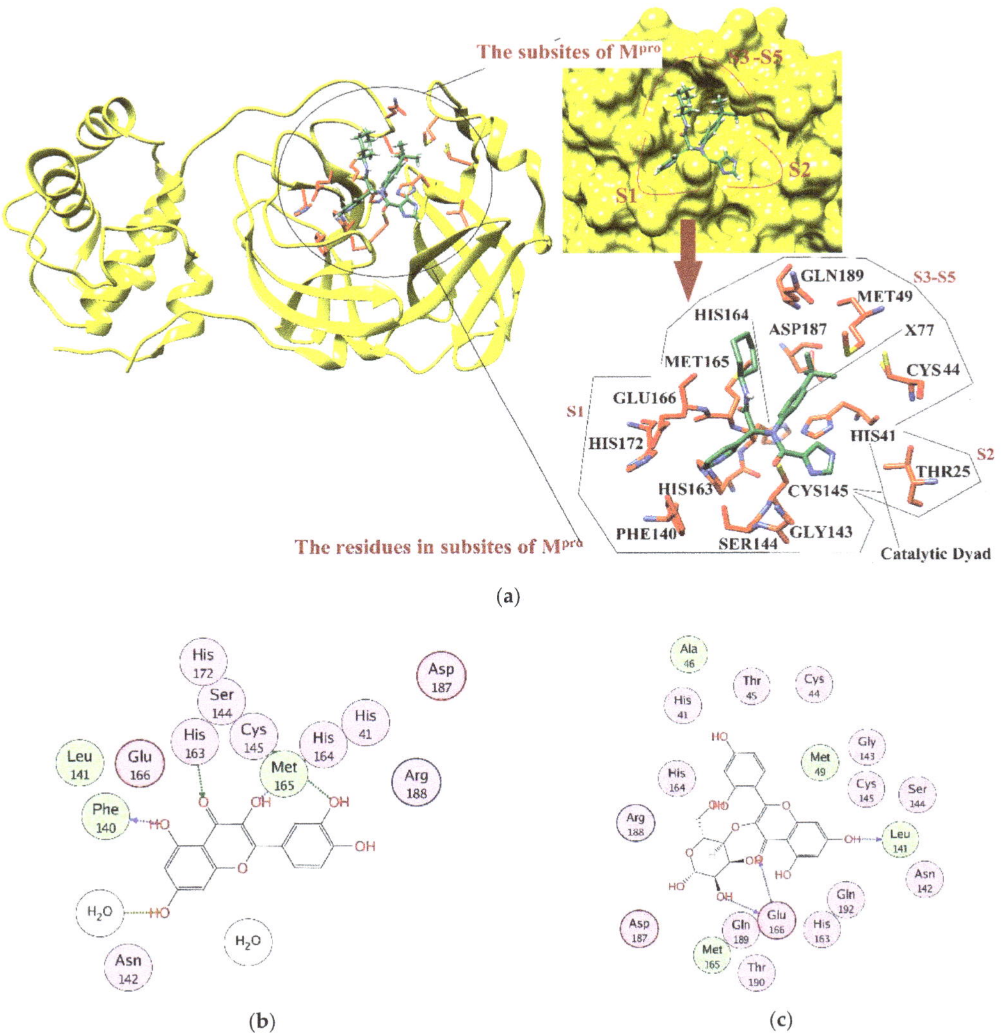

Figure 1. *Cont.*

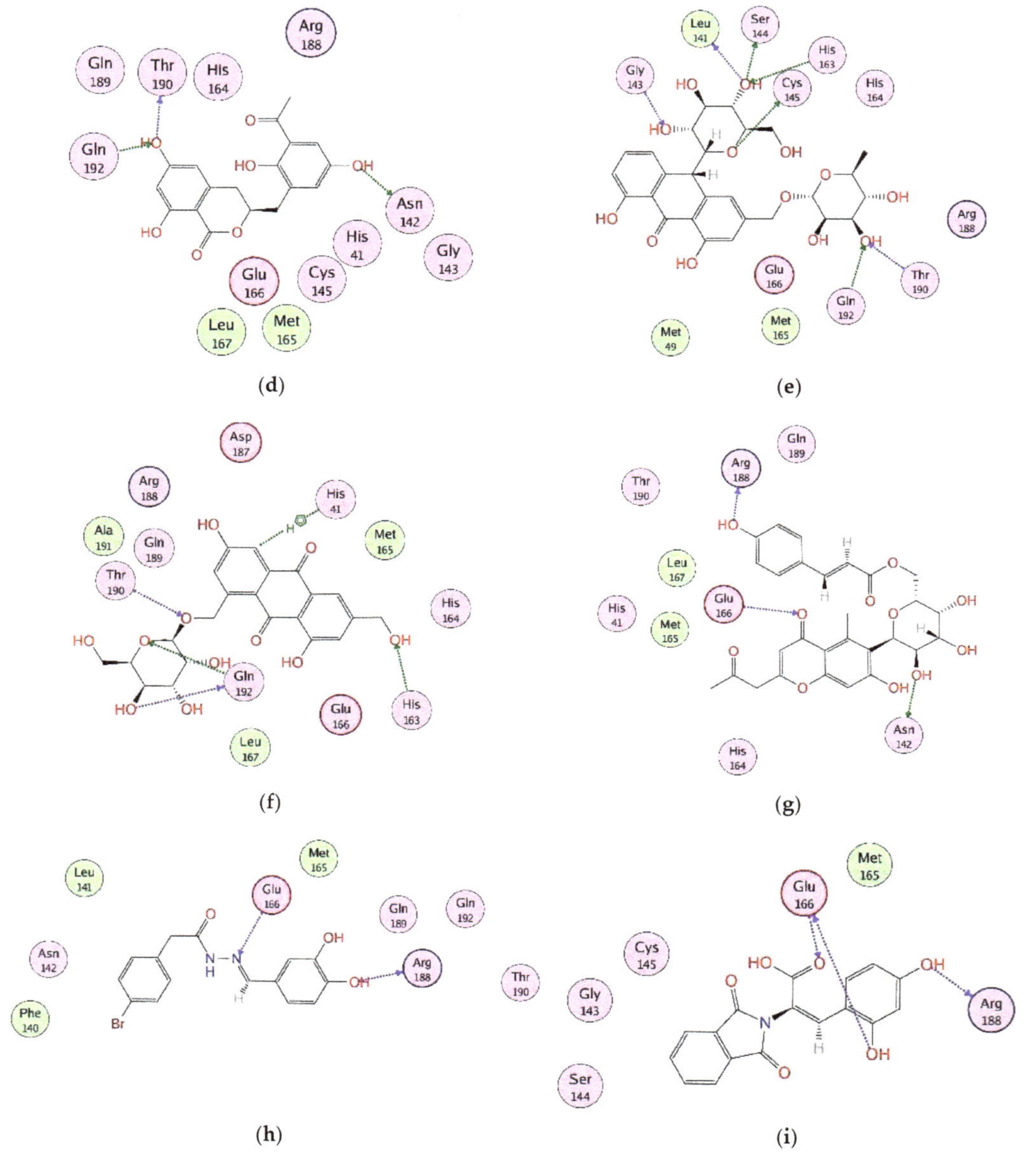

Figure 1. *Cont.*

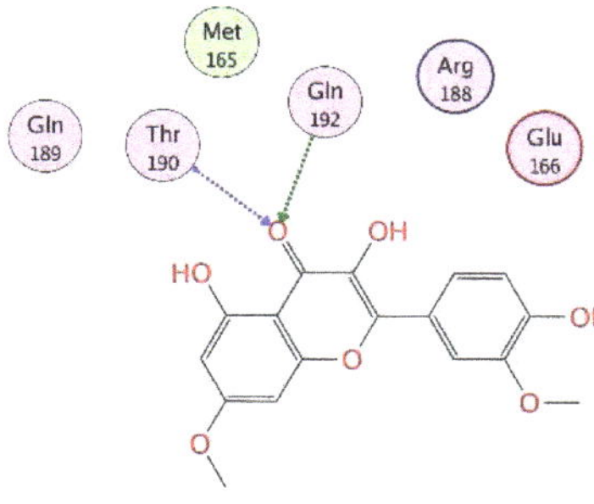

(j)

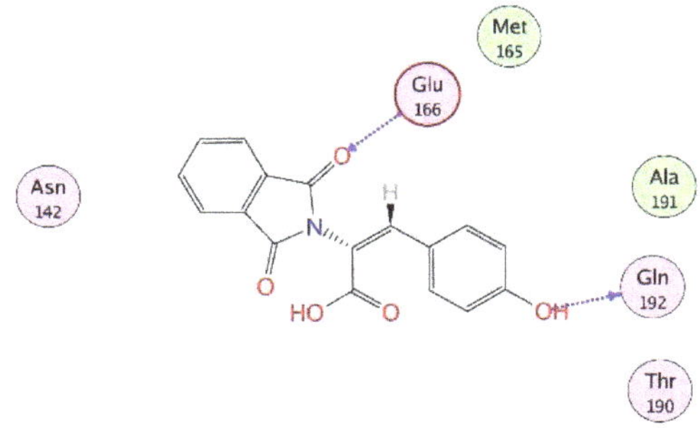

(k)

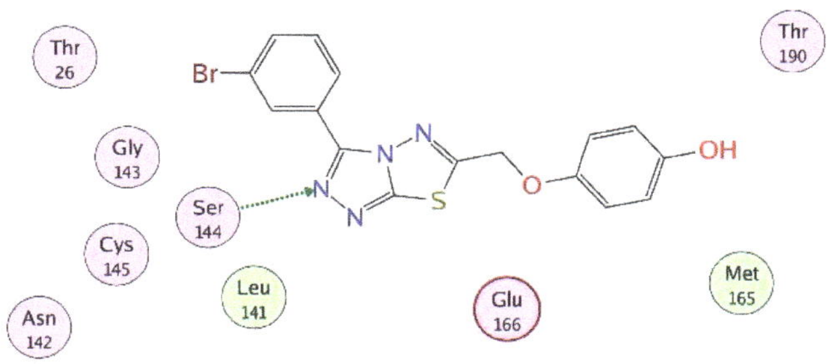

(l)

Figure 1. (**a**) The 3D structure of M^{pro} is shown in complex with **X77** (green stick model). The active site residues are displayed in orange stick models. The S1–S5 subsites are highlighted. The protein–ligand binding interactions of compounds **1**, **3**, **6**, **8**, **10–13**, **17**, **18**, and **28** are shown in 2D format in (**b–l**), respectively. Hydrogen bonds are depicted in dotted arrows. The green and blue colored arrows represent side chain acceptor/donor and backbone acceptor donor atoms, respectively.

2. Results and Discussion

2.1. Validation of Docking Method by Re-Docking and Cross-Docking

Prior to the virtual screening of our in-house database, re-docking and cross-docking of co-crystallized ligands were performed in order to scrutinize the efficiency of the docking method and to select the most appropriate protein file for virtual screening. The re-docking results of twenty protein–ligand complexes showed that 50% of ligands were re-docked with RMSD values of 0.29–1.94 Å, while 30% of ligands were re-docked with RMSD $\leq$ 3 Å. However, only four ligands showed RMSD in the range of 4 to $\geq$7 Å. Therefore, 80% of ligands were correctly re-docked in their X-ray-determined conformations. Thus, the docking method was found efficient in predicting the experimentally determined orientations of compounds. RMSD $\leq$ 3.0 Å is usually considered satisfactory in re-docking experiments; therefore, the results are acceptable. The re-docking results are shown in Table S1.

The cross-docking results (Table S2) showed that 40% of the ligands (ligands in 6Y2F, 6WTK, 6W79, 7BQY, 6ZRT, 7JU7, 6LU7, and 6W63) were correctly ranked between first and third position when docked in their cognate proteins, while two ligands (ligands contained in complexes with PBD codes: 7BRR and 6WNP) were ranked at fifth and seventh position in their X-ray structure. This indicates that MOE accurately ranked 50% of the ligands in good position; therefore, MOE was used in structure-based virtual screening (SB-VS) of our in-house database. The cross-docking results showed that eight proteins (PDB codes: 6Y2F, 6WTK, 6W79, 7BQY, 6ZRT, 7JU7, 6LU7, and 6W63) are appropriate for docking studies; therefore, those proteins were used in the virtual screening experiment.

Analysis of Virtual Screening Accuracy

The predictive accuracy of virtual screening was scrutinized by the ranking or the enrichment of known inhibitors (**KIs**, embedded in the in-house dataset) at the top-ranking position of docked libraries (Table S3). The result was examined by analyzing the percent enrichment factor (%EF) and receiver operating characteristic curves (ROC curves). These matrices are widely used to compare virtual screening results. The results showed that MOE successfully identified **KIs** in 6W79, 7BQY, 6ZRT, 7JU7, and 6W63 with %EF in the range of 33% to 73% at a top-100 position (Table S3), whereas 6W79 showed %EF of 53% at a top-50 position. Moreover, the ROC curve shows an AUC of 0.79–0.84 for 7JU7, 6Y2F, 6WTK, 6LU7, 7BQY, 6W63, and 6ZRT, and 0.90 for 6W79. The %EF and AUC of 6W79 were the highest among all the selected proteins. The ROC curve is displayed in Figure S1.

2.2. Selection of Hits after Consensus Approach

The virtual screening of >800 compounds was carried out on multiple structures of M^{pro} (PDB codes: 6Y2F, 6WTK, 6W79, 7BQY, 6ZRT, 7JU7, 6LU7, and 6W63) with the aim of finding out the most potential inhibitors. Later, the consensus approach was used to select the compounds that are ranked among the top 100 positions in all the proteins. We observed that thirteen (**1–13**) and eight compounds (**14–18**, **28–30**) were mutually ranked at a top-100 position in 8/8 and 7/8 proteins, respectively, whereas nine compounds (**19–27**) were ranked at a top-100 position in $\geq$50% of the proteins. Therefore, a total of thirty compounds were selected, and their pharmacokinetic behavior was studied by SwissADME [37] and ADMETsar [38]. The docking results are tabulated in Table S4.

2.3. Pharmacokinetic Analysis

The physicochemical properties of the selected compounds showed that the molecular weight of compounds is in the range of 290 to 635 g/mol. A total of 19/30 compounds possess $\leq$5 rotatable bonds (RBs), while 11/30 compounds possess 6–10 RBs in their structures. The compounds have 3–13 hydrogen bond acceptor atoms (HBA) and 0–9 hydrogen bond donor atoms (HBD). The molar refractivity (MR) and topological polar surface area (TPSA) of these compounds are in the range of 74.33–169.9 and 62.32–226.83 Å^2, respectively. These results were compared with the physicochemical properties of selected **KIs**. Those **KIs** possess 1–8 HBA atoms, 0–7 HBD atoms, and 1-22 RBs, while 4/15 **KIs** possess a molecular weight in the range of 549 to >681. Similarly, the TPSA of **KIs** was found to be in the range of 20 to >197 Å^2. The **KIs** including remdesivir, lopinavir and ritonavir also have molecular weight > 600, RB = 15–23 and TPSA in the range of 120 to 203 Å^2. According to Veber's rule of drug-likeness [39], TPSA and the number of RBs discriminate between orally active compounds and those that are not orally active for a large dataset of compounds in rats [40]. Therefore, compounds with $\leq$10 RBs and TPSA $\leq$ 140 Å^2 are predicted to have good oral bioavailability [40], while the Ghose filter further improves the predictions of drug-likeness by the following rules: the partition coefficient (LogP) of the compound should be in the range of -0.4 to +5.6, MR = 40 to 130, molecular weight = 180 to 480, and number of atoms from 20 to 70 (including HBDs and HBAs). The predicted partition coefficient (LogP octanol/water) of the selected (30) hits was in the range of +0.25 to 4.74, suggesting their solubility in a hydrophobic medium. The $LogP_{o/w}$ of selected **KIs** is in the range of 0.7 to >5. Similarly, most of the hits demonstrated good to moderate solubility in a water medium.

The predicted pharmacokinetic properties of the selected hits further helped us to choose more appropriate compounds. The admetSAR showed that all the hits passed human intestinal absorption, while SwissADME showed that 17/30 compounds (**1**, **6**, **12–14**, **16–19**, **22–28**, **30**) had high gastrointestinal absorption (GIA) ability. Similarly, all the compounds (except **16** and **27**) exhibited no blood–brain barrier penetration. Additionally, all compounds (except **15**, **22–27**, and **30**) did not have substrate-like properties for P-glycoprotein (P-gp), while compounds **11**, **15**, **19–27**, and **30** displayed inhibitory potential against P-gp. Furthermore, most of the compounds were found to be non-inhibitors of cytochrome p450 enzymes (CYP1A2, CYP2C19, CYP2C9, CYP2D6, and CYP3A4). The skin permeation (LogKp) of ligands was found in the range of −5.30 to −10.61 cm/s, showing that these compounds are not permeable through the skin.

The drug-likeness properties of selected hits were calculated based on the Lipinski rule of five [41] and Ghose [42], Veber's [39], Egan's [43], and Muegge's rules [44]. The compounds **1**, **6**, **12–14**, **16–18**, **26**, **28** and **30** followed all the drug-likeness criteria given by Lipinski, while compounds **1**, **4–6**, **9**, **12–14**, **16–18**, and **28** fulfilled the Ghose rules of drug-likeness. Similarly, compounds **1**, **6**, **12–14**, **16–18**, **26–28**, and **30** followed Veber's, Egan's, and Muegge's rules of drug-likeness. Comparing these results with the drug-likeness of **KIs** shows that 4/15 **KIs** (including O6K, telaprevir, boceprevir and N3) violate two rules of Lipinski's drug-likeness criteria, while the known drug, remdesivir, also showed two violations of Lipinski's rule (MW > 500, HBA > 10), three violations of Ghose rules (MW > 480, MR > 130, number of atoms > 70) and Muegge's rules (MW > 600, TPSA > 150, HBA > 10), two violations of Veber's rules (Rotors > 10, TPSA > 140), and one violation of Egan's rules (TPSA > 131.6). This shows that the selected hits possess comparable drug-likeness with remdesivir. Usually, substrates of biological transporters or natural products do not follow the above-mentioned rules of drug-likeness [45]. Moreover, recently several molecules were approved by the FDA in 2020. Among those approved drugs, several compounds fail on one or the other drug-likeness pharmacokinetic principle, and do not obey Lipinski, Ghose, Veber, Egan, and Muegge's filters, although this does not question the approval of these molecules. Therefore, it is critical to first look for a potent molecule, and once potency is validated, then to look for improved kinetics [46].

The bioavailability score of the compounds was in the range of 0.17–0.56, indicating moderate bioavailability. Among all the selected hits, only a few compounds (**1**, **2**, **4**, **7**, **9**, **10**, **12**, **14**) showed few PAINS alerts, whereas the rest of the compounds did not show any PAINS alerts. Moreover, compounds **1**, **6**, **12–14**, **16–18** passed the lead-likeness criteria, while compounds **2**, **3–5**, **7–11**, **15**, and **19–30** displayed few violations (i.e., MW > 300, rotors > 7, XlogP 3 > 3.5). The calculated synthetic accessibility of the compounds was in the range of 2.70 to 6.30, which reflects that these compounds are synthesizable. The bioavailability score, lead-likeness, and synthetic accessibility of compounds were compared with remdesivir, which showed that the compounds possess comparable scores. The bioavailability score of remdesivir is also 0.17 and synthetic accessibility = 6.33, and remdesivir depicted two violations in lead-likeness (i.e., MW > 350, Rotors > 7). The predicted physiological properties, pharmacokinetic profiles, drug-likeness, and medicinal properties of the selected compounds are tabulated in Tables S5–S9.

2.4. Interaction Analysis

After sequence and structural alignment of eight M^{pro} structures (used in VS), the main pharmacophoric features required for optimal binding were deduced. We observed that His41, Phe140, Gly143, Cys145, His163, His164, Glu166, Gln189, and Thr190 play important roles in the stabilization of protein–ligand binding by providing hydrogen bonds or hydrophobic interactions. Thus, the interactions of the selected ligands with those important residues were scrutinized. The docked view of compound **1** (2-(3,4-dihydroxyphenyl)-3,5,7-trihydroxy-4*H*-chromen-4-one) showed that the compound binds at S1, S2 and S3 subsites, and its hydroxyl groups and the carbonyl moiety formed H-bonds with multiple important residues including Phe140 of S1, Cys145 of S1 and S2, His163 of S1, and His164 of S3. Similarly, the substituted -OH moieties of compound **2** (1R,2R,3*S*,4*S*,6*S*)-6-((E)-3-(3,4-dihydroxyphenyl) acryloyloxy)-2,3,4-trihydroxycyclohexyl 3,4,5-trihydroxybenzoate) formed multiple H-bonds with the side chains of Cys145 (S1 and S2 subsites) and Met165 of S3, and with the main chain carbonyl oxygen of Glu166. Moreover, Glu166 formed bidentate interactions with the -OH group and dihydropyranone oxygen of compound **3** (2-(2,4-dihydroxyphenyl)-5,7-dihydroxy-3-((2R,3*S*,4*S*,5R,6R)-4,5,6-trihydroxy-2-(hydroxy methyl)-tetrahydro-2*H*-pyran-3-yloxy)-4*H*-chromen-4-one), whereas one of the -OH groups of compound **3** mediated H-bonds with Leu141, while the substituted pyran -OH groups of compound **4** (1,3,8-trihydroxy-6-(((2R,3R,4R,5R,6R)-3,4,5-trihydroxy-6-methyl-tetrahydro-2*H*-pyran-2-yloxy) methyl) anthracene-9,10-dione) interacted with Glu166 and Gln192. Similarly, the -OH and the carbonyl oxygen of compound **5** (2-(2,4-dihydroxyphenyl)-5,7-dihydroxy-3-methyl-4*H*-chromen-4-one) mediated H-bonding with Leu141 and Cys145, respectively. However, the substituted -OH groups of compound **6** ((*S*)-3-(3-acetyl-2,5-dihydroxybenzyl)-6,8-dihydroxy-3,4-dihydroisochromen-1-one) formed H-bonds with Asn142, Thr190, and Gln192. Similarly, Thr190 and Glu166 mediated H-bonds with the -OH groups of compound **7** (1,6-dihydroxy-3-methyl-8-((2R,3R,4R,5R,6R)-3,4,5-trihydroxy-6-(hydroxymethyl)-tetrahydro-2*H*-pyran-2-yloxy) anthracene-9,10-dione). Interestingly, compound **8** ((*S*)-4,5-dihydroxy-9-((2R,3R,4R,5*S*,6R)-3,4,5-trihydroxy-6-(hydroxymethyl)-tetrahydro-2*H*-pyran-2-yl)-2-(((2R,3R,4R,5R,6*S*)-3,4,5-trihydroxy-6-methyl-tetrahydro-2*H*-pyran-2-yloxy) methyl) anthracen-10(9*H*)-one) mediated the highest number of H-bonds with the side chains and backbone atoms of Gly143, Leu141, Ser144, His163, Cys145, Thr190, and Gln192. Therefore, this molecule was considered to be the most promising inhibitor. Moreover, compound **9** (1,3,8-trihydroxy-6-(((1R,2R,3R,4S,5*S*)-2,3,4-trihydroxy-5-methylcyclohexyloxy) methyl) anthracene-9,10-dione) formed multiple interactions with Ser144, Thr190, and Gln192. Like compound **8**, compound **10** (1,6-dihydroxy-3-(hydroxymethyl)-8-(2R,3R,4R,5R,6R)-3,4,5-trihydroxy-6-(hydroxymethyl)-tetrahydro-2*H*-pyran-2-yloxy) methyl) anthracene-9,10-dione) also mediated several interactions with key residues including His163, Thr190, and Gln192, whereas His41 provided H–π interaction to the compound. Similarly, compound **11** ((E)-((2R,3R,4R,5R,6R)-3,4,5-trihydroxy-6-(7-hydroxy-5-methyl-4-oxo-2-(2-oxopropyl)-4*H*-chromen-6-yl)-tetrahydro-2*H*-pyran-2-yl) methyl 3-(4-hydroxyphenyl) acrylate) displayed H-bonding with Asn142, Glu166, and Arg188. The compounds **12** ((E)-*N*′-(3,4-dihydroxybenzylidene)-2-phenylacetohydrazide) and **13** ((E)-3-(2,4-dihydroxyphenyl)-2-(1,3-dioxoisoindolin-2-yl) acrylic acid) formed H-bonds with Glu166 and Arg188, while compounds **14** ((2R,3*S*)-2-(3,4-dihydroxyphenyl)-3,4-dihydro-2*H*-chromene-3,5,7-triol) and **16** (4,11-dibutyl 5,10-bis(2-hydroxyphenyl)-3,12-dithiatricyclo[7 .3.0.02,6]dodeca-1,4,6,8,10-pentaene-4,11-dicarboxylate) interacted with Glu166 and Ser144, and Gly143 and Ser144, respectively. The binding mode of compound **15** ((E)-((2R,3R,5R,6R)-3,4,5-trihydroxy-6-(7-methoxy-5-methyl-4-oxo-2-(2-oxopropyl)-4*H*-chromen-6-yl)-tetrahydro-2*H*-pyran-2-yl) methyl 3-(4-hydroxyphenyl) acrylate) demonstrated that Gln192, Thr190, and His163 stabilized the compound in the active site of M^{pro} through multiple H-bonds, while Thr190 and Gln192, and residues Glu166 and Gln192, provided H-bonds to the compounds **17** (3,5-dihydroxy-2-(4-hydroxy-3-methoxyphenyl)-7-methoxy-4*H*-chromen-4-one) and **18** ((E)-2-(1,3-dioxoisoindolin-2-yl)-3-(4-hydroxyphenyl) acrylic acid), respectively. Compound **19** ((R)-3-((R)-6-(2,2-bis(4-fluorophenyl)ethyl)-4-methoxy-5,6,7,8-tetrahydro-[1,3]dioxolo[4,5-g]isoquinolin-5-yl)-6,7-dimethoxyisobenzofuran-1(3*H*)-one) formed a H-bond with the main chain nitrogen of Glu166, while the amino nitrogen and -OH group of Ser144 and main chain nitrogen of Cys145 stabilized compound **20** (3-{4-[2-carboxy-2-(1,3-dioxo-2,3-dihydro-1*H*-isoindol-2-yl)eth-1-en-1-yl]phenyl}-2-(1,3-dioxo-2,3-dihydro-1*H*-isoindol-2-yl)prop-2-enoic acid) through H-bonding, whereas compounds **21** ((E)-((2R,3R,5R,6R)-3,4,5-trihydroxy-6-(7-hydroxy-5-methyl-4-oxo-2-(2-oxopropyl)-4*H*-chromen-8-yl)-tetrahydro-2*H*-pyran-2-yl)methyl 3-(4-hydroxyphenyl)acrylate), **22** ((R)-2-((R)-5-((R)-4,5-dimethoxy-1,3-dihydroisobenzofuran-1-yl)-4-methoxy-7,8-dihydro-[1,3] dioxolo[4,5-g]isoquinolin-6(5*H*)-yl)-2-(9*H*-fluoren-3-yl)ethanamine), **23** ((R)-{6-[2,2-bis(4-fluorophenyl)ethyl]-4-methoxy-2*H*,5*H*,6*H*,7*H*,8*H*-[1,3]dioxolo[4,5-g]isoquinolin-5-yl}[2-(hydroxymethyl)-3,4-dimethoxyphenyl]methanol) and **24** ((*S*)-6-((1-(4-bromobenzyl)-1*H*-1,2,3-triazol-4-yl)methyl)-4-methoxy-5-((R)-5-methoxy-4-methyl-1,3-dihydroisobenzofuran-1-yl)-5,6,7,8-tetrahydro-[1,3]dioxolo[4,5-g]isoquinoline) formed a single H-bond with Cys145, His164, and Glu166, respectively. Moreover, compounds **25** (8-benzyl-*N*-cyclohexyl-14-methyl-7-oxo-5-phenyl-2,3,4,8,18-pentaazatetracyclo [8.8.0.02,6.012,17] octadeca-1(10),3,5,11, 13,15,17-heptaene-9-carboxamide) and **26** ((9R,13R)-4-bromo-*N*9-{[(2R)-oxolan-2-yl]methyl}-14-phenyl-8-oxa-14,15,17-triazatetracyclo [8.7.0.02,7.012,16] heptadeca-1(17),2,4,6,10,15-hexaene-9,13-diamine) were stabilized by Glu166 and His163, and Gly143, respectively, while compounds **27** ((9R,13R)-*N*9-benzyl-4-fluoro-14-phenyl-8-oxa-14,15,17-triazatetracyclo heptadeca-1(17),2(7),3,5,10,15-hexaene-9,13-diamine), **28** (4-((3-(3-bromophenyl)-[1,2,4] triazolo[3,4-b][1,3,4]thiadiazol-6-yl)methoxy)phenol) and **30** (4-[(9R,13R)-13-amino-9-(benzylamino)-8-oxa-14,15,17-triazatetracyclo [8.7.0.02,7.012,16] heptadeca-1(17),2(7),3,5,10,15-hexaen-14-yl]benzoic acid) mediated H-bonds with Glu166, Ser144, and Gly143, respectively. The docked view of compound **29** ((*S*)-4,5,9-trihydroxy-2-(hydroxymethyl)-9-((2R,3*S*,4R,5R,6*S*)-4,5,6-trihydroxy-2-(hydroxymethyl)-tetrahydro-2*H*-pyran-3-yloxy) anthracen-10(9*H*)-one) depicts that Glu166 and Phe140 mediated multiple H-bonds with the -OH moieties of **29**, and His41 mediated π–π interaction with this compound. The protein–ligand interactions of **1–30** hits are tabulated in Table S10. The binding modes of compounds depict that these compounds mainly bind at S1 and S2 subsites of the active site of M^{pro}; however, His164 and Met165 of the S3 subsite, a few residues at the entrance of the active site loop (near S1 subsite including Leu141 and Asn142), and some residues of domain 3 (including Arg188, Thr190, and Gln192) also play important roles in the binding of compounds. Based on the pharmacokinetic profile, drug-likeness, and interaction analysis, eleven compounds (**1**, **3**, **6**, **8**, **10**, **11**, **12**, **13**, **17**, **18**, and **28**) were considered to be good inhibitors; thus, their dynamic behavior was studied by molecular dynamic simulation. The docked orientations and 2D-structures of 11 hits are shown in Figure 1b–l. The chemical structures of compounds **1–30** are shown in Figure S2.

2.5. Molecular Dynamic Simulation

2.5.1. Convergence of M^{pro} Free and Inhibited States

The X-ray structure of M^{pro} (PDB code: 6W79, reported by Mesecar et al. [47]) in complex with the broad-spectrum non-covalent inhibitor (**X77**) was selected for MD simulation as a positive control. The dynamic behavior and structural stability of M^{pro} in the apo form and inhibited states were analyzed through molecular dynamic simulation. The stability of all the complexes was analyzed by calculating the RMSD (alpha carbon, Cα) of all the complexes from the output generated trajectories after 100 ns. The apo–M^{pro} (Figure 2) was stable during the simulation except for the fraction between 96 and 100 ns. The apo–M^{pro} showed an acceptable range of fluctuation and gained stability till 100 ns (showed a smooth and straight graph). This behavior indicates that the free state of the protein was stable. However, the reference complex, M^{pro}–**X77**, showed that the RMSD gains equilibrium after 80 ns and is increased up to 100 ns. On the other hand, compound **1** formed several key interactions with the protein, and therefore showed a considerable increase in the RMSD after 25 ns, which affected the overall stability of the complex. A drastic deviation in the RMSD was observed from 20–80 ns during the simulation, whereas the RMSD for the M^{pro}–compound **3** complex was found stable till 20 ns, excluding the substantial convergence at the 25–45 ns period where the RMSD of the complex increased significantly. Shortly after the increase in the RMSD, no convergence was seen. Similarly, the M^{pro}–compound **6** complex depicted a major stability drift between 20 and 60 ns, while the RMSD remained increased till 100ns. Interestingly, the M^{pro}–**8** complex revealed a substantial convergence in the stability until the simulation time. At different levels, significant convergence was observed in the RMSD of the M^{pro}–**8** complex. The M^{pro}–**10** complex showed a small drift in the convergence at 80 ns; however, the system remained stable. The M^{pro}–**11** complex showed drastic shifts in the stability at several intervals of 15–25, 30–60, and 65–85 ns, which significantly affected the stability of the complex. Moreover, the stability of the M^{pro}–**12** complex was also affected due to a continuous increase in the RMSD after 40 ns. In contrast, the M^{pro}–**13** complex mediated friction between 30 and 40 ns; however, it showed minimal effect on the system's stability. Similarly, the RMSD of the M^{pro}–**17** complex was stable up to 50 ns; however, it increased at 50–60 and 75–90 ns. We observed that the M^{pro}–**8** complex depicted a rapid increase in the RMSD between 20 and 90 ns (and therefore destabilized the system); however, after a drastic increase, the RMSD was stabilized after 90 ns. The M^{pro}–**28** complex remained relaxed until 55 ns; however, the RMSD was increased after 55 ns and remained elevated throughout the simulation. The sudden increase indicates the fluctuation in the stability of the complex. Altogether, the results indicate that M^{pro}–**3**, M^{pro}–**8**, M^{pro}–**11**, M^{pro}–**18**, and M^{pro}–**28** complexes attained more variation as compared to the apo–M^{pro}, while M^{pro}–**8**, M^{pro}–**11**, and M^{pro}–**28** complexes were found unstable till the end of simulation and reached a maximum RMSD of 7 Å, 4 Å, and 3.9 Å, respectively, as compared to apo–M^{pro} and M^{pro}–**X77** complex. During the simulation, no destruction in the simulated complexes (both apo and ligand-bound forms) was observed, which confirms the significance of the simulation. The RMSD graphs of all the complexes are shown in Figure 2.

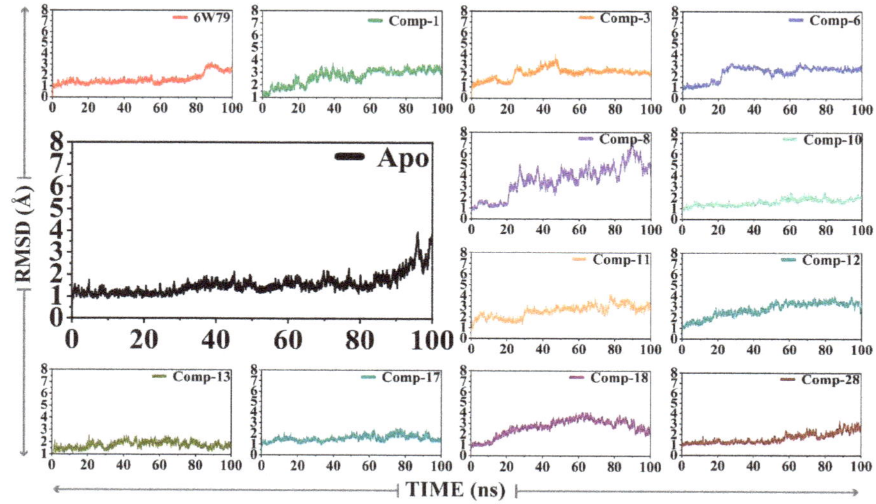

Figure 2. The RMSD plots of apo–M^{pro} and ligand-bound form of M^{pro}. The average RMSD of apo–M^{pro} and inhibited M^{pro} was 2.8 Å and <3.9 Å, respectively.

2.5.2. Root Mean Square Fluctuation (RMSF)

RMSF was calculated to observe the fluctuation in different regions of M^{pro} upon ligand binding during the simulation. The main purpose was to see the effects of ligand binding on the flexibility of each residue of protein. The RMSF graphs of all complexes and apo–M^{pro} are shown in Figure 3. The results show that compound **8** increased the flexibility of all regions of the M^{pro}–**8** complex as compared to the apo–M^{pro}, M^{pro}–**X77** complex, and complexes of the rest of the selected hits from the in-house database. The apo–M^{pro} showed the lowest RMSF as compared to the ligand-bound states, reflecting that the protein is not very flexible in the un-ligated state. The average RMSF of all the systems was found in the range of 1.5 Å. The M^{pro}–**3**, M^{pro}–**8**, M^{pro}–**11**, and M^{pro}–**28** complexes exhibited high flexibility, while the flexibility of M^{pro}–**10** and M^{pro}–**13** complexes was low. The loops in the protein structure fluctuated the RMSF at different regions. The M^{pro}–**1**, M^{pro}–**6**, M^{pro}–**12**, M^{pro}–**17**, and M^{pro}–**18** complexes depicted lower flexibility due to the differential dynamics upon ligand binding. The secondary structures with loops are responsible for the fluctuation in the RMSF at different levels, justifying the residual flexibility. The flexibility of complexes with the selected eleven hits varies as compared to the apo–M^{pro} and **X77**-inhibited states (Figure 3).

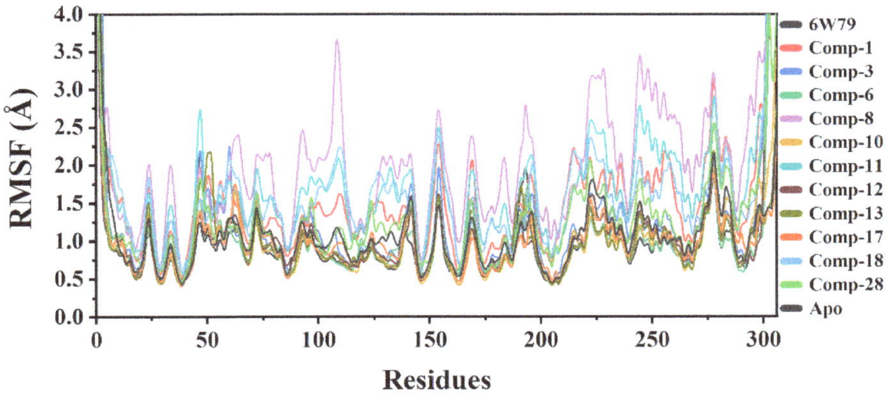

Figure 3. RMSF graphs of apo–M^{pro}, M^{pro}–**X77**, and M^{pro} in complex with selected hits. The RMSF of free state was in range of 0.5 Å to 1.3 Å. Compound **8** attained highest RMSF (between 1.5 Å and 3.5 Å), while the complex with **X77** showed RMSF between 1.0 Å and 1.8 Å.

The total energy of the apo–M^{pro} was stable (energy = −5600 kcal/mol), while the M^{pro}–**X77** exhibited slightly lower energy (−5400 kcal/mol) as compared to apo–M^{pro}. The M^{pro}–**8**, M^{pro}–**11**, M^{pro}–**18**, and M^{pro}–**28** complexes revealed a similar energy pattern (in the range of −5400 kcal/mol to −5200 Kcal/mol), whereas the M^{pro}–**10** and M^{pro}–**13** complexes possess slightly higher total energy (between −5500 kcal/mol and −5700 kcal/mol) than the apo–M^{pro}. The M^{pro}–**1**, M^{pro}–**3**, M^{pro}–**6**, M^{pro}–**12**, and M^{pro}–**17** complexes showed increased total energy ranging from −5600 kcal/mol to −5800 kcal/mol (Figure 4). The inhibited states of M^{pro} shared similar patterns and variations as compared to the apo form, therefore showing the effects of deviation on the structure of the protein created by each inhibitor.

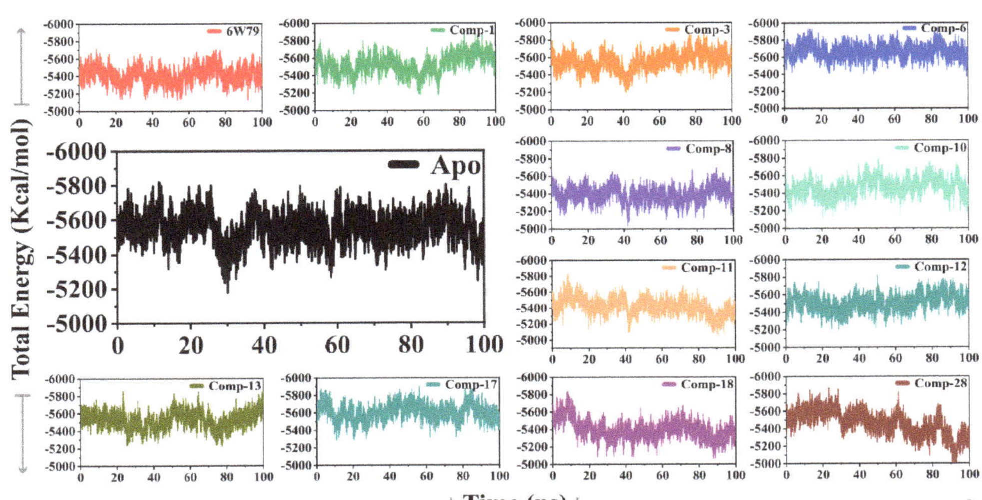

Figure 4. The difference of total energy of M^{pro} is shown in the apo–M^{pro} and inhibited states. The *x*-axis and *y*-axis depict time (nanoseconds) and the total energy of the protein during the simulation (Kcal/mol), respectively.

2.5.3. Protein Motions and Trajectories Clustering

The dynamic impact of eleven hits on the structure of M^{pro} is shown in Figure 5. The structural changes in each complex due to the protein–ligand binding was observed through principal component analysis (PCA). The significant dominant motions (Figure 5) are shown in the first three eigenvectors, while the others indicated localized fluctuation. In the apo–M^{pro}, a total of 48% of variances were contributed by the first three eigenvectors to the total observed motion. Unlike the apo–M^{pro}, the inhibited states showed different behavior of motion. In inhibited states, compounds **8** and **12** showed 60%, compounds **18, 1** and **X77** reflected 57% and 55%, respectively, whereas compounds **6, 28,** and **11** showed 52–50% of total motion. The total motion of compounds **3** and **17** was 40%, while compounds **10** and **13** demonstrated least motion of 38% and 26%, respectively. These structural behavior clearly demonstrated the structural rearrangement of the protein upon ligand binding.

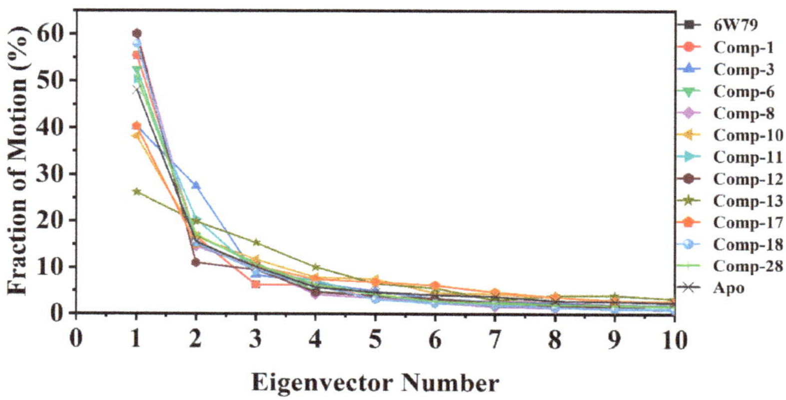

Figure 5. First 10 eigenvector fractions are shown. Each eigenvector contribution (in percentage, %) is acquired from covariance matrix plotted against the corresponding eigenvector from MD trajectory of each complex.

The reliability of attributed motions was achieved by plotting the two initial eigenvectors of each trajectory against each other. During the simulation production run, the flipping over conformation was shown by color blue to red. The dots represented each frame from blue to red. To understand the conformational transformation of the complexes, a 2D subspace was mapped from the trajectories using PC1 and PC2. Figure 6 clearly shows that each complex acquired two conformational states on the subspace differentiated by the colors (blue and red). The unstable conformational state (shown in blue) can be easily separated in neared convergence to obtain a stable conformational state (shown in red). Subsequently, the apo–M^{pro} showed more energetic conformation, while the inhibited states showed stable energy conformation with different periodic jumps. The M^{pro}–**X77** complex reflected very stable lower energy conformation as compared to apo–M^{pro}, while the rest of the inhibitors followed the same pattern and acquired stability with lower energy states.

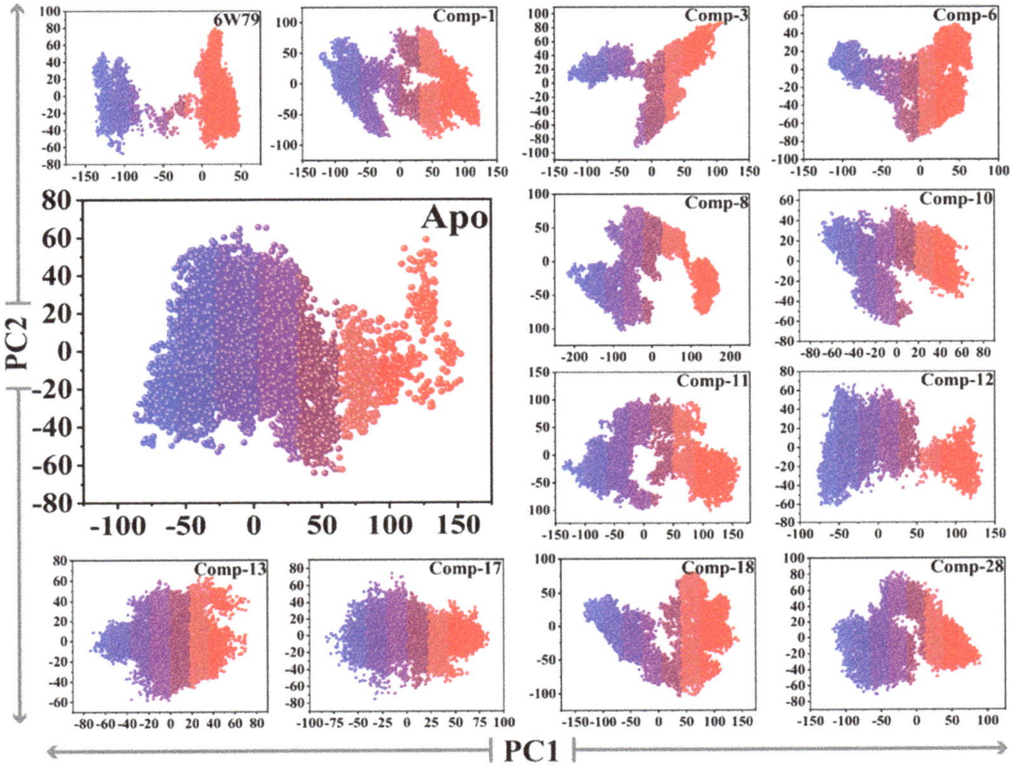

Figure 6. The PCA analysis of apo–M^{pro} and inhibited states of M^{pro}. Principal component 1 (PC1) and principal component 2 (PC2) were plotted against each other using the backbone carbon atoms.

2.5.4. Metastable to Native State Transition Pathway

The transition states of the apo–M^{pro} and inhibited M^{pro} complexes were studied using the free energy landscape (FEL). The FEL plot was constructed from the first two eigenvectors of the trajectory time to explore the transition mechanism from the metastable state to the native state. The lowest energy states of each complex were examined to investigate the structural changes. The apo–M^{pro} showed a significant change in the energy states as compared to the inhibited states (represented by red, yellow, green, and blue in Figure 7). The highest energy levels and the metastable stage in the plots are shown by red and blue colors, respectively. The apo–M^{pro} was stable as compared to the inhibited states because the red color (high energy state) is more prominent in the inhibited states (**X77**, **1**, **3**, **6**, **8**, **10–13**, **17–18**, and **28**). The compounds **3**, **8**, **6**, **11**, **18**, and **28** showed the highest transition states due to the interaction with the active site domain of M^{pro}. The apo–M^{pro} acquired only one state with no energy barriers, and similarly, compound **13** showed a pattern like apo–M^{pro} due to the sliding of compound **13** from the active pocket because of weak interactions. Moreover, compound **10** acquired two states with a stable energy level for the maximum time (shown in yellow). The reference ligand, **X77**, remained mostly in the high energy state, which confirmed the effect on the stability of the protein structure due to the rearrangement of the bonds upon binding with **X77**. Figure 7 depicts that the apo–M^{pro} remains in the green and yellow energy states, while ligand-inhibited complexes are found in the high energy state (red) for most of the simulation time. The inhibition of M^{pro} by the selected hits is evident by FEL, which clearly shows the structural rearrangement of the protein upon binding with small drug-like molecules. The ligand-bound complexes (inhibited states) displayed more conformational transitions as compared to the free state. Various metastable states showed conformational changes in the M^{pro} structure in the ligand-inhibited complexes. The protein structure was ensembled at a distinct nanosecond time scale. In Figure 7, the crucial areas in the structures are shown in shaded form. The X and Y coordinates were obtained from the metastable states from all the trajectories with their respective frame number and time (ns), which are tabulated in Table 1.

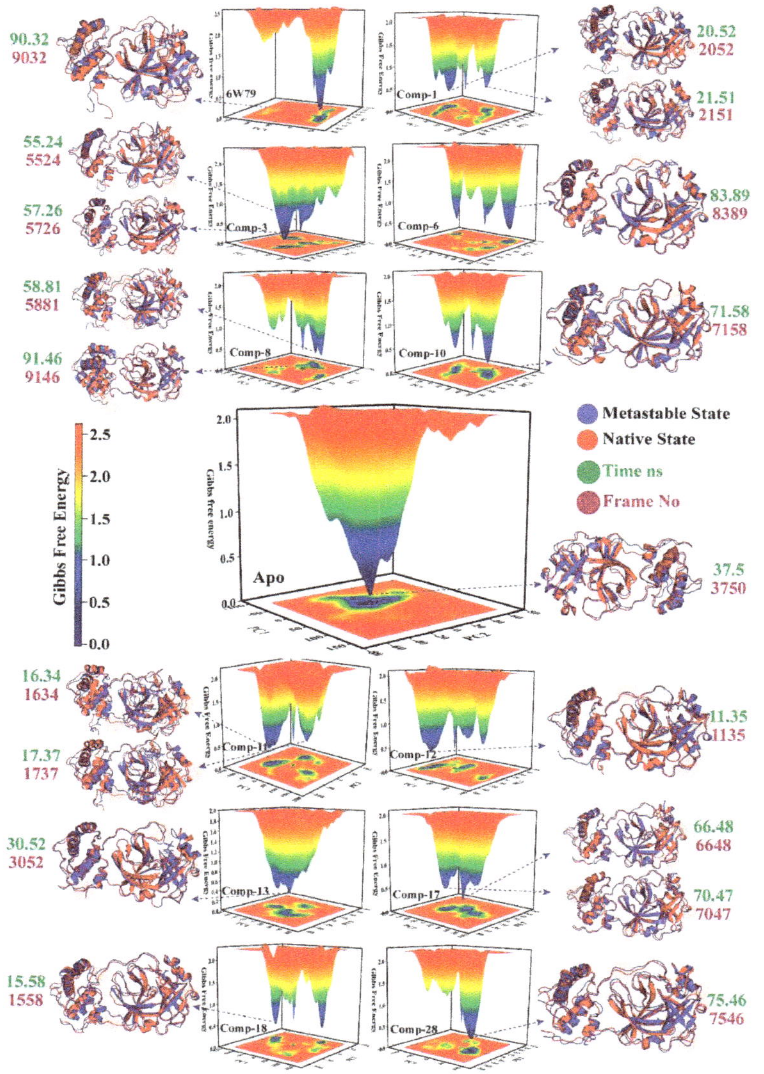

Figure 7. The free energy landscape (FEL) of free state and inhibited states is shown. High and low energy states are shown in distinct colors in the plot. The minimal, intermediate, and the high energy states are presented in dark blue, yellow, and red, respectively. The time of the metastable states (ns) and frame number is presented in green and purple, respectively. The metastable states and the native structures of M^{pro} are depicted in cartoon model in blue and red, respectively.

Table 1. The X and Y coordinates of metastable states with frame number and time (ns).

Complex Name	X Coordinates	Y Coordinates	Frame No	Time ns
Apo–M^{pro}	1.859	−0.699	3750	37.5
M^{pro}–**X77**	29.197	−20.599	9032	90.32
M^{pro}–**1**	−73.840	3.321	2052	20.52
	−71.395	1.503	2151	21.51
M^{pro}–**3**	1.713	−50.468	5524	55.24
	6.430	−46.903	5726	57.26
M^{pro}–**6**	34.503	34.145	8389	83.89
M^{pro}–**8**	7.810	45.191	5881	58.81
	136.017	−19.440	9146	91.46
M^{pro}–**10**	28.891	3.061	7158	71.58
M^{pro}–**11**	−89.371	−31.716	1634	16.34
	−86.385	−25.418	1737	17.37
M^{pro}–**12**	−54.007	−18.018	1135	11.35
M^{pro}–**13**	−29.833	3.606	3052	30.52
M^{pro}–**17**	27.298	−4.897	6648	66.48
	33.972	−6.394	7047	70.47
M^{pro}–**18**	−91.981	0.876	1558	15.58
M^{pro}–**28**	37.636	−1.614	7546	75.46

2.5.5. Dynamic Cross-Correlated Map Analysis

The dynamic cross-correlation matrix (DCCM) was constructed to elaborate the functional displacements of the protein's interactive atoms as a function of time. The apo–M^{pro} reflected more positive correlation motion during 100 ns of simulation, while the dominant-negative correlation motion of the loop was observed. The inhibited M^{pro} demonstrated variation in correlated motion, where maximum residues of the inhibited M^{pro} showed positive correlation motion compared to the apo–M^{pro}. The correlation motion of all the systems is graphically presented in Figure 8. The overall motions in each system are dominated by the correlated motions. In the **X77**-inhibited M^{pro}, the β1 and β2 displayed negative correlation motion and Υ4 and Υ5 loops showed positive correlation motion, while in the M^{pro}–**1** complex, Υ2, Υ3, and Υ4 reflected negative correlation motion, while β1, β2, and β4 displayed positive correlation motion. On the other hand, compounds **8**, **11**, and **18** showed negative high correlation motion in loops Υ3, Υ4, and Υ5, while the β1, β2, β3, and β4 regions acquired apparent positive correlation motion. The compounds **6**, **10**, and **13** showed similar patterns as compared to the apo–M^{pro}, while they displayed insignificant positive correlation motion in Υ4 and Υ5 and negative correlation motion at β1 to β2. However, compound **17** did not show significant positive correlation motion in Υ3, Υ4, and β4 regions of M^{pro}. Furthermore, compound **28** showed a weak negative correlation motion in β1 and Υ1 regions, and slight positive correlation motion at β4. Hence, the internal dynamics of the protein have substitution effects upon ligand binding with the protein. The results indicate that dynamic variability and conformational changes were caused by small inhibitors, therefore revealing the affinity of ligands toward M^{pro}.

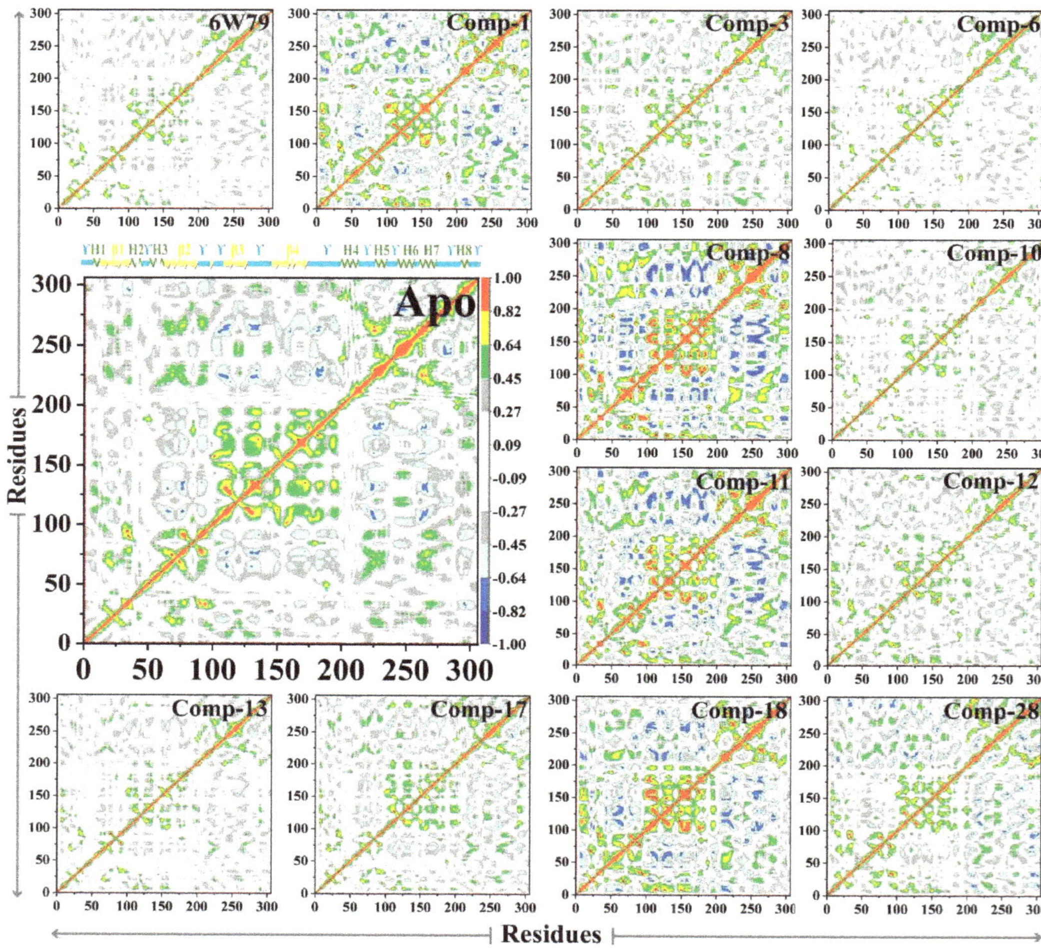

Figure 8. The DCCM plot of apo– and inhibited states of M^{pro} is shown. The positive (green, yellow, and red) and the negative correlation motion (dark blue, light blue, and cyan) are shown in different colors. The incline in color (from one to another) indicates a slow decline in the correlation motion.

2.5.6. Binding Free Energy Calculations

The binding free energy of each ligand was estimated to quantitatively compare the energy differences of the selected hits (from the in-house database) with **X77**. The binding free energy was computed from the last 1000 frames of the 100 ns of MD trajectory. MM-GBSA analysis was performed for each system by calculating each contributing energy, such as van der Waals (ΔVDW), total electrostatic energy (ΔEET), polar and non-polar contributions (ΔEGB), and non-polar solvation energy (SASA) (Table 2). The MM-GBSA results showed variation in energies among **X77** and the eleven molecules. The effect is high in terms of total and electrostatic energies. The reference inhibitor, **X77**, exhibited ΔVDW (−46.7396 Kcal/mol), ΔEEL (−7.2011 Kcal/mol), ΔEGB (22.3537 Kcal/mol), and ΔSASA (−5.6612), with the total energy (ΔG_{TOTAL}) of −37.2483 Kcal/mol, while compounds **11** and **28** reflected total energies of −33.6485 and −33.6723 Kcal/mol, respectively, which varies slightly from **X77**, with a decrease in the ΔVDW (compound **11** = −39.9829, comp. **28** = −41.1238 Kcal/mol) and an increase in the ΔEEL (compound **11** = −15.1839, compound **28** = −7.7362 Kcal/mol). Both **11** and **28** exhibited the highest binding free energy among the eleven hits. Furthermore, compounds **3**, **8**, and **18** showed ΔG_{TOTAL} of −26.9034 Kcal/mol, −26.5848 and −24.7101 Kcal/mol, respectively, which reflects the good affinity of these compounds for M^{pro}. Compounds **1**, **3**, and **17** also showed appropriate binding potential with M^{pro} by making stable complexes with ΔG_{TOTAL} of −22.7848 Kcal/mol, −22.9067 Kcal/mol, and −22.0295 Kcal/mol, respectively. However, compounds **10** and **13** reflected the lowest total binding free energies (compound **10** = −6.4968 Kcal/mol and **13** = −9.4012 Kcal/mol) due to poor binding interactions within the active site of M^{pro}.

Table 2. The MMGBSA analysis of **X77** and eleven hits for M^{pro}.

Complex Name	Kcal/mol				
	Δ_{VDW}	Δ_{EEL}	Δ_{EGB}	Δ_{SASA}	$\Delta_{G\ TOTAL}$
M^{pro}–**X77**	−46.7396	−7.2011	22.3537	−5.6612	−37.2483
M^{pro}–**1**	−27.9473	−11.8236	20.6925	−3.7064	−22.7848
M^{pro}–**3**	−36.3657	−28.7266	43.2732	−5.0843	−26.9034
M^{pro}–**6**	−34.5680	−15.4295	31.3375	−4.2467	−22.9067
M^{pro}–**8**	−41.0277	−15.6216	36.141	−6.0766	−26.5848
M^{pro}–**10**	−10.8292	−5.7753	11.5464	−1.4387	−6.4968
M^{pro}–**11**	−39.9829	−15.1839	25.9731	−4.4549	−33.6485
M^{pro}–**12**	−25.5687	−13.1445	22.4730	−3.8878	−20.1279
M^{pro}–**13**	−15.3599	−5.7322	13.8263	−2.135	−9.4012
M^{pro}–**17**	−25.1406	−18.6810	25.3125	−3.5204	−22.0295
M^{pro}–**18**	−33.2958	−9.3268	22.2269	−4.3144	−24.7101
M^{pro}–**28**	−41.1238	−7.7362	19.6643	−4.4767	−33.6723

The ΔSASA energy of compound **8** was significantly higher than the M^{pro}–**X77** complex, indicating that **8** has greater impact on the structure of the protein. The total energies of compounds **1**, **3**, **6**, **8**, **11–12**, **17–18**, and **28** indicate that these compounds exhibit inhibitory potential by specifically binding with the active site of the SARS-CoV-2 M^{pro}.

3. Materials and Methods

3.1. Preparation of Protein's Structures for Docking

The re-docking and cross-docking experiments were carried out in order to examine the efficiency of the docking method. For re-docking, twenty protein–ligand complexes were taken from Research Collaboratory for Structural Bioinformatics Protein databank (RCSB-PDB). The complexes were chosen based on good resolution (<2.5 Å, Table S11). Only water molecules within the 3 Å of co-crystallized ligand molecule were retained in the protein files, while the rest were removed. Moreover, other heteroatoms (other than ligands) were also deleted from each file. The protein files were imported in MOE interface [48], where proteins were prepared for docking by adding hydrogen atoms and molecular charges using MOE Protonate 3D tool. Each protein was parameterized by MOE Potential setup using Amber12:EHT force field.

Preparation of Compound Database for Docking

For re-docking and cross-docking, the ligands were extracted from the selected proteins (Table S11), their atom types were corrected, hydrogen atoms were added and partial charges were applied using MOE Potential setup (Amber12:EHT force field) [48,49]. Subsequently, each ligand was minimized with Amber12:EHT force field (eps = r, and Cutoff (8, 10)) with RMS gradient of 0.1kcal/mol/Å. Each ligand was imported into MOE database for re-docking, cross-docking, and virtual screening experiments. For virtual screening, the chemical entities were collected from our institute (Natural and Medical Sciences Research Center, University of Nizwa, Oman) [50], which has a diverse set of compounds, originating from natural and synthetic sources. Virtual screening was conducted on our in-house molecular database, comprising >800 chemical compounds. The structures of compounds in the library are given in SMILE format in the Supplementary Materials. Moreover, fifteen known inhibitors (**KIs**) were also added in our in-house database as positive controls (Table S11). The 3D-structure of each ligand (in mol2 format) was imported into MOE compound database, where Wash module of MOE was used to add hydrogen atoms and partial charges (based on Amber12:EHT force field) on each structure, and the structures were minimized with the same parameters as discussed above.

3.2. *Structure-Based Screening by Molecular Docking*

After the preparation of protein and ligand files, molecular docking was performed by Triangle Matcher docking algorithm and London dG scoring function [48,51,52]. The active site/ligand binding site was defined on the co-crystallized ligand in each protein. For re-docking, the ligands were extracted from each protein and re-docked in its cognate binding protein (with the above-mentioned settings), and the results were quantified by calculating root mean square deviation (RMSD) between the docked and X-ray conformation of each ligand. Similarly, cross-docking was performed by docking all the twenty (extracted) ligands in each of twenty proteins and results were examined by ranking (at top position) of compounds in their native X-ray crystal structure. By default, thirty docked conformations of each ligand were obtained. The virtual screening of in-house database was performed on those PDB files that displayed good results in cross-docking experiment.

Analysis Measures and Conformational Sampling after Virtual Screening

The inhibitor with the most potential against SARS-CoV-2 M^{pro} was chosen after virtual screening by consensus approach. The in-house library was docked in eight protein structures individually. Later, each docked library was sorted based on the docking score, and those compounds that were ranked mutually in 'Top-100' position in at least 50% of the structures were declared as potential 'Hits'. The optimal binding modes of the selected compounds were chosen through conformational sampling. The docked orientation of each compound found analogous in all the proteins was considered as the possible binding mode. The interactions of ligand were visualized by Protein–Ligand Interaction Fingerprints (PLIF) [48] of MOE, which calculates several types of interactions between protein and ligands including H-bonds, water-mediated protein–ligand bridging, ionic interactions, surface contacts, metal ligation, and arene attraction in 2D format.

3.3. *Prediction of Pharmacokinetic Properties*

After virtual screening, the pharmacokinetic (ADMET: absorption, distribution, metabolism, excretion, and toxicity) behavior of the selected compounds was studied through SwissADME [37] and admetSAR [38], which predicts ADMET properties and drug-likeness of small molecules by using physicochemical descriptors.

3.4. *Molecular Dynamic Simulation*

The atomic coordinates of PDB ID: 6W79 [47] were chosen for the molecular dynamic simulation studies. Thirteen systems were generated for MD simulation, including apo form of 6W79 (apo–M^{pro}), 6W79 in complex with co-crystallized ligand (M^{pro}–**X77**), and 6W79 in complex with docked conformations of eleven hits. The apo–M^{pro} and M^{pro}–**X77** complex were used as positive controls. The possible overlaps/clashes in the initial structure were eliminated by minimizing the structure with 10,000 cycles of steepest descent [53] (macromolecule was frozen), followed by 20,000 cycles of conjugate gradient method [54]. LEaP module of AMBER20 [55] was used to add the missing hydrogen atoms. To keep the systems neutral, counter-ions from OPC model [56] were added. A truncated octahedral box of the OPC water model [57] was added to all the systems with a 10 Å buffer (8 Å cut-off was used to compute the pairwise interactions, the van der Waals, and direct Coulomb forces). Long-range electrostatic forces were treated with the particle mesh Ewald (PME) algorithm [58]. The intermolecular interactions were calculated by ff19SB [59]. In preparation runs, Langevin thermostat [60] was used with 1 ps^{-1} friction constant, while

Berendsen thermostat [61] was used in the production runs. MD simulation was accelerated using the PMEMD CUDA version in GPU cores. Before running MD production, all the systems were heated for 400 ps, followed by equilibration of up to 2000 ps in the NVT ensemble at 300 K. The conditions applied in the simulation of all systems are given in Table 3.

Table 3. The conditions used in the molecular dynamics of apo– and inhibited states of M^{pro}.

S. No.	System Composition (Complexes)	Temperature (K)	Force Fields	Water Model	Time (ns)
1	Full length apo–M^{pro}	300	FF19SB	Octahedral OPC	100
2	M^{pro}–**X77** (6W79)	300	FF19SB+Gaff2	Octahedral OPC	100
3	M^{pro}–**1**	300	FF19SB+Gaff2	Octahedral OPC	100
4	M^{pro}–**3**	300	FF19SB+Gaff2	Octahedral OPC	100
5	M^{pro}–**6**	300	FF19SB+Gaff2	Octahedral OPC	100
6	M^{pro}–**8**	300	FF19SB+Gaff2	Octahedral OPC	100
7	M^{pro}–**10**	300	FF19SB+Gaff2	Octahedral OPC	100
8	M^{pro}–**11**	300	FF19SB+Gaff2	Octahedral OPC	100
9	M^{pro}–**12**	300	FF19SB+Gaff2	Octahedral OPC	100
10	M^{pro}–**13**	300	FF19SB+Gaff2	Octahedral OPC	100
11	M^{pro}–**17**	300	FF19SB+Gaff2	Octahedral OPC	100
12	M^{pro}–**18**	300	FF19SB+Gaff2	Octahedral OPC	100
13	M^{pro}–**28**	300	FF19SB+Gaff2	Octahedral OPC	100

3.4.1. Post-Dynamic Evaluation

The coordinates of all the simulated systems were extracted from the generated trajectories after every 1 ps and analyzed by PTRAJ [62] module of the AMBER20. The Root Mean Square Deviation (RMSD), Root Mean Square Fluctuation (RMSF), and radius of gyration (Rg) of all the systems were calculated by CPPTRAJ module of AMBER20 on Cα atoms via Equations (1)–(3).

$$\mathrm{RMSD} = \sqrt{\frac{\sum_{i=0}^{N}[m_i * (X_i - Y_i)^2]}{M}} \quad (1)$$

In RMSD calculation, N = the number of atoms, mi = the mass of atoms, Xi = the target atom i vector coordinate, Yi = the reference atom i vector coordinate, and M = the total mass.

$$\mathrm{RMSF(i)} = \sqrt{\langle (x_i - \langle x_i \rangle)^2 \rangle} \quad (2)$$

The RMSF of selected atom i was calculated as: the atomic positions averages over the total input frames (denoted by x).

$$\mathrm{Rg} = \sqrt{\frac{1}{N}\sum_{N}^{i=0}(r_i - r_m)^2} \quad (3)$$

The Rg of N number of atoms was calculated: the atomic position was denoted by ri, and the mean position was denoted by r_m of all the atoms. The Altona and Sundaralingam method [63] was used to calculate the five-membered ring pucker. Standard deviation and averages were reported in the analysis utilities, with proper cyclic averages being computed for periodic values (torsions). Furthermore, the total energy of all the systems (apo– and inhibited states) was calculated.

3.4.2. MD Trajectories Unsupervised Clustering and Free Energy Landscape

Principal component analysis (PCA, focuses on matrix covariance) was used to demonstrate atom movement and protein loop dynamics. The internal motions of the systems were analyzed by PCA approach of CPPTRAJ. The atomic coordinates of eigenvectors and the positional covariance matrix were calculated. The orthogonal coordinate transformation was used to obtain the eigenvalue diagonal matrix by the diagonalizing of the matrix. The principal components were obtained based on eigenvalues and eigenvectors to emphasize the motion of the atoms in MD simulation trajectories. The isolated first principal components, PC1 and PC2, showing the largest variation in the data, were utilized for the free energy landscape (FEL) using Equation (4) from 100 bins of the data population The energies were calculated in kcal/mol at 300 ∘K.

$$G_i = -K_B T\left(\frac{N_i}{N_{Max}}\right) \tag{4}$$

where K_B = Boltzmann's constant, T = specified temperature, N_i = bin_i population, and N_{Max} = most populated bins. The artificial barrier population size of 0.5 was applied to the bins with no population.

3.4.3. Dynamic Cross-Correlation Analysis (DCC)

The dynamic cross-correlation map (DCCM) method was used to obtain the Cα atom's time subordinate movements caused by the attachment of a small molecule (inhibitor) with the protein. The correlation matrix was derived by observing the Cα atoms' correlated and anti-correlated motions of each system. DCCM was calculated by Equation (5).

$$C_{ij} = \langle \Delta r_i \times \Delta r_j \rangle / \left(\langle \Delta r_i^2 \rangle \langle \Delta r_j^2 \rangle\right)^2 \tag{5}$$

where C_{ij} = time correlated data between the atoms i and j in a protein. We used 0.002 ns interval to construct the matrix of Cα from the 10,000 snapshots. The positive and negative values indicate the correlated and anti-correlated motion during the MD simulation, respectively, in the matrix plot.

3.4.4. MM/GBSA Free Energy Calculation

In MD simulation, free energy calculations give quantitative production of protein–ligand binding energies. The binding energy (G_{bind}) was calculated by Equation (6).

$$G_{bind} = G_{R+L} - (G_R + G_L) \tag{6}$$

where G_{R+L} represents the M^{pro} in complex with inhibitors, while G_R and G_L represent the apo–M^{pro} and inhibited M^{pro}, respectively.

In the generalized born surface area (MM/GBSA) approach, each free energy term in Equation (6) was calculated using Equation (7).

$$G = E_{bond} + E_{VDW} + E_{elec} + G_{GB} + G_{SA} - TS_S \tag{7}$$

where E_{bond} represents bond angles and dihedral energy, E_{vdw} and E_{elec} indicate the contribution of van der Waals and electrostatic energy, respectively, while the related polar and non-polar contribution of solvation energy are reported as G_{GB} and G_{SA}. T and S_s show the absolute temperature of the system and the solute entropy, respectively.

The performance of the MMGBSA algorithm is based on the specificity of the forcefield and inhibitor's partial charges, the specificity of protein–inhibitor complex, MD simulation, inner dielectric constant, and the docking pose number based on top scoring. Here, the binding free energies of each system were calculated by MM/PB(GB)SA model of GBSA. The solvent probe of 2 Å radius was used, and the radii were used to optimize the topology files.

3.4.5. Data Analysis

The results were analyzed by MOE [48], UCSF Chimera [64], and Pymol [65]. The average structures were extracted from structure ensembles of the lowest energy. All the analysis graphs were plotted using Origin pro [66] and GnuPlot [67].

4. Conclusions

The main protease or chymotrypsin-like protease of SARS-CoV-2 is considered to be a potential anti-viral drug target. We have employed an efficient structure-based virtual screening protocol to search for novel inhibitors of SARS-CoV-2. The binding potential of several compounds was tested on multiple structures of M^{pro}, and consensus strategy was applied to select the most promising binders. Based on the physiological and pharmacokinetic behavior and protein–ligand binding pattern, eleven compounds were identified as good inhibitors of M^{pro}. Therefore, the structural and dynamic behavior of M^{pro} upon binding with those eleven compounds was further explored through molecular dynamic simulation. Based on the MM-GBSA calculations, two compounds (**11** and **28**) were retrieved with the highest binding affinities for M^{pro}, whereas six compounds (**3**, **8**, **18**, **6**, **1**, and **17**) showed good binding affinities for M^{pro}. Based on our in silico findings, we suggest that these compounds can inhibit the replication of SARS-CoV-2 by specifically inhibiting its M^{pro} enzyme. Therefore, these compounds can act as potential anti-viral candidates against SARS-CoV-2. However, further in vitro testing is required to confirm these in silico results.

Supplementary Materials: The following are available online at https://www.mdpi.com/article/10.3390/ph14090896/s1, Table S1: Re-docking results of MOE, Table S2: The cross-docking analysis of MOE, Calculation of Enrichment Factor (EF) and %EF, Table S3: % Enrichment Factor and AUC of VS, Figure S1: The receiver operating characteristic (ROC) curve of MOE on eight proteins, Table S4: Docking scores and rank of selected hits, Figure S2: The chemical structures of compounds 1–30, Table S5: Physicochemical properties of selected hits (1–30), Table S6: Solubility of selected hits (1–30), Table S7: Pharmacokinetic properties of selected hits, Table S8: Drug-likeness and medicinal properties of selected hits (1–30), Table S9: The ADMET results of admetSAR server, Table S10: Interaction analysis of selected hits (1–30), Table S11. Protein–ligand complexes used in re-docking and cross-docking. The structures of compounds in the in-house library are given in SMILE format in the Supplementary Materials.

Author Contributions: Conceptualization, S.A.H., A.K. and A.A.-H.; methodology, S.A.H. and M.W.; software, S.A.H. and M.W.; validation, S.A.H. and M.W.; formal analysis, S.A.H. and M.W.; investigation, A.K. and A.A.-H.; resources, A.K. and A.A.-H.; data curation, S.A.H. and M.W.; writing—original draft preparation, S.A.H. and M.W.; writing—review and editing, A.K. and A.A.-H.; visualization, S.A.H. and M.W.; supervision, A.K. and A.A.-H.; project administration, A.K. and A.A.-H.; funding acquisition, A.K. and A.A.-H. All authors have read and agreed to the published version of the manuscript.

Funding: The project was supported by a grant from The Oman Research Council (TRC) through the funded project (BFP/RGP/CBS/19/220).

Institutional Review Board Statement: Not applicable.

Informed Consent Statement: Not applicable.

Data Availability Statement: All the data are included in this paper.

Conflicts of Interest: The authors declare no conflict of interest.

References

1. Li, Q.; Guan, X.; Wu, P.; Wang, X.; Zhou, L.; Tong, Y.; Ren, R.; Leung, K.S.M.; Lau, E.H.Y.; Wong, J.Y.; et al. Early Transmission Dynamics in Wuhan, China, of Novel Coronavirus–Infected Pneumonia. *N. Engl. J. Med.* **2020**, *382*, 1199–1207. [CrossRef]
2. Zhu, N.; Zhang, D.; Wang, W.; Li, X.; Yang, B.; Song, J.; Zhao, X.; Huang, B.; Shi, W.; Lu, R.; et al. A novel coronavirus from patients with pneumonia in China, 2019. *N. Engl. J. Med.* **2020**, *382*, 727–733. [CrossRef] [PubMed]
3. Dong, E.; Du, H.; Gardner, L. An interactive web-based dashboard to track COVID-19 in real time. *Lancet Infect. Dis.* **2020**, *20*, 533–534. [CrossRef]
4. Wang, C.; Horby, P.W.; Hayden, F.G.; Gao, G.F. A novel coronavirus outbreak of global health concern. *Lancet* **2020**, *395*, 470–473. [CrossRef]
5. Wu, F.; Zhao, S.; Yu, B.; Chen, Y.-M.; Wang, W.; Song, Z.-G.; Hu, Y.; Tao, Z.-W.; Tian, J.-H.; Pei, Y.-Y.; et al. A new coronavirus associated with human respiratory disease in China. *Nature* **2020**, *579*, 265–269. [CrossRef]

6. Chen, Y.; Liu, Q.; Guo, D. Emerging coronaviruses: Genome structure, replication, and pathogenesis. *J. Med. Virol.* **2020**, *92*, 418–423. [CrossRef] [PubMed]
7. WHO Coronavirus (COVID-19) Dashboard. Available online: https://covid19.who.int/ (accessed on 30 June 2021).
8. Monitoring Knowledge, Risk Perceptions, Preventive Behaviours, and Public Trust in the Current Coronavirus Outbreak in Georgia Analytical Report of the First, Second and Third Wave Studies, WHO Report. May 2020, pp. 1–61. Available online: www.unicef.org/georgia/media/4736/file/COVID-19-Study-Analytical-Report-1-st-2nd-and-3rd-waves-Eng.pdf (accessed on 15 May 2021).
9. Taboada, M.; González, M.; Alvarez, A.; Eiras, M.; Costa, J.; Álvarez, J.; Seoane-Pillado, T. First, second and third wave of COVID-19. What have we changed in the ICU management of these patients? *J. Infect.* **2021**, *82*, e14–e15. [CrossRef] [PubMed]
10. V'kovski, P.; Kratzel, A.; Steiner, S.; Stalder, H.; Thiel, V. Coronavirus biology and replication: Implications for SARS-CoV-2. *Nat. Rev. Microbiol.* **2021**, *19*, 155–170. [CrossRef] [PubMed]
11. Romano, M.; Ruggiero, A.; Squeglia, F.; Maga, G.; Berisio, R. A Structural View of SARS-CoV-2 RNA Replication Machinery: RNA Synthesis, Proofreading and Final Capping. *Cells* **2020**, *9*, 1267. [CrossRef]
12. Pal, M.; Berhanu, G.; Desalegn, C.; Kandi, V. Severe Acute Respiratory Syndrome Coronavirus 2 (SARS-CoV-2): An Update. *Cureus* **2020**, *12*, e7423. [CrossRef]
13. Mousavizadeh, L.; Ghasemi, S. Genotype and phenotype of COVID-19: Their roles in pathogenesis. *J. Microbiol. Immunol. Inf.* **2021**, *54*, 159–163. [CrossRef] [PubMed]
14. Asghari, A.; Naseri, M.; Safari, H.; Saboory, E.; Parsamanesh, N. The novel insight of SARS-CoV-2 molecular biology and pathogenesis and therapeutic options. *DNA Cell Biol.* **2020**, *39*, 1741–1753. [CrossRef] [PubMed]
15. Li, F. Structure, function, and evolution of Coronavirus spike proteins. *Annu. Rev. Virol.* **2016**, *3*, 237–261. [CrossRef]
16. Artika, I.M.; Dewantari, A.K.; Wiyatno, A. Molecular biology of coronaviruses: Current knowledge. *Heliyon* **2020**, *6*, e04743. [CrossRef]
17. Alsobaie, S. Understanding the molecular biology of SARS-CoV2 and the COVID-19 pandemic: A Review. *Infect. Drug Res.* **2021**, *14*, 2259–2268. [CrossRef]
18. Ali, M.J.; Hanif, M.; Haider, M.A.; Ahmed, M.U.; Sundas, F.N.U.; Hirani, A.; Khan, I.A.; Anis, K.; Karim, A.H. Treatment options for COVID-19: A review. *Front. Med.* **2020**, *7*, 480. [CrossRef]
19. Ullrich, S.; Nitsche, C. The SARS-CoV-2 main protease as drug target. *Bioorg. Med. Chem. Lett.* **2020**, *30*, 127377. [CrossRef]
20. Masters, P.S. The molecular biology of coronaviruses. *Adv. Virus Res.* **2006**, *66*, 193–292. [PubMed]
21. Beigel, J.H.; Tomashek, K.M.; Dodd, L.E.; Mehta, A.K.; Zingman, B.S.; Kalil, A.C.; Hohmann, E.; Chu, H.Y.; Luetkemeyer, A.; Kline, S.; et al. Remdesivir for the treatment of Covid-19—Final report. *N. Engl. J. Med.* **2020**, *383*, 1813–1826. [CrossRef]
22. Ferner, R.E.; Aronson, J.K. Chloroquine and hydroxychloroquine in covid-19: Use of these drugs is premature and potentially harmful. *BMJ* **2020**, *369*, m1432. [CrossRef] [PubMed]
23. Shah, R.R. Chloroquine and hydroxychloroquine for COVID-19: Perspectives on their failure in repurposing. *J. Clin. Pharm. Ther.* **2021**, *46*, 17–27. [CrossRef]
24. Samaee, H.; Mohsenzadegan, M.; Ala, S.; Maroufi, S.S.; Moradimaj, P. Tocilizumab for treatment patients with COVID-19: Recommended medication for novel disease. *Int. Immunopharmacol.* **2020**, *89*, 107018. [CrossRef]
25. Rosas, I.O.; Bräu, N.; Waters, M.; Go, R.C.; Hunter, B.D.; Bhagani, S.; Skiest, D.; Aziz, M.S.; Cooper, N.; Douglas, I.S.; et al. Tocilizumab inh patients with severe Covid-19 pneumonia. *N. Engl. J. Med.* **2021**, *384*, 1503–1516. [CrossRef]
26. Cao, B.; Wang, Y.; Wen, D.; Liu, W.; Wang, J.; Fan, G.; Ruan, L.; Song, B.; Cai, Y.; Wei, M.; et al. A trial of Lopinavir–Ritonavir in adults hospitalized with severe Covid-19. *N. Engl. J. Med.* **2020**, *382*, 1787–1799. [CrossRef] [PubMed]
27. Shaffer, L. 15 Drugs Being Tested to Treat COVID-19 and How They Would Work. *Nat. Med.* 2020. Available online: www.nature.com/articles/d41591-020-00019-9 (accessed on 20 May 2021).
28. Sanders, J.M.; Monogue, M.L.; Jodlowski, T.Z.; Cutrell, J.B. Pharmacologic treatments for Coronavirus disease 2019 (COVID-19), A review. *JAMA* **2020**, *323*, 1824–1836. [PubMed]
29. Costanzo, M.; De Giglio, M.A.R.; Roviello, G.N. Anti-Coronavirus Vaccines: Past Investigations on SARS-CoV-1 and MERS-CoV, the Approved Vaccines from BioNTech/Pfizer, Moderna, Oxford/AstraZeneca and others under Development Against SARSCoV-2 Infection. *Curr. Med. Chem.* **2021**, *28*. [CrossRef] [PubMed]
30. Roviello, V.; Musumeci, D.; Mokhir, A.; Roviello, G.N. Evidence of Protein Binding by a Nucleopeptide Based on a Thyminedecorated L-Diaminopropanoic Acid through CD and In Silico Studies. *Curr. Med. Chem.* **2021**, *28*. [CrossRef]
31. Vicidomini, C.; Roviello, V.; Roviello, G.N. In Silico Investigation on the Interaction of Chiral Phytochemicals from Opuntia ficus-indica with SARS-CoV-2 Mpro. *Symmetry* **2021**, *13*, 1041. [CrossRef]
32. Rut, W.; Groborz, K.; Zhang, L.; Sun, X.; Zmudzinski, M.; Pawlik, B.; Wang, X.; Jochmans, D.; Neyts, J.; Młynarski, W.; et al. SARS-CoV-2 M pro inhibitors and activity based probes for patient-sample imaging. *Nat. Chem. Biol.* **2021**, *17*, 222–228. [CrossRef]
33. Zhang, L.; Lin, D.; Sun, X.; Curth, U.; Drosten, C.; Sauerhering, L.; Becker, S.; Rox, K.; Hilgenfeld, R. Crystal structure of SARS-CoV-2 main protease provides a basis for design of improved α-Ketoamide inhibitors. *Science* **2020**, *368*, 409–412. [CrossRef]
34. Jin, Z.; Du, X.; Xu, Y.; Deng, Y.; Liu, M.; Zhao, Y.; Zhang, B.; Li, X.; Zhang, L.; Peng, C.; et al. Structure of M pro from SARS-CoV-2 and discovery of its inhibitors. *Nature* **2020**, *582*, 289–293. [CrossRef]
35. Paasche, A.; Zipper, A.; Schäfer, S.; Ziebuhr, J.; Schirmeister, T.; Engels, B. Evidence for substrate binding-induced zwitterion formation in the catalytic Cys-His dyad of the SARS-CoV main protease. *Biochemistry* **2014**, *53*, 5930–5946. [CrossRef]

36. Dai, W.; Zhang, B.; Jiang, X.-M.; Su, H.; Li, J.; Zhao, Y.; Xie, X.; Jin, Z.; Peng, J.; Liu, F.; et al. Structure-Based design of antiviral drug candidates targeting the SARS-CoV-2 main protease. *Science* **2020**, *368*, 1331–1335. [CrossRef]
37. Daina, A.; Michielin, O.; Zoete, V. SwissADME: A free web tool to evaluate pharmacokinetics, drug-likeness and medicinal chemistry friendliness of small molecules. *Sci. Rep.* **2017**, *7*, 42717. [CrossRef] [PubMed]
38. Cheng, F.; Li, W.; Zhou, Y.; Shen, J.; Wu, Z.; Liu, G.; Lee, P.W.; Tang, Y. admetSAR: A Comprehensive Source and Free Tool for Assessment of Chemical ADMET Properties. *J. Chem. Inf. Model.* **2012**, *52*, 3099–3105. [CrossRef] [PubMed]
39. Veber, D.F.; Johnson, S.R.; Cheng, H.Y.; Smith, B.R.; Ward, K.W.; Kopple, K.D. Molecular properties that influence the oral bioavailability of drug candidates. *J. Med. Chem.* **2002**, *45*, 2615–2623. [CrossRef]
40. Maple, H.J.; Clayden, N.; Baron, A.; Stacey, C.; Felix, R. Developing degraders: Principles and perspectives on design and chemical space. *MedChemComm* **2019**, *10*, 1755–1764. [CrossRef]
41. Lipinski, C.A. Lead- and drug-like compounds: The rule-of-five revolution. *Drug Discov. Today Technol.* **2004**, *1*, 337–341. [CrossRef] [PubMed]
42. Ghose, A.K.; Viswanadhan, V.N.; Wendoloski, J.J. A knowledge-based approach in designing combinatorial or medicinal chemistry libraries for drug discovery. 1. A qualitative and quantitative characterization of known drug databases. *J. Comb. Chem.* **1999**, *1*, 55–68. [CrossRef]
43. Egan, W.J.; Walters, W.P.; Murcko, M.A. Guiding molecules towards drug-likeness. *Curr. Opin. Drug Disc. Dev.* **2002**, *5*, 540–549.
44. Muegge, I.; Heald, S.L.; Brittelli, D. Simple Selection Criteria for Drug-like Chemical Matter. *J. Med. Chem.* **2001**, *44*, 1841–1846. [CrossRef] [PubMed]
45. Bickerton, G.R.; Paolini, G.V.; Besnard, J.; Muresan, S.; Hopkins, A.L. Quantifying the chemical beauty of drugs. *Nat. Chem.* **2012**, *4*, 90–98. [CrossRef]
46. Pathania, S.; Singh, P.K. Analyzing FDA-approved drugs for compliance of pharmacokinetic principles: Should there be a critical screening parameter in drug designing protocols? *Exp. Opin. Drug Metab. Toxicol.* **2021**, *17*, 351–354. [CrossRef]
47. Mesecar, A. A taxonomically driven approach to development of potent, broad-spectrum inhibitors of coronavirus main protease including SARS-CoV-2 (COVID-19). Unpublished work. 2020.
48. *Molecular Operating Environment Version 2014.09*; Chemical Computing Group: Montreal, QC, Canada, 2014.
49. Case, D.A.; Darden, T.A.; Cheatham, T.E.; Simmerling, C.L., III; Wang, J.; Duke, R.E.; Luo, R.; Walker, R.C.; Zhang, W.; Merz, K.M.; et al. *AMBER 12*; University of California: San Francisco, CA, USA, 2012.
50. Available online: https://www.unizwa.edu.om/index.php?contentid=1038 (accessed on 5 January 2021).
51. Edelsbrunner, H. *Weighted Alpha Shapes*; Report UIUCDCS-R-92-1760; Department of Computer Science, University of Illinois, Urbana Champagne: Champaign, IL, USA, 1992.
52. Naïm, M.; Bhat, S.; Rankin, K.N.; Dennis, S.; Chowdhury, S.F.; Siddiqi, I.; Drabik, P.; Sulea, T.; Bayly, C.I.; Jakalian, A.; et al. Solvated interaction energy (SIE) for scoring protein-ligand binding affinities. 1. Exploring the parameter space. *J. Chem. Inf. Model.* **2007**, *47*, 122–133. [CrossRef] [PubMed]
53. Fletcher, R.; Powell, M.J. A rapidly convergent descent method for minimization. *Comput. J.* **1963**, *6*, 163–168. [CrossRef]
54. Shewchuk, J.R. *An Introduction to the Conjugate Gradient Method without the Agonizing Pain*; Department of Computer Science, Carnegie-Mellon University: Pittsburgh, PA, USA, 1994.
55. Case, D.A.; Aktulga, H.M.; Belfon, K.; Ben-Shalom, I.Y.; Brozell, S.R.; Cerutti, D.S.; Cheatham, T.E.; Cruzeiro, V.W.D., III; Darden, T.A.; Duke, R.E. *Amber 2021*; University of California: San Francisco, CA, USA, 2021.
56. Sengupta, A.; Li, Z.; Song, L.F.; Li, P.; Merz, K.M., Jr. Parameterization of Monovalent Ions for the OPC3, OPC, TIP3P-FB, and TIP4P-FB Water Models. *J. Chem. Inf. Model.* **2021**, *61*, 869–880. [CrossRef] [PubMed]
57. Izadi, S.; Anandakrishnan, R.; Onufriev, A.V. Building water models: A different approach. *J. Phys. Chem. Lett.* **2014**, *5*, 3863–3871. [CrossRef]
58. Allaire, G.; Dapogny, C.; Frey, P. A mesh evolution algorithm based on the level set method for geometry and topology optimization. *Struct. Multidiscip. Optim.* **2013**, *48*, 711–715. [CrossRef]
59. Tian, C.; Kasavajhala, K.; Belfon, K.A.A.; Raguette, L.; Huang, H.; Migues, A.N.; Bickel, J.; Wang, Y.; Pincay, J.; Wu, Q.; et al. ff19SB: Amino-acid-specific protein backbone parameters trained against quantum mechanics energy surfaces in solution. *J. Chem. Theory Comput.* **2020**, *16*, 528–552. [CrossRef]
60. Davidchack, R.L.; Handel, R.; Tretyakov, M. Langevin thermostat for rigid body dynamics. *J. Chem. Phys.* **2009**, *130*, 234101. [CrossRef]
61. Hunenberger, P.H. Thermostat algorithms for molecular dynamics simulations. *Adv. Polym. Sci.* **2005**, *173*, 105–149.
62. Roe, D.R.; Cheatham, T.E., III. PTRAJ and CPPTRAJ: Software for processing and analysis of molecular dynamics trajectory data. *J. Chem. Theory Comput.* **2013**, *9*, 3084–3095. [CrossRef] [PubMed]
63. Altona, C.T.; Sundaralingam, M. Conformational analysis of the sugar ring in nucleosides and nucleotides. New description using the concept of pseudo rotation. *J. Am. Chem. Soc.* **1972**, *94*, 8205–8212.
64. Pettersen, E.F.; Goddard, T.D.; Huang, C.C.; Couch, G.S.; Greenblatt, D.M.; Meng, E.C.; Ferrin, T.E.J. UCSF Chimera- A visualization system for exploratory research and analysis. *Comput. Chem.* **2004**, *13*, 1605–1612. [CrossRef] [PubMed]
65. *The PyMOL Molecular Graphics System, Version 2.0*; Schrödinger, LLC.: New York, NY, USA. Available online: https://pymol.org/ (accessed on 15 March 2021).

66. Origin (Pro), OriginLab Corporation, Northampton, Massachusetts, United States of America. 2021. Available online: www.originlab.com (accessed on 15 March 2021).
67. Williams, T.; Kelley, C. Gnuplot 5.4, An Interactive Plotting Program, User Manual. 2020. Available online: www.gnuplot.info (accessed on 15 March 2021).

pharmaceuticals MDPI

Article

Predicting the Skin Sensitization Potential of Small Molecules with Machine Learning Models Trained on Biologically Meaningful Descriptors

Anke Wilm [1,2], Marina Garcia de Lomana [3], Conrad Stork [1], Neann Mathai [4], Steffen Hirte [3], Ulf Norinder [5,6,7], Jochen Kühnl [8] and Johannes Kirchmair [1,3,*]

1 Center for Bioinformatics (ZBH), Department of Informatics, Universität Hamburg, 20146 Hamburg, Germany; wilm@zbh.uni-hamburg.de (A.W.); stork@zbh.uni-hamburg.de (C.S.)
2 HITeC e.V., 22527 Hamburg, Germany
3 Department of Pharmaceutical Sciences, Faculty of Life Sciences, University of Vienna, 1090 Vienna, Austria; a11853333@unet.univie.ac.at (M.G.d.L.); steffen.hirte@univie.ac.at (S.H.)
4 Computational Biology Unit (CBU), Department of Chemistry, University of Bergen, N-5020 Bergen, Norway; neann.mathai@uib.no
5 MTM Research Centre, School of Science and Technology, Örebro University, SE-70182 Örebro, Sweden; ulf.norinder@farmbio.uu.se
6 Department of Computer and Systems Sciences, Stockholm University, SE-16407 Kista, Sweden
7 Department of Pharmaceutical Biosciences, Uppsala University, SE-75124 Uppsala, Sweden
8 Front End Innovation, Beiersdorf AG, 22529 Hamburg, Germany; Jochen.Kuehnl@Beiersdorf.com
* Correspondence: johannes.kirchmair@univie.ac.at; Tel.: +43-1-4277-55104

Citation: Wilm, A.; Garcia de Lomana, M.; Stork, C.; Mathai, N.; Hirte, S.; Norinder, U.; Kühnl, J.; Kirchmair, J. Predicting the Skin Sensitization Potential of Small Molecules with Machine Learning Models Trained on Biologically Meaningful Descriptors. *Pharmaceuticals* **2021**, *14*, 790. https://doi.org/10.3390/ph14080790

Academic Editor: Osvaldo Andrade Santos-Filho

Received: 14 July 2021
Accepted: 6 August 2021
Published: 11 August 2021

Abstract: In recent years, a number of machine learning models for the prediction of the skin sensitization potential of small organic molecules have been reported and become available. These models generally perform well within their applicability domains but, as a result of the use of molecular fingerprints and other non-intuitive descriptors, the interpretability of the existing models is limited. The aim of this work is to develop a strategy to replace the non-intuitive features by predicted outcomes of bioassays. We show that such replacement is indeed possible and that as few as ten interpretable, predicted bioactivities are sufficient to reach competitive performance. On a holdout data set of 257 compounds, the best model ("Skin Doctor CP:Bio") obtained an efficiency of 0.82 and an MCC of 0.52 (at the significance level of 0.20). Skin Doctor CP:Bio is available free of charge for academic research. The modeling strategies explored in this work are easily transferable and could be adopted for the development of more interpretable machine learning models for the prediction of the bioactivity and toxicity of small organic compounds.

Keywords: skin sensitization; toxicity prediction; in silico prediction; machine learning; random forest; conformal prediction; bioactivity descriptors

1. Introduction

Substances that can induce allergic contact dermatitis after repeated contact to the skin are called skin sensitizers [1,2]. In order to prevent the induction of skin sensitization, exposure to skin sensitizers must be minimized [3–8]. The ability to detect and predict skin sensitizers is therefore of significant importance for several sectors of industry to develop safe and efficacious functional small molecules [9].

Until recent years, strategies to assess the risk of small molecules to induce skin sensitization relied on animal experiments. Historically, an important animal experiment to address skin sensitization potential is the guinea pig maximization test (GPMT), which was used to determine the percentage of test animals that develop contact allergy symptoms after repeated exposure to the test substance. Typically, a substance was classified as a sensitizer if at least 15% of the guinea pigs developed allergic symptoms. The GPMT was later replaced by the murine local lymph node assay (LLNA) [10], an animal model measuring the proliferation rate of cells in the draining lymph node in mice. The LLNA is still regarded as the gold standard among the animal experiments to assess skin sensitization potential as it provides advantages concerning animal welfare (compared to other animal models) and additional information to quantify the skin sensitization potency of compounds (based on the EC3 value, defined as the substance concentration that induces a 3-fold stimulation of proliferation) [11,12].

Ambitious efforts are ongoing to fully replace animal experiments, and a diverse set of alternative experimental and theoretical methods have been developed [13,14] to assess skin sensitization potential and, to a limited degree, skin sensitization potency [15]. Among others, these approaches include non-animal testing methods (i.e., in vitro and in chemico assays) [16–19] and in silico methods [18–21].

Several OECD-validated non-animal testing methods address three out of four key events of the adverse outcome pathway of skin sensitization induction: The first key event, or molecular initiating event, describes the so-called haptenization, which is the covalent binding of the substance to skin proteins or peptides. This is experimentally assessed by the direct peptide reactivity assay (DPRA) [22]. The second key event, which is the activation of keratinocytes [23], is covered by the KeratinoSens and LuSens assays, while the third key event, which is the activation of the skin's dendritic cells [24], is addressed, among others, by the U937 cell line activation test (U-SENS) and the human cell line activation test (h-CLAT). As all of these assays cover certain aspects of the adverse outcome pathway; none of them is suitable as a standalone methodology for the prediction of the skin sensitization potential of small molecules.

Computational methods that predict skin sensitization can be classified into expert systems, similarity-based approaches, and (quantitative) structure–activity relationship (QSAR) approaches [20]. These approaches offer fast predictions at low cost, enabling their use also in early stages of research and development, where a large number of candidate compounds may be under investigation. To be accepted as a component of regulatory risk assessment, computational methods have to fulfill certain quality criteria. For example, according to the OECD [25], a model should have a defined endpoint, an unambiguous algorithm, a defined applicability domain, appropriate measures of goodness-of–fit, robustness, and predictivity, and, if possible, a mechanistic interpretation.

No particular non-animal testing method or individual computational model has so far yielded a level of performance, robustness, interpretability, and coverage to be accepted as a standalone approach for skin sensitization prediction in the regulatory context. The most promising strategy to advance alternative testing methods is the combination of experimental and computational tools [26] within defined approaches, integrated approaches for testing and assessment (IATAs; for a review of IATAs and defined approaches see Ref. [27]), or in "weight of evidence" considerations [28].

In our previous work [29], we presented Skin Doctor CP, a random forest (RF) model for the prediction of LLNA outcomes for small molecules that complies with the above-mentioned OECD principles to the furthest possible extent. The Skin Doctor CP model is trained on a set of 1278 compounds annotated with binary LLNA outcomes (i.e., skin sensitizer and skin non-sensitizer). To the best knowledge of the authors, this data set represents the largest collection of high-quality LLNA data in the public domain at present. The data set has been characterized regarding its composition and chemical space coverage [29]. The RF model derived from this data set is wrapped into an aggregated Mondrian conformal prediction (CP) framework, which ensures predictivity and robustness by a mathematically founded measure of reliability [30–32]. More specifically, the CP framework guarantees an observed prediction error of the model close to the error rate ε set by the user (this is as long as the randomness assumption of the samples holds true; an assumption that is also made for any classical machine learning model). The CP framework will only return a predicted class membership for a substance if the prediction lies within the desired confidence level $1-\varepsilon$. The measure of reliability offered by the CP approach can guide the use of Safety

Assessment Factors of different levels and serve as a powerful, mathematically founded alternative to applicability domain definitions [33].

Depending on the available data and computational capacities, different variants of CP may be developed [34]. In the case of LLNA prediction, the data available for model development are limited and imbalanced; hence, the use of an aggregated CP framework is advised. The aggregated CP framework repeats the framework several times with different proper training and calibration sets [35]. This reduces the variance in the model predictions and allows every datapoint of the training set to be used for model development. It is therefore best suited for modeling small data sets.

To address data imbalance in addition to data scarcity (such as in the case of the LLNA data modeled in our previous study), the combination of the aggregated CP framework with Mondrian CP is advised. Mondrian CP is tailored to describe imbalanced data as it treats each of the classes independently and ensures the validity of their predictions [36–38]. This is especially beneficial in toxicity prediction, where the toxic class is usually the minority class and therefore more difficult to predict [39].

In addition to the OECD requirement for a model to produce results with defined reliability (which we address by using a CP framework), model interpretability is a further key factor to consider. Model interpretability depends on the types of descriptors employed in model building. Most of the existing models for the prediction of the skin sensitization potential of compounds, including our Skin Doctor CP models, rely on molecular fingerprints [29,40–42]. Interpreting these fingerprints can prove challenging, but in general, some links between chemical patterns and the biological outcomes can be identified [43].

In an attempt to generate predictive models from physically meaningful (and hence more intuitive) descriptors, we previously investigated the capacity of physicochemical property descriptors to produce predictive models for the prediction of the skin sensitization potential [44]. However, the models trained on physicochemical property descriptors do not perform as well as those trained on molecular fingerprints, and their interpretation is still challenging due to the high number of descriptors required to obtain models with an acceptable performance.

Recent studies have shown that in silico models for the prediction of complex in vivo endpoints can benefit from the inclusion of measured or predicted biological data (i.e., in vivo and/or in vitro data) into the feature set. More specifically, descriptive models have been built on small sets of hand-picked biological descriptors relevant to the endpoint of interest [45], as well as on large sets of screening data that may or may not be directly related to the endpoint of interest [46–50]. There are several examples of in silico models, nearest neighbor approaches in particular, that are trained on predicted bioactivities [51,52]. For example, the RASAR models [53] are RF models that predict nine health hazard endpoints (including the skin sensitization potential) based on the distances of a compound of interest to its nearest active and inactive neighbors in reference data sets for 19 toxicological outcomes. Another computational approach utilizes a reasoning framework to build an information-rich network based on assay knowledge, assay data, and predicted bioactivities [54]. The visualization of this network can provide guidance to researchers for the assessment of the safety profile of small molecules.

Recently, Norinder et al. [55] presented a CP framework that utilizes predicted bioactivities as input for in silico models for bioactivity and cytotoxicity prediction. This approach has the advantage of improving a model's predictivity by the use of bioactivity data without the need to perform additional experimental testing for a compound of interest. A similar methodological framework was successfully applied to three in vivo toxicological endpoints (i.e., genotoxicity, drug-induced liver injury, and cardiological complications) by some of us [56].

The aim of this work is to investigate the capacity of predicted bioactivities to produce simple, interpretable machine learning models for the prediction of the skin sensitization potential of small organic compounds without compromising on performance. In order to reach this goal, we explored strategies to replace the molecular fingerprints (MACCS keys) used in Skin Doctor CP by a small set of predicted bioactivities. We selected these predicted bioactivities using Lasso regression from a panel of 372 published CP models for compound toxicity prediction [56] plus three new, additional models for assays of direct relevance to skin sensitization (i.e., DPRA, KeratinoSens assay, and h-CLAT). The final classifiers for the prediction of the skin sensitization potential of compounds were trained on 1021 compounds. They utilize only 10 predicted bioactivity descriptors but perform comparably to the Skin Doctor CP models. The best model ("Skin Doctor CP:Bio") is available free of charge for academic research purposes.

2. Materials and Methods

2.1. Data Sets and Data Processing

2.1.1. Binary LLNA Data

This work is based on the identical LLNA data set that was used for the development of Skin Doctor CP [29]. The random split into a training set (80%) and a test set (20%) was also preserved. The chemical structures were processed with a refined preprocessing protocol that was developed by Garcia de Lomana et al. [56]. This protocol includes the removal of solvents and salts, annotation of aromaticity, neutralization of charges, and mesomerization. Substances containing (i) different components with non-identical SMILES or (ii) fewer than four heavy atoms or (iii) elements other than H, B, C, N, O, F, Si, P, S, Cl, Se, Br, and I were removed from the data set.

The use of the new structure preprocessing protocol led to the rejection of 7 compounds of the training set (and none of the test set) because they do not fulfill the requirements for molecules to be composed of at least one carbon atom and to consist of at least four heavy atoms. The processed training set consists of 1021 compounds and the test set of 257 compounds.

2.1.2. Non-Animal Data on Skin Sensitization

For the calculation of additional bioactivity descriptors, chemical information, and binary assay data for 194 compounds measured in the DPRA, 190 compounds measured in the KeratinoSens assay and 160 compounds measured in the h-CLAT were collected from Alves et al. [57]. The chemical structures were preprocessed following the protocol described above. Preprocessing resulted in the removal of one particular substance (formaldehyde) that is present in all three data sets. The final KeratinoSens assay, h-CLAT, and DPRA data sets comprised 189, 159, and 193 compounds, respectively.

2.1.3. Data for Chemical Space Analysis

In preparation for chemical space comparison, the 7030 cosmetics and 4036 agrochemicals included in the CompTox Chemicals Dashboard [58] and the 2509 approved drugs included in DrugBank [59] were downloaded and processed following the protocol described above. This resulted in a data set of 4488 cosmetics, 2433 agrochemicals, and 2227 approved drugs (the significant reductions are related to the fact that many of the listed cosmetics and agrochemicals are either inorganic salts or without a defined molecular structure).

2.2. Descriptor Calculation and Normalisation

A set of 750 bioactivity descriptors related to 375 predicted binary assay outcomes was calculated for all compounds of the LLNA data set and the three reference data sets (the number of bioactivity descriptors is double that of the predicted binary assay outcomes because the predicted class probabilities of the active and the inactive class were included in the descriptor set independently from each other). More specifically, class probabilities for 372 bioactivity assays were calculated with aggregated Mondrian CP models that we trained on bioactivity assay data collected from ToxCast [60], eMolTox [61], the eChemPortal [62], and literature, following the identical protocol published by Garcia de Lomana et al. [56]. In addition, predicted class probabilities for three assays relevant to skin sensitization prediction (i.e., DPRA, KeratinoSens assay, h-CLAT) were computed using Mondrian CP models generated by applying the identical model generation framework as described for the other assays [56] to the three corresponding data sets retrieved from Alves et al. Prior to modeling, the standard scaler of the preprocessing module of scikit-learn [63] was used (with default settings) to normalize all bioactivity descriptors. The standard scaler was trained on the LLNA training set only and applied to the full LLNA data set (training and test set). In addition, MACCS keys were calculated with RDKit version 2020.09.1 [64] for all compounds in the LLNA data set.

2.3. Model Development

2.3.1. Aggregated Mondrian Conformal Prediction Modeling

In preparation for model generation, each training set was divided into a proper training set (80%) and a calibration set (20%) by stratified random splitting utilizing the train_test_split function of the Model_selection module of scikit-learn (data shuffling was enabled prior to data set splitting). Then, a RF model was generated (with the RandomForestClassifier function of scikit-learn; all parameters kept default, except for n_estimators = 500 and random_state = 43) and applied to the corresponding calibration and test set.

From the prediction probabilities obtained for the calibration set and the test set, non-conformity scores (α-values) were calculated following Equation (1):

$$\alpha_i = 0.5 - \frac{\hat{P}(y_i|x_i) - max_{y \neq y_i}\hat{P}(y|x_i)}{2} \quad (1)$$

where $\hat{P}(y_i|x_i)$ is the class probability for class i returned by the model, and $max_{y \neq y_i}\hat{P}(y|x_i)$ is the maximum class probability for any other class returned by the model.

The non-conformity scores of the calibration set were sorted class-wise (following the Mondrian conformal prediction protocol), and the relative ranks of the non-conformity scores of each compound of the test set in relation to these lists were retrieved as so-called p-values.

Within the aggregated CP framework, the procedure was repeated for 20 times with different stratified random splits into a proper training and calibration set, altering the random state of the train_test_split function from 0 to 19. For every compound in the test set, a p-value was derived during each run. The median over the p-values obtained during all 20 runs was processed as the final p-value of the compound. The p-values denote the probability of a compound belonging to the corresponding activity class. The model assigns a compound to a specific activity class if the corresponding p-value exceeds the selected error significance level ε.

2.3.2. Measurement of Model Performance

In this work, the classical performance measures (i.e., accuracy (ACC), Matthews correlation coefficient (MCC) [65], correct classification rate (CCR), sensitivity (Sens), specificity (Spec), negative predictive rate (NPV), and positive predictive rate (PPV)) are calculated based exclusively on compounds that were assigned by the CP models to exactly one activity class, i.e., "sensitizer" or "non-sensitizer". This is to enable the application of classic performance measures to CP and, at the same time, to ensure the comparability of the classical performance measures and the results reported for classical non-CP models elsewhere.

In contrast, the CP-specific performance measures (i.e., validity and efficiency) are calculated for all models based on the full sets of compounds to fulfill the common definition of these measures and enable the comparison with other CP models. Validity is defined as the percentage of predictions that include the true class, independently of the prediction of the other class (i.e., it includes "true" predictions as well as "both" predictions). A model is deemed to be valid if the validity is close or equal to the expected value of 1-ε. Efficiency can be understood as an equivalent to the term coverage for non-CP models. It is defined as the percentage of distinct predictions (i.e., predictions that predict exactly one class to be true).

2.3.3. Feature Selection and Parameter Optimization

For feature selection (Figure 1), 10-fold cross-validation (CV) was performed on the training set using the scikit-learn StratifiedKFold function (Model_selection module; n_splits = 10, shuffle = True, random_state = 43).

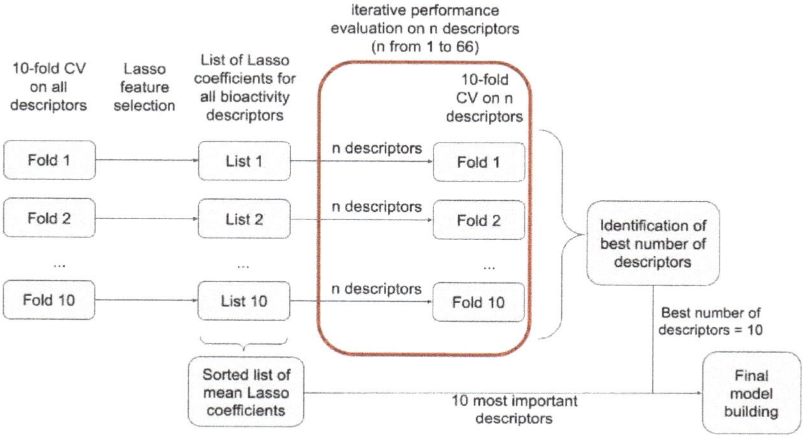

Figure 1. Schematic representation of the workflow for feature selection.

First, the relative importance of each feature within each fold of the CV was investigated. Therefore, hyperparameters for a Lasso classifier were optimized by a 10-fold CV within each fold of the outer CV. This was achieved with the scikit-learn LassoCV function (Linear_model module; random_state = 43, cv = 10, max_iter = 3000, n_alphas = 200). The optimized Lasso classifier was then used to obtain the Lasso coefficients of all bioactivity descriptors within the corresponding fold. The relative importance of each descriptor was calculated as the absolute value of the mean Lasso coefficient calculated over all folds of the CV run.

Second, the optimum number of bioactivity descriptors for model generation was determined. To do so, the 10-fold CV on the training data was repeated, this time without feature selection with Lasso. Instead, a varying number of the most important bioactivity descriptors (i.e., 1 to 66 descriptors; selected based on their coefficients obtained with Lasso) were selected for model building. The mean performance during 10-fold CV in dependence of the number of descriptors was used to select the number of features for the final model.

3. Results and Discussion

3.1. *Identification of the Optimum Number of Bioactivity Descriptors for Model Building*

In order to identify the most suitable number of bioactivity descriptors n for model building, we investigated, within a 10-fold CV framework, the performance of models as a function of the number of descriptors used (reflecting model interpretability/complexity). Within each CV fold, we performed Lasso regression to rank the descriptors by their corresponding Lasso coefficients (Table S1) and selected the n most important descriptors for model building. In Figure 2, we show the improvement of model performance as more bioactivity descriptors are added. In particular, for the first 10 descriptors, a steep increase in MCC and efficiency is observed (see section "Measurement of model performance" of the Methods for important information on how, and in particular on what data, the individual performance measures are calculated). Beyond 10 descriptors, the improvements in model performance are minor and reach a plateau at approximately 25 descriptors. This led us to the conclusion that models based on the 10 most relevant bioactivity descriptors offer the best balance between model performance and complexity (Table 1). Validity is close to the expected value of 1-ε for all the significance levels (i.e., ε = 0.05, 0.10, 0.20, and 0.30) and numbers of descriptors (in this experiment, 1 to 66) investigated.

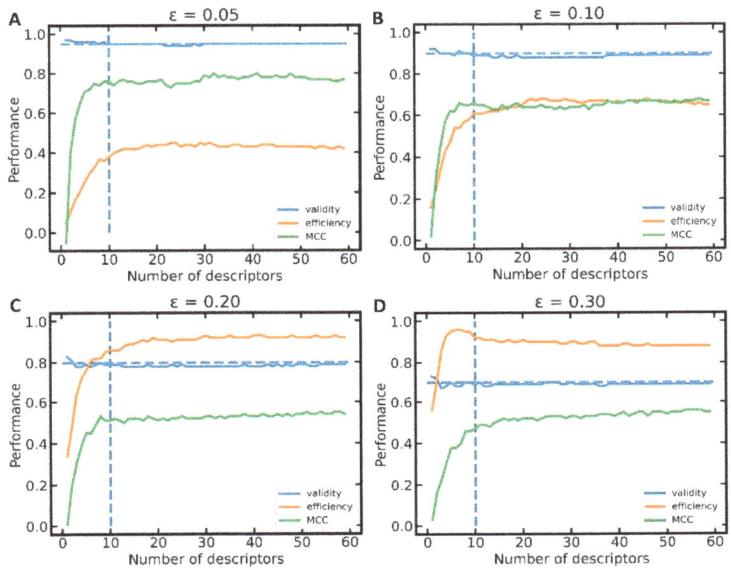

Figure 2. Mean performance of 10-fold CV as a function of the number of bioactivity descriptors selected for model building at the significance level (**A**) ε = 0.05, (**B**) ε = 0.10, (**C**) ε = 0.20, (**D**) ε = 0.30. The horizontal, dashed line indicates the validity expected from the selected significance level ε; the vertical, dashed line marks the performance of models trained on 10 descriptors.

Table 1. Ten-fold CV Performance of Models Based on 10 Bioactivity Descriptors [1].

Error Significance ε	Validity	Efficiency	ACC	MCC	CCR	Sens	Spec	NPV	PPV
0.05	0.95 (0.03)	0.38 (0.06)	0.88 (0.06)	0.76 (0.12)	0.88 (0.05)	0.87 (0.08)	0.89 (0.08)	0.92 (0.06)	0.85 (0.11)
0.10	0.89 (0.03)	0.61 (0.06)	0.83 (0.05)	0.66 (0.10)	0.83 (0.05)	0.83 (0.10)	0.83 (0.08)	0.88 (0.07)	0.77 (0.09)
0.20	0.79 (0.05)	0.86 (0.04)	0.76 (0.06)	0.51 (0.12)	0.76 (0.06)	0.75 (0.09)	0.77 (0.08)	0.82 (0.07)	0.69 (0.07)
0.30	0.69 (0.07)	0.92 (0.03)	0.74 (0.06)	0.47 (0.11)	0.74 (0.06)	0.72 (0.08)	0.75 (0.07)	0.79 (0.06)	0.67 (0.06)

[1] Standard deviation in parentheses.

3.2. Investigation of the Ten Most Relevant Bioactivity Descriptors

With 10 identified as the optimum number of bioactivity descriptors for model building, we reiterated the above-mentioned descriptor selection process on the full training set and analyzed the relevance and biological meaning of the 10 descriptors with the highest absolute Lasso coefficients averaged over the 10 folds of the CV (Table 2).

Table 2. Overview of the Top-10 Bioactivity Descriptors.

Descriptor Name	Assay Title	Mean Lasso Coefficient [1]	σ (Lasso Coefficient)	Correlation to Positive LLNA Outcome [2]	5-Fold CV Performance at Significance Level of 0.20			Most Correlating Assays [3]
					Validity	Efficiency	MCC	
p0 BSK KF3CT ICAM1 down	Bioseek human keratinocytes and foreskin fibroblasts intercellular adhesion molecule 1 assay	0.074	0.009	positive	0.80	0.83	0.41	BSK KF3CT SRB down (0.79) BSK KF3CT TGFb1 down (0.78) BSK KF3CT MCP1 down (0.78) BSK KF3CT uPA down (0.78) BSK hDFCGF TIMP1 down (0.77)
p1 BSK 4H uPAR down	Bioseek human umbilical vein endothelium plasminogen activator, urokinase receptor assay	0.051	0.045	negative	0.81	0.82	0.46	BSK 3C uPAR down (0.83) BSK LPS SRB down (0.81) BSK 3C MCP1 down (0.81) BSK 4H SRB down (0.8) BSK SAg MCP1 down (0.8)
p0 Chromosome aberration	Chromosome aberration assay	0.049	0.010	positive	0.79	0.70	0.30	Mammalian cell gene mutation (0.47) AMES (0.41) Inhibitors of Hepatocyte nuclear factor 4 (HNF4) dimerization (0.35) Modulator of Muscarinic acetylcholine receptor M4 (−0.33) Modulator of Bradykinin B2 receptor (−0.33)
p1 DPRA	Direct peptide reactivity assay	0.047	0.013	positive	0.74	0.71	0.30	h-CLAT (0.42) Inhibitors of Hepatocyte nuclear factor 4 (HNF4) dimerization (0.31) KeratinoSens (0.31) Inhibit CYP2C19 Activity (−0.29) Modulator of Peroxisome proliferator-activated receptor gamma (−0.29)
p1 Modulator of Dopamine D1 receptor	Modulator of Dopamine D1 receptor assay	0.045	0.006	positive	0.81	0.81	0.98	Modulator of Alpha-2b adrenergic receptor (0.37) Modulator of Serotonin 1a (5-HT1a) receptor (0.32) Modulator of Alpha-2a adrenergic receptor (0.31) Modulator of Serotonin 2a (5-HT2a) receptor (0.31) Modulators of myocardial damage (0.3)
p1 h-CLAT	Human cell line activation test	0.043	0.013	positive	0.87	0.56	0.54	PGPinhibition (−0.48) Caco2 (0.46) LTEA HepaRG DDIT3 up (−0.46) ATG TA CIS up (−0.46) Modulator of P2X purinoceptor 3 (−0.45)

Table 2. *Cont.*

Descriptor Name	Assay Title	Mean Lasso Coefficient [1]	σ (Lasso Coefficient)	Correlation to Positive LLNA Outcome [2]	5-Fold CV Performance at Significance Level of 0.20			Most Correlating Assays [3]
					Validity	Efficiency	MCC	
p1 BSK 3C E-selectin down	Bioseek human umbilical vein endothelium selectin E assay	0.043	0.021	positive	0.79	0.77	0.41	BSK 3C VCAM1 down (0.82) BSK 4H Pselectin down (0.81) BSK 4H VCAM1 down (0.81) BSK 3C MCP1 down (0.81) BSK 4H SRB down (0.79)
p1 LTEA HepaRG APOA5 dn	LifeTech/Expression Analysis human HepaRG apolipoprotein A-V assay	0.040	0.012	negative	0.82	0.77	0.51	LTEA HepaRG CYP4A22 dn (0.78) LTEA HepaRG CYP4A11 dn (0.77) LTEA HepaRG FMO3 dn (0.76) LTEA HepaRG HMGCS2 dn (0.76) LTEA HepaRG GSTA2 dn (0.75)
p1 KeratinoSens	ARE-Nrf2 Luciferase test method	0.039	0.004	positive	0.82	0.51	0.31	DPRA (0.31) h-CLAT (0.31) Inhibitors of Hepatocyte nuclear factor 4 (HNF4) dimerization (0.29) Inhibit CYP1A2 Activity (0.27) Modulator of Monoamine oxidase A (0.27)
p0 ATG NRF2 ARE CIS up	Attagene human HepG2 nuclear factor, erythroid 2-like 2 assay	0.036	0.014	positive	0.81	0.87	0.55	ATG PPARg TRANS up (0.67) ATG VDRE CIS up (0.66) ATG MRE CIS up (0.65) ATG PXR TRANS up (0.64) ATG AP 1 CIS up (0.64)

[1] Mean over the 10 folds of the CV. Note that the feature importance rankings of the Lasso model and the RF model may differ. [2] Correlation of the positive assay outcomes and the skin sensitization potentials measured in the LLNA. Since the probability of a compound to belong to the inactive class (p0) or the active class (p1) in a given assay are strongly correlated, either p0 or p1 is selected as an important descriptor by the Lasso model for that assay. Depending on whether p0 or p1 has been selected, and depending on the algebraic sign of the mean Lasso coefficient, a positive predicted assay outcome can either be associated with a positive or a negative LLNA result (i.e., if p0 has a positive correlation with the LLNA result this describes anticorrelation between the positive outcome of both endpoints). [3] Numbers in parentheses report the Kendall τ correlation coefficients between the descriptor and the (most) correlated assay. The full names of the assays are provided in Table S2.

The bioactivity descriptor ranked first by the Lasso model is the ToxCast assay "BSK KF3CT ICAM1 down" (Lasso coefficient 0.074). This feature describes the expression of ICAM1 in human keratinocytes. This ToxCast assay is observed to correlate with predictions for other keratinocytes and foreskin assays from the ToxCast BSK family (Kendall τ correlation coefficients between 0.77 and 0.79). The ICAM1 readout is also known as CD54, which is a readout of the skin sensitization-related h-CLAT. The underlying model shows good predictivity (validity = 0.80, efficiency = 0.83, MCC = 0.41 at the significance level of 0.20) The nine further bioactivity descriptors all have similar Lasso coefficients, between 0.036 and 0.051 (validities between 0.74 and 0.87; efficiencies between 0.51 and 0.87; MCCs between 0.30 and 0.98, respectively). Among these are the three assays that we added to the descriptor set because of their direct relevance to skin sensitization: DPRA, KeratinoSens assay, and h-CLAT. As expected, a direct correlation between a positive outcome in any of these three assays and the probability of a compound being a skin sensitizer is identified by the Lasso model. The fact that these assays do not show a high correlation with any other bioactivity descriptors within our full set of descriptors underlines the fact that these descriptors may add important additional information on the skin sensitization potential of compounds. The models predicting these bioactivity descriptors are built on comparably small data sets (<200 compounds). This is reflected by a higher deviation of the significance of these models from the expected value of 0.80 at the investigated significance level of 0.20, compared to the other models. The MCCs of these models are between 0.30 and 0.54.

The ToxCast assay "ATG NRF2 ARE CIS up" describes the activation of NRF2 in human liver cells. Being the fundamental concept of keratinocyte activation analysis via KeratinoSens and LuSens assay, Nrf2 activation is known to play a vital role in the regulation of cellular cytoprotective responses, metabolism, and immune regulation. Included in the top-10 features are also the ToxCast assays "BSK 3C E-selectin down" and "BSK 4H uPAR down", both of which describe inflammation-related biological processes in the endothelium environment. As such, these assays might encode aspects of the immunological response of the human body. "BSK 3C E-selectin down" correlates with other assays associated with inflammation and immune reaction and which are often located in the endothelium. While it shows a positive correlation with the skin sensitization potential (which might indicate an activation of compounds or increased bioavailability), "BSK 4H uPAR down" is one out of only two bioactivity descriptors (among the top-10 features) that show negative correlation with the skin sensitization potential. This assay may therefore report processes involving the deactivation of a compound or the reduction of its bioavailability.

The chromosome aberration assay may not be directly linked to skin sensitization, but it may be relevant to the detection of reactive compounds. The feature is weakly correlated with other assays that are linked to the detection of reactive molecules (e.g., mammalian cell gene mutation assay or AMES mutagenicity assay). Chromosome aberration predictions show no strong correlation with any other descriptors in the set of models.

3.3. Coverage of the Chemical Space Relevant to the Development of Cosmetics, Drugs and Agrochemicals

In order to develop an understanding of to what extent the LLNA data set, which we will use to develop the in silico models, represents drugs, cosmetics, and agrochemicals in the feature space defined by the ten selected bioactivity descriptors, a principal component analysis (PCA) was performed on the LLNA data set and the reference sets. As shown in the PCA scatter plot in Figure 3 (PCA loadings plot provided in Figure S1), the LLNA data set covers well the areas in feature space populated by cosmetics, approved drugs, and agrochemicals.

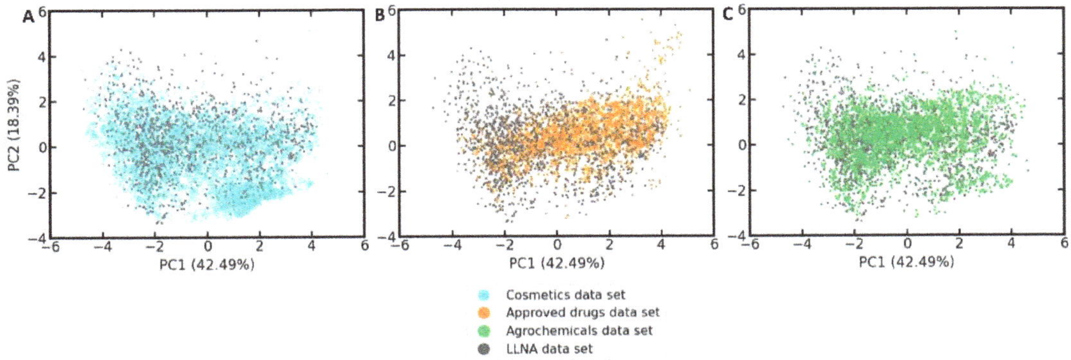

Figure 3. PCA quantifying the coverage of the LLNA data by the reference sets of (**A**) cosmetics, (**B**) approved drugs, and (**C**) agrochemicals in the feature space of the 10 selected bioactivity descriptors. The percentages in parentheses report the variance explained by the respective principal component (PC).

3.4. Analysis of the Distribution of Sensitizers and Non-Sensitizers in the Feature Space of the Ten Selected Bioactivity Descriptors

To investigate the distribution of sensitizers and non-sensitizers within the feature space of the ten selected bioactivity descriptors, another PCA was performed, this time exclusively on the compounds of the LLNA data set (Figure 4). Three characteristic areas can be identified in the scatter plot resulting from this PCA (Figure 4A): Area 1, covering mainly sensitizers; Area 2, covering mainly non-sensitizers; and Area 3, showing intense mixing of sensitizers and non-sensitizers.

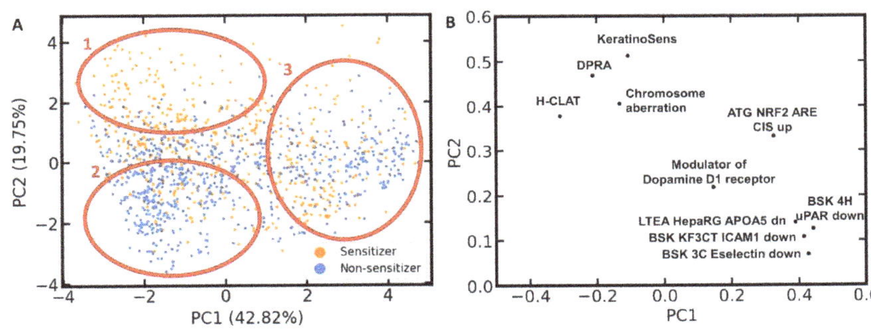

Figure 4. LLNA data set analyzed by PCA in the feature space of the ten selected bioactivity descriptors. (**A**) Scatter plot colored by the binary skin sensitization potential; (**B**) loadings plot of the ten descriptors. The percentages in parentheses report the variance explained by the respective principal component (PC). Note that the axis sections differ for panels (**A**,**B**).

The corresponding loadings plot (Figure 4B) places the bioactivity descriptors for the three skin sensitization assays (h-CLAT, DPRA, and KeratinoSens assay) and the chromosome aberration assay in quadrant 2 (upper left). All four of these assays contribute positively to PC2 and, to a lower degree, negatively to PC1. Since a positive outcome in one or several of the skin sensitization assays should be correlated with a positive skin sensitization potential, this is in agreement with the PCA scatter plot showing a high accumulation of sensitizers in the upper left region. Since a positive outcome in the chromosome aberration assay is likely correlated with a reactive compound, it is also within the expectations that it will shift a compound towards this Area 1 in the PCA scatter plot.

For the remaining six bioactivity descriptors, higher PC1 and PC2 values are expected for compounds that are active in the corresponding assay. Thus, all ten bioactivity descriptors contribute positively to PC2. This means that every compound predicted to be positive in those bioactivity assays is moved towards Area 1 or 3 in the scatter plot. This comes along with the increased probability of a compound to be a skin sensitizer (i.e., to be located in Area 1). At the same time, every negative predicted assay outcome moves the compound towards Area 2, where we mainly expect non-sensitizers to be located, or Area 3, where no prevalence in activity is detected. This positive contribution to PC2 is higher for KeratinoSens, DPRA, chromosome aberration, h-CLAT, and ATG NRF2 than for the other five bioactivity descriptors. In Area 3, we observe intense mixing of skin sensitizers and non-sensitizers, hence posing a significant challenge to classification.

3.5. Model Based on Ten Selected Bioactivity Descriptors

Following the identification of the optimum model setup, a final, aggregated Mondrian CP model based on the ten selected bioactivity descriptors was derived from the full training set and evaluated on the holdout data set. From here on, we refer to this model as the SkinDoctor CP:Bio model.

3.5.1. Performance on the Test Set

Within the standard deviation expected from CV, the SkinDoctor CP:Bio model was valid at all four significance levels investigated (Table 3). The efficiencies of the model ranged from 0.39 to 0.95 and the MCCs ranged from 0.72 to 0.49, depending on the significance level.

Table 3. Performance of the model based on ten selected bioactivity descriptors on the test set.

Error Significance ε	Validity	Efficiency	ACC	MCC	CCR	Sens	Spec	NPV	PPV
0.05	0.95	0.39	0.86	0.72	0.86	0.84	0.88	0.88	0.84
0.10	0.89	0.56	0.81	0.62	0.81	0.85	0.77	0.88	0.74
0.20	0.81	0.82	0.76	0.53	0.77	0.80	0.74	0.83	0.69
0.30	0.70	0.95	0.74	0.49	0.75	0.78	0.72	0.82	0.67

Class-wise performance analysis (Table 4) showed that the SkinDoctor CP:Bio model was valid for sensitizers and non-sensitizers at all significance levels investigated. The largest difference in validity between the two classes (0.08) was observed at the significance level of 0.30. Efficiency was in general similar for both classes (largest difference 0.04).

Table 4. Class-wise performance of the model based on ten selected bioactivity descriptors on the test set.

Error Significance ε	Class	Validity	Efficiency
0.05	Non-sensitizer	0.95	0.38
	Sensitizer	0.93	0.41
0.10	Non-sensitizer	0.87	0.55
	Sensitizer	0.92	0.58
0.20	Non-sensitizer	0.79	0.82
	Sensitizer	0.83	0.82
0.30	Non-sensitizer	0.67	0.94
	Sensitizer	0.75	0.95

3.5.2. Comparison of the New Model with the Skin Doctor CP Model

The previously developed Skin Doctor CP model [29] is trained on MACCS keys (166 features), whereas the Skin Doctor CP:Bio model is trained on ten selected bioactivity descriptors. All other differences in the data and protocols used for model building and testing are minor (Table S3), thus enabling a direct, comparative assessment of the two feature types and their impact on model performance and behavior.

On the holdout data set of 257 compounds measured in the LLNA (none of these compounds is part of the training set of either model), both the Skin Doctor CP model and the Skin Doctor CP:Bio model were valid at all significance levels investigated. For the sake of clarity, we focus our discussion here on the commonly applied significance level of 0.20; performance data on all significance levels are provided in Table S4. At the significance level of 0.20, the Skin Doctor CP and Skin Doctor CP:Bio models yielded validities of 0.82 and 0.81, respectively. The efficiencies (0.78 vs. 0.82) and MCCs (0.55 vs. 0.53) obtained for the Skin Doctor CP and Skin Doctor CP:Bio models were also comparable. The differences in performance between the two models are slightly above the standard deviation observed for the 10-fold CV experiments but small enough to consider the performance of the two models similar.

3.6. Combination of Bioactivity Descriptors with MACCS Keys in an Attempt to Improve Model Performance

MACCS keys encode structural patterns of molecules and thus information that is very different from that encoded by the bioactivity descriptors. The use of MACCS keys in combination with the ten selected bioactivity descriptors could hence yield better models. However, a RF model derived from the combined set of MACCS keys and the ten selected bioactivity descriptors (n_estimators = 500; all other parameters default) did not yield better performance on the test set.

Therefore, we generated a model trained exclusively on MACCS keys plus a model trained exclusively on the ten selected bioactivity descriptors (both models with n_estimators = 500; all other parameters default), and, based on a simple set of rules (see Figure 5), combined both models to form a consensus model. This set of rules follows the idea that only unambiguous predictions by the single models (i.e., predictions assigning a compound to exactly one class) are considered. If one model returns an unambiguous prediction or if both models return an unambiguous prediction and are in agreement, the unambiguous prediction is reported as the final result. In all other cases, the consensus model does not return a prediction.

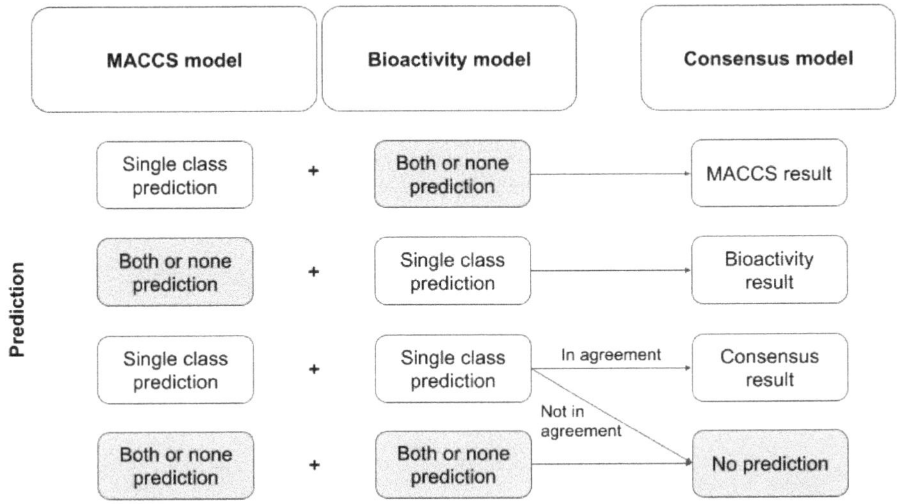

Figure 5. Architecture of the consensus model.

Table 5 reports on the performance of this consensus model at different error significance levels. Note that because the consensus model does not fulfill the definitions of a pure CP model, validity and efficiency cannot be calculated for this model.

Table 5. Performance of the consensus and the combined models on the test set.

		Consensus Model Based on a Set of Rules							
Error significance ε [1]		**Coverage**	**ACC**	**MCC**	**CCR**	**Sens**	**Spec**	**NPV**	**PPV**
0.05		0.51	0.86	0.72	0.86	0.84	0.88	0.88	0.84
0.10		0.71	0.79	0.59	0.80	0.83	0.77	0.88	0.70
0.20		0.89	0.77	0.54	0.78	0.82	0.73	0.85	0.68
0.30		0.83	0.78	0.56	0.79	0.85	0.72	0.88	0.68
		Combined Model Based on Mean *p*-Values							
Error significance ε	**Validity**	**Efficiency**	**ACC**	**MCC**	**CCR**	**Sens**	**Spec**	**NPV**	**PPV**
0.05	0.97	0.24	0.89	0.77	0.89	0.92	0.86	0.94	0.82
0.10	0.93	0.46	0.86	0.72	0.87	0.94	0.80	0.95	0.76
0.20	0.82	0.79	0.77	0.56	0.78	0.85	0.72	0.87	0.69
0.30	0.71	0.95	0.75	0.50	0.76	0.80	0.72	0.84	0.66

[1] Error significance of the underlying model, not of the combined model itself.

When running the two CP models underlying the consensus approach at a significance level of 0.20, the consensus approach reached a coverage of 0.89 and an MMC of 0.54. Hence, compared to the Skin Doctor CP:Bio model (efficiency 0.82 and MCC 0.53 at a significance level of 0.20), the consensus model obtained only slightly better coverage while maintaining the MCC.

A second, combined, model was constructed by averaging the *p*-values returned for each class by the model based on MACCS keys and the model based on bioactivity descriptors. The model was valid to over-predictive at the four significance levels investigated. At the significance level of 0.20, the validity was 0.82. The efficiency at this significance level was 0.79 (vs. 0.82 for the Skin Doctor CP:Bio model) and the MCC was 0.56 (vs. 0.53 for the Skin Doctor CP:Bio model). Hence, compared to the Skin Doctor CP:Bio model, this combined model obtains a slightly higher MCC, at the cost of efficiency.

In order to obtain a better understanding of the advantages and disadvantages of the two combined models over the single models, we investigated the relationship between classification performance (MCC) and coverage. From Figure 6, it can be seen that the combined models tend to obtain better MCC values at a given coverage than the single models. At higher coverages, the combined model based on averaged *p*-values has slightly better MCCs than the combined model based on the set of rules. A further advantage of the combined model based on *p*-value averaging is that users can select a confidence level; this is not possible with the combined model based on the set of rules.

Overall, the *p*-value averaging approach seems to be preferable over the rule-based approach. Compared to the single model (i.e., the Skin Doctor CP:Bio model), the advantages of the combined approach with respect to performance are outweighed by the fact that the single model has much lower complexity and, hence, better interpretability.

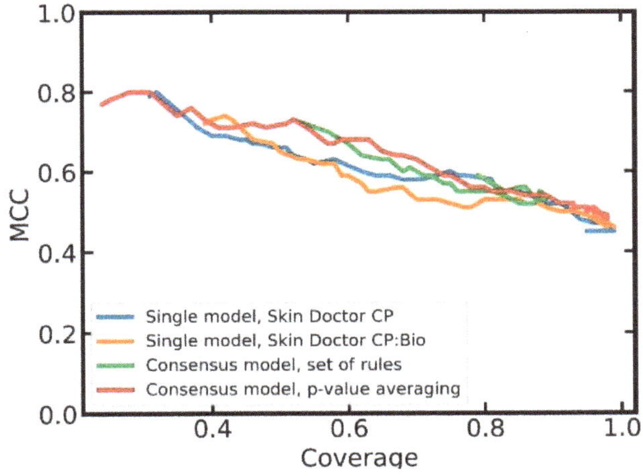

Figure 6. Relationship between MCC and coverage for the individual and the combined models.

3.7. Investigation of the Influence of Experimental Skin Sensitization Assay Results on Predictivity

Feature selection with Lasso and the RF algorithm identified the three bioactivity descriptors derived from the three skin sensitization-specific assays (i.e., DPRA, KeratinoSens assay, h-CLAT) as important for modeling the LLNA. In order to obtain a better understanding of the role and significance of these three bioactivity descriptors, we investigated them from different perspectives.

First, we determined the (5-fold) CV performance of the CP models for the DPRA, KeratinoSens assay, and h-CLAT descriptors on the (i) 194 compounds measured in the DPRA, (ii) 190 compounds measured in the KeratinoSens assay, and (iii) 160 compounds measured in the h-CLAT. The KeratinoSens and h-CLAT models (Table 6) were valid at a significance level of 0.2 (validities of 0.82 and 0.87, respectively) while the DPRA model showed a slight underperformance (validity 0.74). The efficiencies of the models were fairly low (0.51 to 0.71) in comparison to most of the other CP models for bioactivity prediction. We assume that the low efficiency is related to the fact that the training sets for these CP models are small (<200 compounds). The other evaluated performance measures are within expectations (e.g., MCC between 0.30 and 0.54). Overall, we conclude from these results that the predicted assay outcomes from these three models could make a substantial contribution to models predicting the skin sensitization potential.

Table 6. Five-fold CV performance of the CP models for DPRA, KeratinoSens assay, and h-CLAT at the significance level of 0.20 [1].

Assay to be Predicted	No. Compounds in Data Set	Validity	Efficiency	ACC	ACC (Sensitizers)	ACC (Non-Sensitizers)	F1 Score	MCC
DPRA	194	0.74 (0.09)	0.71 (0.14)	0.64 (0.07)	0.60 (0.06)	0.69 (0.20)	0.64 (0.07)	0.30 (0.18)
KeratinoSens	190	0.82 (0.11)	0.51 (0.08)	0.67 (0.19)	0.66 (0.24)	0.68 (0.23)	0.64 (0.19)	0.31 (0.35)
h-CLAT	160	0.87 (0.03)	0.56 (0.56)	0.78 (0.05)	0.76 (0.15)	0.75 (0.29)	0.74 (0.06)	0.54 (0.08)

[1] Standard deviation in parentheses.

Second, we investigated (by 10-fold CV on the full LLNA data set) whether the high importance attributed by Lasso to the skin sensitization-specific assays could be a result of overlaps in the training or test data of the LLNA model (SkinDoctor CP:Bio model) and the training data of the DPRA/KeratinoSens assay/h-CLAT models. For the overlapping compounds, the p-values used as bioactivity descriptors should be accurate (since the experimental value of the in vitro assays is known) and therefore more informative. In order to investigate this, we determined the performance of the SkinDoctor CP:Bio model in dependence of the number of compounds overlapping between the LLNA data set (i.e., the test data within each fold) and the training data of the DPRA/KeratinoSens assay/h-CLAT models. We found that six compounds of the LLNA data set were present also in exactly one of the DPRA/KeratinoSens assay/h-CLAT training sets, 45 compounds were present in exactly two of these assays, and 132 compounds in each of these three assays. Note that the number of compounds present in the LLNA data set and in exactly one of the three non-animal assay data sets is too low to make any meaningful observations, for which reason this case was not further pursued. For the remaining two subsets of compounds, the performances of the models were comparable to each other as well as to the subset containing the compounds that are not present in any of three assay data sets (Table 7). For this reason, we are confident that the importance attributed to the predicted DPRA, KeratinoSens assay, and h-CLAT outcomes is genuine and not a result of a bias in the data.

Table 7. Performance of the SkinDoctor CP:Bio model during 10-fold CV on the full LLNA data set in dependence of the number of skin sensitization assays for which experimental data are available.

Error Significance ε	Validity	Efficiency	MCC	Validity	Efficiency	MCC	Validity	Efficiency	MCC
	For Compounds Exclusive to the LLNA Data Set			For Compounds Present in the LLNA Data Set Plus Exactly Two of the DPRA/KeratinoSens Assay/h-CLAT Training Sets			For Compounds Present in the LLNA Data Set Plus Exactly Three of the DPRA/KeratinoSens Assay/h-CLAT Training Sets		
0.05	0.97	0.33	0.77	0.98	0.44	0.79	0.98	0.45	0.77
0.10	0.91	0.56	0.64	0.96	0.62	0.74	0.93	0.65	0.67
0.20	0.81	0.83	0.52	0.91	0.84	0.66	0.86	0.81	0.51
0.30	0.69	0.94	0.45	0.82	0.93	0.68	0.73	0.93	0.42

Third, we tested the capacity of a model trained only on DPRA, KeratinoSens assay, and h-CLAT assay data to predict the outcomes of the LLNA. This experiment is particularly interesting because a number of existing in silico models for the prediction of the skin sensitization potential are trained exclusively on data from these three assays [66–68].

In five-fold CV, our CP model trained exclusively on DPRA, KeratinoSens assay, and h-CLAT assay data descriptors (n_estimators = 500; all other parameters default) was valid at all error significance levels investigated (Table 8), but its efficiency (0.21 at $\varepsilon = 0.05$; 0.88 at $\varepsilon = 0.30$) and MCC (0.48 at $\varepsilon = 0.05$; 0.37 at $\varepsilon = 0.30$) were substantially lower than those of the CP model derived from the ten selected bioactivity descriptors. These results indicate that the bioactivity descriptors derived from other assays add relevant, additional information to the models that is needed to obtain good classifiers.

Table 8. Test set performance of the classifier trained exclusively on predicted values of the DPRA, KeratinoSens and h-CLAT assays.

Error Significance ε	Validity	Efficiency	ACC	MCC	CCR	Sens	Spec	NPV	PPV
0.05	0.94	0.21	0.71	0.48	0.72	0.92	0.52	0.88	0.63
0.10	0.90	0.40	0.75	0.51	0.76	0.82	0.69	0.84	0.67
0.20	0.80	0.70	0.72	0.44	0.72	0.76	0.69	0.81	0.61
0.30	0.72	0.88	0.68	0.37	0.69	0.71	0.66	0.78	0.59

3.8. Impact of the Limitation of the Available Experimental Data on Model Performance

Most of the freely available models for the prediction of the skin sensitization potential of small molecules are trained on LLNA data, and the evaluation reports for many of these models indicate that their performance is comparable [29,40,44,57]. It is plausible that the observed plateauing of model performance is related to the limited quantity and quality of the data available for model development. In order to investigate whether our classifiers could benefit from additional LLNA data, we investigated the relationship between model performance and the size of the training data.

As expected, and shown in Figure 7, the performance of models increases with the number of training instances, regardless of the type of descriptors used. The MCCs of the models based on bioactivity descriptors improve from an average of 0.41 to an average of 0.50, respectively. Consistent with our initial CV experiments, the use of more than ten bioactivity descriptors yields minor improvements in model performance that we believe are outweighed by higher model complexity.

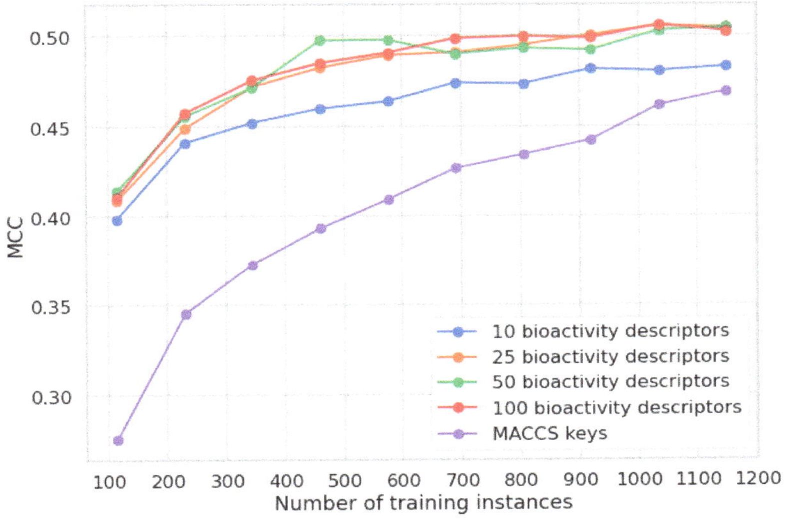

Figure 7. Performance of the RF classifier (n_estimators = 500; all other parameters default) underlying the CP model as a function of the number of instances the model was trained on.

The MCC of the model based on MACCS keys improves from 0.28 (when trained on 115 compounds) to 0.47 (when trained on 1150 compounds), indicating that the models trained on MACCS keys require substantially more training data than the models trained on bioactivity descriptors to obtain good performance. In this particular case, the MACCS keys model reaches a comparable performance to the model based on bioactivity descriptors only when all the available LLNA data are used for modeling. This leaves the MACCS keys model clearly more data-hungry than the models based on predicted bioactivities, with the benefit of showing the potential to surpass the model based on predicted bioactivities given the availability of sufficient amounts of data.

4. Conclusions

In this work, we report on the development and validation of a new machine learning model for the prediction of the skin sensitization potential of small organic molecules: Skin Doctor CP:Bio. Whereas the previously reported models are mostly based on molecular fingerprints (which in general are difficult to interpret), Skin Doctor CP:Bio utilizes just ten bioactivity descriptors to reach competitive performance. Most of these bioactivity descriptors are known to be directly or indirectly linked to skin sensitization, which adds to the interpretability of the model and supports its meaningfulness.

At the significance level of 0.20, Skin Doctor CP:Bio obtained an efficiency of 0.82 and an MCC of 0.53 on the holdout data set of 257 compounds. These results demonstrate the good performance of the model and, hence, the relevance of the selected bioactivity descriptors. Analysis of the LLNA training data projected into the new feature space proves that cosmetics, drugs, and agrochemicals are well embedded in the data, hence corroborating the relevance of the model to different industries.

In an attempt to further improve model performance and coverage, we explored different strategies to exploit the information contained in molecular fingerprints (MACCS keys) and biological descriptors. The models obtained from these experiments showed minor improvements in performance that are outweighed by the costs of higher model complexity and limited interpretability.

An important observation to make was that models based on MACCS keys are clearly more data-hungry than models based on predicted bioactivities. Only when using all of the available LLNA data, the model based on MACCs keys was able to catch up with the model based on predicted bioactivities. This highlights the relevance of the presented approach to the development of strategies to address the many questions in biology, pharmacology, and toxicology where measured data are scarce. We believe that the modeling strategies presented in this work could be easily adopted to address many of these research questions. The Skin Doctor CP:Bio model is available free of charge for academic research purposes.

Supplementary Materials: The following are available online at https://www.mdpi.com/article/10.3390/ph14080790/s1. Figure S1. Loadings plot for the PCA on the LLNA and the three reference data sets, based on the ten selected bioactivity descriptors; Table S1: Mean absolute lasso coefficients and standard deviation σ retrieved from the 10-fold CV; Table S2: Full name of the assays with high correlation to the ten selected bioactivity descriptors; Table S3: Comparison of the Skin Doctor CP and Skin Doctor CP:Bio approaches; Table S4: Results of Skin Doctor CP on the test set.

Author Contributions: Conceptualization, A.W., U.N., J.K. (Jochen Kühnl) and J.K. (Johannes Kirchmair); methodology, A.W., M.G.d.L., N.M., J.K. (Jochen Kühnl), and J.K. (Johannes Kirchmair); software, A.W., M.G.d.L., N.M., C.S., and S.H.; validation, A.W., J.K. (Jochen Kühnl), and J.K. (Johannes Kirchmair); resources, J.K. (Jochen Kühnl) and J.K. (Johannes Kirchmair); data curation, A.W., N.M., and M.G.d.L.; writing—original draft preparation, A.W., M.G.d.L., C.S., N.M., S.H., U.N., J.K. (Jochen Kühnl), and J.K. (Johannes Kirchmair); visualization, A.W. and S.H.; supervision, J.K. (Jochen Kühnl), J.K. (Johannes Kirchmair), and U.N.; project administration, J.K. (Jochen Kühnl) and J.K. (Johannes Kirchmair); funding acquisition, J.K. (Jochen Kühnl) and J.K. (Johannes Kirchmair). All authors have read and agreed to the published version of the manuscript.

Funding: N.M. and J.K. (Johannes Kirchmair) are supported by the Trond Mohn Foundation (BFS2017TMT01). C.S. and J.K. (Johannes Kirchmair) are supported by the Deutsche Forschungsgemeinschaft (DFG, German Research Foundation)-project number KI 2085/1-1. A.W. is supported by Beiersdorf AG through HITeC e.V.

Institutional Review Board Statement: Not applicable.

Informed Consent Statement: Not applicable.

Data Availability Statement: The models for generating the ten bioactivity descriptors as well as the final LLNA model are available free of charge for academic research from https://doi.org/10.5281/zenodo.5101594, accessed on 7 August 2021 [69]. The LLNA data set used for model development and evaluation was published earlier [29].

Conflicts of Interest: A.W. is funded by Beiersdorf AG through HITeC e.V and J.K. (Jochen Kühnl) is employed at Beiersdorf AG.

Abbreviations

ACC	accuracy
CCR	correct classification rate
CP	conformal prediction
CV	cross validation
DPRA	direct peptide reactivity assay
GPMT	guinea pig maximization test
h-CLAT	human cell line activation test
IATA	integrated approach for testing and assessment
LLNA	local lymph node assay
MCC	Matthews correlation coefficient
NPV	negative predictive rate
PC	principal component
PCA	principal component analysis
PPV	positive predictive rate
(Q)SAR	(quantitative) structure activity relationship
RF	random forest
Sens	sensitivity
Spec	specificity

References

1. Kimber, I.; Basketter, D.A.; Gerberick, G.F.; Ryan, C.A.; Dearman, R.J. Chemical Allergy: Translating Biology into Hazard Characterization. *Toxicol. Sci.* **2011**, *120* (Suppl. 1), S238–S268. [CrossRef]
2. Olusegun, O.A.; Martincigh, B.S. Allergic Contact Dermatitis: A Significant Environmental and Occupational Skin Disease. *Int. J. Dermatol.* **2021**. [CrossRef] [PubMed]
3. Lushniak, B.D. Occupational Contact Dermatitis. *Dermatol. Ther.* **2004**, *17*, 272–277. [CrossRef] [PubMed]
4. Thyssen, J.P.; Linneberg, A.; Menné, T.; Johansen, J.D. The Epidemiology of Contact Allergy in the General Population—Prevalence and Main Findings. *Contact Dermat.* **2007**, *57*, 287–299. [CrossRef] [PubMed]
5. van Amerongen, C.C.A.; Ofenloch, R.F.; Cazzaniga, S.; Elsner, P.; Gonçalo, M.; Naldi, L.; Svensson, Å.; Bruze, M.; Schuttelaar, M.L.A. Skin Exposure to Scented Products Used in Daily Life and Fragrance Contact Allergy in the European General Population—The EDEN Fragrance Study. *Contact Dermat.* **2021**, *84*, 385–394. [CrossRef]
6. Aalto-Korte, K.; Suuronen, K. Ten Years of Contact Allergy from Acrylic Compounds in an Occupational Dermatology Clinic. *Contact Dermat.* **2021**, *84*, 240–246. [CrossRef]
7. Nedorost, S.; Hammond, M. Art of Prevention: Allergic Sensitization through Damaged Skin: Atopic, Occupational, and Stasis Dermatitis. *Int. J. Women's Dermatol.* **2020**, *6*, 381–383. [CrossRef]
8. Salah, S.; Taieb, C.; Demessant, A.L.; Haftek, M. Prevalence of Skin Reactions and Self-Reported Allergies in 5 Countries with Their Social Impact Measured through Quality of Life Impairment. *Int. J. Environ. Res. Public Health* **2021**, *18*, 4501. [CrossRef]
9. Felter, S.; Kern, P.; Ryan, C. Allergic Contact Dermatitis: Adequacy of the Default 10X Assessment Factor for Human Variability to Protect Infants and Children. *Regul. Toxicol. Pharmacol.* **2018**, *99*, 116–121. [CrossRef]
10. OECD. *OECD Guidelines for the Testing of Chemicals, Section 4 Test No. 429: Skin Sensitisation Local Lymph Node Assay: Local Lymph Node Assay*; OECD Publishing: Paris, France, 2010; ISBN 9789264071100.
11. Anderson, S.E.; Siegel, P.D.; Meade, B.J. The LLNA: A Brief Review of Recent Advances and Limitations. *J. Allergy* **2011**, *2011*, 424203–424213. [CrossRef]
12. Gerberick, G.F.; House, R.V.; Fletcher, E.R.; Ryan, C.A. Examination of the Local Lymph Node Assay for Use in Contact Sensitization Risk Assessment. *Fundam. Appl. Toxicol.* **1992**, *19*, 438–445. [CrossRef]
13. Santín, E.P.; Solana, R.R.; García, M.G.; Del Mar García Suárez, M.; Díaz, G.D.B.; Cabal, M.D.C.; Rojas, J.M.M.; Sánchez, J.I.L. Toxicity Prediction Based on Artificial Intelligence: A Multidisciplinary Overview. *WIREs Comput. Mol. Sci.* **2021**, *11*, e1516. [CrossRef]
14. Pistollato, F.; Madia, F.; Corvi, R.; Munn, S.; Grignard, E.; Paini, A.; Worth, A.; Bal-Price, A.; Prieto, P.; Casati, S.; et al. Current EU Regulatory Requirements for the Assessment of Chemicals and Cosmetic Products: Challenges and Opportunities for Introducing New Approach Methodologies. *Arch. Toxicol.* **2021**, *95*, 1867–1897. [CrossRef] [PubMed]
15. Ta, G.H.; Weng, C.F.; Leong, M. In Silico Prediction of Skin Sensitization: Quo Vadis? *Front. Pharmacol.* **2021**, *12*, 1052. [CrossRef] [PubMed]
16. Mehling, A.; Eriksson, T.; Eltze, T.; Kolle, S.; Ramirez, T.; Teubner, W.; van Ravenzwaay, B.; Landsiedel, R. Non-Animal Test Methods for Predicting Skin Sensitization Potentials. *Arch. Toxicol.* **2012**, *86*, 1273–1295. [CrossRef]
17. Reisinger, K.; Hoffmann, S.; Alépée, N.; Ashikaga, T.; Barroso, J.; Elcombe, C.; Gellatly, N.; Galbiati, V.; Gibbs, S.; Groux, H.; et al. Systematic Evaluation of Non-Animal Test Methods for Skin Sensitisation Safety Assessment. *Toxicol. Vitro* **2015**, *29*, 259–270. [CrossRef]

18. Ezendam, J.; Braakhuis, H.M.; Vandebriel, R.J. State of the Art in Non-Animal Approaches for Skin Sensitization Testing: From Individual Test Methods towards Testing Strategies. *Arch. Toxicol.* **2016**, *90*, 2861–2883. [CrossRef]
19. Thyssen, J.P.; Giménez-Arnau, E.; Lepoittevin, J.-P.; Menné, T.; Boman, A.; Schnuch, A. The Critical Review of Methodologies and Approaches to Assess the Inherent Skin Sensitization Potential (skin Allergies) of Chemicals. Part I. *Contact Dermat.* **2012**, *66* (Suppl. 1), 11–24. [CrossRef] [PubMed]
20. Wilm, A.; Kühnl, J.; Kirchmair, J. Computational Approaches for Skin Sensitization Prediction. *Crit. Rev. Toxicol.* **2018**, *48*, 738–760. [CrossRef]
21. ECHA (European Chemicals Agency). The Use of Alternatives to Testing on Animals for the REACH Regulation, Third Report under Article 117(3) of the REACH Regulation. Available online: https://echa.europa.eu/documents/10162/13639/alternatives_test_animals_2017_en.pdf (accessed on 10 July 2019).
22. OECD. Test No. 442C: In Chemico Skin Sensitisation. Available online: http://www.oecd.org/env/test-no-442c-in-chemico-skin-sensitisation-9789264229709-en.htm (accessed on 10 July 2019).
23. OECD. Test No. 442D: In Vitro Skin Sensitisation. Available online: http://www.oecd.org/env/test-no-442d-in-vitro-skin-sensitisation-9789264229822-en.htm (accessed on 17 April 2018).
24. OECD. Test No. 442E: In Vitro Skin Sensitisation. Available online: http://www.oecd.org/env/test-no-442e-in-vitro-skin-sensitisation-9789264264359-en.htm (accessed on 17 April 2018).
25. OECD. OECD Principles for the Validation, for Regulatory Purposes, of (Quantitative) Structure-Activity Relationship Models. Available online: https://www.oecd.org/chemicalsafety/risk-assessment/37849783.pdf (accessed on 10 July 2019).
26. Jowsey, I.R.; Basketter, D.A.; Westmoreland, C.; Kimber, I. A Future Approach to Measuring Relative Skin Sensitising Potency: A Proposal. *J. Appl. Toxicol.* **2006**, *26*, 341–350. [CrossRef]
27. Hoffmann, S.; Kleinstreuer, N.; Alépée, N.; Allen, D.; Api, A.M.; Ashikaga, T.; Clouet, E.; Cluzel, M.; Desprez, B.; Gellatly, N.; et al. Non-Animal Methods to Predict Skin Sensitization (I): The Cosmetics Europe Database. *Crit. Rev. Toxicol.* **2018**, *48*, 344–358. [CrossRef] [PubMed]
28. Safford, R.J.; Api, A.M.; Roberts, D.W.; Lalko, J.F. Extension of the Dermal Sensitisation Threshold (DST) Approach to Incorporate Chemicals Classified as Reactive. *Regul. Toxicol. Pharmacol.* **2015**, *72*, 694–701. [CrossRef]
29. Wilm, A.; Norinder, U.; Agea, M.I.; de Bruyn Kops, C.; Stork, C.; Kühnl, J.; Kirchmair, J. Skin Doctor CP: Conformal Prediction of the Skin Sensitization Potential of Small Organic Molecules. *Chem. Res. Toxicol.* **2020**, *34*, 330–344. [CrossRef] [PubMed]
30. Vovk, V.; Gammerman, A.; Shafer, G. *Algorithmic Learning in a Random World*; Springer Science & Business Media: New York, NY, USA, 2005; ISBN 9780387001524.
31. Norinder, U.; Carlsson, L.; Boyer, S.; Eklund, M. Introducing Conformal Prediction in Predictive Modeling for Regulatory Purposes. A Transparent and Flexible Alternative to Applicability Domain Determination. *Regul. Toxicol. Pharmacol.* **2015**, *71*, 279–284. [CrossRef]
32. Norinder, U.; Rybacka, A.; Andersson, P.L. Conformal Prediction to Define Applicability Domain—A Case Study on Predicting ER and AR Binding. *SAR QSAR Environ. Res.* **2016**, *27*, 303–316. [CrossRef]
33. Vovk, V. Conditional Validity of Inductive Conformal Predictors. *Mach. Learn.* **2013**, *92*, 349–376. [CrossRef]
34. Concepts and Applications of Conformal Prediction in Computational Drug Discovery. Available online: https://arxiv.org/pdf/1908.03569.pdf (accessed on 17 March 2020).
35. Carlsson, L.; Eklund, M.; Norinder, U. Aggregated Conformal Prediction. In Proceedings of the IFIP International Conference on Artificial Intelligence Applications and Innovations, Rhodes, Greece, 19–21 September 2014; pp. 231–240.
36. Svensson, F.; Afzal, A.M.; Norinder, U.; Bender, A. Maximizing Gain in High-Throughput Screening Using Conformal Prediction. *J. Cheminform.* **2018**, *10*, 7. [CrossRef]
37. Norinder, U.; Svensson, F. Multitask Modeling with Confidence Using Matrix Factorization and Conformal Prediction. *J. Chem. Inf. Model.* **2019**, *59*, 1598–1604. [CrossRef]
38. Norinder, U.; Ahlberg, E.; Carlsson, L. Predicting Ames Mutagenicity Using Conformal Prediction in the Ames/QSAR International Challenge Project. *Mutagenesis* **2019**, *34*, 33–40. [CrossRef]
39. Zhang, J.; Norinder, U.; Svensson, F. Deep Learning-Based Conformal Prediction of Toxicity. *J. Chem. Inf. Model.* **2021**. [CrossRef]
40. Di, P.; Yin, Y.; Jiang, C.; Cai, Y.; Li, W.; Tang, Y.; Liu, G. Prediction of the Skin Sensitising Potential and Potency of Compounds via Mechanism-Based Binary and Ternary Classification Models. *Toxicol. Vitro* **2019**, *59*, 204–214. [CrossRef]
41. Borba, J.V.B.; Braga, R.C.; Alves, V.M.; Muratov, E.N.; Kleinstreuer, N.; Tropsha, A.; Andrade, C.H. Pred-Skin: A Web Portal for Accurate Prediction of Human Skin Sensitizers. *Chem. Res. Toxicol.* **2021**, *34*, 258–267. [CrossRef]
42. Liu, J.; Kern, P.S.; Gerberick, G.F.; Santos-Filho, O.A.; Esposito, E.X.; Hopfinger, A.J.; Tseng, Y.J. Categorical QSAR Models for Skin Sensitization Based on Local Lymph Node Assay Measures and Both Ground and Excited State 4D-Fingerprint Descriptors. *J. Comput. Aided Mol. Des.* **2008**, *22*, 345–366. [CrossRef] [PubMed]
43. Riniker, S.; Landrum, G.A. Similarity Maps—A Visualization Strategy for Molecular Fingerprints and Machine-Learning Methods. *J. Cheminform.* **2013**, *5*, 43. [CrossRef] [PubMed]
44. Wilm, A.; Stork, C.; Bauer, C.; Schepky, A.; Kühnl, J.; Kirchmair, J. Skin Doctor: Machine Learning Models for Skin Sensitization Prediction That Provide Estimates and Indicators of Prediction Reliability. *Int. J. Mol. Sci.* **2019**, *20*, 4833. [CrossRef]

45. Kleinstreuer, N.C.; Hoffmann, S.; Alépée, N.; Allen, D.; Ashikaga, T.; Casey, W.; Clouet, E.; Cluzel, M.; Desprez, B.; Gellatly, N.; et al. Non-Animal Methods to Predict Skin Sensitization (II): An Assessment of Defined Approaches. *Crit. Rev. Toxicol.* **2018**, *48*, 359–374. [CrossRef]
46. Zhang, J.; Hsieh, J.-H.; Zhu, H. Profiling Animal Toxicants by Automatically Mining Public Bioassay Data: A Big Data Approach for Computational Toxicology. *PLoS ONE* **2014**, *9*, e99863. [CrossRef]
47. Ribay, K.; Kim, M.T.; Wang, W.; Pinolini, D.; Zhu, H. Predictive Modeling of Estrogen Receptor Binding Agents Using Advanced Cheminformatics Tools and Massive Public Data. *Front. Environ. Sci.* **2016**, *4*, 12. [CrossRef]
48. Zhu, H.; Zhang, J.; Kim, M.T.; Boison, A.; Sedykh, A.; Moran, K. Big Data in Chemical Toxicity Research: The Use of High-Throughput Screening Assays to Identify Potential Toxicants. *Chem. Res. Toxicol.* **2014**, *27*, 1643–1651. [CrossRef]
49. Kim, M.T.; Huang, R.; Sedykh, A.; Wang, W.; Xia, M.; Zhu, H. Mechanism Profiling of Hepatotoxicity Caused by Oxidative Stress Using Antioxidant Response Element Reporter Gene Assay Models and Big Data. *Environ. Health Perspect.* **2016**, *124*, 634–641. [CrossRef]
50. Riniker, S.; Wang, Y.; Jenkins, J.L.; Landrum, G.A. Using Information from Historical High-Throughput Screens to Predict Active Compounds. *J. Chem. Inf. Model.* **2014**, *54*, 1880–1891. [CrossRef]
51. Guo, Y.; Zhao, L.; Zhang, X.; Zhu, H. Using a Hybrid Read-across Method to Evaluate Chemical Toxicity Based on Chemical Structure and Biological Data. *Ecotoxicol. Environ. Saf.* **2019**, *178*, 178–187. [CrossRef]
52. Zhu, H.; Bouhifd, M.; Donley, E.; Egnash, L.; Kleinstreuer, N.; Kroese, E.D.; Liu, Z.; Luechtefeld, T.; Palmer, J.; Pamies, D.; et al. Supporting Read-across Using Biological Data. *ALTEX* **2016**, *33*, 167–182. [CrossRef] [PubMed]
53. Luechtefeld, T.; Marsh, D.; Rowlands, C.; Hartung, T. Machine Learning of Toxicological Big Data Enables Read-Across Structure Activity Relationships (RASAR) Outperforming Animal Test Reproducibility. *Toxicol. Sci.* **2018**, *165*, 198–212. [CrossRef]
54. Ball, T.; Barber, C.G.; Cayley, A.; Chilton, M.L.; Foster, R.; Fowkes, A.; Heghes, C.; Hill, E.; Hill, N.; Kane, S.; et al. Beyond Adverse Outcome Pathways: Making Toxicity Predictions from Event Networks, SAR Models, Data and Knowledge. *Toxicol. Res.* **2021**, *10*, 102–122. [CrossRef] [PubMed]
55. Norinder, U.; Spjuth, O.; Svensson, F. Using Predicted Bioactivity Profiles to Improve Predictive Modeling. *J. Chem. Inf. Model.* **2020**, *60*, 2830–2837. [CrossRef] [PubMed]
56. Garcia de Lomana, M.; Morger, A.; Norinder, U.; Buesen, R.; Landsiedel, R.; Volkamer, A.; Kirchmair, J.; Mathea, M. ChemBioSim: Enhancing Conformal Prediction of In Vivo Toxicity by Use of Predicted Bioactivities. *J. Chem. Inf. Model.* **2021**, *61*, 3255–3272. [CrossRef] [PubMed]
57. Alves, V.M.; Capuzzi, S.J.; Braga, R.C.; Borba, J.V.B.; Silva, A.C.; Luechtefeld, T.; Hartung, T.; Andrade, C.H.; Muratov, E.N.; Tropsha, A. A Perspective and a New Integrated Computational Strategy for Skin Sensitization Assessment. *ACS Sustain. Chem. Eng.* **2018**, *6*, 2845–2859. [CrossRef]
58. CompTox Chemicals Dashboard. Available online: https://comptox.epa.gov/dashboard/ (accessed on 20 February 2021).
59. DrugBank Release Version 5.1.8. Available online: https://go.drugbank.com/releases/latest (accessed on 20 February 2021).
60. Epa, U.S. ToxCast & Tox21 Data Spreadsheet from Invitrodb_v3.3. Available online: https://www.epa.gov/chemical-research/toxicity-forecaster-toxcasttm-data (accessed on 7 September 2020).
61. Ji, C.; Svensson, F.; Zoufir, A.; Bender, A. eMolTox: Prediction of Molecular Toxicity with Confidence. *Bioinformatics* **2018**, *34*, 2508–2509. [CrossRef]
62. eChemPortal. Available online: https://www.echemportal.org/echemportal/ (accessed on 6 August 2020).
63. Scikit-Learn. Available online: https://scikit-learn.org/stable/ (accessed on 20 February 2021).
64. Landrum, G. RDKit. Available online: http://www.rdkit.org (accessed on 20 February 2021).
65. Matthews, B.W. Comparison of the Predicted and Observed Secondary Structure of T4 Phage Lysozyme. *Biochim. Biophys. Acta* **1975**, *405*, 442–451. [CrossRef]
66. Otsubo, Y.; Nishijo, T.; Miyazawa, M.; Saito, K.; Mizumachi, H.; Sakaguchi, H. Binary Test Battery with KeratinoSens^{TM} and H-CLAT as Part of a Bottom-up Approach for Skin Sensitization Hazard Prediction. *Regul. Toxicol. Pharmacol.* **2017**, *88*, 118–124. [CrossRef]
67. Asturiol, D.; Casati, S.; Worth, A. Consensus of Classification Trees for Skin Sensitisation Hazard Prediction. *Toxicol. Vitro* **2016**, *36*, 197–209. [CrossRef]
68. Roberts, D.W.; Patlewicz, G. Non-Animal Assessment of Skin Sensitization Hazard: Is an Integrated Testing Strategy Needed, and If so What Should Be Integrated? *J. Appl. Toxicol.* **2018**, *38*, 41–50. [CrossRef]
69. Wilm, A.; Garcia de Lomana, M.; Stork, C.; Mathai, N.; Hirte, S.; Norinder, U.; Kühnl, J.; Kirchmair, J. Predicting the skin sensitization potential of small molecules with machine learning models trained on biologically meaningful descriptors. *Zenodo* **2021**. [CrossRef]

pharmaceuticals

Article

Should We Embed in Chemistry? A Comparison of Unsupervised Transfer Learning with PCA, UMAP, and VAE on Molecular Fingerprints

Mario Lovrić [1,2], Tomislav Đuričić [1,3], Han T. N. Tran [1], Hussain Hussain [1,3], Emanuel Lacić [1], Morten A. Rasmussen [4,5] and Roman Kern [1,3,*]

1 Know-Center, Inffeldgasse 13, 8010 Graz, Austria; mlovric@know-center.at (M.L.); tduricic@tugraz.at (T.Đ.); htran@know-center.at (H.T.N.T.); hhussain@know-center.at (H.H.); elacic@know-center.at (E.L.)
2 Centre for Applied Bioanthropology, Institute for Anthropological Research, 10000 Zagreb, Croatia
3 Institute of Interactive Systems and Data Science, Graz University of Technology, Inffeldgasse 16C, 8010 Graz, Austria
4 Copenhagen Studies on Asthma in Childhood, Herlev-Gentofte Hospital, University of Copenhagen, Ledreborg Alle 34, 2820 Gentofte, Denmark; morten.arendt@dbac.dk
5 Department of Food Science, University of Copenhagen, Rolighedsvej 26, 1958 Frederiksberg, Denmark
* Correspondence: rkern@know-center.at; Tel.: +43-316-873-30860

Abstract: Methods for dimensionality reduction are showing significant contributions to knowledge generation in high-dimensional modeling scenarios throughout many disciplines. By achieving a lower dimensional representation (also called embedding), fewer computing resources are needed in downstream machine learning tasks, thus leading to a faster training time, lower complexity, and statistical flexibility. In this work, we investigate the utility of three prominent unsupervised embedding techniques (principal component analysis—PCA, uniform manifold approximation and projection—UMAP, and variational autoencoders—VAEs) for solving classification tasks in the domain of toxicology. To this end, we compare these embedding techniques against a set of molecular fingerprint-based models that do not utilize additional pre-preprocessing of features. Inspired by the success of transfer learning in several fields, we further study the performance of embedders when trained on an external dataset of chemical compounds. To gain a better understanding of their characteristics, we evaluate the embedders with different embedding dimensionalities, and with different sizes of the external dataset. Our findings show that the recently popularized UMAP approach can be utilized alongside known techniques such as PCA and VAE as a pre-compression technique in the toxicology domain. Nevertheless, the generative model of VAE shows an advantage in pre-compressing the data with respect to classification accuracy.

Keywords: manifold learning; machine learning; rdkit; embeddings; Tox21; principal component analysis; autoencoder

Citation: Lovrić, M.; Đuričić, T.; Tran, H.T.N.; Hussain, H.; Lacić, E.; Rasmussen, M.A.; Kern, R. Should We Embed in Chemistry? A Comparison of Unsupervised Transfer Learning with PCA, UMAP, and VAE on Molecular Fingerprints. *Pharmaceuticals* **2021**, *14*, 758. https://doi.org/10.3390/ph14080758

Academic Editor: Osvaldo Andrade Santos-Filho

Received: 30 June 2021
Accepted: 22 July 2021
Published: 2 August 2021

1. Introduction

Chemical (or molecular) representation is an important topic in cheminformatics [1] and quantitative structure–activity relationships (QSARs), as QSAR model quality depends largely on the predictive features defined by the task at hand, i.e., mapping a feature space (X) onto a target chemical or biological activity (y). Besides using molecular descriptors, which are numerous and sometimes hard to explain [2], the development of deep learning [3–5] and big data [6–9] gave rise to the utilization of various representations such as molecular fingerprints [10] and NLP-based methods like Mol2Vec [11]. With the advent of graph neural networks, researchers also started to learn from molecular images themselves [12]. More and more researchers are utilizing diverse representations to compare and find suitable features for solving the modeling problem [13–16] as no single feature set appears to be the optimal one. Hence, sometimes, combinations of features are also utilized [16]. Another difficulty in machine learning (and consequently cheminformatics) is the so-called curse of dimensionality, a term coined by Richard Bellman [17], which refers to various problems that arise when working with high-dimensional data (such as fingerprints) including increased chances of overfitting and spurious results. With high dimensionality, distances and densities (such as neighborhoods) might no longer be representative [18]. A well-established strategy, besides feature selection, to cope with this issue is dimensionality reduction, i.e., transforming the data into a low-dimensional space such that the resulting low-dimensional representation preserves certain properties of the original data. Such an approach has proven to be highly useful for numerous downstream machine learning tasks like classification [19], anomaly detection [20], and recommender systems [21]. Generally speaking, algorithms for dimensionality reduction can be categorized into three main groups, namely, matrix factorization, neighbor graphs, and deep learning-based approaches. Matrix factorization algorithms include approaches such as latent Dirichlet allocation [22], non-negative matrix factorization [23], and linear autoencoders [24]. However, the most commonly used approach is principal component analysis (PCA) [25]. It is founded on eigenvalue and eigenvector decomposition of symmetric semipositive definite matrices, and hence constitutes a clean linear orthogonal basis transformation to maximize variance explanation of both samples and variables. Indeed, the derived low-dimensional space—often referred to as scores—is a linear mapping of the original features. However, the systematic part of the original data is furthermore a linear mapping of the scores. In this way, PCA is a mathematically transparent and chemically interpretable tool for mapping data to a low-dimensional space and translating between this space and the original feature space. The linearity of PCA is what makes the method mathematically more concise than some nonlinear methods, but at the price of variance maximization as well as the inability to capture nonlinear phenomena in single dimensions. When it comes to nonlinear methods for dimensionality reduction, there are a number of noteworthy approaches, such as locally linear embedding [26], Laplacian eigenmaps [27], or t-SNE [26]. One of the most effective and commonly used methods that also falls into this category is uniform manifold approximation and projection for dimension reduction or UMAP [28]. It is a nonlinear method that works by utilizing local manifold approximations and combining their local fuzzy simplicial set representations in order to create a topological representation of the high-dimensional data. It then minimizes the cross-entropy between topological representations, thus optimizing the layout of the data representation. UMAP was employed already in understanding patterns in chemical/structural [29,30] and biological data [31,32] by transferring them to a lower dimensional space. More recently however, the category of nonlinear dimensionality reduction approaches has been extended with deep learning-based algorithms. The most prominent approach here is the traditional autoencoder model [33]. Autoencoders are (typically nonlinear) neural network architectures that learn to copy their input onto their output by passing the input through an intermediate bottleneck layer. As they were originally proposed, there has been a number of adaptations of the original autoencoder with variational autoencoders or VAEs [34] as one of the latest state-of-the-art methods. Autoencoders are often applied in cheminformatics for tasks like chemical space navigation and de novo molecular generation [4,29,35] or prediction [36]. The aim of this work is thus to evaluate chemical space information generated from fingerprints and investigate the impact of generating embeddings in an unsupervised manner using prominent linear and nonlinear methods. That is, we specifically look into the utility of PCA, UMAP, and VAE (hereinafter embedders) as pre-compression techniques for solving classification tasks with 12 binary toxic outcomes.

2. Results and Discussion

2.1. Setting the Baseline

Before presenting the results of embeddings as predictive features, we present here the baseline models trained on raw fingerprints. The results are shown in Table 1. Furthermore, we compared the results to recent work [37] where the results are also presented by means of MCC and trained on fingerprints (like in the present study). The limitations of this comparison are as follows: (a) the train–test splits are not the same; (b) there is a difference in fingerprint parameters; (c) we limited hyperparameter optimization, as our aim was to compare the results of the embeddings; (d) we used average values of the predictions on the test set for several random states; and (e) Zhang et al. use a Bayesian optimization instead of the grid-search we used. We also want to note that the classification results from Zhang et al. [37] show higher MCC values than the results in this work. Besides the mentioned differences, in our work, instead of using nested-CV, we report on a true external test set. The purpose of this comparison is to present the expectations towards the individual labels in Tox21.

Table 1. A comparison of our baseline results trained on fingerprints to a similar study from Zhang et al. [37]. The results from Zhang are denoted with a "Z", while the respective classifiers are as follows: L—lightGBM, R—random forests, S—support vector machines, X—XGBM, D—deep neural networks. The classifiers from this work are k-nearest neighbor classifier (KNN), logistic regression (LR), and random forests classifier (RFC), which are represented by their mean values per classifier, respectively. Additionally, the mean and max of all classifiers in this work are compared. The best baseline models in our work are marked with an superscript "a", while the best models from Zhang are marked with an superscript "b".

Label (endpoint)	Mean (all)	Max (all)	KNN	LR	RFC	Z-L	Z-R	Z-S	Z-X	Z-D
NR-AR	0.52	0.62	^{a}0.59	0.4	0.56	0.50	0.62	0.43	0.60	^{b}0.68
NR-AR-LBD	0.57	0.63	0.61	0.48	^{a}0.62	0.60	0.71	0.60	^{b}0.73	0.72
NR-AhR	0.44	0.47	^{a}0.45	0.44	0.43	0.52	^{b}0.61	0.47	0.54	0.59
NR-Aromatase	0.29	0.35	^{a}0.32	0.25	0.29	0.28	^{b}0.52	0.32	0.50	0.48
NR-ER	0.29	0.34	^{a}0.33	0.24	0.29	0.37	0.42	0.32	0.40	^{b}0.44
NR-ER-LBD	0.35	0.47	0.37	0.26	^{a}0.42	0.45	0.56	0.36	^{b}0.59	0.58
NR-PPAR-gamma	0.18	0.26	0.14	0.18	^{a}0.22	0.32	0.50	0.30	^{b}0.52	0.47
SR-ARE	0.28	0.36	0.25	^{a}0.31	0.29	0.46	0.49	0.36	0.46	0.48
SR-ATAD5	0.24	0.26	^{a}0.25	0.22	0.24	0.37	^{b}0.59	0.36	0.53	0.55
SR-HSE	0.18	0.25	0.15	0.18	^{a}0.20	0.31	^{b}0.37	0.21	0.40	^{b}0.37
SR-MMP	0.44	0.47	0.44	^{a}0.47	0.43	0.63	^{b}0.65	0.54	0.64	0.63
SR-p53	0.22	0.26	0.21	^{a}0.24	0.23	0.42	^{b}0.57	0.37	0.52	0.55

2.2. Embedding Chemical Spaces

In this section, the classification results of models trained on embeddings (internal/external) are presented and discussed. For the purpose of training the models, the fingerprints were subjected to transformations into low-dimensional spaces by either PCA, UMAP, or VAE. Visual examples of the transformations (CS1 and CS2) are shown in Figure 1 for both data sets.

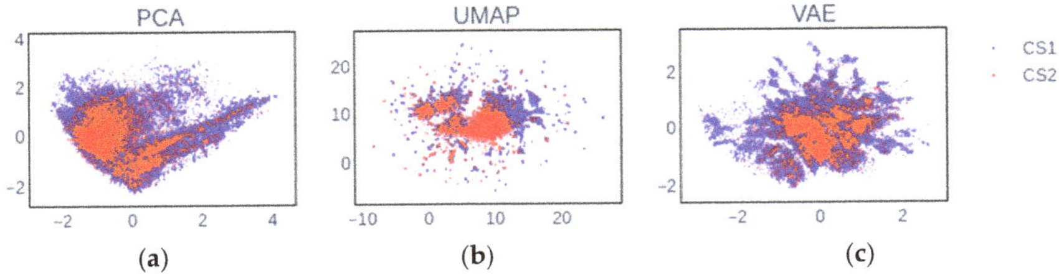

Figure 1. Exemplary visualization of CS1 (red) and CS2 (blue) show in 2D embedded space generated from molecular fingerprints by means of (**a**) principal component analysis (PCA), (**b**) uniform manifold approximation and projection (UMAP), and (**c**) variational autoencoders (VAEs).

Our first observation by visually inspecting Figure 1 is that the three studied embedding algorithms produce greatly different data representations owing to the underlying differences in how they operate. Furthermore, we observe that CS1 covers a larger chemical space in comparison with CS2 owing to the difference in data set size. Additionally, some areas of CS1 data space are barely covered in CS2, making it harder to transfer knowledge for these compounds. This behavior appears more pronounced in UMAP and VAE data representations. Finally, UMAP and VAE appear to produce a number of smaller observable clusters in comparison with PCA. This is an inherent consequence of UMAP, where indeed the underlying graphs of the samples are pruned, while PCA is a linear mapping, making it impossible to introduce discrete clusters if they are not directly present in the raw data.

2.3. Impact of Embedding Size and Information Content

In this section, we want to evaluate the contribution of the number of latent variables (dimensions) and the data input size for creating embeddings from the external data set prior to solving the classification tasks (see Figure 2). The embedding approaches were varied in input size (200–30,000 compounds from CS1) and number of dimensions (2–15 latent variables) and evaluated for three random states, three different classifiers (RFC, KNN, LR), and three embedders (PCA, UMAP, VAE) as described in the Materials and Methods section. The results are depicted in Figures 2–4.

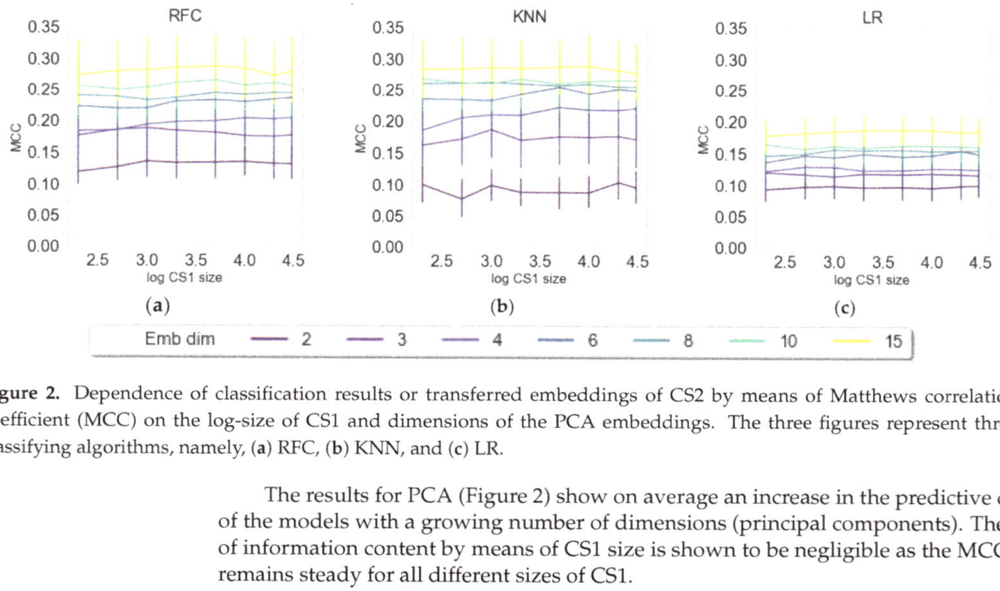

Figure 2. Dependence of classification results or transferred embeddings of CS2 by means of Matthews correlation coefficient (MCC) on the log-size of CS1 and dimensions of the PCA embeddings. The three figures represent three classifying algorithms, namely, (**a**) RFC, (**b**) KNN, and (**c**) LR.

The results for PCA (Figure 2) show on average an increase in the predictive quality of the models with a growing number of dimensions (principal components). The effect of information content by means of CS1 size is shown to be negligible as the MCC score remains steady for all different sizes of CS1.

Models embedded with UMAP (Figure 3) show distinctively different patterns compared with PCA. For KNN and RFC, there is a clear trend for increasing dimensions and information content, while there seems to be some randomness in LR with an existing trend for model improvement when increasing dimensions and information content. The third embedding algorithm, VAE, shows similar patterns to UMAP (see Figure 4). An observable difference to UMAP is that, for RFC and KNN, it seems to approach a plateau, while UMAP shows a steady increase. All machine learning methods show a clear increase of model quality with an increase of dimensions and CS1 data size.

PCA by definition only extracts linear features, and the ability to capture nonlinear behavior relies on the upstream use of nonlinear classifiers. Here, we indeed see that nonlinear phenomena are captured using kNN or RFC in contrast to logistic regression.

On the other hand, PCA is powerful in filtering off stochastic white noise, simply because of the nature of white noise where there is no dependency across features. Indeed, this phenomenon is observed for the PCA embedding as the performance is insensitive towards the size of training data as well as classifier type, simply pointing out that the principal components' directions are well defined even for small data set. It is interesting to observe that, with UMAP, we see a saturation regarding the number of dimensions (6, 8, 10, and 15 perform similarly), while with VAE, we observe the effect, but to a lesser extent. VAE seems to benefit more from input data size in comparison with UMAP, which we attribute to deep learning methods typically requiring larger data sizes for learning [38]. In further evaluations, we compared only the results on maximum dimension size (15) and maximum set size (30,000 compounds in CS1).

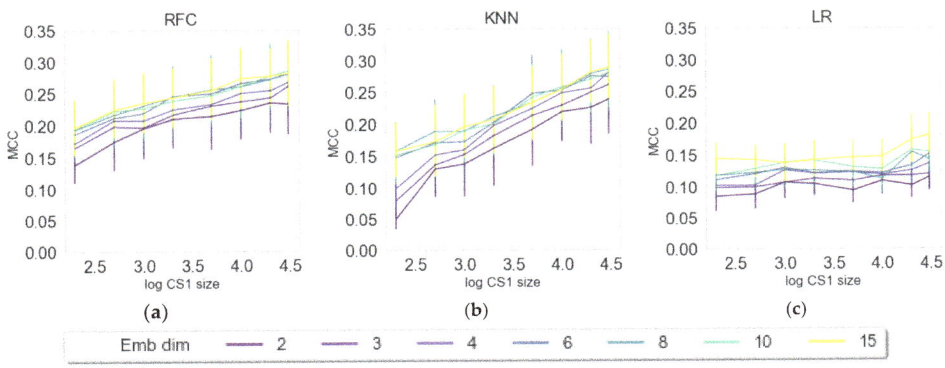

Figure 3. Dependence of classification results or transferred embeddings of CS2 by means of MCC on the log-size of CS1 and dimensions of the UMAP embeddings. The three figures represent three classifying algorithms, namely, (**a**) RFC, (**b**) KNN, and (**c**) LR.

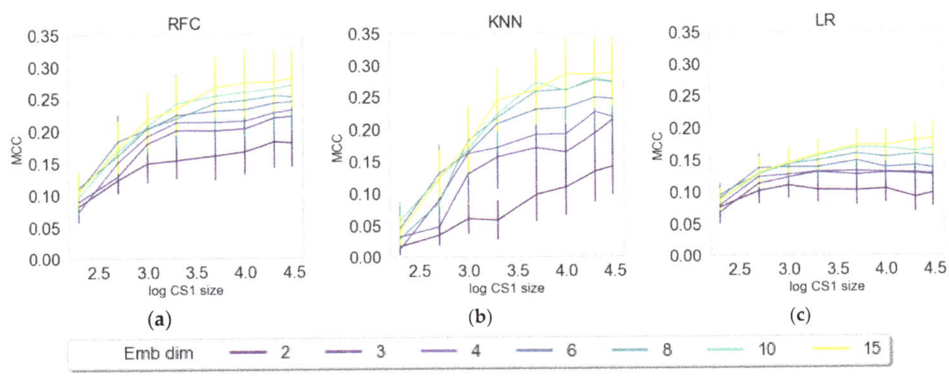

Figure 4. Dependence of classification results or transferred embeddings of CS2 by means of MCC on the log-size of CS1 and dimensions of the VAE embeddings. The three figures represent three classifying algorithms, namely, (**a**) RFC, (**b**) KNN, and (**c**) LR.

2.4. Internal versus External Knowledge

To evaluate whether the external knowledge (from CS1) is beneficial for the classification task in CS2, we list the MCC score of each embedding algorithm, trained (a) on external data from CS1 and (b) on internal data from CS2, in Table 2. One has to keep in mind that CS1 size was varied, while CS2 is fixed.

Table 2. Comparison of external and internal embeddings for PCA, UMAP, and VAE. Each cell represents the mean MCC score across nine different machine learning models (three random states × three classifiers). Values marked with an asterisk (*) highlight cases where, on average, models trained using external knowledge outperformed models trained on internal knowledge. Additionally results marked with a quotation mark (') highlight cases where using external or internal knowledge yielded equal results (when rounded off to two decimal places).

Label	PCA		UMAP		VAE	
	IN	EX	IN	EX	IN	EX
NR-AR	0.45	0.43	' 0.47	' 0.47	0.45	0.44
NR-AR-LBD	0.45	0.43	* 0.45	* 0.53	' 0.43	' 0.43
NR-AhR	' 0.33	' 0.33	* 0.34	* 0.35	' 0.34	' 0.34
NR-Aromatase	0.22	0.18	0.18	0.15	' 0.21	' 0.21
NR-ER	0.22	0.21	' 0.23	' 0.23	' 0.27	0.24
NR-ER-LBD	0.31	0.26	' 0.26	' 0.26	' 0.28	' 0.28
NR-PPAR-gamma	' 0.14	' 0.14	* 0.09	* 0.11	0.11	0.09
SR-ARE	* 0.19	* 0.21	* 0.19	* 0.2	* 0.19	* 0.2
SR-ATAD5	0.16	0.13	* 0.12	* 0.16	* 0.14	* 0.15
SR-HSE	* 0.09	* 0.11	' 0.08	' 0.08	* 0.07	* 0.1
SR-MMP	' 0.36	' 0.36	' 0.32	' 0.32	* 0.35	* 0.36
SR-p53	0.19	0.18	0.16	0.14	* 0.15	* 0.17

Our results have a few important takeaways. In comparison with PCA, both UMAP and VAE were able to achieve better results overall when fitted on external knowledge versus fitting on internal knowledge. With external knowledge, PCA achieved better results on two labels and equal results (rounded on two decimals) on three. UMAP and VAE performed similarly as both approaches performed better when trained on external knowledge on five labels and performed equally to respective models trained on internal knowledge on five labels (out of 12 labels in total). It is important to note that, even though UMAP and VAE showed similar performance overall, they performed differently for different labels. For example, UMAP showed a strong improvement in MCC score for NR-AR-LBD when using external knowledge, whereas VAE did not improve in comparison with VAE trained on internal knowledge. There was only one label (SR-ARE) for which all three embedding algorithms yielded better results when trained on external knowledge.

2.5. *Should We Embed? Does Embedding Win over Baseline?*

Figure 5 and Table 3 compare the MCC score of all embedders (internal and external) to the fingerprint baseline model (FPR-BL) on each classification task. From Figure 5, it is clear that the fingerprint baseline model performs better overall for most of the labels.

Table 3 shows that the embedders do not increase in the score in general. However, for the NR-ER label, VAE embedders show an increase in MCC score. To present embedding capabilities, we compared the maximum values per embedder in Table 3. Each value is the maximum of nine machine learning experiments (three classifiers × three random states). For easier comparison, we set the FPR-BL maximum per label to 100%. The results show that 3 out of 12 labels embedded features can reach or surpass the baseline, namely, NR-AR, NR-AR-LBD, and NR-ER. With PCA, both internally and externally, the maximum value never reached those of the baseline, while with externally trained UMAP, only one target performed on par with the baseline. With the variational autoencoder, the baseline was reached three times. This shows the dominance of VAE over other embedders given the constraints in our experiments. In conclusion, by embedding molecular fingerprints, we can obtain a comparable and sometimes improved classification accuracy with toxicological models compared with no embedding. The main advantage in applying embedding techniques on the molecular fingerprints in this way is a reduced model complexity, by utilizing smaller feature sets, without the need to sacrifice predictive accuracy.

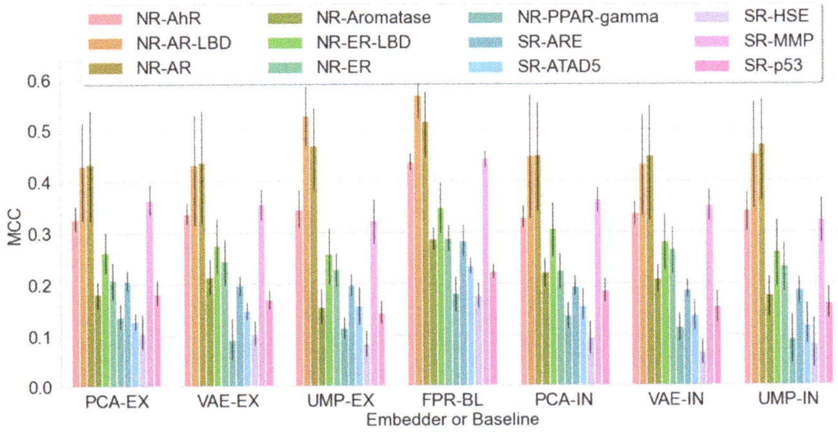

Figure 5. Comparison of machine learning classifications mean + error bar across all feature sets: FPR-BL = fingerprint baseline, PCA = principal component analysis (EX = external, IN = internal), UMP = uniform manifold approximation and projection, VAE = variational autoencoders. Each bar present nine runs (three classifiers × three random states).

Table 3. Classification results across all data sets and labels expressed by maximum values of the MCC. The fingerprint-based model maxima (FPR-BL) were set as 100%, while the embedding models referred to these 100%. Results assigned with an asterisk (*) outperformed baseline.

Label (endpoint)	FPR-BL	PCA-EX	PCA-IN	UMAP-EX	UMAP-IN	VAE-EX	VAE-IN
NR-AR	100	95	99	96	96	97	* 100
NR-AR-LBD	100	92	98	* 100	97	98	* 102
NR-AhR	100	84	85	90	86	83	85
NR-Aromatase	100	65	82	75	74	84	75
NR-ER	100	83	85	86	95	* 103	* 101
NR-ER-LBD	100	70	90	79	88	90	83
NR-PPAR-gamma	100	81	82	68	81	78	75
SR-ARE	100	74	69	70	69	63	63
SR-ATAD5	100	63	99	92	84	75	88
SR-HSE	100	82	77	56	90	65	55
SR-MMP	100	92	87	83	83	93	89
SR-p53	100	99	95	79	87	85	93

2.6. Insights into Latent Representations

The embedders compress information in an unsupervised way, thus the resulting output is based on the efficacy of the utilized approach; underlying data; and, to an extent, how well the hyperparameters are tuned. Therefore, it is difficult to predict whether utilizing the same compression techniques would be beneficial for use cases that are different from our problem of predicting 12 toxic outcomes. To better understand how the classification tasks can profit from compression, we calculated silhouette coefficients on the calculated embeddings within the data sets, s (Equation (1)), in the latent space (for 2D and 3D latent spaces as well as using external embeddings):

$$s(i) = \frac{b(i)-a(i)}{\max\{a(i), b(i)\}}, if\ |C_i| > 1 \qquad s(i) = 0, if\ |C_i| = 0 \tag{1}$$

In this equation, *a(i)* is the mean distance between a molecule *i* and all other molecules in the same cluster and *b(i)* is the mean distance of molecule *i* to all molecules in any other cluster. For each label, the coefficients are plotted in Figure 6. The average silhouette coefficients per label were correlated to the predictive quality (MCC), as shown in Table 4. Besides that, we compared the baseline models (raw fingerprints) and the imbalance ratio with respect to the MCC results of the classifiers that utilize embeddings. The results show that the predictive quality correlates almost perfectly (0.98+) with the baseline models, which means that achieving a good classification on raw data (i.e., fingerprints) will most likely also lead to good results after embedding.

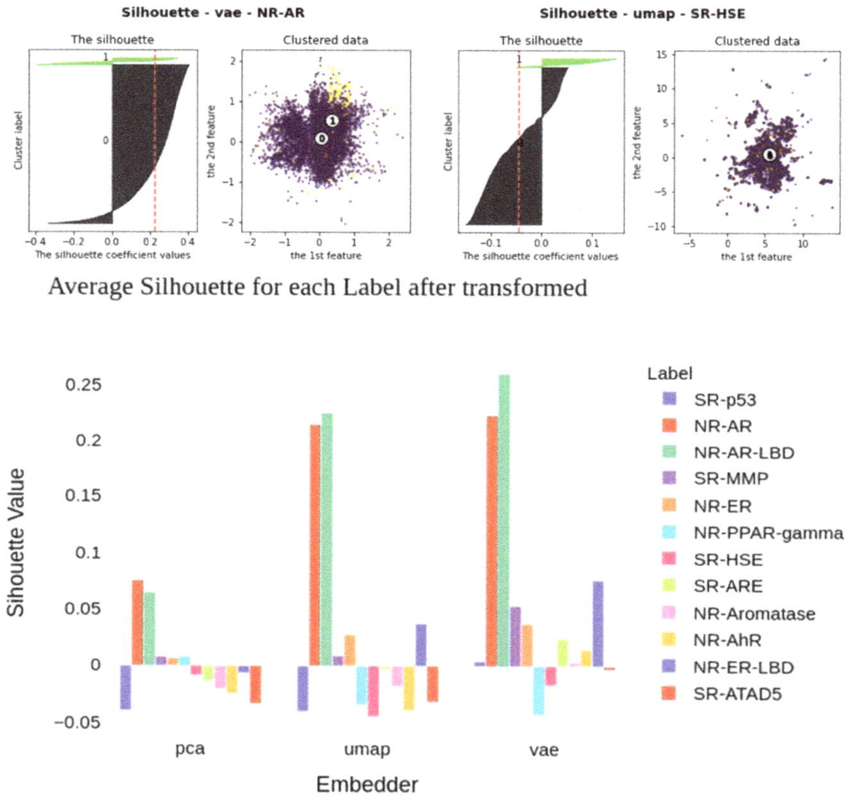

Figure 6. Top: Silhouette plots for best (top left) and worst (top right) performing clustering, which are VAE with NR-AR and UMAP with SR-HSE, respectively. The gray and green masses are points in two classes (0 and 1) with their silhouette coefficients, respectively. The dashed red line is the average value of both. The scatter plot visualizes their coordinates in the 2D embedded space. The number is their center points for each class (0 and 1). We notice that, for the best clustering, the silhouette coefficient tends to be higher, and points that belong to NR-AR label visually agglomerate together. Conversely, the silhouette coefficient seems to be negative for the worst clustering, and the points belonging to SR-HSE label are visually indistinguishable from other points. Silhouette coefficients for externally embedded CS2 data (bottom) by means of the three embedders (PCA, UMAP, VAE) calculated per label, which are presented by the color map. We see that VAE gains a higher silhouette coefficient on most tasks than UMAP or PCA, indicating a better separation.

Table 4. Correlation of average classification results of the embedded classifiers (PCA-EX, UMAP-EX. VAE-EX) with the imbalance ratio (Pos class %) and baseline fingerprints classifiers (FPR-BL) with their respective silhouette coefficients—s(PCA), s(UMAP), and s(VAE).

	PCA-EX	UMAP-EX	VAE-EX
s(PCA)	0.74		
s(UMAP)		0.86	
s(VAE)			0.85
Pos class %	0.11	0.02	0.13
FPR-BL	0.98	0.98	0.99

Nevertheless, there is also a high correlation between the calculated silhouette coefficients and the predictive quality of embedded classifiers. This indicates that, even though the embedders distribute the classes without prior knowledge, they still seem to keep more relevant information regarding the given classification task. This turned out to be more relevant for the nonlinear methods (i.e., UMAP and VAE) than for PCA.

3. Materials and Methods

In this section, we present the data for conducting the study, the machine learning methods used for solving the classification tasks, the embedding techniques utilized, and the overall modeling pipeline.

3.1. Data

The data for the classification experiment (here named compound set 2 or CS2) were downloaded from the Tox21 public repository [39]. The chosen set is the 2014 Tox21 challenge subset with 12 toxicological endpoints related to stress response and nuclear receptor panels. This dataset was studied in many works and was subject to a plethora of reports on the outcomes [3,15,40,41]. Hence, it represents a baseline dataset for QSAR classification as it is imbalanced, chemically diverse, and large (~10k compounds), but has also several endpoints with different predictive capabilities (modeling challenges). Owing to the mentioned challenges this dataset offers, it has been subject to numerous studies in advanced machine learning methods [3,40], balancing methods [15,42], as well as novelties in chemical representation such as conformational resampling [41] and multitask learning [3]. We subjected the data to preprocessing as they consist of duplicated structures, which was reported previously [15]. During preprocessing, we removed structures that did not have valid SMILES or identifiers [7] and they were additionally converted to their canonical SMILES. Furthermore, we removed duplicates by both their IDs and SMILES. We removed inorganic compounds and metal-containing compounds as well as fragments. The procedure is inspired by [15,43] to keep the active part of the compounds. For the predictive tasks, Morgan fingerprints (FPR) were calculated for the 8314 structures by means of the RDKit library [44]. Owing to the possibility of colliding bits in fingerprints [45,46], we set the fingerprint vector length to 5120 bits and the radius to 2. In order to foster reproducibility, we made the scripts that are used for data preprocessing and feature engineering available already in our recent work [16].

The compounds used for generating external embeddings were retrieved from [47] and consist of 68,679 compounds. This compound set 1 (i.e., CS1) was preprocessed in the same manner as the Tox21 dataset described above. After preprocessing and duplicate removal, a total of 54,820 structures remained. During modeling, the structures present in both sets (CS1 and CS2) were removed from CS2 to avoid a target leak.

3.2. Machine Learning Methods

The task at hand is to predict the labels in Tox21, which are binary classes. For this, we employed three common classifiers, namely a random forests classifier (RFC) [48], logistic regression (LR) [49], and a k-nearest neighbor classifier (kNN) [50]. These algorithms are conventional tools when conducting machine learning studies and represent different inductive biases (e.g., assuming that the relationship between input attributes and the output of a LR algorithm is linear)). As the datasets are imbalanced, which makes them challenging when trying to avoid random classification issues [51], we employed penalization and optimization techniques to improve classification outcomes. In our experiments, we first randomly split the data into a train and test set with a 3:1 ratio (i.e., 75% of the data are part of the train set). To penalize the models for misclassification of the minor class (active compounds), we employed the Matthews correlation coefficient (MCC) [52] as a scoring function, as it was shown in our previous studies to work well for imbalanced sets [13,53]. MCC is defined by Equation (2), where TP, TN, FN, and FP are the elements of the confusion matrix given in Table 5.

$$\text{MCC} = \frac{TP \cdot TN - FP \cdot FN}{\sqrt{(TP + FP) \cdot (TP + FN) \cdot (TN + FP) \cdot (TN + FN)}} \quad (2)$$

Table 5. Elements of the confusion matrix that show the possible outcomes when predicting labels in Tox21.

Experimental/Model	Positive (Model) (1)	Negative (Model) (0)
Positive (Experimental) (1)	TP (experimentally active and predicted active)	FN (experimentally active, but predicted as inactive)
Negative (Experimental) (0)	FP (experimentally inactive, but predicted as active)	TN (inactive experimentally and predicted)

The models were tuned with respect to their hyperparameters, which were found using exhaustive grid-search evaluated by cross-validation [54]. All models were trained with the scikit-learn library for Python [55].

3.3. Transfer Learning with Embeddings

3.3.1. Principal Component Analysis (PCA)

PCA [25] is an algorithm for dimensionality reduction based on the maximization of variance in a lower-dimensional projected space. In that regard, PCA can be perceived as a linear autoencoder [56]. The mathematics of PCA is described in many textbooks, but in short, the original data (**X**~(n,p)) are represented by the product of two matrices, namely the scores (**T**~(n,k)) and the loadings (**P**~(p,k)), Equation (3):

$$X = TP^T + E \quad (3)$$

where **E**~(n,p) is the residual matrix and n, p, and k are the number of samples, variables, and components, respectively. The parameters are estimated to capture as much of the variance in the original data in a least squares sense, and further to be orthogonal matrices, i.e.,

$$\{T, P\} = argmax_{T,P}\left(\|X - TP^T\|_2^2\right) \quad (4)$$

The combination of vectors of **T** and **P** are referred to as principal components, and used in various ways in, e.g., exploratory data analysis to map the multivariate sample distribution as well as interrogating feature2feature correlation structure, as well as—like in this work—to represent the data in a few meaningful features used for further analysis. A rewrite of Equation (4) above shows that the score space (**T**) is a linear mapping by the orthogonal basis represented by **P**: **T** = **XP**, and hence a rotation of the coordinate system as depicted in Figure 7.

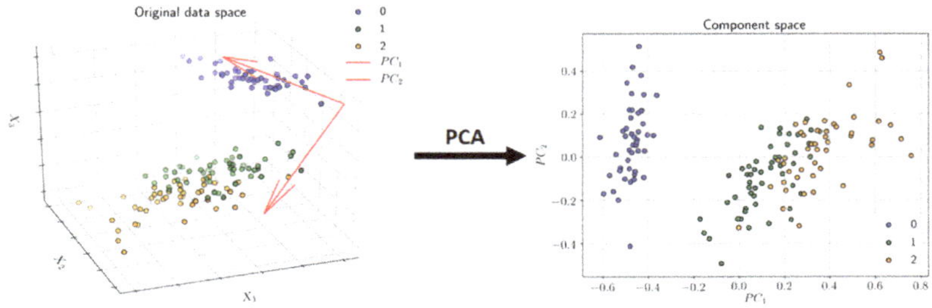

Figure 7. An example of dimensionality reduction by means of PCA. Instances/points in a 3D space (original space) are transformed into a 2D space of two latent variables called principal components (PC1 and PC2).

3.3.2. Uniform Manifold Approximation and Projection (UMAP)

The recent work of McInnes et al. [28] has tackled the problem of dimensionality reduction by generalizing linear approaches like PCA in order to be sensitive to a possible nonlinear structure in data. By applying a completely new field of mathematics, which is based on Riemannian geometry and algebraic topology, they developed the uniform manifold approximation and projection (UMAP) algorithm.

Using every available data point, UMAP first creates a graph with respect to the distances on the underlying topology and to the k-neighborhood of each element (as seen in Figure 8). The Laplacian eigenmaps dimensionality reduction method is then applied on that graph. The resulting graph is further modified by a forced directed graph layout algorithm, which minimizes the cross-entropy between this modified graph and the original one. In this manner, the resulting low-dimensional data representation is optimized to well preserve both the local and global structure of the original data. The main advantage of UMAP over PCA is that it is able to capture a more complex (nonlinear) structure in high-dimensional data, which is a desirable characteristic in our use-case. UMAP is able to achieve this by initially constructing a high-dimensional graph representation of the original data, followed by optimizing a low-dimensional graph to be as structurally similar to the original as possible. In this manner, the resulting low-dimensional data representation is able to well preserve both the local and global structure of the original data.

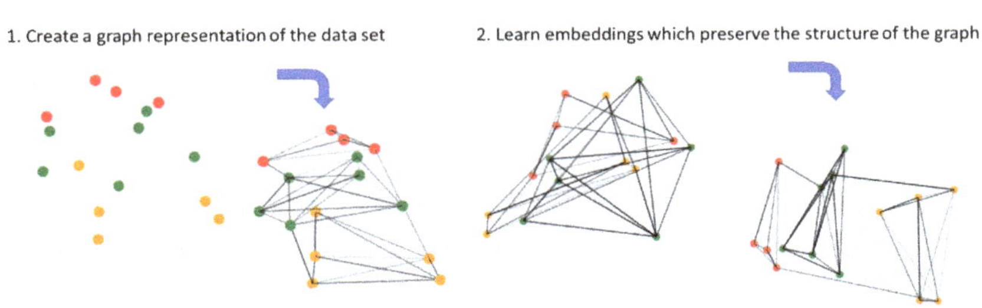

Figure 8. Visual explanation of how UMAP works. It first computes a graph representation of the input data, which is then used to learn embeddings that preserve the structure of the graph representation. Figures is redrawn based on ref. [57].

3.3.3. Variational Autoencoders (VAE)

Since the work of Kramer [58], autoencoders have become a popular alternative to PCA in providing an effective method to reduce the dimensionality of data. This type of neural network is defined by a two-part architecture, which consists of an encoder and a decoder. In its simplest form, it has only one hidden layer (i.e., the information bottleneck), which is a low-dimensional representation of the original data. It is trained in an unsupervised manner to encode the data in a way that keeps the information loss minimal when the decoder attempts to recreate the input from the hidden layer. One popular extension of this approach is to use variational inference when extracting the latent representation [59]. The main difference lies in the fact that the network does not encode the input as a single point. Rather, it makes strong assumptions that the input data can be represented as a probability distribution like Gaussian and encodes the mean and variance of the data separately. As seen in Figure 9, the decoder of the variational autoencoder then samples the latent representation to produce a probability distribution of the low-dimensional representation. Such a probabilistic approach allows the variational autoencoder to be a generative model, i.e., the decoder is capable of creating completely new data that are similar to the observed data used for training the model.

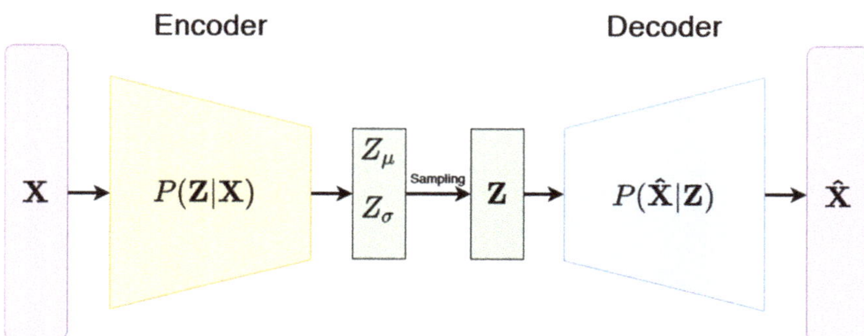

Figure 9. Architecture illustration of the variational autoencoder. Encoder compresses the input X into a latent representation Z. VAE is different to a standard autoencoder as it assumes that the input data have an underlying probability distribution (e.g., Gaussian) for which they try to optimize parameters. The decoder then attempts to reconstruct the original input from the representation by minimizing the reconstruction loss.

3.3.4. Embedder Training

The embedders are trained on molecular fingerprints. For this purpose, we created two sets of embedders: (1) embedders created with the external data set (CS1), which are then consecutively used to encode CS2, which results in the transformed representation of CS2 (hereinafter, external embeddings (EX)); and (2) embedders that were created on the respective pre-split train set of CS2 and used to encode the pre-split test set of CS2 (hereinafter, internal embeddings (IN)). Both procedures are shown in Figure 10. The two sets of embeddings were used for solving the classification task of the 12 toxicological labels alongside commonly used fingerprints. We have fitted the three embedding techniques (i.e., PCA, UMAP, VAE) on the fingerprints from the CS1 set in eight different data sizes of randomly selected compounds (200, 500, 1000, 2000, 5000, 10,000, 20,000, and 30,000 compounds) and embedding dimensions (i.e., number of latent variables: 2, 4, 6, 8, 10, and 15). The concept of how to train and apply embedders on chemical spaces is shown in Figure 11. The Tox21 dataset was transformed with each of the embedders subsequently and used in the machine learning prediction for each of the 12 toxicological endpoints. The full experimental matrix consists of 18,288 individual machine learning experiments (see Table 6).

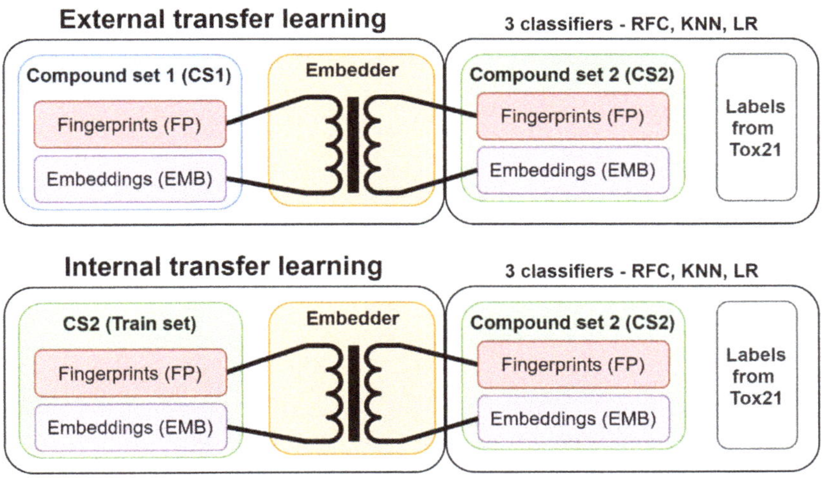

Figure 10. In external transfer learning, an embedder (PCA, UMAP, VAE) is fit on fingerprints on an external set of fingerprints (CS1). The same model (pre-trained embedder) is then utilized to encode fingerprints from CS2. In internal transfer learning, the embedder is fit on the pre-split train set of CS2 and used to encode the test set of CS2. The embeddings of CS2 were utilized for training predictive classification tasks.

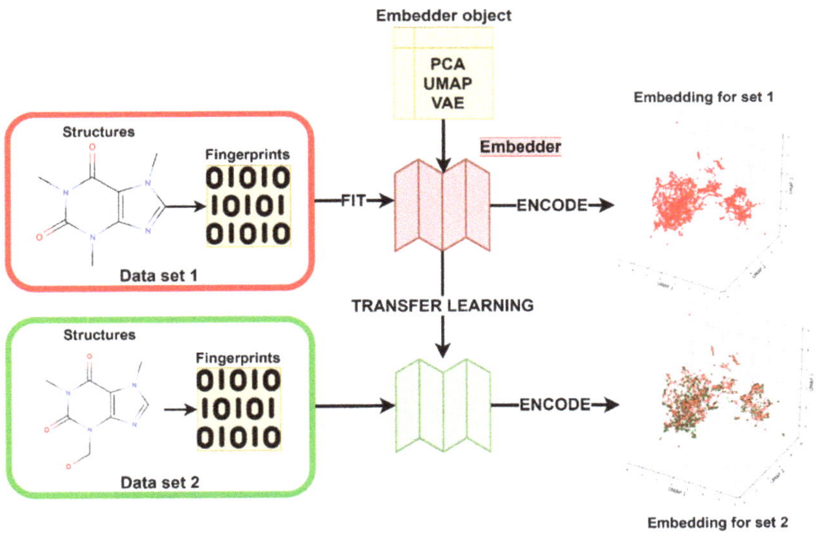

Figure 11. Schematics of chemical space transformation from fingerprint through a pre-trained embedder model. The transformation can either be conducted from an external data set to the data set of interest or within the data set of interest, but split into the train and test set.

Table 6. Experimental matrix. See abbreviations below the table.

Predictive Variables	Classifier	Seed	Embedder	Emb. Dim.	CS1 Data Size	N Models
Fingerprints (raw data)	RFC, KNN, LR	1–3	N/A	N/A	N/A	144
Internal emb.	RFC, KNN, LR	1–3	PCA, UMAP, VAE	2–15	N/A	9072
External emb.	RFC, KNN, LR	1–3	PCA, UMAP, VAE	2–15	200–30,000	9072

CS1—compound set 1, Seed—random state in machine learning, RFC—random forests classifier, KNN—k-nearest neighbours classifier, LR—logistic regression, emb—Embeddings.

3.3.5. Modeling

A modeling pipeline was created and written in the programming language Python (v3.6.0). The pipeline is set as follows: **(1)** data for CS1 and CS2 are loaded, where CS2 involves the Tox21 modeling data (fingerprints—FPs, labels/endpoints) and CS2 fingerprints; **(2)** FPs columns for both CS1 and CS2 below 5% variance are removed; **(3)** removal of structures from CS2 which appear in CS1; **(4)** train and apply embedders; and **(5)** optimize classification models and apply them on embedded data, as shown in Table 6.

4. Limitations and Future Outlook

This study includes several limitations. First there are many other chemical representations besides fingerprints. Among those, interesting results may be revealed from approaches such as Mol2Vec [11] or graph-based methods [12]. The fingerprints parameters (5120-bit length and radius 3) do not have an optimal representation, but are rather based on suggestions from past research [46]. We limited also the embedded data set sizes owing to computational performance issues in training thousands of models. Therefore, with just a few latent variables uses compared with fingerprint, we might have experienced some information loss. Furthermore, there is a plethora of machine learning methods; here, we used only three that are well described and different by their paradigms in learning. The hyperparameters space for either machine learning or embedding algorithms can also be further explored for each individual method as well as the methods for choosing them, like Bayesian optimization [16,37]. These methods can also be applied to smaller labeled datasets, which is one of our aims in future research.

5. Conclusions

In this work, we evaluated the effects of pre-compression techniques on chemical space information generated from fingerprints and utilized in the domain of toxicology. Specifically, we focused on prominent linear and nonlinear techniques like PCA, UMAP, and VAE and showed their utility when using QSAR models, which are related to stress response and nuclear receptors. We showed that, with external knowledge that is transferred via a pre-trained embedder, we can classify toxicity outcomes with a reasonable model quality. The quality of the prediction, however, depends to a large extent on the class separation within each of the 12 toxic outcomes. The results of the silhouette coefficients suggest that nonlinear methods can achieve a much higher performance than PCA. Moreover, our research revealed that, for the utilized data sets, VAE exhibits much better results when compared with PCA and UMAP. Nevertheless, the recently popularized UMAP approach can still be employed for pre-compression as it shows the ability to maintain high-dimensional relationships.

Author Contributions: Conceptualization M.L., T.D. and H.H.; Data curation M.L.; Formal analysis H.T.N.T.; Funding acquisition E.L. and R.K.; Investigation M.L.; Methodology T.D., H.H., E.L. and M.A.R.; Project administration R.K.; Software H.T.N.T.; Supervision E.L. and R.K.; Visualization H.T.N.T.; Writing—original draft M.L., T.D., H.H., E.L. and M.A.R.; Writing—review & editing M.A.R. and R.K. All authors have read and agreed to the published version of the manuscript.

Funding: The Know-Center is funded within the Austrian COMET Program-Competence Centers for Excellent Technologies under the auspices of the Austrian Federal Ministry of Transport, Innovation, and Technology; the Austrian Federal Ministry of Economy, Family, and Youth; and by the State of Styria. COMET is managed by the Austrian Research Promotion Agency FFG. This work is partially supported by the H2020 project TRUSTS (GA: 871481) and the "DDAI" COMET Module within the COMET.

Institutional Review Board Statement: Not applicable.

Informed Consent Statement: Not applicable.

Data Availability Statement: The datasets were retrieved from https://tripod.nih.gov/tox21/assays/index.html (compound set 2) and https://zenodo.org/record/4248826 (compound set 1).

Acknowledgments: We thank Esben Jannik Bjerrum, PhD D for fruitful discussions that helped improve the quality of our research. Open Access Funding by the Graz University of Technology.

Conflicts of Interest: The authors declare no conflict of interest.

References

1. David, L.; Thakkar, A.; Mercado, R.; Engkvist, O. Molecular representations in AI-driven drug discovery: A review and practical guide. *J. Cheminform.* **2020**, *12*, 56. [CrossRef] [PubMed]
2. Ghasemi, F.; Mehridehnavi, A.; Pérez-Garrido, A.; Pérez-Sánchez, H. Neural network and deep-learning algorithms used in QSAR studies: Merits and drawbacks. *Drug Discov. Today* **2018**, *23*, 1784–1790. [CrossRef] [PubMed]
3. Mayr, A.; Klambauer, G.; Unterthiner, T.; Hochreiter, S. DeepTox: Toxicity prediction using deep learning. *Front. Environ. Sci.* **2016**, *3*. [CrossRef]
4. Prykhodko, O.; Johansson, S.V.; Kotsias, P.-C.; Arús-Pous, J.; Bjerrum, E.J.; Engkvist, O.; Chen, H. A de novo molecular generation method using latent vector based generative adversarial network. *J. Cheminform.* **2019**, *11*, 74. [CrossRef]
5. Lusci, A.; Pollastri, G.; Baldi, P. Deep architectures and deep learning in chemoinformatics: The prediction of aqueous solubility for drug-like molecules. *J. Chem. Inf. Model.* **2013**, *53*, 1563–1575. [CrossRef] [PubMed]
6. Capuccini, M.; Ahmed, L.; Schaal, W.; Laure, E.; Spjuth, O. Large-scale virtual screening on public cloud resources with Apache Spark. *J. Cheminformatics* **2017**, *9*, 15. [CrossRef]
7. Lovrić, M.; Molero, J.M.; Kern, R. PySpark and RDKit: Moving towards big data in cheminformatics. *Mol. Inform.* **2019**, *38*, e1800082. [CrossRef]
8. Tetko, I.V.; Engkvist, O.; Chen, H. Does "Big Data" exist in medicinal chemistry, and if so, how can it be harnessed? *Future Med. Chem.* **2016**, *8*, 1801–1806. [CrossRef]
9. Chen, H.; Kogej, T.; Engkvist, O. Cheminformatics in drug discovery, an industrial perspective. *Mol. Inform.* **2018**, *37*. [CrossRef]
10. Rogers, D.; Hahn, M. Extended-connectivity fingerprints. *J. Chem. Inf. Model.* **2010**, *50*, 742–754. [CrossRef]
11. Jaeger, S.; Fulle, S.; Turk, S. Mol2vec: Unsupervised machine learning approach with chemical intuition. *J. Chem. Inf. Model.* **2018**, *58*, 27–35. [CrossRef] [PubMed]
12. Jiang, D.; Wu, Z.; Hsieh, C.-Y.; Chen, G.; Liao, B.; Wang, Z.; Shen, C.; Cao, D.; Wu, J.; Hou, T. Could graph neural networks learn better molecular representation for drug discovery? A comparison study of descriptor-based and graph-based models. *J. Cheminform.* **2021**, *13*, 12. [CrossRef] [PubMed]
13. Lovrić, M.; Malev, O.; Klobučar, G.; Kern, R.; Liu, J.; Lučić, B. Predictive capability of QSAR models based on the CompTox zebrafish embryo assays: An imbalanced classification problem. *Molecules* **2021**, *26*, 1617. [CrossRef] [PubMed]
14. Abdelaziz, A.; Spahn-Langguth, H.; Schramm, K.-W.; Tetko, I.V. Consensus modeling for HTS assays using in silico descriptors calculates the best balanced accuracy in Tox21 challenge. *Front. Environ. Sci.* **2016**, *4*, 2. [CrossRef]
15. Idakwo, G.; Thangapandian, S.; Luttrell, J.; Li, Y.; Wang, N.; Zhou, Z.; Hong, H.; Yang, B.; Zhang, C.; Gong, P. Structure–Activity relationship-based chemical classification of highly imbalanced Tox21 datasets. *J. Cheminform.* **2020**, *12*, 66. [CrossRef] [PubMed]
16. Lovrić, M.; Pavlović, K.; Žuvela, P.; Spataru, A.; Lučić, B.; Kern, R.; Wong, M.W. Machine learning in prediction of intrinsic aqueous solubility of drug-like compounds: Generalization, complexity, or predictive ability? *J. Chemom.* **2021**, e3349. [CrossRef]
17. Bellman, R.E. Dynamic programming. *Science* **1966**, *153*, 34–37. [CrossRef] [PubMed]
18. Aggarwal, C.C.; Hinneburg, A.; Keim, D.A. On the surprising behavior of distance metrics in high dimensional space. In *Database Theory—ICDT 2001. Lecture Notes in Computer Science*; van den Bussche, J., Vianu, V., Eds.; Springer: Berlin/Heidelberg, Germany, 2001; Volume 1973. [CrossRef]
19. Geng, X.; Zhan, D.-C.; Zhou, Z.-H. Supervised nonlinear dimensionality reduction for visualization and classification. *IEEE Trans. Syst. Man Cybern. Part B* **2005**, *35*, 1098–1107. [CrossRef] [PubMed]
20. Sakurada, M.; Yairi, T. Anomaly detection using autoencoders with nonlinear dimensionality reduction. In Proceedings of the MLSDA 2014 2nd Workshop on Machine Learning for Sensory Data Analysis—MLSDA'14, Gold Coast, QLD, Australia, 2 December 2014; p. 4.

21. Duricic, T.; Hussain, H.; Lacic, E.; Kowald, D.; Helic, D.; Lex, E. Empirical comparison of graph embeddings for trust-based collaborative filtering. In Proceedings of the 25th International Symposium on Methodologies for Intelligent Systems, Graz, Austria, 23–25 September 2020.
22. Blei, D.M.; Ng, A.Y.; Jordan, M.I. Latent Dirichlet allocation. *J. Mach. Learn. Res* **2003**, *3*, 993–1022.
23. Choi, S. Algorithms for orthogonal nonnegative matrix factorization. In Proceedings of the 2008 IEEE International Joint Conference on Neural Networks (IEEE World Congress on Computational Intelligence), Hong Kong, China, 1–6 June 2008; pp. 1828–1832.
24. Sampson, G.; Rumelhart, D.E.; McClelland, J.L. The PDP research group parallel distributed processing: Explorations in the microstructures of cognition. *Language* **1987**, *63*, 871. [CrossRef]
25. Hotelling, H. Analysis of a complex of statistical variables into principal components. *J. Educ. Psychol.* **1933**, *24*, 417–441. [CrossRef]
26. Van der Maaten, L. Hinton G visualizing data using t-SNE. *J. Mach. Learn. Res.* **2008**, *9*, 2579–2605.
27. Belkin, M.; Niyogi, P. Laplacian Eigenmaps for dimensionality reduction and data representation. *Neural Comput.* **2003**, *15*, 1373–1396. [CrossRef]
28. McInnes, L.; Healy, J.; Melville, J. UMAP: Uniform Manifold Approximation and Projection for dimension reduction. *J. Open Source Softw.* **2018**, *3*, 861. [CrossRef]
29. Shrivastava, A.; Kell, D. FragNet, a contrastive learning-based transformer model for clustering, interpreting, visualizing, and navigating chemical space. *Molecules* **2021**, *26*, 2065. [CrossRef]
30. Probst, D.; Reymond, J.-L. Visualization of very large high-dimensional data sets as minimum spanning trees. *J. Cheminformatics* **2020**, *12*, 12. [CrossRef] [PubMed]
31. Becht, E.; McInnes, L.; Healy, J.; Dutertre, C.-A.; Kwok, I.W.H.; Ng, L.G.; Ginhoux, F.; Newell, E.W. Dimensionality reduction for visualizing single-cell data using UMAP. *Nat. Biotechnol.* **2019**, *37*, 38–44. [CrossRef] [PubMed]
32. Obermeier, M.M.; Wicaksono, W.A.; Taffner, J.; Bergna, A.; Poehlein, A.; Cernava, T.; Lindstaedt, S.; Lovric, M.; Bogotá, C.A.M.; Be1rg, G. Plant resistome profiling in evolutionary old bog vegetation provides new clues to understand emergence of multi-resistance. *ISME J.* **2021**, *15*, 921–937. [CrossRef] [PubMed]
33. Bengio, Y.; Lamblin, P.; Popovici, D.; Larochelle, H. Greedy layer-wise training of deep networks. *Adv. Neural. Inf. Process. Syst.* **2007**, 153–160. [CrossRef]
34. Kingma, D.P.; Welling, M. Auto-encoding variational bayes. In Proceedings of the 2nd International Conference on Learning Representations, ICLR 2014, Banff, AB, Canada, 14–16 April 2014.
35. Kwon, Y.; Yoo, J.; Choi, Y.-S.; Son, W.-J.; Lee, D.; Kang, S. Efficient learning of non-autoregressive graph variational autoencoders for molecular graph generation. *J. Cheminformatics* **2019**, *11*, 70. [CrossRef] [PubMed]
36. Bjerrum, E.J.; Sattarov, B. Improving chemical autoencoder latent space and molecular de novo generation diversity with heteroencoders. *Biomolecules* **2018**, *8*, 131. [CrossRef]
37. Zhang, J.; Mucs, D.; Norinder, U.; Svensson, F. LightGBM: An effective and scalable algorithm for prediction of chemical toxicity–application to the Tox21 and mutagenicity data sets. *J. Chem. Inf. Model.* **2019**, *59*, 4150–4158. [CrossRef] [PubMed]
38. Ding, J.; Li, X.; Gudivada, V.N. Augmentation and evaluation of training data for deep learning. In Proceedings of the 2017 IEEE International Conference on Big Data (IEEE Big Data 2017), Boston, MA, USA, 11–14 December 2017; pp. 2603–2611.
39. Ehuang, R.; Exia, M.; Nguyen, D.-T.; Ezhao, T.; Esakamuru, S.; Ezhao, J.; Shahane, S.A.; Erossoshek, A.; Esimeonov, A. Tox21Challenge to build predictive models of nuclear receptor and stress response pathways as mediated by exposure to environmental chemicals and drugs. *Front. Environ. Sci.* **2016**, *3*, 85. [CrossRef]
40. Fernandez, M.; Ban, F.; Woo, G.; Hsing, M.; Yamazaki, T.; Leblanc, E.; Rennie, P.S.; Welch, W.J.; Cherkasov, A. Toxic colors: The use of deep learning for predicting toxicity of compounds merely from their graphic images. *J. Chem. Inf. Model.* **2018**, *58*, 1533–1543. [CrossRef] [PubMed]
41. Hemmerich, J.; Asilar, E.; Ecker, G. Conformational oversampling as data augmentation for molecules. In *Transactions on Petri Nets and Other Models of Concurrency XV*; Springer Science and Business Media LLC: Berlin/Heidelberg, Germany, 2019; pp. 788–792.
42. Klimenko, K.; Rosenberg, S.A.; Dybdahl, M.; Wedebye, E.B.; Nikolov, N.G. QSAR modelling of a large imbalanced aryl hydrocarbon activation dataset by rational and random sampling and screening of 80,086 REACH pre-registered and/or registered substances. *PLoS ONE* **2019**, *14*, e0213848. [CrossRef] [PubMed]
43. Fourches, D.; Muratov, E.; Tropsha, A. Trust, but verify: On the importance of chemical structure curation in cheminformatics and QSAR modeling research. *J. Chem. Inf. Model.* **2010**, *50*, 1189–1204. [CrossRef]
44. Greg Landrum, RDKit. Available online: http://rdkit.org (accessed on 21 May 2020).
45. Gütlein, M.; Kramer, S. Filtered circular fingerprints improve either prediction or runtime performance while retaining interpretability. *J. Cheminform.* **2016**, *8*, 60. [CrossRef] [PubMed]
46. Landrum G RDKit: Colliding Bits III. Available online: http://rdkit.blogspot.com/2016/02/colliding-bits-iii.html (accessed on 23 December 2019).
47. Alygizakis, N.; Slobodnik, J. S32 | REACH2017 | >68,600 REACH Chemicals. 2018. Available online: https://zenodo.org/record/4248826 (accessed on 23 December 2020).
48. Breiman, L. Random forests. *Mach. Learn.* **2001**, *45*, 5–32. [CrossRef]

49. Hastie, T.; Tibshirani, R.; Friedman, J. *The Elements of Statistical Learning*; Springer: New York, NY, USA, 2009.
50. Cover, T.; Hart, P. Nearest neighbor pattern classfication. *IEEE Trans. Inf. Theory* **1967**, *13*, 21–27. [CrossRef]
51. Lučić, B.; Batista, J.; Bojović, V.; Lovrić, M.; Kržić, A.S.; Bešlo, D.; Nadramija, D.; Vikić-Topić, D. Estimation of random accuracy and its use in validation of predictive quality of classification models within predictive challenges. *Croat. Chem. Acta* **2019**, *92*, 379–391. [CrossRef]
52. Boughorbel, S.; Jarray, F.; El Anbari, M. Optimal classifier for imbalanced data using Matthews Correlation Coefficient metric. *PLoS ONE* **2017**, *12*, e0177678. [CrossRef]
53. Žuvela, P.; Lovrić, M.; Yousefian-Jazi, A.; Liu, J.J. Ensemble learning approaches to data imbalance and competing objectives in design of an industrial machine vision system. *Ind. Eng. Chem. Res.* **2020**, *59*, 4636–4645. [CrossRef]
54. Lerman, P.M. Fitting segmented regression models by Grid Search. *J. R. Stat. Soc. Ser. C Appl. Stat.* **1980**, *29*, 77. [CrossRef]
55. Pedregosa, F.; Varoquaux, G.; Gramfort, A.; Michel, V.; Thirion, B.; Grisel, O.; Blondel, M.; Prettenhofer, P.; Weiss, R.; Dubourg, V.; et al. Scikit-learn: Machine Learning in Python. *J. Mach. Learn Res.* **2011**, *12*, 2825–2830. [CrossRef]
56. Deisenroth, M.P.; Faisal, A.A.; Ong, C.S. *Mathematics for Machine Learning*; Cambridge University Press: Cambridge, UK, 2020; p. 391.
57. Sainburg, T.; McInnes, L.; Gentner, T.Q. Parametric UMAP embeddings for representation and semi-supervised learning. *arXiv* **2020**, arXiv:2009.12981.
58. Kramer, M.A. Nonlinear principal component analysis using autoassociative neural networks. *AIChE J.* **1991**, *37*, 233–243. [CrossRef]
59. Jordan, M.I.; Ghahramani, Z.; Jaakkola, T.S.; Saul, L.K. An introduction to variational methods for graphical models. *Mach. Learn.* **1999**, *37*, 183–233. [CrossRef]

pharmaceuticals

Article

Rational Design of Novel Inhibitors of α-Glucosidase: An Application of Quantitative Structure Activity Relationship and Structure-Based Virtual Screening

Sobia Ahsan Halim [1], Sumaira Jabeen [2], Ajmal Khan [1,*] and Ahmed Al-Harrasi [1,*]

[1] Natural and Medical Sciences Research Center, University of Nizwa, P.O. Box 33, Birkat Al Mauz 616, Nizwa, Oman; sobia_halim@unizwa.edu.om

[2] Department of Chemistry, Government Post-Graduate College for Women, Shadbagh, Lahore 54950, Pakistan; sumairabhatti23@gmail.com

* Correspondence: ajmalchemist@yahoo.com (A.K.); aharrasi@unizwa.edu.om (A.A.-H.); Tel.: +96-825-446-328 (A.A.-H.)

Abstract: α-Glucosidase is considered a prime drug target for Diabetes Mellitus and its inhibitors are used to delay carbohydrate digestion for the treatment of diabetes mellitus. With the aim to design α-glucosidase inhibitors with novel chemical scaffolds, three folds ligand and structure based virtual screening was applied. Initially linear quantitative structure activity relationship (QSAR) model was developed by a molecular operating environment (MOE) using a training set of thirty-two known inhibitors, which showed good correlation coefficient (r^2 = 0.88), low root mean square error (RMSE = 0.23), and cross-validated correlation coefficient r^2 (q^2 = 0.71 and RMSE = 0.31). The model was validated by predicting the biological activities of the test set which depicted r^2 value of 0.82, indicating the robustness of the model. For virtual screening, compounds were retrieved from zinc is not commercial (ZINC) database and screened by molecular docking. The best docked compounds were chosen to assess their pharmacokinetic behavior. Later, the α-glucosidase inhibitory potential of the selected compounds was predicted by their mode of binding interactions. The predicted pharmacokinetic profile, docking scores and protein-ligand interactions revealed that eight compounds preferentially target the catalytic site of α-glucosidase thus exhibit potential α-glucosidase inhibition *in silico*. The α-glucosidase inhibitory activities of those Hits were predicted by QSAR model, which reflect good inhibitory activities of these compounds. These results serve as a guidelines for the rational drug design and development of potential novel anti-diabetic agents.

Keywords: α-Glucosidase; QSAR modeling; homology modeling; molecular docking; ADMET profiling

Citation: Halim, S.A.; Jabeen, S.; Khan, A.; Al-Harrasi, A. Rational Design of Novel Inhibitors of α-Glucosidase: An Application of Quantitative Structure Activity Relationship and Structure-Based Virtual Screening. *Pharmaceuticals* **2021**, *14*, 482. https://doi.org/10.3390/ph14050482

Academic Editor: Osvaldo Andrade Santos-Filho

Received: 3 March 2021
Accepted: 2 April 2021
Published: 19 May 2021

Publisher's Note: MDPI stays neutral with regard to jurisdictional claims in published maps and institutional affiliations.

1. Introduction

Diabetes mellitus (DM) is one of the most prominent metabolic, chronic and persistent diseases illustrated by hyperglycemia, which itself poses a great global health challenge [1,2]. The morbidity rate of DM is expected to exceed up to 10.4% by 2040 globally [3]. DM is linked with impaired production of insulin or due to improper response of body cells towards insulin. Several complications including hypertension, kidney failure, loss of vision, neuropathy, cardiovascular diseases (CVDs) and atherosclerosis are associated with inadequate production of insulin or due to prolonged hyperglycemia. DM is classified into Type I DM (T1DM) and Type II DM (T2DM). T1DM is also known as insulin dependent DM, which is caused by environmental, genetic and autoimmune factors. T-cell mediated autoimmune damage of β-cells of the pancreas is responsible for this type and illustrated by complete scarcity of insulin. One of the significant complications of this disease is ketoacidosis. Patients are susceptible to other diseases like Grave's disease, Addison's disease, Celiac sprain and autoimmune hepatitis [3]. T2DM is non-insulin dependent diabetes or adult onset diabetes associated with insulin resistance in peripheral tissues or relative deficiency of insulin. It is a progressive and most common type of disease. β-Cells are not damaged in this case; however, obesity is associated in most individuals and ketoacidosis rarely occurs. Most of the time, patients remain asymptomatic and have an enhanced risk of serious macrovascular and microvascular complications. Moreover, autooxidation of glucose and enhanced oxidative stress are also associated with T2DM. The risk of T2DM increases due to increased age, weight, improper physical activity and sedentary lifestyle [4]. In the advance stage of T2DM more complications occur as free radicals are formed, which cause insulin resistance and the dysfunction of β-cells.

Enhanced production of glucose is directed by α-glucosidase in the body; therefore, its level can be controlled by discovering its inhibitors [5,6]. α-Glucosidase is a lysosomal exo-glycosidase that catalyzes the breakdown of complex sugar like starch and disaccharides to glucose that are further absorbed by gut and subsequently raises postprandial hyperglycemia. Thus, α-glucosidase is the pathological hallmark of this disease. Furthermore, this enzyme has been linked in tumor metastasis in association with collagen type I and IV. In DM patients, inhibition of α-glucosidase efficiently lowers the risk of colorectal cancer and cerebrovascular events [7,8].

Many drugs like sulfonylureas, meglitinides, biguanides and thiazolidinediones and α-glucosidase inhibitors are most potent hypoglycemic agents [9]. Metformin, miglitol, acarbose, voglibose and glibenclamide are clinically used drugs for the management of diabetes. They are highly expensive and put a financial burden on patients, which results in huge economic loss. Their detrimental side effects also created an alarming situation like dropsy, increase in weight, resistance against drug, liver disorder, renal tumors, acute hepatitis, hepatic injury and hypoglycemia [10]. Thus, design and discovery of novel α-glucosidase inhibitors with reduced cost and lower side effects are urgently needed to control DM [11–13].

Computational drug designing approaches have proven effective in delivering novel chemical scaffolds in the market against several drug targets [14–16]. Due to our interest in finding novel leads against α-glucosidase [17–19], ligand and structure based virtual screening strategies were applied in this study to target α-glucosidase enzyme. The study comprises of ligand based QSAR modeling, structure-based virtual screening, pharmacokinetic profiling, and QSAR-based prediction of biological activities of new scaffolds against α-glucosidase. In-silico techniques have proven effective in the discovery of chemical agents against specific drug target with high binding affinity and specificity [15]. Several potent drugs including Captopril (Angiotensin-converting enzyme inhibitor, treats congestive heart failure and hypertension), Nelfinavir (HIV-protease inhibitor), Zanamivir (neuraminidase inhibitor of influenza viruses), Dorzolamide (carbonic anhydrase inhibitor), Cinanserin (potent inhibitor of 3C-like protease of SARS), Saquinavir, Indinavir, and Ritonavir (anti-HIV/AIDS drugs) were successfully designed by computational methods which are available on the market [20–23]. In addition, computer-aided drug designing (CADD) has delivered numerous novel anti-cancer compounds such as Erlotinib (EGFR kinase inhibitor, suppresses Non-small cell lung carcinoma and pancreatic cancer), Sorafenib (VEGFR inhibitor, treat thyroid, renal and liver cancer), Lapatinib (for the management of ERBB2-postive breast cancer), Abiraterone (inhibits androgen production to treat metastatic castration-resistant prostate cancer or hormone-refractory prostate cancer) and Crizotinib (ALK inhibitor, to treat Non-small cell lung carcinoma) [24–39].

Keeping the successful applications of CADD in mind, we employed both ligand and structure-based methods to design novel α-glucosidase inhibitors.

2. Results and Discussion

2.1. QSAR Modeling

QSAR models are widely used to predict the biological activities of compounds in silico [40,41]. Molecular Operating Environment (MOE) use descriptor-based technique to develop linear QSAR model and give two values, i.e., predicted pIC_{50} and residual value. Initially 192 2D-descriptors were calculated for thirty-two known α-glucosidase inhibitors (**αGI1-αGI4, αGI6-αGI15, αGI17-αGI20, αGI22-αGI24, αGI26-αGI31, αGI33-αGI34, αGI36-αGI38**) via QuaSAR-Descriptor module and QuaSAR-contingency was used to select the appropriate descriptors. Out of 192, nine descriptors (apol, bpol, a_acc, a_heavy, logP(o/w), logS, TPSA, Weight and wienerPol) were suggested as best descriptors for our data by contingency analysis. Partial least square (PLS) regression method was applied on training set to develop model. Model adequacy was measured as the square of correlation coefficient (r^2), root mean square error (RMSE), cross–validated r^2 (r^2_{LOO} or q^2) and cross–validated RMSE. The developed model showed good correlation coefficient ($r^2 = 0.88$) and low root mean square error (RMSE = 0.23), suggesting the strength of the model. Cross validation was performed using leave-one-out (LOO) cross validations scheme which resulted acceptable cross-validated correlation coefficient ($q^2 = 0.71$ and RMSE = 0.31). The biological activities of the test set [six molecules (**αGI5, αGI16, αGI21, αGI25, αGI32, αGI35**)] were predicted by the model which showed r^2 value of 0.82. The model accurately predicted the activities of test set. The chemical structures, biological activities, predicted activities and residual values of **αGIs** are summarized in Table 1. The correlation plots of training and test set are shown in Figure 1. The 2D linear regression model is shown in the equation below, which is statistically significant and explain 88% of the variability of the IC_{50} coefficient, characterized by usefulness of the model to predict the α-glucosidase inhibitory activity of test set compounds.

Table 1. The chemical structures, α-Glucosidase inhibitory activities, QSAR-predicted activities, and residual values of [α-Glucosidase known Inhibitors (**αGIs**)] used in QSAR modeling.

αGIs	R1	R2	IC_{50} (μM)	pIC_{50}	Predicted	Residual
		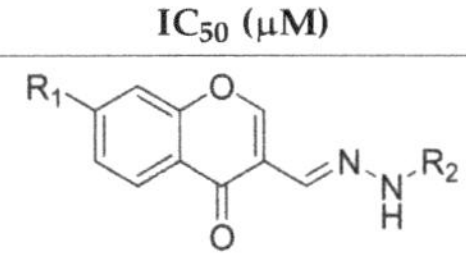				
αGI1	H	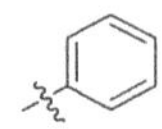	26.7	4.57	4.46	0.11
αGI2	H	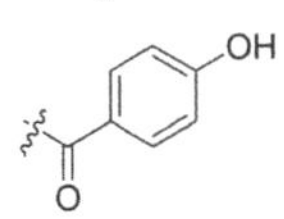	39.8	4.40	4.33	0.07
αGI3	H	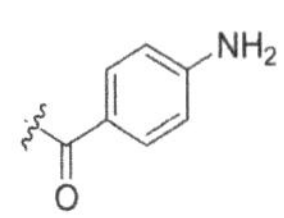	96.9	4.01	4.02	−0.01
αGI4	H	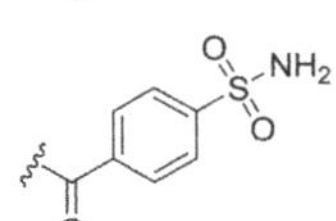	20.1	4.69	4.65	0.04
αGI5 *	H	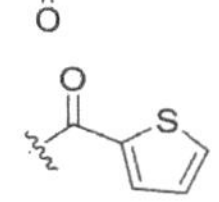	100	4.00	3.83	0.17
αGI6	H	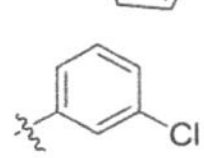	100	4.00	3.88	0.12

Table 1. *Cont.*

αGIs	R1	R2	IC_{50} (μM)	pIC_{50}	Predicted	Residual
αGI**7**	H	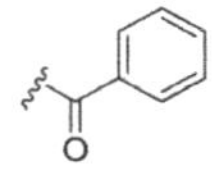	100	4.00	4.07	−0.07
αGI**8**	H	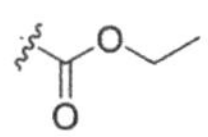	100	4.00	3.89	0.11
αGI**9**	OH	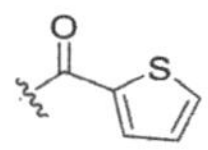	60.8	4.21	4.11	0.10
αGI**10**	H	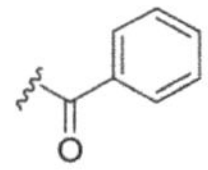	45.7	4.34	4.35	−0.01
αGI**11**	OH	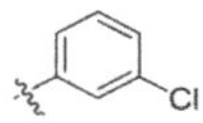	96.7	4.01	4.15	−0.14
αGI**12**	OH	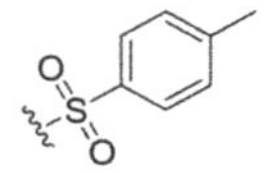	100	4.00	4.09	−0.09
αGI**13**	OH	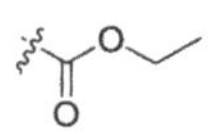	95.4	4.02	4.02	0.00
αGI**14**	OH	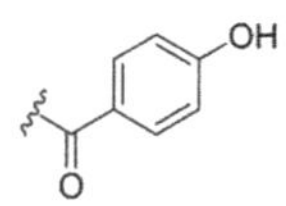	86.3	4.06	4.01	0.05
αGI**15**	H	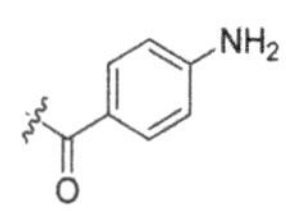	30.8	4.51	4.29	0.22
αGI**16** *	OH	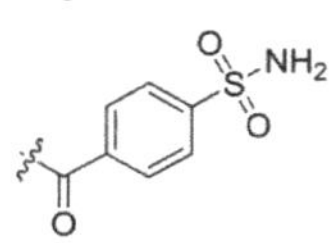	25.2	4.59	4.90	−0.31

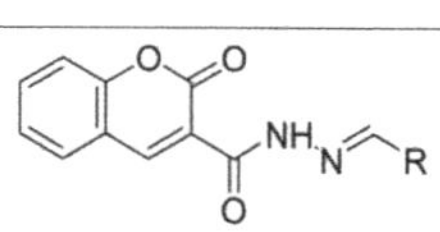

αGIs	R	IC_{50} (μM)	pIC_{50}	Predicted	Residual
αGI**17**	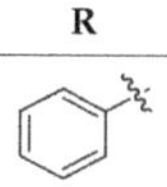	29.14	4.53	4.99	−0.46
αGI**18**	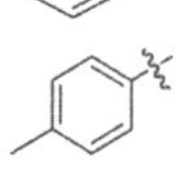	7.58	5.12	4.85	0.27
αGI**19**	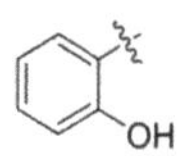	1.1	5.95	5.60	0.35

Table 1. *Cont.*

αGIs	R1	R2	IC_{50} (μM)	pIC_{50}	Predicted	Residual
αGI20	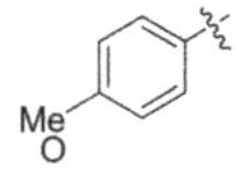		4.26	5.37	4.99	0.38
αGI21 *	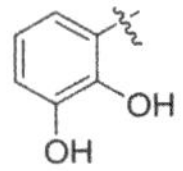		3.15	5.50	5.01	0.49
αGI22	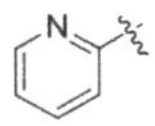		6.1	5.21	5.00	0.21
αGI23	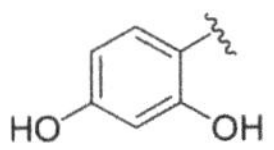		4.58	5.33	5.35	−0.02
αGI24	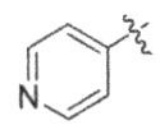		16.1	4.79	4.95	−0.16
αGI25 *	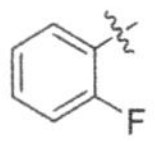		36.46	4.43	4.01	0.42
αGI26	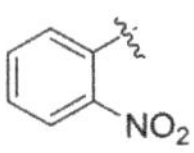		24.14	4.61	4.87	−0.26
αGI27	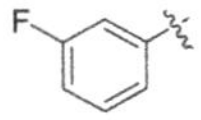		29.14	4.53	4.71	−0.18
αGI28	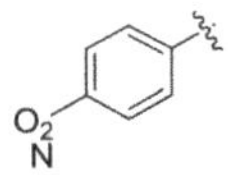		4.58	5.33	5.08	0.25
αGI29	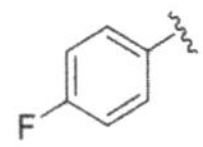		16.1	4.79	4.70	0.09
αGI30	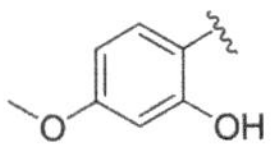		6.46	5.18	5.06	0.12
αGI31	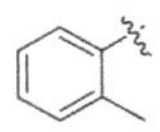		34.14	4.46	4.64	−0.18
αGI32 *	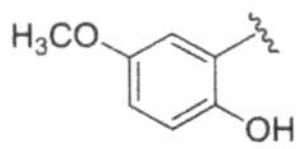		11.14	4.95	5.09	−0.14
αGI33	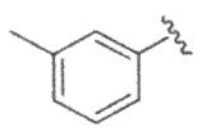		10.58	4.97	4.87	0.10

Table 1. *Cont.*

αGIs	R1	R2	IC_{50} (μM)	pIC_{50}	Predicted	Residual
			αGIs 34–38			
αGI**34**	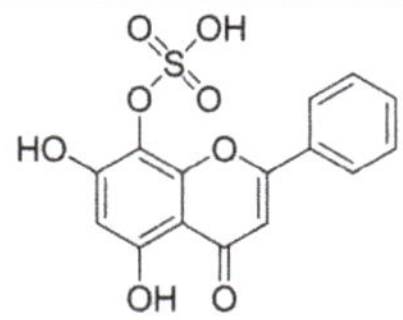		133.57	3.87	3.72	0.15
αGI**35** *	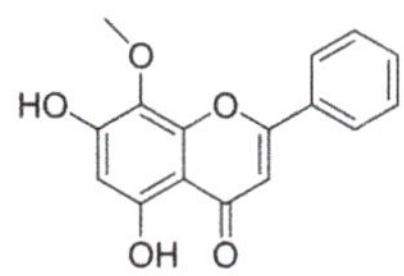		500	3.30	3.40	−0.10
αGI**36**	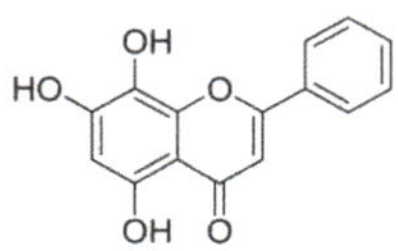		500	3.30	3.68	−0.38
αGI**37**	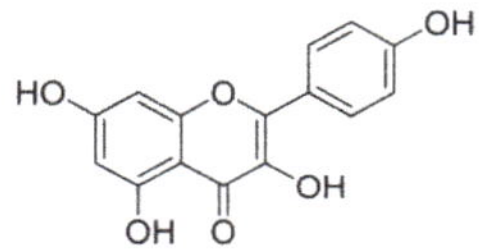		68.46	4.16	3.93	0.23
αGI**38**	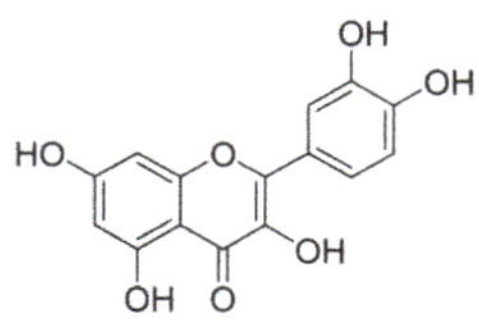		61.86	4.20	4.00	0.20

* Test Set Compounds.

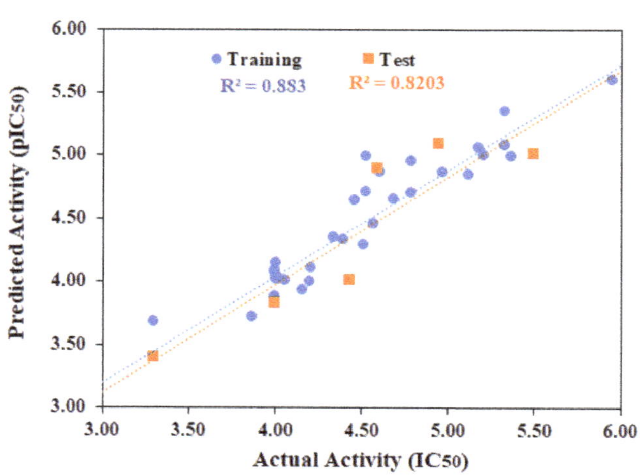

Figure 1. Graphical presentation of correlation between actual and predicted α-glucosidase inhibitory activities of training and test set compounds. R^2 of training and test set are 0.883 and 0.820, respectively.

One metric to measure a descriptor's relative importance in a QSAR model is to compute the product of the magnitude of a regression coefficient times the range in values adopted by its descriptor across the training set. This metric is a measure of the variability of dependent variable of the QSAR upon the descriptor. The relative importance of descriptors is: a_heavy = 1.000, Weight = 0.773, and wienerPol = 0.718, TPSA = 0.471, a_acc = 0.424, logP(*o/w*) = 0.355, logS = 0.244, apol = 0.242, bpol = 0.207. The data shows that the weight, and wienerPol descriptors are the most important factor because of their correlation coefficient > 0.5, followed by TPSA, a_acc and logP.

The positive coefficient of descriptor in model reflects that increasing the number of heavy (polar) atoms, hydrogen bond acceptor atoms, logP(o/w), bpol (Sum of the absolute value of the difference between atomic polarizabilities of all bonded atoms in the molecule (including implicit hydrogens) with polarizabilities) and topological polar surface area ($Å^2$) will increase the activity of compounds. The descriptors a_heavy, logP(o/w), bpol and TPSA are physical properties which can be calculated from the connection table (with no dependence on conformation) of a molecule while a_acc belongs to pharmacophore feature/atom type descriptors.

The negative coefficient of descriptors shows that decreasing some of the physical properties including apol, logS, molecular weight and one of the adjacency and distance matrix descriptors, i.e., wiener polarity number will be beneficial to enhance the activity of the compounds.

$$\begin{aligned} \text{pIC50} = {} & 3.39574 - 0.08965\ (\text{apol}) + 0.09305\ (\text{bpol}) + 0.49740\ (\text{a\_acc}) \\ & + 0.71639\ (\text{a\_heavy}) + 0.40979\ (\text{logP(o/w)}) - 0.37591\ (\text{logS}) \\ & + 0.02502\ (\text{TPSA}) - 0.03659\ (\text{Weight}) - 0.24818\ (\text{wienerPol}) \end{aligned} \quad (1)$$

r2 = 0.88, RMSE = 0.23, q2 = 0.71, RMSE(LOO) = 0.31, N(train) = 32; N (test) = 6

where apol = Sum of the atomic polarizabilities (including implicit hydrogens) with polarizabilities, bpol = Sum of the absolute value of the difference between atomic polarizabilities of all bonded atoms in the molecule (including implicit hydrogens) with polarizabilities, a_acc = hydrogen bond acceptor atoms (not counting acidic atoms but counting atoms that are both hydrogen bond donors and acceptors such as –OH), a_heavy = number of heavy atoms, logP(*o/w*) = Log of the octanol/water partition coefficient (including implicit hydrogens), logS = Log of the aqueous solubility (mol/L), TPSA = Polar surface area ($Å^2$) calculated using group contributions to approximate the polar surface area from connection table information only, Weight = molecular weight (including implicit hydrogens) in atomic mass units with atomic weights, wienerPol = wiener polarity number (half the sum of distance matrix entries with a value of 3), r^2 = Correlation coefficient, RMSE = Root mean square error, q^2 = Cross-validated r^2, $RMSE_{(LOO)}$ = Cross-validated RMSE.

2.2. Structure-Based Screening of Filtered Compounds against α-Glucosidase

Previously we have generated the 3D-coordinates of *S. cerevisiae* α-glucosidase by homology modeling [17–19], which is composed of 579 residues. According to Ramachandran plot, the model possesses excellent stereochemical properties. Out of 579, 444 (86.7%), 63 (12.3%) and 3 (0.6%) residues lied in the most favored, additionally allowed and generously allowed regions, respectively. While two residues (0.4%) (Ala278 and Thr566) are present in disallowed regions which are not a part of active site. ERRAT showed 93.52 quality factor of the model, while in verify3D plot, 95.5% residues showed average 3D-1D score of 0.2. The stereochemical and geometric properties of the model is good and can be used in the structure-based filtration of compounds. The structural geometry and topology of the model was found to be similar to the structural topology of its template (Figure 2). The catalytic residues are conserved among *S. cerevisiae* isomaltase and *S. cerevisiae* α-glucosidase. The sequence alignment of the model and the template is shown in (Figure S1, Supporting Information). The substrate molecule (isomaltose taken from PDB ID 3AXH [22]) was manually docked to deduce the important catalytic residues of protein. Asp214, Glu276, and Asp349 constitutes the catalytic triad for substrate catalysis, where Asp214 and Glu276 serves as nucleophile and proton donor, respectively and Asp349 stabilized the transition state of substrate molecule. The lining of the active site is composed to Asp68, Tyr71, Val108, His111, Phe157, Phe158, Phe177, Gln181, Arg212, Thr215, Ala278, Phe300, Arg312, His348, Gln350, Asp408, Arg439, and Arg443 that mediates multiple hydrophilic and hydrophobic interactions with the substrate and the competitive inhibitor of α-glucosidase 'acarbose'. Moreover, we have recognized that ten water molecules (1021,1026, 1056, 1058, 1061, 1087, 1102, 1122, 1174, and 1228) in the active site play important role in protein-substrate/protein-inhibitor bridging (Figure 3).

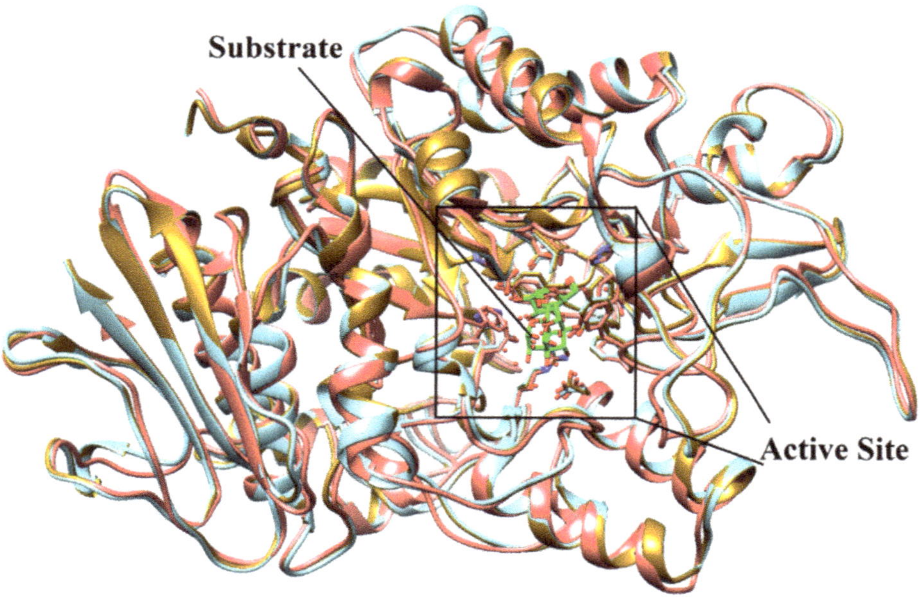

Figure 2. The superimposed view of model (coral ribbons) and templates [3AXH (golden ribbon) and 3A47 (Cyan ribbon)] shows the structural topology of the model is similar to its templates. The active site residues are shown in stick model. The substrate molecule (isomaltose) is depicted in green stick model.

For structure-based screening, ZINC database [22] was filtered according to the physicochemical properties of the substrate molecule (isomaltose) and 6609 compounds were matched with the given parameters. A dataset of 6609 compounds with 38 known inhibitors (αGIs used in QSAR modeling) was docked in the active site of *S. cerevisiae* α-glucosidase to determine their binding potential with α-glucosidase enzyme. The known inhibitors (αGIs) were embedded in the screening library to test the screening accuracy of docking method. The virtual screening accuracy was tested by using two metrics namely enrichment factor (EF) and Receiver operating characteristic-curve (ROC-curve). The analysis of EF and ROC-curve is discussed in Supporting Information. MOE showed >7, >47 and >78%EF in top 1%, 5% and 10% screened library. Additionally, ROC-curve shows area under the curve (AUC) value of 0.94, reflecting good virtual screening performance of MOE. The ROC-curve and the correlation of inhibitory activities of known inhibitors with their docking score is displayed in Figures S2 and S3, Supporting Information.

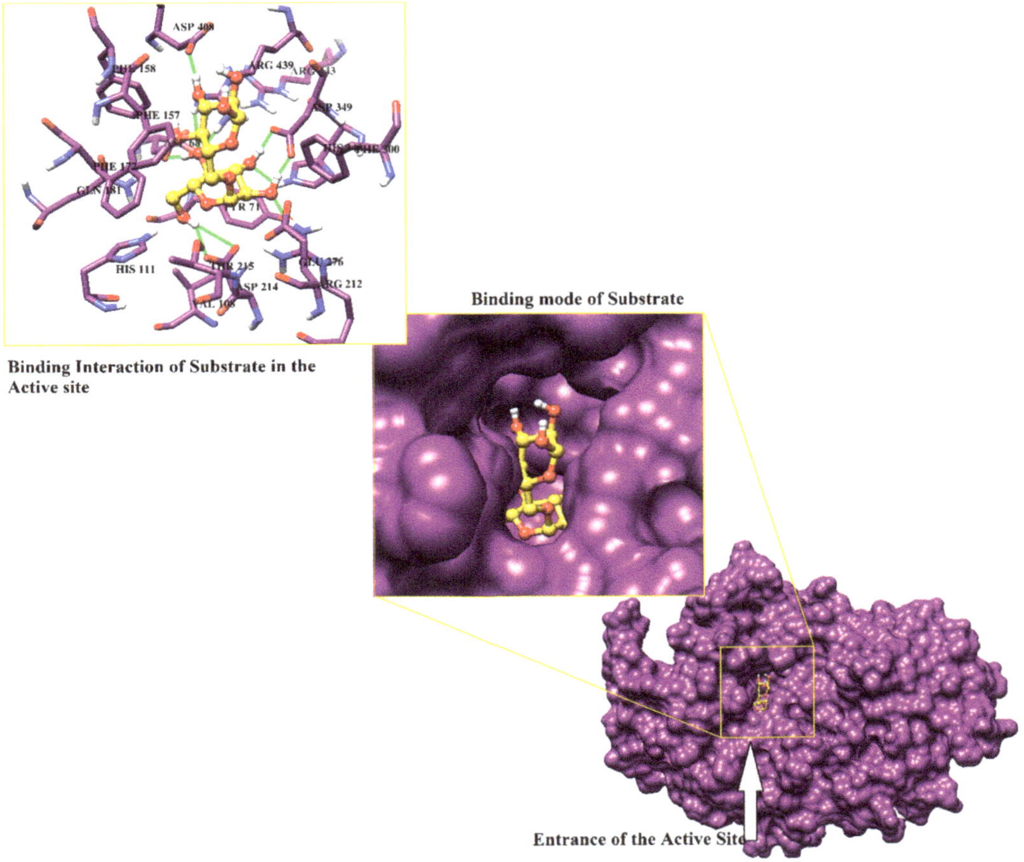

Figure 3. The binding mode of substrate is shown in the active site of enzyme. The binding interactions are highlighted in box. Hydrogen bonds are shown in green lines.

The docked library was ranked according to the docking score and top 10% of the screened compounds (>600) were selected for post-docking filtration. Based on docking ranks, scores and calculated protein-ligand interaction fingerprints (PLIF), 202 compounds were considered 'best' and their pharmacokinetics (absorption, distribution, metabolism, excretion and toxicity) profiling was carried out by computational tools [SwissADME (http://www.swissadme.ch/ accessed on 15 December 2020) and admetSAR (http://lmmd.ecust.edu.cn/admetsar2 accessed on 15 December 2020)].

2.3. ADMET Analysis of Selected Hits

The top ranked docked compounds (202 best hits) were selected for their ADMET prediction which showed that 142/202 compounds exhibited acceptable pharmacokinetic properties (named as compounds **1–142**, Table S1, Supporting Information). Those compounds do not penetrate blood brain barrier (BBB), display high human intestinal absorption (HIA), revealed no AMES toxicity and carcinogenicity. The calculated oral toxicity showed that these compounds fall in category III of acute oral toxicity (LD_{50} = >500 mg/kg to <5000 mg/kg), indicating that the compounds are non-toxic. The predicted RAT acute toxicity reflect that the compounds show low in vivo toxicity up to the dose of ≥2 mol/kg. The synthetic accessibility (SA) values of these compounds are also ≤5 indicating that these compounds are easily synthesizable.

2.4. Protein-Ligand Interaction Analysis of 142 Compounds

According to ADMET profile, compounds **1–142** were retrieved as good inhibitors. The modes of binding of all those (142) compounds were analyzed in the active site of α-glucosidase to select the potential inhibitors of α-glucosidase. The compounds were sorted on the basis of higher number of hydrogen bonding pattern within the active site, and compounds with number of hydrogen bonds ≥ 3, were selected. Subsequently eight molecules (**20, 28, 48, 63, 94, 112, 135 and 140**) were retrieved as 'Hits' which specifically interacted with one or two residues of catalytic triad (Asp214-Glu276-Asp349). Therefore, based on docking scores and binding interactions, those 'Hits' were considered as most active inhibitors. The predicted protein-ligand interactions of 142 compounds are shown in Figure 4. The docking ranks, scores, and molecular interactions of each compound are summarized in Table S2 (Supporting Information).

Comps	HB	II	WB	Comps	HB	II	WB	Comps	HB	II	WB	Comps	HB	II	WB
1	1	5	0	37	1	0	0	73	2	4	0	109	1	0	0
2	1	4	1	38	0	2	1	74	2	2	0	110	0	1	1
3	2	4	1	39	1	3	0	75	0	0	1	111	0	2	0
4	0	9	0	40	0	1	1	76	0	1	2	112	3	2	0
5	0	5	0	41	2	3	0	77	0	2	1	113	1	3	0
6	2	0	0	42	0	2	0	78	2	8	1	114	0	2	1
7	0	2	1	43	0	2	1	79	0	1	0	115	1	1	2
8	0	4	0	44	0	2	0	80	0	6	0	116	0	0	0
9	0	6	0	45	1	1	0	81	1	2	1	117	0	3	0
10	1	5	0	46	1	2	0	82	0	2	1	118	0	0	0
11	0	6	0	47	1	5	0	83	1	0	2	119	0	0	0
12	2	5	0	48	3	0	0	84	1	0	0	120	0	0	0
13	1	3	0	49	1	3	1	85	0	6	0	121	0	3	1
14	1	0	0	50	1	5	0	86	2	2	1	122	1	2	0
15	1	2	0	51	2	4	1	87	2	2	0	123	1	2	0
16	0	2	2	52	0	4	0	88	1	1	0	124	2	0	1
17	1	2	2	53	0	3	0	89	0	5	1	125	0	2	1
18	0	1	0	54	1	3	0	90	0	3	0	126	0	2	0
19	2	2	0	55	0	0	1	91	1	2	0	127	1	5	0
20	3	6	1	56	1	7	0	92	1	7	1	128	1	2	0
21	0	3	1	57	2	4	1	93	2	2	1	129	2	2	0
22	1	6	0	58	1	2	1	94	4	0	2	130	1	3	0
23	1	2	1	59	1	2	0	95	0	1	0	131	0	2	0
24	0	7	0	60	1	3	0	96	1	4	0	132	0	5	0
25	1	5	0	61	1	1	1	97	0	3	0	133	2	1	0
26	1	4	0	62	2	0	0	98	1	6	1	134	1	3	1
27	0	3	0	63	3	0	0	99	0	3	1	135	4	4	2
28	4	2	0	64	0	2	0	100	0	7	0	136	0	2	0
29	2	2	1	65	1	5	0	101	1	4	0	137	1	2	0
30	2	7	1	66	0	3	1	102	1	2	0	138	1	2	0
31	1	3	0	67	0	2	0	103	2	6	2	139	1	2	0
32	2	3	1	68	1	3	1	104	2	1	2	140	6	0	0
33	0	7	0	69	0	1	0	105	1	2	1	141	0	3	0
34	0	3	0	70	0	4	0	106	0	0	0	142	2	0	0
35	1	5	0	71	0	0	0	107	1	3	0				
36	2	2	1	72	2	3	0	108	1	3	0				

Figure 4. The predicted interaction pattern of compounds **1–142.** The binding interactions are shown in 3-color-scale (green through red colour scheme) where red and green indicates least and high number of bonds, respectively, HB = Hydrogen bonds, II = ionic interactions, WB = water bridging.

2.5. The Binding Potential of High Active Hits

The analysis of binding interactions reflect that eight compounds (**20, 28, 48, 63, 94, 112, 135** and **140**) can act as potential inhibitors of α-glucosidase enzyme. Those compounds exhibited good binding interactions within the active site of enzyme. The docked view of compound **20** showed that Glu276 and Asp214 of catalytic triad (CT) and Thr215 formed hydrogen bonds with the amino group of the compound. Moreover, the side chains of Asp68, Asp214 and Glu276 mediated ionic interaction with the amino and the nitrile groups of the compound. Additionally, a water molecule was involved in the protein-ligand bridging. These interactions are responsible for the higher binding affinity of the compound [docking score (DS) = −18.35 kcal/mol and docking rank (DR) = 34). The triazolopyrimidine ring of compound **28** (DS= −18.04 kcal/mol, DR = 46) interacted with the side chain of Asp349 of CT, while the hydroxyl group of the compound formed H-bonds with the side chains of Asp214 and Arg212. Moreover, Asp349 and Phe157 provide ionic and π-π interactions to the compound, respectively. The morpholine ring of **48** (DR = 77, and DS = −17.50 kcal/mol) interacted with Asp214 and Arg439 through H-bonds, while Asp214 also mediated ionic interaction with the compound. The amino group of the compound **63** (DR = 99, and DS = −16.99 kcal/mol) formed H-bonds with the side chains of Asp214 and Thr215, while the sulfone moiety of **63** interacted with the amino group of Thr215 via H-bond. The docked view of compound **94** (DS = 16.47 kcal/mol, DR = 143) showed that the thioxoimidazolidinone moeity of **94** interacts with multiple residues including Asp68, Asp214 and His111 through H-bonds. Additionally, two water molecules also stabilize the compound by H-bonding. The binding mode of compound **112** showed that the triazolopyridine ring of the compound mediated ionic interactions with Asp349, while the substituted hydroxyl group of the compound formed H-bonds with Glu276 and Arg212. The compound depicted DS and DR of −16.27 kcal/mol and 167, respectively. The docked view of **135** showed that one of the nitrile group formed H-bond with His348, while amino group and piperidine nitrogen of the compound mediated H-bonds Asp68 and Glu276, respectively. Moreover, the side chains of Asp68 and Glu276 also offered ionic interaction to the compound. The compound exhibited DS = −16.02 kcal/mol and DR =194. The binding mode of compound **140** (DS = −15.95 kcal/mol, DR = 200) depicted that the hydroxytetrahydropyrimidinone ring of **140** binds with Asp214, Asp349, Arg212 and His348 through H-bonds.

The binding interactions reflect that these compounds possess strong binding potential with α-glucosidase. The chemical structures of the selected hits, and their binding interactions with the active site residues are shown in Table 2 and docking results are tabulated in Table S2. The 3D-structures of selected hits are given in Table S3. The binding modes of the selected hits are depicted in Figure 5. Therefore, by using virtual screening, we selected most appropriate binders of α-Glucosidase enzyme. Thus, this study will be useful in the identification of novel and more potent anti-diabetic compounds.

Table 2. The Chemical Structures and Binding Interactions of Eight Hits.

Comp	Chemical Formula	Chemical Structure	Interactions with Active Site Residues		
			HB	II	WB
20	C25H31N5O2	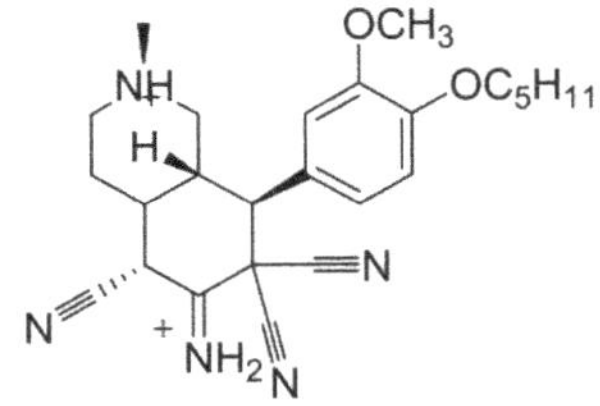	ASP214, GLU276, THR215	ASP68, ASP214, GLU276	HOH1174

Table 2. *Cont.*

Comp	Chemical Formula	Chemical Structure	Interactions with Active Site Residues		
			HB	II	WB
28	C23H23ClN5O4	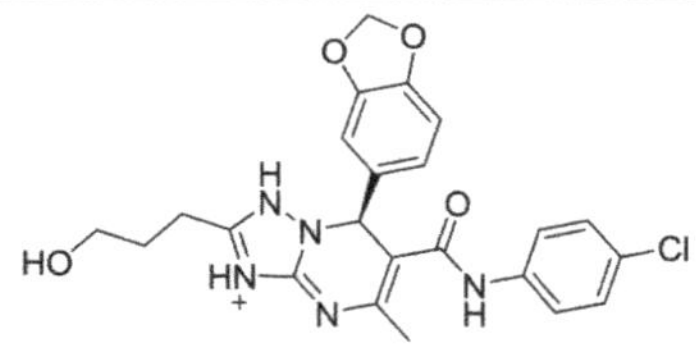	ASP349, ASP214, ARG212	ASP349	none
48	C19H21BrN3O2S	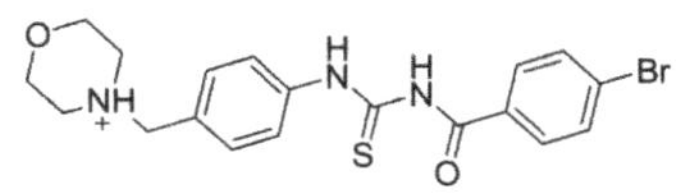	ASP214, ARG439	ASP214	HOH1026
63	C18H20F2N2O4S	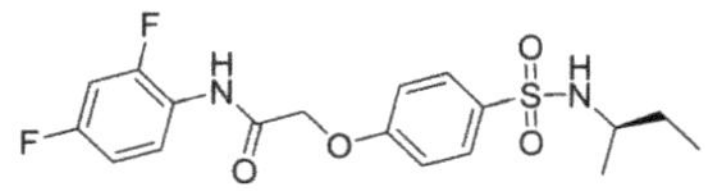	ASP214, THR215	none	none
94	C17H14BrN3O3S	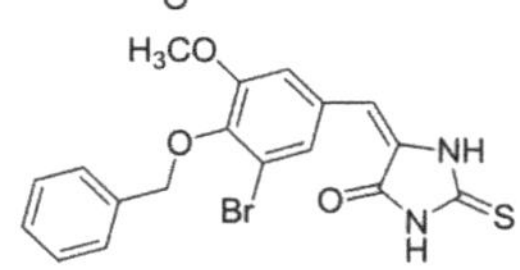	ASP68, ASP214, THR215, HIS111,	none	HOH1102, HOH1174
112	C24H27FN5O4	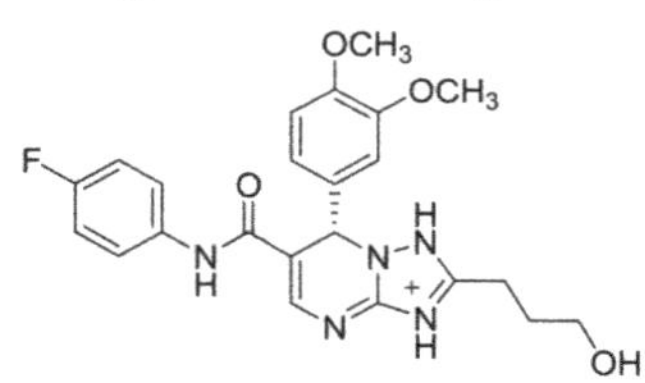	GLU276, ARG212	ASP349	none
135	C20H19BrFN5	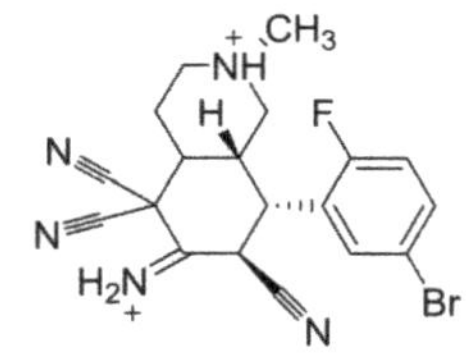	GLU276, ASP68, HIS348	GLU276, ASP68	HOH1026, HOH1228
140	C21H20ClF3N2O5	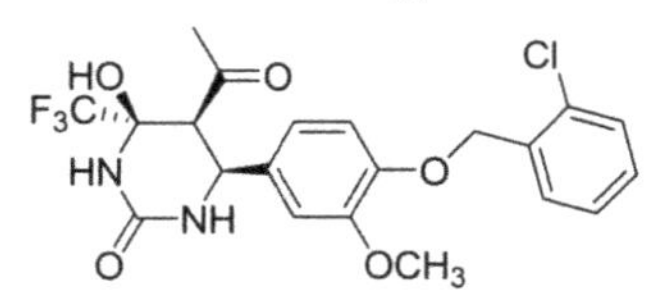	ASP349, ASP214, ARG212, HIS348	none	none

HB= Hydrogen bonds, II = Ionic interactions, WB = water bridging.

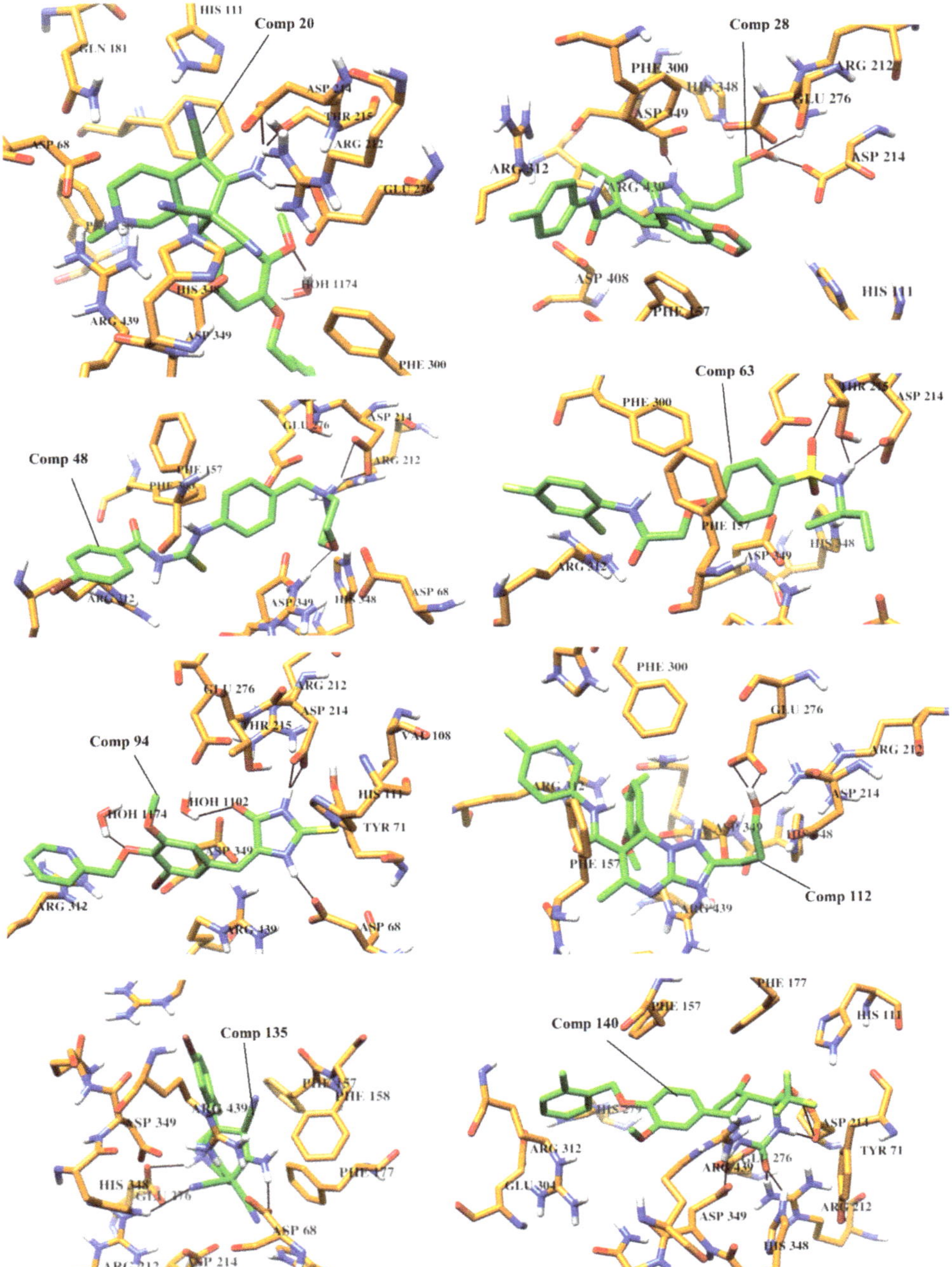

Figure 5. The binding modes of compounds **20, 28, 48, 63, 94, 112, 135** and **140** are depicted in the active site of α-glucosidase. Ligands are shown in green stick model, H-bonds are displayed in black lines, the active site residues are presented in orange stick model.

*2.6. Prediction of α-Glucosidase Inhibitory Activities of Compounds (**20, 28, 48, 63, 94, 112, 135** and **140**) by QSAR Model*

The ADMET profile, and predicted binding interactions of compounds 1-142, led us to identify eight new compounds as good inhibitors of α-glucosidase, therefore their α-glucosidase inhibitory activities were predicted by QSAR model. Prior to the prediction, the model was validated by a set of thirty-two compounds (regarded as Test set 2). The compounds in Test set 2 were randomly selected from literature with α-glucosidase inhibitory activities. The developed QSAR model predicted their activities with r^2 value of 0.62, indicating that the QSAR model can accurately predict the α-glucosidase inhibitory potential of compounds. The results are shown in Table S4 and Figure S4.

The predicted activities (pIC_{50} values) of compounds **20, 28, 48, 63, 94, 112, 135** and **140** are 5.57, 6.79, 4.04, 4.53, 4.71, 5.85, 5.39, and 4.72, respectively. It reflects that these compounds will serve as better inhibitors when tested in vitro.

3. Methods and Materials

3.1. Selection of Data Set for QSAR Analysis

A set of thirty-eight structurally diverse compounds (**αGIs**) with α-glucosidase inhibitory activities was retrieved from literature [42–45]. **αGIs** covers a good range of inhibitory activities. **αGI1- αGI16**, **αGI17- αGI33**, and **αGI34- αGI38**, are reported by Wang et al. 2017, Taha et al. 2008, and Alhassan et al. 2018, respectively [42–45]. Based on the diversity of structure and the activity, the data was segregated into training and test sets of 32 and 6 compounds, respectively. The training set was used to develop QSAR model whereas test set was used for the validation of the generated model. The range of biological activities and chemical diversity of compounds was evenly spanned in both sets. The IC_{50} values were converted into negative logarithmic scale ($pIC_{50}= -logIC_{50}$) which cover an interval of 3 log units (Table 1). The 3D-cordinates of compounds were built by MOE [46]. Partial charges were applied on compounds and their structures were minimized by MMFF94 force field until gradient was reached to 0.1 kcal/mol/Å^2 [46].

The Generation and Validation of QSAR Model

QSAR modeling was performed on MOE. Initially 192 2D-descriptors were calculated for each compound of training set. The best descriptors were selected by using MOE "QuaSAR-Contingency" applications. Descriptors with contingency coefficient above 0.6 and Cramer's, uncertainty, and correlation coefficients above 0.2 were selected for QSAR which proposed nine 2D-descriptors including apol (Sum of the atomic polarizabilities), bpol (Sum of the absolute value of the difference between atomic polarizabilities of all bonded atoms in the molecule), a_acc (Number of hydrogen bond acceptor atoms), a_heavy (Number of heavy atoms), logP(o/w) (Log of the octanol/water partition coefficient), logS (Log of the aqueous solubility (mol/L)), TPSA (topological polar surface area (Å2) c), Weight (molecular weight) and wienerPol (Wiener polarity number) as "best" for our dataset. These descriptors are widely used to predict biological activity and ADMET properties of dataset [46]. QSAR model was built by selecting the inhibitory activities of compounds (as descriptor variable) and calculated descriptors as model fields. Regression analysis was performed on the training set, and r^2 and RMSE values of the fit were obtained. The generated QSAR model was validated by cross validation by leave-one-out method. QSAR fit was used to validate the model by cross validation method. The predictive activities and the residual values of each compound of training set was assessed. Residual value, Z-score and predicted values were calculated for validation and cross-validation of model. The results were interpreted by drawing correlation plot between predicted values (actual activity) on x-axis versus predicted IC_{50} values on y-axis. The developed model was used to predict the biological activities of test set and test set 2 compounds in terms of correlation coefficient (r^2) between the experimental and predicted activities of test set. The developed QSAR model was used for the prediction of biological activities of selected Hits.

3.2. Filtration of ZINC Database for Virtual Screening

A dataset from ZINC database [47] was selected for virtual screening against α-glucosidase. Compounds were searched by using filter parameters calculated by the physicochemical properties of substrate molecule (molecular weight = 150–500, range of xlogP= −4 to 5, number of rotatable bonds = 0–8, maximum topological surface area = 150, number of hydrogen bond donor and acceptor = 0–10, polar desolvation = −400 to 1 kcal/mol, apolar desolvation = −100 to 40 kcal/mol and net charge = −4 to 5). 6609 compounds were matched with the filter parameters that were selected and imported into MOE database, their protonation states were set according to neutral pH, partial charges were applied, and energy was minimized (as described above).

3.3. Docking Based Screening

The crystallographic structure of *Saccharomyces cerevisiae* α-glucosidase is unavailable. Thus, α-glucosidase model was generated in our previous studies [17–19]. The homology model was used in the screening of 6609 compounds (collected from ZINC database) and 38 known inhibitors by MOE docking suit [46]. The protonation state of protein model was assigned according to neutral pH, partial charges were applied, and 3D-coordinates of the model was minimized by MMFF94x force field by retaining all heavy atoms fixed until RMSD gradient was reached to 0.1 kcal/mol/Å^2. Triangle matcher docking algorithm was used with London dG scoring function and GBVI/WSA rescoring method. Force-field based scoring function was applied for post-docking refinement. Later, protein-ligand interaction fingerprint (PLIF) of MOE was used to calculate the binding interactions of compounds within the active site of α-glucosidase. PLIF calculates hydrogen bonding, ionic and hydrophobic interactions [46].

3.4. Pharmacokinetic (ADMET) Analysis

Pharmacokinetic properties of compounds were calculated by SwissADME (http://www.swissadme.ch/ (accessed on 15 December 2020)) and admetSAR servers (http://lmmd.ecust.edu.cn/ (accessed on 15 December 2020)). These servers are widely used to calculate the absorption, distribution, metabolism, excretion and toxicity (ADMET) of compounds. They predict the drug likeness, lead likeness and synthetic feasibility of compounds. These servers predict the ADMET/drug likeness/lead likeness/pharmacokinetics of compounds via different similarity searching methods or ADMET-QSAR models which are developed by the structures of several drugs or drug like compounds (curated from literature). For ADMET calculation, SMILE format of each compound was uploaded on servers and the obtained results were saved in tabular form.

4. Conclusions

α-Glucosidase inhibitors are class of oral medications which have a promising role in the management of glycemic control in T2DM. In the present study, computational techniques including QSAR modeling and structure-based virtual screening were used to identify potent inhibitors of α-glucosidase. The developed linear QSAR model displayed high predictability with correlation coefficient value (r^2 = 0.88). The test set validated the model with significant r^2 (0.82) values. Additionally, virtual screening of 6609 compounds was performed by molecular docking on *S. cerevisiae* α-glucosidase homology model. The best binders were further screened by ADMET profiling and interaction analysis. Eventually eight compounds were selected with high binding affinity for α-glucosidase. Results indicates that those in-silico identified α-glucosidase inhibitors can block the biological activity of α-glucosidase when tested in vitro.

Supplementary Materials: The following are available online at https://www.mdpi.com/article/10.3390/ph14050482/s1, Procedure of Homology Modeling and Calculation of Enrichment Factor (EF) and Receiver operating characteristic-curve (ROC-curve), Figure S1: The sequence alignment of S. cerevisiae α-glucosidase model and templates, Figure S2: Receiver Operating Curve (ROC) for α-glucosidase obtained from MOE, Figure S3: correlation of inhibitory activities of known inhibitors with their docking score, Table S1: ADMET Properties of Selected 142 Hits, Table S2: Docking scores, docking ranks and protein-ligand interactions of 142 Hits, Table S3: 3D-structures of selected hits, Table S4: The predicted activities of thirty-two compounds (Test set 2), Figure S4: The correlation plot of Test set 2.

Author Contributions: Conceptualization, S.A.H. and A.A.-H.; Methodology, S.A.H. and S.J.; Software, S.J.; Formal Analysis, A.K.; Writing—Original Draft Preparation, S.A.H. and A.K.; Writing—Review & Editing, S.A.H. and A.K.; Supervision, A.A.-H.; Funding Acquisition, A.A.-H. All authors have read and agreed to the published version of the manuscript.

Funding: The project was supported by grant from The Oman Research Council (TRC) through the funded project BFP/RGP/HSS/18/018).

Institutional Review Board Statement: Not applicable.

Informed Consent Statement: Not applicable.

Data Availability Statement: Data is contained within the article or Supplementary Materials.

Acknowledgments: The authors would like to thank the University of Nizwa for the generous support of this project.

Conflicts of Interest: The authors declare no conflict of interest.

References

1. International Diabetes Federation. *IDF Diabetes Atlas*, 8th ed.; International Diabetes Federation: Brussels, Belgium, 2017.
2. Roglic, G. WHO Global report on diabetes: A summary. *Int. J. Noncommun. Dis.* **2016**, *1*, 3. [CrossRef]
3. Okur, M.E.; Karantas, I.D.; Siafaka, P.I. Diabetes mellitus: A review on pathophysiology, current status of oral medica-tions and future perspectives. *Acta Pharm. Sci.* **2017**, *55*, 61–82.
4. Colberg, S.R.; Sigal, R.J.; Yardley, J.E.; Riddell, M.C.; Dunstan, D.W.; Dempsey, P.C.; Horton, E.S.; Castorino, K.; Tate, D.F. Physical activity/exercise and diabetes: A position statement of the American Diabetes Association. *Diabetes Care* **2016**, *39*, 2065–2079. [CrossRef]
5. Moelands, S.V.; Lucassen, P.L.; Akkermans, R.P.; De Grauw, W.J.; Van de Laar, F.A. Alpha-glucosidase inhibitors for pre-vention or delay of type 2 diabetes mellitus and its associated complications in people at increased risk of develop-ing type 2 diabetes mellitus. *Cochrane Database Syst. Rev.* **2018**, *12*, CD005061.
6. Damsud, T.; Chanwun, T.; Kaewpiboon, C. Antidiabetic agents with α-glucosidase inhibition and antioxidant capacity from the shoots of Clausena cambodiana Guill. *Int. J. Agric. Technol.* **2017**, *13*, 449–456.
7. Saltos, M.B.V.; Puente, B.F.N.; Faraone, I.; Milella, L.; De Tommasi, N.; Braca, A. Inhibitors of α-amylase and α-glucosidase from Andromachia igniaria Humb. & Bonpl. *Phytochem. Lett.* **2015**, *14*, 45–50.
8. Patel, S.S. Cerebrovascular Complications of Diabetes: Alpha Glucosidase Inhibitor as Potential Therapy. *Horm. Metab. Res.* **2016**, *48*, 83–91. [CrossRef]
9. Chaudhury, A.; Duvoor, C.; Dendi, V.S.R.; Kraleti, S.; Chada, A.; Ravilla, R.; Marco, A.; Shekhawat, N.S.; Montales, M.T.; Kuriakose, K.; et al. Clinical Review of Antidiabetic Drugs: Implications for Type 2 Diabetes Mellitus Management. *Front. Endocrinol.* **2017**, *8*, 6. [CrossRef] [PubMed]
10. Stein, S.A.; Lamos, E.M.; Davis, S.N. A review of the efficacy and safety of oral antidiabetic drugs. *Expert Opin. Drug Saf.* **2013**, *12*, 153–175. [CrossRef] [PubMed]
11. Proença, C.; Freitas, M.; Ribeiro, D.; Oliveira, E.F.T.; Sousa, J.L.C.; Tomé, S.M.; Ramos, M.J.; Silva, A.M.S.; Fernandes, P.A.; Fernandes, E. α-Glucosidase inhibition by flavonoids: An in vitro and in silico structure–activity relationship study. *J. Enzym. Inhib. Med. Chem.* **2017**, *32*, 1216–1228. [CrossRef]
12. Li, W.; Yuan, G.; Pan, Y.; Wang, C.; Chen, H. Network Pharmacology Studies on the Bioactive Compounds and Action Mechanisms of Natural Products for the Treatment of Diabetes Mellitus: A Review. *Front. Pharmacol.* **2017**, *8*, 74. [CrossRef]
13. Wu, P.-P.; Zhang, B.-J.; Cui, X.-P.; Yang, Y.; Jiang, Z.-Y.; Zhou, Z.-H.; Zhong, Y.-Y.; Mai, Y.-Y.; Ouyang, Z.; Chen, H.-S.; et al. Synthesis and biological evaluation of novel ursolic acid analogues as potential α-glucosidase inhibitors. *Sci. Rep.* **2017**, *7*, 45578. [CrossRef]
14. Hassan Baig, M.; Ahmad, K.; Roy, S.; Mohammad Ashraf, J.; Adil, M.; Haris Siddiqui, M.; Khan, S.; Amjad Kamal, M.; Provazník, I.; Choi, I. Computer aided drug design: Success and limitations. *Curr. Pharm. Des.* **2016**, *22*, 572–581. [CrossRef]

15. Prada-Gracia, D.; Huerta-Yépez, S.; Moreno-Vargas, L.M. Application of computational methods for anticancer drug discovery, design, and optimization. *Bol. Med. Hosp. Infant. México* **2016**, *73*, 411–423.
16. Lu, W.; Zhang, R.; Jiang, H.; Zhang, H.; Luo, C. Computer-Aided Drug Design in Epigenetics. *Front. Chem.* **2018**, *6*, 57. [CrossRef] [PubMed]
17. Avula, S.K.; Khan, A.; Halim, S.A.; Al-Abri, Z.; Anwar, M.U.; Al-Rawahi, A.; Csuk, R.; Al-Harrasi, A. Synthesis of novel (R)-4-fluorophenyl-1H-1,2,3-triazoles: A new class of α-glucosidase inhibitors. *Bioorg. Chem.* **2019**, *91*, 103182. [CrossRef] [PubMed]
18. Rizvi, T.; Hussain, I.; Ali, L.; Mabood, F.; Khan, A.; Shujah, S.; Rehman, N.; Al-Harrasi, A.; Hussain, J.; Khan, A.; et al. New gorgonane sesquiterpenoid from Teucrium mascatense Boiss, as α-glucosidase inhibitor. *S. Afr. J. Bot.* **2019**, *124*, 218–222. [CrossRef]
19. Ur Rehman, N.; Rafiq, K.; Khan, A.; Ahsan Halim, S.; Ali, L.; Al-Saady, N.; Hilal Al-Balushi, A.; Al-Busaidi, H.K.; Al-Harrasi, A. α-Glucosidase Inhibition and Molecular Docking Studies of Natural Bromin-ated Metabolites from Marine Macro Brown Alga Dictyopteris hoytii. *Mar. Drugs* **2019**, *17*, 666. [CrossRef]
20. Lüthy, R.; Bowie, J.U.; Eisenberg, D. Assessment of protein models with three-dimensional profiles. *Nature* **1992**, *356*, 83–85. [CrossRef]
21. Pettersen, E.F.; Goddard, T.D.; Huang, C.C.; Couch, G.S.; Greenblatt, D.M.; Meng, E.C.; Ferrin, T.E. UCSF Chimera—a visualization system for exploratory research and analysis. *J. Comput. Chem.* **2004**, *25*, 1605–1612. [CrossRef] [PubMed]
22. Yamamoto, K.; Miyake, H.; Kusunoki, M.; Osaki, S. Steric hindrance by 2 amino acid residues determines the substrate specificity of isomaltase from *Saccharomyces cerevisiae*. *J. Biosci. Bioeng.* **2011**, *112*, 545–550. [CrossRef]
23. Elliott, M. Zanamivir: From drug design to the clinic. *Philos. Trans. R. Soc. B Biol. Sci.* **2001**, *356*, 1885–1893. [CrossRef] [PubMed]
24. Cushman, D.W.; Ondetti, M.A. Design of angiotensin converting enzyme inhibitors. *Nat. Med.* **1999**, *5*, 1110–1112. [CrossRef] [PubMed]
25. Chen, L.; Gui, C.; Luo, X.; Yang, Q.; Günther, S.; Scandella, E.; Drosten, C.; Bai, D.; He, X.; Ludewig, B.; et al. Cinanserin Is an Inhibitor of the 3C-Like Proteinase of Severe Acute Respiratory Syndrome Coronavirus and Strongly Reduces Virus Replication In Vitro. *J. Virol.* **2005**, *79*, 7095–7103. [CrossRef]
26. Graves, B.J.; Hatada, M.H.; Miller, J.K.; Graves, M.C.; Roy, S.; Cook, M.C.; Krohn, A.; Martin, J.A.; Roberts, N.A. The Three-Dimensional X-Ray Crystal Structure of HIV-1 Protease Complexed with a Hydroxyethylene Inhibitor. In *Structure and Function of the Aspartic Proteinases*; Springer: Berlin, Germany, 1991; pp. 455–460.
27. Pollack, V.A.; Savage, D.M.; Baker, D.A.; Tsaparikos, K.E.; Sloan, D.E.; Moyer, J.D.; Barbacci, E.G.; Pustilnik, L.R.; Smolarek, T.A.; Davis, J.A.; et al. Inhibition of epidermal growth factor receptor-associated tyrosine phos-phorylation in human carcinomas with CP-358,774: Dynamics of receptor inhibition in situ and antitumor effects in athymic mice. *J. Pharmacol. Exp. Ther.* **1999**, *291*, 739–748.
28. Ng, S.S.; Tsao, M.-S.; Nicklee, T.; Hedley, D.W. Effects of the epidermal growth factor receptor inhibitor OSI-774, Tarceva, on downstream signaling pathways and apoptosis in human pancreatic adenocarcinoma 1 supported by the Na-tional Cancer Institute of Canada and the Pat Myhal Fund for Pancreatic Cancer Research. 1. *Mol. Cancer Ther.* **2002**, *1*, 777–783. [PubMed]
29. Bulgaru, A.M.; Mani, S.; Goel, S.; Perez-Soler, R. Erlotinib (Tarceva®): A promising drug targeting epidermal growth fac-tor receptor tyrosine kinase. *Expert Rev. Anticancer Ther.* **2003**, *3*, 269–279. [CrossRef]
30. Heim, M.; Sharifi, M.; Hilger, R.; Scheulen, M.; Seeber, S.; Strumberg, D. Antitumor effect and potentiation or reduction in cytotoxic drug activity in human colon carcinoma cells by the Raf kinase inhibitor (RKI) BAY 43-9006. *Int. J. Clin. Pharmacol. Ther.* **2003**, *41*, 616–617. [CrossRef]
31. Ahmad, T.; Eisen, T. Kinase Inhibition with BAY 43–9006 in Renal Cell Carcinoma. *Clin. Cancer Res.* **2004**, *10*, 6388S–6392S. [CrossRef]
32. Wilhelm, S.M.; Carter, C.; Tang, L.; Wilkie, D.; McNabola, A.; Rong, H.; Chen, C.; Zhang, X.; Vincent, P.; McHugh, M.; et al. BAY 43-9006 Exhibits Broad Spectrum Oral Antitumor Activity and Targets the RAF/MEK/ERK Pathway and Receptor Tyrosine Kinases Involved in Tumor Progression and Angiogenesis. *Cancer Res.* **2004**, *64*, 7099–7109. [CrossRef]
33. Xia, W.; Liu, L.-H.; Ho, P.; Spector, N.L. Truncated ErbB2 receptor (p95 ErbB2) is regulated by heregulin through hetero-dimer formation with ErbB3 yet remains sensitive to the dual EGFR/ErbB2 kinase inhibitor GW572016. *Oncogene* **2004**, *23*, 646–653. [CrossRef] [PubMed]
34. Wood, E.R.; Truesdale, A.T.; McDonald, O.B.; Yuan, D.; Hassell, A.; Dickerson, S.H.; Ellis, B.; Pennisi, C.; Horne, E.; Lackey, K.; et al. A unique structure for epidermal growth factor receptor bound to GW572016 (Lapatinib): Relationships among protein confor-mation, inhibitor off-rate, and receptor activity in tumor cells. *Cancer Res.* **2004**, *64*, 6652–6659. [CrossRef] [PubMed]
35. Jarman, M.; Barrie, S.E.; Llera, J.M. The 16, 17-double bond is needed for irreversible inhibition of human cytochrome P45017α by abiraterone (17-(3-Pyridyl) androsta-5, 16-dien-3β-ol) and related steroidal inhibitors. *J. Med. Chem.* **1998**, *41*, 5375–5381. [CrossRef] [PubMed]
36. O'Donnel, A.; Judson, I.; Dowsett, M.; Raynaud, F.; Dearnaley, D.; Mason, M.; Harland, S.; Robbins, A.; Halbert, G.; Nutley, B.; et al. Hormonal impact of the 17alpha-hydroxylase/C (17, 20)-lyase inhibitor abi-raterone acetate (CB7630) in patients with prostatic cancer. *Br. J. Cancer* **2004**, *90*, 2317–2325. [CrossRef] [PubMed]

37. Jagusch, C.; Negri, M.; Hille, U.E.; Hu, Q.; Bartels, M.; Jahn-Hoffmann, K.; Mendieta, M.A.; Rodenwaldt, B.; Müller-Vieira, U. Schmidt, D.; et al. Synthesis, biological evaluation and molecular modelling studies of methylene-imidazole substituted biaryls as inhibitors of human 17α-hydroxylase-17, 20-lyase (CYP17). Part I: Heterocyclic modifications of the core structure. *Bioorg. Med Chem.* **2008**, *16*, 1992–2010. [CrossRef]
38. Butrynski, J.E.; D'Adamo, D.R.; Hornick, J.L.; Cin, P.D.; Antonescu, C.R.; Jhanwar, S.C.; Ladanyi, M.; Capelletti, M.; Rodig, S.J. Ramaiya, N.; et al. Crizotinib inALK-Rearranged Inflammatory Myofibroblastic Tumor. *N. Engl. J. Med.* **2010**, *363*, 1727–1733 [CrossRef] [PubMed]
39. Rodig, S.J.; Shapiro, G.I. Crizotinib, a small-molecule dual inhibitor of the c-Met and ALK receptor tyrosine kinases. *Curr. Opin. Investig. Drugs* **2010**, *11*, 1477–1490.
40. Neves, B.J.; Braga, R.C.; Melo-Filho, C.C.; Moreira-Filho, J.T.; Muratov, E.N.; Andrade, C.H. QSAR-based virtual screening: Advances and applications in drug discovery. *Front. Pharmacol.* **2018**, *9*, 1275. [CrossRef]
41. Kwon, S.; Bae, H.; Jo, J.; Yoon, S. Comprehensive ensemble in QSAR prediction for drug discovery. *BMC Bioinform.* **2019**, *20*, 521. [CrossRef]
42. Taha, M.; Shah, S.A.A.; Afifi, M.; Imran, S.; Sultan, S.; Rahim, F.; Khan, K.M. Synthesis, α-glucosidase inhibition and molecular docking study of coumarin based derivatives. *Bioorg. Chem.* **2018**, *77*, 586–592. [CrossRef]
43. Wang, G.; Chen, M.; Wang, J.; Peng, Y.; Li, L.; Xie, Z.; Deng, B.; Chen, S.; Li, W. Synthesis, biological evaluation and molecular docking studies of chromone hydra-zone derivatives as α-glucosidase inhibitors. *Bioorg. Med. Chem. Lett.* **2017**, *27*, 2957–2961. [CrossRef] [PubMed]
44. Alhassan, A.M.; Ahmed, Q.U.; Latip, J.; Shah, S.A.A. A new sulphated flavone and other phytoconstituents from the leaves of Tetracera indica Merr. and their alpha-glucosidase inhibitory activity. *Nat. Prod. Res.* **2019**, *33*, 1–8. [CrossRef] [PubMed]
45. Gong, Z.; Peng, Y.; Qiu, J.; Cao, A.; Wang, G.; Peng, Z. Synthesis, In Vitro α-Glucosidase Inhibitory Activity and Molecular Docking Studies of Novel Benzothiazole-Triazole Derivatives. *Molecules* **2017**, *22*, 1555. [CrossRef] [PubMed]
46. MOE. *Molecular Operating Environment (MOE), 2013.08*; Chemical Computing Group: Montreal, QC, Canada, 2019.
47. Irwin, J.J.; Shoichet, B.K. ZINC—A Free Database of Commercially Available Compounds for Virtual Screening. *J. Chem. Inf. Model.* **2005**, *45*, 177–182. [CrossRef] [PubMed]

pharmaceuticals

Article

Marine-Derived Natural Products as ATP-Competitive mTOR Kinase Inhibitors for Cancer Therapeutics

Shraddha Parate [1], Vikas Kumar [2], Gihwan Lee [1], Shailima Rampogu [2], Jong Chan Hong [1,*] and Keun Woo Lee [2,*]

1 Division of Applied Life Science, Plant Molecular Biology and Biotechnology Research Center (PMBBRC), Gyeongsang National University (GNU), 501 Jinju-daero, Jinju 52828, Korea; parateshraddha@gmail.com (S.P.); pika890131@gmail.com (G.L.)
2 Division of Life Sciences, Department of Bio & Medical Big Data (BK21 Program), Research Institute of Natural Science (RINS), Gyeongsang National University (GNU), 501 Jinju-daero, Jinju 52828, Korea; vikaspathania777@gmail.com (V.K.); shailima.rampogu@gmail.com (S.R.)
* Correspondence: jchong@gnu.ac.kr (J.C.H.); kwlee@gnu.ac.kr (K.W.L.); Tel.: +82-55-772-1360 (K.W.L.)

Abstract: The mammalian target of rapamycin (mTOR) is a serine/threonine kinase portraying a quintessential role in cellular proliferation and survival. Aberrations in the mTOR signaling pathway have been reported in numerous cancers including thyroid, lung, gastric and ovarian cancer, thus making it a therapeutic target. To attain this objective, an in silico investigation was designed, employing a pharmacophore modeling approach. A structure-based pharmacophore (SBP) model exploiting the key features of a selective mTOR inhibitor, Torkinib directed at the ATP-binding pocket was generated. A Marine Natural Products (MNP) library was screened using SBP model as a query. The retrieved compounds after consequent drug-likeness filtration were subjected to molecular docking with mTOR, thus revealing four MNPs with better scores than Torkinib. Successive refinement via molecular dynamics simulations demonstrated that the hits formed crucial interactions with key residues of the pocket. Furthermore, the four identified hits exhibited good binding free energy scores through MM-PBSA calculations and the subsequent in silico toxicity assessments displayed three hits deemed essentially non-carcinogenic and non-mutagenic. The hits presented in this investigation could act as potent ATP-competitive mTOR inhibitors, representing a platform for the future discovery of drugs from marine natural origin.

Keywords: mTOR kinase; marine natural products; ATP-competitive inhibitors; structure-based pharmacophore modeling; virtual screening; molecular docking; molecular dynamics simulations; binding free energy; in silico ADMET

Citation: Parate, S.; Kumar, V.; Lee, G.; Rampogu, S.; Hong, J.C.; Lee, K.W. Marine-Derived Natural Products as ATP-Competitive mTOR Kinase Inhibitors for Cancer Therapeutics. *Pharmaceuticals* **2021**, *14*, 282. https://doi.org/10.3390/ph14030282

Academic Editor: Osvaldo Andrade Santos-Filho

Received: 15 February 2021
Accepted: 18 March 2021
Published: 21 March 2021

1. Introduction

The growth factors, nutrients and energy levels in cells are key determining factors of cellular growth and proliferation [1]. Dysregulation of the phosphoinositide 3-kinase (PI3K)/AKT/mammalian target of rapamycin (mTOR) axis has been heavily implicated in tumorigenesis and the progression of numerous cancers, including lung, thyroid, ovarian and gastric cancer [2–5]. Therefore, targeting mTOR signaling represents an attractive therapy in cancer. mTOR is a serine/threonine kinase (UniProt ID: P42345), first discovered in budding yeast Saccharomyces cerevisiae [6] and functions as a cardinal regulator of cell growth, proliferation, metabolism, energy homeostasis, angiogenesis and survival [7,8]. In mammalian cells, mTOR exists in two evolutionarily conserved complexes: mTORC1, which regulates protein synthesis through the phosphorylation of p70S6K1, and 4E-BP1 and mTORC2, which regulate cell survival and proliferation through the phosphorylation of AKT/PKB [9,10]. The mTORC1 comprises regulatory-associated protein of mTOR (RAPTOR), lethal with SEC13 protein 8 (LST8), proline-rich substrate of 40 kDa (PRAS40) and domain-containing mTOR-interacting protein (DEPTOR), while mTORC2 consists of rapamycin-insensitive companion of mTOR (RICTOR), LST8, stress-activated protein kinase interacting protein 1 (SIN1), DEPTOR and protein observed with RICTOR (PROTOR) [6]. Deregulation of mTORC1/ mTORC2 both upstream and downstream is implicated in various cancers, including breast, ovarian, prostate and lung cancer [11].

Currently, numerous pharmacological possibilities have been developed to inhibit mTOR, resulting in three generations of mTOR inhibitors. Rapamycin and its analogs (rapalogs) belong to the first generation of mTORC1 inhibitors, approved for different cancer treatments [12]. In spite of being approved, these inhibitors cause the stabilization of the disease and not tumor regression, thereby behaving as cytostatic and not as cytotoxic. Additionally, their continued use results in copious adverse effects causing suppression of the immune system, reduction in male fertility and hematological toxicity [13]. The second generation of mTOR inhibitors act as ATP-competitive inhibitors of the catalytic kinase domain controlling the activity of both mTORC1 and mTORC2 [14]. Various resistant mutations interfering with mTOR drug binding are observed in rapalogs as well as ATP-competitive kinase domain inhibitors. The third generation of mTOR inhibitors consist of bivalent drugs binding simultaneously to the regulator and mTOR catalytic sites thereby supplementing to eliminate the resistant mutations [15,16]. In recent years, several second generation of mTOR inhibitors were identified as selective ATP-competitive kinase domain inhibitors including INK-128, OSI-027 and CC-223. Moreover, dual mTOR/PI3K inhibitors, including BEZ235, PF-04691502 and GSK2126458, were also discovered as effective inhibitors. Nevertheless, these inhibitors exhibit detrimental effects including thrombocytopenia, depression, weight loss, skin rash and mucositis [17,18]. Hence, there is an emergent need to discover potent mTOR kinase domain inhibitors as therapeutic candidates for cancerous ailments.

Natural products are predominant sources of active ingredients in medicine, demonstrating varying structural diversity and exhibiting greater potential druggable pharmacophores than synthetic molecules [19,20]. Moreover, lead compounds of natural origin have proven to show significant inhibitory activities on mTOR kinase domain in the past and this provided a structural basis for identifying natural products as potent mTOR inhibitors [21–23]. Natural products from marine resources have recently shown therapeutic potential in the development of anti-cancer drugs [24–30]. It is noteworthy to mention that 7 compounds from marine organisms have been approved as pharmaceuticals for marketing, 23 compounds are in various phases of clinical trials and about 1000 compounds are undergoing preclinical studies [25]. Four marine compounds, namely cytarabine (Cytosars), trabectedin (Yondeliss), eribulin mesylate (Halavens) and the conjugated antibody brentuximab vedotin (Acentriss), are currently utilized as anti-cancer therapeutics [25]. Marine natural extracts have also exhibited significant anti-cancer effects in recent years [24,31–34].

The aforementioned perspectives prompted us to identify natural compounds from marine resources as potential therapeutics targeted to mTOR for treatment in cancer. In accordance with it, we have carried out an in silico study to identify mTOR inhibitors via structure-based pharmacophore modeling approach. We have used pharmacophore-based virtual screening followed by molecular docking to select candidates from a Marine Natural Product (MNP) library. Subsequently, the drug-like marine compounds showing the best docking scores and molecular interactions with the kinase domain of mTOR were further refined by molecular dynamics (MD) simulations and Molecular Mechanics Poisson–Boltzmann Surface Area (MM-PBSA) analysis. The compounds demonstrating good binding affinity scores, as revealed by MM-PBSA were confirmed as final hits and reported in this study as potential ATP-competitive mTOR kinase domain inhibitors for cancer therapeutic treatment.

2. Results

2.1. Structure-Based Pharmacophore Model

A structure-based pharmacophore was generated from the crystallographic structure of mTOR kinase complexed with PP242 inhibitor, in which the key features of PP242 binding with mTOR were exploited. Accordingly, a total of six pharmacophore models were generated with hydrogen bond donbr (HBD), hydrogen bond acceptor (HBA) and hydrophobic (Hy) as common indispensable features (Table 1). The *Pharmacophore_01* with five features (1 HBA, 2 HBD and 2 Hy) and with the highest selectivity score of 9.2973 was observed to be the best pharmacophore model among the six generated pharmacophores and hence selected for further analysis. Upon meticulous examination, *Pharmacophore_01* displayed requisite features complementing the key residues for binding—Asp2195, Gly2238, Val2240 and Ile2356. The HBA feature complements with the essential residue Val2240, where PP242 is responsible for forming a hydrogen bond. The pyrazolopyrimidine scaffold of PP242 also maps on to the two HBD features by hydrogen bonding with two vital residues—Asp2195 and Gly2238. A previously published study suggests HBA and HBD as crucial features required for mTOR inhibition [21]. Moreover, the two Hy features complement the PP242 binding with Ile2356 residue via π-alkyl interactions. The Hy pharmacophoric feature was also reported as an essential feature in an earlier study on nanomolar mTOR inhibitors [35]. Therefore, *Pharmacophore_01* was escalated for further analysis (Figure 1).

Table 1. Structure-based pharmacophore models with their generated features.

Pharmacophore Models	Number of Features	Feature Set *	Selectivity Score
Pharmacophore_01	5	ADDHH	9.2973
Pharmacophore_02	4	DDHH	7.7825
Pharmacophore_03	4	ADDH	7.7825
Pharmacophore_04	4	ADDH	7.7825
Pharmacophore_05	4	ADHH	6.8689
Pharmacophore_06	4	ADHH	6.8689

* A: hydrogen bond acceptor (HBA); D: hydrogen bond donor (HBD); H: hydrophobic (Hy).

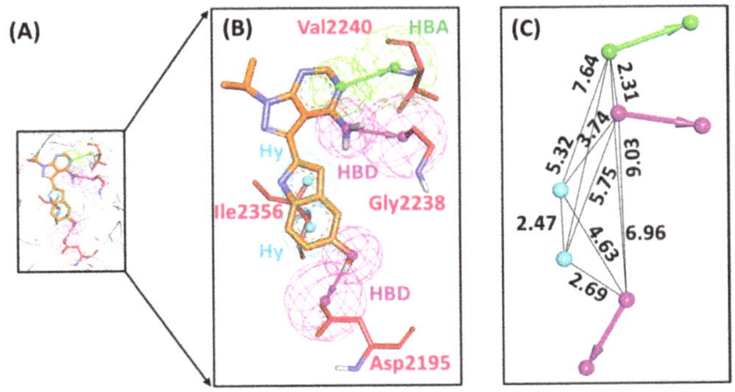

Figure 1. Structure-based pharmacophore model- *Pharmacophore_01*. (**A**) Pharmacophore model generated at the catalytic site of mTOR with co-crystallized ligand, PP242. (**B**) Pharmacophore features mapped with the key residues of the binding pocket. (**C**) Interfeature distance between the mapped pharmacophore features. HBA (hydrogen bond acceptor); HBD (hydrogen bond donor) and Hy (hydrophobic).

2.2. Decoy Set Validation of the Structure-Based Pharmacophore Model

The selected model *Pharmacophore_01* was evaluated for its efficiency in retrieving active mTOR compounds from a given database of active and inactive molecules. This validation was prompted by screening an external database (D) of 300 compounds, with 50 active compounds (A). With 61 hits retrieved from the database (Ht), active compounds obtained were 49 (Ha). The goodness of fit (GF) score was calculated as 0.80, thereby confirming that *Pharmacophore_01* can predict active compounds from a given dataset reasonably well (Table 2).

Table 2. Decoy set validation of *Pharmacophore_01* from an external database composed of active and inactive mTOR inhibitors.

S. No.	Parameters	Values
1	Total number of compounds in the database (D)	300
2	Total number of active compounds in the database (A)	50
3	Total number of hits retrieved by pharmacophore model from the database (Ht)	61
4	Total number of active compounds in the hit list (Ha)	49
5	% Yield of active ((Ha/Ht) × 100)	80
6	% Ratio of actives ((Ha/A) × 100)	98
7	False negatives (A-Ha)	1
8	False positives (Ht-Ha)	12
9	Goodness of fit score (GF)	0.80

2.3. Drug-Like Marine Compounds Retrieved by Virtual Screening

The validated model *Pharmacophore_01* mapped 3019 compounds from the Marine Natural Products (MNP) library of 14,492 compounds. Subsequent filtering of mapped compounds by Lipinski's Rule of Five (Ro5) and absorption, distribution, metabolism, excretion and toxicity (ADMET) properties led to further reducing the amount to 135 compounds. These 135 marine drug-like compounds along with reference inhibitor PP242 were escalated for molecular docking with mTOR crystallographic structure and their interactions with residues Leu2185, Asp2195, Ile2237, Gly2238, Trp2239, Val2240, Thr2245, Met2345, Leu2354, Ile2356, and Asp2357 were scrutinized (Figure 2).

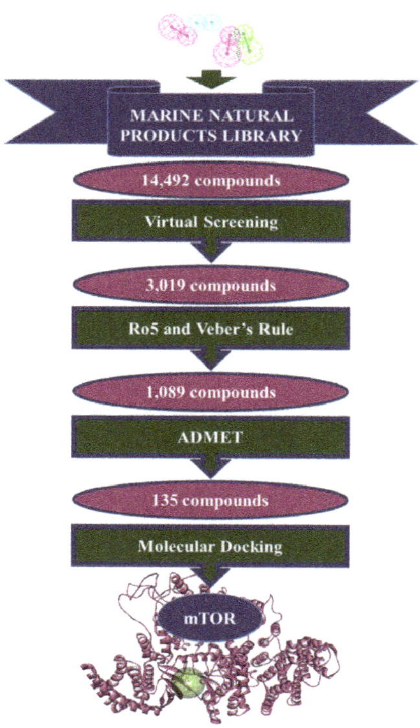

Figure 2. Illustration of the stages involved in the retrieval of potential drug-like compounds from Marine Natural Products (MNP) library using the structure-based pharmacophore model.

2.4. Molecular Docking of Retrieved Marine Drug-Like Compounds with mTOR Kinase

The molecular docking process demarcates on the binding affinity, mode of ligand binding in the target protein pocket and also elucidates the interactions of compounds with essential residues. The performance of GOLD software was evaluated by re-docking the co-crystallized ligand PP242 into mTOR binding pocket, resulting in an acceptable RMSD of 0.71 Å (Figure S1). Docking of screened 135 marine drug-like compounds with mTOR kinase domain was then carried out along with reference inhibitor PP242. A total of four marine compounds demonstrated higher Gold scores than PP242 reference inhibitor. The reference compound displayed a lower Gold score of 63.20 as compared with marine compounds hereafter referred to as MNP1, MNP2, MNP3 and MNP4 exhibiting higher Gold scores of 65.48, 65.41, 64.72 and 63.75, respectively (Table 3). The four compounds also demonstrated interactions with the aforementioned residues of the ATP-binding pocket of mTOR kinase domain. A total of 15 molecules exhibited lower docking scores than Torkinib and, therefore, were not considered for further evaluation. However, it was observed that these 15 marine molecules also target similar residues of the mTOR pocket, as seen for the above four compounds (Table S1). Therefore, these four marine compounds and the reference PP242 inhibitor were taken forward for MD simulations to confirm on their stabilities with the mTOR binding pocket.

Table 3. The docking scores and intermolecular interactions of reference PP242 and Marine Natural Product (MNP) library compounds with mTOR kinase domain (PDB ID: 4JT5).

Compound No.	MNP ID (CAS No *)	Gold Score	Hydrogen Bond Interactions	Hydrophobic and van der Waals Interactions
1 (MNP1)	200936-85-2	65.48	Val2240, Asp2357	Leu2185, Lys2187, Leu2192, Asp2195, Tyr2225, Val2227, Ile2237, Gly2238, Trp2239, His2242, Cys2243, Asp2244, Thr2245, Met2345, Arg2348, Ile2356, Phe2358
2 (MNP2)	230295-94-0	65.41	Asp2195, Trp2239, Val2240	Leu2185, Lys2187, Leu2192, Met2199, Tyr2225, Val2227, Ile2237, Pro2241, His2242, Cys2243, Met2345, Arg2348, Ile2356, Asp2357, Phe2358
3 (MNP3)	149636-93-1	64.72	Trp2239, Val2240	Leu2185, Lys2187, Glu2190, Leu2192, Asp2195, Tyr2225, Ile2237, Trp2239, Val2240, Pro2241, His2242, Cys2243, Met2345, Arg2348, Ile2356, Asp2357, Phe2358
4 (MNP4)	200936-84-1	63.75	Asp2195, Val2240, Asp2357	Ile2163, Leu2185, Leu2192, Met2199, Tyr2225, Val2227, Ile2237, Trp2239, Pro2241, His2242, Cys2243, Asp2244, Thr2245, Met2345, Arg2348, Ile2356
5 (PP242)	Reference (1092351-67-1)	63.20	Asp2195, Gly2238, Val2240	Ile2163, Leu2185, Lys2187, Met2199, Tyr2225, Ile2237, Trp2239, Cys2243, Thr2245, Met2345, Ile2356, Asp2357, Phe2358

* CAS: Chemical Abstracts Service.

2.5. Binding Mode and Binding Free Energy Analysis of Identified Marine Compounds by Molecular Dynamics Simulations

MD simulations employing GROningen Machine for Chemical Simulations (GROMACS) package were executed for the four identified marine compounds docked with the mTOR kinase to comprehend the dynamic behavior at the atomistic level. Simulations were also supplemented with the calculation of binding free energies for the identified hits by MM-PBSA methodology and the compounds were ranked as hits accordingly (Table S2). To gain insight into the binding mode of identified compounds inside the mTOR ATP-binding pocket, the representative structures from the last 5 ns of stable MD trajectories were extracted and subsequently superimposed. Upon scrupulous analysis, it was observed that the identified compounds exhibited a similar binding mode as the PP242 co-crystallized ligand of mTOR (Figure 3).

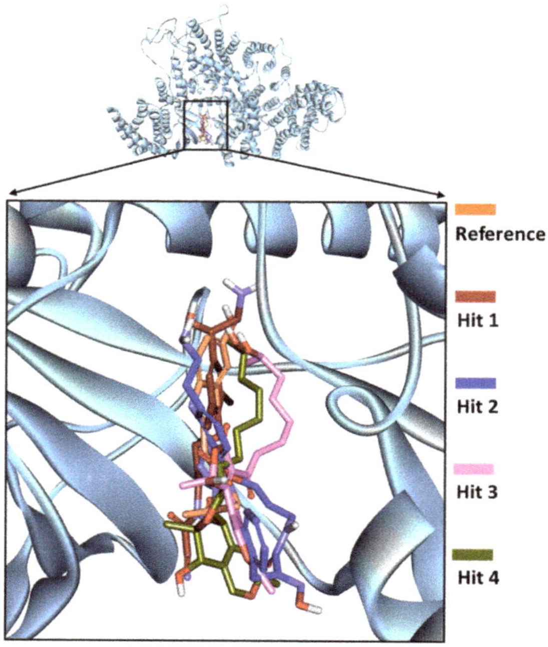

Figure 3. Binding mode of reference PP242 and identified Marine Natural Product (MNP) library hits within the ATP-binding pocket of mTOR kinase domain.

2.6. Characteristic Binding Interaction and Binding Free Energy Analysis of the Confirmed Marine Hits with mTOR ATP-Binding Pocket Residues

2.6.1. mTOR-Hit1 Interaction

The marine compound MNP2 acquired from the docking analysis (Table 3) exhibited the highest BFE of −101.187 ± 17.842 kJ/mol, as investigated by MM-PBSA calculations and, therefore, referred to as Hit1 (Table S2). The estimated BFE gives insight on the diverse components of interaction energy contributing to Hit1 binding. Both electrostatic and van der Waals components contribute a major role in the binding of Hit1 with the ATP-binding pocket of mTOR, where the van der Waals contribution (−151.961 ± 11.779 kJ/mol) is higher than the electrostatic component (−101.485 ± 16.574 kJ/mol). The solvent accessible surface area (SASA) provides a slightly favorable contribution towards the binding of Hit1 with mTOR (−17.534 ± 0.909 kJ/mol). Energy decomposition analysis led to the identification of vital residues contributing to the binding of Hit1 with mTOR (Figures 4A and 5A, Table S2). It was observed that the major contribution for Hit1 binding was from van der Waals interaction with residue Trp2239 (−8.5 kJ/mol) and hydrophobic interaction with residue Ile2356 (−7.9 kJ/mol) which was consistent with its binding mode (Figure 5B). The binding of Hit1 in the mTOR ATP-binding pocket is rendered by hydrogen bond interactions (Figures 4A and 5B) with Asp2195 (bond length: 1.72 Å) and Asp2357 (bond length: 1.96 Å). Additionally, the benzene ring of Hit1 interacted with key residues Tyr2225 (bond length: 4.25 Å), Ile2237 (bond length: 4.70 Å), Val2240 (bond length: 4.94 Å) and Ile2356 (bond length: 4.47 Å) via π-alkyl hydrophobic interactions. Moreover, mTOR residues Ile2163, Leu2185, Lys2187, Val2198, Gly2238, Trp2239, Met2345 and Phe2358 form van der Waals interactions with Hit1 (Figure 5B).

2.6.2. mTOR-Hit2 Interaction

The marine compound MNP3 (hereafter referred to as Hit2) attained from docking analysis (Table 3), demonstrated with BFE of −101.041 ± 20.457 kJ/mol, was observed to be comparable with the BFE of Hit1 (Table S2). Similar to Hit1, contribution of van der Waals (-165.824 ± 15.257 kJ/mol) and electrostatic (-70.466 ± 12.892 kJ/mol) components for the binding of Hit2 with mTOR played a major role than the corresponding SASA energy. The contribution of SASA energy component (-21.107 ± 0.998 kJ/mol) for Hit2 binding was observed to be higher than that of Hit1 with mTOR ATP-binding pocket. The major residues contributing to Hit2 binding with mTOR were also observed to be similar to Hit1 contributing residues (Figure 5C), with Trp2239 (−9.3 kJ/mol) and Ile2356 (−7.0 kJ/mol) forming hydrophobic bonds with Hit2 (Figure 5D). Elucidating on the binding interaction of Hit2 predicted by MD analysis, it was noticed that Hit2 formed three hydrogen bonds (Figures 4B and 5D) with residues Lys2187 (bond length: 1.75 Å), Thr2245 (bond length: 1.80 Å) and Asp2357 (bond length: 2.45 Å). Moreover, the bromo-phenoxy group interacts with residues Leu2185 (bond length: 4.50 Å), Ile2237 (bond length: 3.77 Å) and Trp2239 (bond length: 5.45 Å) via alkyl and π-alkyl hydrophobic interactions. Additional interactions with residues Ala2248 (bond length: 5.18 Å) and Ile2356 (bond length: 4.37 Å) also hold Hit2 in the mTOR hydrophobic pocket via π-alkyl bonds. Furthermore, the residues Ile2163, Thr2164, Glu2190, Asp2195, Gly2238, Val2240, Cys2243, Asp2244, Met2345 and Phe2358 assist in holding Hit2 in the mTOR binding pocket firmly via van der Waals interactions (Figure 5D).

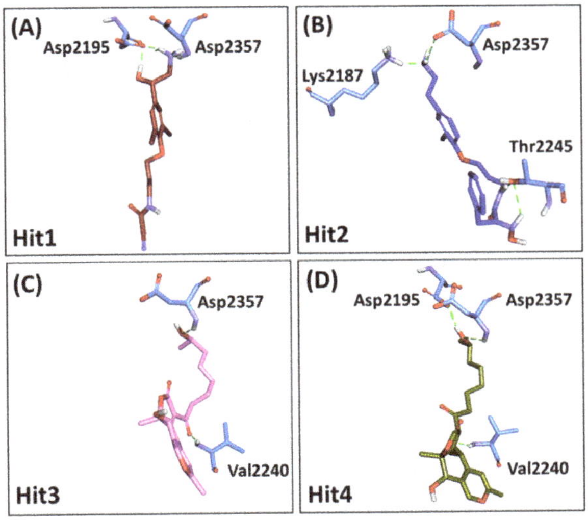

Figure 4. Interactions of (**A**) Hit1, (**B**) Hit2, (**C**) Hit3 and (**D**) Hit4 from Marine Natural Product (MNP) library with key residues of mTOR ATP-binding pocket via hydrogen bonds. The compounds and interacting residues are represented as sticks while the hydrogen bonding interactions are shown as green dashed lines.

2.6.3. mTOR-Hit3 Interaction

The marine compound MNP1, exhibiting the highest dock score of 65.48 (Table 3) presented with the BFE of -91.924 ± 12.264 kJ/mol (Table S2) and, therefore, ranked and referred as Hit3. It was observed that the van der Waals component was responsible for majorly contributing (-171.314 ± 11.172 kJ/mol) to Hit3 binding with mTOR than electrostatic (-17.958 ± 10.086 kJ/mol) and SASA (-19.290 ± 1.055 kJ/mol) energy components. The van der Waals contribution was observed to be the highest for Hit3-mTOR interaction than mTOR interactions with other hits (Table S2). Additionally, the contribution of this component is 10-fold higher than electrostatic component (-17.958 ± 10.086 kJ/mol) for Hit3-mTOR binding. Emphasizing the major residues contributing to the binding energy of Hit3 with mTOR, van der Waals interaction via Ile2356 (-9.2 kJ/mol) and hydrophobic interactions via Trp2239 (−11.1 kJ/mol) and Met2345 (8.9 kJ/mol) were seen to have a greater impact on binding (Figure 5E,F). Hydrogen bond analysis of the predicted binding mode demonstrated with Hit3 forming two bonds (Figures 4C and 5F) with residues Val2240 (bond length: 2.05 Å) and Asp2357 (bond length: 2.37 Å). Moreover, Hit3 interacts with Leu2185 (bond length: 5.0 Å) from the inner hydrophobic pocket and with Met2345 (bond length: 5.13 Å) of mTOR hydrophobic chamber via alkyl interactions. Two π-alkyl bonds are formed with residue Trp2239 (bond length: 4.32 Å and 4.90 Å) of the hydrophobic chamber. Besides above interactions, van der Waals bonds with residues Ile2163, Met2199, Tyr2225, Val2227, Ile2237, Gly2238, Thr2245, Leu2354, His2355, Ile2356 and Phe2358 contribute to the BFE obtained for Hit3 (Figure 5F).

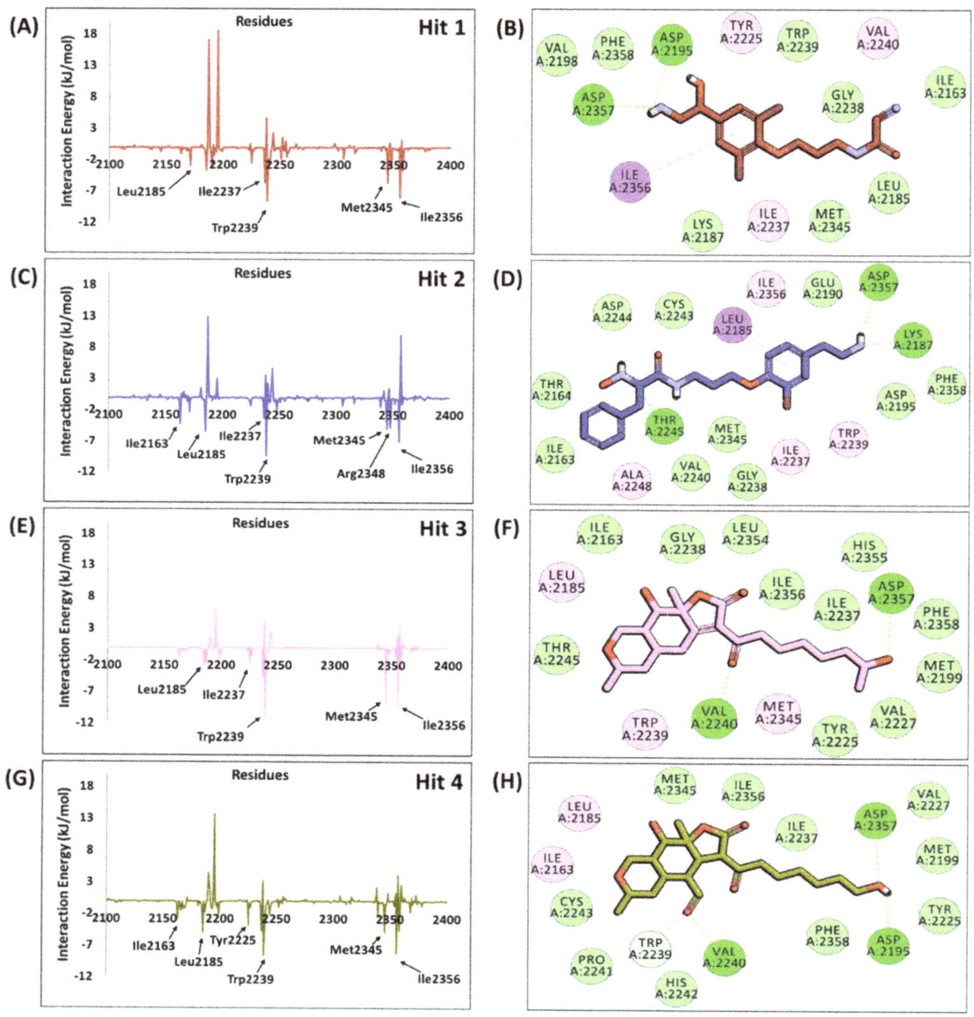

Figure 5. Energy decomposition of individual residues from MM-PBSA contributing to total binding free energy (BFE) for (**A**) Hit1, (**C**) Hit2, (**E**) Hit3 and (**G**) Hit4, and 2D interaction of (**B**) Hit1, (**D**) Hit2, (**F**) Hit3 and (H) Hit4 with residues of mTOR ATP-binding pocket. The hydrogen bonding interactions are shown as green dashed lines, the hydrophobic interactions are shown as pink and purple spheres and the van der Waals interactions are displayed as light green spheres.

2.6.4. mTOR-Hit4 Interaction

The marine compound MNP4 (hereafter referred to as Hit4) with lowest dock score among obtained hits (Table 3) demonstrated a BFE of −86.049 ± 14.961 kJ/mol (Table S2). Similar to other hit compounds, the van der Waals component of BFE also contributed greatly to Hit4-mTOR binding (−169.882 ± 11.839 kJ/mol). Correspondingly, the contribution of SASA energy component for Hit4 binding (−19.569 ± 0.780 kJ/mol) was in comparable range with SASA energy for Hit3 binding (−19.290 ± 1.055 kJ/mol). The interaction energy of individual residues towards Hit4-mTOR binding revealed Trp2239 (−8.5 kJ/mol) and Ile2356 (−8.1 kJ/mol) as the major contributing residues via hydrophobic and van der Waals interactions, respectively, as also observed in the above hits (Figure 5G,H). The binding interaction of Hit4 with mTOR revealed that Hit4 interacts with Asp2195 (bond length: 2.03 Å), Val2240 (bond length: 2.40 Å) and Asp2357 (bond length: 2.83 Å) via hydrogen bonds (Figures 4D and 5H). Similar interactions with Asp2195 and Val2240 via hydrogen bonds were also observed in reference structure bonding with mTOR kinase (Figure S2). Elucidating on the hydrophobic interactions of Hit4 with mTOR kinase domain residues, it was observed that Hit4 interacts with hydrophobic chamber residue Ile2163 (bond length: 4.69 Å) and inner hydrophobic pocket residue Leu2185 (bond length: 4.52 Å) via alkyl bonds. Moreover, three π-alkyl bonds (bond lengths: 4.82 Å, 5.22 Å and 5.24 Å) and one π-sigma bond (bond length: 3.73 Å) with hydrophobic chamber residue Trp2239 also contribute to Hit4-mTOR interaction. Furthermore, residues Met2199, Tyr2225, Val2227, Ile2237, Pro2241, His2242, Cys2243, Met2345, Ile2356 and Phe2358 also participate in positioning Hit4 firmly in mTOR binding pocket via van der Waals interactions (Figure 5H).

2.7. Evaluation of Drug-Likeness, ADME and Toxicity Properties of Identified mTOR Hits

Knowledge of the drug-likeness and ADME properties of final hits is vital, prior to their consideration as a lead candidate in drug development and/or their usage as anti-cancer drugs. These properties for the final hits were assessed using DS and tabulated. Furthermore, the *Toxicity Prediction (TOPKAT)* module in DS was used to evaluate the toxicity properties of identified hits. Given the structural information of a compound as a query, TOPKAT relies on the concept of Quantitative Structure–Toxicity Relationship (QSTR) models for computing toxicity properties, including AMES mutagenicity and rodent carcinogenicity, based on the National Toxicology Program (NTP) dataset. According to the U.S. NTP protocol, a compound's carcinogenicity is assessed by testing it in female and male sexes of mouse as well as rat. As per the calculations, all hits were observed to obey the Lipinski's Ro5 and displayed molecular weight of less than 500 Da with predicted octanol/water partition coefficient logP of less than 5.0 and estimated hydrogen bond donors and acceptors of less than 5 and 10, respectively (Table S2). The hits also followed the Veber's rule except for Hit2 with 10 rotatable bonds. Additionally, the identified hits satisfied the ADME properties demonstrating low blood–brain barrier (BBB) penetration, no inhibition of CYP2D6, good human intestinal absorption (HIA) as well as good aqueous solubility (Table S3). The results from TOPKAT analysis suggested that our identified hits demonstrated non-carcinogenicity in both sexes of rat models, while Hit2 appeared to be carcinogenic in mouse male (Table S4). According to the TOPKAT AMES mutagenicity analysis, Hit2 was displayed as being a mutagen while other hits were observed to be non-mutagenic (Table S4).

2.8. Novelty and Source Documentation of Identified mTOR Inhibitors

As a final assessment, the source of the identified marine hits was evaluated. For this purpose, the PubChem chemistry database (https://pubchem.ncbi.nlm.nih.gov/, (accessed on 11 February 2021)) was searched with Chemical Abstracts Service (CAS) numbers/MNP IDs of the respective hits as queries to identify if our hits have already been reported in the literature for mTOR kinase or other target proteins. From PubChem literature analysis, it was found that the compound Hit1 (7-Hydroxyceratinamine) is a cyanoformamide-containing metabolite originating from a Micronesian sponge, *Aplysinella* sp [36]. In addition, Hit2 was found to be a marine alkaloid isolated from the sponge *Psammaplysilla purpurea* [37]. The source for Hit3 could not be identified while Hit4 was recognized as a phytolide of the *Colletotrichum boninense* fungal origin [38]. As per the literature analysis, the four identified hits have not been reported as inhibitors of mTOR kinase. Therefore, the identified hits in the present study provide valuable alternatives as therapeutic candidates for further lead optimization.

3. Discussion

Kinase proteins act as chief regulatory entities in cellular biology. Moreover, their hyperactivation leads to several pathologies, including cancer. Therefore, kinases have become essential pharmacological targets and the discovery of small molecule drugs is a predominant scientific activity to mitigate the cancerous ailments. The mammalian target of rapamycin, mTOR is a dual specificity protein kinase which phosphorylates serine/threonine as well as tyrosine residues. The deregulation of mTOR is associated with diabetes, obesity, aging and various types of cancer [39–43]. The PI3K/AKT/mTOR pathway has been largely implicated in the tumorigenesis and progression of aforementioned cancers. Specific mTOR inhibitors are currently in various stages of clinical trials [44]. The mTOR inhibitors appear to be well tolerated combined with adverse effects, including myelosuppression, metabolic abnormalities, stomatitis and skin reactions, among other abnormalities [45]. These inhibitors can be classified into first generation allosteric inhibitors such as rapamycin and its analogues [46] and second generation ATP-competitive inhibitors. Several ATP-competitive mTOR inhibitors have been discovered and being tested in clinical trials including selective inhibitors like CC-223, INK-128 and OSI-027 [47] Unlike the former category of inhibitors, the ATP-competitive mTOR inhibitors block the ATP-binding catalytic site as well as reduce the activity of mTORC1 and mTORC2 complexes and hence has become an effective strategy to suppress both the ATP and allosteric sites. Encouraged from these efforts, we pursued our research strategy to identify natural product compounds as mTOR ATP-competitive inhibitors by applying structure-based pharmacophore modelling. Such a pharmacophore strategy works towards exploiting the key interactions between the protein residues and the bound co-crystallized ligand [48].

Marine extracts have displayed a great potential as an essential source of new drugs. Marine environments remain extensively unexplored despite being a huge source of bioactive compounds against cancer. Aquatic habitats have produced a variety of marine-derived alkaloids, triterpenoids and peptides. Intriguingly, a purple sponge extract of Turkish marine origin was shown to display promising activity against a panel of tyrosine kinases and cell lines including A549, A375, KMS-12PE and K562 cancer cell lines [32]. Similarly, the brown algae-derived polysaccharide, Fucoidan, was shown to exert anti-cancer effects not only through cell cycle arrest but also by indirectly killing cancerous cells by activation of natural killer cells and macrophages. Fucoidan was also shown to demonstrate inhibitory activity against cancer A549, MCF-7, PC-3 and SMMC-7721 cells [31]. In addition, Fascaplysin which is a bis-indole of a marine sponge demonstrated anticancer activity as CDK4 inhibitor in lung cancer cell line [46]. The antitumor potential of marine algae-derived compounds has also been extensively reviewed recently [24]. We therefore designed our study to target the mTOR dysregulation in cancer using marine-derived bioactive natural products employing a series of computational methods. Using a structure-based pharmacophore approach, we have developed a pharmacophore model from mTOR protein structure co-crystallized with ligand PP242 (Figure 1). Torkinib/PP242 is a selective ATP-competitive inhibitor of mTOR with promising anti-cancer activity over numerous cancer types [49]. A total of 14,492 compounds of marine origin were screened with the pharmacophore model as a query, deriving 3019 compounds as candidates mapping the pharmacophore model. Subsequently, a drug-like database was prepared employing Lipinski's Ro5 and ADMET rules, thereby retrieving 135 compounds (Figure 2). Molecular docking-based interaction screening of these 135 compounds resulted in the identification of four compounds with higher docking scores than PP242 and similar interactions with the ATP-binding pocket of mTOR (Table 3). Escalating the identified four compounds to molecular dynamics simulations for observing their behavior at the atomistic level gave insights into the critical residues required for the specific mTOR inhibition.

The structure-based pharmacophore and MD analysis of the mTOR-PP242 crystal structure revealed that the inhibitor targets key residues Asp2195, Gly2238 and Val2240 via hydrogen bonds entailing essential pharmacophoric features including HBD and HBA (Figure 1B and Figure S2A). It has been elucidated in previous studies that hydrogen bonds with Asp2195 and Val2240 are indispensable for mTOR inhibitory activity [50–56]. In the current study, Hit1 was observed to retain the hydrogen bonding interaction with Asp2195 (Table 3, Figure 4A), while Hit4 interaction with both residues was preserved even after 30 ns of production simulation run (Table 3, Figure 4D). Additionally, our hits formed hydrogen bonds with catalytic hydrophilic residue Asp2357 of the mTOR ATP-binding site which offers a level of specificity for our hits towards mTOR than PI3K (Figure 4) [51–55]. The compound Hit2 also formed additional hydrogen bonds with residues Lys2187 and Thr2245 (Figure 4B) and interactions with these residues were also reported in previously published studies [22,51,52,55]. A recent study reported natural products as mTOR ATP-binding site and rapamycin binding site inhibitors derived from three databases—Marine Natural Products Library, SuperNatural II and ZINC natural products—and also provided experimental evidence against mTOR for eleven compounds [23]. However, the marine compounds identified from their studies as mTOR inhibitors are distinct from our proposed marine natural product hits. In addition to the aforementioned hydrogen bonds, our hits are also characterized by several hydrophobic and van der Waals interactions (Figure 5). In particular, interaction with residue Trp2239 of the hydrophobic chamber was observed via π-stacking bonds or van der Waals interaction for our hits, similar to Torkinib interaction with mTOR (Figure 5 and Figure S2B). Earlier studies reported that Trp2239 is not present in canonical protein kinases such as PI3K and interaction with this residue provides for mTOR inhibitor specificity over PI3K [56,57]. All of these results suggest that our hits may be selective mTOR inhibitors. From our per-residue contribution analysis, Trp2239 was observed to contribute the highest for Hit3 binding (−11.1 kJ/mol) (Figure 5E) followed by Hit2 (−9.3 kJ/mol) (Figure 5C), Hit1 (−8.53 kJ/mol) (Figure 5A) and Hit4 (−8.52 kJ/mol) (Figure 5G) binding with mTOR. The Trp2239 contributed the highest energy for binding of Hit3 among the four identified hits forming strong interactions via π hydrophobic bonds as observed (Figure 5F), thus suggesting a higher level of selectivity of Hit3 binding with mTOR. In a recently published review, the significant residues involved in ligand selectivity towards mTOR over PI3K were reviewed in detail and reported as Arg770, Glu2190 and Cys2243 [50]. Our identified Hit2 displayed bonds with Glu2190 and Cys2243 via van der Waals interactions (Figure 5D), while Cys2243 was also observed to support Hit4 via van der Waals interactions in the ATP-binding pocket of mTOR (Figure 5H). The above-mentioned analyses indicate that our identified marine hits have better binding affinity, as computed from MM-PBSA binding free energy scores, and also seem to confer comparable selectivity towards mTOR as the previously identified selective inhibitor, Torkinib. Correspondingly, the identified hits also portray the essential pharmacophoric features required for mTOR inhibition, similar to Torkinib (Figures 1 and 6).

As a final analysis, the four identified marine hits were scrutinized for their physicochemical, pharmacokinetic and toxicity properties to evaluate their in vivo disposition prior to their consideration as therapeutic anti-cancer drugs. The drug-likeness properties and ADME results demonstrated that the identified hits satisfied the Ro5 criteria, could be absorbed easily in the human intestine, show good aqueous solubility, do not inhibit the CYP2D6 enzyme and do not penetrate the BBB (Table S3). Despite presenting with good Ro5 properties, Hit2 displayed with the upper limit value (i.e., 10) in the case of Veber's rule of rotatable bonds. In addition, the hits were identified as non-carcinogenic in rodent NTP models and non-AMES mutagenic, except for Hit2, which showed carcinogenicity in the mouse male NTP model and also showed AMES mutagenicity (Table S4). Although Hit2 exhibited with a BFE of −101.041 kJ/mol (Table S2) and presented with key intermolecular interactions with mTOR (Figures 4B and 5D), it cannot be considered as a therapeutic candidate for further drug optimization, owing to its toxicity properties. Overall, we believe the potentiality of Hit1, Hit3 and Hit4 as alternatives and their scaffolds can be further explored for developing efficient ATP-binding site mTOR inhibitors for cancer therapeutics. Though the in vitro studies of our identified marine hits are further required to clinically substantiate these findings, structure-based pharmacophore modeling and virtual screening strategy can be very useful to design potent molecules as mTOR inhibitors in future drug discovery studies. In addition, our study characterizes a platform for future discovery of novel natural chemotherapeutic drugs from marine natural habitat

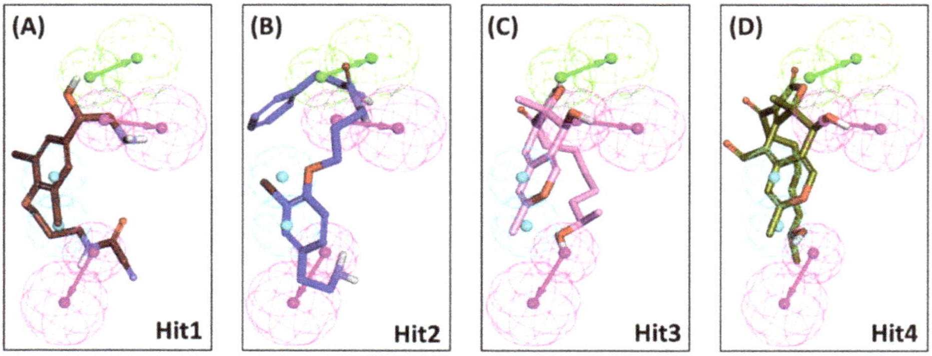

Figure 6. Alignment of the (**A**) Hit1, (**B**) Hit2, (**C**) Hit3 and (**D**) Hit4 with the pharmacophoric features. All hits represent the HBA (hydrogen bond acceptor), HBD (hydrogen bond donor) and Hy (hydrophobic) features of *Pharmacophore_01*.

4. Materials and Methods

4.1. Structure-Based Pharmacophore Model Generation

Receptor-based pharmacophore model delves into the catalytic site of the target protein bound with its inhibitor to identify essential pharmacophoric features effective for inhibition [58]. The structure of mTOR target protein bound with its ATP-site inhibitor PP242 (PDB ID: 4JT5, 3.45 Å) was retrieved from Research Collaboratory for Structural Bioinformatics (RCSB) Protein Data Bank (PDB) and considered for the generation of a structure-based pharmacophore model [56]. PP242 (also known as Torkinib) is a potent and specific inhibitor of mTOR kinase domain proven to be more effective than traditional mTOR inhibitor rapamycin [14,59]. Subsequently, the residues within 9 Å around PP242 were considered and *Receptor-Ligand Pharmacophore Generation* module embedded in Discovery Studio (DS) v.2018 was employed for model generation. The model with the highest selectivity score was chosen for subsequent validation.

4.2. Validation of Generated Pharmacophore Model

Given a particular dataset, pharmacophore validation is a quintessential criterion for ensuring efficient retrieval of active target protein compounds. Accordingly, the model chosen from the above-mentioned criteria was validated by Güner–Henry approach (decoy set) approach [60] for evaluating the robustness of the pharmacophore model on the basis of goodness of fit (GF) score in the range of 0 (null model) and 1 (ideal model) [58,61,62].

$$GF = \left(\frac{Ha}{4HtA}\right)(3A + Ht) \times \left\{1 - \frac{Ht - Ha}{D - A}\right\}$$

The decoy set approach was instigated by evaluating the selected pharmacophore model on an external dataset (D) of 300 compounds obtained from the same biological assay [63]. This dataset was divided into 50 compounds exhibiting $IC_{50} < 100$ nmol/L, referred to as active (A) mTOR inhibitors, with the remaining compounds being inactive. The *Ligand Pharmacophore Mapping* was executed for dataset screening, complemented with *FAST* algorithm and the GF score was calculated.

4.3. Virtual Screening of Marine Natural Product Library

The validated pharmacophore model was escalated to screen the Marine Natural Product (MNP) library composed of 14,492 compounds (http://docking.umh.es/downloaddb, (accessed on 11 December 2020). The DS module *Ligand Pharmacophore Mapping* was employed in pursuit of identifying scaffolds mapping the pharmacophoric features. The compounds obtained from screening were further subjected to filtering by Lipinski's Rule of Five (Ro5) [64], Veber's rules [65] and pharmacokinetics by absorption, distribution, metabolism, excretion and toxicity (ADMET) for retrieval of drug-like compounds. Accordingly, the *Filter by Lipinski and Veber Rules* and *ADMET Descriptors* modules within DS were recruited for evaluation. The Ro5 and Veber's rules collectively oversee the physiochemical properties for efficient retrieval of compounds with molecular weight $\leq$500 kDa, number of hydrogen bond donors $\leq$5, compound's lipophilicity (log*P*) $\leq$5, number of hydrogen bond acceptors $\leq$10 and the number of rotatable bonds $\leq$10. The drug-like compounds so obtained were subjected to molecular docking with the mTOR kinase domain along with PP242 as reference inhibitor.

4.4. Molecular Docking of Drug-Like Compounds with mTOR Kinase Domain

Molecular docking methods explore the binding conformations adopted within the catalytic sites of macromolecular protein targets, thereby evaluating the vital phenomena for the intermolecular recognition process [66]. The drug-like compounds obtained from the above filtering criterion were subjected to molecular docking in Genetic Optimisation for Ligand Docking (GOLD) v5.2.2 automated docking software [67]. The compounds were evaluated on the basis of the GOLD default scoring function—Gold score [68]. This fitness score functions by scoring the summation of protein-ligand van der Waals interaction energy and hydrogen-bonding energy. The retrieved 3D crystallographic structure of mTOR (PDB ID: 4JT5) complexed with PP242 ATP-competitive inhibitor was prepared by utilizing the *Clean Protein* module in DS. Protein preparation was further carried out by adding the missing residues and hydrogen atoms. The water molecules were removed along with the bound PP242 ligand. Prior to docking, the performance of GOLD docking was assessed by re-docking the native PP242 ligand into mTOR. The drug-like compounds were subjected to minimization employing *Minimize Ligands* module in DS, preceding docking. Subsequently, molecular docking of drug-like compounds with mTOR was followed by applying the same docking parameters utilized for PP242 docking allowing for generation of 50 conformers per ligand. Clustering of the obtained conformations was carried out to obtain the largest cluster and each compound in the cluster was examined on the basis of higher Gold score than reference compound PP242, binding mode within the mTOR catalytic site and molecular interactions with the key residues of the mTOR kinase domain. The selected potential compounds acquired from this strategy were refined by MD simulations.

4.5. Molecular Dynamics Simulation of Identified Hits

MD simulation studies of compounds identified from above docking were extensively carried out to decipher the molecular dynamics in water and comprehend the interaction of hit compounds with vital residues of mTOR active site at the atomistic level. The docked structures of these marine hits in complex with mTOR were used as initial coordinates for simulations with GROMACS v2018 [69]. The mTOR and hit compounds were applied with CHARMm27 force field [70] and topologies generated with SwissParam [71] fast force field generation tool, respectively. The dodecahedron water box was utilized to solvate the systems with TIP3P water model and further neutralized with Na^{+} counter ions. The steepest descent energy minimization was performed to dodge bad contacts and this was followed by a two-fold equilibration. The NVT (constant number of particles, volume and temperature) equilibration at 300 K with a V-rescale thermostat supplemented with NPT (constant number of particles, pressure and temperature) equilibration at 1 bar pressure with a Parrinello-Rahman barostat [72] was orchestrated, each for 1000 ps. The LINear Constraint Solver (LINCS) [73] and SETTLE algorithms [74] were applied to monitor bond constrains and the geometry of water molecules. The long-range electrostatic interactions were calculated by means of Particle Mesh Ewald (PME) [75] and the equilibrated systems were subjected to production simulation runs of 30 ns. The acquired MD results were visualized and interpreted manually in visual molecular dynamics (VMD) [76] and DS. The binding free energy (BFE) scores were further computed for hit compounds by MM-PBSA executing *g_mmpbsa* tool implemented in GROMACS [77]. For this purpose, 40 frames of mTOR-ligand complexes were selected evenly from the last 10 ns of MD trajectories and the BFE ΔG_{bind} was computed as per the below equation.

$$\Delta G_{bind} = G_{complex} - \left(G_{protein} + G_{ligand}\right)$$

5. Conclusions

A structure-based pharmacophore model, exploiting the crystal structure of mTOR serine/threonine kinase with its bound selective inhibitor Torkinib revealed fundamental pharmacophoric features required for mTOR inhibition at its ATP-binding pocket. A systematic virtual screening strategy with the model as a query, retrieved 3019 compounds from the Marine Natural Products library and subsequent filtering via Lipinski's Ro5, Veber's rule, and ADMET was able to acquire 135 drug-like compounds. Molecular docking of these compounds at the ATP-binding site of mTOR procured four marine compounds with higher dock scores than Torkinib and significant binding interactions with key residues of the pocket. These compounds also presented with good binding free energy scores and the energy contribution of essential residues unveiled that our hits can inhibit mTOR via Glu2190, Trp2239 and Cys2243 deemed requisite for selective inhibition over PI3K. The in silico ADME and toxicity analysis suggests three out of the four identified hits with acceptable pharmacokinetic profile for their in vivo disposition. Additionally, the biological origin of these hits was identified as marine fungus and sponge. Overall, we believe that our hits provide scaffolds for future drug optimization studies and, therefore, recommend these hit compounds from marine natural habitat as therapeutics for the treatment of cancer. The identification of marine-derived natural compounds embodies an essential platform for future drug discovery studies against various protein targets implicated in cancers.

Supplementary Materials: The following are available online at https://www.mdpi.com/1424-8247/14/3/282/s1, Figure S1: Overlay of the docked pose (orange) PP242 inhibitor of mTOR kinase with its crystal structure conformation (green) in PDB ID: 4JT5. Figure S2. (A) 3D and (B) representation of interaction between PP242 and catalytic residues of the ATP-binding pocket of mTOR. The compounds and interacting residues are represented as sticks. The hydrogen bonding interactions are shown as green dashed lines, the hydrophobic interactions are shown as pink and purple spheres and the van der Waals interactions are displayed as light green spheres. Table S1. The docking scores and intermolecular interactions of reference PP242 and Marine Natural Product (MNP) library compounds with mTOR kinase domain (PDB ID: 4JT5). Table S2. Binding free energy scores of identified Marine Natural Product (MNP) library hits with mTOR calculated through MM-PBSA methodology. Table S3. Lipinski's and ADME properties of identified marine hits to determine their drug-likeness. Table S4. Toxicity properties of identified marine hits to determine their drug likeness.

Author Contributions: Conceptualization, S.P.; methodology, S.P.; software, S.P.; validation, S.P.; formal analysis, S.P., V.K., S.R. and G.L.; investigation, S.P.; resources, K.W.L.; data curation, S.P., V.K. and K.W.L.; writing—original draft preparation, S.P.; writing—review and editing, S.P. and K.W.L.; visualization, S.P.; supervision, K.W.L.; project administration, K.W.L.; funding acquisition, J.C.H. All authors have read and agreed to the published version of the manuscript.

Funding: This research was supported by Basic Science Research Program through the National Research Foundation of Korea (NRF) funded by the Ministry of Education (2020R1A6A1A03044344).

Institutional Review Board Statement: Not applicable.

Informed Consent Statement: Not applicable.

Data Availability Statement: Data are contained within the article.

Acknowledgments: This research was supported by the Bio & Medical Technology Development Program of the National Research Foundation (NRF) and funded by the Korean government (MSIT) (No. NRF-2018M3A9A70-57263).

Conflicts of Interest: The authors declare no conflict of interest.

References

1. Kim, Y.C.; Guan, K.L. MTOR: A pharmacologic target for autophagy regulation. *J. Clin. Investig.* **2015**, *125*, 25–32. [CrossRef] [PubMed]
2. Tan, A.C. Targeting the PI3K/Akt/mTOR pathway in non-small cell lung cancer (NSCLC). *Thorac. Cancer* **2020**, *11*, 511–518. [CrossRef] [PubMed]
3. Fattahi, S.; Amjadi-Moheb, F.; Tabaripour, R.; Ashrafi, G.H.; Akhavan-Niaki, H. PI3K/AKT/mTOR signaling in gastric cancer: Epigenetics and beyond. *Life Sci.* **2020**, *262*, 118513. [CrossRef]
4. Ediriweera, M.K.; Tennekoon, K.H.; Samarakoon, S.R. Role of the PI3K/AKT/mTOR signaling pathway in ovarian cancer: Biological and therapeutic significance. *Semin. Cancer Biol.* **2019**, *59*, 147–160. [CrossRef]
5. Tirrò, E.; Martorana, F.; Romano, C.; Vitale, S.R.; Motta, G.; Di Gregorio, S.; Massimino, M.; Pennisi, M.S.; Stella, S.; Puma, A.; et al. Molecular alterations in thyroid cancer: From bench to clinical practice. *Genes* **2019**, *10*, 709. [CrossRef]
6. Tian, T.; Li, X.; Zhang, J. mTOR signaling in cancer and mtor inhibitors in solid tumor targeting therapy. *Int. J. Mol. Sci.* **2019**, *20*, 755. [CrossRef]
7. Guertin, D.A.; Sabatini, D.M. Defining the Role of mTOR in Cancer. *Cancer Cell* **2007**, *12*, 9–22. [CrossRef] [PubMed]
8. Meric-Bernstam, F.; Gonzalez-Angulo, A.M. Targeting the mTOR signaling network for cancer therapy. *J. Clin. Oncol.* **2009**, *27*, 2278–2287. [CrossRef] [PubMed]
9. Sabatini, D.M. mTOR and cancer: Insights into a complex relationship. *Nat. Rev. Cancer* **2006**, *6*, 729–734. [CrossRef]
10. Abraham, R.T.; Gibbons, J.J. The mammalian target of rapamycin signaling pathway: Twists and turns in the road to cancer therapy. *Clin. Cancer Res.* **2007**, *13*, 3109–3114. [CrossRef]
11. Kim, L.C.; Cook, R.S.; Chen, J. mTORC1 and mTORC2 in cancer and the tumor microenvironment. *Oncogene* **2017**, *36*, 2191–2201. [CrossRef] [PubMed]
12. Zheng, Y.; Jiang, Y. mTOR inhibitors at a glance. *Mol. Cell. Pharmacol.* **2015**, *7*, 15–20. [CrossRef] [PubMed]
13. Faes, S.; Demartines, N.; Dormond, O. Resistance to mTORC1 Inhibitors in Cancer Therapy: From Kinase Mutations to Intratumoral Heterogeneity of Kinase Activity. *Oxid. Med. Cell. Longev.* **2017**, *2017*. [CrossRef] [PubMed]
14. Zhou, H.Y.; Huang, S. Le Current development of the second generation of mTOR inhibitors as anticancer agents. *Chin. J. Cancer* **2012**, *31*, 8–18.
15. Rodrik-Outmezguine, V.S.; Okaniwa, M.; Yao, Z.; Novotny, C.J.; McWhirter, C.; Banaji, A.; Won, H.; Wong, W.; Berger, M.; De Stanchina, E.; et al. Overcoming mTOR resistance mutations with a new-generation mTOR inhibitor. *Nature* **2016**, *534*, 272–276. [CrossRef] [PubMed]
16. Flemming, A. Cancer: Bivalent mTOR inhibitors—The next generation. *Nat. Rev. Drug Discov.* **2016**, *15*, 455. [CrossRef]
17. Xu, J.; Tian, D. Hematologic toxicities associated with mTOR inhibitors temsirolimus and everolimus in cancer patients: A systematic review and meta-analysis. *Curr. Med. Res. Opin.* **2014**, *30*, 67–74. [CrossRef]
18. Calvo, A.S.; Rochefort, J.; Javelot, M.J.; Descroix, V.; Lescaille, G. Management of mTOR inhibitors oral mucositis: Current state of knowledge. *J. Oral Med. Oral Surg.* **2019**, *25*, 11. [CrossRef]
19. Bauer, R.A.; Wurst, J.M.; Tan, D.S. Expanding the range of "druggable" targets with natural product-based libraries: An academic perspective. *Curr. Opin. Chem. Biol.* **2010**, *14*, 308–314. [CrossRef]
20. Harvey, A.L.; Edrada-Ebel, R.; Quinn, R.J. The re-emergence of natural products for drug discovery in the genomics era. *Nat. Rev. Drug Discov.* **2015**, *14*, 111–129. [CrossRef]
21. Chen, L.; Wang, L.; Gu, Q.; Xu, J. An in silico protocol for identifying mTOR inhibitors from natural products. *Mol. Divers.* **2014**, *18*, 841–852. [CrossRef]
22. Park, H.; Choe, H.; Hong, S. Virtual screening and biochemical evaluation to identify new inhibitors of mammalian target of rapamycin (mTOR). *Bioorganic Med. Chem. Lett.* **2014**, *24*, 835–838. [CrossRef] [PubMed]
23. Ruiz-Torres, V.; Losada-Echeberría, M.; Herranz-López, M.; Barrajón-Catalán, E.; Galiano, V.; Micol, V.; Encinar, J.A. New mammalian target of rapamycin (mTOR) modulators derived from natural product databases and marine extracts by using molecular docking techniques. *Mar. Drugs* **2018**, *16*, 385. [CrossRef] [PubMed]

24. Alves, C.; Silva, J.; Pinteus, S.; Gaspar, H.; Alpoim, M.C.; Botana, L.M.; Pedrosa, R. From marine origin to therapeutics: The antitumor potential of marine algae-derived compounds. *Front. Pharmacol.* **2018**, *9*, 777. [CrossRef] [PubMed]
25. Jimenez, P.C.; Wilke, D.V.; Costa-Lotufo, L.V. Marine drugs for cancer: Surfacing biotechnological innovations from the oceans. *Clinics* **2018**, *73*, e482s. [CrossRef] [PubMed]
26. Dyshlovoy, S.A.; Honecker, F. Marine compounds and cancer: 2017 updates. *Mar. Drugs* **2018**, *16*, 41. [CrossRef]
27. Sarfaraj, H.M.; Sheeba, F.; Saba, A.; Khan, M.S. Marine natural products: A lead for anti-cancer. *Indian J. Geo-Marine Sci.* **2012**, *41*, 27–39.
28. Carroll, A.R.; Copp, B.R.; Davis, R.A.; Keyzers, R.A.; Prinsep, M.R. Marine natural products. *Nat. Prod. Rep.* **2019**, *36*, 122–173 [CrossRef]
29. Blunt, J.W.; Carroll, A.R.; Copp, B.R.; Davis, R.A.; Keyzers, R.A.; Prinsep, M.R. Marine natural products. *Nat. Prod. Rep.* **2018**, *35*, 8–53. [CrossRef]
30. Cragg, G.M.; Pezzuto, J.M. Natural Products as a Vital Source for the Discovery of Cancer Chemotherapeutic and Chemopreventive Agents. *Med. Princ. Pract.* **2016**, *25*, 41–59. [CrossRef]
31. Lin, Y.; Qi, X.; Liu, H.; Xue, K.; Xu, S.; Tian, Z. The anti-cancer effects of fucoidan: A review of both in vivo and in vitro investigations. *Cancer Cell Int.* **2020**, *20*, 1–14. [CrossRef] [PubMed]
32. Ciftci, H.I.; Can, M.; Ellakwa, D.E.; Suner, S.C.; Ibrahim, M.A.; Oral, A.; Sekeroglu, N.; Özalp, B.; Otsuka, M.; Fujita, M.; et al. Anticancer activity of Turkish marine extracts: A purple sponge extract induces apoptosis with multitarget kinase inhibition activity. *Investig. New Drugs* **2020**, *38*, 1326–1333. [CrossRef] [PubMed]
33. Kauffmann-Guerrero, D.; Huber, R.M. Orphan drugs in development for the treatment of small-cell lung cancer: Emerging data on lurbinectedin. *Lung Cancer Targets Ther.* **2020**, *11*, 27–31. [CrossRef] [PubMed]
34. Lauritano, C.; Martínez, K.A.; Battaglia, P.; Granata, A.; de la Cruz, M.; Cautain, B.; Martín, J.; Reyes, F.; Ianora, A.; Guglielmo, L. First evidence of anticancer and antimicrobial activity in Mediterranean mesopelagic species. *Sci. Rep.* **2020**, *10*, 4929. [CrossRef]
35. Khanfar, M.A.; Taha, M.O. Elaborate ligand-based modeling coupled with multiple linear regression and k nearest neighbor QSAR analyses unveiled new nanomolar mTOR inhibitors. *J. Chem. Inf. Model.* **2013**, *53*, 2587–2612. [CrossRef]
36. Fu, X.; Schmitz, F.J. 7-Hydroxyceratinamine, a new cyanoformamide-containing metabolite from a sponge, Aplysinella sp. *J. Nat. Prod.* **1999**, *62*, 1072–1073. [CrossRef]
37. Dictionary of Alkaloids with CD-ROM—Google Books. Available online: https://books.google.co.kr/books?id=mynNBQAAQBAJ&pg=PA1601&dq=149636-93-1&hl=en&sa=X&ved=2ahUKEwjdjN36y7vuAhUBc3AKHZyGC8sQ6AEwAHoECAAQAg#v=onepage&q=149636-93-1&f=false (accessed on 27 January 2021).
38. Caraballo Rodriguez, A.M. Acesso a Produtos Naturais Mediante a Estrategia de Cultivos Mistos de Endofiticos: O Fungo Colletotrichum boninense FLe 8.1 e a Actinobacteria Streptomyces albospinus Rle 7. Master's Thesis, Universidade de São Paulo, São Paulo, Brazil, 2013. [CrossRef]
39. Papadopoli, D.; Boulay, K.; Kazak, L.; Pollak, M.; Mallette, F.A.; Topisirovic, I.; Hulea, L. Mtor as a central regulator of lifespan and aging. *F1000Research* **2019**, *8*. [CrossRef]
40. Tuo, Y.; Xiang, M. mTOR: A double-edged sword for diabetes. *J. Leukoc. Biol.* **2019**, *106*, 385–395. [CrossRef]
41. Costa, R.L.B.; Han, H.S.; Gradishar, W.J. Targeting the PI3K/AKT/mTOR pathway in triple-negative breast cancer: A review. *Breast Cancer Res. Treat.* **2018**, *169*, 397–406. [CrossRef]
42. Marquard, F.E.; Jücker, M. PI3K/AKT/mTOR signaling as a molecular target in head and neck cancer. *Biochem. Pharmacol.* **2020**, *172*, 113729. [CrossRef]
43. Shorning, B.Y.; Dass, M.S.; Smalley, M.J.; Pearson, H.B. The PI3K-AKT-mTOR pathway and prostate cancer: At the crossroads of AR, MAPK, and WNT signaling. *Int. J. Mol. Sci.* **2020**, *21*, 4507. [CrossRef] [PubMed]
44. Arachchige Don, A.S.; Zheng, F.S.X. Recent Clinical Trials of mTOR-Targeted Cancer Therapies. *Rev. Recent Clin. Trials* **2010**, *6*, 24–35. [CrossRef] [PubMed]
45. Gridelli, C.; Maione, P.; Rossi, A. The Potential Role of mTOR Inhibitors in Non-Small Cell Lung Cancer. *Oncologist* **2008**, *13*, 139–147. [CrossRef] [PubMed]
46. Rath, B.; Hochmair, M.; Plangger, A.; Hamilton, G. Anticancer activity of fascaplysin against lung cancer cell and small cell lung cancer circulating tumor cell lines. *Mar. Drugs* **2018**, *16*, 383. [CrossRef] [PubMed]
47. Schenone, S.; Brullo, C.; Musumeci, F.; Radi, M.; Botta, M. ATP-Competitive Inhibitors of mTOR: An Update. *Curr. Med. Chem.* **2011**, *18*, 2995–3014. [CrossRef]
48. Rana, R.M.; Rampogu, S.; Bin Abid, N.; Zeb, A.; Parate, S.; Lee, G.; Yoon, S.; Kim, Y.; Kim, D.; Woo Lee, K. In silico study identified methotrexate analog as potential inhibitor of drug resistant human dihydrofolate reductase for cancer therapeutics. *Molecules* **2020**, *25*, 3510. [CrossRef] [PubMed]
49. Hua, H.; Kong, Q.; Zhang, H.; Wang, J.; Luo, T.; Jiang, Y. Targeting mTOR for cancer therapy. *J. Hematol. Oncol.* **2019**, *12*, 1–19. [CrossRef] [PubMed]
50. Luo, Y.; Wang, L. Discovery and Development of ATP-Competitive mTOR Inhibitors Using Computational Approaches. *Curr. Pharm. Des.* **2017**, *23*, 4321–4331. [CrossRef]
51. Naveed, M. Molecular Docking and Pharmacokinetic of Highly Specific Novel Pan-Mtor Inhibitors against Solid Tumors. *MOJ Proteom. Bioinform.* **2017**, *5*, 13–16. [CrossRef]

52. Wang, L.; Chen, L.; Yu, M.; Xu, L.H.; Cheng, B.; Lin, Y.S.; Gu, Q.; He, X.H.; Xu, J. Discovering new mTOR inhibitors for cancer treatment through virtual screening methods and in vitro assays. *Sci. Rep.* **2016**, *6*, 18987. [CrossRef]
53. Khanfar, M.A.; Abukhader, M.M.; Alqtaishat, S.; Taha, M.O. Pharmacophore modeling, homology modeling, and in silico screening reveal mammalian target of rapamycin inhibitory activities for sotalol, glyburide, metipranolol, sulfamethizole, glipizide, and pioglitazone. *J. Mol. Graph. Model.* **2013**, *42*, 39–49. [CrossRef]
54. Wu, F.; Hou, X.; Luo, H.; Zhou, M.; Zhang, W.; Ding, Z.; Li, R. Exploring the selectivity of PI3Kα and mTOR inhibitors by 3D-QSAR, molecular dynamics simulations and MM/GBSA binding free energy decomposition. *MedChemComm* **2013**, *4*, 1482–1496. [CrossRef]
55. Tanneeru, K.; Guruprasad, L. Ligand-based 3-D pharmacophore generation and molecular docking of mTOR kinase inhibitors. *J. Mol. Model.* **2012**, *18*, 1611–1624. [CrossRef] [PubMed]
56. Yang, H.; Rudge, D.G.; Koos, J.D.; Vaidialingam, B.; Yang, H.J.; Pavletich, N.P. MTOR kinase structure, mechanism and regulation. *Nature* **2013**, *497*, 217–223. [CrossRef] [PubMed]
57. Liu, Q.; Wang, J.; Kang, S.A.; Thoreen, C.C.; Hur, W.; Ahmed, T.; Sabatini, D.M.; Gray, N.S. Discovery of 9-(6-aminopyridin-3-yl)-1-(3-(trifluoromethyl)phenyl)benzo[h][1,6]naphthyridin-2(1 H)-one (torin2) as a potent, selective, and orally available mammalian target of rapamycin (mTOR) inhibitor for treatment of cancer. *J. Med. Chem.* **2011**, *54*, 1473–1480. [CrossRef] [PubMed]
58. Rampogu, S.; Parate, S.; Parameswaran, S.; Park, C.; Baek, A.; Son, M.; Park, Y.; Park, S.J.; Lee, K.W. Natural compounds as potential Hsp90 inhibitors for breast cancer-Pharmacophore guided molecular modelling studies. *Comput. Biol. Chem.* **2019**, *83*, 107113. [CrossRef]
59. Feldman, M.E.; Apsel, B.; Uotila, A.; Loewith, R.; Knight, Z.A.; Ruggero, D.; Shokat, K.M. Active-site inhibitors of mTOR target rapamycin-resistant outputs of mTORC1 and mTORC2. *PLoS Biol.* **2009**, *7*, e1000038. [CrossRef]
60. Lin, S.-K. Pharmacophore Perception, Development and Use in Drug Design. Edited by Osman F. Güner. *Molecules* **2000**, *5*, 987–989. [CrossRef]
61. Zeb, A.; Kim, D.; Alam, S.I.; Son, M.; Kumar, R.; Rampogu, S.; Parameswaran, S.; Shelake, R.M.; Rana, R.M.; Parate, S.; et al. Computational Simulations Identify Pyrrolidine-2,3-Dione Derivatives as Novel Inhibitors of Cdk5/p25 Complex to Attenuate Alzheimer's Pathology. *J. Clin. Med.* **2019**, *8*, 746. [CrossRef]
62. Rampogu, S.; Park, C.; Ravinder, D.; Son, M.; Baek, A.; Zeb, A.; Bavi, R.; Kumar, R.; Lee, G.; Parate, S.; et al. Pharmacotherapeutics and molecular mechanism of phytochemicals in alleviating hormone-responsive breast cancer. *Oxid. Med. Cell. Longev.* **2019**, *2019*. [CrossRef] [PubMed]
63. Rampogu, S.; Baek, A.; Park, C.; Parate, S.; Parameswaran, S.; Park, Y.; Shaik, B.; Kim, J.H.; Park, S.J.; Lee, K.W.; et al. Discovery of Small Molecules that Target Vascular Endothelial Growth Factor Receptor-2 Signalling Pathway Employing Molecular Modelling Studies. *Cells* **2019**, *8*, 269. [CrossRef] [PubMed]
64. Lipinski, C.A. Lead- and drug-like compounds: The rule-of-five revolution. *Drug Discov. Today Technol.* **2004**, *1*, 337–341. [CrossRef] [PubMed]
65. Veber, D.F.; Johnson, S.R.; Cheng, H.Y.; Smith, B.R.; Ward, K.W.; Kopple, K.D. Molecular properties that influence the oral bioavailability of drug candidates. *J. Med. Chem.* **2002**, *45*, 2615–2623. [CrossRef] [PubMed]
66. Ferreira, L.G.; Dos Santos, R.N.; Oliva, G.; Andricopulo, A.D. Molecular docking and structure-based drug design strategies. *Molecules* **2015**, *20*, 13384–13421. [CrossRef] [PubMed]
67. Jones, G.; Willett, P.; Glen, R.C.; Leach, A.R.; Taylor, R. Development and validation of a genetic algorithm for flexible docking. *J. Mol. Biol.* **1997**, *267*, 727–748. [CrossRef] [PubMed]
68. Verdonk, M.L.; Cole, J.C.; Hartshorn, M.J.; Murray, C.W.; Taylor, R.D. Improved protein-ligand docking using GOLD. *Proteins Struct. Funct. Bioinform.* **2003**, *52*, 609–623. [CrossRef]
69. Abraham, M.J.; Murtola, T.; Schulz, R.; Páll, S.; Smith, J.C.; Hess, B.; Lindah, E. Gromacs: High performance molecular simulations through multi-level parallelism from laptops to supercomputers. *SoftwareX* **2015**, *1–2*, 19–25. [CrossRef]
70. Zhu, X.; Lopes, P.E.M.; Mackerell, A.D., Jr. Recent developments and applications of the CHARMM force fields. *Wiley Interdiscip. Rev. Comput. Mol. Sci.* **2012**, *2*, 167–185. [CrossRef] [PubMed]
71. Zoete, V.; Cuendet, M.A.; Grosdidier, A.; Michielin, O. SwissParam: A fast force field generation tool for small organic molecules. *J. Comput. Chem.* **2011**, *32*, 2359–2368. [CrossRef]
72. Parrinello, M.; Rahman, A. Polymorphic transitions in single crystals: A new molecular dynamics method. *J. Appl. Phys.* **1981**, *52*, 7182–7190. [CrossRef]
73. Hess, B.; Bekker, H.; Berendsen, H.J.C.; Fraaije, J.G.E.M. LINCS: A Linear Constraint Solver for molecular simulations. *J. Comput. Chem.* **1997**, *18*, 1463–1472. [CrossRef]
74. Miyamoto, S.; Kollman, P.A. Settle: An analytical version of the SHAKE and RATTLE algorithm for rigid water models. *J. Comput. Chem.* **1992**, *13*, 952–962. [CrossRef]
75. Darden, T.; York, D.; Pedersen, L. Particle mesh Ewald: An N·log(N) method for Ewald sums in large systems. *J. Chem. Phys.* **1993**, *98*, 10089–10092. [CrossRef]
76. Humphrey, W.; Dalke, A.; Schulten, K. VMD: Visual molecular dynamics. *J. Mol. Graph.* **1996**, *14*, 33–38. [CrossRef]
77. Kumari, R.; Kumar, R.; Lynn, A.; Open Source Drug Discovery Consortium. G-mmpbsa—A GROMACS tool for high-throughput MM-PBSA calculations. *J. Chem. Inf. Model.* **2014**, *54*, 1951–1962. [CrossRef] [PubMed]

pharmaceuticals

Article

A New Computer Model for Evaluating the Selective Binding Affinity of Phenylalkylamines to T-Type Ca^{2+} Channels

You Lu [1] and Ming Li [2,*]

1 Center for Aging, School of Medicine, Tulane University, New Orleans, LA 70112, USA; ylu6@tulane.edu
2 Department of Physiology, School of Medicine, Tulane University, New Orleans, LA 70112, USA
* Correspondence: mli@tulane.edu; Tel.: +1-504-988-8207

Abstract: To establish a computer model for evaluating the binding affinity of phenylalkylamines (PAAs) to T-type Ca^{2+} channels (TCCs), we created new homology models for both TCCs and a L-type calcium channel (LCC). We found that PAAs have a high affinity for domains I and IV of TCCs and a low affinity for domains III and IV of the LCC. Therefore, they should be considered as favorable candidates for TCC blockers. The new homology models were validated with some commonly recognized TCC blockers that are well characterized. Additionally, examples of the TCC blockers created were also evaluated using these models.

Keywords: T-type calcium channel blocker; homology modeling; computer-aid drug design; virtual drug screening; L-type calcium channel

Citation: Lu, Y.; Li, M. A New Computer Model for Evaluating the Selective Binding Affinity of Phenylalkylamines to T-Type Ca^{2+} Channels. *Pharmaceuticals* **2021**, *14*, 141. https://doi.org/10.3390/ph14020141

Academic Editor: Osvaldo Andrade Santos-Filho
Received: 27 January 2021
Accepted: 8 February 2021
Published: 10 February 2021

1. Introduction

As the only type of voltage-gated Ca^{2+} channels that are activated at or near resting membrane potentials, T-type Ca^{2+} channels (TCCs) play an important role in regulating $[Ca^{2+}]_i$ homeostasis in a variety of tissues, including pancreatic β-cells and tumor cells [1–4]. Therefore, TCC antagonists could be potentially useful for the treatment of chronic diseases associated with Ca^{2+} dysregulation [5–7]. For this reason, it is imperative to develop more selective TCC antagonists for prospective clinical applications. Since many existing TCC blockers, such as mibefradil, also show inhibitory effects on L-type calcium channels (LCCs), the most important task in developing new TCC blockers is to enhance their selectivity to TCCs over LCCs. To achieve this, we established TCC–phenylalkylamine interaction models based on the specific amino acid sequences in the P-loop of TCCs, and α_1C LCCs for characterizing the drug molecules' affinities for TCCs and LCCs, respectively.

TCCs have a close evolutional relationship with LCCs. A recent report from a cryo-electron microscopy study reveals that the frame of the α_1G (Ca_v3.1) pore domain structure is similar to that of α_1S (Ca_v1.1) [8]. This similarity allowed us to confidently adopt the global structure of the calcium channel Ca_vAb model, constructed based upon Arcobacter butzleri crystallization [9], in the establishment of our TCC model. One of the most remarkable differences between all types of TCCs and LCCs is a lysine residue located adjacent to the critical glutamic acid/aspartic acid residue in domain III. The existence of a positively charged lysine (K^{3p49}) may swing the aspartic acid (D^{3p50}) away from the center of the calcium filter and change the preferred calcium ion and drug binding sites from domains III and IV for LCCs to domains I and IV for TCCs. Therefore, we used the ZMM molecule modeling program [10–12] to create four-domain TCC models, in which the binding affinities of drugs to TCCs and α_1C LCC were determined by scoring their free energy in binding to the channels [13].

The new TCC models are adopted from a drug–protein interaction framework for modeling Ca_vAb blocking by phenylalkylamines (PAAs) [9]. This is rational because many TCC blockers are PAAs or their derivatives, and because PAAs block Ca_vAb [9,14].

It is proposed that PAAs bind to LCCs in an inverse V-shaped configuration, with the ammonium group towards the P-helices, and the nitrile group bound to the calcium ion coordinated by the selectivity filter glutamates in domains III and IV of the LCC [15]. We reason that this is also true for TCC blockers, except that the calcium ion is coordinated in the cavity between domains I and IV, since the depolarization confirmed that the pore domains of $Ca_V3.1$ and $Ca_V1.1$ are superimposed [8]. As a result, the two rings of the flexible PAA molecule [15] will make hydrogen bonding contacts with the mobile side chains of relevant amino acids from domains I and IV of TCCs. This strategy allowed us to create computer models for simulating the interactions between drugs and channel receptors for LCC and TCCs, respectively.

2. Results

2.1. Homology Modeling of TCCs and α_1C LCC

Using the bacterial calcium Ca_VAb open channel 3D structure as the input, ZMM generated the first template of the calcium channel, which was then modified with S5-P-loop-S6 segments of α_1C, and α_1G, α_1H, and α_1I (Table 1) to create corresponding protein structures of $Ca_v1.2$ LCC and $Ca_v3.1$, $Ca_v3.2$, and $Ca_v3.3$ TCCs, respectively (Figure 1A–D). For cross-validation of ZMM-generated 3D structure models, we also performed ab initio modeling of α_1C and α_1G calcium channels. Since there is a considerable overlap of PAA inhibition between LCC and TCCs [9], the allosteric structures of LCC and TCCs are more likely to be similar. Comparing two different homology modeling tools, ZMM generates more consistent 3D models of the domain III S5-P-loop-S6 segment of α_1C and α_1G (Figure 1E,F) than the ab initio method (Figure 1G,H).

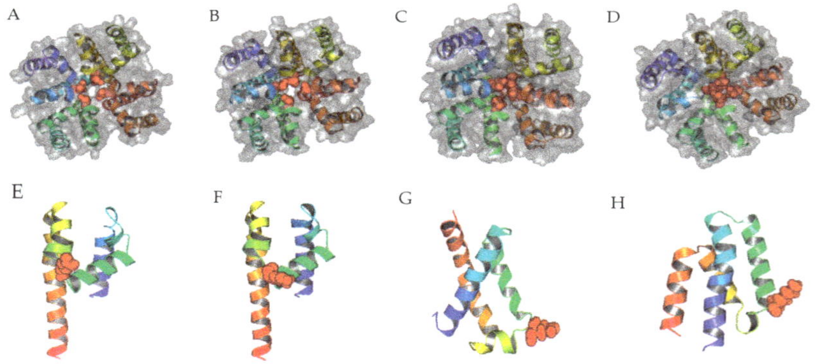

Figure 1. Top views of homology modeling results from ZMM for α_1C, α_1G, α_1H, and α_1I. (**A–D**) The structures of α_1C, α_1G, α_1H, and α_1I, respectively; blue, green, brown, and yellow represent domains I, II, III, and IV, respectively; the four selectivity-determining amino acids (glutamic acid or aspartic acid) in the P-loop are colored red and displayed as spheres; ZMM generates more consistent 3D structure than the ab initio modeling method for α_1C and α_1G; (**E**) the predicted 3D structure of the α_1C domain III generated by ZMM, the glutamic acid is represented by red spheres; (**F**) the predicted 3D structure of the α_1G domain III generated by ZMM, the lysine is represented by red spheres; (**G**) the most representative structure selected by Calibur clustering analysis [16] of α_1C domain III, the glutamic acid is represented by red spheres; (**H**) the most representative structure selected by Calibur clustering analysis of α_1G domain III, the lysine is represented by red spheres.

2.2. Further P-Loop Remodeling of TCCs

After determining the globe structure of TCC 3D models, we focused on the variability of the P-loop structure, which is the major drug–ligand interaction segment. The Rosetta P-loop remodeling module [17] was utilized to estimate the variability of P-loop 3D structures on every domain of TCCs. After inputting a perturbation to the original structure, the remodeling process was conducted by sampling the possible locations of a given length of an amino acid sequence in three-dimensional space. Using the ZMM generated α_1G structure as the reference, the energy-based clustering method [18] was used to determine the P-loop remodeling results with the lowest root-mean-square-displacement (RMSD) score. We found that for α_1G, domain II had a clear variation between two different homology modeling methods in sample sizes 500 and 20,000 (Figure 2). It showed that the central P-loop helix segment is in the horizontal position rather than the diagonal position found in other domains. As a result, the selectivity-determining glutamic acids E^{2p50} may have a larger vertical distance from other glutamic acids/aspartic acids (E^{1p50}, D^{3p50}, and D^{4p50}) in α_1G TCCs. This may exclude glutamic acid E^{2p50} as a Ca^{2+} binding candidate, leaving the Ca^{2+} to bind either E^{1p50} to D^{4p50} or D^{3p50} to D^{4p50} in TCCs. Additionally, to validate the normality of the remodeling data, we conducted a nonparametric test for the α_1G P-loop remodeling data and confirmed that all the sampling processes (500 and 20,000) came from the same distribution (see Supplementary Table S2, Supplementary Figure S2 for statistical results).

Table 1. Comparison of numerical results of P-loop electrostatic potential at the four different domains with different lengths of amino acid sequences. TCC: T-type calcium channel.

Channel Domain	Channel Type	AA Sequence Alignment	PyGBe [19] (*Esol, Ecoul*)
Domain I	α_1G	I T L E G W V D	−11, −407
	α_1H	I T L E G W V D	−110, −408
	α_1I	I T L E G W V E	−116, −409
	Reduced TCC	T L E G W V	−87, −323
Domain II	α_1G	L T Q E D W N K	−217, −631
	α_1H	L T Q E D W N V	−262, −631
	α_1I	L T Q E D W N V	−487, −633
	Reduced TCC	T Q E D W	−164, −425
Domain III	α_1G	A S K D G W V D	−107, −392
	α_1H	S S K D G W V N	−113, −425
	α_1I	A S K D G W V N	−105, −394
	Reduced TCC	S K D G W	−101, −303
Domain IV	α_1G	S T G D N W N G	−132, −568
	α_1H	S T G D N W N G	−164, −574
	α_1I	S T G D N W N G	−177, −574
	Reduced TCC	T G D N W	−86, −393

2.3. *Local Electrostatic Potentials of the Selective P-Loop of TCC Domains and the Impact of K^{3p49}*

A previous study indicated that when a calcium ion enters the selectivity filter region of a LCC, it binds to the selectivity-determining glutamic acids (E^{3p50}, E^{4p50}) in domains III and IV [15]. Consequently, the phenylalkylamine molecules will bind to domains III and IV due to the interaction between the nitrile nitrogen and Ca^{2+} [15]. In contrast, all TCCs have a lysine (K^{3p49}) located at the 5′ end adjacent to D^{3p50} in domain III. It is reported that the replacement of lysine (K^{3p49}) with Phe or Gly causes the activation curve to shift to the right [8], which indicates that the lysine in the position adjacent to aspartic acid (D^{3p50}) plays a significant role in the kinetic/dynamic mechanism of Ca^{2+} interaction with the inner environment of the central cavity of TCCs. This positively charged lysine alters the negative charge field distribution of D^{3p50} to attract Ca^{2+} (Supplementary Figure S1). It is possible that the lysine (K^{3p49}) swings aspartic acid (D^{3p50}) away from the original Ca^{2+} binding position, thus causing the Ca^{2+} to bind glutamic acid or aspartic acid in other domains, probably to domains I and IV since domain II has a configuration deviation. As a result, the phenylalkylamine may also switch its binding region from domains III and IV to domains I and IV.

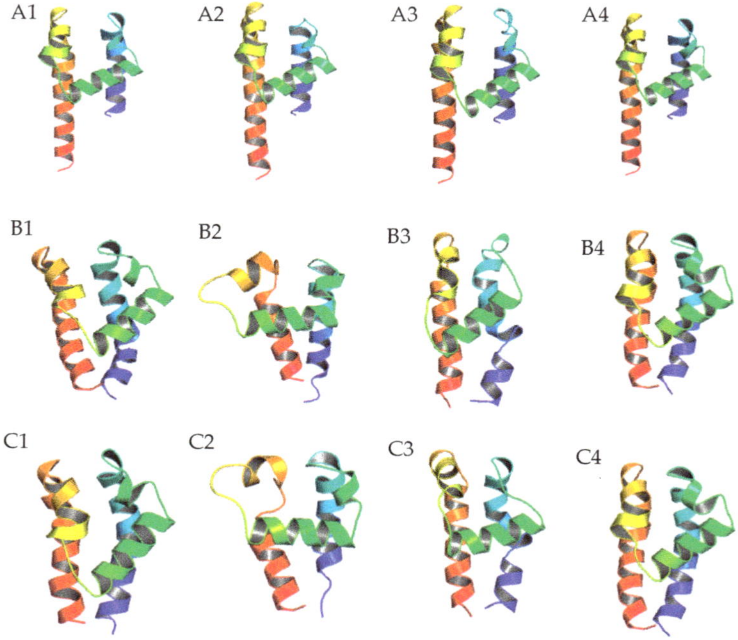

Figure 2. Comparison of the P-loop conformation differences before and after Rosetta P-loop remodeling. (**A**) Homology modeling of P-loop structures of α_1G domain I (**A1**), domain II (**A2**), domain III (**A3**), and domain IV (**A4**) generated by ZMM; (**B**) Rosetta P-loop remodeling results of α_1G domain I (**B1**), domain II (**B2**), domain III (**B3**), and domain IV (**B4**) with the sampling size equal to 500; (**C**) Rosetta P-loop remodeling results of α_1G domain I (**C1**), domain II (**C2**), domain III (**C3**), and domain IV (**C4**) with the sampling size equal to 20,000.

To determine the effect of lysine (K^{3p49}) on overall electrostatic potential (E) for given TCC homology models, we calculated the electrostatic potential (E) for the tailed P-loop of domain I to IV. Table 1 shows that the combined electrostatic potential (E_{coul}) becomes more negative in each domain as the number of testing amino acids is reduced from seven to five. In TCCs, E_{coul} for domain I is more negative than that for domain IV in the five amino acid-reduced sequence, indicating a possible switching of the Ca^{2+} binding site from domains III and IV to domains I and IV.

We used Coulomb's electric force equation to quantitively analyze the influence of lysine on the electrical attraction force between Ca^{2+} and aspartic acid (D^{3p50}). According to the equation in Section 4.2, lysine (K^{3p49}) has the least effect on the Ca^{2+}-D^{3p50} attraction when K^{3p49} is located on the opposite side of the Ca^{2+} and when D^{3p50} is at the center. When a = 4.3 Å and b = 3.8 Å [8] (calculated in PyMOL.2.3.3 for ZMM results), Coulomb's force equation (found in Section 4) yields: $F_{(Ca,\ D,\ attraction)} = 2.489 \times 10^{-9}$ N and $F_{(Ca,\ K,\ repellent)} = 0.702 \times 10^{-9}$ N; thus, lysine, at a minimum, reduces the attraction force between Ca^{2+} and aspartic acid by more than 28%. The attraction force between Ca^{2+} and D^{3p50} will reduce further or reverse into a repellent force as the distance from the Ca^{2+} to K^{3p49} decreases; therefore, the preferred binding position of Ca^{2+} will likely be switched to domains I and IV in TCCs. This limits the PAA binding region on TCCs to domains I and IV. We could use the amino acid structure of domains I and IV to evaluate the affinities of the PAAs (and their derivatives) for TCCs (using models established for α_1G, α_1H, and α_1I) and use the amino acid structure of domains III and IV for evaluating their binding affinities to LCC (using the model of α_1C).

2.4. Model Predictions and Vina Screening Output of Some Current T-Type Ca^{2+} Channel Blockers

Mibefradil is reported to have an inhibitory effect on both LCC and TCCs [20]. The α_1C model predicts that one hydrogen atom from the nitrogen (N_3) on the cyclopentadiene connects to methionine (M^{4i27}) on domain IV of α_1C LCC, as shown in Figure 3A,B. This is consistent with the prediction of another model in a previous study [9]. In contrast, the α_1C homology model does not predict that hydrogen bonds to NNC 55-0396. NNC 55-0395 inhibits both L- and T-type calcium channels [14]. The α_1C homology model predicts that NNC 55-0395 has one hydrogen bond that connects nitrogen (N_3) to the glycine (G^{3p49}) on P-loop domain IV. For NNC 55-0397, the α_1C homology model also predicts that RO 40-5966, a hydrolyzed metabolite of mibefradil [20], has one hydrogen atom from the hydroxy group of the benzene ring bound to the glycine (G^{4p49}) at domain IV. No hydrogen bond has been found between the LCC and the TCC blocker SKF-96365.

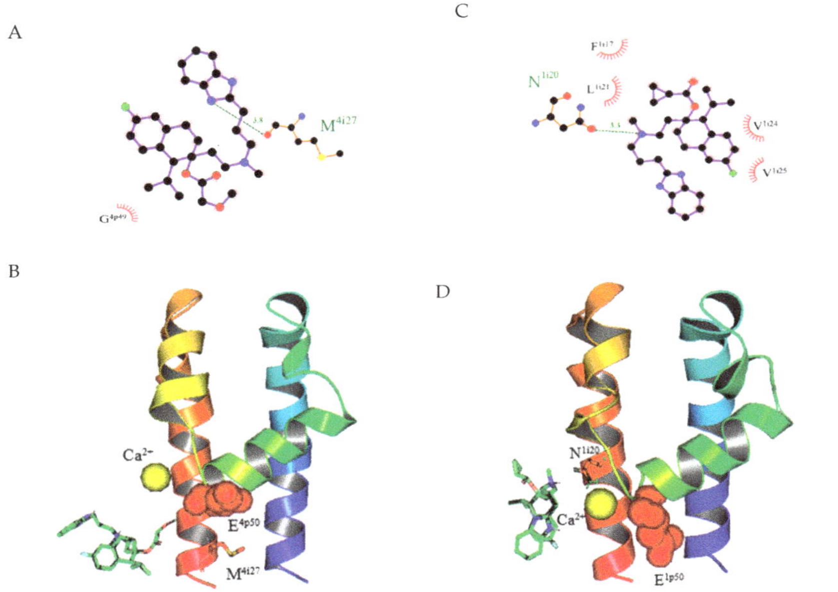

Figure 3. Models of ligand–receptor interactions of mibefradil and NNC 55-0396. (**A**) The predicted binding sites of mibefradil on α_1C. The H-bond formed between the ammonia (N_3) on the cyclopentadiene of mibefradil and methionine (M^{4i27}) on domain IV. The relative locations of surrounding amino acid residues of the α_1C L-type calcium channel (LCC) are shown by the arch–dash symbols. (**B**) The predicted 3D binding sites of mibefradil on α_1C domain IV from a side view. Red spheres represent the position of glutamic acid E^{4p50}. Mibefradil is represented by the green ring structure. (**C**) The predicted binding sites of NNC 55-0396 on α_1G domain IV. The H-bond formed between the central ammonium of NNC 55-0396 and asparagine (N^{1i20}) on domain I. (**D**) The predicted 3D binding sites of NNC 55-0396 on α_1G. NNC 55-0396 is represented by the green ring structure. Red spheres represent the position of glutamic acid E^{4p50}. For A and C, carbon, nitrogen, oxygen, and fluorine elements are represented by black, blue, red, and green, respectively; for B and D, the blue and orange ribbon helices represent S5 and S6, respectively. The ribbon helix structures linking S5 and S6 are P-loops. The yellow ball represents the position of the calcium ion.

Using TCCs as templates, we have revealed some current TCC blockers of α_1G, α_1H, and α_1I. The α_1G model predicts that the fluorine atom from the compound NNC 55-0395 forms a halogen bond to glycine (G^{1p51}) in domain I. Our α_1G model also predicts a binding site of NNC 55-0396 to asparagine (N^{1i20}) in domain I (Figure 3C,D). For NNC 55-0397, the fluorine atom from the compound forms a halogen bond with valine (V^{1p46}) at the P-loop of domain I. For mibefradil, one oxygen atom from the side chain of the compound forms hydrogen bonds with asparagine (N^{1o4}) at S5 of domain I. For RO 40-5966, one hydrogen atom from the nitrogen (N_3) on the cyclopentadiene forms a hydrogen bond with alanine (A^{1i27}) in domain I. For SKF-96365, the center oxygen atom forms a hydrogen bond with asparagine (N^{1o4}) at S5 of domain I.

Our α_1H model predicts that one hydrogen atom from the nitrogen (N_3) on the cyclopentadiene of NNC 55-0395 interacts with valine (V^{1p46}) at the P-loop of domain I to form a bond. The fluorine atom from NNC 55-0396 forms a halogen bond with isoleucine (I^{1i8}) from the α_1H S6 of domain I. For NNC 55-0397, one hydrogen atom from the nitrogen (N_3) on the cyclopentadiene forms a bond to asparagine (N^{4p51}) at the P-loop of domain IV. The hydrogen atom from the nitrogen (N_3) on the cyclopentadiene of mibefradil finds asparagine (N^{1o4}) to form a bond at S5 of domain I. For RO 40-5966, the fluorine atom from the compound forms a halogen bond with histidine (H^{4i29}) at S6 of domain IV. One oxygen atom from the side chain of SKF-96365 forms a hydrogen bond with asparagine (N^{1o4}) at S5 of domain I.

Our α_1I homology model predicts that NNC 55-0395 forms a halogen bond between the fluorine atom from the compound and isoleucine (I^{1i8}) at S6 of domain I. The hydrogen atom from NNC 55-0396 forms a bond to asparagine (N^{1o4}) at S5 of domain I. For NNC 55-0397, one hydrogen atom from the nitrogen (N_3) on the cyclopentadiene interacts with valine (V^{1p46}) at the P-loop of domain I to form a bond. For mibefradil, there is a halogen bond formed between a fluorine atom from the compound and a hydrogen atom from asparagine (N^{4p53}) at the P-loop of domain IV. For RO 40-5966, one hydrogen atom from the ammonia on the cyclopentadiene interacts with asparagine (N^{1o4}) at S5 of domain I to form a bond. Our model does not predict the hydrogen bond formed when docking SKF-96365 to α_1I.

A comparison of the predicted binding affinity K_d and experimental measurements of IC_{50} for given TCC blockers are listed in Supplementary Table S4. Table 2 summarizes the predicted binding affinity results for all existing TCC blockers.

2.5. Evaluation of New Compounds

The Vina [13] models were employed for evaluating the binding affinity of the testing compounds. We randomly selected 300,000 compounds from PubChem and used these as the database to train our recurrent neural networks (RNNs) [21] with the given compound properties.

After performing virtual screening, we found that the compounds TC 7, TC 4, and TC 2 satisfied our screening criteria for α_1G, α_1H, and α_1I, respectively. Compound TC 7 has the highest binding affinity, as well as a lower (water–octanol partition coefficient) logP and a higher Quantitative Estimation of Drug-likeness (QED) than existing TCC blockers. The 3D binding plots between TC 7 and α_1G are shown in Supplementary Figure S3. The predicted binding affinities between existing TCC blockers and screened compounds on TCCs and α_1C LCC are shown in Figure 4. Our results show that these screened compounds have smaller logP and Synthetic Accessibility Scores (SAS) but larger QED values than those of selected TCC blockers (as seen in Table 3). More structures and chemical properties for the 13 identified compounds can be found in Supplementary Figures S5–S17.

Table 2. Predicted Gibbs free energy ΔG of phenylalkylamines (PAAs) on calcium channels (N/A: not available).

Receptor	Drug ID	ΔG (kcal/mol)	Binding Domain
α_1C	NNC 55-0395	−6.0	IV
	NNC 55-0396	N/A	N/A
	NNC 55-0397	−6.4	IV
	Mibefradil	−6.4	IV
	RO 40-5966	−5.7	IV
	SKF-96365	N/A	IV
α_1G	NNC 55-0395	−6.5	I
	NNC 55-0396	−8.1	I
	NNC 55-0397	−7.4	I
	Mibefradil	−6.8	I
	RO 40-5966	−7.3	I
	SKF-96365	−5.6	I
α_1H	NNC 55-0395	−6.6	I
	NNC 55-0396	−7.7	I
	NNC 55-0397	−7.0	IV
	Mibefradil	−7.4	I
	RO 40-5966	−7.4	IV
	SKF-96365	−5.4	I
α_1I	NNC 55-0395	−6.6	I
	NNC 55-0396	−7.7	I
	NNC 55-0397	−7.5	I
	Mibefradil	−6.5	IV
	RO 40-5966	−6.9	I
	SKF-96365	N/A	N/A

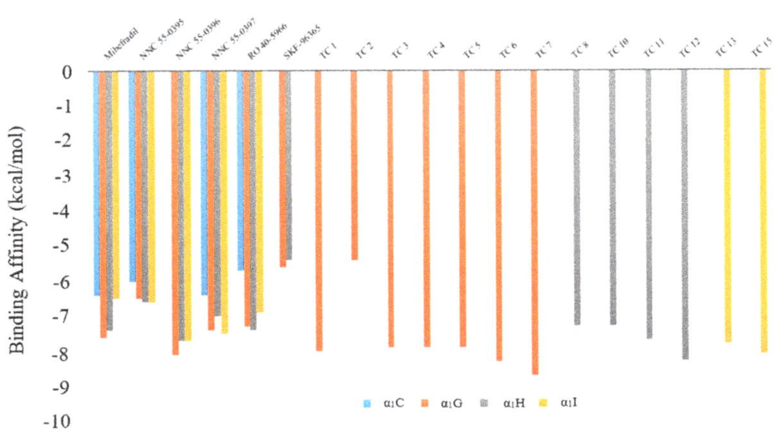

Figure 4. Predicted Gibbs free energy of select T-type Ca^{2+} channel (TCC) blockers and computer-designed compounds of different receptors. Blue—α_1C, brown—α_1G, gray—α_1H, and yellow—α_1I.

Table 3. The chemical properties of computer-designed compounds and selected TCC blockers. SAS: Synthetic Accessibility Scores, QED: Quantitative Estimation of Drug-likeness.

Compound Name	logP	SAS	QED
NNC 55-0365	6.8147	3.678636	0.273518
NNC 55-0396	6.0345	3.716436	0.351695
NNC 55-0397	6.2805	3.718535	0.337773
Mibefradil	5.2709	3.71918	0.367183
TC 1	6.1671	4.433975	0.402836
TC 2	5.3351	5.24865	0.408449
TC 3	4.8963	4.777741	0.474028
TC 4	5.0404	4.731275	0.441386
TC 5	5.5879	4.951457	0.415026
TC 6	4.4585	4.79633	0.469604
TC 7	3.6902	4.806084	0.63381
TC 8	6.2697	4.851381	0.242332
TC 10	4.1891	4.542497	0.312353
TC 11	5.372	3.089346	0.276759
TC 12	4.9472	3.971406	0.248549
TC 13	5.7028	4.449589	0.406663
TC 15	4.73	3.921747	0.368816

3. Discussion

A TCC ($Ca_v3.1$) 3D structure has already been modeled with cryo-electron microscopy [8], however, this structure is constructed based on a splice variant containing a deletion of 133 amino acids within the I-II linker. Electrophysiological characterization of these variants ($Ca_v3.1$-Δ8b) shows 1.5-2-fold conductance increases when compared with the full-length form in human and rat preparations. Both activation and steady-state inactivation curves are shifted in the human preparation [8]. In addition, the pore diameter estimated from $Ca_v3.1$-Δ8b is smaller than the biophysical measurement [8]. These alterations in TCC electrophysiological properties suggest that the conformation of the cryo-electron microscopy structure is not the same as the full-length $Ca_v3.1$ TCC. Therefore, the 3D structure of $Ca_v3.1$-Δ8b may not be the most suitable template for the general modeling of TCCs, especially for PAA binding, which is highly dependent on the position of Ca^{2+} interacting with the selectivity filter of TCCs. In this study, we chose to use Ca_vAb as the model template since this channel is blocked by PAA and therefore is suitable for establishing a model for evaluating PAAs that inhibit TCCs selectively over LCCs.

Increasing evidence indicates the pathological role of TCCs in the progression of different diseases [6]. It is crucial to develop selective TCC blockers to establish new treatments for these diseases. Unfortunately, lacking the TCC X-ray crystallization structure hampers the progress of creating new TCC blockers. In practice, it is very difficult to find or design a compound that selectively blocks TCCs but not LCCs, since most current TCC blockers exhibit a certain level of inhibitory effects on LCCs. For example, mibefradil, the first launched TCC inhibitor, was quickly recognized to cross inhibit LCC [20]. Here, we provide a new strategy by which the specificity of candidate compounds for binding TCCs but not LCCs can be pre-screened with new computer-based models. This is desirable for designing and developing compounds that more selectively block TCCs than LCCs.

We chose to build models for the interaction between TCCs and PAAs since the binding mechanism of these compounds to LCCs has been studied extensively [9,15,22–26]. Based upon the critical single amino acid lysine (K^{3p49}) difference between LCCs and TCCs, we have created a strategy that can distinguish the affinity of PAAs to TCCs and LCCs, respectively. The models have been validated by measuring the affinities of existing TCC blockers to LCCs and TCCs. We also used these models for evaluating the specificities of novel PAAs and phenylalkylamine derivatives in terms of their binding affinities to TCCs and LCCs.

Using ZMM, we simultaneously created α_1G, α_1H, and α_1I TCC and a_1C LCC structures with four domains, each containing three segments: segment 5, a P-loop, and segment 6. In contrast, the ab initio modeling method failed to produce a suitable calcium channel structure compared to ZMM.

The selectivity of the calcium channel is dependent on the critical glutamate residues located in the selectivity filter of the P-loop of the α_1 subunit in each domain. In this region, there are two negatively charged glutamic acid residues likely to attract one Ca^{2+} in the space close to domains III and IV [15]. When a phenylalkylamine molecule approaches a calcium channel from the cytoplasmic side, its nucleophilic nitrile nitrogen reaches the Ca^{2+}, while the other parts of the molecule form affiliated interactions with the amino acids in the P-loop and segments 5 and 6 in domains III and IV of the calcium channel. This causes a physical blockage of ion flow through the channel. In the case of TCCs, there is a lysine (K^{3p49}) located adjacent to D^{3p50} in domain III, and the ionized electric potential distribution of the aspartic acid is altered by lysine, which attenuates the electric attraction of aspartic acid (K^{3p49}) to Ca^{2+} at the minimum binding distance (4.3 angstroms) and may swing K^{3p49} away from the selectivity filter. Based on this analysis, we suggest that Ca^{2+} will not bind to domain III but to domain I of TCCs. This prediction is consistent with the Ca_v3.1 structure estimated with cryo-electron microscopy [8], which showed the electron density of the top Ca^{2+} ion is closest to Glu354 of Ca_v3.1 (E^{1p50}, Table 4). Additionally, Rosetta P-loop remodeling shows that the P-loop of domain II is in a more horizontal confirmation than that of other domains, rendering the glutamic acid (E^{2p50}) further away from the Ca^{2+} binding site. Since the movements of PAAs will follow the location of Ca^{2+} docking, our models are built for evaluating the affinity of candidate compounds binding to domains I and IV. The compounds that are predicted to have a higher affinity to bind domains I and IV of TCCs but not domains III–IV of LCC (α_1C) are considered to be ideal selective TCC blocker candidates. This strategy screens out the compounds that are unlikely to bind LCC and TCCs as well as the compounds that are likely to bind both LCC and TCCs. To test whether Ca^{2+} docking is consistent on domains I and II across different TCCs, a molecular dynamics study should be conducted with modified membrane conditions and simulation environments [27].

Table 4. Amino acid sequences of α_1G used for searching the homology modeling template.

Channel	Domain/Segment	Residue Label Prefix [a]	Selected Key Amino Acid Sequence [b]
			1 11 21
α_1C	1S5	1o	PLLHIALLVL FVIIIYAIIG LELFMGK
α_1G	1S5	1o	MLGNVLLLCF FVFFIFGIVG VQLWAGL
α_1C	2S5	2o	SIASLLLLLF LFIIIFSLLG MQLFGGK
α_1G	2S5	2o	NVATFCMLLM LFIFIFSILG MHLFGCK
α_1C	3S5	3o	TIGNIVIVTT LLQFMFACIG VALFKGK
α_1G	3S5	3o	PIGNIVVICC AFFIIFGILG VQLFKGK
α_1C	4S5	4o	ALPYVALLIV MLFFIYAVII GMQVFGK
α_1G	4S5	4o	QVGNLGLLFM LLFFIFAALG VELFGDL
			33 43 53
α_1C	1p	1p	FDNFAFAMLT VFQCITMEGW TDVLY
α_1G	1p	1p	FDNIGYAWIA IFQVITLEGW VDIMY
α_1C	2p	2p	FDNFPQSLLT VFQILTGEDW NSVMY
α_1G	2p	2p	FDSLLWAIVT VFQILTQEDW NKVLY
α_1C	3p	3p	FDNVLAAMMA LFTVSTFEGW PELLY
α_1G	3p	3p	FDNLGQALMS LFVLASKDGW VDIMY
α_1C	4p	4p	FQTFPQAVLL LFRCATGEAW QDIML
α_1G	4p	4p	FRNFGMAFLT LFRVSTGDNW NGIMK
			1 11 21
α_1C	1S6	1i	ELPWVYFVSL VIFGSFFVLN LVLGVLSGEF
α_1G	1S6	1i	FYNFIYFILL IIVGSFFMIN LCLVVIATQF
α_1C	2S6	2i	MLVCIYFIIL FICGNYILLN VFLAIAYDNL
α_1G	2S6	2i	SWAALYFIAL MTFGNYVLFN LLVAILVEGF
α_1C	3S6	3i	VEISIFFIIY IIIIAFFMMN IFVGFVIVTF
α_1G	3S6	3i	PWMLLYFISF LLIVAFFVLN MFVGVVVENF
α_1C	4S6	4i	SFAVFYFISF YMLCAFLIIN LFVAVIMDNF
α_1G	4S6	4i	VISPIYFVSF VLTAQFVLVN VVIAVLMKHL

Notes: The difference in amino acid sequences among α_1G, α_1H, and α_1I are underlined. H: L^{3o7}, $Y4^{o16}$, $R4^{o29}$, V^{2p54}, S^{3p47}, N^{3p54}, V^{2i8}, S^{3i15}, A^{4i1}, L^{4i2}, V^{4i5}, T^{4i9}, V^{4i13}, V^{4i23}. I: I^{1o19}, V^{1p42}, E^{1p54}, V^{2p54}, P^{2i1}, S^{2i4}, V^{2i8}, L^{3o7}, N^{3p54}, S^{3i15}, Y^{4o16}, K^{4o29}, Q^{4p45}, F^{4i1}, V^{4i2}, I^{4i19}, V^{4i23}. [a,b] Residue sequences are labeled according to the alignment of the outer helix, the P-loop, and the inner helix of the KcsA structure [15].

Previous studies suggest that the nitrile and isopropyl groups in devapamil and some other PAAs serve to guide the drug to the position of Ca^{2+}; this function persists if the nitrile is replaced with other elements with high electronegative potentials, such as oxygen or sulfur [15]. In many molecules discussed here, including mibefradil, the nitrile is replaced with a methoxy acetyl side chain or a similar side chain with a high electronegative potential. These molecules behave presumably like those of molecules with nitrile in their alkaline chain. Some of the molecules, such as RO 40-5966 and SKF-96365, do not share the binding mechanism described by our model, and therefore their inhibitory effects on Ca^{2+} channels may not be explained by our new models. For example, by using the input template SKF-96365, we obtained 14 unique structures (as seen in Supplementary Table S3, Figure S4), which had negative binding affinities to our TCC models.

Although our models are designed to select compounds that are likely to bind domains I and IV of TCCs, this does not exclude the possibility that PAAs or their derivatives might inhibit TCCs via binding to domains I and II, domains II and III, or even domains III and IV. The goal of our models was to increase the likelihood of success in screening selective TCC blockers based on their chemical structures.

Our α_1C model has a similar channel pore size (selectivity filter region) as Ca_VAb [9]; however, α_1G, α_1H, and α_1I may have smaller diameters than Ca_VAb, since the unitary conductance of TCC currents is smaller than that of LCC. Further statistical analyses of P-loop remodeling data show that a minimal structural difference exists in the P-loop region remodeling data (see Supplementary Materials for details of the statistical analysis).

The Vina screening results of α_1C identify no binding location for NNC 55-0396 or SKF-96365. The predicted α_1C binding amino acid for NNC 55-0397, as well as mibefradil, matches the experimental results, which show the inhibitory effect of NNC 55-0397 and mibefradil on LCCs. Although RO 40-5966 has a lower ΔG than mibefradil when binding to α_1C, the predicted binding location is closer to the center of the channel filter region than mibefradil, which indicates a stronger blocking effect on the rate of Ca^{2+} influx than mibefradil.

Although the K_d values predicted by Vina have some gaps compared to the experiment data, they do follow the same order of magnitude (Supplementary Table S4). To obtain a more accurate Gibbs free energy for PAAs binding to TCCs, at least two consecutive steps must be conducted: first, the flexible docking process [28]; second, the free energy calculation between ligand and receptor [29]. These two steps require an extensive computational cost and the final K_d value is very sensitive to the initial input of the receptor structures. Recently deposited human α_1G structures offer a good template for developing TCC blockers [8]; however, they have some uncommon regions missing, which could affect PAA binding. Therefore, we argue that it is less likely that the Gibbs free energy of mibefradil/NNC 55-00396 between the prediction and the experiment is matched by choosing different docking programs or conducting a molecular dynamics simulation to find the free energy.

Our work only focuses on the first step of the drug development process in silico, providing a strategy for predicting the comparative potency of candidate compounds to TCCs versus LCCs. Neither are used for evaluating the pharmacological effects of these compounds on other types of cation channels. Since the strength of the pharmacological effects of PAAs and their derivatives on blocking calcium channels are increased by the appearance of a calcium cation in the channel pore [15], it is unlikely that these PAAs and their derivatives will exhibit a strong inhibitory effect on other cation channels.

4. Materials and Methods

4.1. Homology Modeling of the α_1 Subunit

Three classes of calcium channel families have been discovered: Ca_V1.X, Ca_V2.X, and Ca_V3.X. The X represents the subdivisions of the sequence homology of the α_1 subunit in each class. The models of drug–channel interactions built upon the structural differences in the relevant S5, P-loop, and S6 regions of α_1G, α_1H, α_1I TCCs, and α_1C LCC, respectively.

The protein templates were obtained from BAM [30] using truncated inputs of human α_1G α_1H, α_1I, and α_1C (UniProt id: O43497) amino acid sequences (see Table 4 for details The crystallization structure (PDB id: 5kmh) for the depolarization status of the calcium channel protein, originally extracted from Arcobacter butzleri [9], was employed as the structure template of our model. The multi-domain protein structures of human α_1G, α_1H α_1I, and α_1C were built using the ZMM molecular modeling software. The forcefield of specific amino acids was simulated by using the Assisted Model Building with Energy Refinement (AMBER) program. The final structure of the target peptides was optimized by using the Monte Carlo minimization protocol. The maximum iteration time for finding the global minimum was set to 5000. During the energy optimization, structural similarity between target and template was maintained by a flat-bottom parabolic energy penalty function that allows for penalty-free deviations of alpha-carbons up to 1 atom distance from their respective positions in the template, and a penalty was imposed with a force constant of 10 kcal mol-1A-2 for larger deviations [15]. The homology models for human α_1H (UniProt id: O95180), α_1I (UniProt id: Q9P0X4), and α_1C (UniProt id: Q13936) were also built with this method.

4.2. Local Electrostatic Potential Calculation

To calculate the electric double layer-related local electrostatic potential while a channel protein interacted with a surrounding water molecule, we generated the corresponding meshes using MSMS (v2.6.1) [31] and set the probe radius to 1.4 and the density to 3.0 for quality control. For truncated amino acid sequences, the local electrostatic potential/binding energy is derived from the summation of the solvation energy and Coulomb energy, i.e., $G_{complex} = G_{solution} + G_{Coulomb}$. The $G_{Coulomb}$ for LCC and TCCs in the P-loop region was calculated by using PyGBe with pre-defined parameters (Supplementary Table S1). To compare the influence provided by a single lysine, we used Coulomb's law to calculate the electric attracting force between Ca^{2+} and aspartic acid:

$$F_{(Ca,D)} = k_e \frac{q_{Ca} q_D}{a^2},$$

where k_e is Coulomb's constant 8.99×109 $N \cdot m^2 \cdot C^{-2}$; a is the distance between Ca^{2+} and aspartic acid; q is the point charge for Ca^{2+}, aspartic acid (D), and lysine (K), respectively The effect of the repellent force on Ca^{2+} by lysine in the direction of the Ca^{2+} and the aspartic acid attracting force is defined by

$$F_{(Ca,K)} = k_e \frac{q_{Ca} q_K}{r^2} \cdot \cos\theta,$$

where θ is the angle between the lines from Ca^{2+} to aspartic acid and from Ca^{2+} to lysine; r is the distance between Ca^{2+} and lysine, which is calculated by

$$r = a \cdot \cos\theta \pm \sqrt{b^2 - (a \cdot \sin\theta)^2},$$

where b is the distance from aspartic acid to lysine. When the angle between Ca^{2+} and aspartic acid, and lysine and aspartic acid (ϕ) is less than 90°, $r = a \cdot \cos\theta + \sqrt{b^2 - (a \cdot \sin\theta)^2}$; when ϕ is equal to 90°, $r = a \cdot \cos\theta$; when ϕ is larger than 90°, $r = a \cdot \cos\theta - \sqrt{b^2 - (a \cdot \sin\theta)^2}$ Therefore, the electric force between Ca^{2+} and aspartic acid is

$$F_{(Ca,\,D,\,K)} = F_{(Ca,D)} - F_{(Ca,K)} = k_e \frac{q_{Ca} q_D}{a^2} - k_e \frac{q_{Ca} q_K}{r^2} \cdot \cos\theta.$$

4.3. Ab Initio Modeling

The ab initio modeling modules from Rosetta were employed to find the three-dimensional structure of target fragmental peptides by sampling and assembling a large candidate pool containing 22,000–27,000 decoy structures for every inputted amino acid sequence [32]. The output results of ab initio modeling were analyzed using the Calibur and energy-based clustering methods.

4.4. P-Loop Remodeling

The P-loop region of α_1G was remodeled using a Rosetta loop modeling module combined with the FastRelax protocol. Twenty-seven amino acids in the P-loop were selected from domains I, II, III, and IV of the TCCs. The modeling used phenylalanine as the starting amino acid and tyrosine, tryptophan, proline, and isoleucine as the ending amino acids. The effective sample size used for subsequent statistical analysis was validated by two groups of data for every remodeled domain. The first group contained 500 output structures, and the second group had 20,000 output structures. The results were analyzed using the Calibur and energy-based clustering methods.

4.5. Compound Generation

We used the de novo drug generation package "chemical vae" developed by Gomez-Bombarelli et al. [21] to create a data-driven RNN for new compound production. The dataset we used to train the RNN was prepared by randomly sampling approximately 250,000 compounds from PubChem. The maximum length of encoding for the SMILES-based compounds was set to 120 characters. To analyze the compounds using the RNN, one fully connected layer of width 200 was used. To convert a predicted compound back to the original data type, three layers of gated recurrent units with a hidden dimension of 500 were used. The variational loss of the RNN was annealed according to a sigmoid schedule after 35 epochs, running for 130 epochs while property prediction training the RNN, such that the RNN trained on the PubChem data set with objective properties including: logP, SAS [33], and QED [34]. We kept the other hyperparameters to train the RNN unchanged from the reference [21]. To transfer the predicted compound back to SMILES-based data, we set the Gaussian noise value to 5 and the iteration time to 1000. Once the 2D structure had been obtained, we converted it into a 3D structure via the online program Frog 2.1 [35,36]. The program OpenBabel 2.4.1 [37] was used to add the hydrogen atom and set the pH equal to 7.35 for select compounds.

The 2D structure of mibefradil was employed as a redesigned template for new compounds. Based on its structure, we recreated 129 PAAs and their derivatives. Their corresponding 3D structures (involving up to 800 isomers) were created by Frog 2.1. We used the same program to find the 3D structures for NNC 55-0395, NNC 55-0396, and NNC 55-0397, and combined them with SKF96365 and RO 40-5966, whose 3D structures were downloaded from PubChem, for use as reference compounds for testing and validating the faithfulness of our TCC models.

Some of the candidates of screening compounds may contain oxygen, which replaces the role of nitrile; this structural formula has been reported in certain PAAs such as falipamil, BRL-32872, and tiapamil [15].

4.6. Virtual Drug Screening

Virtual drug screening was conducted by using AutoDock Vina [13] with user-defined configuration scripts on the Tulane supercomputer Cypress. The search box was placed in the center of the protein model. The number of mesh elements in the X, Y, and Z directions was set to 60, 124, and 102 for α_1C and 58, 48, and 50 for α_1G, α_1H, and α_1I, respectively, when simulating the ligand–receptor interaction for existing TCC blockers. The number of mesh elements in the X, Y, and Z directions was increased to 126 when conducting virtual screening for newly designed compounds. To achieve repeatable docking results using Vina, the seed number was fixed at −1460306363. As the grid number for every direction was set to the maximum, Vina had to search a very large three-dimensional space. To find the local minimum, the exhaustiveness was set to 2000 for new compound screening cases and 8 for existing TCC blocker screening cases. The number of predictable binding models expressed as the output was limited to 3 for new compound screening cases and 20 for existing TCC cases.

The Vina output results were checked using PyMOL to ensure the binding locations for existing and newly designed compounds. The predicted binding affinity for the testing compound was calculated as:

$$K_d = \exp\left(\frac{-\Delta G \cdot \text{kcal} \cdot \text{mol}^{-1}}{0.001986 \cdot \text{kcal} \cdot \text{mol}^{-1} \cdot \text{K}^{-1} \cdot 310\ \text{K}}\right),$$

where ΔG is the Gibbs free energy predicted by Vina.

The 2D ligand–receptor interaction plot was created using LigPlot^{+} [38].

4.7. Data Analysis

The Anderson–Darling normality test and the Kruskal–Wallis one-way ANOVA test (Supplementary Table S2) were conducted on the generated homology modeling data from Rosetta ab initio modeling and P-loop remodeling in Anaconda Spyder (3.2.8) using a Python 3.6 environment.

5. Patents

All the new identified compounds in this study are patented by the Office of Technology Transfer and Intellectual Property Development at Tulane University (Patent ID: US62/859,519).

Supplementary Materials: The following are available online at https://www.mdpi.com/1424-8247/14/2/141/s1. Figure S1. The negatively charged lysine affects the electric potential distribution of aspartic acid in the x-y plane. (A) The Dist. of E_D (0,0) without K; (B) the Dist. of E_D (0,0) after adding the lysine E_K (3.8, 0), Figure S2. The predicted versus theoretical RMSD plots for group sampling size 500 and 20,000. (A,B,C,D) Domains I to IV for 500 sampling size group; (E,F,G,H) Domains I to IV for 20,000 sampling size group Figure S3. The predicted 3D binding plots between TC 7 and α_1G. An alkyl bond (4.31 angstroms) has been formed between TC 7 (green) and the sidechain of V^{1i24} (red) at domain I. The sidechain of E^{1p50} is colored as blue and one Ca^{2+} is colored as yellow; Figure S4. Based on the 2D structure of SKF-96365, 10 structures have been found using the Deep-Learning based de novo drug design approach, Figure S5. 2D structure and chemical properties of the redesigned phenylalkylamine analog, TC 1, Figure S6. 2D structure and chemical properties of the redesigned phenylalkylamine analog, TC 2, Figure S7. 2D structure and chemical properties of the redesigned phenylalkylamine analog, TC 3, Figure S8. 2D structure and chemical properties of the redesigned phenylalkylamine analog, TC 4, Figure S9. 2D structure and chemical properties of the redesigned phenylalkylamine analog, TC 5, Figure S10. 2D structure and chemical properties of the redesigned phenylalkylamine analog, TC 6, Figure S11. 2D structure and chemical properties of the redesigned phenylalkylamine analog, TC 7, Figure S12. 2D structure and chemical properties of the redesigned phenylalkylamine analog, TC 8, Figure S13. 2D structure and chemical properties of redesigned phenylalkylamine analog, TC 10, Figure S14. 2D structure and chemical properties of the redesigned phenylalkylamine analog, TC 11, Figure S15. 2D structure and chemical properties of the redesigned phenylalkylamine analog, TC 12, Figure S16. 2D structure and chemical properties of the redesigned phenylalkylamine analog, TC 13, Figure S17. 2D structure and chemical properties of the redesigned phenylalkylamine analog, TC 15. Table S1. Numerical parameter settings for running PyGbe, Table S2. Normality test for P-loop remodeling data (α_1G) from two groups with different sampling sizes, Table S3. The structures and properties of computer-designed compounds using Deep-Learning (D: distance; C: count; F: frequency). Table S4. Predicted binding affinity (K_d) by Vina versus experimental measurement of IC_{50} of given TCC blockers (unit: micromolar).

Author Contributions: Conceptualization, Y.L. and M.L.; methodology, Y.L. and M.L.; software, Y.L.; validation, Y.L. and M.L.; formal analysis, Y.L.; investigation, Y.L.; resources, Y.L.; data curation, Y.L.; writing—original draft preparation, Y.L.; writing—review and editing, Y.L. and M.L.; visualization, Y.L.; supervision, M.L.; project administration, M.L.; funding acquisition, M.L. All authors have read and agreed to the published version of the manuscript.

Funding: This research was supported, in part, through the use of high-performance computing (HPC) resources and services provided by Technology Services at Tulane University, New Orleans, LA.

Institutional Review Board Statement: Not applicable.

Informed Consent Statement: Not applicable.

Data Availability Statement: The data presented in this study are available on request from the corresponding author.

Acknowledgments: Y.L. thanks the interdisciplinary Ph.D. Program in Aging Studies at Tulane University for their support of this research.

Conflicts of Interest: The authors declare no conflict of interest.

References

1. Taylor, J.T.; Huang, L.; Pottle, J.E.; Liu, K.; Yang, Y.; Zeng, X.; Keyser, B.M.; Agrawal, K.C.; Hansen, J.B.; Li, M. Selective blockade of T-type Ca2+ channels suppresses human breast cancer cell proliferation. *Cancer Lett.* **2008**, *267*, 116–124. [CrossRef]
2. Keyser, B.M.; Taylor, J.T.; Choi, S.K.; Lu, Y.; Bhattacharjee, A. Role of T-type Ca 2+ channels in basal [Ca 2+] i regulation and basal insulin secretion in rat islet cells. *Curr. Trend Endocrinol.* **2014**, *7*, 35–44.
3. Lu, Y.; Long, M.; Zhou, S.; Xu, Z.; Hu, F.; Li, M. Mibefradil reduces blood glucose concentration in db/db mice. *Clinics* **2014**, *69*, 61–67. [CrossRef]
4. Pottle, J.; Sun, C.; Gray, L.; Li, M. Exploiting MCF-7 Cells' Calcium Dependence with Interlaced Therapy. *J. Cancer Ther.* **2013**, *4*, 32–40. [CrossRef]
5. Dogrul, A.; Gardell, L.R.; Ossipov, M.H.; Tulunay, F.C.; Lai, J.; Porreca, F. Reversal of experimental neuropathic pain by T-type calcium channel blockers. *Pain* **2003**, *105*, 159–168. [CrossRef]
6. Li, M. Role of T-Type Ca2+ Channels in Basal Insulin Release. In *T-Type Calcium Channels in Basic and Clinical Science*; Springer: Berlin/Heidelberg, Germany, 2015; pp. 137–150.
7. Cribbs, L. T-type calcium channel expression and function in the diseased heart. *Channels (Austin)* **2010**, *4*, 447–452. [CrossRef]
8. Zhao, Y.; Huang, G.; Wu, Q.; Wu, K.; Li, R.; Lei, J.; Pan, X.; Yan, N. Cryo-EM structures of apo and antagonist-bound human Ca v 3.1. *Nature* **2019**, *576*, 492–497. [CrossRef] [PubMed]
9. Tang, L.; El-Din, T.M.G.; Swanson, T.M.; Pryde, D.C.; Scheuer, T.; Zheng, N.; Catterall, W.A. Structural basis for inhibition of a voltage-gated Ca(2+) channel by Ca(2+) antagonist drugs. *Nature* **2016**, *537*, 117–121. [CrossRef]
10. Li, Z.Q.; Scheraga, H.A. Monte-Carlo-Minimization Approach to the Multiple-Minima Problem in Protein Folding. *Prac. Natl. Acad. Sci. USA* **1987**, *84*, 6611–6615. [CrossRef]
11. Zhorov, B.S. Vector Method for Calculating the Derivatives of the Energy of Deformation of the Valence Angles and the Torsional Energy of Complex-Molecules with Respect to Generalized Coordinates. *J. Struct. Chem.* **1982**, *23*, 649–655. [CrossRef]
12. Zhorov, B.S. A Vector Method for Calculating the Derivatives of the Energy of the Atom-Atom Interactions of Complex-Molecules with Respect to Generalized Coordinates. *J. Struct. Chem.* **1981**, *22*, 4–8. [CrossRef]
13. Trott, O.; Olson, A.J. Software News and Update AutoDock Vina: Improving the Speed and Accuracy of Docking with a New Scoring Function, Efficient Optimization, and Multithreading. *J. Comput. Chem.* **2010**, *31*, 455–461. [PubMed]
14. Li, M.; Hansen, J.B.; Huang, L.; Keyser, B.M.; Taylor, J.T. Towards selective antagonists of T-type calcium channels: Design, characterization and potential applications of NNC 55-0396. *Cardiovasc. Drug Rev.* **2005**, *23*, 173–196. [CrossRef] [PubMed]
15. Cheng, R.C.K.; Tikhonov, D.B.; Zhorov, B.S. Structural Model for Phenylalkylamine Binding to L-type Calcium Channels. *J. Biol. Chem.* **2009**, *284*, 28332–28342. [CrossRef] [PubMed]
16. Li, S.C.; Ng, Y.K. Calibur: A tool for clustering large numbers of protein decoys. *BMC Bioinform.* **2010**, *11*, 25. [CrossRef] [PubMed]
17. Song, Y.; DiMaio, F.; Wang, R.Y.-R.; Kim, D.; Miles, C.; Brunette, T.; Thompson, J.; Baker, D. High-resolution comparative modeling with RosettaCM. *Structure* **2013**, *21*, 1735–1742. [CrossRef]
18. Hosseinzadeh, P.; Bhardwaj, G.; Mulligan, V.K.; Shortridge, M.D.; Craven, T.W.; Pardo-Avila, F.; Retti, S.A.; Kim, D.E.; Silva, D.A.; Ibrahim, Y.M.; et al. Comprehensive computational design of ordered peptide macrocycles. *Science* **2017**, *358*, 1461–1466. [CrossRef]
19. Cooper, C.D.; Barba, L.A. Poisson–Boltzmann model for protein–surface electrostatic interactions and grid-convergence study using the PyGBe code. *Comput. Phys. Commun.* **2016**, *202*, 23–32. [CrossRef]
20. Wu, S.W.; Zhang, M.; Vest, P.A.; Bhattacharjee, A.; Liu, L.; Li, M. A mibefradil metabolite is a potent intracellular blocker of L-type Ca2+ currents in pancreatic beta-cells. *J. Pharmacol. Exp. Ther.* **2000**, *292*, 939–943.
21. Gomez-Bombarelli, R.; Wei, J.N.; Duvenaud, D.; Hernandez-Lobato, J.M.; Sanchez-Lengeling, B.; Sheberla, D.; Aguilera-Iparraguirre, J.; Hirzel, T.D.; Adams, R.P.; Aspuru-Guzik, A. Automatic Chemical Design Using a Data-Driven Continuous Representation of Molecules. *ACS Central Sci.* **2018**, *4*, 268–276. [CrossRef]
22. Tang, L.; Gamal El-Din, T.M.; Payandeh, J.; Martinez, G.Q.; Heard, T.M.; Scheuer, T.; Zheng, N.; Catterall, W.A. Structural basis for Ca2+ selectivity of a voltage-gated calcium channel. *Nature* **2014**, *505*, 56–61. [CrossRef] [PubMed]

23. Hockerman, G.H.; Peterson, B.Z.; Johnson, B.D.; Catterall, W.A. Molecular determinants of drug binding and action on L-typ calcium channels. *Annu. Rev. Pharmacol. Toxicol.* **1997**, *37*, 361–396. [CrossRef]
24. Peterson, B.Z.; Tanada, T.N.; Catterall, W.A. Molecular determinants of high affinity dihydropyridine binding in L-type calciu channels. *J. Biol. Chem.* **1996**, *271*, 5293–5296. [CrossRef] [PubMed]
25. Hockerman, G.H.; Johnson, B.D.; Scheuer, T.; Catterall, W.A. Molecular Determinants of High-Affinity Phenylalkylamine Block o L-Type Calcium Channels. *J. Biol. Chem.* **1995**, *270*, 22119–22122. [CrossRef]
26. Catterall, W.A.; Striessnig, J. Receptor-Sites for Ca2+ Channel Antagonists. *Trends Pharmacol. Sci.* **1992**, *13*, 256–262. [CrossRef]
27. Barreiro, G.; Guimarães, C.R.W.; de Alencastro, R.B. A molecular dynamics study of an L-type calcium channel model. *Protei Eng.* **2002**, *15*, 109–122. [CrossRef] [PubMed]
28. Chodera, J.D.; Mobley, D.L.; Shirts, M.R.; Dixon, R.W.; Branson, K.; Pande, V.S. Alchemical free energy methods for dru discovery: Progress and challenges. *Curr. Opin. Struct. Biol.* **2011**, *21*, 150–160. [CrossRef] [PubMed]
29. Wang, E.; Sun, H.; Wang, J.; Wang, Z.; Liu, H.; Zhang, J.Z.H.; Hou, T. End-Point Binding Free Energy Calculation with MM/PBS and MM/GBSA: Strategies and Applications in Drug Design. *Chem. Rev.* **2019**, *119*, 9478–9508. [CrossRef]
30. Shapovalov, M.V.; Wang, Q.; Xu, Q.F.; Andrake, M.; Dunbrack, R.L. BioAssemblyModeler (BAM): User-Friendly Homolog Modeling of Protein Homo- and Heterooligomers. *PLoS ONE* **2014**, *9*, e98309. [CrossRef]
31. Sanner, M.F.; Olson, A.J.; Spehner, J.C. Reduced surface: An efficient way to compute molecular surfaces. *Biopolymers* **1996**, *3* 305–320. [CrossRef]
32. Kim, D.E.; Chivian, D.; Baker, D. Protein structure prediction and analysis using the Robetta server. *Nucleic Acids Res.* **2004**, *3* W526–W531. [CrossRef]
33. Ertl, P.; Schuffenhauer, A. Estimation of synthetic accessibility score of drug-like molecules based on molecular complexity an fragment contributions. *J. Cheminformatics* **2009**, *1*, 8. [CrossRef] [PubMed]
34. Bickerton, G.R.; Paolini, G.V.; Besnard, J.; Muresan, S.; Hopkins, A.L. Quantifying the chemical beauty of drugs. *Nat. Chem.* **201** *4*, 90–98. [CrossRef] [PubMed]
35. Leite, T.B.; Gomes, D.; Miteva, M.A.; Chomilier, J.; Villoutreix, B.O.; Tuffery, P. Frog: A FRee Online druG 3D conformatio generator. *Nucleic Acids Res.* **2007**, *35*, W568–W572. [CrossRef] [PubMed]
36. Miteva, M.A.; Guyon, F.; Tuffery, P. Frog2: Efficient 3D conformation ensemble generator for small compounds. *Nucleic Acids Re* **2010**, *38*, W622–W627. [CrossRef]
37. O'Boyle, N.M.; Banck, M.; James, C.A.; Morley, C.; Vandermeersch, T.; Hutchison, G.R. Open Babel: An open chemical toolbox. *Cheminformatics* **2011**, *3*, 33. [CrossRef]
38. Laskowski, R.A.; Swindells, M.B. LigPlot+: Multiple Ligand-Protein Interaction Diagrams for Drug Discovery. *J. Chem. Inf. Mode* **2011**, *51*, 2778–2786. [CrossRef]

MDPI
St. Alban-Anlage 66
4052 Basel
Switzerland
Tel. +41 61 683 77 34
Fax +41 61 302 89 18
www.mdpi.com

Pharmaceuticals Editorial Office
E-mail: pharmaceuticals@mdpi.com
www.mdpi.com/journal/pharmaceuticals

www.ingramcontent.com/pod-product-compliance
Lightning Source LLC
Chambersburg PA
CBHW061445220926
51850CB00004B/18
* 9 7 8 3 0 3 6 5 5 3 8 4 9 *